618.1/HIL

Scientific Essentials of Reproductive Medicine

Scientific Essentials of Reproductive Medicine

Edited by

SG Hillier
PhD DSc MRCPath
Professor of Reproductive Endocrinology
Centre for Reproductive Biology
University of Edinburgh
Edinburgh, UK

HC Kitchener
MD MB ChB FRCS FRCOG
Professor of Gynaecologic Oncology
University of Manchester
Manchester, UK

JP Neilson
MD MB ChB MRCOG
Professor of Obstetrics and Gynaecology
University of Liverpool
Liverpool, UK

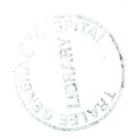
W B Saunders Company Ltd
London • Philadelphia • Toronto • Sydney • Tokyo

W. B. Saunders Company Ltd   24–28 Oval Road
London NW1 7DX, UK

The Curtis Center
Independence Square West
Philadelphia, PA 19106-3399, USA

Harcourt Brace & Company
55 Horner Avenue
Toronto, Ontario M8Z 4X6, Canada

Harcourt Brace & Company, Australia
30–52 Smidmore Street
Marrickville, NSW 2204, Australia

Harcourt Brace & Company, Japan
Ichibancho Central Building, 22-1 Ichibancho
Chiyoda-ku, Tokyo 102, Japan

A catalogue record for this book is available from the British Library

ISBN 0-7020-1826-0

Typeset by Phoenix Photosetting, Chatham, Kent
Printed in Great Britain by The Bath Press, Avon

Contents

Section 1 – Basic Sciences

Section 2 – Development and Function of the Genital Tract

Contents \

Section 3 – Fetal Development and Pregnancy

Section 4 – Reproductive Cancers

Section 5 – Applied Science

Contributors

RJ Aitken PhD, Honorary Professor, MRC Reproductive Biology Unit, University of Edinburgh Centre for Reproductive Biology, Edinburgh, UK.

L Allan PhD, Research Fellow, Department of Medical Genetics, University of Aberdeen, Foresterhill, Aberdeen, UK.

C Yding Anderson MSc, Senior Research Fellow, Laboratory of Reproductive Biology, Department of Obstetrics and Gynaecology, Rigshospitalet, University of Copenhagen, Copenhagen, Denmark.

D Ashby BSc, MSc PhD Hon MFPHM CStat, Reader in Medical Statistics, Department of Public Health and Department of Statistics and Computational Mathematics, The University of Liverpool, Liverpool, UK.

JBL Bard BA PhD, Senior Lecturer, Department of Anatomy, Edinburgh University Medical School, Edinburgh, UK.

JMS Bartlett BSc (Hons) PhD, Lecturer, University of Glasgow Department of Surgery, Glasgow Royal Infirmary, Glasgow, UK.

F Beck MD DSc, Senior Principal Research Fellow, Howard Florey Institute of Experimental Physiology and Medicine, University of Melbourne, Parkville, Victoria, Australia.

L Bennet BA MA PhD, Postdoctoral Research Fellow, Department of Obstetrics and Gynecology, University College London Medical School, London, UK.

Y Ben-Yoseph PhD FACMG, Professor of Pediatrics, Biochemistry, Obstetrics and Gynecology, Department of Pediatrics, Obstetrics and Gynecology and Biochemistry, Wayne State University School of Medicine, Detroit, Michigan, USA.

DT Bonthron MA BM Bch MRCP (UK), Senior Lecturer, Human Genetics Unit, University of Edinburgh, Western General Hospital, Edinburgh, UK.

TA Bramley BSc PhD, Senior Lecturer, Department of Obstetrics and Gynaecology, University of Edinburgh Centre for Reproductive Biology, Edinburgh, UK.

AG Byskov PhD, Dr Science, Chief of Clinic, Laboratory of Reproductive Biology, Juliane Marie Center for Children, Women and Reproduction, Rigshospitalet, University Hospital of Copenhagen, Copenhagen, Denmark.

IT Cameron BSc MA MD MRCOG MRACOG, Regius Professor of Obstetrics and Gynaecology, Department of Obstetrics and Gynaecology, University of Glasgow, The Queen Mother's Hospital, Yorkhill, Glasgow, UK.

J Cassidy MD FRCP MSc, Professor of Oncology, Department of Medicine, Medical School, University of Aberdeen, Foresterhill, Aberdeen, UK.

KJ Catt MD FRCP MSc, Professor of Oncology, Chief, Endocrinology and Reproduction Research Branch, National Institute of Child Health and Human Development, National Institutes of Health, Bethesda, Maryland, USA.

Contributors \

SE Christmas	MA DPhil, Lecturer in Immunology, Department of Immunology, University of Liverpool Medical School, Liverpool, UK.
IJ Clarke	PhD, Associate Professor, Prince Henry's Institute of Medical Research, Clayton, Victoria, Australia.
J-A Clyma	BSc, Research Associate, Centre for Cancer Epidemiology, University of Manchester, Christie Hospital NHS Trust, Withington, Manchester, UK.
HOD Critchley	BSc (Hons) MBChB (Hons) MD MRCOG FRACOG, Senior Lecturer, Department of Obstetrics and Gynaecology, University of Edinburgh Centre for Reproductive Biology, Edinburgh, UK.
GB Cutler Jr	MD, Chief, Section on Developmental Endocrinology, National Institute of Child Health and Human Development, National Institutes of Health, Bethesda, Maryland, USA.
C Davidson	Scientific Officer, MRC Human Genetics Unit, Western General Hospital, Edinburgh, UK.
NAM De Clercq	PhD, Research Associate, Institute of Obstetrics and Gynaecology, Royal Postgraduate Medical School, Hammersmith Hospital, London, UK.
P Devroey	Professor, Clinical Director, Centre for Reproductive Medicine, Dutch-Speaking Brussels Free University (Vrije Universiteit Brussel), Brussels, Belgium.
SAD Ebrahim	MD, Assistant Professor in Pathology, Department of Obstetrics and Gynecology, Molecular Medicine and Genetics, Pathology and Pediatrics, Wayne State University School of Medicine, Detroit, Michigan, USA.
DL Economides	MBBS MD MRCOG, Consultant and Senior Lecturer, Department of Obstetrics and Gynaecology, Royal Free Hospital, London, UK.
D Elbourne	BSc (Soc) Dip Stats MSc (Stats) PhD CStat, Child Statistician, Acting Director of Perinatal Trials Service, National Perinatal Epidemiology Unit, Radcliffe Infirmary, Oxford, UK.
JJ Eppig	PhD, Senior Staff Specialist, The Jackson Laboratory, Bar Harbour, Maine, USA.
MI Evans	MD FACOG FACMG, Professor and Vice-Chief of Obstetrics and Gynecology, Professor of Molecular Medicine and Genetics, Professor of Pathology, Department of Obstetrics and Gynaecology, Molecular Medicine and Genetics and Pathology, Wayne State University School of Medicine, Detroit, Michigan, USA.
H Fox	MD FRCPath FRCOG, Emeritus Professor of Reproductive Pathology, Department of Pathological Services, University of Manchester, Manchester, UK.
S Franks	MD SRCP Hon MD Uppsala, Professor of Reproductive Endocrinology, Department of Obstetrics and Gynaecology and Unit of Metabolic Medicine, Imperial College of Science and Technology and Medicine, St Mary's Hospital Medical School, London, UK.
CM Gosden	PhD MRCPath, Professor of Medical Genetics, Department of Obstetrics and Gynaecology, University of Liverpool, Liverpool, UK.
A Grant	DM MSc FRCOG MFPHM, Professor and Director of Health Services Research Unit, Health Services Research Unit, University of Aberdeen, Foresterhill, Aberdeen, UK.
JA Grootegoed	Professor-Dr, Department of Endocrinology and Reproduction, Faculty of Medicine and Health Sciences, Erasmus University, Rotterdam, The Netherlands.

DA Guissani	BSc PhD, Postdoctoral Research Fellow, Department of Obstetrics and Gynaecology, University College London Medical School, London, UK.
N Haites	MB ChB PhD, Reader in Clinical Genetics, Medical Genetics, University of Aberdeen, Foresterhill, Aberdeen, UK.
MA Hanson	MA DPhil Cert Ed, Professor of Fetal and Neonatal Physiology, Department of Obstetrics and Gynaecology, University College London Medical School, London, UK.
SG Hillier	PhD DSc MRCPath, Professor of Reproductive Endocrinology, Department of Obstetrics and Gynaecology, University of Edinburgh Centre for Reproductive Biology, Edinburgh, UK.
AG Howatson	BSc MB ChB FRCS (Edin) MRCPath, Consultant Paediatric and Perinatal Pathologist, Department of Pathology, Royal Hospital for Sick Children and Queen Mother's Hospital, The Yorkhill NHS Trust, Glasgow, UK.
R Hume	BSc MBChB PhD FRCP (Edin), Reader in Developmental Medicine, Centre for Research into Human Development, Departments of Child Health, Obstetric and Gynaecology and Biochemical Medicine, University of Dundee, Dundee, UK.
G Irvine	MBChB MRCOG, Lecturer, Department of Obstetrics and Gynaecology, University of Glasgow, The Queen Mother's Hospital, Yorkhill, Glasgow, UK.
PM Johnson	DSc FRCPath, Professor of Immunology, Department of Immunology, University of Liverpool, Liverpool, UK.
SB Kaye	MD FRCP BSc, Professor of Medical Oncology, CRC Department of Medical Oncology, Beatson Oncology Centre, Western Infirmary, Glasgow, UK.
J Kingdom	MD MRCP MRCOG, Consultant/Senior Lecturer, Department of Obstetrics and Gynaecology, University College London Medical School, London, UK.
WD Lawrence	MD, Chief of Pathology, Hutzell Hospital/Institute for Women's Medicine, Professor of Pathology, Wayne State University, School of Medicine, Detroit, Michigan, USA.
R Leake	MA DPhil, Reader in Biochemistry and Molecular Biology, Division of Biochemistry and Molecular Biology, Institute of Biomedical and Life Sciences, University of Glasgow, Glasgow, UK.
I Liebaers	Professor, Director, Centre for Medical Genetics, Dutch-Speaking Brussels Free University (Vrije Universiteit Brussel), Brussels, Belgium.
A López Bernal	MA DPhil DMC EOG (Murcia), University Research Lecturer, Nuffield Department of Obstetrics and Gynaecology, University of Oxford, The John Radcliffe Hospital, Headington, Oxford, UK.
LS Martin	MD FAAP FACMG, Assistant Professor in Pathology, Pediatrics, Obstetrics and Gynecology, Department of Obstetrics and Gynecology, Molecular Medicine and Genetics, Pathology and Pediatrics, Wayne State University School of Medicine, Detroit, Michigan, USA.
WN McDicken	BSc PhD, Professor of Medical Physics and Medical Engineering, Department of Medical Physics and Medical Engineering, The University of Edinburgh, Royal Infirmary, Edinburgh, UK.
B Milner	PhD, Research Fellow, Department of Medical Genetics, University of Aberdeen, Foresterhill, Aberdeen, UK.

ID Morris	BPharm (Hon) PhD DSc, Reader, Pharmacology, Physiology and Toxicology, School of Biological Sciences, University of Manchester, Manchester, UK.
JG Nijhuis	MD PhD, Associate Professor of Perinatology, University Hospital St Radboud, Department of Obstetrics and Gynaecology, Nijmegen, The Netherlands.
JE Norman	MD MRCOG, Senior Lecturer, Department of Obstetrics and Gynaecology, University of Glasgow, The Queen Mother's Hospital, Yorkhill, Glasgow, UK.
K Oerter Klein	MD, Pediatric Endocrinology, Clinical Research Scientist, Alfred I. duPont Institute, A Children's Hospital, Wilmington, Delaware, USA.
JA Owens	PhD, NHMRC Research Fellow, Department of Obstetrics and Gynaecology, University of Adelaide, South Australia, Australia.
DW Purdie	MD FRCOG, Honorary Consultant Gynaecologist, Centre for Metabolic Bone Disease, Hull Royal Infirmary, Hull, UK.
M Robertson	Scientific Officer, MRC Human Genetics Unit, Western General Hospital, Edinburgh, UK.
JS Robinson	BSc MBCh BAO FRCOG FRACOG, Professor of Obstetrics and Gynaecology, Department of Obstetrics and Gynaecology, University of Adelaide, South Australia, Australia.
PA Robinson	PhD, Senior Research Fellow, Molecular Medicine Unit and Division of Dental Surgery, St James's University Hospital, Leeds, UK.
S Robinson	MA MB BChir MRCP, Senior Lecturer in Metabolic Medicine, Department of Obstetrics and Gynaecology and Unit of Metabolic Medicine, Imperial College of Science and Technology and Medicine, St Mary's Hospital Medical School, London, UK.
SC Robson	MD MRCOG, Professor of Fetal Medicine, Royal Victoria Infirmary, University of Newcastle upon Tyne, Newcastle, UK.
TP Rollason	BSc MBChB FRCPath, Consultant Histopathologist, Histopathology Department, Birmingham Maternity Hospital, Edgbaston, Birmingham, UK.
S Shaunak	PhD MRCP, Senior Lecturer, Human Retrovirus Group, Department of Infectious Diseases, Royal Postgraduate Medical School, Hammersmith Hospital, London, UK.
C Sibley	PhD, Reader in Child Health and Physiology, Department of Child Health, University of Manchester, St Mary's Hospital, Manchester, UK.
RA Silver	MD, Neonatal Fellow, Department of Pediatrics, University of Vermont College of Medicine, Burlington, Vermont, USA.
F Smaill	MB ChB FRACP FRCPC, Associate Professor, Departments of Pathology and Medicine, Faculty of Health Sciences, McMaster University Hamilton, Ontario, Canada.
RF Soll	MD, Associate Professor of Pediatrics, Department of Pediatrics, University of Vermont College of Medicine, Burlington, Vermont, USA.
CM Steel	MBchB PhD DSc FRCPE FRCSE FRCPath FRSE, Professor of Medical Sciences, School of Biological and Medical Sciences, University of St Andrews, St Andrews, Fife, UK.

RP Symonds   MD FRCP FRCR, Consultant Clinical Oncologist, Beatson Oncology Centre, Western Infirmary, Glasgow, UK.

A Van Steirteghem   Professor, Scientific Director, Centre for Reproductive Medicine, Dutch-Speaking Brussels Free University (Vrije Universiteit Brussel), Brussels, Belgium.

DW Visscher   MD, Associate Professor of Pathology, Department of Pathology, Harper Hospital, Detroit, Michigan, USA.

SE Wedden   MA PhD, Lecturer, Department of Anatomy, Edinburgh University Medical School, Edinburgh, UK.

M Wells   BSc MD FRCPath, Consultant Pathologist, Centre for Molecular Medicine and Department of Pathology, St James's University Hospital, Leeds, UK.

JO White   PhD, Senior Lecturer, Institute of Obstetrics and Gynaecology, Royal Postgraduate Medical School, Hammersmith Hospital, London, UK.

S Wilson   BA, Deputy Director, Centre for Cancer Epidemiology, University of Manchester, Christie Hospital NHS Trust, Withington, Manchester, UK.

H Winter   MD MRCOG, Lecturer, Department of Public Health and Epidemiology, The Health Services Research Centre, The Medical School, University of Birmingham, Edgbaston, Birmingham, UK.

CBJ Woodman   MD MRCOG MFPHM, Professor of Cancer Epidemiology, Centre for Cancer Epidemiology, University of Manchester, Christie Hospital NHS Trust, Withington, Manchester, UK.

AJ Zeleznik   PhD, Professor of Cell Biology, Physiology, Obstetrics, Gynecology and Reproductive Sciences, Department of Obstetrics and Gynecology, University of Pittsburgh School of Medicine, Pittsburgh, Pennsylvania, USA.

Preface

In 1953 Crick and Watson described the double-helix structure of DNA. Since then a steady stream of major discoveries and technological progress has yielded much greater insight into the molecular functions of normal cells. Our understanding of these complex events holds the key to unraveling the abnormal functions responsible for disease and, in turn, the possibility of revolutionary new treatments. Because of the emphasis in the undergraduate curriculum on the traditional preclinical subjects, students have learned too little of this new molecular and cellular science, and it can be very difficult for the uninitiated medical graduate to become familiar with these important advances.

We see reproductive medicine as a broad subject encompassing the development and maturation of reproductive function, pregnancy and parturition, and the malignant changes that may affect the reproductive organs. The scientific basis of this field forms the bedrock of clinical Obstetrics and Gynecology and it is therefore important for clinicians to keep abreast of developments. It is the prime purpose of this book to enable doctors who do not have a scientific background, to understand the rapid progress that is being made in reproductive medicine. Any reader of the leading medical journals will realize that an understanding of the traditional undergraduate basic sciences is no longer sufficient to be able to read critically much of what is now published.

The book is restricted to scientific matters, and deliberately avoids description of clinical management and traditional preclinical subject material which is well covered in other texts.

Scientific Essentials is set out in five sections. Section 1 covers important basic topics such as gene expression, immunology and genetics. Sections 2–4 cover in systematic fashion, development and function of the reproductive organs, fetal development and pregnancy, and reproductive cancers. The final section deals with clinical trials and statistics. The book has been designed to be understood by those with no prior knowledge of molecular biology and is generously illustrated.

We hope that *Scientific Essentials of Reproductive Medicine* will benefit several groups. In addition to those studying for specialist examinations in Obstetrics and Gynecology, many trained postgraduates will feel the need to update themselves and those embarking on research will be able to acquire a solid background in their chosen subject. The authorship comprises a mix of scientists and clinicians and wherever possible jargon has been avoided. Scientific expression inevitably involves a galaxy of unfamiliar terms, but gaining an understanding of these alone will leave the reader feeling more empowered.

Stephen G Hillier
Henry C Kitchener
James P Neilson

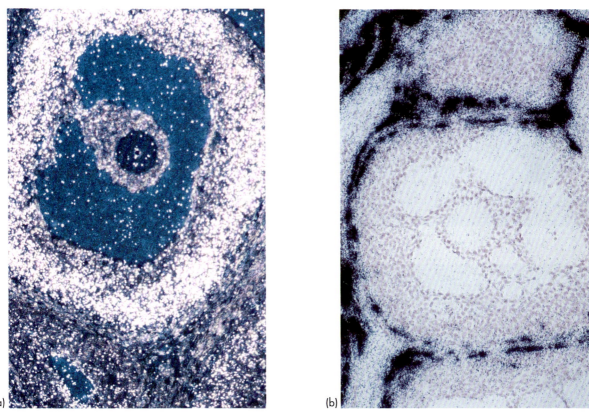

Plate 1. *Cell-specific localization of steroidogenic enzymes necessary for androgen and estrogen synthesis in the rat Graafian follicle, revealed by in situ hybridization. (a) Selective localization of P450arom mRNA in granulosa cells[39] (dark-field view, ×70); (b) selective localization of P450c17 mRNA to thecal cells[59] (bright-field view, ×70).* **(Fig. 2.3.6)**

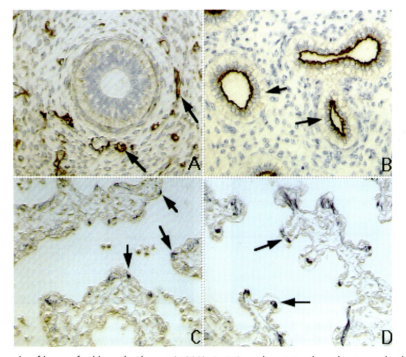

Plate 2. *Light photomicrographs of human fetal lung develpment (×230). A, A 9-week gestation lung showing a developing bronchial airway and extensive mesenchymal blood vessel development immunostained with vimentin antibody (arrows). B, A 16-week gestation lung showing distal airways lined with partially differentiated columnar cells filled with glycogen (arrows) and apically immunostained with epithelial membrane antigen. C, A 23-week gestation lung showing that the distal airways are dilating, that the epithelium is flattening and foci of elastin, stained histochemically, are being deposited (arrows). D, A 27-week gestation lung showing the formation of secondary-alveolar crests subdividing the distal airsac at sites of elastin deposition (arrows).* **(Fig. 3.9.1)**

Gene Expression

CM Steel

GENERAL INTRODUCTION

The central dogma

For many decades argument raged about whether DNA or protein was the true repository of genetic information and once the debate ended in a clear victory for the former, an awkward problem remained. It was accepted that genes specified proteins ('one gene, one enzyme') yet DNA was, for practical purposes, confined to the cell nucleus while proteins were synthesized in the cytoplasm. So how was the message conveyed from one site to the other? The answer had to be a chemical intermediary, eventually shown to be RNA. The sequence of events in gene expression is thus DNA → RNA ('transcription') then RNA → Protein ('translation') and that unidirectional progression is some-times termed the central dogma of molecular biology.[1] All dogma invites disproof and indeed exceptions have been found to this one. In some instances an RNA molecule can be the end product of gene expression, that is, translation is not required since no protein is synthesized. Very rarely, transcription operates in reverse. This applies mainly to the replication cycle of the small RNA viruses which undergo reverse transcription to generate a DNA 'provirus' copy for insertion into the genome of the infected cell.[2] There is also evidence that, in the course of evolution, some DNA sequences in higher organisms, including man, have undergone transcription followed by reverse transcription and re-insertion so that extra copies are now carried.[3] For most practical purposes, however, the central dogma holds true; gene expression requires the sequential operation of two processes, transcription and translation.

The genetic code

Since DNA is composed of only four bases (Fig. 1.1.1) but proteins comprise 20 amino acids (plus others that are derived from these 20 by chemical modification) there has to be some means of conveying at least 20 separate pieces of information through combinations and permutations of four variables. The problem is comparable to that of expressing the alphabet in dots and dashes which Samuel Morse solved with his Morse Code. The Genetic Code is, in some respects, simpler since all the 'letters' are of the same length, namely three bases. There are however $4 \times 4 \times 4$ (=64) possible permutations of the bases in these triplets so that the genetic code is 'redundant', that is, the same amino acid can be specified by two or more triplets (Fig 1.1.2). Variation is seen particularly in the third base of the triplet, for reasons that will be discussed later. It follows that the effect of a mutation substituting one base for another in the DNA will depend very much on chance. For example, changing the triplet CCG to CCA will not alter the protein product since both encode proline. On the other hand, if CGG becomes GGG, glycine is substituted for arginine and since these amino acids have very different chemical properties the characteristics and function of the protein may be altered significantly. There is no mech-anism for recognizing the 'correct' division into triplets once the process of transcription has started; thus if the DNA base sequence gets out of phase by the insertion or deletion of nucleotides other than in multiples of three, all the triplets beyond the point of change will be misread. The usual effect of such a 'frame-shift' mutation is to generate a string of incorrect amino acids in the protein chain which is also shortened because one of the altered triplets is likely to specify 'stop'.

Gene expression in context

Germ cells apart, all the body's cells contain the same DNA. Therefore everything that distinguishes one cell from another – the specification of different tissues, the varying states of cellular maturity, activation and prolifera-tion within a single tissue – depends on selective gene

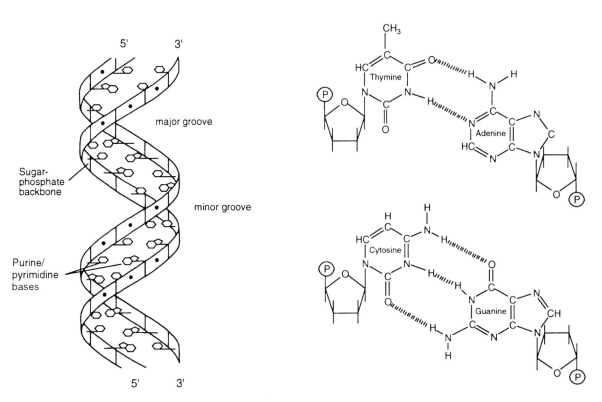

a) DNA structure

b) Base - pairing in DNA

Fig. 1.1.1 *The DNA double helix (a) and the base-pairing (b) that underlies its structure.*

expression. Regulation of gene expression is thus among the most fundamental processes of life and assumes increasing importance as the complexity of living organisms increases. Not surprisingly, there are multiple levels of regulation, each showing evidence of growing sophistication throughout the course of evolution.

Transcription itself can be started, stopped and up- or down-regulated. The RNA transcript is subject to processing in the nucleus while its half-life depends on the activity of ribonucleases and on factors that modulate sensitivity of the RNA to digestion. Translation into protein is subject to control at several points and post-translational modification of proteins can determine subcellular localization, biological activity, route and rate of catabolism. In many instances function is dependent on precise interactions between two or more proteins so that regulating the quantity or conformation of just one can affect a range of biological processes. Later sections cover the mechanics of gene expression and its regulation in more detail but an important concept to grasp at the outset is that the response of a cell to its environment usually requires a chain of events culminating in a change in gene expression.[4,5] Thus availability of nutrients, hormone and growth factor levels, contact with adjacent cells or with extracellular matrix, infections, drugs and even changing temperature all evoke signals that ultimately impinge on transcription and/or post-transcriptional events that reflect

the activity of specific genes. It follows that the ability of the whole organism (or person) to survive in anything but a constant environment is, to some extent, a measure of the efficiency with which its cells can achieve appropriate regulation of gene expression.

CURRENT CONCEPTS

The mechanics of gene expression

Transcription

In a few situations, for example in the salivary glands of fruit flies, transcription can actually be observed as a series of 'puffs' on the polytene chromosomes, implying that there is a physical change in the conformation of the DNA protein complex while genes are being expressed.[6] This happens to be an exception to the rule that chromosomes are visible only during metaphase, when transcription does not occur. Nevertheless there is a very definite structure to the interphase chromatin of all cells, which does have a bearing on the process of transcription. The DNA double helix is wrapped twice round a core of basic proteins, forming a unit termed a 'nucleosome' (Fig 1.1.3) and repetition of this unit at intervals of about 200 base-

SECOND BASE

FIRST BASE		U	C	A	G
	U	UUU ⎫ Phe UUC ⎭ UUA ⎫ Leu UUG ⎭	UCU ⎫ UCC ⎬ Ala UCA ⎪ UCG ⎭	UAU ⎫ Tyr UAC ⎭ ⌀UAA⌀ ⎫ TERM ⌀UAG⌀ ⎭	UGU ⎫ Cys UGC ⎭ ⌀UGA⌀ TERM UGG ⎬ Trp
	C	CUU ⎫ CUC ⎬ Leu CUA ⎪ CUG ⎭	CCU ⎫ CCC ⎬ Thr CCA ⎪ CCG ⎭	CAU ⎫ His CAC ⎭ CAA ⎫ Gln CAG ⎭	CGU ⎫ CGC ⎬ Arg CGA ⎪ CGG ⎭
	A	AUU ⎫ Ile AUC ⎬ AUA ⎭ AUG ⎬ Met	ACU ⎫ ACC ⎬ Pro ACA ⎪ ACG ⎭	AAU ⎫ Asn AAC ⎭ AAA ⎫ Lys AAG ⎭	AGU ⎫ Ser AGC ⎭ AGA ⎫ Arg AGG ⎭
	G	GUU ⎫ GUC ⎬ Val GUA ⎪ GUG ⎭	GCU ⎫ GCC ⎬ Ser GCA ⎪ GCG ⎭	GAU ⎫ Asp GAC ⎭ GAA ⎫ Glu GAG ⎭	GGU ⎫ GGC ⎬ Gly GGA ⎪ GGG ⎭

TERM = Termination ("STOP codon")

Fig. 1.1.2 *The genetic code: RNA triplet codons and the amino acids they specify.*

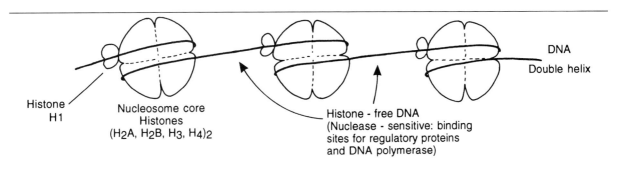

Fig. 1.1.3 *Nucleosome structure of chromatin.*

pairs gives dispersed chromatin the appearance of a string of beads when viewed under the highest magnification of the electron microscope. Tight association with the histone core serves to protect the DNA from enzymic degradation so that when endogenous nucleases are released, for example, in cells undergoing apoptosis, the DNA fragments are initially generated by cleavage between nucleosomes and thus form a size 'ladder' in multiples of 200 bases. The association also tends to inhibit other biochemical activity, including DNA replication and transcription, during both of which the nucleosome structure has to be relaxed, though it never breaks down completely.[7]

Transcription begins when a complex of RNA polymerase II and associated proteins attaches itself to the DNA helix just upstream (i.e. in the 5′ direction) of the start of a structural gene. The complex then moves down the gene in the 3′ direction, reading off the base sequence from one strand (the 'template' strand) and generating a complementary RNA sequence, using the same rules of base-pairing that apply to DNA replication, except that uracil replaces the thymine of DNA.[8] As a result, the RNA sequence generated corresponds to that of the non-copied DNA strand which is therefore known as the 'coding' strand. The key to *selective* transcription lies in regulation of the attachment of the complex to the upstream recognition site. In fact this usually consists of multiple elements, variously termed 'promoters' and 'enhancers', which are simply small blocks of DNA with characteristic base sequences and often occupying positions that are quite precisely related to the transcription start point. They are never transcribed themselves since their function is to bind nuclear proteins that regulate transcription.[9] The most ubiquitous is the 'TATA box', so named because the characteristic DNA sequence is TATAATA or some minor variant of that. It is found 25 bases 5′ of the first transcribed codon and some 45 bases further away there is usually another recognition sequence GGTCAATCT (the 'CAAT box'). Some genes, particularly those with so-called 'housekeeping' functions, that are transcribed in all tissues at similar rates, seem to dispense with these promoter elements but have, instead, the upstream sequence GGGCGG. The TATA box binds a protein called the 'general transcription factor' (or TFIID) which forms part of the transcription initiation and regulation apparatus. RNA polymerase II is one component of this apparatus but further accessory proteins which bind to other recognition sequences also play a part. For example the sequence TGACTCA binds the *fos/jun* dimer which has important effects on the rate of transcription of adjacent genes. Some of the 'enhancer' binding sites can be located a long way from the structural gene, upstream or downstream and in either orientation. It is probable that the DNA becomes folded in such a way that these regulatory sites and the proteins bound to them can interact physically, all contributing to the complex that regulates transcription.[10] In cells where a particular gene is expressed, it seems that the regulatory elements for that gene are located in the internucleosomal 'accessible' regions of the chromatin so that the protein transcription factors can bind to them (Fig. 1.1.4). In fact it is likely that binding of these proteins to the nascent DNA chain as it is synthesized during cell division determines the exclusion of these regions from the tightly wound nucleosome.[7,11,12] Some of the regulatory elements show a degree of tissue specificity in their sequence and these Locus Control Regions (LCR) offer scope for tissue specific regulation of transfected genes – a potentially important consideration in gene therapy.[13] Cells also differ in their content of various transcription factors and hence will differ in the positioning of nucleosomes in relation to particular structural genes. Besides the accessibility of regulatory elements, levels of gene expression appear to be influenced, in some instances, by the degree of methylation of upstream clusters of cytidine residues ('CpG

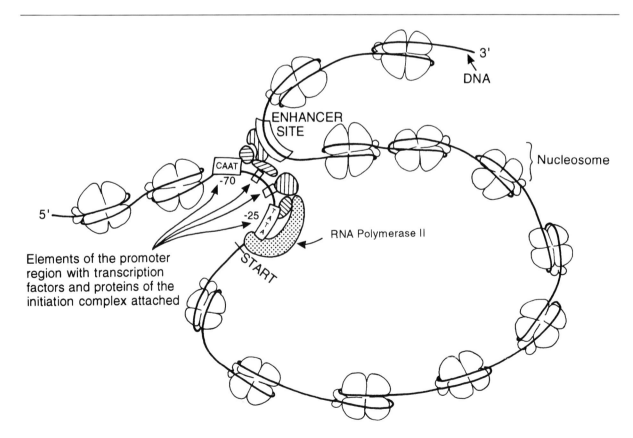

Fig. 1.1.4 *Binding of transcription factors, RNA polymerase II and other accessory proteins, to form the initiation complex at an accessible internucleosomal site. Note that proteins bound to an enhancer site far downstream are involved in the initiation complex.*

islands'); the less methylation the more actively expressed the adjacent structural gene but quite how this control is exercised remains to be explained.[14]

Proteins that bind to promoter and enhancer sites can have either positive or negative effects on transcription ('induction' or 'repression') and they interact with other nuclear proteins, generating scope for very subtle regulation of gene expression.[4] The receptors for steroid hormones, including the sex hormones, are transcription factors and the underlying mechanisms whereby these hormones influence cellular function are now well understood. They are discussed in a later section.

The primary transcript and messenger RNA

Once the transcription apparatus has been assembled and bound to the promoter sites, the DNA starts to unwind to allow separation of the strands of the double helix and to accommodate the RNA polymerase II moving along the template strand. This unwinding is purely local and the double helix re-forms rapidly in the wake of the 'transcription bubble' (Fig. 1.1.5). The transcription start site is recognized by its relation to the TATA box. Once transcription is under way, it continues until a termination site is reached at the 3' end of the gene. Close to the 3' end the transcript almost always contains the sequence AAUAAA which is recognized by a poly(A) polymerase and leads to the addition of a string of adenine residues (about 150) to the 3' end of the RNA chain.[15] While one

polymerase progresses along the gene, another may join the initiation complex so that a very actively expressed gene may be generating several RNA copies simultaneously, at different stages of completion. The RNA representing a copy of the complete DNA sequence between initiation and termination, with its poly(A) tail, is termed the 'primary transcript' or 'heterogeneous nuclear' RNA (hnRNA), and must undergo considerable further processing within the nucleus before it can pass to the cytoplasm as 'messenger' RNA (mRNA). An important purpose of this processing is to excise the portions that do not represent coding regions of the original DNA. The great majority of eukaryotic genes (as distinct from those of bacteria or other simple organisms) are arranged in blocks of coding sequences ('exons') interspersed with non-coding blocks ('introns'). A collection of small nuclear molecules that comprise both RNA and protein ('snRNPs') work on the primary transcript, recognizing the sequences GU and AG that denote the beginning and end of each intron as well as at least one moderately conserved heptamer, related to the yeast sequence UACUAAC, that occurs about 40 bases upstream of the 3' end of the intron.[16] The complex that undertakes the cleavage and looping out of intronic sequences and re-joining of the RNA to form a contiguous series of exons is termed a 'spliceosome' (Fig. 1.1.6). Some genes can undergo further modification at this stage through a process of 'alternative splicing'. Certain exons may be excluded completely from the final transcript so that, by varying the set of exons represented, different

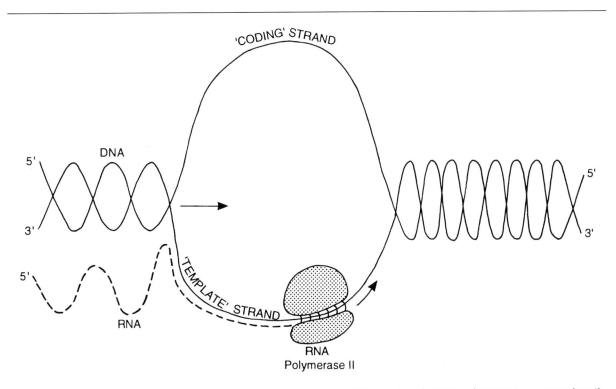

Fig. 1.1.5 *Transcription: The 'transcription bubble' allows separation of the DNA strands so that RNA polymerase II can move along the template strand making an RNA copy of the coding strand. The DNA double helix becomes more tightly coiled in advance of the bubble and association with histones in the nucleosome is relaxed as the bubble passes.*

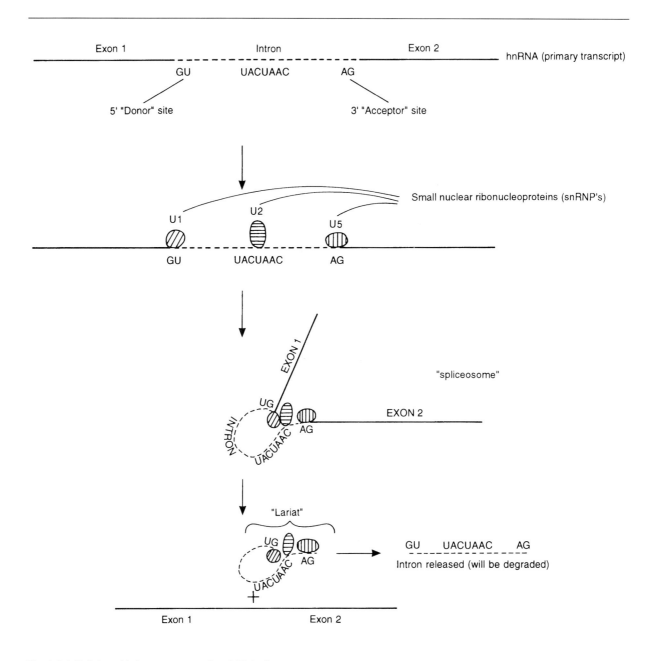

Fig. 1.1.6 *Splicing of heterogeneous nuclear RNA to form messenger RNA.*

peptides may be synthesized though the same gene is being expressed. One further important modification before the RNA leaves the nucleus is addition of 7-methylguanosine, as a 'cap', to the 5′ end of the molecule. Thus, having been spliced, capped and tailed, the messenger RNA is ready to convey its information to the protein synthesis machinery.

Translation

Messenger RNA leaves the nucleus and enters the cyto-plasm through the nuclear pores, by an active transport process in which the poly(A) tail probably plays some part.

It finds its way rapidly to the sites of protein synthesis, the 'ribosomes', which are themselves complexes of RNA and protein, forming structures large enough to be visible as granules on electron microscopy. In cells synthesizing large amounts of protein for export (e.g. plasma cells making antibodies) ribosomes form the 'rough' component of rough endoplasmic reticulum but they also exist as free organelles in the cytoplasm.

The genes that encode ribosomal RNA (rRNA) are located on the short arms of the acrocentric chromosomes and, in interphase, are found in the nucleolus.[17] Two large rRNA molecules are generated by cleavage of a single precursor transcript and these form the core elements of the two subunits of the ribosome itself (Fig 1.1.7). The mRNA winds itself between the two subunits where a series of enzymes, which also form part of the ribosome complex, read off the triplet code and assemble a corresponding peptide chain. This process of translation involves several distinct biochemical reactions some of which are now understood in some detail.

The active site of the ribosome engages mRNA by recognizing the 7-methylguanosine cap on the 5′ end. The ribosome then slides in the 3′ direction until it encounters the first codon to be translated, which is always AUG (specifying methionine). From then on, each triplet of bases is read and translated in turn.[18] Amino acids are ferried to the ribosome on carrier molecules which represent yet another form of RNA, 'transfer' RNA (tRNA).[1,19] They comprise only 70–80 bases folded into a 'clover leaf' form by internal base pairing. On one face is a triplet 'anticodon' complementary to the triplet codon of mRNA and at the other end of the tRNA molecule is a sequence of seven or eight bases that specifies the covalent attachment of an amino acid (Fig. 1.1.8). Thus tRNA serves as the 'adaptor' that converts a nucleotide sequence into an amino acid sequence. Any given tRNA molecule will transfer only one

specific amino acid and it is clearly essential that the specificities of the anticodon and the amino acid attachment sequence are co-ordinated, for example the tRNA bearing the anticodon UAC (which is complementary to the codon AUG) *must* carry methionine and no other amino acid, otherwise the peptide synthesized on the mRNA template will not correspond to the genetic code as set out in Fig. 1.1.2. So important is this matching of anticodon to amino acid attachment sequence on the tRNA, it is sometimes referred to as the 'second genetic code'. The ribosome moves along the mRNA in the 3′ direction, one triplet at a time and as each codon in turn enters the active site a tRNA molecule with the complementary anticodon 'plugs in' and the amino acid it is carrying is added to the growing peptide chain (Fig. 1.1.9). Because the folding of tRNA produces a convex anticodon face, the fit between codon and anticodon is imperfect, particularly at the third ('wobble') base. This accounts for some of the redundancy of the genetic code and explains why redundancy is greatest at the third base position. The peptide chain always starts with the N terminal amino acid and elongates towards the C terminus, which is reached when the mRNA specifies 'stop' (UAA, UAG or UGA). The peptide is then released and the two ribosomal subunits detach from the

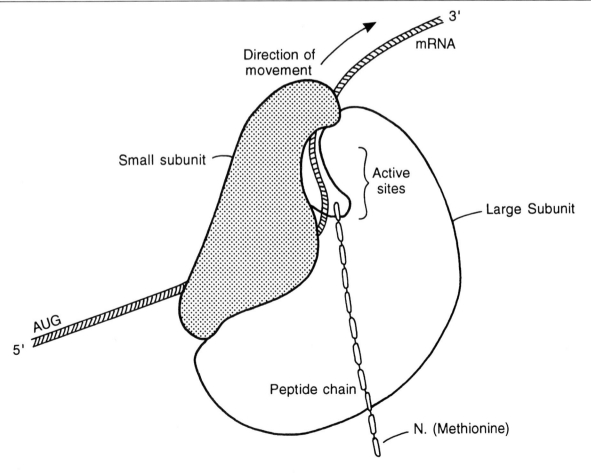

Fig. 1.1.7 *Ribosome structure.*

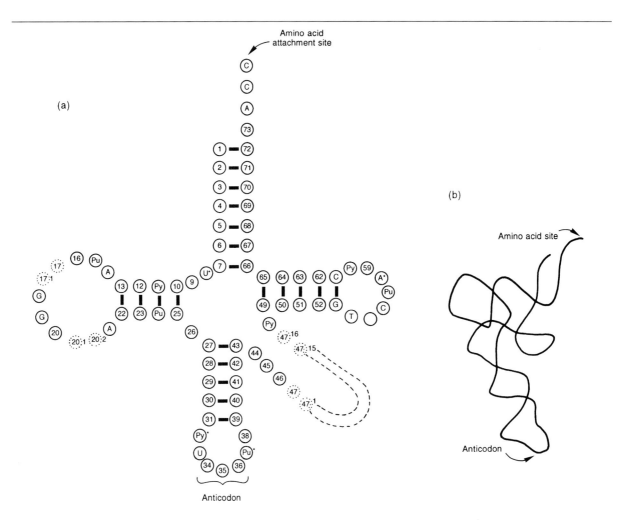

Fig. 1.1.8 *Structure of transfer RNA (tRNA). (a) Stylized diagram; note 'hairpin loops' formed by internal base-pairing G–C and A–U. (b) Actual shape of folded molecule.*

mRNA chain and from each other. Further ribosomes may attach in succession to the 5′ cap site before the preceding ones have reached the terminus so that the message may be undergoing simultaneous translation at several points and multiple peptide chains, each at a different stage of completion, may be issuing from it.

The whole process of translation requires not only the mRNA template, ribosomes and tRNA but also several

Table 1.1.1 Inhibitors of transcription and translation

Inhibitor	Function affected	Notes
Alpha Amanatin	Transcription in higher organisms	This is the 'death cap' mushroom toxin
Rifamycin	Transcription in bacteria	
Actinomycin D	Transcription of ribosomal RNA	Also inhibits translation through lack of ribosomes
Diphtheria toxin	Elongation phase of translation	Toxin is an enzyme, hence extremely potent
Puromycin	Elongation phase of translation	Affects bacteria and higher organisms
Cycloheximide	Translation	Affects bacteria and higher organisms
Neomycin Tetracyclines Chloramphenicol Erythromycin Kanamycin Fusidic acid	Various phases of translation	Affect principally bacteria (hence clinical value)
Interferons	Translation (among other effects)	May account for some antitumor activity

soluble protein factors[20] that are specifically involved at different phases (initiation, elongation, termination). In addition, the covalent bonding of amino acids with their tRNA partners is an energy-requiring reaction catalyzed by aminoacyl tRNA synthetases each of which is specific for a given amino acid/tRNA combination.[21] This complexity affords considerable scope for interference and a number of naturally occurring inhibitors of translation are known

(Table 1.1.1). The amount of a given protein being synthesized at any point is influenced by the rates of synthesis and degradation of the corresponding mRNA. The half-life of mRNA is normally brief but it can be stabilized by a number of factors, including, in some instances, hormones.[22] Translation is also subject to regulation, for example through alterations in the activity of some of the accessory proteins mentioned above.

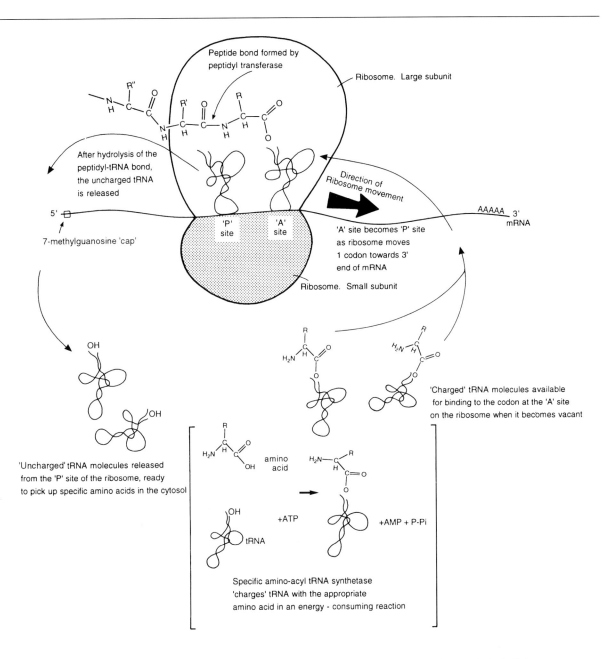

NB more than a dozen soluble proteins (initiation, elongation and termination factors) are required to facilitate the reactions occurring at the active sites of the ribosome during protein synthesis

Fig. 1.1.9 *The translation process.*

Post-transcriptional modification of proteins

As the peptide chain elongates and even before separation from the ribosome, the N-terminal methionine is removed and, in most cases, the protein rapidly undergoes folding to adopt a three-dimensional conformation determined simply by the amino acid sequence. In some cases non-covalent associations between two or more copies of the same molecule (homo-multimers) or between different molecules (hetero-multimers) also form spontaneously (e.g. the formation of heterodimers between transcription factors *jun* and *fos* by their 'leucine zipper' domains, as discussed later). Many other processes which lead to modification of newly synthesized proteins are enzyme catalyzed. They include cleavage by specific peptidases, for example in the generation of hormones from pro-hormones and of digestive enzymes from zymogens. Some of these reactions may take place very close to the site of synthesis (e.g. the mature insulin molecule is manufactured in the islet beta cell which synthesizes pre-proinsulin and carries out two subsequent peptidase reactions. Immunoglobulin heavy and light chains are linked by disulphide bonds within the B lymphoid cell); others are carried out in a different setting (e.g. the pancreatic enzymes are secreted in inactive form and are activated by proteolytic cleavage in the duodenum).

Glycosylation, conjugation with lipids or polysaccharides and the covalent attachment of prosthetic groups are further examples of post-translational modifications that can be essential to protein function and hence to physiological gene expression. These modifications are undertaken, as a rule, in specialized cellular organelles, glycosylation for example, principally in the endoplasmic reticulum. Bacteria are therefore unable to carry out most of the reactions so that 'recombinant' proteins synthesized in cultures of prokaryotes may be non-functional. Some modern bio-engineering processes make use of yeasts, insect or other cultured eukaryotic cells and even transgenic animals (mice or sheep, for example) in order to manufacture proteins that have undergone appropriate post-transcriptional modification. Those proteins that are secreted from the cell incorporate a specialized 'signal' sequence that docks with a signal recognition particle and is then directed to the endoplasmic reticulum where a further series of interacting proteins create a pore through which the newly synthesized protein slides. The signal peptide is usually cleaved, left behind and degraded.[23]

Thus the generation of a completely functional protein often requires the expression of several genes, not simply the one that encodes the information for its amino acid sequence. Even more genes are likely to be implicated in regulating the timing and rate of its synthesis.

Regulation of gene expression

How does a cell decide when to bring the above processes into play and how does it determine which of its 50 000+ genes will be expressed at any given time? These questions have taxed the ingenuity of scientists throughout much of the past decade for they represent the essential bridge between molecular and cell biology. It would be misleading to suggest that we now have a complete understanding of the regulation of gene expression but it is certainly not the black box it once was. In the case of bacteria, the first clues to the nature of the underlying mechanisms came from studies of changes in gene expression that followed changes in the availability of nutrients. For the cells of higher organisms in tissue culture, the simplest signals that could be shown to alter gene expression in a consistent fashion were exposure to brief periods of heating ('heat shock'), manipulating the amount of serum in the culture medium or addition of appropriate hormones. In each case it was found that the effects on gene expression were mediated via changes in the amounts and/or properties of specific DNA-binding proteins in the nucleus.

The mode of action of the steroid hormones[24,25] serves as a good illustration of the general principle (Fig. 1.1.10) (see Chapter 1.4). Within the cytoplasm there are steroid-binding proteins (receptors) non-covalently associated with another protein. When a steroid hormone (the term includes glucocorticoids, mineralocorticoids, estrogens, progestogens, thyroid hormone and retinoic acid) enters the cell, it displaces its specific receptor from the associated protein and the steroid–receptor complex passes into the nucleus where it binds, through its N-terminal region, to a specific DNA sequence. Although each steroid has its own unique receptor, these are structurally related, forming a family of proteins that have probably evolved from a common precursor. Similarly, the DNA sequences recognized by each of the steroid receptor binding domains are clearly related to each other. The glucocorticoid receptor, for example, binds to the 15 base-pair sequence GGTACANNNTGTTCT (where N is any base). Occupation of the steroid-binding C-terminal domain of the receptor protein by the appropriate hormone not only releases it from the cytoplasmic complex and permits binding to DNA, it also triggers functional 'activation' of the receptor so that it now drives expression of an adjacent 'steroid inducible' gene. 4-OH-Tamoxifen binds to the estrogen receptor but cannot activate it and thus functions as a competitive antagonist of estrogen. When the steroid–receptor complex binds to the target DNA sequence, it induces a change in the conformation of the chromatin, probably displacing a nucleosome and making an adjacent promoter site accessible to 'constitutive' transcription factors (i.e. those already present in the nucleus). In addition, it is likely that direct interactions occur between the DNA-bound steroid–receptor complex and other transcription factors so that a complicated network of interconnected regulatory proteins can be created to exert subtle control over transcription of a given gene or set of genes. In some instances a steroid–receptor combination may inhibit rather than enhance transcription. It appears that the 'inhibitory' DNA binding site differs from the corresponding 'positive' one at only a few of the 15 positions, mainly at the beginning and end of the base sequence.

A somewhat different mechanism of transcriptional control is illustrated by the transcription factor AP1 which binds to the DNA sequence TGAGTCAG. This 'AP1 site' is found upstream of a large number of genes, including many that are involved in cell growth and mobility. AP1 itself has been found to comprise a heterodimer of proteins *jun* and *fos*, already identified as oncogenes and known to be produced in increased amounts in response to several growth factors and tumor promoters such as phorbol esters. The C-terminal ends of the proteins associate strongly with each other by interdigitating a series of leucine residues repeating at intervals of eight amino acids. This 'leucine zipper' then presents paired basic domains towards the N terminus of the proteins which 'grip' the DNA double helix wherever the AP1 binding sequence occurs and drives transcription of the downstream genes (Fig. 1.1.11). Other transcription factors also tend to have recognizable structural motifs (such as 'helix-turn-helix' or 'zinc finger') that are particularly well adapted for interaction with specific short DNA sequences.[9,24]

Rather less is known at present about general transcription repressors in higher organisms, though they are clearly important in the control of cell growth and may well figure

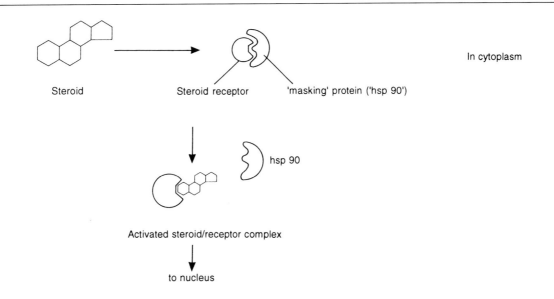

Steroid Steroid receptor 'masking' protein ('hsp 90')

In cytoplasm

hsp 90

Activated steroid/receptor complex

to nucleus

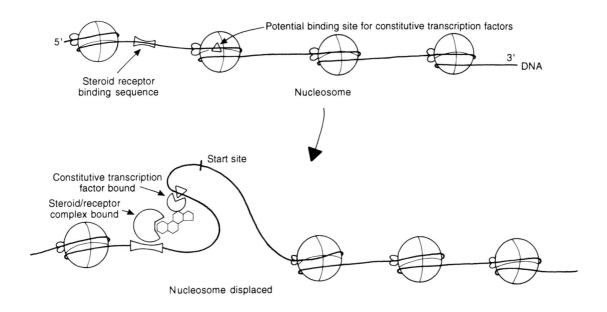

Potential binding site for constitutive transcription factors

5'

3' DNA

Steroid receptor binding sequence

Nucleosome

Start site

Constitutive transcription factor bound

Steroid/receptor complex bound

Nucleosome displaced

Sites for binding of constitutive transcription factor - and for start of transcription - exposed

Fig. 1.1.10 *Regulation of transcription by steroid hormones.*

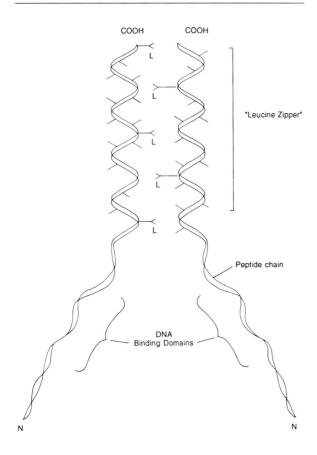

COOH   COOH

L

"Leucine Zipper"

L

L

L

Peptide chain

DNA
Binding Domains

N   N

Fig. 1.1.11 *Schematic diagram of an AP1 type transcription factor, e.g.* fos/jun *heterodimer.*

prominently among genes designated 'tumor suppressors'.[26,27] One of the most intensively studied physiological regulators of growth is transforming growth factor beta (TGF-β).[28] Its effects include reduced transcription of *c-myc* and blockade of phosphorylation of Rb, the nuclear retinoblastoma protein (a definitive 'tumor suppressor'). The latter mode of action is consistent with the observation that phosphorylation of Rb permits cells to progress through the replicative cycle.[29] Nevertheless the inhibitory actions of TGF-β require transcription and translation of some (as yet unidentified) TGF-β-dependent genes so that it is certainly not just a transcription-repressor. Likely candidates as TGF-β targets include inhibitors of cyclin dependent kinases, particularly p15, which influence cell cycle progression. Similarly, the major role of p53 appears to be preventing replication of damaged DNA (i.e. growth arrest until the damage has been repaired), but this effect is probably a consequence of its demonstrable activity as a transcription factor, affecting particularly the p21 cyclin-dependent kinase inhibitor.[30–32]

Apoptosis

The mode of cell death characterized by a distinct sequence of morphological changes (Fig. 1.1.12) – rounding up of the cell, condensation and fragmentation of the nucleus, dilatation of the endoplasmic reticulum and finally 'explosion' of the cell into membrane-bound vesicles which are ingested by phagocytes – was first delineated by Kerr *et al.* in 1972[33] who proposed the term 'apoptosis'. It is commonly observed in development of the organism, at the stage of

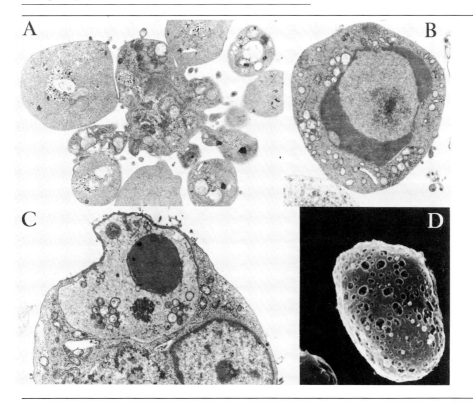

Fig. 1.1.12 *Apoptosis. A. Apoptotic cell in the course of explosion into multiple membrane-bounded bodies. B. Characteristic nuclear changes: margination of chromatin under the nuclear membrane and dispersion of the nucleolar transcription complexes. C. Part of a viable cell (nucleus visible, bottom right) which has engulfed an apoptotic neighbor whose nucleus is the conspicuous dense body, top centre. D. Scanning electron microscope picture of an apoptotic cell, showing the blister-like regions where the dilated endoplasmic reticulum has fused with the cell surface. Figure generously provided by Professor Andrew Wyllie, Edinburgh, from* Cancer Metast Rev 1992 **11**: 95–103. *Reprinted with permission of Kluwer Academic Publishers.*

tissue modeling, when it corresponds to 'programmed cell death' but it can also be induced by cytotoxic drugs, withdrawal of essential nutrients and a variety of physical stimuli. Apoptotic cells can often be observed within tumors and the process, which is quite different from coagulative necrosis or infarction, can evidently have a major influence on the overall growth rate of many tumours. Though it is the antithesis of growth, it is an active process requiring the expression of a number of specific genes plus a source of energy and in some situations apoptosis is prevented by blocking synthesis of RNA or protein.[34,35] The actual mechanisms involved in the initiation and implementation of apoptosis are not fully understood but early events include a rise in free cytosolic calcium levels and increased transcription of the gene encoding the calcium-binding protein calmodulin. As the chromatin undergoes visible condensation, the DNA is found to be undergoing fragmentation through activation of one or more endogenous nucleases. As described earlier, the cleavage-sensitive sites are internucleosomal so that DNA fragment sizes tend to be multiples of 180–200 base pairs. Over-expression of the oncogene *bcl-2*, particularly in lymphoid cells, is a powerful blocker of apoptosis. In fact it is the only oncogene currently known with this primary function and there is intense interest in the mode of its action, which has so far proved elusive. Two other genes that play some part in the process are the famil-

iar *c-myc* and p53. Expression of the former is associated with rapid proliferation except when essential nutrients or growth factors are deficient. Under these conditions, *myc* induces apoptosis. In cells that have undergone DNA damage, normal 'wild type' (as distinct from mutant) p53 arrests proliferation and, if the damage is irreparable, it directs them down the apoptotic pathway.

Measuring gene expression

To estimate the expression of a given gene, we can measure rate of mRNA production or ambient level of mRNA (which reflects the balance between synthesis and degradation) and we can do the same for the protein product. Alternatively, we can apply some functional measure (e.g. of hormone activity). It is, in fact, quite rare for all of these approaches to give concordant results since, as discussed above, transcription and translation are both subject to a variety of independent controls and since physiological activity of a protein may be partially or totally dependent on post-translational modification. It is important to keep these caveats in mind when undertaking or interpreting gene expression studies.

Isolation of mRNA from tissue is technically demanding because ribonucleases are activated very readily when cells

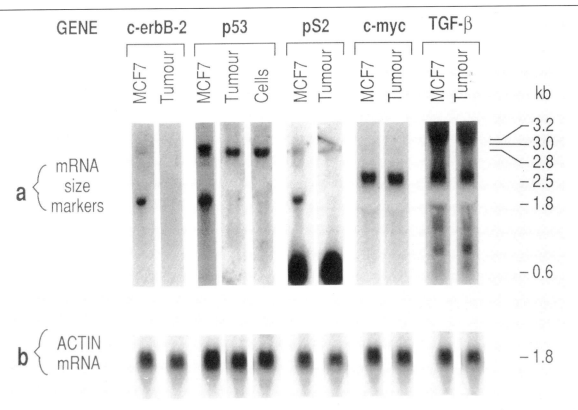

Fig. 1.1.13 *Detection of gene expression by measurement of mRNA levels. 'Northern' blots of mRNA extracted from experimental tumors and transferred to a nylon membrane after gel electrophoresis, have been probed with labeled oligonucleotides specific for a number of genes believed to be implicated in breast cancer. (The particular gene being assayed is indicated above each set of tracks.) The level and molecular mass of each mRNA species detected is indicated by the intensity and position of the corresponding autoradiograph band. Actin mRNA serves as a control for the loading of each gel track. Figure reprinted from AM Thompson et al. Br J Cancer 1990, **62**: 78–84, with permission of the authors and of Macmillan Press Ltd.*

are handled. The skin is also an abundant source of exogenous RNA-degrading enzymes and elaborate precautions must be taken to inhibit them. On the other hand, the poly(A) tail of mRNA provides a convenient means of purifying it (via immobilized poly(T), under conditions that encourage A–T base pairing). Once isolated, the mRNA is allowed to bind to a nylon membrane which is then probed with a labeled single-stranded nucleotide sequence that recognizes the gene in question. This can be preceded by electrophoresis of the RNA so that the identity of the gene transcript can be confirmed by its size but that step is not always necessary (Fig. 1.1.13).

With an appropriate internal control (such as beta actin which is transcribed at a steady state in many cell types) semiquantitative information can be obtained from these procedures. The same principles can be applied to measuring rates of transcription and mRNA degradation. A radiolabeled nucleotide is made available to the cells for a period and is then replaced with the unlabeled equivalent. Messenger RNA is isolated from cells harvested after various intervals and the fate of the label can be followed in any specific transcript, giving an indication of how rapidly it is being produced and replaced. Detection of mRNA *in situ* is becoming an increasingly practical proposition. It carries the advantage that transcription of a given gene can be localized to a specific region of a tissue and even to individual cells (Fig. 1.1.14). Rapid freezing or fixation of tissue usually preserves the RNA well though access to the molecule

for hybridization with a complementary probe can be difficult in formalin fixed material. Until recently, only radiolabelled probes gave a sufficiently strong signal for *in situ* use and accuracy of localization was limited by the autoradiographic procedure which deposits grains of silver within a photographic emulsion overlying the tissue section. Within the past few years, however, colorimetric and fluorescence labeling techniques for DNA/RNA hybridization have improved to the point where they are often the methods of first choice for *in situ* work (Fig. 1.1.15).

Protein identification, by means of specific staining reactions and, more recently, by immunohistochemistry, is a very long established practice in histology and was not originally considered a measure of gene expression (though, of course, it always was precisely that). The range of its applications seems endless, particularly since the development of monoclonal antibodies which gives the technique such exquisite specificity. There is a wide choice of signal detection systems available and the sensitivity of the reaction can often be enhanced by coupling the primary antibody to an enzyme (peroxidase or alkaline phosphatase, for example) then using the enzyme to generate the final signal (Fig. 1.1.15).

The methods outlined for detection of mRNA or protein product *in situ* often provide semiquantitative information, particularly if a fluorescence or luminometric signal is generated since these are amenable to quite accurate measurement with the appropriate equipment.[36-38]

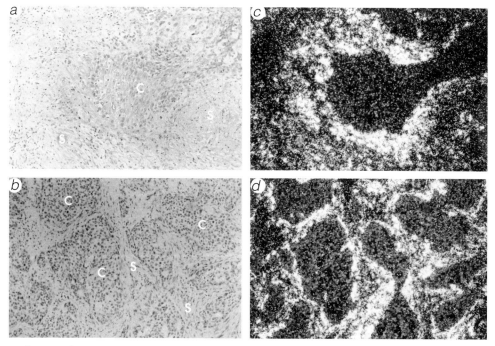

Fig. 1.1.14 *Localization of gene expression by* in situ *RNA hybridization. Comparison of H&E stained histological sections of breast cancer (a,b) with brightfield microscopy of adjacent sections (c,d) after autoradiography shows that the mRNA for a stromelysin gene is expressed exclusively in the stromal cells. The silver grains generated by the radioactivity in the oligonucleotide probe show up as white areas with this technique. Figure kindly provided by Professor Pierre Chambon, Strasbourg. Reprinted from Basset et al. Nature 1990* **348**: *699–704 with permission from Macmillan Magazines Ltd.*

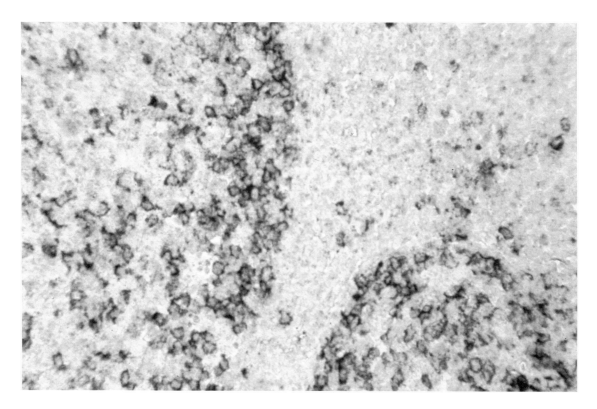

Fig. 1.1.15 *Colorimetric demonstration of mRNA by* in situ *hybridization. Histone mRNA is detected in dividing cells within the germinal centres of normal tonsil, using a digoxigenin-labelled oligonucleotide 'cocktail' subsequently visualized by anti-digoxigenin antibody coupled to alkaline phosphatase which is used to generate a dark red precipitate from a soluble substrate. Thus this technique combines* in situ *DNA/RNA hybridization with immunohistochemistry. Figure kindly provided by Hybaid Ltd and Novocastra Laboratories.*

FUTURE PERSPECTIVES

New insights on the regulation of gene expression (e.g. Reference 39) will eventually allow us to dissect the molecular machinery of the entire body. Such knowledge has applications in all branches of medicine but especially perhaps in genetic and metabolic disorders, oncology, infectious diseases and endocrinology. The challenge is to recognize the limitations and the potential of the current wave of technological advances and to assemble the mass of new facts being generated into a coherent framework so that they contribute to a real advance in our understanding of the fundamental basis of disease and hence to new methods of prevention and treatment.

SUMMARY

- Genetic information is encoded as DNA from which it is *transcribed* into RNA and *translated* into protein.
- The process of transcription is controlled by modification of chromatin structure, specifically by changes in the physical relationship between the DNA and associated histones forming the nucleosome unit. Further control is exercised by the binding of protein *transcription factors* to specific short 'promoter' and 'enhancer' sequences of DNA that flank genes.
- An RNA copy of the DNA 'coding' strand is made by RNA polymerase II which moves along the 'template' strand, the two strands separating in the transcription 'bubble'. The RNA chain elongates in the 5′ to 3′ direction and as it terminates a poly-adenine tail is added.
- Heterogeneous nuclear RNA is modified in the nucleus by splicing out intron sequences and by addition of a 5′-methylguanosine cap. As

messenger RNA (mRNA) it enters the cytoplasm. Translation takes place within the ribosomes which are complexes of RNA and protein. The 'adaptor' that converts the nucleotide code into amino acids is transfer RNA (tRNA).

- The genetic code is read in triplets ('codons'). Most amino acids can be specified by more than one codon and three triplets are used as 'stop' signals. One face of each tRNA molecule has a triplet 'anticodon' that docks with the complementary mRNA sequence in the active site of the ribosome.
- As the ribosome moves along the mRNA from 5' to 3', the amino acid chain elongates from N terminus to C until a stop codon is reached. The peptide is then released.
- Post-transcriptional modification of proteins (glycosylation, conjugation, cleavage etc.) may be required before they become fully functional. The enzymes involved in these processes therefore play a part in the regulation of gene expression.
- Gene expression can be measured at the level of mRNA (by 'Northern blotting' or by *in situ* hybridization) or at the level of protein (e.g. by immunohistochemistry or in functional assays).

REFERENCES

1. Piel J (ed.). The molecules of life. *Sci Am* 1985 **253**: 34–157.
2. Varmus H. Retroviruses. *Science* 1988 **242**: 1427–1435.
3. Fink GR, Bocke JD, Garfinkel DJ. The mechanism and consequences of retrotransposition. *Trends Genet* 1985 **1**: 250–254.
4. Nigg EA. Mechanisms of signal transduction to the cell nucleus. *Adv Cancer Res* 1990 **55**: 271–309.
5. Ptashne M. How gene activators work. *Sci Am* 1989 **260**: 24–31.
6. Bradbury EM, Maclean N, Matthews HR. Transcriptionally active chromosomes. In *DNA, Chromatin and Chromosomes*. Oxford: Blackwell, 1981: 203–229.
7. Morse RH. Transcribed chromatin. *Trends Biochem Sci* 1992 **17**: 23–26.
8. Woychik NA, Young RA. RNA polymerase II: subunit structure and function. *Trends Biochem Sci* 1990 **15**: 347–351.
9. Mitchell PJ, Tjian R. Transcription regulation in mammalian cells by sequence-specific DNA binding proteins. *Science* 1989 **245**: 371–378.
10. Muller H–P, Schaffner W. Transcriptional enhancers can act in trans. *Trends Genet* 1990 **6**: 300–304.
11. Svaren J, Chalkley R. The structure and assembly of active chromatin. *Trends Genet* 1990 **6**: 52–56.
12. Grunstein M. Nucleosomes: regulators of transcription. *Trends Genet* 1990; **6**: 395–400.
13. Moran N. A snap shot of Britain's sole gene therapy company. *Nature Med* 1995 **1**: 502–503.
14. Bird AP. CpG-rich islands and the function of DNA methylation. *Nature* 1986 **321**: 209–213.
15. Wickens M. How the messenger got its tail: addition of poly(A) in the nucleus. *Trends Biochem Sci* 1990 **15**: 277–281.
16. Grabowski PJ, Konarska MN, Sharp PA. Splicing messenger RNA precursors: branch sites and lariat RNAs. *Trends Biochem Sci* 1985 **10**: 154–157.
17. Sommerville J. Nucleolar structure and ribosome biogenesis. *Trends Biochem Sci* 1986 **11**: 438–442.
18. Rhoads RE. Cap recognition and the entry of mRNA into the protein synthesis initiation cycle. *Trends Biochem Sci* 1988 **13**: 52–56.
19. Normanly J, Abelson J. tRNA identity. *Annu Rev Biochem* 1989 **58**: 1029–1049.
20. Riis B, Rattan SIS, Clark BFC, Merrick WC. Eukaryotic protein elongation factors. *Trends Biochem Sci* 1990 **15**: 420–424.
21. Schimmel P. Aminoacyl tRNA synthetases: general scheme of structure–function relationships in the polypeptides and recognition of transfer RNAs. *Annu Rev Biochem* 1987 **56**: 125–158.
22. Ross J. The turnover of messenger RNA. *Sci Am* 1989 **260**: 28–35.
23. Rapoport TA. Protein transport across the ER membrane. *Trends Biochem Sci* 1990 **15**: 355–358.
24. Latchman DS. *Eukaryotic Transcription Factors* London: Academic Press, 1991: 270pp.
25. Parker MG (ed.). Growth regulation by nuclear hormone receptors. *Cancer Surv* 1992 **14**: 1–240.
26. Weinberg RA. Oncogenes, anti-oncogenes and the molecular basis of multistep carcinogenesis. *Cancer Res* 1989 **49**: 3713–3721.
27. Bishop JM. Molecular themes in oncogenesis. *Cell* 1991 **64**: 235–248.
28. Moses HL, Yang EY, Pietenpol JA. TGF-β stimulation and inhibition of cell proliferation: new mechanistic insights. *Cell* 1990 **63**: 245–247.
29. Cobrinik D, Dowdy SF, Hinds PW, Mittnacht S, Weinberg RA. The retinoblastoma protein and the regulation of cell cycling. *Trends Biochem Sci* 1992 **17**: 312–315.
30. Lane DP. p53, guardian of the genome. *Nature* 1992 **358**: 15–16.
31. Oliner JD. Discerning the function of p53 by examining its molecular interactions. *BioEssays* 1993 **15**: 703–707.
32. Karp JE, Brooler S. Molecular foundations of cancer: new targets for intervention. *Nature Med* 1995 **1**: 309–320.
33. Kerr JFK, Wyllie AH, Currie AH. Apoptosis, a basic biological phenomenon with wider implications in tissue kinetics. *Br J Cancer* 1972 **26**: 239–245.
34. Wyllie AH. Apoptosis. (The 1992 Frank Rose memorial lecture). *Br J Cancer* 1993 **67**: 205–208.
35. Martin SJ, Green DR, Cotter TG. Dicing with death: dissecting the components of the apoptosis machinery. *Trends Biochem Sci* 1994 **19**: 26–30.
36. Radinsky R, Bucana CD, Ellis LM *et al.* A rapid colorimetric *in situ* messenger RNA hybridisation technique for analysis of epidermal growth factor receptor in paraffin-embedded surgical specimens of human colon carcinomas. *Cancer Res* 1993 **53**: 937–943.
37. Le Beau MM. Detecting genetic changes in human tumor cells: have scientists 'gone fishing'? *Blood* 1993 **81**: 1979–1983.
38. Mason WT (ed.). *Fluorescent and Luminescent Probes for Biological Activity: A Practical Guide to Technology for Quantitative Real-time Analysis*. London: Academic Press, 1993.
39. Moore MJ. When the junk isn't junk. *Nature* 1996 **379**: 402–403.

Cell Structure and Function

TA Bramley

INTRODUCTION

cell (sel). 1. In biology, a unit from which living organisms and tissues are built. At some stage of its existence it is capable of reproduction by mitotic division. Each is a highly organized structure containing a nucleus (karyoplasm) surrounded by protoplasm (cytoplasm) and limited externally by a cell membrane. The cytoplasm contains organoids such as mitochondria and the reticular apparatus of Golgi, and in many cases such inclusions as secretory granules, pigment, fat droplets, glycogen etc. In multicellular organisms, cells are differentiated in relation to different functions (e.g. secretory cells, nerve cells, germ cells etc.). They are also classified according to their shape (e.g. columnar, cubical, squamous, etc.), or arrangement (e.g. stratified cells), or cytoplasmic inclusions (e.g. pigment cells, fat cells, etc.), or presence in a particular tissue (e.g. connective-tissue cells, cartilage cells), or from the possession of some special structural feature (e.g. ciliated cell, hair cell). Butterworth's Medical Dictionary, 2nd edition.

In recent years, there has been an information explosion concerning the molecular biology of the cell.[1,2] As a background to other chapters in this volume, I shall briefly review the general structure of the eukaryotic cell, the functions of the major organelles and the process of protein hormone secretion.

CURRENT CONCEPTS

Cell structure and function

The basic structure of a eukaryotic cell is shown in Fig. 1.2.1. The *cell surface* or *plasma membrane* (pm) consists of a continuous, two-dimensional lipid bilayer (composed mainly of phospholipids and cholesterol, with other minor but important lipids) arranged as a fluid but stable bilayer, studded with a diverse array of membrane-associated or transmembrane-spanning proteins (fluid mosaic). Lipids and proteins are distributed asymmetrically between inner and outer membrane layers.

The lipid bilayer acts as both a physical barrier and permeability seal, yet is a very dynamic structure. Transmembrane proteins anchored to the contractile cytoskeletal network of the cell can undergo large-scale active reorganization (patching, capping, cell membrane folding and ruffling), whilst membrane proteins not anchored to the cytoskeleton can diffuse laterally in the plane of the membrane. The plasma membrane plays a vital role in nutrient supply and maintenance of cell homeostasis by the actions of transmembrane pumps or channels which transport specific molecules (ions, nutrients) passively or actively into or out of the cell. Other transmembrane proteins act as highly specific receptors for soluble hormones and growth factors. Ligand binding induces a change in receptor conformation, generating one or more intracellular signals (opening of ion channels, activation of heterotrimeric G-proteins or receptor-enzyme cascades) which alter the behavior of the target cell (see Chapters 1.4. and 1.5).

Cell responses have been categorized as: *endocrine* (activation by hormones or factors secreted by a cell type remote from the responsive cell, usually requiring hormone transport to the target tissue via the circulation), *paracrine* (factor secreted by one cell type acts locally via receptors on adjacent cells of a different type) or *autocrine* (cells have receptors which respond to factors that they also secrete).[3]

Cell adhesion

Plasma membranes of adjacent cells may be physically anchored to one another or to the basement membrane (bm) by three types of specialized cell junctions: occluding junctions, anchoring junctions and communicating junctions.

Occluding (tight) junctions encircle the apical end of

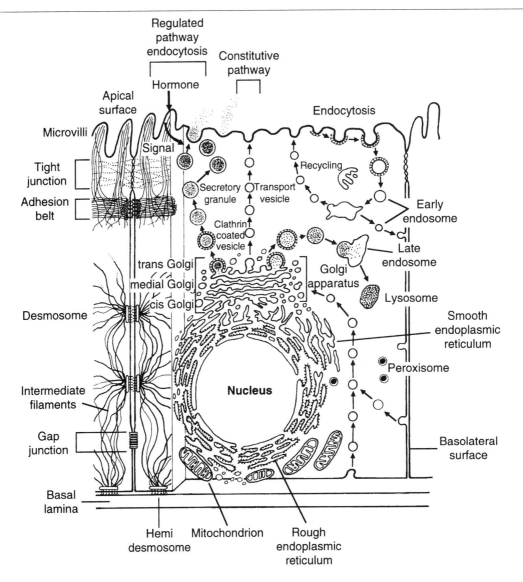

Fig. 1.2.1 *The basic structure of a eukaryotic cell.*

epithelial cells, sealing adjacent cells in a continuous epithelial sheet, and preventing exchange of even small hydrophilic molecules and ions across the cell layer. They maintain the unique compositions of intercellular and luminal fluids, and prevent exchange of membrane lipids and proteins between apical and basolateral surfaces of the cell.[4]

Anchoring junctions connect cytoskeletal elements of the cell to those of adjacent cells or underlying extracellular matrix (ECM). There are three main types of structural junctions in mammalian cells which each utilize different transmembrane linker and extracellular binding proteins, coupled via specific attachment proteins to distinct cytoskeletal proteins (Table 1.2.1): (a) adherens junctions (cell–cell or cell–ECM), (b) desmosomes (molecular 'rivets' joining adjacent cells) and (c) hemi-desmosomes (which anchor epithelial cells to the basal lamina).[5]

Communicating (gap) junctions consist of hexagonal arrays of channel proteins (connexins) which create a pore (connexon), permitting free diffusion of ions and other small molecules between the cytoplasm of adjacent cells.[6] Thus, cells connected by GJs are electrically and biochemically coupled, and can respond coordinately to external signals.

Non-junctional adhesion mechanisms

Besides the highly organized specialized junctional complexes described, cells interact with one another and with the ECM in other ways. The selectins (carbohydrate-binding transmembrane proteins) mediate transient heterotypic cellular interactions with surface-membrane glycoproteins and glycolipids. Similarly, membrane-associated proteoglycans and integrins can bind to one another and to ECM

Table 1.2.1 Properties of anchoring junctions

Junction type	Transmembrane linker proteins	Extracellular binding protein	Intracellular cytoskeletal attachment	Attachment proteins
Cell–cell adherens	Cadherin	Cadherin in adjacent cell	Actin filaments	Catenins, vinculin α-actinin
Cell–matrix adherens	Integrin	ECM proteins	Actin filaments	Talin, vinculin, α-actinin
Desmosome	Cadherins	Cadherin in adjacent cell	Intermediate filaments	Desmoplakins, γ-catenin
Hemi-desmosome	Integrin	ECM (basal lamina) proteins	Intermediate filaments	Desmoplakin-like proteins

Adapted from Reference 1.

proteins. Although of low affinity, the sum total of multiple 'receptors' binding to multiple 'ligands' on adjacent cells or ECM is enormous – the so-called 'Velcro principle'. Multipoint surface binding is greatly stabilized by lateral clustering interactions and by associations with the cytoskeleton.

Cell organelles

Organelles are discrete, membrane-bounded subcellular structures which create distinct metabolic compartments within the cell. Each organelle performs the same basic biochemical functions in all cell types, but organelles vary in abundance and may have additional specialized functions in differentiated cells.

The nucleus

The nucleus is the most prominent organelle of the cell. It is surrounded by the nuclear envelope, the outer membrane bilayer of which is continuous with the endoplasmic reticulum network. Inner and outer nuclear membranes are connected by nuclear pores which can actively transport selected molecules between nucleus and cytoplasm.[7] The nucleus contains almost all the genetic material of the cell packaged into chromosomes. Actively transcribed chromosomes are decondensed into more accessible looped structures,[8] and their histones are distinct from those in 'inactive' chromatin in several respects (less phosphorylated, highly acetylated, variant forms, etc). These 'active' DNA loops may be attached to the nuclear matrix,[9] an intranuclear cytoskeletal framework which not only organizes the chromosomes, but is thought to be the site of DNA replication, transcription and pre-mRNA splicing.[10]

Cytoplasm

The *cytoplasm* (cytosol plus cytosolic organelles) is the site of most of the intermediary metabolism of the cell. Cytosol is highly organized, and three distinct cytoskeletal networks are present in all cells: (1) microtubules, (2) intermediate filaments and (3) actin filaments.

Microtubules

Microtubules (MTs) form a rigid scaffolding within the cytoplasm of the cell, consisting of tubulin monomers (α and β) arranged side-by-side in long, hollow cylindrical structures.[11] These alternately grow steadily at one end (the *plus* end), then shrink catastrophically by the loss of subunits at the *minus* end (dependent on GTP-hydrolysis) unless stabilized. The *minus* ends of MTs in most cells radiate from the 'microtubule organizing centre' (MTOC or centrosome) which usually lies close to the cell nucleus. Microtubule-associated proteins (MAPs) stabilize MT structures and can also attach MTs to cell organelles, enabling active organelle movement within the cell by interactions with two distinct myosin-like motor proteins, the kinesins (which move away from the MTOC) and the dyneins (which move towards the MTOC).[12]

Intermediate filaments

Intermediate filaments (IFs) constitute the framework of the cell and determine its shape. They consist of highly elongated, fibrous proteins which form rope-like dimers. These are then assembled into more complex filaments. IFs are tissue-specific;[13] epithelial cells express cytokeratin, heart cells express desmin and mesenchymal cells, vimentin, whereas neuronal and glial cells express unique IFs. The nuclear lamins, which form a filamentous meshwork beneath the nuclear membrane, are also IFs.

Microfilaments

Microfilaments (MFs) are polarized α-helical double-stranded polymers of the abundant cytosol protein, actin. Actin exists in a wide variety of different structures at different locations in the cell (monomers, parallel bundles, contractile bundles, gel networks).[14] Actin polymerization is a dynamic process, occurring at the *plus* end of the filament. Actin structure, dynamics and function are regulated by interactions with over 70 different actin-binding proteins (ABPs).[15] Just beneath the plasma membrane lies a layer of actin filaments and actin-binding proteins (the cortex of the cell) which controls the shape and movement of most animal cells. These microfilaments can interact with motor proteins linked to the cell membrane or intracellular organelles (myosin-I, responsible for localized ruffling of membranes or movement of organelles within the cell, or myosin-II, which generates cell surface movements and cell locomotion[16,17]). The three types of cytoskeletal filament are connected to one another and their functions are coordinated.[17]

Mitochondria

The mitochondrion has a smooth outer membrane (which is permeable to molecules ca. 5000 daltons) and an impermeable inner membrane which is folded extensively into numerous tubulovesicular or lamelliform cristae. Mitochondria can undergo rapid changes in volume and shape. They are the power plants of the cell. Reduced nicotine adenine dinucleotide (NAD) and flavin adenine dinucleotide (FAD) formed during oxidation of carbohydrates deliver electrons to an elaborate electron-transport chain in the inner membrane. The large drop in redox potential at the NADH dehydrogenase complex, the cytochrome b–c_1 complex and at cytochrome oxidase is efficiently coupled to a proton (H^+) pump which generates an electrochemical gradient across the inner membrane. The backflow of protons down this gradient is utilized to drive ATP synthase[18] and for a variety of other mitochondrial functions.

Peroxisomes

Peroxisomes are electron-dense organelles (~300 nm diameter), bounded by a single membrane.[1] Like mitochondria, they are also major sites of oxygen utilization, generating high concentrations of hydrogen peroxide (used to oxidize fatty acids and other molecules), and have such high levels of oxidative enzymes (e.g. catalase, peroxidase and urate oxidase) that they may crystallize as a paracrystalline core. Peroxisomal proteins are synthesized in the cytoplasm and actively imported across the peroxisomal membrane. Peroxisomes divide by fission.[19]

Protein secretion

The endoplasmic reticulum

The smooth endoplasmic reticulum (SER) consistutes an elaborate labyrinth of interconnected branching tubules and flattened sacs extending throughout the cytoplasm which encloses the cisternal space. The ER is the site of production of transmembrane proteins and lipids, as well as proteins destined for secretion or for other organelles. Membrane components pass from the ER to the Golgi where they are processed, then delivered to the appropriate region of the cell by specific transport vesicles. This apparatus is therefore essential in all active cells. However, cells whose principal function is the synthesis and export of protein hormones usually have highly developed abundant endoplasmic reticulum and Golgi for the translocation of secreted proteins and their packaging into secretory granules.

Protein synthesis

Synthesis of the N-terminal 15–30 hydrophobic amino acids of a secreted protein (the signal sequence) on a ribosome results in binding of the nascent peptide to the signal recognition particle (SRP), targeting the polyribosomes to an SRP-docking protein on the cytosolic surface of the ER and creating regions termed 'rough' endoplasmic reticulum (RER). The growing peptide chain is actively extruded through a transient gated ER-membrane channel into the lumen of the RER where the signal peptide is cleaved off.[20,21] (A few proteins are synthesized entirely in the cytosol, then translocated into the ER lumen.) The newly synthesized polypeptide is folded and oligomers assembled with the assistance of molecular-folding proteins (chaperone proteins[22-24]) and RER-resident enzymes which catalyze disulphide bond formation and peptide chain bending (cyclophilins). N-glycosylation of peptides begins in the ER. Transport of correctly folded proteins from the lumen of the ER to the cis-face of the Golgi apparatus is mediated (at least in part) by transport vesicles which bud from the transitional regions of the ER.[25] Incorrectly or incompletely folded proteins are retained in the ER and degraded.[24] ER-resident proteins are selectively retrieved from the Golgi and returned to the ER by special transport vesicles.

The Golgi complex

The *Golgi complex* is a dynamic organelle, usually located close to the nucleus, consisting of an orderly stack (usually 4–6) of plate-like membrane-bound cisternae. Both *cis* and *trans* faces are closely linked to interconnected tubular and cisternal networks.[26] Luminal proteins move through the Golgi in specific transport vesicles which bud from one cisternum of the Golgi and fuse with the next. Post-translational modification of proteins (*O*-linked glycosylation, proteoglycan formation and sulphation of sugars and tyrosine residues) occurs in specific Golgi compartments. Proteins leaving the *trans*-Golgi network (TGN) are distributed by one of a number of distinct routes.

Protein transport to lysosomes

Proteins tagged with an oligosaccharide bearing a mannose 6-phosphate (M-6-P) group (destining them for the *lysosomes*) bind to M-6-P receptors in the TGN.[27] The cytoplasmic surface of the M-6-P receptor binds clathrin, which drives the budding and pinching off of clathrin-coated vesicles from the TGN. The vesicles rapidly lose their clathrin coat and subsequently fuse with the late endosomes, delivering their contents into the lumen.

Mature lysosomes form from late endosomes.[28] Lysosomes are extraordinarily diverse in size and shape. They are the major site of intracellular digestion, and contain a wide range of hydrolytic enzymes (proteases, lipases, nucleases, phosphatases, sulphatases, etc.) optimal at acid pH. Luminal pH (pH 5) is maintained by a proton pump in the lysosomal membrane. The membrane also contains proteins which specifically transport the final products of lysosomal digestion into the cytosol.

Constitutive protein secretion

Other TGN-derived transport vesicles carry surface membrane lipids and proteins for insertion into the plasmamembrane.[25,29] These vesicles are coated, not by clathrin, but by a number of coatomer proteins (COPs). In contrast to clathrin coats, coatomers do not self-assemble but require ATP and various specific monomeric GTP-binding proteins to drive their formation and docking.[29,30] Each stage of vesicle budding and fusion may require the participation of specific monomeric[31,32] and trimeric[33] GTP-binding proteins as well as nucleotides and other factors. Soluble proteins enclosed within these TGN-derived vesicles are released from the cell rapidly (typically 10–20 min) by fusion of vesicles with the cell surface-membrane – the constitutive ('default') secretory pathway. In polarized cells, transport mechanisms from the TGN operate selectively to ensure the delivery of proteins destined for either the apical or basolateral surface membrane.

Regulated protein secretion

Whereas the constitutive secretory pathway exists in all cell types, the regulated secretion pathway operates only in specialized secretory cells. Secretory proteins are segregated and concentrated into clathrin-coated vesicles[34,35] which bud from the TGN,[25,29] lose their coat and condense to form 'dense core' secretory granules. Many secreted proteins and peptides are synthesized as inactive precursors and are proteolytically processed in the TGN and maturing secretory granule. Granules are transported along the cytoskeleton and accumulate just below the plasma membrane (often only at the apical surface of the cell), where they are stored (typically one to several hours until release). An appropriate signal (e.g. activation of a cell-surface receptor by binding of its hormone ligand) then either directly activates voltage-gated calcium channels or generates an intracellular signal (second message) which causes a rise in intracellular calcium concentrations $[Ca^{2+}]_i$, disruption of the actin filament network beneath the plasma membrane, fusion of granule membrane with the cell membrane, and release of vesicle contents into the extracellular space by exocytosis – the 'regulated' secretory pathway.[30,36]

Endocytosis

Continued fusion of secretory vesicle membrane with the cell membrane would result in inexorable expansion of the cell surface. However, plasma membrane is continually recovered by endocytosis. Internalization of membrane and receptor-bound ligands can occur by at least two mechanisms. Some ligands (e.g. low-density lipoprotein, LDL) bind to specific receptors which cluster in clathrin-coated pits and pinch off to form clathrin-coated vesicles (receptor-mediated endocytosis[37]). (Note that, although clathrin-coated vesicles are formed both at the cell membrane during endocytosis and in the TGN, different clathrin-binding adapter proteins are involved in the two processes.[34,35] The clathrin cage is rapidly removed, the uncoated vesicles fuse with early endosomes (dissociating ligand from its receptor for delivery to lysosomes), whilst receptors are returned via transport vesicles to the cell surface membrane for re-use (recycling), or to a different plasma-membrane domain (transcytosis; e.g. IgA transport in mammary epithelial cells). In some circumstances, both ligand and receptor are degraded in the lysosomes ('receptor down-regulation': see Chapter 1.5). However, other cell surface components are internalized by a clathrin-independent mechanism, and are probably targeted to a non-degradative compartment.[38]

FUTURE PERSPECTIVES

Complex cell responses (differentiation, proliferation, programmed cell death) are generally stimulated by specific combinations of signals that the cell must integrate in order to respond appropriately. Contact with substratum and with other cells can profoundly influence cell structure and function, effects mediated by cell–cell and cell–ECM adhesion molecules.[39–41] On the other hand, it has long been appreciated that changes in cell shape (often mediated by ECM) can regulate gene expression,[41–43] and that malignant transformation often leads to decreased cell attachment and spreading on ECM and poor cell differentiation.[44] Hence, the molecules involved in cell–cell and cell–matrix adhesion (CAMs, cadherins, integrins) and the nature of their interactions with the cell cytoskeleton will be an area of major current research activity. There is particular interest in understanding how the various cell adhesion molecules can affect intracellular processes and, conversely, how changes in cell state are signaled through these same molecules to affect cell surface adhesiveness and responsiveness.[43–47]

ECM and cell adhesion molecules can also act synergistically with soluble growth factors to produce cellular responses which neither can induce alone. Research is beginning to define the detailed biochemical pathways activated by different hormones, and to outline the ways in which the enormous variety of intracellular signals generated by different hormones, growth factors, cell–ECM and cell–cell contacts interact[48–51] to induce stimulation of cell growth, cell differentiation or programmed cell death.

The processes whereby newly synthesized proteins are correctly folded and assembled in the lumen of the ER are beginning to be understood.[22–24] There is currently much debate about the mechanisms which segregate secretory proteins from other proteins in the Golgi and specifically package them into regulated secretory granules in the TGN.[52,53] Future work will undoubtedly seek to clarify the molecular signals which efficiently sequester proteins into the secretory granule.

Studies indicate that each stage of vesicle budding and

fusion requires the participation of specific components.[31-33] Further studies will elucidate the roles of Rab proteins, and of the various GTP-GDP exchange, GTPase activating proteins (GAPs)[31,32] and heterotrimeric G proteins[33] involved in driving transport vesicle formation and docking, and of the molecular 'ligands' of transport vesicles and the 'receptor' proteins (SNAPs and NSFs) of their target membranes which direct vesicle–acceptor membrane fusion in such a specific fashion.[25,30,54,55]

SUMMARY

- Eukaryotic cells are structurally and functionally highly organized and compartmentalized. Most cells grow and differentiate in intimate contact with other cells and/or extracellular matrix. Specific adhesion molecules link attached cell surfaces to the cytoskeleton.
- The cell surface membrane acts as a dynamic physical and electrochemical barrier. Transmembrane pumps and channels maintain cell homeostasis, and receptors enable the cell to sense and respond to changes in its environment.
- The prominent nucleus contains most of the genetic information of the cell (DNA) packaged as chromosomes, and has the necessary enzymes for replication and transcription of DNA, and splicing and processing of RNA.
- Mitochondria supply the energy of the cell by oxidative phosphorylation.
- Synthesis of proteins for secretion begins on the ribosome. Newly synthesized proteins are extruded into the lumen of the endoplasmic reticulum where they are actively assembled into their correctly folded configuration.

- Proteins are transported from the ER lumen to the Golgi apparatus where they are further processed by enzymes present in each subsequent Golgi stack. In the *trans*-Golgi network, protein for secretion is packaged into secretory granules, whereas other transport vesicles target proteins for delivery to the lysosomes, or to the cell surface membranes (the constitutive secretion pathway).
- Budding and fusion of transport vesicles is highly specific and closely regulated.
- Mature secretory granules are transported to the cell cortex where they are stored. Further processing of hormone may occur within the secretory granule.
- Receipt of a secretory stimulus triggers a rise in intracellular calcium levels, fusion of secretory granule membrane with the cell surface membrane, and release of granule contents into the extracellular space.
- Surface membrane and secretory granule membrane components are continuously recovered by endocytosis and recycled to the cell surface or delivered to lysosomes for degradation.

REFERENCES

1. Alberts B, Bray D, Lewis J, Raff M, Roberts K, Watson JD. *Molecular Biology of the Cell*, 3rd edition, New York and London: Garland Publishing, 1994.
2. Darnell J, Lodish H, Baltimore D. *Molecular Cell Biology*. New York: Scientific American Books, 1986.
3. Heath JK. *Growth Factors: In Focus*. Oxford: IRL Press, 1993.
4. Anderson JM, Balda MS, Fanning AS. The structure and regulation of tight junctions. *Curr Opin Cell Biol* 1993 5: 772–778.
5. Schwartz MA, Owaribe K, Kartenbeck J, Franke WW. Desmosomes and hemidesmosomes: constitutive molecular components. *Annu Rev Cell Biol* 1990 6: 461–491.
6. Beyer EC. Gap junctions. *Int Rev Cytol* 1993 137: 1–38.
7. Gerace L, Burke B. Functional organisation of the nuclear envelope. *Annu Rev Cell Biol* 1988 4: 335–374.
8. Bradbury EM. Reversible histone modifications and the chromosome cell cycle. *BioEssays* 1992 14: 9–16.
9. Gerace L, Burke B. Functional organisation of the nuclear envelope. *Annu Rev Cell Biol* 1988 4: 335–374.
10. Fakan S. Perichromatin fibrils are *in situ* forms of nascent transcripts. *Trends Cell Biol* 1994 4: 86–90.
11. Gelfand VI, Bershadsky AD. Microtubule dynamics: mechanism, regulation and function. *Annu Rev Cell Biol* 1991 7: 93–116.
12. Skoufias DA, Scholey JM. Cytoplasmic microtubule-based motor proteins. *Curr Opin Cell Biol* 1993 5: 95–104.
13. Stewart M. Intermediate filament structure and assembly. *Curr Opin Cell Biol* 1993 5: 3–11.
14. Bretscher A. Microfilament structure and function in the cortical cytoskeleton. *Annu Rev Cell Biol* 1991 7: 337–374.
15. Vanderkerkhove J, Vancompernolle K. Structural relationships of actin-binding proteins. *Curr Opin Cell Biol* 1992 4: 36–42.
16. Cooper JA. The role of actin polymerization in cell motility. *Annu Rev Physiol* 1991 53: 585–605.
17. Langford GM. Actin- and microtubule-dependent organelle motors: interrelationships between the two motility systems. *Curr Opin Cell Biol* 1995 7: 82–88.
18. Nicholls DG, Ferguson SJ. *Bioenergetics 2*. London: Academic Press, 1992.
19. Lazarow PB. Biogenesis of peroxisomes. *Trends Cell Biol* 1993 3: 89–93.
20. Sanders SL, Schekman R. Polypeptide translocation across the endoplasmic reticulum membrane. *J Biol Chem* 1992 267: 13791–13794.
21. Habener JF. Genetic control of hormone formation. In

Wilson JD, Foster DW (eds) *Williams Textbook of Endocrinology*, 8th edition. London: WB Saunders, 1992; 9–33.

22. Shinde U, Inouye M. Intramolecular chaperones and protein folding. *Trends Biochem Sci* 1993 **18**, 442–446.

23. Hartl F-U, Hlodan R, Langer T. Molecular chaperones in protein folding: the art of avoiding sticky situations. *Trends Biochem Sci* 1994 **19**: 20–25.

24. Bergeron JJM, Brenner MB, Thomas DY, Williams DB. Calnexin: a membrane-bound chaperone of the endoplasmic reticulum. *Trends Biochem Sci* 1994 **19**: 124–128.

25. Sztul ES, Melancon P, Howell KE. Targetting and fusion in vesicular transport. *Trends Cell Biol* 1992 **2**: 381–386.

26. Rambourg A, Clermont Y. Three-dimensional electron microscopy: structure of the Golgi apparatus. *Eur J Cell Biol* 1990 **51**: 189–200.

27. von Figura K. Molecular recognition and targeting of lysosomal proteins. *Curr Opin Cell Biol* 1991 **3**: 642–646.

28. Kornfeld S, Mellman I. The biogenesis of lysosomes. *Annu Rev Cell Biol* 1989 **5**: 483–525.

29. Gruenberg J, Clague MJ. Regulation of intracellular membrane transport. *Curr Opin Cell Biol* 1992 **4**: 593–599.

30. Pryer NK, Wuesthube LJ, Schekman R. Vesicle-mediated protein sorting. *Annu Rev Biochem* 1992 **61**: 471–516.

31. Pfeffer SR. GTP-binding proteins in intracellular transport. *Trends Cell Biol* 1992 **2**: 41–46.

32. Goud B, McCaffrey M. Small GTP-binding proteins and their role in transport. *Curr Opin Cell Biol* 1993 **3**: 626–633.

33. Barr FA, Leyte A, Huttner WB. Trimeric G proteins and vesicle formation. *Trends Cell Biol* 1992 **2**: 91–94.

34. Morris S, Ahle S, Ungewickell E. Clathrin-coated vesicles. *Curr Opin Cell Biol* 1989 **1**: 684–690.

35. Brodsky FM, Hill BL, Acton SL et al. Clathrin light chains: arrays of protein motifs that regulate coated-vesicle dynamics. *Trends Biochem Sci* 1991 **16**: 208–213.

36. White JM. Membrane fusion. *Science* 1992 **258**: 917–924.

37. Vallee RB, Okamoto PM. The regulation of endocytosis: identifying dynamin's binding partners. *Trends Cell Biol* 1995 **5**: 43–47.

38. Sandvig K, van Deurs B. Endocytosis without clathrin. *Trends Cell Biol* 1994 **4**: 275–277.

39. Kuhn K, Eble J. The structural bases of integrin–ligand interaction. *Trends Cell Biol* 1994 **4**: 256–261.

40. Tuckwell DS, Weston S, Humphries MJ. Integrins: a review of their structure and mechanisms of binding. In Jones G, Wigley C, Warn R (eds) *Cell Behaviour: Adhesion and Motility* Cambridge, UK: The Company of Biologists Ltd, 1993: 107–136.

41. Williams J, Kieffer N. Adhesion molecules in cellular interactions. *Trends Cell Biol* 1994 **4**: 102–104.

42. Hogg N, Landis RC, Bates PA, Stanley P, Randi AM. The sticking point: how integrins bind to their ligands. *Trends Cell Biol* 1994 **4**: 379–382.

43. Hynes RO. Integrins: versatility, modulation and signalling in cell adhesion. *Cell* 1992 **69**: 11–25.

44. Van Roy F, Mareel M. Tumour invasion: effects of cell adhesion and motility. *Trends Cell Biol* 1992 **2**: 163–169.

45. Quaranta V, Jones JCR. The internal affairs of an integrin. *Trends Cell Biol* 1991 **1**: 2–4.

46. Schwartz MA. Transmembrane signalling by integrins. *Trends Cell Biol* 1992 **2**: 304–308.

47. Williams MJ, Hughes PE, O'Toole TE, Ginsberg MH. The inner world of cell adhesion: integrin cytoplasmic domains. *Trends Cell Biol* 1994 **4**: 109–112.

48. Inagaki N, Ito M, Nakano T, Inagaki M. Spatiotemporal distribution of protein kinase and phosphatase activities. *Trends Biochem Sci* 1994 **19**: 448–452.

49. Wilson C. Receptor tyrosine kinase signalling: not so complex after all? *Trends Cell Biol* 1994 **4**: 409–414.

50. Sun H, Tonks NK. The coordinated action of protein tyrosine phosphatases and kinases in cell signalling. *Trends Biochem Sci* 1994 **19**: 480–485.

51. Daum G, Eizenmann-Tappe I, Fries H-W, Troppmair J, Rapp UR. The ins and outs of Raf kinases. *Trends Biochem Sci* 1994 **19**: 474–480.

52. Griffiths G, Doms RW, Mayhew T, Lucocq J. The bulk flow hypothesis: not quite the end. *Trends Cell Biol* 1995 **5**: 9–13.

53. Balch WE, Farquhar MG. Beyond bulk flow. *Trends Cell Biol* 1995 **4**: 16–19.

54. Whiteheart SW, Kubalek EW. SNAPs and NSF: general members of the fusion apparatus. *Trends Cell Biol* 1995 **5**: 64–68.

55. Warren G, Levine T, Misteli T. Mitotic disassembly of the mammalian Golgi apparatus. *Trends Cell Biol* 1995 **5**: 413–416.

1.3

Cell Cycle

R Leake

INTRODUCTION

To understand both the development and differentiation of normal tissues and to approach therapy of tissues which have adopted abnormal growth patterns, such as in hyperplasia, dysplasia and cancer, it is necessary to have a good understanding of the nature and regulation of the normal cell cycle. There is also increasing evidence that the growth of tissues in both health and disease is a balance of cell division and programmed cell death (apoptosis). This chapter describes the biological basis of the cell cycle, then goes on to review some of the mechanisms involved in control of the cell cycle and, finally, discusses some of the points of breakdown which can lead to clinical disease in reproductive tissues.

Cells can, of course, grow without dividing. They may simply absorb more liquid or increase the amount of intracellular protein etc. However, most reproductive cells will begin the processes that lead to cell division, once they reach a critical size and/or receive an appropriate signal. The prin-

cipal objective of a dividing cell is to achieve the production of a pair of identical daughter cells, both of which contain exact and complete copies of the genetic information present in the parent cell. In other words, the total DNA content of the parent cell must be accurately replicated and then the replicated chromosomes must be segregated into two separate cells. Thus, the simplest version of the cell cycle is that shown in Fig. 1.3.1, in which the only feature is the accurate replication of the full DNA complement of the parent cell. However, in practice, reproductive cells are also going to require that the cell mass is doubled and all the subcellular organelles (mitochondria, Golgi bodies etc.) are doubled so that the daughter cells have exactly the same functional potential as does the parent cell.

CURRENT CONCEPTS

The cell cycle

The length of the cell cycle can vary considerably. Bone marrow cells have a cycle time of about 18 h, whereas colon crypt cells have a cycle length of about 450 h.[1] When human cells are grown *in vitro*, they have a cycle length of around 24 h.[2] The cycle is divided up into different phases, each to represent a period with a particular function. An obvious starting point is the phase of mitosis (the M phase). The overall process involves the segregation of the daughter chromosomes and the division of the nucleus into two approximately equal halves. In *prophase* the genetic material condenses into visible chromosomes. The microtubules of the cell reorganize themselves into the mitotic spindle. During *metaphase* the chromosomes, already duplicated, line up on the mitotic spindle, ready for segregation. Segregation of the chromosome sets marks the beginning of *anaphase*. In *telophase*, the two daughter nuclei begin to separate from each other. The process of *cytokinesis* involves the separation of the two daughter cells and marks the end of the

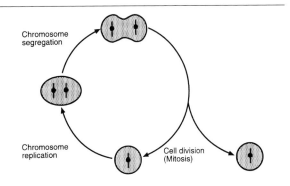

Fig. 1.3.1 *The simplest form of the cell cycle is one in which the genetic material of a parent cell is replicated and divided in such a way that each daughter cell receives a complete and identical copy of each of the parent chromosomes.*

M phase. The whole of the M phase only occupies about one hour in dividing reproductive cells.

The two daughter cells can either go into a resting phase or they can plan to divide again at the earliest opportunity. If they are programmed to go straight into another round of cell division, then DNA synthesis cannot begin immediately. There has to be a period of gene transcription and protein synthesis to provide the necessary enzymes to drive the replication of all the DNA in the nucleus. Because this phase is a period of growth, it is known as the G_1 phase. If the cells have entered a sustained resting period (as in terminal differentiation), then this is known as the G_0 phase. At the end of the G_1 phase cells enter a period of DNA synthesis known as the S phase. Once S phase is completed, there is then another period of growth before mitosis can begin again. This is known as the G_2 phase. A typical cell cycle, based on an overall time of 24 h is shown in Fig. 1.3.2.

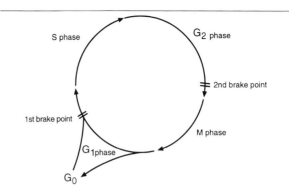

Fig. 1.3.2 *A diagram of a typical cell cycle, showing mitosis (M), the possibility to enter a resting phase (G_0), the first growth phase (G_1), the period of DNA synthesis (S) and the second period of growth in preparation for cell division (G_2). Note the positions of the two brake points, which must be overcome for cell division to be achieved.*

Regulation of the cell cycle

There are two principal brake points, at which progress through the cell cycle can either be stopped or promoted. The first brake point is in late G_1 phase and the second is immediately prior to entry into the M phase. Exogenous factors (hormones, growth factors and cytokines, see later section), which are designed to increase or decrease the rate of cell division, are most likely to act during the G_1 phase. It is a combination of endogenous factors (size, protein content, calcium concentration[3]) together with the exogenous regulators that push the cell through the critical phase of G_1 such that it will enter S phase. Once cells have entered S phase they are normally committed to go and divide. Determination of the length of S phase can be determined using a brief pulse of [3H]thymidine to label the newly synthesized DNA. The number of cells is then determined by autoradiography. Similarly, newly synthesized DNA can be determined with a pulse of bromodeoxyuridine (BrdU), which can be detected with an anti-BrdU antibody. Alternatively, the proportion of cells in G_1, S or $G_2 + M$ can be determined in the flow cytometer after treating cells with fluorescent dyes such as propidium iodide. Various computer programs are available to analyze the data but it is essential to incorporate the necessary controls.[4] Further details of these methods can be found in ref. 2.

Growth, as measured by increasing protein and RNA content occurs throughout the cell cycle, apart from the M phase when the chromosomes are too tightly packed to allow transcription. However, as already mentioned, in dividing cells the critical point in committing a cell to enter the cycle is late in G_1 when the balance of exogenous and endogenous factors decides whether the cell shall enter DNA synthesis. There is also a second point which decides whether or not the cell will enter M phase.

The regulatory molecules

There are two closely related families of proteins which are involved in regulating the cell cycle. These are the *cyclin-dependent protein kinases* (the CdKs) and the *cyclins* themselves. The CdKs are serine/threonine protein kinases. The cyclins regulate the activities of the CdKs and so control their ability to modulate the enzymes involved in driving the cell cycle. The CdKs are only functional when combined with one of the cyclins. Thus, the assembly, activation and disassembly of the cyclin–CdK complex are the critical events in controlling the cell cycle. As their name implies, cyclins undergo synthesis and degradation during each cycle of the cell. There are two main classes of cyclins, the G_1 cyclins which bind to CdKs during the G_1 phase and are required for entry into S phase, and the mitotic cyclins which bind CdK during G_2 to permit the entry of the cell into M phase. In mammalian cells, there are at least two different families of CdKs, one for each of the two critical regulatory points. The destruction of cyclin is as important as its synthesis. For example, in mitosis, cyclin is suddenly destroyed by proteolysis at the metaphase–anaphase boundary and without this step the daughter cells will not emerge from mitosis.

Much of the work on understanding the molecular roles of the cyclin–CdK complexes in regulating the animal cell cycle has come from study of the *Xenopus* oocyte, though the mechanisms involved seem to be almost identical in human cells (see Chapter 2.4). When cytoplasm from M phase is injected into a G_2 phase oocyte, the oocyte then enters M phase and completes its maturation – hence the factor involved was given the name maturation-promoting factor or MPF. Later experiments[5] showed that MPF was the same factor which drove G_2 phase cells into M phase. Once purified, MPF was found to consist of a CdK called Cdc2 complexed with the mitosis cyclin (Fig. 1.3.3) (in mammalian cells the mitosis cyclin is known as cyclin B). The details of the activation of the Cdc2–cyclin complex have been carefully reviewed.[6] A CdK-activating kinase stimulates the activity of Cdc2 by phosphorylating it on threonine residue 161. However, there is further regulation through inhibitory phosphorylation of tyrosine 15 (achieved through a balance of activity of the Cdc2-specific

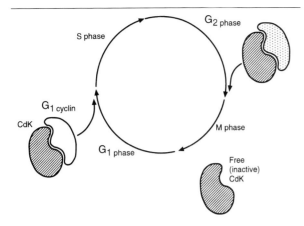

Fig. 1.3.3 *Different cyclins complex with and activate the cyclin-dependent kinase in order to push the cell through the two brake points of the cell cycle.*

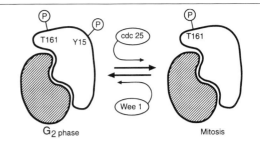

Fig. 1.3.4 *Activation of cyclin-dependent kinase requires not only formation of a complex with cyclin but also phosphorylation of threonine-161 and dephosphorylation of tyrosine-15. The phosphorylation state of tyrosine-15 is very tightly regulated by the two enzymes Cdc 25 (a highly specific phosphatase) and wee 1 (a Cdc-2-specific tyrosine kinase).*

tyrosine kinase *wee 1* and a competing phosphatase (Cdc25), which is extremely specific and closely regulated). Once the cyclin–Cdc2 complex is formed, the *wee 1* protein phosphorylates tyrosine 15 and keeps the complex in the inactive form. Phosphorylation of threonine 161 potentially activates MPF but it only acquires the necessary activity to push the cell into M phase, once the tyrosine 15 has been dephosphorylated by the Cdc25 enzyme. For more details, see reference 7. A simplified diagram is shown in Fig. 1.3.4.

The same Cdc2 molecule (and, in mammalian cells the closely related CdK2 molecule) is involved in the push past the brake point in G_1. However, in this case, it needs to form a complex with a different cyclin, the G_1 cyclin. The situation is complex in that there are several cyclins (those named so far are A, B, C, D, E and F). When the Cdc2 forms a complex with the first G_1 cyclin, the complex induces transcription of the genes for the other G_1 cyclins, such that a cascade effect rapidly pushes the cell through the brake point. Cdc2–cyclin E is thought to be the complex which initially pushes the cell through the brake point and Cdc2–cyclin A then activates the DNA synthesis machinery (Fig. 1.3.5). Although there is increasing evidence that the Cdc–G_1 cyclin complex is involved in the activation of the enzymes involved in DNA synthesis (DNA polymerases, ligase, topoisomerase, enzymes for nucleotide synthesis, initiation factors), most of these enzymes are present throughout the cell cycle and the complex must simply activate them through phosphorylation. There is also evidence however, to suggest that it can additionally increase transcription of the relevant genes. Once the cell enters S phase, the G_1 cyclins are degraded and cannot be detected again until a similar stage in the G_1 phase of the next cycle. When hormones regulate cell growth, it can be shown that the levels of the G_1 cyclins become elevated so the evidence is consistent with the concept that activity of the Cdc–cyclin complex is critical to both endogenously and exogenously activated cell division.

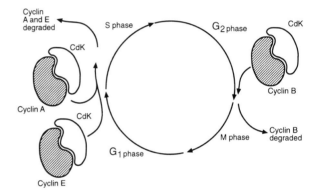

Fig. 1.3.5 *Human dividing cells contain a family of cyclins. The sites of action of the major representatives are shown.*

Growth factors

Mammalian cells in serum-free culture medium, or in quiescent states *in vivo*, enter a resting phase known as G_0. They are typically pushed back into the cell cycle by one of a variety of polypeptide growth factors. Each growth factor works through a specific receptor on the plasma membrane of the cell and the many steps involved between activation of the receptor and activation of the cyclin–CdK2 complex to push the cell towards S phase have now been worked out. These steps are largely outside the scope of this review but details can be found in reference 8. However, it is worthwhile to summarize models of the interaction of different growth factors in the regulation of reproductive cells. It is now recognized that at least some of the growth regulatory actions of both steroid and peptide hormones on reproductive cells are, in fact, mediated by local growth factors. In both endometrium and ovary, there is evidence for hormonal stimulation of the transforming growth factor TGF-α,[9] of platelet-derived growth factor (PDGF), of fibroblast growth factors (FGFs)[10] and of insulin-like growth factors (IGFs).[11] Additionally, growth of epithelial cells in reproductive tissues can be down-regulated by TGF-β and there is also increasing evidence for roles for cytokines such as tumour necrosis factor, interleukin-1, interleukin-6, etc. Models of the complex interaction of these growth factors are outside the scope of this review but details of their interaction in reproductive tissues can be found in references 12 and 13.

When hormones[14] and growth factors[15] stimulate target cells, early response genes such as *myc, fos,* and *jun* are activated well before the genes for CdKs and cyclins. Indeed, the product of the *myc* gene is essential for the increase in CdKs and cyclins that occurs prior to the passage of the G$_1$ brake point. Thus, the *myc* gene product has an important role to play in growth factor-induced cell growth and this is relevant to the roles of growth factors in promotion of gynecological tumors (see later). The whole control mechanism is summarized in Fig. 1.3.6.

Inhibitory regulators

So far, we have discussed stimulators of the cell cycle. However, in the same way that tyrosine dephosphorylation was the last, critical step before the CdK–cyclin complex could push the cell through the brake point, there are specific proteins which positively inhibit the entry of the cell into S phase. Perhaps the best known of these inhibitory proteins is the product of the retinoblastoma (*Rb*) gene. The *Rb* gene was first detected because patients who suffer loss of both copies, then show very rapid and excessive proliferation of the cells in the immature retina.[16] From this observation, it became clear that the Rb product plays an important role in inhibiting cell proliferation in all tissues. The Rb protein acts by binding to and neutralizing other proteins.[17] This ability to bind other proteins depends on its state of phosphorylation. When dephosphorylated, it binds several of the proteins required to promote cell proliferation. The dephosphorylated Rb binds to and inactivates transcription factors which directly induce expression of the genes for *myc, fos* and other, related nuclear proteins. Once Rb becomes phosphorylated, for example as a result

of growth factor action, the transcription factors are released and *myc* protein and related proteins are then able to induce an increase in CdK which, in turn, causes the push through the G$_1$ brake. Rb protein remains phosphorylated through S phase and into G$_2$ (at least partly, due to the kinase activity of the CdK) but then becomes dephosphorylated until the next G$_1$ phase. Indeed, it is probably the action of Rb protein in neutralizing cell growth promoting proteins such as the *myc* protein that allows cells to enter G$_0$. These processes are summarized in Fig. 1.3.7.

Another protein which plays an important role in monitoring the cell cycle is the p53 protein. p53, like Rb, was originally discovered because mutations to the gene were found in various cancers.[18] In fact, it turns out that p53 monitors the quality of the DNA in the cell before replication can take place and, indeed, p53 is only detected in cells which contain damaged DNA. Thus, if the p53 protein locates any faults in the DNA, S phase is blocked (by both inducing genes whose protein products inhibit cell growth and by suppressing genes whose products stimulate cell growth[19]) until the repair enzymes have restored the DNA to its original state.[20] If the amount of damage is too great, the cell is pushed into programmed cell death, rather than allowed to divide. Hence loss of the p53 protein, through an inactivating mutation within the gene, can lead to cancer because cells with seriously mutated or translocated DNA can now proliferate. p53 binds to DNA and induces transcription of a gene which results in synthesis of a protein that binds to and neutralizes the CdK–cyclin complex. Hence inactivation of p53 means that the cell can now push through the cell cycle brakes. The molecular basis of the ability of HPV 16 and 18 to induce cervical cancer is thought to be because the proteins E6 and E7, coded by the virus, bind to and inactivate both Rb and p53 proteins.[21]

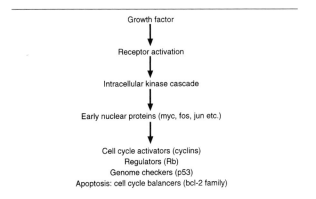

Growth factor
↓
Receptor activation
↓
Intracellular kinase cascade
↓
Early nuclear proteins (myc, fos, jun etc.)
↓
Cell cycle activators (cyclins)
Regulators (Rb)
Genome checkers (p53)
Apoptosis: cell cycle balancers (bcl-2 family)

Fig. 1.3.6 *A highly simplified summary of the critical steps in growth factor-driven changes in cell division rates.*

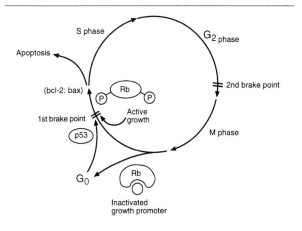

Fig. 1.3.7 *A summary of the molecules involved in the critical balance between entry into the cell cycle or commitment to programmed cell death (apoptosis). The retinoblastoma protein can hold essential nuclear growth promoters in an inactive form but these are released when Rb is phosphorylated. The p53 protein will only allow the cell to enter S-phase if the genome is undamaged. The ratio of active bcl-2:bax makes the critical decision over whether the cell should replicate DNA or die.*

Apoptosis

As mentioned earlier, when cells reach the G_1 brake, they can be directed either to go into S phase or, if there is evidence of damaged DNA, they can be sent into programmed cell death. This latter process is known as apoptosis.[22] Similarly, cells which are likely to be damaged, and so pushed into apoptosis because of oxidative stress, are thought to be protected from apoptosis by the bcl-2 protein.[23] bcl-2 protein functions as a dimer and is a member of a family of closely related proteins which includes the *bax* gene product. bcl-2/bcl-2 protein dimers promote cell survival, bax/bax dimers promote cell death and the heterodimer has intermediate effects.[24]

It follows from the foregoing that there must be interaction between Rb, p53, myc, bcl-2 and bax proteins, in addition to the roles that growth factors have in regulating the amounts and activities of these nuclear proteins. To try to summarize these interactions: high myc+high growth factors will lead to cell growth; low myc+low growth factors will lead to growth arrest; high myc+low growth factors will lead to apoptosis. p53 is thought to influence the relative amounts of bcl-2 and bax, thereby influencing the nature of the active dimer and so pushing either for cell division or apoptosis.[25] Similarly growth factors control the activity of Rb protein by governing its phosphorylation state, thereby controlling whether or not there is enough cyclin–CdK complex to push the cell into S phase, given that the p53/bcl2-bax combination has given the green light for growth rather than apoptosis. Thus, if transformed reproductive cells suffer from either inactivation of Rb or p53 or overexpression of bcl-2 or myc, then there will be increased cell division and loss of cell death, such that tumor growth and progression will be favored.

Conclusions

The length of the cell cycle for mammalian cells can be as little as a few hours in embryonic cells or cells can move into a resting or G_0 phase in which the next round of cell division does not occur for weeks or months. Depending on the conditions (presence of serum and/or added hormones or growth factors; presence of basement membrane), human cells grown *in vitro* have a cell cycle length of about 24 h.

There are two important points at which the brakes can be applied to stop cell division. The first brake point occurs late in G_1 phase and must be passed in order to enter S phase. The second brake point occurs immediately prior to entry into mitosis. A complex of cyclin and cyclin-dependent kinase (CdK) is essential to pass either of these brake points. This complex is initially held in an inactive state. However, as a result of the downstream responses to extracellular growth factors, acting through their receptor-linked second messenger systems, phosphorylation of a specific threonine on the complex is followed by dephosphorylation of a specific tryosine. The cyclin–CdK complex can now push the cell through the brake point. This induction of the cyclin–CdK complex involves nuclear proteins such as the products of the genes *myc* and *fos*. These genes are only expressed once the Rb protein has been phosphorylated and released the necessary transcription factors.

The cellular decision to enter proliferation is only partly made in response to exogenous factors such as hormones or growth factors. It can also be influenced by the calcium/calmodulin balance, by the state of the DNA, as reflected in the activity of the p53 protein or by metabolic stress. If there is DNA damage or oxidative stress (measured by the bcl-2 protein), then the cellular policing mechanism may decide on cell death (apoptosis). The decision to go for proliferation or apoptosis is dependent on the relative levels of various nuclear proteins (myc, bcl-2, bax etc.). The success of this policing mechanism ensures that most tissues remain healthy throughout life. Clinical complications in reproductive tissues (hyperplasia, cancer etc.) reflect a breakdown in this policing system.

FUTURE PERSPECTIVES

As our understanding of the control of entry into the cell cycle increases[26], it may be possible to rescue cells which appear to have lost the ability to divide. Conversely, for some clinical conditions (dysplasia, cancer), it may soon be possible to promote natural cell death (apoptosis) and so avoid the use of highly toxic, non-specific cell poisons. It is experimentally possible to target specific members of the cyclin and cyclin-dependent kinase families, so it should be realistic to introduce therapies which act by blocking cell division. Equally, more knowledge of the mechanisms of phosphorylation and de-phosphorylation of critical molecules such as the retinoblastoma protein and an ability to alter the ratio of different members of the *bcl-2* family should both lead to new therapies for the control of abnormal cell growth. Specific tyrosine and serine/threonine kinase inhibitors are being developed for clinical use. Clincally effective, specific phosphatases should also be considered.

SUMMARY

- There are two points (brake points) through which the cell must pass before it can enter cell division.
- Progress through each brake point requires the presence of an active cyclin-dependent kinase (CdK).
- There are specific cyclins to activate the CdKs at different parts of the cell cycle.

- Activation of the cyclin–CdK complex is tightly regulated by the phosphorylation state of the CdK.

- Exogenous (hormones, growth factors and cytokines) growth stimulators all work through an intracellular kinase cascade which drives the production and activation of *early* nuclear proteins which, in turn, induce transcription of the genes for cyclins, CdKs and other cell cycle regulators.

- Retinoblastoma protein regulates cell division by inactivating specific growth-promoting proteins. Thus mutation of the Rb gene can lead to uncontrolled cell division and so promotion of transformed cells.

- p53 protein will prevent replication of cells with damaged DNA. Hence, transformed cells can only readily progress to tumors if the p53 gene is mutated in a manner which inactivates the protein product.

- Members of the bcl-2 family act, in homo- and heterodimers, to shunt cells into either cell division or into apoptosis.

- Understanding the mechanisms by which the balance of cell cycle:apoptosis can be manipulated will lead to new ways of controlling abnormal cellular growth.

- Most aspects of cellular function reflect changes in phosphorylation of critical serine, threonine and tyrosine residues on the relevant regulatory proteins. The kinases and phosphatases involved are themselves under tight control.

REFERENCES

1. Baserga R. *The Biology of Cell Reproduction*. Cambridge, MA.: Harvard University Press, 1985.

2. O'Farrell MK, Dealtry GB. In Dealtry GB, Rickwood D (eds) *Cell Biology Labfax*. Oxford: Bios Blackwell, 1992: 205–210.

3. Lu KP, Means AR. Regulation of the cell cycle by calcium and calmodulin. *Endocr Rev* 1993 **14**: 40–58.

4. Watson JV. *Introduction to Flow Cytometry*. Cambridge: Cambridge University Press, 1991.

5. Nakamura T, Matsumoto K. *Growth Factors, Cell Growth, Morphogenesis and Transformation*. New York: CRC Press, 1994.

6. Lohka MJ, Hayes MK, Maller JL. Purification of maturation-promoting factor, an intracellular regulator of early mitotic events. *Proc Natl Acad Sci USA* 1988 **85**: 3009–3013.

7. Draetta G. cdc2 activation: the interplay of cyclin binding and Thr 161 phosphorylation. *Trends Cell Biol* 1993 **3**: 287–289.

8. Dunphy WG. The decision to enter mitosis. *Trends Cell Biol* 1994 4: 202–207.

9. Owens OJ, Stewart C, Leake RE. Growth factor concentration and distribution in ovarian cancer. *Br J Cancer* 1991 **64**: 1177–1181.

10. Leake R, Barber A, Owens O, Langdon S, Miller WR. Growth factors and receptors in ovarian cancer. In: Sharp F, Mason P, Blackett T, Berek J (eds) *Ovarian Cancer-3*. London: Chapman & Hall Medical, 1995: 99–109.

11. Westley BR, May FEB. Role of insulin-like growth factors in steroid-modulated proliferation. *J Steroid Biochem* 1994 **51**: 1–12.

12. Murphy LJ. Growth factors and steroid hormone action in endometrial cancer. *J Steroid Biochem* 1994 **48**: 419–423.

13. Leake R, Carr L, Rinaldi F. Autocrine and paracrine effects in the endometrium. *Ann NY Acad Sci* 1991 **622**: 145–148.

14. Schuchard M, Landers JP, Punkay N, Spelsburg TC. Steroid hormone regulation of nuclear proto-oncogenes. *Endocr Rev* 1993 **14**: 659–669.

15. Alvarez NG, Northwood IC, Gonzalez FA, *et al.* Pro-Leu-Ser/Thr-Pro is a consensus primary sequence for substrate protein phosphorylation. Characterization of the phosphorylation of c-*myc* and c-*jun* proteins by an epidermal growth factor receptor threonine 669 protein kinase. *J Biol Chem* 1991 **266**: 15277–15285.

16. Cobrinik D, Dowdy SF, Hinds PW, Mittnacht S, Weinberg RA. The retinoblastoma protein and regulation of the cell cycle. *Trends Biochem Sci* 1992 **17**: 312–315.

17. Hollingsworth RE, Chen PL, Lee WH. Integration of cell cycle control with transcriptional regulation by the retinoblastoma protein. *Curr Opin Cell Biol* 1993 **5**: 194–200.

18. Lane DP. Worrying about p53. *Curr Biol* 1992 **2**: 581–583.

19. Brown R. p53 as a potential target for anticancer drugs. *Cancer Topics* 1993 **9**: 102–104.

20. Perry ME, Levine AJ. Tumour suppressor p53 and the cell cycle. *Curr Opin Genet Dev* 1993 **3**: 50–54.

21. Schwartzman W, Cidlowski JA. Apoptosis: The biochemistry and molecular biology of programmed cell death. *Endocr Rev* 1993 **14**: 133–151.

22. Gissman L. Papilloma viruses and human oncogenesis. *Curr Opin Genet Dev* 1992 **2**: 97–102.

23. Hall PA, Lane DP. Genetics of growth arrest and cell death: key determinants of tissue homeostasis. *Eur J Cancer* 1994 **30A**: 2001–2012.

24. Oltvai ZN, Millman CL, Korsemeyer SJ. bcl-2 heterodimerises *in vivo* with a conserved homolog bax which accelerates cell death. *Cell* 1993 **74**: 609–619.

25. Selvakumaran M, Lin HK, Miyashita T et al. Immediate early up regulation of bax expression by p53 but not by TGFβ1: a paradigm for distinct apoptotic pathways. *Oncogene* 1994 **9**: 1791–1798.

26. Massagné J, Roberts JM. Cell cycle 1995: constructing cell physiology with molecular building blocks. *Curr Opin Cell Biol* 1995 **7**: 769–772.

1.4

Hormone Receptors

KJ Catt

INTRODUCTION

Many hormones and other ligands that regulate cell function circulate at subnanomolar concentrations and exert their actions by binding to specific receptors located on the cell surface or within the cell. In general, peptide hormones are bound by receptors residing on the plasma membrane and activate processes that release molecular signals (second messengers) into the cytoplasm of the cell. On the other hand, steroid hormones diffuse into the cell and are bound by receptor proteins in the cytoplasm and/or nucleus. Once occupied by the hormone, steroid receptors undergo activation and translocation to the nucleus, where they influence gene transcription and the expression of specific proteins. An outline of the manner in which ligands bind to the two major classes of receptors and activate signaling pathways in the cytoplasm and nucleus of their target cells is shown in Fig 1.4.1.

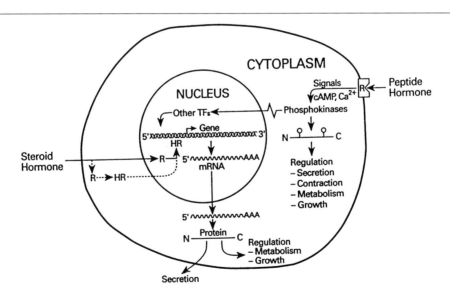

Fig. 1.4.1 Receptors and signaling pathways of peptide and steroid hormones. Peptide hormones bind to plasma-membrane receptors and stimulate the formation of intracellular signals, including cyclic nucleotides and calcium, that activate protein kinases. These in turn phosphorylate proteins that are involved in a variety of cellular responses, including metabolism, secretion, contraction, neurotransmission, and growth. Many peptide hormones also stimulate a cascade of phosphorylation that extends into the nucleus and activates transcription factors (TFs) that in turn influence gene transcription. Steroid hormones diffuse into their target cells and bind to receptors located in the cytoplasm or nucleus. The hormone–receptor complexes (HR) undergo conformational changes followed by association with nuclear chromatin and binding to hormone response elements in the promoters of hormone-regulated genes. The protein products of these genes act on growth and metabolic pathways in the cell, and in some cases are secreted and exert local actions, as in the reproductive tract.

CURRENT CONCEPTS

Peptide hormone receptors

The existence of receptors was first proposed to explain the actions of drugs on specific cell responses, and the application of the concept to hormone action is a relatively recent development. The first evidence that peptide hormones and transmitters generate intracellular signals by binding to cell-surface receptors was the demonstration that catecholamines stimulate the formation of the second messenger, cyclic AMP, by increasing the enzymatic activity of adenylyl cyclase in the plasma membrane.[1] Since 1960, hundreds of hormone receptors have been identified, at first functionally in terms of their ability to bind hormones and elicit specific responses, and more recently by molecular cloning and elucidation of their amino acid sequences and structural arrangements in relation to the plasma membrane. As described in the following chapter, cell-surface receptors control the activities of numerous membrane-associated enzymes and channels involved in the generation of intracellular signals. Such signals in turn activate or inhibit pathways that regulate a variety of specific cellular responses, including secretion, contraction, neurotransmission, and growth. The major plasma-membrane receptors and their proximate effector systems are shown in Table 1.4.1.

The numerous peptide and protein hormones that influence target-cell function can be subdivided into several major groups according to their major physiological actions, and are further classified by their amino acid sequences and structural properties. Likewise, the receptors for such hormones fall into several families that possess common structural features and mediate similar functional responses.[2] All peptide hormone receptors possess specific binding domains that interact with the nanomolar or lower concentrations of their ligands that are present in the extracellular fluid. Such domains are of high affinity and specificity, and often depend on disulfide bridges between cysteine residues for the maintenance of their specific binding conformations. The external regions of receptors, like other cell-surface proteins, are usually glycosylated and are correspondingly hydrophilic. In most receptors the carbohydrate groups are not directly involved in the binding site, but contribute to the expression and general conformation of the receptor protein. The extracellular domain varies greatly in size among peptide hormone receptors, and often contains the ligand binding site. However, in some cases the binding site also involves the transmembrane domain(s) of the receptor.

All cell-surface receptors are anchored in the plasma membrane by one or more stretches of hydrophobic amino acids. Such membrane-spanning domains are composed of about 23 amino acids, corresponding to the number of residues required to form an α-helix of the length required to cross the membrane bilayer. The transmembrane domains are often flanked by charged amino acids that help to lock the hydrophobic regions into the plasma membrane. Many receptors, especially those for growth

Table 1.4.1 Plasma membrane receptors and effector systems

Receptors	Primary effector systems
CRF, GHRH, ACTH, TSH, MSH, LH, FSH, VIP, glucagon, PACAP, PTH, calcitonin, vasopressin V_2, β-adrenergic, dopamine D_1, serotonin 5-HT$_3$	Adenylyl cyclase: activation
α_2-Adrenergic, somatostatin, opiate, muscarinic M_2, M_4, adenosine A_1, angiotensin II, serotonin 5HT$_1$	Adenylyl cyclase: inhibition
ANP	Guanylyl cyclase: activation
α_1-Adrenergic, muscarinic M_1, M_3, histamine H_1, vasopressin V_1, TRH, GnRH, angiotensin II, serotonin 5-HT$_2$, PDGF, thrombin	Phospholipase C: activation Calcium: mobilization
EGF, insulin, IGF-1, PDGF, FGF	Intrinsic receptor tyrosine kinase: activation
Growth hormone, prolactin, other cytokines	Cytoplasmic tyrosine kinase: activation
Activin, TGF-β	Serine/threonine phosphorylation: activation
Nicotinic acetylcholine	Sodium channel: activation
NMDA, AMPA, kainate	Sodium/calcium channel: activation
GABA, glycine	Chloride channel: activation
Muscarinic M_2	Potassium channel: inhibition

Abbreviations: ACTH, adrenocorticotropin; CRF, corticotropin releasing factor; EGF, epidermal growth factor; FGF, fibroblast growth factor; FSH, follicle-stimulating hormone; GABA, gamma-aminobutyric acid; GnRH, gonadotropin releasing hormone; GHRH, growth hormone releasing hormone; 5-HT, 5-hydroxy-tryptamine; IGF, insulin-like growth factor; LH, luteinizing hormone; MSH, melanocyte stimulating hormone; TGF, transforming growth factors; PACAP, pituitary adenylate cyclase activating peptide; PDGF, platelet-derived growth factor; PTH, parathyroid hormone; TRH, thyrotropin releasing hormone; TSH, thyrotropin; VIP, vasoactive intestinal peptide. NMDA, *N*-methyl-D-aspartic acid; AMPA, α-amino-3-hydroxy-5-methyl-isoxazale 4-propionic acid.

factors and cytokines, contain a single transmembrane domain located between the large extra- and intracellular regions of the receptor protein. Other major groups of receptors contain multiple membrane-spanning domains, either four or seven in number, that form bundles of α-helices within the plasma membrane. The seven transmembrane domain receptors, like those with a single transmembrane domain, are formed by monomeric proteins that have extracellular N-terminal and intracellular C-terminal regions. In contrast, the receptor proteins with four transmembrane regions are subunits of large multimeric protein complexes, each composed of several peptide chains. Such subunits typically have a large extracellular N-terminal domain and a C-terminal extracellular domain.

The three major types of cell-surface receptors are exemplified by growth factor/cytokine receptors with one transmembrane domain;[3] transmitter and peptide hormone receptors coupled to signaling proteins in the plasma membrane, with seven transmembrane domains;[4] and the subunits of ligand-gated channels, with four transmembrane domains.[5] The general structures of these receptors are shown in Fig 1.4.2, and are described in more detail below. Their common features, in addition to their cell-surface location, are their abilities to bind selectively to hormones and transmitters with high affinity, and to transmit signals across the plasma membrane by undergoing conformational changes that promote their interactions with other proteins located in the plasma membrane. In the case of growth factor receptors, such interactions typically involve other receptors of the same type, leading to dimerization of the ligand-activated receptors within the cell membrane.[6] In the seven transmembrane domain receptors, ligand binding promotes the interaction of the occupied receptors with transducing proteins, termed guanine nucleotide regulatory proteins or G proteins, located on the inner surface of the plasma membrane.[7] In ligand-regulated channels, activation alters the interactions between the several subunits of the receptor channel and increases its permeability to ions.

In addition to their extracellular binding domains and transmembrane regions, certain types of peptide hormone receptors possess signaling domains within their cytoplasmic regions. These motifs are activated by hormone-induced changes in receptor conformation, and either produce intracellular signals or interact with coupling proteins that in turn activate signal-generating enzymes located in the plasma membrane. In some receptors, hormone binding promotes the activation of intrinsic enzyme activities, such as protein kinase or guanylyl cyclase, that are located within the intracellular region of the receptor itself. By these various mechanisms, the binding of hormones to the extracellular region of the receptor leads to changes in cyclic nucleotide formation, phospholipid turnover, calcium mobilization, ion fluxes, and protein phosphorylation, and these changes in turn activate specific intracellular signaling pathways (Table 1.4.1).

General properties

In addition to the properties described earlier, there are several features of peptide hormone receptors that are common to many members of this large receptor family. These include high specificity for hormone agonists and antagonists, high binding affinity with (usually) rapid kinetics of association and dissociation, equilibrium dissociation constants (K_d) of nanomolar or below, and saturability. As opposed to transport processes, receptor binding is a saturable process and hormone binding reaches a maximum at concentrations of about five times the K_d. This corresponds to the number of receptor sites expressed on the cell surface, which is measurable as the molar equivalent of the maximum number of ligand molecules bound under saturating conditions. This assumes that each receptor binds one molecule of hormone, which is frequently the case. The number of receptors expressed per cell is determined by the concurrent rates of receptor synthesis and degradation, and varies during development and at stages of the cell cycle. Cell stimulation by the homologous hormone often leads to changes in receptor expression, due to changes in the rates of receptor formation and degradation. In many cell types, the initial binding of hormone to receptor is followed by internalization of the hormone–receptor complexes at specialized regions of the plasma membrane, termed coated pits.[8] If extensive, this process can lead to significant changes in the number of receptors available for further hormone binding, and could thereby alter the responsiveness of the cell to subsequent agonist stimulation. Once internalized, the receptors may undergo processing and degradation within lysosomes, or in some cases are recycled to the plasma membrane.

Many cells show decreased responses to repeated hormonal stimulation, and this has been termed desensitization or refractoriness. This phenomenon is sometimes observed during *in vivo* treatment with certain hormones, and often after *in vitro* exposure of tissues and cells to drugs and hormones, and is most evident after frequent and/or intensive stimulation. The nature of desensitization has been extensively studied in hormone-treated cells, and has

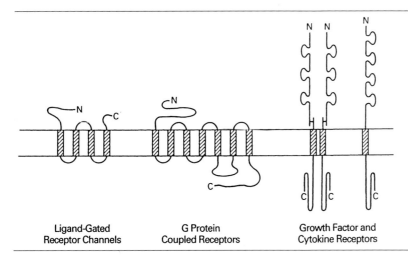

Fig. 1.4.2 *General structural organization of the major groups of plasma-membrane receptors. Ligand-gated receptor channels are composed of several of the four transmembrane domain units shown on the left, arranged to form a channel that is lined by the second transmembrane domains of the subunits. The seven transmembrane domain receptors exist as single entities that bind ligands and activate G proteins. The growth factor receptors either exist as dimers (insulin, IGF-I) or undergo dimerization during receptor activation.*

Ligand-Gated Receptor Channels

G Protein Coupled Receptors

Growth Factor and Cytokine Receptors

at least two components. The most rapid and important of these is a loss of ability of the receptor molecule to generate further intracellular signals, resulting from a change in the receptor itself. This usually results from phosphorylation of the receptor protein by kinases that become stimulated during receptor activation, and serves to limit the response of the cell to repetitive or excessive hormonal stimulation.[9] The second component is internalization of the receptor–hormone complex, which is slower and probably less important than receptor phosphorylation except under conditions of extensive receptor occupancy and endocytosis.

G-protein-coupled receptors

Numerous cell stimuli, including peptide and glycoprotein hormones, biogenic amines, alkaloids, and odorants, exert their actions by binding to plasma-membrane receptors that are structurally related to the visual rhodopsins (Table 1.4.2). Almost all members of this large superfamily of

Table 1.4.2 The G-protein-coupled seven-transmembrane domain receptor superfamily

Peptide hormones	Neurotransmitters
Hypothalamic hormones	*Adrenergic agents*
CRF, GnRH, GHRH, TRH	α_1-adrenergic (α_{1A}–α_{1D})
	α_2-adrenergic (α_{2A}–α_{2C})
Pituitary hormones	β-adrenergic (β_1–β_3)
ACTH, MSH; LH, FSH, TSH	
	Other amines
Neurohypophysial peptides	Dopamine (D_1–D_5)
Oxytocin, vasopressin (V_{1A}, V_{1B}, V_2)	Histamine (H_1–H_3)
	Octopamine
Vasoactive peptides	Serotonin ($5HT_{1,2,4-7}$)
Angiotensin (AT_1)	
Endothelin (ET_A, ET_B)	*Purines*
Atrial natriuretic peptides	Adenosine (A_1, A_2) (P_1)
(ANP A, B, C)	ATP (P_2)
Gut hormones	*Ion channel ligands*
Gastrin	$GABA_B$
Glucagon	Metabotropic glutamate
Secretin	Muscarinic ACh (M_1–M_5)
Kinins	*Sensory transduction*
Bradykinin (B_1, B_2)	Olfaction: odorants
Tachykinin (NK_1–NK_3)	Taste: tastants
	Vision: photons
Calcium-regulating hormones	
Calcitonin	**Other ligands**
Parathyroid hormone	
	Lipid derivatives
Others	Platelet-activating factor
Bombesin	Prostaglandins
Neurotensin	Leukotrienes
Opiates	
Somatostatin	*Miscellaneous*
	Calcium
	Cannabinoids
	f-met-leu-phe
	Thrombin

receptors are coupled to heterotrimeric guanine nucleotide regulatory proteins that in turn activate plasma membrane effector systems to initiate the release of messenger molecules into the cytoplasm. The visual rhodopsins, a group of seven-transmembrane domain proteins that subserve photoreception in the retinal rod cells, were the first G-protein-coupled receptors to be identified.[10] Each rhodopsin molecule contains a molecule of the light-sensitive chromophobe, retinal, and in the absence of light remains in a constrained inactive form. When photons act on retinal, rhodopsin undergoes a conformational change to its activated form, which interacts with the G protein, transducin. Transducin then binds GTP and activates a cyclic GMP-specific phosphodiesterase, causing a fall in cyclic GMP levels and closure of cation channels in the plasma membrane. This leads to hyperpolarization of the rod cells and activation of neuronal signaling to the visual cortex.[11] The discovery that the β-adrenergic receptor was a seven transmembrane domain protein gave the first indication that rhodopsin-like receptors transduce other intracellular stimuli by triggering G proteins to activate intracellular signaling responses.[12] The G-protein-coupled receptor (GPCR) superfamily is characterized by the presence of seven hydrophobic segments that form α-helices within the plasma membrane. The helices are grouped into a bundle surrounding a central cavity within which the polar residues of the constituent amino acids are exposed, and their hydrophobic surfaces face into the membrane lipids. The integrity of the receptor probably depends on an invariant disulfide bond that links the first and second extracellular loops. In general, the most conserved residues are located in the transmembrane and cytoplasmic regions of the receptor, rather than in the extracellular regions, and are clustered together in the core and cytoplasmic surface of the receptor in its three-dimensional state.[13]

Other conserved residues that are present in most members of the GPCR family include proline residues in TM segments 5, 6, and 7, which contribute to the structure of the ligand binding site; tryptophan in TM segments 4 and 6 and phenylalanine in TM segment 6 that may form the aromatic base of the ligand binding site; aspartic acid in TM segment 2 and the Asn-Pro-X-X-Tyr sequence in helix 7, which are adjacent in the helix bundle and could form hydrogen bonds with the ligand; and an Asp-Arg-Tyr sequence at the end of helix 3, which with a trysosine residue at the end of helix 5 has been implicated in the activation of G proteins.[14]

The extracellular N-terminal portion of the receptor usually contains two or three sites for the attachment of N-linked carbohydrate chains. These do not appear to be necessary for hormone binding or transmembrane signaling in most receptors, but may be involved in the intracellular trafficking and expression of receptors during their biosynthesis. The intracellular loops of the receptor, and its carboxyterminal cytoplasmic region, contain several potential sites for phosphorylation by various protein kinases that influence the properties and activity of the receptor. Such phosphorylations typically occur on serine or threonine residues, and are catalyzed by protein kinase A, protein kinase C, or specific receptor kinases.[15]

Many of the predictions about the conformations of GPCRs are based on the structure of bacteriorhodopsin or mammalian rhodopsin, the retinal receptor for light. This includes the proposed assembly of the transmembrane helices to form a cluster around a central pocket within which small hormonal ligands are bound to the receptor.[16] In rhodopsin, retinal is bound within the pocket by its association with a conserved lysine group in the seventh transmembrane domain. In receptors for neurotransmitter ligands, the positively charged nitrogen group appears to interact with a negatively charged aspartate residue in the third transmembrane domain.[17] Such charge interactions, as well as hydrogen bonding and hydrophobic effects, are responsible for the binding of many natural and synthetic ligands to their specific receptor sites.

In addition to their interaction with the negatively charged Asp residue in helix 3, the amine transmitters also interact with a hydrophobic pocket formed by conserved aromatic residues (tyrosine and phenylalanine) located on helices 4, 5, 6, and 7. The seventh transmembrane domain is often less helical than the other six, and appears to be close to helices 3 and 5 in the packing arrangement of these domains. There is growing evidence for the participation of hydrophobic side chains and/or aromatic residues located deep in helices 6 and 7 in the formation of the binding site for agonist and antagonist ligands.[18] The binding of agonist ligands to the receptor pocket perturbs the conformation of the receptor, leading to exposure of domains in the cytoplasmic aspect (mainly in the third intracellular loop) which interact with intermediate G proteins that in turn activate intracellular signaling pathway(s). Two regions in the third intracellular loop, located at its amino- and carboxy-terminal ends adjacent to the fifth and sixth transmembrane domains, are known to be involved in G-protein coupling.[19] In many receptors, regions in the carboxy-terminal cytoplasmic domain have also been implicated in coupling to G proteins. However, this is not universal since receptors with truncated cytoplasmic tails, such as those for GnRH, exhibit effective G-protein-coupled responses during ligand activation.[20] A small group of seven transmembrane domain receptors, including subtypes of the dopamine, angiotensin II (AT$_2$), and somatostatin receptors, do not appear to be coupled to G proteins.[21]

Much of our current knowledge about GPCR structure and function has come from studies on the receptors for amine ligands, including epinephrine (adrenaline) and norepinephrine (noradrenaline), dopamine, acetylcholine (muscarinic), and serotonin. More recent work has begun to define the manner in which peptides and protein hormones interact with their receptors and switch them from their inactive to active conformations. In receptors for small peptide hormones, residues located in surface regions of the receptor protein, as well as in its hydrophobic intramembrane pocket, participate in ligand binding. In receptors for luteinizing hormone (LH), follicle stimulating hormone (FSH), and thyroid stimulating hormone (TSH), which have very large N-terminal regions, high-affinity binding sites are present in the bulky external domain of the receptor protein.[22] However, the bound hormone also interacts with a site within the bundle of transmembrane domains to bring about activation of the receptor and its coupling to G proteins and signal generation. Activation of the thrombin receptor also involves a two-step process, in which thrombin cleaves off an N-terminal sequence from the extracellular region of the receptor protein, exposing a new N-terminus in which the first 14 amino acids act as a tethered agonist peptide and activates the receptor by binding to its transmembrane regions.

Antagonists of G-protein-coupled receptors

In addition to the well-known antagonists of amine transmitters, antagonists to several peptide hormones have been developed by modification of the native peptide agonist. In the case of angiotensin II, for example, potent and specific peptide antagonists have been synthesized by replacing the C-terminal phenylalanine residue of the octapeptide with a non-aromatic hydrophobic residue, typically alanine or isoleucine.[23] Such antagonists have been of value for blockade of AII receptors *in vitro*, as well as *in vivo* when administered parenterally. The peptide antagonists were crucial in revealing the extent to which AII participates in physiological regulation of blood pressure, and is involved in several forms of hypertension. However, the need for parenteral treatment precluded their use in the treatment of essential hypertension, the commonest form of elevated blood pressure.

This obstacle to the use of receptor blockade in the clinical management of hypertensive patients was removed by the recent development of orally active non-peptide AII antagonists. These agents are exemplified by the compound losartan, an imidazole derivative with potent inhibitory activity at the AII receptor in man and other species.[24] This specific antagonist, and others developed for blockade of substance P and cholecystokinin B/gastrin receptors, bind to groups of amino acids situated in the transmembrane helices of the receptor. Interestingly, the residues that form the antagonist binding site are less important for binding of the peptide ligands, which appear to bind to a distinct but partially overlapping site.[25] The non-peptide antagonists may thus act as allosteric inhibitors of agonist binding by driving the receptor into an inactive conformation that is associated with loss of the agonist binding site. Such specific non-peptide inhibitors that bind in the pocket between the transmembrane helices could be developed for a variety of peptide hormone receptors if the requisite conformations for interaction with their individual interhelical domains can be designed.

Abnormalities of receptor function

The molecular cloning of GPCRs has revealed many aspects of their structural requirements for ligand binding, coupling to G proteins and activation of signal transduction systems. Elucidation of the amino acid sequences of hormone receptors has been rapidly followed by the discovery of several receptor mutations in conditions associated with hormone resistance or autonomous overactivity of endocrine cells. Those include several forms of familial endocrine insensitivity or overactivity in which inactivating or activating mutations of single amino acids have been demonstrated. Inactivating mutations are present in the V_2 vasopressin receptor of patients with X-linked diabetes insipidus, the adrenocorticotropin (ACTH) receptor of patients with hereditary glucocorticoid deficiency, and the growth hormone releasing hormone (GHRH) receptor of one variety of dwarf mice.[26] Activating mutations have been found in the LH receptor in familial male precocious puberty, in rhodopsin in some forms of retinal degeneration, and in the TSH receptors of some hyperplastic thyroid nodules.[27] Whereas the inactivating mutations are usually associated with loss of hormone binding activity, the activating mutations affect residues located in the transmembrane and cytoplasmic regions of the receptor that are probably important in maintaining the receptor in its inactive conformation.

Ligand-gated ion channels

Cell membrane receptors for neurotransmitters are essential elements in the process of neurotransmission. Many of these receptors, including the nicotinic acetylcholine receptors and those for excitatory (glutamate and aspartate) and inhibitory (GABA and glycine) amino acids, are ionotropic complexes that contain an integral ion pore or channel.[28] The activities of such channels are controlled by ligands that bind to the complex and regulate the open or closed state of the channel. There is a large superfamily of neurotransmitter receptors that are composed of multiple subunits which share considerable amino acid homology and several structural features. All subunits have four transmembrane domains, with a large amino-terminal extracellular region and a smaller carboxy-terminal region that is also extracellular. The extracellular regions are glycosylated and hydrophilic, and contain loop structures and hydrophobic domains for interaction with the ligand. The ion channels are lined by the second transmembrane domains, which contain hydrophilic uncharged residues that permit the rapid influx of hydrated ions when the channels are activated. Although the native receptor channels are composed of several different subunits, some of the individual subunits can form functional channels when expressed as homoligomers in transfected cells. It should be noted that in addition to their typical actions on ligand-gated channels, most neurotransmitters also activate receptor subtypes of the seven transmembrane domain type that are coupled to G proteins. These include the muscarinic cholinergic, metabotropic glutaminergic, serotonin $5HT_3$, and $GABA_B$ receptors.

Among the ligand-gated receptor channels, the nicotinic acetylcholine (ACh) receptors were the first to be extensively studied and to have their structures determined.[29] They form a large family of receptor channels located in muscle and nerve cells, where they mediate synaptic neurotransmission by ACh by controlling sodium influx and consequent depolarization of the cell membrane. Normal ACh receptors are pentameric complexes of four individual subunits that combine in the ratio $\alpha_2\beta\gamma\delta$ (or $\alpha_2\beta\epsilon$) to form pentameric 250 kDa receptors that contain a central ion channel and an external ligand binding site for acetylcholine and other cholinergic ligands. Binding of ACh to the receptor causes the channel to open for a few milliseconds and to admit a rapid and transient flow of sodium ions. The ion channel is lined by the M2 domains of the subunits, and its external region contains rings of negatively charged amino acids to exclude anions. Neuronal ACh receptors differ from muscle receptors in their higher permeability to calcium and their sensitivity to extracellular calcium, which increases their opening frequency and their ion currents during activation by ACh.[30] They are composed largely of α and β subunits, of which seven α and four β isoforms have been identified.

The receptors for excitatory amino acids (glutamate and aspartate) mediate excitatory synaptic activity in the majority of cerebral neurones and are also involved in neuromuscular transmission in vertebrates.[31] These receptor channels convey sodium ions and varying amounts of calcium into the cell, and exist as three major subtypes that are defined by their sensitivities to agonist activation by specific amino·acid analogs. These are: AMPA (α-amino-3-hydroxy-5-methyl-isoxazale 4-propionic acid), kainate and NMDA (N-methyl-D-aspartic acid). Each of the pharmacologically defined receptor subtypes is composed of several subunits, each with four transmembrane domains, that form the multimeric assemblies which make up the individual receptors. Several agonist subunit families have been identified based on their functional properties and amino acid sequences. AMPA receptors are composed of four subunits termed GluR1–GluR4; kainate receptors of two subunits, KA1 and KA2; and NMDA receptors of a major NMDAR1 subunit and four NMDR2 (A–D) subunits that modulate the activity of the ion channels formed by the R1 subunits.[32] Many of the subunits are transcribed as alternatively spliced forms and some are modified by RNA editing of their messenger transcripts. The vast array of complexes that can be formed from the numerous subunits is responsible for the formation of channels with specific pharmacological properties, calcium permeabilities, and sensitivity to modulation by co-factors such as Mg^{2+} and glycine. Such subunits are distributed within anatomically discrete and functionally distinct cell types within the brain. In addition to their major role in excitatory synaptic transmission in the hippocampus and neocortex, the EAA receptors are also involved in cell-dependent modification of synaptic efficacy, excitotoxicity, and cell death.[33]

Growth factor receptors

Growth factors differ from peptide hormones that stimulate signaling through G protein-coupled receptors in several respects. Their actions are concerned mainly with regulation of cell growth and proliferation, and their receptors and signaling pathways are largely distinct from those of other peptides and transmitters. The major growth factors are insulin and insulin-like growth factor I (IGF-I), epidermal growth factor (EGF), platelet-derived growth factor (PDGF), and fibroblast growth factor (FGF). Those and many other types of growth factors are responsible for controlling the growth and proliferation of numerous specific cell types and target tissues.[6] Several growth factors have been found to exert actions in endocrine and reproductive tissues that are primarily responsive to peptide and steroid hormones.

Growth factor receptors possess a characteristic structure that is quite unlike that of the GPCRs (Fig.1.4.3). The receptor protein contains only one transmembrane domain, and typically has large N-terminal extracellular and C-terminal intracellular regions that respectively subserve hormone binding and signal generation. Whereas GPCRs bind small ligands within their transmembrane domains, and peptide hormones in their extracellular regions as well, binding to growth factor receptors occurs entirely to a site formed by the large extracellular domain. Such receptors are activated not by direct ligand-induced changes in their normally constrained signaling domain, but by ligand-induced dimerization that is followed by transphosphorylation of tyrosine residues located in the cytoplasmic region.[34] Growth factor receptors possess intrinsic tyrosine kinase domains in their cytoplasmic regions, and these are activated by dimerization to transphosphorylate specific tyrosine residues in their adjacent receptor and subsequently in associated proteins. For this reason, growth factor receptors are often termed 'receptor tyrosine kinases', and tyrosine phosphorylation is regarded as a characteristic early feature of numerous intra-

cellular growth signaling pathways. The initial step of ligand-induced dimerization of growth factor receptors is essential for the subsequent activation of their intracellular signaling domains, and is dependent on the exposure of interacting surfaces of the receptor upon ligand binding. Following dimerization and activation, many growth factor receptors undergo clustering and subsequent endocytosis of the receptor–hormone complex.[35]

Receptor serine kinases

An important family of proteins that exert prominent actions on growth and differentiation has been identified as a subset of growth factors which act on receptors that contain an intracellular protein kinase domain which phosphorylates serine and threonine residues.[36] This contrasts with the majority of the growth factor receptor kinases, including insulin, IGF-I, EGF, PDGF, and FGF, in which the kinase entities are specific for tyrosine phosphorylation. The ligands that activate the receptor serine kinases include activins, inhibins, TGF-β, and other molecules of diverse origin that participate in embryogenesis and development. These are: Müllerian-inhibiting factor (MIF), involved in male sexual development; the *Vg-1* gene product, which

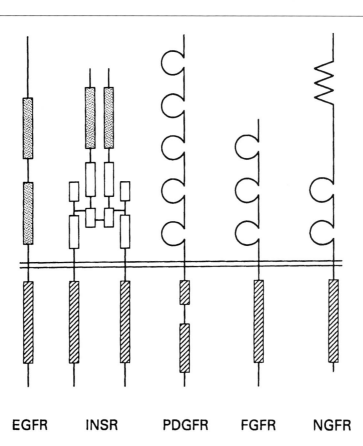

EGFR **INSR** **PDGFR** **FGFR** **NGFR**

Fig. 1.4.3 *Structures of the major growth factor receptors. The stippled boxes represent cysteine-rich domains, and the loops represent immunoglobulin-like regions. The hatched boxes indicate the intracellular catalytic domains. The receptors for epidermal growth factor (EGF), insulin (INS), platelet-derived growth factor (PDGF), fibroblast growth factor (FGF), and nerve growth factor (NGF) are shown. Modified from reference 34.*

controls early embryonic development in *Xenopus*, two proteins involved in *Drosophila* development; dorsalis and nodal, involved in neuronal tube development and gastrulation, respectively; bone morphogenetic proteins; and others of yet undefined function.

These proteins are related in terms of their biosynthesis, structure, and functions. All are disulfide-linked dimers that are formed by cleavage from the C-terminal regions of larger precursor proteins, and contain seven or more cysteine residues. The two monomers are linked by a single disulfide bond to form an extended conformation which contains a 'knot' motif that involves the several cysteines and other conserved residues.[37] Similar cysteine knots are present in PDGF and nerve growth factor (NGF), which are also extended rather than globular in their three-dimensional structure.

The receptors for this group of developmentally active proteins are characterized by a relatively small extracellular domain, a single transmembrane domain, and an intracellular region containing a serine–threonine kinase domain. Each of the receptor subtypes exists in two forms, termed type I and type II. Both contain serine kinase domains, and are believed to form a heterodimeric complex in the presence of the ligand. Whereas type I receptors bind a variety of ligands, type II receptors are specific for each ligand family. Ligand binding to type I receptors requires the presence of type II receptors, which determine the specificity of binding, and both receptors are required for the activation of intracellular signaling responses.[38] These features of the receptor serine kinases have been most extensively studied in receptors for TGF-β and activin, but also appear to apply to the other membrane of this family. Whereas the type II receptors bind the ligands independently of type I, the type I receptors must be associated with type II for ligand binding. Neither receptor can generate a signaling response alone, but only in the heterodimeric complex formed by association with the ligand and the other receptor.

Guanylyl cyclase receptors

A small but important group of receptors that carry a guanylyl cyclase domain in their intracellular regions is responsible for the generation of cyclic GMP in response to cell stimulation by hormones and neurotransmitters. Guanylyl cyclase also exists as soluble forms within the cells, and those are activated by the diffusible intercellular messenger, nitric oxide. This system is described in more detail in the following chapter. The membrane-bound guanylyl cyclases were first identified as in sea urchin sperm receptors for sea urchin egg peptides that stimulate sperm mobility and directional movement.[39] Such receptors were also found to mediate the actions of the atrial natriuretic peptides (ANPs) that are produced in the heart and other tissues, and exert prominent hypotensive actions. Three groups of ANPs have been identified, termed types A, B, and C, and range in size from 22 to 32 amino acids. Their actions include vasodilatation, natriuresis, diuresis, and inhibition of the renin–angiotensin–aldosterone system.

Two forms of ANP receptors possess protein kinase and guanylyl cyclase domains within their cytoplasmic regions,

and are known as guanylyl cyclase-A and guanylyl cyclase-B. Guanylyl cyclase-A is sensitive to the type A and type B natriuretic peptides, and guanylyl cyclase B is sensitive only to the type C natriuretic peptide. A particulate form of guanylyl cyclase is abundant in the large and small intestines, and is activated by heat-stable enterotoxins produced by certain strains of pathogenic bacteria.[40] These are termed STa receptors, and mediate the induction of diarrhea by the common types of heat-stable toxins. Such toxins, and the related peptide guanylin that is produced in the gut, act on a third form of receptor termed guanylyl cyclase-C.

Cytokine receptors

Cytokines are small proteins that are produced by activated cells of the immune and hematopoietic systems and mediate the transfer of information between the cells that comprise these systems. Unlike the traditional hormones of the endocrine system, cytokines usually exert local rather than systemic actions, and exert a wide range of overlapping biological actions in a variety of tissues and cell types. Thus, cytokines are important regulators of the immune response, hematopoiesis, inflammatory reactions, cell proliferation, and tumor growth.[41] In addition to such pleiotropic actions, cytokines are also characterized by their redundancy, in that multiple cytokines can elicit similar responses from the same cell type. The pleiotropic nature of cytokines is exemplified by interleukin 6 (IL-6), which acts not only to promote B cell maturation in the immune system but also has effects in the endocrine, hematopoietic, hepatic, and nervous systems. Their redundancy is illustrated by the ability of not only IL-6 but also of several other interleukins and cytokines to induce antibody production in B cells.[42] The cytokines include several subgroups, termed hematopoietins, interferons, tumor necrosis factor (TNF)-like factors, and others.

The classification of cytokines has been further influenced by the elucidation of the structures of the ligands and their receptors. The three-dimensional structure of many cytokines is characterized by the presence of four long α-helices arranged in an anti-parallel fashion. This structural feature is common to numerous cytokines, even though the hormones differ in their primary sequences. These 'helix bundle' hormones fall into several groups of homologous proteins, including GH, PRL, HPL, and their relatives; IL-6, IL-11, granulocyte colony stimulating factor (G-CSF), and macrophage-colony stimulating factor (M-CSF); and IL-4 and granulocyte/macrophage-colony stimulating factor (GM-CSF). Second, elucidation of the structures of their receptors (R) led to the recognition that GH-R, PRL-R, IL-2-R, IL-6-R, and erythropoietin-R form a family of cytokine/hematopoietic receptors. This family now includes more than 20 members, all of which influence the growth and differentiation of cells of the lymphatic and hematopoietic lineages.

The cytokine receptors possess several common structural fixtures, including a single transmembrane domain and a 200-amino acid extracellular region that contains two sequential 100-amino acid domains. The outermost domain contains two pairs of cysteine residues that may frame the ligand binding site, and the inner domain contains a conserved sequence (WSXWS) near the transmembrane domain that is probably required for receptor dimerization. The cytoplasmic regions of the cytosine receptors vary considerably in length and do not possess identifiable enzymatic motifs that could act as mediators of signal generation. However, all contain proline-rich motifs located about 10–20 residues from the cell membrane that may be involved in binding to SH3 (Src homology 3) domains of downstream signaling molecules.[44] In addition to these shared structural features, many of the cytosine receptors exist as soluble forms that are shed from the cell membrane or translated from differentially spliced mRNAs that encode proteins lacking transmembrane and cytoplasmic domains, and are released as soluble binding proteins with high affinity for their ligands.[45]

The pleiotropic actions and redundancy of cytokines are attributable to some unusual properties of this receptor superfamily. First, cytokine receptors often exist as complexes formed by homo- or heterodimerization, or by association with other protein subunits. In the case of GH and PRL, one hormone molecule is bound by two receptor molecules, but other ligand-receptor ratios (1:1, 2:1, and 3:3) are observed among the various cytokines and their receptors. Second, several of the receptors that exist as multichain complexes share common subunits, some of which are involved in signal generation. This can account for the ability of different cytokines to elicit similar responses in a given cell type, due to the activation of a common signaling unit. The presence of such common chains is often required for high-affinity ligand binding, as well as for signal transduction. In some receptors the ligand binding subunit cannot activate intracellular signaling pathways, and is only functional when associated with a transducer subunit with the capacity for inducing downstream signaling.

Steroid hormone receptors

The nuclear receptor superfamily

The steroid hormones secreted by the gonads and adrenal glands (estrogen, progesterone, androgens, glucocorticoids, and mineralocorticoids) belong to a large group of circulating or locally formed ligands that influence gene activity in their target cells. After diffusing into cells, these ligands bind to highly selective receptors present in the cytoplasm or nucleus of their target cells. These hormone receptors, which are actually dormant transcription factors, become activated by steroid binding and interact with hormone response elements (HRE) located in the upstream DNA sequence of genes encoding a wide variety of cellular proteins. This general mechanism of action of steroid hormones is shared with thyroid hormone, vitamin D, ecdysone, retinoic acid, and 9-cis retinoic acid, all of which bind to and activate specific receptor proteins that act as nuclear transcription factors in their respective target cells.[46] The ligands were originally thought to interact with their receptors in the cytoplasm and to promote their translocation to the nucleus. However, most of the steroid receptor subtypes are now believed to be associated with the nucleus even in the absence of hormone and to undergo much tighter binding to DNA once activated by the ligand.

Heat shock proteins

Several of the unliganded receptors are inactive because they exist as complexes with other proteins, including the heat shock proteins hsp 90 and hsp 70, and their potential DNA binding domains are inaccessible. This applies to the steroid hormone receptors (ER, PR, AR, GR, MR), which are 8–10 S complexes when associated with heat shock proteins, and are converted into their non-associated 4 S forms after binding hormone. The liganded receptors rapidly form dimers that bind tightly to their respective HREs and activate the associated genes. Other intracellular receptors, including those for thyroid hormone, vitamin D, retinoic acid, and 9-cis retinoic acid (TR, VDR, RAR, and RXR) are not associated with heat shock proteins and are able to bind to DNA in the absence of hormone. These receptors are activated upon ligand binding and form homodimers (or heterodimers with RXR) that bind to HREs with high affinity and stimulate gene transcription (see below). These two groups of receptors thus differ in their initial locations and modes of activation by hormones, but act similarly to initiate transcription in their target genes.[47]

Receptor phosphorylation

Although the inactive receptors that are complexed with heat shock proteins must dissociate from the complex in order to become activated, additional actions of the hormone are necessary for receptor activation. The most important of these is the conformational change caused by the bound ligand, which includes a more compact arrangement of the large ligand-binding domain, with exposure of the dimerization domains. Once formed, the dimeric receptors attach to HREs by their DNA binding domains and induce gene transcription.

In addition to this crucial change in conformation, many receptors become phosphorylated in the course of ligand-induced activation by their respective hormones. Such ligand-dependent phosphorylation does not seem to be necessary for the activation of receptors but often enhances their capacity for gene activation.[48] Whereas hormone-induced phosphorylation may precede receptor translocation, it also occurs after binding of the activated receptor to DNA and is catalyzed by a DNA-dependent protein kinase. In addition to modulating the ligand-dependent activation of receptors, phosphorylation may be an important factor in the continuous energy-dependent exchange of receptors between the cytoplasm and the nucleus.

Several hormone receptors have been found to undergo ligand-independent phosphorylation by agonists and other agents that increase intracellular cyclic AMP levels. Furthermore, such phosphorylations can activate certain receptors in the absence of steroid hormone. Thus, estrogen and progesterone receptors are activated in dopamine-treated cells, and this could account for the central actions of dopamine on sexual behavior in female rats.[49] In addition to hormones that activate cyclic AMP-dependent protein kinase, several growth factors (EGF, IGF-I, TGF-β) have been found to activate estrogen receptors and stimulate gene transcription in the absence of estrogen. Whether this involves tyrosine phosphorylation of the receptor is not yet known, but it is clear that multiple hormonal mechanisms can lead to similar conformational changes in steroid hormone receptors that are required for DNA binding and induction of gene transcription.[50] The recognition of this interaction between peptide and steroid hormone receptors is a new and important development in the area of intracellular signaling. Such 'cross-talk' extends the purview of the growth signaling pathways through which plasma membrane receptors can influence gene transcription. Conversely, steroid hormones have been found to influence some of the signaling responses mediated by plasma membrane receptors, indicating that each of the traditionally distinct major signaling pathways can modulate the activity of the other under appropriate conditions.[51]

Functional domains

The steroid hormone receptors are modular proteins in which several functional domains have been shown to be responsible for ligand binding, dimerization, DNA binding, and transactivation. As shown in Fig. 1.4.4, the several domains vary considerably in size, and in some cases a given function involves more than a single domain. The N-terminal region of the receptor is concerned largely with transactivation and the C-terminal region with ligand binding. The ligand binding domain is large, and occupies most of the C-terminal half of the molecule. This region also participates in the association with heat shock proteins, as well as in dimerization, nuclear localization, transactivation, and intramolecular silencing and repression.

Some of these functions involve only small regions of the molecule, but others require almost the entire stretch of amino acids within the C-terminal section of the receptor. The dimerization domain, which includes leucine-rich sequences that favor coil–coil interactions between receptors, is located towards the C-terminal end of the ligand binding domain. The interaction of the ligand binding domain with heat shock proteins seems to maintain the unliganded receptor in its inactive state.[52]

A small region N-terminal to the ligand-binding domain (the hinge region) is involved in nuclear localization and sometimes transactivation, and in folding of the receptor. Adjacent to the hinge region is the DNA-binding domain, which contains two specialized amino acid sequences, termed zinc fingers, that participate in DNA binding and dimerization.[53] The remaining N-terminal portion of the receptor varies considerably in size and amino acid sequence among members of the steroid receptor superfamily. It is required for efficient transactivation of genes that specifically bind the receptor, and is believed to interact with the complex of transcription factors that interact with the TATA box or other initiator elements at which transcription commences. Other regions of the receptor molecule, including the ligand- and DNA-binding domains, have also been implicated in the process of transactivation. The mechanisms by which steroid hormone receptors bind to DNA and activate transcription is described in Chapter 1.5.

Ligand binding and receptor activation

The traditional steroid hormone receptors (ER, PR, AR, GR, MR) are believed to be maintained in an inactive state when complexed with heat shock proteins, and appear to be devoid of function. However, some of the receptors that do not form such complexes may act as constitutive repressors of their target genes in the absence of ligand. These include the TR, VDR, RAR and RXR, which have relatively short N-terminal transactivation domains and do

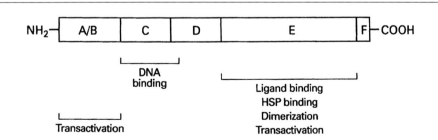

Fig. 1.4.4 *Domain structure of steroid hormone receptors. The receptors are subdivided into six domains (A–F) according to their conserved sequences and functional properties. The DNA binding domain (C) is the most highly conserved region of the receptors, and encodes two zinc finger motifs that interact with specific recognition sequences in the major groove of the DNA helix. The E domain is less highly conserved and participates in ligand binding, interaction with heat shock proteins, dimerization, and transactivation. The A/B domain is poorly conserved and contains residues that influence cell-specific transcriptional activation. The D domain is variable and may serve as a hinge during changes in receptor conformation. It is also involved in nuclear localization and transactivation functions in some receptors. The F domain is the variable and its function is not known.*

not interact with heat shock proteins. These receptors bind to DNA in the absence of hormone, either as monomers or dimers, and this is facilitated by their ability to form homodimers in the unliganded state. This group of receptors is also notable for the formation of heterodimers, especially with RXR, that can also participate in the regulation of target genes by activation or repression of their transcriptional activity.[54]

The extent to which the bound hormone is required for subsequent actions of the dimeric receptor is not known, but the presence of agonist seems to be necessary for optimal transactivation, as well as for rapid dissociation of the receptor from its DNA binding element[55,56]. In contrast, hormone antagonists can also promote binding of receptors to their response elements but do not cause efficient transactivation. This, and the relatively slow dissociation of the antagonist-receptor complex from the HRE, favor their competition with hormone-activated receptors for DNA binding and are major factors in the inhibitory action of steroid hormone antagonists.[57]

The fact that some antagonists not only promote DNA binding and sometimes phosphorylation of receptors, but can also act as partial agonists, is consistent with their abilities to cause major conformational changes when bound to the receptor. These include exposure of the dimerization domain and the formation of dimeric receptors with high affinity for the HRE. However, the conformation of the antagonist-bound receptor differs significantly from that of the agonist-receptor complex by several criteria, and its C-terminal region appears to be less compact. This has been attributed to the presence of a repressor function in the extreme C-terminal region of the steroid receptors that inhibits the activation domain(s) of the native receptor, and is sequestered into a compacted structure during agonist binding.[58] Whereas the incomplete conformational change during antagonist binding leads to exposure of the dimerization domain and DNA binding, it does not change the repressor function of the C-terminal domain upon transactivation, and the DNA-bound inactive complex competitively inhibits the binding of agonist-activated receptors to the HRE and prevents gene transcription. The ability of some antagonists to act as partial agonists may reflect the presence of other activation functions in the C-terminal domain or elsewhere in the receptor that are not subject to the inhibitory control of the suppressor C-terminal sequence.

It is interesting to note that several parallels exist between the actions of antagonists on steroid hormone receptors and GPCRs. In both cases, antagonists bind to a region near the C-terminal of the activating domain of the receptor, and interact with a site that may overlap the agonist binding site but is largely distinct from it. The antagonist ligands do not compete for identical sites, but for mutually exclusive ligand-induced conformations of the receptor. Finally, the slow dissociation rates of antagonists from GPCRs is analogous to the slow dissociation of antagonist-receptor complexes from the HREs of their target genes.

FUTURE PERSPECTIVES

The classic concept that receptors mediate selective actions of drugs on individual cell types has been extended to explain diverse physiological and pathological responses to hormones and growth factors throughout the body. Recent advances in molecular biology have permitted the characterization of receptor structure and function at the molecular level, and have revealed an extraordinary level of diversity among receptors and their associate signal transduction proteins.

It is now clear that large numbers of cell membrane-associated and nuclear receptors exist in or on individual cells, reflecting their histogenetic origins and specific functions within the body. Intriguingly, many of these recently discovered receptors have no known function or their ligands are as yet unidentified. Such 'orphan' receptors are presumed to have physiological relevance based on structural homologies with other proteins that are known to be receptors for hormones or growth factors. At the time of writing, over 100 members of the nuclear transcription factor family that includes steroid hormone/thyroid hormone/vitamin D/ecdysone/retinoic acid receptors, etc., are known to exist. Similarly, there are numerous examples of orphan G-protein-coupled receptors. Given the fundamental processes controlled by receptors with known physiological functions, it is likely that major new insights into the cellular basis of health and disease will be gained from the elucidation of roles played by these yet uncharacterized receptor molecules.

SUMMARY

- Hormones regulate cellular function by binding to highly specific receptor proteins that in turn activate biochemical signaling pathways leading to phenotypic cell responses – metabolic, secretory, contractile, growth, etc.
- Hormone receptors are broadly subdivided into two major groups, for peptide and steroid hormones, that are located on the cell surface or in the cytoplasm/nucleus, respectively.

- Peptide hormone receptors are locked into the plasma membrane by their hydrophobic transmembrane domains. They possess unique recognition sites in their extracellular regions, and signal transducing or activating domains in their cytoplasmic regions.
- Plasma-membrane hormone receptors are of two major types – the seven transmembrane domain group that couple to G proteins, and

the single transmembrane variety that possess or acquire intrinsic enzymatic activity in their cytoplasmic domains.

- Hormone binding causes conformational changes in the receptor, with exposure of its signal transducing domains or initiation of its intrinsic enzymatic activity. In many receptors, agonist activation is followed by desensitization and/or internalization of the hormone–receptor complex.
- Receptor activation usually involves interactions between individual receptors or among their subdomains. Growth factor receptors often undergo dimerization upon ligand binding as the initial step to activation. A few receptors are dimeric to begin with (e.g. insulin) and some (e.g. cytokines) form clusters of subunits upon ligand binding. The seven transmembrane domains of G-protein-coupled receptors are in a sense already clustered, and undergo conformational changes after agonist binding.
- Peptide hormone antagonists compete with

the physiological agonists for binding to the receptor. In G-protein-coupled receptors, antagonists may bind either to the extracellular domain or within the cleft between the transmembrane domains. The recently developed non-peptide receptor antagonists bind to epitopes between the transmembrane regions that are largely distinct from the peptide binding domain.

- Steroid hormones diffuse into cells and bind to specific receptor proteins located in the cytoplasm or loosely associated with the nucleus.
- Steroid hormone receptors are quiescent transcriptional regulatory proteins (transcription factors) that undergo dimerization and bind tightly to specialized regions of the DNA to activate gene expression.
- Steroid hormone antagonists bind to receptors at sites that are largely distinct from the agonist binding site, and cause conformational changes that favor dimerization and DNA binding of the inactive antagonist–receptor complex.

REFERENCES

1. Sutherland EW, Robinson GA. The role of cyclic-3′-5′-AMP in responses to catecholamines and other hormones. *Pharmacol Rev* 1966 **18**: 145–161.
2. Catt KJ. Molecular mechanisms of hormone action: Control of target cell function by peptide and catecholamine hormones. In Felig P, Baxter J, Frohman L (eds) *Endocrinology and Metabolism* 3rd edition New York: McGraw-Hill; 1995: 91–167.
3. Carpenter GW. Receptors for growth factors and other polypeptide mitogens. *Annu Rev Biochem* 1987 **56**: 881 914.
4. Collins S, Lohse MJ, O'Dowd B, Caron MG, Lefkowitz RJ. Structure and regulation of G protein-coupled receptors: the beta-2 adrenergic receptor as a model. *Vitam Horm* 1991 **49**: 1–39.
5. Numa S. A molecular view of neurotransmitter receptors and ionic channels. *Harvey Lect* 1987–88 **83**: 121–165.
6. White MF. Structure and function of tyrosine kinase receptors. *J Bioenerg Biomembr* 1991 **23**: 63–82.
7. Taylor CW. The role of G proteins in transmembrane signalling. *Biochem J* 1990 **J272**: 1–13.
8. Pley U, Parham P. Clathrin: its role in receptor-mediated vesicular transport and specialized functions in neurons. *Crit Rev Biochem Mol Biol* 1993 **28**: 431–464.
9. Hausdorff WP, Caron MG, Lefkowitz RJ. Turning off the signal: desensitization of β-adrenergic receptor function. *FASEB J* 1990 **4**: 2881–2889.
10. Khorana HG. Bacteriorhodopsin, a membrane protein that uses light to translocate protons. *J Biol Chem* 1988 **236**: 7439–7442.
11. Applebury ML. Molecular determinants of visual pigment function. *Curr Opin Neurobiol* 1991 **1**: 263–269.
12. Dixon RAF, Kobilka BK, Strader DJ, Benovic JL, Dohlman HG. Cloning of the gene and cDNA for mammalian β-adrenergic receptor and homology with rhodopsin. *Nature* 1986 **321**: 75–79.
13. Saverese TM, Fraser CM. *In vitro* mutagenesis and the search for structure–function relationships among G pro-

tein-coupled receptors. *Biochem J* 1992 **283**: 1–19.
14. Donnelly D, Findlay JBC, Blundell TM. The evolution and structure of aminergic G protein-coupled receptors. *Receptors Channels* 1994 **2**: 61–78.
15. Inglese J, Freedman NJ, Koch WJ, Lefkowitz RJ. Structure and mechanism of the G protein-coupled receptor kinases. *J Biol Chem* 1993 **268**: 23735–23738.
16. Schertler GF, Villa C, Henderson R. Projection structure of rhodopsin. *Nature* 1993 **362**: 770–772.
17. Collins S, Lohse MJ, O'Dowd B, Caron MG, Lefkowitz RJ. Structure and regulation of G protein-coupled receptors: the beta-2 adrenergic receptor as a model. *Vitam Horm* 1991 **49**: 1–39.
18. Gether U, Johanson TE, Snider RM, Low JA, Nakanishi S, Schwartz TW. Different binding epitopes on the NK₁ receptor for substance P and a non-peptide antagonist. *Nature* 1993 345–348.
19. Hedin KE, Duerson K, Clapham DE. Specificity of receptor-G protein interactions: searching for the structure behind the signal. *Cell Signal* 1993 **5**: 505–518.
20. Reinhart J, Mertz LM, Catt KJ. Molecular cloning and expression of cDNA encoding the murine gonadotropin-releasing hormone receptor. *J Biol Chem* 1992 **267**: 21281–21284.
21. Mukoyama M, Nakajima M, Horiuchi M, Sasamura H, Pratt RE, Dzau VJ. Expression cloning of type 2 angiotensin II receptor reveals a unique class of seven-transmembrane receptors. *J Biol Chem* 1993 **268**: 24539–24542.
22. Tsai-Morris CH, Buczko E, Wang W, Dufau ML. Intronic nature of the rat luteinizing hormone receptor gene defines a soluble receptor subspecies with hormone binding activity. *J Biol Chem* 1990 **265**: 19385–19388.
23. Streeten DHP, Anderson GH, Freiberg JM, Dalakos TG. Use of an angiotensin II antagonist (Saralasin) in the recognition of 'angiotensinogenic' hypertension. *N Engl J Med* 1975 **292**: 657–662.
24. Wexler RR, Carini DJ, Duncia JV *et al*. Rationale for the chemical development of angiotensin II receptor antagonists. *Am J Hypertens* 1992 **5**: 209–220.
25. Ji H, Leung M, Zhang Y, Catt KJ, Sandberg K. Differential

structural requirements for specific binding of nonpeptide and peptide antagonists to the AT$_1$ receptor. *J Biol Chem* 1994 **269**: 16533–16566.

26. Pan Y, Metzenberg A, Das S, Jing B, Gitschier J. Mutations in the V2 vasopressin receptor gene are associated with X-linked nephrogenic diabetes insipidus. *Nat Genet* 1992 **2**: 103–106.

27. Lefkowitz RJ. Turned on to ill effect. *Nature* 1993 **365**: 603–604.

28. Reddy GL, Iwamoto T, Tomich JM, Montal M. Synthetic peptides and four-helix bundle proteins as model systems for the pore-forming structure of channel proteins. II. Transmembrane segment M2 of the brain glycine receptor is a plausible candidate for the pore-lining structure. *J Biol Chem* 1993 **268**: 14608–14615.

29. Galzi J-L, Revah F, Bessis A, Changeux J-P. Functional architecture of the nicotinic acetylcholine receptor: from electric organ to brain. *Annu Rev Pharmacol Toxicol* 1991 **31**: 37–72.

30. Deneris ES, Connoly J, Rogers S, Duvoison R. Pharmacological and functional diversity of neuronal nicotinic acetylcholine receptors. *Trends Pharmacol Sci* 1991 **12**: 34–40.

31. Seeburg PH. The molecular biology of mammalian glutamate receptor channels. *Trends Pharmacol Sci* 1993 **14**: 297–303.

32. Ishii T, Moriyoshi K, Sugihara H, Sakurada K, Kadotani H, Yokoi M, Akazawa C, Shigemoto R, Mizuno N, Masu M, Nakanishi S. Molecular characterization of the family of the *N*-methyl-*D*-aspartate receptor subunits. *J Biol Chem* 1993 **268**: 2836–2843.

33. Huntley GW, Vickers JC, Morrison JH. Cellular and synaptic localization of NMDA and non-NMDA receptor subunits in neocortex: organizational features related to cortical circuitry, function, and disease. *Trends Neurosci* 1994 **17**: 536–543.

34. Van der Geer P, Hunter T, Lindberg RA. Receptor protein-tyrosine kinases and their signal transduction pathways. *Int Res Cell Biol* 1994 **10**: 251–337.

35. Sorkin A, Waters CM. Endocytosis of growth factor receptors. *Bioessays* 1993 **15**: 375–382.

36. Lin HY, Wang XF, Ng-Eaton E, Weinberg RA, Lodish HF. Expression cloning of the TGF-β type II receptor, a functional transmembrane serine/threonine kinase. *Cell* 1992 **68**: 1–20.

37. McDonald NQ, Hendrickson WA. A structural superfamily of growth factors containing a cystine knot motif. *Cell* 1993 **73**: 421–424.

38. Matthews LS. Activin receptors and cellular signaling by the receptor serine kinase family. *Endocr Rev* 1994 **15**: 310–325.

39. Drewett J, Garbers DL. The family of guanylyl cyclase receptors and their ligands. *Endocr Rev* 1994 **15**: 135–162.

40. Schulz S, Green CK, Yuen PST, Garbers DL. Guanyl cyclase is a heat-stable enterotoxin receptor. *Cell* 1990 **63**: 941–948.

41. Bazan JF. Structural design and molecular evolution of a cytokine receptor superfamily. *Proc Natl Acad Sci USA* 1990 **87**: 6934–6938.

42. Kishimoto T, Taga T, Akira S. Cytokine signal transduction. *Cell* 1994 **76**: 253–262.

43. Miyajima A, Kitamura T, Harada N, Yokota T, Arai K-I. Cytokine receptors and signal transduction. *Annu Rev Immunol* 1992 **10**: 295–331.

44. Horseman ND, Yu-Lee L-Y. Transcriptional regulation by the helix bundle peptide hormones: growth hormone, prolactin, and the hematopoietic cytokines. *Endocr Rev* 1994 **15**: 627–649.

45. Rose-John S, Heinrich PC. Soluble receptors for cytokines and growth factors: generation and biological function. *Biochem J* 1994 **300**: 281–290.

46. Carlstedt-Duke J, Wright A, Göttlicher M, Okret S, Gustaffson J-A. Regulation of target cell function by the steroid hormone receptor supergene family. In Felig P, Baxter J, Frohman L (eds) *Endocrinology and Metabolism*, 3rd edition. New York: McGraw-Hill, 1995: 169–199.

47. Tsai M-J, O'Malley BW. Molecular mechanisms of action of steroid/thyroid receptor superfamily members. *Annu Rev Biochem* 1994 **63**: 451–486.

48. Truss M, Beato M. Steroid hormone receptors: Interaction with deoxyribonucleic acids and transcription factors. *Endocr Rev* 1993 **14**: 459–479.

49. Power RF, Mani SK, Codina J, Conneely OM, O'Malley BJ. Dopaminergic and ligand-independent activation of steroid hormone receptors. *Science* 1991 **254**: 1636–1639.

50. Denton RR, Koszewski NJ, Notides AC. Estrogen receptor phosphorylation: hormonal dependence and consequence on specific DNA binding. *J Biol Chem* 1992 **267**: 7263–7268.

51. Nemere I, Zhou LX, Norman AW. Nontranscriptional effects of steroid hormones. *Receptor* 1993 **3**: 277–291.

52. Godowski PJ, Picard D. Steroid receptors. How to be both a receptor and a transcription factor. *Biochem Pharmacol* 1989 **38**: 3135–3143.

53. Evans RM, Hollenberg SM. Zinc fingers: gilt by association. *Cell* 1988 **52**: 1–3.

54. Glass CK. Differential recognition of target genes by nuclear receptor monomers, dimers, and heterodimers. *Endocr Rev* 1994 **15**: 391–407.

55. Renaud J-P, Rochel N, Ruff M, Vivat V, Chambon P, Gronemeyer H, Moras D. Crystal structure of the RAR-γ ligand-binding domain bound to *all*-trans retinoic acid. *Nature* 1995 **378**: 681–689.

56. Wagner RL, Apriletti JW, McGrath ME, West BL, Baxter JD, Fletterick RJ. A structural role for hormone in the thyroid hormone receptor. *Nature* 1995 **378**: 690–696.

57. Pham TA, Elliston NJ, Nawaz J, McDonnell DP, Tsai MJ, O'Malley BW. Antiestrogen can establish non-productive receptor complexes and alter chromatin structure at target genes. *Proc Natl Acad Sci USA* 1991 **88**: 3125–3129.

58. Vegeto E, Allen GF, Schrader WT, Tsai M-J, McDonnell D, O'Malley BW. The mechanism of RU486 antagonism is dependent on the conformation of the carboxy-terminal tail of the human progesterone receptor. *Cell* 1992 **69**: 703–713.

Intracellular Signaling

KJ Catt

INTRODUCTION

The regulation of cellular function by hormones and growth factors depends on the ability of target cells to recognize and display appropriate responses to individual effector molecules in the extracellular milieu. Such responses can be rapid (e.g. contraction, transmission, secretion, etc.) or long-term (e.g. differentiation, proliferation, death, etc.). Chapter 1.4 summarizes how response 'specificity' is governed by the structural properties of the receptors to which hormone and growth factors bind on the cell surface or within the nucleus. The purpose of this chapter is to consider how the subcellular mechanisms activated by receptor occupancy are relayed within the cell to determine how it will respond.

CURRENT CONCEPTS

The signaling pathways activated by hormones and growth factors are prominent in the cytoplasm and its organelles, but also reach into the nucleus and regulate gene expression. In contrast, most of the responses elicited by steroid hormones originate in the nucleus, since the receptors that bind steroid hormones are essentially inactive transcriptional regulatory proteins that control the activities of a wide variety of genes. The non-nuclear actions of steroid hormones are less prominent but are nevertheless important in mediating certain rapid effects of steroids at the plasma membrane level. This chapter focuses on the major signal transduction pathways that mediate the actions of gonadotropins and steroid hormones following their binding to receptors located in the plasma membrane and nucleus.

Transmembrane signaling mechanisms

The incoming hormonal stimuli that activate plasma-membrane receptors are conveyed into the cytoplasm and nucleus by transduction into second messenger molecules that activate intracellular enzymes, or into cascades of protein kinases initiated by tyrosine phosphorylation. Early studies on the adenylyl cyclase/cyclic AMP (cAMP) system led to the proposal that peptide hormone receptors contain external ligand binding sites and intracellular enzymatic domains that generate potent signals such as cAMP from inactive precursors such as ATP. This concept has been modified with the recognition that many hormone receptors interact with transducing proteins that in turn activate or inhibit plasma-membrane and cytoplasmic effector pathways.[1,2]

G proteins and signal transduction

Hormonal activation of cAMP formation involves the sequential action of three proteins: the receptor, a guanine nucleotide coupling protein (G protein) termed G_s, and adenylyl cyclase. This signaling pathway is characteristic of the seven-transmembrane domain receptor family that includes the gonadotropin receptors (Chapter 1.4). The G_s proteins that mediate signaling from seven transmembrane domain receptors are composed of three subunits (α, β, and γ) that are tightly associated as inactive heterotrimeric $\alpha\beta\gamma$ complexes in their basal state.[3-5] These complexes rapidly dissociate into α- and $\beta\gamma$-subunits during agonist stimulation, and subsequently re-associate into the inactive $\alpha\beta\gamma$ form (Fig. 1.5.1). In this manner, the heterotrimeric G proteins undergo repeated cycles of activation and inactivation that depend upon their interaction with agonist-occupied receptors. Such interactions promote the release of bound GDP from the α subunits of the G proteins, and its replacement by GTP. This leads to the formation of transiently activated α-subunits that in turn regulate the activities of signal-generating enzymes and channels in the plasma membrane.

The ability of G protein α-subunits to shuttle between their active and inactive states enables them to act as molecular switches that control the activities of their effector systems. This property depends on their intrinsic GTPase

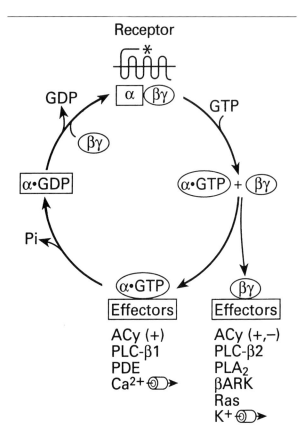

Receptor

Fig. 1.5.1 *The G protein cycle through which activated hormone receptors initiate signaling through multiple effector systems. Hormone binding and receptor activation accelerate GTP binding to the inactive αβγ complex, promoting its dissociation into α-GTP and βγ-subunits. When the bound GTP is hydrolyzed to GDP by the intrinsic GTPase activity of the α-subunit, the latter reassociates with βγ to form the inactive heterotrimeric complex. As indicated below, both α-GTP and βγ-subunits can stimulate a variety of effector enzymes and channels which generate the intracellular second messengers that stimulate (or inhibit) cellular responses.*

activity, which slowly catalyzes the hydrolysis of bound GTP to GDP and thus causes their reversion to the inactive basal state.[4] Hormones that bind to seven transmembrane domain receptors activate their associated G proteins by promoting GTP binding to their α-subunits, which in turn activate effector systems. Subsequently, GTP hydrolysis terminates the transiently activated state of the α-subunit and consequently of the activated effectors.

Many G protein-regulated processes in permeabilized cells and membrane fractions can be stimulated by GTP through G_s-mediated activation of adenylyl cyclase. However, in cells stimulated by certain receptors, GTP causes suppression rather than stimulation of adenylyl cyclase activity because the enzyme is also regulated by an inhibitory (G_i) protein. G_i is activated by receptors for opiates, somatostatin, α_2 agonists, and other agents that reduce intracellular cAMP levels. At least 20 heterotrimeric G proteins are involved in the coupling of cell-surface receptors of the seven transmembrane domain superfamily to their effector systems (Table 1.5.1).

Molecular structure of G-proteins

In their inactive states, heterotrimeric G proteins exist as 80–90 kDa αβγ complexes with considerable heterogeneity in their subunit structures. There are at least 17 distinct α-subunits, four β-subunits, and eight γ-subunits. The α-subunits range in molecular mass from 39 to 50 kDa and contain sequences that are highly homologous with those required for GTP binding and hydrolysis in other important G proteins, such as the proto-oncogene product, ras.[6]

The β- and γ-subunits of the G proteins, which exist as tightly bound βγ dimers after GTP-induced dissociation of the heterotrimeric αβγ complex, also occur in several forms. The masses of the four β-subunits and eight γ-subunits are 35–36 kDa and 6–10 kDa, respectively. The βγ dimers were formerly believed to serve largely as ligand-independent suppressors of receptor activity, since the reassociation of βγ with α-GDP subunits reconstitutes the

Table 1.5.1 G Proteins: expression, receptors, and signal transduction pathways

G Protein	Toxin	Expression	Receptors	Effectors	Signals
G_s	CT	General	Adrenergic (β), glucagon, PTH, calcitonin vasopressin V_2, GHRH, VIP, CRF ACTH, LH, FSH, TSH	Adenylyl cyclase L-type channels	↑ cAMP ↑ Ca^{2+} influx
G_{olf}	CT	Olfactory cilia	Odorant	Adenylyl cyclase	↑ cAMP (olfaction)
G_{t1}	CT/PT	Rods	Rhodopsin	cGMP phosphodiesterase	↓ cGMP (vision)
G_{t2}	CT/PT	Cones	Rhodopsin	cGMP phosphodiesterase	↓ cGMP (colour)
G_{i1}	PT	Neural	Noradrenaline (α_2), $5HT_1$	Adenylyl cyclase	↓ cAMP
G_{i2}	PT	General	Muscarinic (M2, M4), opiates, angiotensin AT_1, somatostatin	Phospholipase C-β2 Phospholipase A_2	↑ $InsP_3$, DAG, Ca^{2+} ↑ Arachidonate
G_{i3}	PT	General		K^+ channels	↑ Membrane potential
G_0	PT	Neural Endocrine	Not defined	Phospholipase C L-type channels	↑ $InsP_3$, DAG, Ca^{2+} ↓ Ca^{2+} influx
G_q	–	General	Adrenergic (α_1), angiotensin AT_1,	Phospholipase C-β1	↑ $InsP_3$, DAG, Ca^{2+}
G_{11}	–	General	bombesin, bradykinin, cholecystokinin,		
G_{14}	–	Liver, lung, kidney	GnRH, histamine, leukotrienes, metabotropic glutamate, muscarinic (M1,3,5), oxytocin, tachykinins, thrombin, TRH, vasopressin, $5HT_2$, PTH, CT, LH, TSH		

Abbreviations: CT, cholera toxin; 5HT, serotonin; PT, pertussis toxin; PTH, parathyroid hormone. For others see Table 1.4.1, page 33.

inactive heterotrimeric complexes to be utilized during subsequent agonist activation. However, βγ is now known to inhibit the activity of at least one form of adenylyl cyclase. In addition, βγ-subunits exert positive regulatory actions on several effector proteins, including muscarinic potassium channels, phospholipase-A$_2$ (PLA$_2$) and phospholipase C-β (PLC-β), β-adrenergic receptor kinase, and ras.[7] Also, two of the six forms of adenylyl cyclase are markedly stimulated by βγ-subunits in the presence of activated α-subunits, an effect referred to as 'conditional' activation of the enzyme.[8] This action of βγ explains the ability of certain hormones that are unable to activate adenylyl cyclase to potentiate the action of agents that can. In certain cell types, PLC activity is stimulated by βγ-subunits released from G$_i$ or G$_o$ during agonist stimulation. This effect of βγ appears to be responsible for the pertussis toxin-sensitive activation of PLC observed in several hematopoietic tissues.[9]

Members of the G protein γ-subunit family are important in the selectivity of receptor–G protein interactions, and in some cases are specific to certain tissues or cell types. Most γ-subunits contain lipid chains attached to cysteine residues near their carboxy-terminus that tether them to the plasma membrane, together with their associated β-subunits. The γ-subunits probably serve as determinants of the specificity with which receptors bind to individual G proteins.

Abnormalities of G protein function

Several endocrine disorders are caused by reduced expression or constitutive activation of the α-subunits of the G proteins that regulate adenylyl cyclase activity. A deficiency of G$_s$ is found in patients with pseudohypoparathyroidism, who are resistant to several of the hormones (parathyroid hormone (PTH), TSH, gonadotropins, and glucagon) that normally stimulate cyclic AMP production.[10] Conversely, activating *gsp* mutations are present in the G$_s$ α-subunit gene in certain somatotrope adenomas and thyroid tumors, and in certain tissues of patients with the McCune–Albright syndrome. In somatotrope adenomas, constitutive activation of the mutant α$_s$-subunits causes overproduction of cAMP, which induces the expression of the transcriptional regulatory protein Pit-1 and stimulates cell hyperplasia.[11] In the McCune–Albright syndrome, a form of mosaicism that results from a somatic mutation of α$_s$ in the endocrine glands, melanotrophs, and osteoblasts, overproduction of cyclic AMP leads to cell proliferation and/or overactivity of the affected tissues. Another type of activating mutation (termed *gip2*) is found in the G$_{i2}$ α-subunit in some adrenal and ovarian tumors, and is associated with constitutive activation of G$_i$ and inhibition of cAMP production. This mutation also leads to cell proliferation because G$_i$ mediates mitogenic responses to activation of G protein-coupled receptors in certain cell types.

The GTP-binding protein superfamily

The heterotrimeric G proteins belong to a large superfamily of regulatory proteins that bind and hydrolyze GTP, and function as molecular switches that control a wide range of intracellular functions. The general mechanism of GTP binding and activation, followed by GTP hydrolysis and inactivation, is utilized by a wide variety of proteins that control transmembrane signaling, ribosomal protein synthesis, protein translocation into the endoplasmic reticulum, and intracellular vesicular transport, as well as cell differentiation and proliferation. These GTP-binding proteins (or GTPase proteins) are extremely diverse in size and function, but all are characterized by the ability to assume an active conformation after binding GTP. The activated G proteins then interact with their target molecules for a period that depends on their intrinsic GTP-hydrolyzing activity. Since their basal enzymatic activity is relatively weak, the effects of modulator proteins that influence GTPase activity and the rate of exchange of GTP and GDP are important determinants of G protein activation. In the heterotrimeric G proteins, the ligand-activated receptors promote the exchange of GTP for GDP on the α-subunit and the consequent dissociation of the complex into α-GTP and βγ-subunits.

Small GTP-binding proteins

A growing family of small GTP-binding proteins (or small GTPases) that range in size from 20 to 35 kDa has been found to participate in numerous aspects of cell regulation. These are exemplified by the ras proteins, which are associated with the cell membrane and participate in the regulation of cell growth and proliferation.[12] The ras protein is anchored to the plasma membrane by lipid groups attached to cysteine residues near its carboxy-terminus, and contains conserved regions that participate in guanine nucleotide binding and hydrolysis. Mutations of specific amino acids within these regions can endow ras with transforming activity as a result of persistent activation by bound GTP, and are present in a significant proportion of mammalian tumors.

The activities of ras and other small GTPases are regulated by GTPase activating and inhibitory proteins, and also by exchange proteins that accelerate or inhibit the exchange of bound GDP for GTP. In this way, the rates at which the small G proteins cycle between their 'on' and 'off' conformations are determined by factors that control their kinetics of GTP binding and hydrolysis. Some of the proteins that inhibit GTPase activity and promote G protein activation are regulated by phospholipid breakdown products. The GTPase activating proteins (GAPs) act largely as negative regulators by accelerating GTP hydrolysis and keeping the proteins in their inactive forms.[13] These several forms of regulation enable small G proteins to act not only as molecular switches but also as timers that operate a wide variety of effectors for periods that are determined by the rates of association, dissociation, and hydrolysis of their bound GTP.[14]

Other small G proteins include the rab family, which participates in the control of vesicular transport within the cell and in the processes of endocytosis and exocytosis.[15] Also membrane-associated are the ARF (ADP ribosylation factor) proteins that influence protein transport within the Golgi system, and also participate in the activation of phospholipase-D.[16] Cytoplasmic small G proteins include the rho proteins, which act in the Golgi apparatus and regulate actin filament formation, and the rac proteins, which mediate the effects of growth factors on actin filaments and pinocytic vesicle formation.[17] The effects of growth factors on the cytoskeleton appear to be mediated through ras, which in turn controls the activities of rho and rac.

Cyclic nucleotide signaling pathways

Numerous G-protein-coupled receptors are coupled through G_s to the activation of adenylyl cyclase and the formation of cAMP, which acts predominantly through cAMP-dependent protein kinase (PKA) to control multiple aspects of cell function through phosphorylation of protein substrates.[18]

Adenylyl cyclases

Several structurally related types of adenylyl cyclase have been identified in animal cells, and in general contain two hydrophobic domains composed of six transmembrane helices that are associated with the plasma membrane.[19] Type I adenylyl cyclase is expressed in neural tissues, type II in brain and lung, type III in olfactory tissue, type IV in the brain and elsewhere, and types V and VI in heart, brain, and other tissues. All six enzymes are stimulated by G_{sa} and forskolin, and types I and III are also activated by Ca^{2+}-calmodulin (CaM). The Ca^{2+}-CaM regulated adenylyl cyclases are abundant in neural tissue and are sensitive to transmitter-induced changes in cytoplasmic calcium concentration. In several cell types, including pituitary somatotropes, Ca^{2+} exerts a direct inhibitory effect on the activity of the type III enzyme. Since Ca^{2+}-mobilizing hormones usually act through stimulation of phosphoinositide hydrolysis, G_q is indirectly responsible for regulating the activities of the Ca^{2+}- and CaM-sensitive adenylyl cyclases.

The membrane-bound adenylyl cyclases are regulated by G_s or G_i α-subunits that activate or inhibit enzyme activity (see above). However, some of the enzymes are also controlled by βγ-subunits.[7] Type I adenylyl cyclase activity, when stimulated by $α_s$ or Ca^{2+}-CaM, is inhibited by βγ. Conversely, the stimulation of type II and type IV enzymes by $α_s$ is potentiated by βγ-subunits. The βγ-subunits that modulate adenylyl cyclase activity are probably derived from G_i and G_o, which are abundant in the brain and elsewhere. The basal and $α_s$-stimulated activities of the type II enzyme are also increased by calcium-dependent protein kinase (PKC) during activation of G_q by calcium-mobilizing hormones. Thus, the activation of adenylyl cyclases by G_s can be potentiated or inhibited by other receptor-mediated pathways that operate through G_i, G_o, or G_q in the same cell type.[20]

Cyclic nucleotide phosphodiesterases

The cyclic nucleotides produced in agonist-stimulated cells are rapidly inactivated by phosphodiesterases (PDEs), and are often released into the extracellular fluid. Intracellular cyclic nucleotide levels are usually governed by changes in their rates of production, but in some tissues (e.g. the retina) activation of PDEs is the major determinant of their concentration. Another important function of PDEs is to coordinate the activities of the cyclic nucleotide and phosphoinositide signaling pathways, largely through the regulatory action of Ca^{2+}-CaM on PDE activity.

Mammalian cells contain about 20 PDEs that are classified into five main types according to their physical and functional properties.[21] All possess a central catalytic domain and an N-terminal regulatory domain that binds Ca^{2+}-CaM and also contains binding sites for cyclic guanosine monophosphate. Type I PDEs are stimulated by Ca^{2+}-CaM, and are activated by calcium-mobilizing agonists and inhibited by methylxanthines. Type II PDEs are stimulated by cAMP and are activated by atrial natriuretic peptides. Type III PDEs are inhibited by cGMP, which competes with cAMP at the catalytic site, and are regulated by insulin, glucagon, and dexamethasone. Type IV PDEs are specific for cAMP and are activated by cAMP-stimulating agonists. Type V PDEs are specific for cGMP and include rod and cone isoforms that are activated by transducin during visual transduction.

Agonist-induced increases in cAMP are accompanied by increased activity of the cGMP-inhibited PDEs as a result of their cAMP-dependent phosphorylation, and by a transient decrease in the activity of the Ca^{2+}-CaM PDEs. Several hormones that stimulate cAMP production also increase the expression of the high-affinity cAMP-specific PDEs. This occurs in Sertoli cells treated with follicle-stimulating hormone (FSH) and probably accounts for their progressive loss of responsiveness to FSH during sexual maturation.[22]

Cyclic AMP-dependent protein kinases

Cyclic AMP-dependent protein kinases (PKAs) are present in all eukaryotic cells and are the major mediators of the effects of cAMP on cellular function.[23] Cyclic nucleotide-dependent protein kinases are rapidly activated by the micromolar concentrations of cAMP or cGMP that occur in hormone-stimulated cells. The cyclic nucleotides bind to specific regulatory sites on the enzymes, which share several common structural features. In PKA, the regulatory and catalytic domains are expressed as two separate molecules that associate to form an inactive complex. In the cGMP-dependent enzyme (PKG), these domains are present in a single molecule.

The inactive form of PKA is a tetramer ($R_2.C_2$) composed of two regulatory (R) subunits and two catalytic (C) subunits (Fig. 1.5.2). In the absence of cAMP, the subunits bind to each other with high affinity and sequences in the regulatory subunits interact with the catalytic site and maintain the holoenzymes in their basal inactive state. Binding of cAMP to the R subunits dissociates the inactive holoenzyme and releases catalytic subunits that phosphorylate intracellular substrates.[24] The regulatory subunits released by cAMP-induced dissociation of protein kinase remain as an R_2 dimer and later undergo reassociation with free catalytic subunits. This sequence can be represented by

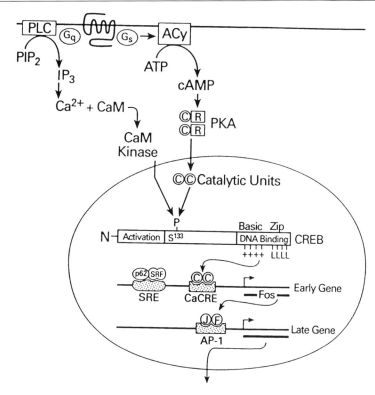

Fig. 1.5.2 *Receptor-mediated activation of signaling to CREB via the cAMP and calcium/CaM pathways. Both PKA and CaM kinase can phosphorylate and activate CREB, which binds to the CaCRE present in the promoter region of early response genes such as* fos. *The increased expression of* fos, *and the formation of* fos-jun *heterodimers, leads to activation of AP-1 sites in the promoter regions of a variety of intermediate and late response genes.*

the equation: $R_2.C_2 + 4cAMP \leftrightarrow R_2.cAMP_4 + 2C$. The catalytic subunit is common to both major forms of PKA, but the regulatory subunits show several differences. Two forms of protein kinase are present in most tissues, but their proportions vary in each cell type. The holoenzymes are generally similar in subunit composition ($R_2.C_2$) and molecular mass (about 170 kDa). The regulatory subunits differ in their molecular masses, R_I being smaller (49 kDa) and more uniform in size than RII (52–56 kDa).

The RI and RII subunits exist in α and β isoforms that differ in size and tissue distribution. The α isoforms are expressed constitutively in many tissues, but the β isoforms have a more limited distribution and are most abundant in the nervous system. The selective regulation of these isoforms during differentiation and hormonal stimulation could mediate specific responses to the cAMP pathway. In some tissues, free RI and RII subunits are present in excess over the catalytic subunit and interact with other cellular proteins or structures. Selective increases in the RII subunit occur in several tissues during cAMP-induced differentiation, as in the developing follicles of the FSH-stimulated ovary. The C subunits are also encoded by multiple genes, giving rise to α, β, and γ isoforms (the latter confined to the testis). Since each R subunit can associate with any of the C subunits, a wide variety of $R_2.C_2$ holoenzymes could exist in various tissues. The presence of at least 12 forms of PKA provides for a considerable degree of diversity in the tissue-specific expression, intracellular localization, and activation properties of the individual enzymes.

Nuclear signaling by the cAMP/PKA pathway

The receptor-mediated activation of adenylyl cyclase activity is often followed by cAMP-mediated stimulation of gene transcription. This results from the phosphorylation by PKA of transcriptional regulatory proteins that bind to cAMP-responsive enhancer elements (CREs) located in the promoter regions of cAMP-regulated genes. The CRE binding (CREB) proteins that mediate transcriptional activation during stimulation of cAMP production are members of a family that includes both activators and inhibitors of gene expression.[25] The CREBs belong to a superfamily of transcription factors that are characterized structurally as basic region-leucine zipper (bZip) proteins. Such proteins interact via their leucine zipper domains to form specific homodimers and heterodimers with other family members. In some CREBs, the phosphorylation of a specific serine residue by PKA promotes their transcriptional activation potential and stimulates gene expression. The same residue is also phosphorylated by Ca^{2+}-CaM-dependent protein kinases, and thus serves to integrate signals from two distinct signaling pathways (Fig. 1.5.2).

An important subset of the CREB family are termed CRE modulator (CREM) proteins, which are derived from a single gene by a variety of transcriptional and translational processes. CREM proteins possess specific activator or inhibitory functions and tissue localizations, and are important mediators of physiological and neuroendocrine responses, including FSH-stimulated spermatogenesis in the testis.[26] CREMs are phosphorylated by PKA and Ca^{2+}-CaM-dependent kinases at the same serine residue as CREB, as well as by protein kinase C and the mitogen-activated S6 kinase. The CREM proteins are thus responsive to multiple signal transduction pathways, including those responsible for mitogen-induced gene expression.

Guanylyl cyclase

Cyclic GMP is a major physiologic regulator of vasodilatation induced by atrial natriuretic peptides (atriopeptins or ANPs), which activate membrane-associated guanylyl cyclase in smooth muscle, kidney, endothelial cells, and adrenal glands.[27] Several hormones that stimulate phospholipid turnover also increase cGMP production, probably reflecting activation of guanylyl cyclase by PKC and/or arachidonic acid metabolites. The resulting increases in cGMP production are responsible for smooth muscle relaxation and vasodilatation, via activation of PKG and phosphorylation of specific proteins involved in the contractile mechanism.

In vertebrates, cGMP serves as the intracellular messenger mediating visual transduction by modulating the activity of a cation channel in the plasma membrane of rod photoreceptors of the retina.[28] The guanylyl cyclases that catalyze the formation of cGMP from GTP are present in most mammalian cells as membrane-associated and soluble forms.[29] The membrane-associated enzymes are located within the cytoplasmic portions of cell-surface receptors with a single transmembrane domain and an extracellular hormone-binding domain. These receptors are activated by ANPs, heat-stable *Escherichia coli* enterotoxins, and sea urchin egg peptides that stimulate sperm motility. The three major forms of receptor-guanylyl cyclase (termed GC-A, GC-B, and GC-C) contain a cysteine-rich extracellular domain for ligand binding and an intracellular catalytic domain that is highly conserved in guanylyl and adenylyl cyclases.[30] The ANPs produced by the heart and brain act on GC-A and GC-B receptors, and enterotoxins probably act on the GC-C receptor.

Soluble guanylyl cyclases are present in most tissues and are abundant in lung and smooth muscle. They contain no membrane-spanning domains and are activated by nitric oxide, which interacts with a potential heme-binding region of the molecule. This effect of nitric oxide is responsible for the vasodilator actions of nitroglycerin and related compounds. It also accounts for the actions of endogenous vasodilators such as acetylcholine, bradykinin, and substance P, which stimulate nitric oxide synthesis in endothelial cells. The gaseous messenger diffuses into the adjacent cells and activates soluble guanylate cyclase, leading to smooth muscle relaxation.[31]

PKGs are abundant in invertebrates but have a more limited distribution in mammalian tissues. Whereas PKAs regulate the activities of major metabolic pathways including lipolysis, glycogenolysis, and steroidogenesis, the cGMP-dependent enzymes are involved in the control of gene expression, neuronal function, vascular tone, and platelet aggregation. Since PKGs are single molecules, their activation does not involve the subunit dissociation that is typical of the cAMP-dependent enzyme. There are marked amino acid sequence homologies between cGMP- and cAMP-dependent PKs, suggesting that the two enzymes have evolved from an ancestral phosphotransferase.

Calcium and calcium-dependent enzyme systems

Many cells are regulated by calcium-mobilizing receptors that promote the movement of calcium ions into their cytoplasm.[32-34] The calcium involved in such movements is derived from the extracellular fluid and from intracellular stores in microsomes and other organelles. The cytosolic free calcium concentration is about 100 nM under basal conditions, and increases to levels of up to 1500 nM during hormonal stimulation. Although calcium entry is favored by the large calcium gradient across the plasma membrane, the rate of calcium influx is low in the absence of cell stimulation. However, membrane permeability to calcium is frequently increased during agonist stimulation by mechanisms that differ in excitable and non-excitable cells. Activation of calcium-mobilizing receptors causes an immediate release of Ca^{2+} from intracellular stores in the endoplasmic reticulum, leading to a rapid increase in cytoplasmic calcium concentration (Fig. 1.5.3).

Although calcium is a major intracellular messenger, excessive or prolonged elevations of cytoplasmic calcium concentration exert deleterious effects on cell function and viability. In all cells, agonist-induced Ca^{2+} elevations are accompanied by rapid increases in calcium sequestration and efflux from the cell. Much of the Ca^{2+} that enters the cytoplasm during agonist stimulation is pumped back into the endoplasmic reticulum by a Ca^{2+}-ATPase that is inhibited by the tumor promoter, thapsigargin. In addition, agonist-induced elevations of cytoplasmic Ca^{2+} often activate the Ca^{2+}-CaM-sensitive enzyme, Ca^{2+}, Mg^{2+}-ATPase, which pumps Ca^{2+} out through the plasma membrane. This leads to calcium efflux that promotes restoration of the normal cytoplasmic calcium concentration but tends to reduce intracellular Ca^{2+} stores. This is usually compensated by subsequent increases in Ca^{2+} entry through plasma membrane calcium channels and other influx mechanisms.

Most of the signaling actions of calcium are dependent on its interaction with binding proteins such as CaM and regulatory enzymes such as PKC. The calcium–CaM complex regulates the activities of numerous enzyme systems, including adenylyl and guanylyl cyclase, cyclic nucleotide phosphodiesterase, Ca^{2+}, Mg^{2+}-ATPase, and calcineurin. By influencing the cytoplasmic levels of cyclic nucleotides and calcium, CaM links the intracellular messenger systems as well as controlling enzymes involved in signaling, secretion, and contractility.

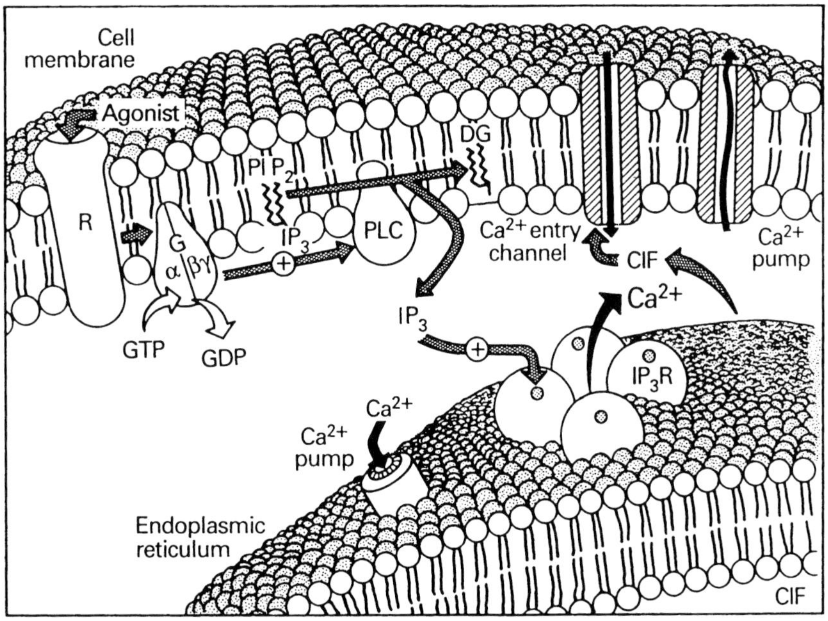

Fig. 1.5.3 *Agonist-induced mobilization of intracellular calcium from stores in the endoplasmic reticulum, and from the extracellular fluid. The release of a diffusible calcium influx factor (CIF) during depletion of calcium stores leads to the opening of plasma-membrane ion channels through which calcium enters the cell and is pumped back into the endoplasmic reticulum. The activation of phospho-inositide hydrolysis to produce inositol 1,4,5-triphosphate (IP₃) and diacylglycerol (DG) from phosphatidylinositol bisphosphate (PIP₂) is followed by the opening of IP₃ receptor channels through which calcium enters the cytoplasm from the endoplasmic reticulum storage pool. The subsequent depletion of the calcium store is a major stimulus to calcium entry through the plasma membrane, which is mediated by CIF or a related influx factor (modified from reference 33).*

Calcium–calmodulin and enzyme activation

Calmodulin is structurally and functionally similar to troponin C and other calcium-binding proteins, and subserves numerous regulatory functions in eukaryotic cells.[35] It is one of a family of small, acidic proteins that contain multiple copies of a helix–loop–helix motif that binds calcium with high affinity. These domains contain a loop of 12 amino acids, five of which have carboxyl or hydroxyl groups that coordinate the calcium molecule. Multiple copies of this calcium-binding structure are present in CaM, troponin C, myosin light chains, calcineurin, and at least 200 other calcium-binding proteins.[36] The functional role of CaM in non-contractile tissues is to mediate the actions of calcium on regulatory enzyme systems. By serving as an intracellular calcium receptor, CaM modifies calcium transport, the calcium-dependent regulation of cyclic nucleotide and glycogen metabolism, and processes such as secretion and cell motility. It also regulates the activity of calcineurin, an important phosphoprotein phosphatase with broad specificity for neuronal and other phosphoproteins, including tyrosyl phosphoproteins. Calcineurin is an intracellular target for immunosuppressive drugs such as cyclosporin, and is involved in signal transduction pathways that regulate interleukin production in T cells.[37]

Protein kinase C

Calcium also binds directly to several calcium-dependent enzymes, the most important of which is PKC, a calcium- and phospholipid-dependent phosphokinase that depends for its activity on calcium and phosphatidylserine (PS).[38]

In several cell types, PKC also acts as a negative feedback regulator of agonist-induced signaling responses.[39] Activation of PKC can inhibit phosphoinositide hydrolysis formation, leading to reduced calcium mobilization, and can stimulate calcium extrusion by activation of plasma membrane calcium pumps. Such effects probably contribute to the decreased duration of the calcium signal and the attenuation of secretory responses sometimes observed in target cells exposed to high hormone concentrations. PKC also inhibits signal transduction by phosphorylating certain plasma-membrane receptors, including those for EGF and insulin. Prolonged activation of PKC can cause loss of receptors and impaired coupling between receptors and adenylyl cyclase, possibly through an action on the intermediate G protein.

The PKC superfamily

At least nine distinct PKC isoenzymes have been identified, and differ in their tissue expression as well as in their mode of activation and their substrate specificities. The individual enzymes will probably prove to have distinct functions in signal transduction and in the control of metabolism, secretion, differentiation, and proliferation.[40] The nine isoenzymes can be subdivided into the conventional Ca²⁺-dependent isoforms (α, βI, βII, and γ) and the Ca²⁺-independent isoforms (δ, ε, η, θ, and ζ). The former are single polypeptide chains with catalytic domains containing the ATP and substrate binding sites located in the carboxy-terminal half of the molecule, and regulatory domains containing the Ca^{2+}, phospholipid, and diacylglycerol (DAG)/phorbol ester binding sites in the amino-terminal half. The regulatory domains are similar among the calcium-dependent α, β, and γ enzymes, but the Ca^{2+}-independent δ–ζ enzymes lack the Ca^{2+} binding domain, and ζ is not activated by DAG or phorbol ester.

The major lipid activator of PKCs is DAG, acting in conjunction with PS as a cofactor. In ligand-stimulated cells, the Ca^{2+} released from inositol 1,4,5-triphosphate (IP_3)-sensitive stores binds to the conventional PKC isoenzymes and promotes their translocation to the plasma membrane, where they are activated by the PS present in the lipid bilayer and the DAG produced from phosphoinositide hydrolysis. Phorbol esters act by mimicking the action of DAG, and lowering the Ca^{2+} requirement for enzyme activation. In the case of the Ca^{2+}-independent PKCs, PS and DAG or other lipid derivatives are required for activation. Several of the PKC isoenzymes are activated by other phospholipid metabolites including *cis*-unsaturated fatty acids, arachidonic acid and its derivatives, and phosphatidylinositol 4,5-bisphosphate (PIP_2). Differential activation can also result from DAG produced during phosphatidylcholine breakdown stimulated by certain hormones and cytokines, and from the PIP_3 formed during activation of growth factor receptors.[41] In this way the several PKCs could be differentially activated by specific stimuli to phosphorylate their substrates at defined cellular locations.

Hormone action and phospholipid signaling

Plasma membrane phospholipids are major components of the signal transduction pathways that mediate the actions of many hormones and other ligands that regulate cellular function. Their hydrolysis by receptor-activated phospholipases produces a variety of intracellular signaling molecules with diverse actions on cell metabolism, secretion, transmission, and growth. In the plasma membrane, the predominant phospholipid is phosphatidylcholine, with lesser quantities of phosphatidylinositol and PS. Phosphatidylcholine is synthesized largely by the enzymatic transfer of phosphocholine from CDP-choline to DAG. Phosphoinositides are synthesized by sequential phosphorylation of phosphatidylinositol to form phosphatidylinositol 4-phosphate and PIP_2. Although PIP_2 constitutes only a small fraction of the total inositol phospholipids, it is of primary importance in the activation of cells by calcium-mobilizing hormones.

Agonist-induced phosphoinositide hydrolysis

The breakdown of PIP_2 to form DAG and IP_3 is catalyzed by PLC, which is activated by agonist binding to both G-protein-coupled receptors and receptor tyrosine kinases[42] (Fig. 1.5.4). The actions of calcium-mobilizing agonists that bind to about 30 G-protein-coupled receptors are mediated by PLC-β, which is activated not only by α-subunits of the G_q family (PLC-β1) but also by $\beta\gamma$-subunits

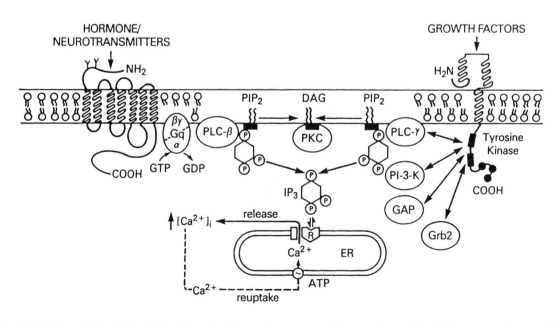

Fig. 1.5.4 *Activation of phosphoinositide-calcium signaling by G-protein-coupled receptors and tyrosine kinase receptors. In addition to the well-defined actions of hormones and transmitters that activate G protein-coupled receptors and phospholipid hydrolysis through PLC-β, many growth factors and other tyrosine kinase receptors stimulate PLC-γ. The latter enzyme is activated after binding to tyrosine phosphorylated receptors via its SH2 domains, and catalyzes the production of signaling molecules such as DAG and IP₃ from plasma-membrane phospholipids. The production of lipid second messengers, and in some cases of IP₃ and calcium signaling, is a common accompaniment to the activation of growth factor and other tyrosine kinase receptors.*

produced from *Bordetella pertussis*-sensitive G proteins (PLC-β2). On the other hand, the actions of growth factors and other agonists that bind to receptors coupled to tyrosine kinase are mediated by PLC-γ, which becomes physically associated with the activated receptors and is tyrosine-phosphorylated during cell stimulation by numerous growth factors and cytokines.[43]

The IP₃ produced during phosphoinositide hydrolysis binds to IP₃ receptor channels in the endoplasmic reticulum and releases stored Ca^{2+}, and is rapidly degraded to inositol. IP₃ is also metabolized to multiple inositol phosphates but none of these, with the possible exception of I(1,3,4,5)P₄, has a significant role in calcium mobilization.[44] The I(1,4,5)P₃ receptor is a complex of four large subunits surrounding a central ion channel and is structurally related to the ryanodine receptor of excitable muscle and neuronal cells.[45] I(1,4,5)P₃ does not activate the ryanodine receptor, for which the second messenger is probably cyclic ADP-ribose, a recently discovered compound that releases Ca^{2+} in sea urchin eggs. In some cells, cyclic ADP-ribose levels are regulated by cGMP. One form of the ryanodine receptor is as widely distributed as the IP₃ receptor, and probably acts in conjunction with the IP₃ receptor to generate some of the oscillatory calcium responses that occur in various agonist-stimulated cells.[46] Both IP₃ receptors and ryanodine receptors are influenced by the prevailing intracellular calcium concentration. The IP₃ receptor shows biphasic sensitivity to calcium, being least sensitive at high and low calcium levels. The ryanodine receptor in muscle and other excitable cells can be directly activated by calcium entering through voltage sensitive channels or released from ER stores, leading to the development of calcium-induced calcium release.[47]

Phosphatidylcholine signaling

In addition to the lipid second messengers derived from phosphoinositides, agonist stimulation is also associated with the hydrolysis of phosphatidylcholine by PLA₂, PLC, and PLD to form DAG, phosphatidic acid and arachidonic acid. Both G proteins and PKC have been implicated in the activation of PLD, leading to the release of phosphatidic acid and its subsequent conversion (via phosphatidic acid phosphohydrolase) to DAG.[48] In a given cell type, various agonists can stimulate the activation of PLC and/or PLD, and the proportion of DAG generated from phosphatidylcholine versus phosphoinositide hydrolysis can range from zero to 100%. During agonist activation of G-protein coupled receptors, the DAG produced from phosphoinositide breakdown can lead to secondary activation of PLD through PKC, causing a further increase in DAG production from the hydrolysis of phosphatidylcholine and metabolism of phosphatidic acid.

Production and metabolism of arachidonic acid

Many peptide hormones stimulate the production of arachidonic acid, the precursor of numerous active metabolites that exert secondary effects on vascular and cellular responses during hormone action. Arachidonic acid is the most abundant unsaturated fatty acid in tissue phospholipids, and is converted into a variety of eicosanoids by the cyclooxygenase and lipoxygenase pathways. Its production during receptor-mediated cell activation depends on membrane-bound phospholipases that catalyze the hydrolysis of ester linkages in glycerophospholipids. Phospholipase A₂, which releases fatty acids esterified at the *sn2* position of diacyl-glycerophospholipids, is the major source of arachidonic acid in many cell types.[49] Arachidonic acid is also produced by the action of diglyceride lipase on the diacylglycerol released during hydrolysis of phosphoinositides by PLC. The formation of arachidonic acid is the rate-limiting step in the synthesis of prostaglandins, leukotrienes, lipoxins, and platelet activating factor.

Growth factor action

In contrast to the signaling mode of G protein-coupled receptors, with formation of small second messenger molecules that activate potent serine/threonine protein kinases located throughout the cell, receptors for growth factors and cytokines operate through a network of enzymatic proteins that act directly or indirectly on sets of transduction molecules that form several signaling pathways to the nucleus. These pathways are initiated at the cell surface by ligand-induced dimerization or oligomerization of several types of receptors, leading to activation of their intrinsic tyrosine or serine/threonine kinase activity or to interaction with other proteins that possess tyrosine kinase activity or activate such enzymes in the cytoplasm. Some of the protein tyrosine kinase receptors in the plasma membrane, including those for epidermal growth factor (EGF) and fibroblast growth factor (FGF), are monomeric proteins that dimerize upon ligand binding.[50] However, receptors for other cytokines exist as either disulfide-bonded dimers (platelet-derived growth factor (PDGF), colony stimulating factor (CSF) or heterotetramers (insulin, insulin-like growth factor-I (IGF-I), or as oligomers bound by noncovalent forces (stem cell factor (SCF), tumor necrosis factor (TNF), and antigen receptors). The ligand-induced dimerization of tyrosine kinase receptors, or ligand binding to the preformed oligomeric receptors, leads to tyrosine phosphorylation of the receptor molecules (for growth factor receptors) or recruitment of cytoplasmic tyrosine kinases in the case of cytokine and related receptors. This is followed by the activation of several major cellular signaling pathways, the best defined of which is dependent on the activity of ras and its regulation by G nucleotide exchange proteins and GTPase activating proteins (GAPs) (Fig. 1.5.5).

The tyrosine residues that are autophosphorylated after ligand binding to the receptor fall into two groups in terms of their function and location. One group is related to the tyrosine kinase catalytic activity of the receptor, and their phosphorylation promotes enzyme activity and additional phosphorylation of the receptor and other protein substrates. The other set of phosphotyrosine residues does not

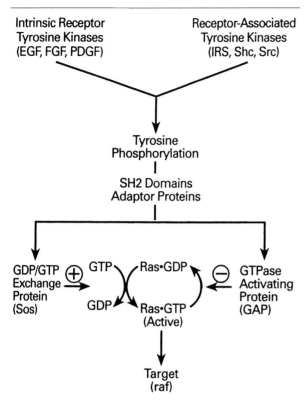

Fig. 1.5.5 *The convergent activation pathway of tyrosine phosphorylation from receptor tyrosine kinases and receptors that associate with cytoplasmic tyrosine kinases. Tyrosine phosphorylation by both types of receptors initiates a series of protein–protein interactions and protein phosphorylation cascades, exemplified by the manner in which ras activation by Grb.SoS leads to stimulation of raf and ultimately of MAP kinase. Many receptors that lack tyrosine kinase activity, and some that possess it, utilize cytoplasmic tyrosine kinases (such as IRS, Shc, Src) to activate a variety of growth-related and other signal transduction pathways.*

influence kinase activity but provides binding sites for signal transduction proteins that possess specific recognition domains for phosphotyrosine-containing sequences. These regions are known as SH2 (Src homology 2) domains, based on their similarity to a sequence in the *src* oncogene product, the original tyrosine kinase to be identified.[51] The SH2 domain facilitates the binding of src and other soluble tyrosine kinases to signaling proteins that are phosphorylated on specific tyrosine residues. Similar domains are present in several of the downstream signaling proteins, including PLC-γ, PI-3-kinase, Src-related kinases, and ras-GAP, that became associated with activated receptors (Fig. 1.5.4).

Some of the autophosphorylation sites that participate in protein–protein interactions are located in a non-catalytic region of the kinase domain, as in PDGF and CSF receptors, and others are near the plasma membrane or in the C-terminal region (as in the EGF receptor). In the PDGF receptor, several autophosphorylated tyrosine residues participate in specific interactions with about eight individual signal transduction molecules.[52] However, this orderly arrangement of the docking sites may not be gen-

eral, since it does not apply to the EGF receptor. The selectivity of the binding between individual SH2 domains and tyrosine phosphorylated receptors is dependent on the amino acid sequence surrounding the phosphorylated tyrosine residue. Several tyrosine kinases also possess another src homology domain (SH3) that binds to other cellular proteins, including the GAPs that regulate the activities of the small G proteins. Thus, SH3 domains can connect the tyrosine kinase and small G protein signaling pathways, and in general mediate protein–protein interactions that serve to organize enzyme–substrate interactions and facilitate information transfer within the cell.

The signaling molecules that are recruited to receptors by binding via their SH2 domains to autophosphorylated tyrosine residues undergo activation by several mechanisms. The most obvious is by tyrosine phosphorylation, as in the case of PLC-γ recruitment to growth factor receptors, and the STATs (signal transducers and activators of transcription) that are bound by activated cytokine receptors and their associated JAK kinases (see below). Others are conformational changes, as in the activation of PI-3-kinase by binding to growth factor receptors, and the translocation of Grb.Sos to the plasma membrane that triggers the activation of ras by stimulation of guanine nucleotide exchange.[53]

Activation of signaling pathways by receptor tyrosine kinases

Almost all tyrosine kinase signaling pathways appear to operate through the adaptor protein Grb2, which contains both SH2 and SH3 domains that enable it to link tyrosine-phosphorylated receptors with regulators of small G protein activity. Thus, Grb2 binds directly to receptors for EGF and other growth factors and thereby brings Sos to the plasma membrane where it activates ras.[54] Such a change in location is also important for the activation of PLC-γ1, PI-3-kinase, and ras-GAP, which likewise become associated with the EGF receptor through their SH2 domains. In some cases Grb2 does not bind directly to the receptor but to an associated protein (Syp for the PDGF receptor; shc for the NGF receptor; IRS for the insulin receptor) that in turn serves to bring the Grb.Sos complex in proximity to ras at the plasma membrane. Once activated by Sos, ras links the receptor tyrosine kinase to a cascade of enzymatic proteins that carries signals from the cell membrane into the cytoplasm and nucleus. Major among these is the three-component pathway formed by raf, a serine/threonine protein kinase that activates MEK, a tyrosine and serine/threonine kinase that in turn activates the central signaling molecule, mitogen-activated protein kinase (MAPK). The ras/raf/MEK/MAPK pathway, and the subsequent actions of MAPK, are shown in Fig. 1.5.6. This pathway is also activated by calcium-mobilizing receptors via βγ-subunits and PKC, and can be inhibited by adenylyl cyclase-coupled receptors through the action of cAMP.

Another important tyrosine kinase signaling pathway is activated by cytokine receptors, which lack intrinsic

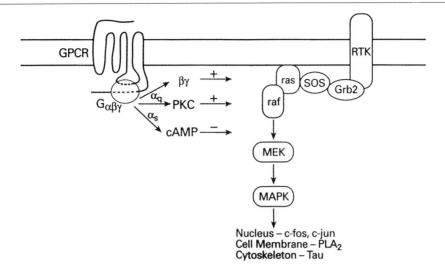

Fig. 1.5.6 *Dual control of the MAP kinase pathway by tyrosine kinase and G-protein-coupled receptors. The major activation route to MAP kinase is initiated by ligand binding to tyrosine kinase receptors and subsequent activation of ras by the binding of Grb2.SoS via SH2 domains to the receptor. This initiates a cascade of ras-dependent phosphorylations that extend to MAP kinase, a multifunctional enzyme with target proteins located in all regions of the cell. Recent work has shown that numerous G-protein-coupled receptors also influence MAP kinase activity, with activation through βγ-subunits and protein kinase C, and inhibition via cyclic AMP-dependent mechanisms.*

tyrosine kinase activity but upon activation by dimerization or oligomerization become associated with cytoplasmic tyrosine kinases that bind to the juxtamembrane region of their intracellular domains. These include members of the Janus kinase (JAK) family, which possess two tyrosine kinase and two SH2 domains.[55] The JAKs in turn phosphorylate the signal transduction proteins termed STATs, which form dimers and undergo translocation into the nucleus where they act as transcriptional regulatory proteins. The ability of several cytokine receptors to activate the same JAKs, as well as their sharing of receptor subunits for oligomerization, accounts for the redundancy and pleiotropy that are features of the cytokines.[56] The JAKs may also phosphorylate their associated cytokine receptors, creating sites whereby these receptors can interact with SH2 domain signaling proteins to activate some of the pathways, such as ras and PI-3-kinase, that mediate the actions of tyrosine kinase receptors for growth factors.

Steroid hormone action

The receptors that mediate steroid hormone action are ligand-inducible transcriptional regulatory proteins that bind to specific hormone response elements (HREs) located in the 5′ promoter regions of their target genes.[57] A few such genes are rapidly activated by steroid hormones and express mRNA within 15–30 min, but the majority are more slowly activated and produce specific mRNAs and proteins during the first few hours after hormone stimulation.

Steroid hormone receptors form one of the largest families of transcription factors, and possess specific domains for ligand binding and DNA binding as described in Chapter 1.4. They include the well-characterized receptors for gonadal and adrenal steroids, thyroid hormone, vitamin D, and retinoids, as well as numerous isoforms and structurally similar proteins ('orphan receptors') of unknown function. Such receptors modulate gene expression by binding as dimers to the oligonucleotide sequences that form response elements. The DNA sequences of individual response elements and the spaces between them determine their selectivity for particular types of receptor[58,59] (Fig. 1.5.7).

The ligand-binding domain of steroid receptors is an extensive region located in the carboxy-terminal half of the receptor molecule. The more compact and highly conserved DNA binding domain contains two so-called zinc finger motifs that interact with the HRE. The DNA-binding domains of the receptors interact with their response elements through two zinc finger conformations that are separated by several amino acids.[60] Each finger contains four cysteine residues that form a zinc coordination center, as shown in Fig. 1.5.7. The first finger contains an alpha-helical region between the second pair of zinc-coordinating cysteines that binds to the major groove of the DNA double helix by interacting with the individual base pairs of their response elements. The binding specificity of each receptor is determined by three critical amino acids located within this five residue stretch. Thus, the GR, MR, PR, MR group contains the sequence -C*GSCKV*-, the ER contains -C*EGCKA*-, and the TR, VDR, RAR, RXR group contains -C*EGCKG*-. The amino acids in the second zinc finger are important for receptor dimerization and for interaction with the phosphate backbone of the DNA helix in the region of the HRE. These features of the receptor molecules, and the nature of their individual DNA

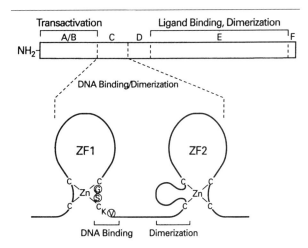

Fig. 1.5.7 *Modular structure, DNA binding domain, and response elements of steroid hormone receptors. The DNA binding and dimerization domain (C) of a typical steroid hormone receptor (above) is shown in diagrammatic form (center) to illustrate the formation of zinc fingers by the amino acids of the binding domain. The zinc fingers in turn interact with DNA response elements and activate transcription. The major DNA binding domains and their response elements are shown below.*

Receptors	DNA Binding Domains	Response Elements
GR, MR, PR, AR	-Cys-**Gly**-**Ser**-Cys-Lys-**Val**-	AGAACAnnnTATXCX
ER	-Cys-**Asn**-**Gly**-Cys-Lys-**Ala**-	AGGTCAnnnTGACCT
TR, VDR, RAR, RXR	-Cys-**Asn**-**Gly**-Cys-Lys-**Gly**-	AGTTCA(n$_x$)AGTTCA

response elements, are largely responsible for the specificity of steroid hormone action upon activation of gene transcription. Although the steroid hormone receptors bind to their DNA response elements only when dimerized by their respective ligands, the TR, VDR, and RAR and RXR group can dimerize in the absence of ligand activation and bind to DNA in a ligand-independent manner.

Regulation of gene expression

After binding as homo- or heterodimers to the DNA sequences of their cognate HREs (Fig. 1.5.8), steroid receptors activate or inhibit gene expression in their various target tissues.[59] This is brought about by their actions on the preinitiation complex of transcription factors (TFs) and RNA polymerase that become assembled at the TATA box (or other initiator elements) in the promoter region of the target gene. This complex is formed by the sequential binding of TFs to the initiation site and to one another, followed by the entry of RNA polymerase and other TFs to activate gene expression. The binding of steroid hormone receptors to their upstream response elements leads to either activation or silencing of their target genes. The ligand-induced binding of the classical steroid receptors (ER, PR, AR, GR, MR) to DNA is followed by their interaction with one of the TFs (specifically TFIIB) that is a rate-limiting factor in preinitiation complex formation, and is essential for positioning RNA polymerase at the site of transcription initiation.[59] In the absence of hormones this group of receptors remains inactive and neither binds to DNA nor influences gene transcription.

The other major subgroup of nuclear receptors (TR, VDR, RAR, RXR) bind to DNA in their unliganded state, but do not activate transcription until they are occupied by the respective ligands. The unoccupied receptors can exert silencing activity on basal promoter activity until ligand binding occurs, when they are converted into activators of transcription. Additional mechanisms for repression of gene activity by receptors include their interaction with other factors (such as c-*jun* and c-*fos*) that prevent transcription, and their binding to specific DNA sequences (negative HREs) that induce receptor conformations with silencing rather than stimulating activity on the core transcriptional machinery.

FUTURE PERSPECTIVES

The intracellular signaling pathways that subserve hormone action are now known to include numerous primary messengers that in turn activate cytoplasmic and nuclear

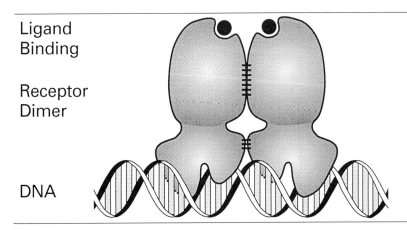

Ligand Binding

Receptor Dimer

DNA

Fig. 1.5.8 *Interaction of ligand-activated hormone receptors with DNA. The dimeric receptor complex formed after agonist occupancy binds with high affinity to the bases within the hormone response element. Dimerization involves at least two regions of the receptor, one of which is adjacent to the DNA binding domain. The zinc finger region of the dimer binds within the major groove of the DNA comprising the hormone response element.*

enzymes, most commonly protein phosphokinases and phosphatases, that regulate the activities of target proteins engaged in secretion, metabolism, contraction, transmission growth, and other cellular responses. In the near future, it is likely that the mechanism by which the known hormones activate these signaling pathways will be fully clarified. In particular, the structural biology of hormone action will be advanced by crystallographic analysis of the major signaling proteins, combined with molecular biology to evaluate the residues and sequences involved in the expression of molecular conformations that permit specific protein interactions and enzymatic activities.[61] In addition, the manner in which different types of receptor-activated pathways converge on common final steps, such as the ability of both G-protein-coupled receptors and growth factor/cytokine receptors to elicit growth signaling and

nuclear responses, will be more fully understood.[62] The role of hormones in early development is being increasingly clarified by gene knockout studies, many of which are revealing unexpected and important functions of hormones hitherto defined by their roles in the control of cell responses in post-embryonic life. Likewise, the identification of molecular defects responsible for specific genetic disorders of metabolism will provide compelling evidence for the importance of known or proposed protein regulators and pathways in defined biosynthetic and other metabolic processes. Advances in the analysis of steroid hormone action will depend on more complete understanding of the basic mechanisms of transcriptional regulation, and the manner in which these are influenced by the nuclear actions of steroid hormone receptors during binding to their DNA response elements.

SUMMARY

- The coupling of agonist-activated receptors to plasma-membrane and other intracellular effector systems generates a wide variety of messenger molecules that subsequently initiate cytoplasmic and nuclear responses. Many of these responses depend on protein–protein interactions and on protein phosphorylations that are mediated by a variety of protein kinases.

- Seven transmembrane domain receptors are coupled through a family of heterotrimeric G proteins to plasma membrane enzymes and channels – typically, adenylyl cyclase, phospholipases, and ion channels. Each of these effector proteins exists in a number of subtypes, isoenzymes, and subunits, providing for great diversity within the signaling pathways of individual cells during hormonal stimulation.

- Receptors for growth factors and cytokines signal through tyrosine and serine/threonine protein kinases that form cascades extending to the nucleus, leading to activation of gene expression.

- The cAMP/PKA system forms a major signaling pathway that controls numerous metabolic reactions, biosynthetic steps, and differentiation programs. It is less frequently involved in growth regulation, and sometimes mediates negative effects of hormones on growth stimulatory pathways.

- The phosphoinositide/calcium system has rapid stimulatory effects on many secretory pathways, in particular exocytosis, as well as on contractile processes and neurotransmission. It is also involved in the growth-stimulating actions of several hormones that activate G-protein-coupled receptors.

- Tyrosine phosphorylation is a cardinal feature of mitogenic signaling from receptors for growth factors and cytokines. Some of these receptors dimerize and activate their own cytoplasmic tyrosine kinase domains, while others associate with cytoplasmic tyrosine kinases that initiate their phosphorylation signaling cascades.

- Many tyrosine phosphorylation pathways operate through recruitment of signal transduction proteins with SH2 domains – PLC-γ, PI-3 kinase, Grb2 – that in turn activate a variety of intracellular signaling pathways.

- Many growth-stimulating pathways operate through activation of MAP kinase, which in turn activates cytoplasmic, plasma-membrane, and nuclear responses. In the nucleus, MAP kinase stimulates the expression of early response genes, such as c-*fos*, and c-*jun*, that encode transcriptional regulatory proteins which form homo- or heterodimers and promote the expression of numerous intermediate and late response genes.

- Ligand-activated steroid hormone receptors bind to specific response elements in the promoter region of their target genes and activate or inhibit gene expression by acting on the pre-initiation complex of transcription factors and RNA polymerase.

- The classical steroid hormone receptors remain inactive in the absence of agonists and do not bind to DNA, whereas the TR, VDR, RAR, and RXR bind to DNA in their unliganded state and can exert silencing effects on basal promoter activity.

REFERENCES

1. Dohlman HG, Thorner J, Caron MC, Lefkowitz RJ. Model systems for the study of seven-transmembrane-segment receptors. *Annu Rev Biochem* 1991 **267**: 653–688.
2. Watson S, Arkinsall S. *The G-Protein Linked Receptor Facts Book*. London: Academic Press, 1994: 427pp.
3. Hepler JR, Gilman AG. G proteins. *Trends Biochem Sci* 1992 **17**: 383–387.
4. Bourne HR, Sanders DA, McCormick F. The GTPase superfamily: conserved structure and molecular mechanism. *Nature* 1991 **349**: 117–127.
5. Neer, E. Heterotrimeric G proteins: organizers of transmembrane signals. *Cell* 1995 **80**: 249–257.
6. Markby DW, Onrust R, Bourne HR. Separate GTPase activating domains of a G alpha subunit. *Science* 1993 **262**: 1895–1901.
7. Clapham DE, Neer E. New roles for G protein β-dimers in transmembrane signaling. *Nature* 1993 **365**: 403–406.
8. Tang W-J, Gilman AG. Type-specific regulation of adenylyl cyclase by G protein β-subunits. *Science* 1991 **254**: 1500–1503.
9. Katz A, Wu D, Simon MI. Subunits βγ of heterotrimeric G protein activate β2 isoform of phospholipase C. *Nature* 1992 **360**: 686–689.
10. Spiegel AM, Shenker A, Weinstein LS. Receptor–effector coupling by G proteins: implications for normal and abnormal signal transduction. *Endocr Rev* 1992 **13**: 536–565.
11. Lyons J, Landis CA, Harsh G, Vallar L, Grünewald K, Feichtinger H, Duh Q-Y, Clark OH, Kawasaki E, Bourne HR, McCormick F. Two G protein oncogenes in human endocrine tumors. *Science* 1990 **249**: 655–659.
12. Barbacid M. Ras genes. *Annu Rev Biochem* 1987 **56**: 779–827.
13. Polakis P, McCormick F. Structural requirements for the interaction of p21ʳᵃˢ with GAP, exchange factors, and its biological effector target. *J Biol Chem* 1993 **268**: 9157–9160.
14. Neer EJ. G proteins: critical control points for transmembrane signals. *Protein Sci* 1994 **3**: 3–14.
15. Bucci, C, Parton RG, Mather IH, Stunnenberg H, Simons K, Hoflack B, Zerial M. The small GTPase rab5 functions as a regulatory factor in the early endocytic pathway. *Cell* 1992 **70**: 715–728.
16. Cockcroft S, Thomas GMH, Fensome A, Geny B, Cunningham E, Gout I, Hiles I, Totty NF, Truong O, Hsuan JJ. Phospholipase D: A downstream effector of ARF in granulocytes. *Science* 1994 **263**: 523–526.
17. Hall A. The cellular functions of small GTP-binding proteins. *Science* 1990 **249**: 635–640.
18. Scott JD. Cyclic nucleotide-dependent protein kinases. In Taylor CW (ed.) *Intracellular Messengers*. Oxford: Pergamon Press, 1993: 137–146.
19. Tang WD, Gilman AG Adenylyl cyclases. *Cell* 1992 **70**: 869–872.
20. Lustig KD, Conklin BR, Herzmark P, Taussig R, Bourne HR. Type II adenylyl cyclase integrates coincident signals from G_s, G_i and G_q. *J Biol Chem* **268**: 13900–13905.
21. Conti M, Jin SL, Monaco L, Repaske DR, Swinnen JV. Hormonal regulation of cyclic nucleotide phosphodiesterases. *Endocr Rev* 1991 **12**: 218–234.
22. Conti M, Toscano MV, Petrelli L, Geremia R, Stefanini M. Involvement of phosphodiesterase in the refractoriness of the Sertoli cell. *Endocrinology* 1983 **113**: 1845–1853.
23. Døkeland SO, Maronde E, Gjertsen BT. The genetic subtypes of cAMP-dependent protein kinase – functionally different or redundant? *Biochim Biophys Acta* 1993 **1178**: 249–258.
24. Hanks SM, Quinn AM, Hunter T. The protein kinase family: conserved features and deduced phylogeny of the catalytic domains. *Science* 1988 **241**: 42–52.
25. Lalli E, Sassone-Corsi P. Signal transduction and gene regulation: the nuclear response to cAMP. *J Biol Chem* 1994 **269**: 17359–17362.

26. Foulkes NS, Schotter F, Pevet P, Sassone-Corsi P. Pituitary hormone FSH directs the CREM functional switch during spermatogenesis. *Nature* 1993 **362**: 264–267.
27. Inagami T. Atrial natriuretic factor. *J Biol Chem* 1989 **264**: 3043–3046.
28. Lolley RN, Lee RH. Cyclic GMP and photoreceptor function. *FASEB J* 1990 **4**: 3001–3008.
29. Schulz S, Yuen PST, Garbers DL. The expanding family of guanylyl cyclases. *Trends Pharmacol Sci* 1991 **12**: 116–120.
30. Garbers DL. Guanylyl cyclase receptors and their endocrine, paracrine, and autocrine ligand. *Cell* 1992 **71**: 1–4.
31. Ignarro LJ. Biosynthesis and metabolism of endothelium-derived nitric oxide. *Annu Rev Pharmacol Toxicol* 1990 **30**: 535–560.
32. Berridge MJ. Inositol trisphosphate and calcium signaling. *Nature* 1993 **361**: 315–325.
33. Clapham DE. A mysterious new influx factor? *Nature* 1994 **364**: 763–764.
34. Bertolino M, Llinas RR. The control role of voltage-activated and receptor-operated calcium channels in neuronal cells. *Annu Rev Pharmacol Toxicol* 1992 **32**: 399–421.
35. Means AR, VanBerkum MFA, Bagchi I, Ping Lu K, Rasmussen CD. Regulatory functions of calmodulin. In Taylor CW (ed.) *Intracellular Messengers*, Oxford: Pergamon Press, 1993: 265–285.
36. Heizmann CW, Hunziker W. Intracellular calcium-binding proteins: more sites than insights. *Trends Biochem Sci* 1991 **16**: 98–103.
37. Fruman DA, Klee CB, Bierer BE, Burakoff SJ. Calcineurin phosphatase activity in T lymphocytes is inhibited by FK 506 and cyclosporin A. *Proc Natl Acad Sci* 1992 **89**: 3686–3690.
38. Nishizuka Y. The molecular heterogeneity of protein kinase C and its implications for cellular regulation. *Nature* 1988 **334**: 661–665.
39. Drummond AH, Macintyre DE. Protein kinase C as a bidirectional regulator of cell function. *Trends Pharmacol Sci* 1985 **6**: 233–237.
40. Hug H, Sarre TF. Protein kinase C isoenzymes: divergence in signal transduction? *Biochem J* 1993 **291**: 329–343.
41. Nakanishi H, Brewer KA, Exton JH. Activation of the isozyme of protein kinase C by phosphatidylinositol 3,4,5-triphosphate. *J Biol Chem* 1993 **268**: 13–16.
42. Rhee SG, Choi KD. Multiple forms of phospholipase C and their activation mechanisms. *Adv Second Mess Phosphopr Res* 1992 **26**: 35–61.
43. Whitman M, Cantley L. Phosphoinositide metabolism and the control of cell proliferation. *Biochim Biophys Acta* 1988 **948**: 327–344.
44. Mennitis FS, Oliver KG, Putney JW, Shears SB. Inositol phosphates and cell signaling: new views of InsP_5 and InsP_6. *Trends Biochem Sci* 1993 **18**: 53–56.
45. Mikoshiba K. Inositol 1,4,5-triphosphate receptor. *Trends Pharmacol Sci* 1993 **14**: 86–89.
46. Sorrentino V, Volpe P. Ryanodine receptors: how many, where and why? *Trends Pharmacol Sci* 1993 **14**: 98–103.
47. McPherson PS, Campbell KP. The ryanodine receptor/Ca²⁺ release channel. *J Biol Chem* 1993 **268**: 13765–13768.
48. Exton JH. Phosphatidylcholine breakdown and signal transduction. *Biochim Biophys Acta* 1994 **1212**: 26–42.
49. Glaser KB, Mobilio D, Chang JY, Senko N. Phospholipase A₂ enzymes: regulation and inhibition. *Trends Pharmacol Sci* 1993 **14**: 92–96.
50. Schlessinger J, Ullrich A. Growth factor signaling by receptor tyrosine kinases. *Neuron* 1992 **9**: 383–391.
51. Cohen GB, Ren R, Baltimore D. Modular binding domains in signal transduction proteins. *Cell* 1995 **80**: 237–248.
52. Claesson-Welsh L. Platelet-derived growth factor signals. *J Biol Chem* 1994 **269**: 32023–32026.
53. Marshall J. Specificity of receptor tyrosine kinase signaling: transient versus sustained extracellular signal-regulated kinase activation. *Cell* 1995 **80**: 174–185.

54. Schlessinger J. SH2/SH3 signaling proteins. *Curr Opin Genet Dev* 1994 **4**: 25–30.
55. Darnell JE, Kerr IM, Stark GR. Jak-STAT pathways and transcriptional activation in response to INFs and other extracellular signaling proteins. *Science* 1994 **264**: 1415–1421.
56. Heldin C-H. Dimerization of cell-surface receptors in signal transduction. *Cell* 1995 **80**: 213–223.
57. Godowski PJ, Picard D. Steroid receptors. How to be both a receptor and a transcription factor. *Biol Pharmacol* 1989 **38**: 3135–3143.
58. Umesono K, Murakami KK, Thompson CC, Evans RM. Direct repeats as selective response elements for the thyroid hormone, retinoic acid, and vitamin D_3 receptors. *Cell* 1991 **65**: 1255–1266.
59. Tsai M-J, O'Malley BW. Molecular mechanisms of action of steroid/thyroid receptor superfamily members. *Annu Rev Biochem* 1994 **63**: 451–486.
60. Freedman LP. Anatomy of the steroid receptor zinc finger regions. *Endocr Rev* 1992 **13**: 129–145.
61. Clapham DE. The G-protein nanomachine. *Nature* 1996 **379**: 297–299.
62. Eisenman RN, Cooper JA. Beating a path to Myc. *Nature* 1995 **378**: 438–439.

1.6

Fundamental Immunology

SE Christmas and PM Johnson

GENERAL INTRODUCTION

The primary function of the immune system is the recognition and elimination from the body of potentially pathogenic organisms. This requires an exquisitely sensitive and specific means of discriminating between self and what is foreign (non-self) and therefore potentially the target of an immune response. A second important requirement of the immune response is that it should have memory so that re-exposure of an immune individual to a foreign antigen will lead to a greater and more rapid reaction. Specificity and memory are features of the adaptive immune response, whereas the innate response lacks both of these characteristics but is immediately active.[1,2] In these respects, the two types of response are complementary, the innate immune system providing a rapid but relatively weak and non-specific antimicrobial response until the adaptive immune system has had sufficient time to generate a specific response.

CURRENT CONCEPTS

Innate and adaptive immunity

The innate immune response encompasses non-specific soluble products such as lysozyme and acute phase proteins, as well as cellular components including macrophages and natural killer (NK) cells. Lymphocytes are the cells providing specificity of the adaptive immune system, which can be divided into two distinct but interdependent components, humoral and cellular immune responses.[1,2] B lymphocytes are the effector cells of the humoral response, whereas T lymphocytes (T cells) are responsible for cell-mediated immunity and are also essential for B lymphocyte function. The humoral response is mediated by soluble antibody molecules, whose primary function is to bind and facilitate the elimination of free or cell-bound microorganisms.

Antibodies are produced by plasma cells (differentiated B lymphocytes) and recognize intact antigen molecules which may be either in soluble or particulate form. In contrast, T lymphocytes do not respond to free intact protein antigens, but instead recognize only short peptides presented to them by association with cell-surface structures on host cells. In the case of bacterial phagocytosis by macrophages (i.e. innate host defence), this can then lead to T cell-dependent activation of the host cell to lyse the intracellular microorganisms.

For virus-infected host cells, the cellular immune system detects and destroys these cells before they can release large numbers of infective virus. This concerted attack by the immune system facilitates the elimination of both extracellular and intracellular pathogens.

Immunoglobulin structure and function

The basic structural model of an antibody (i.e. immunoglobulin, Ig) molecule comprises two identical light chains and two identical heavy chains held together by disulfide bonds (Fig. 1.6.1).[1,2] The N-terminal region of each chain has three hypervariable regions, which contribute to the the two identical antigen-binding sites in the so-called Fab (fragment antigen-binding) fragments of any single four-chain unit. It is this particular region of both heavy and light chains which varies extensively in amino acid sequence between individual Ig molecules, giving the wide differences in antigen specificity within the normal serum immunoglobulin (antibody) pool. The major part of each heavy chain (the Fc region) is structurally almost invariant for each Ig class and includes the so-called effector sites for interaction with host phagocyte clearance systems, amongst which are the cellular Fc receptors and the binding site for the first protein component of the complement system. The latter is a cascade

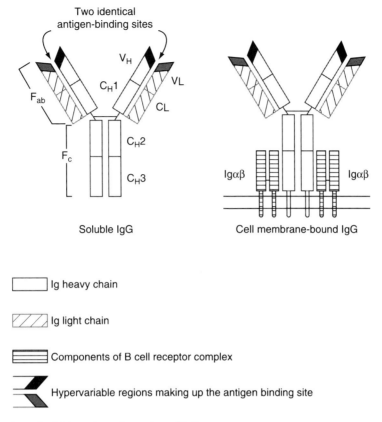

Two identical
antigen-binding sites

Soluble IgG

Cell membrane-bound IgG

Ig heavy chain

Ig light chain

Components of B cell receptor complex

Hypervariable regions making up the antigen binding site

Fig. 1.6.1 *Molecular structure of soluble and membrane-bound IgG.*

of plasma proteins activated following antigen–antibody binding (classical pathway) or interaction with particular microbial surfaces or enzymes (alternative pathway), leading to cleavage of the key complement component C3.[3]

Some bacteria are susceptible to direct complement-mediated lysis in the presence of specific antibody. In the case of resistant bacteria, the presence of receptors for C3b (the activated form of C3) on macrophages and neutrophils greatly facilitates phagocytosis of microorganisms, enhancing their clearance and elimination, a process known as opsonization.

There are five different classes of Ig, each based on the same common four-chain structural model but differing in specific heavy chain amino-acid sequence (Fig. 1.6.2).[1,2] IgM is commonly a pentamer of the basic four-chain unit and is the main component of the primary humoral response. Each antigen-binding site is generally of low affinity but, in view of its ten potential antigen binding sites, has a high overall antigen-binding and cross-linking capacity. This enables IgM to immobilize infections until higher affinity IgG responses have been generated towards the end of the primary response; IgG then constitutes the main component of the secondary response in all body fluids other than at secretory surfaces. There are four IgG subclasses which differ mostly in their ability to bind complement (Table 1.6.1). IgG, a monomer of the basic

Table 1.6.1 Functions of human serum immunoglobulins

Immunoglobulin	IgG	IgA	IgM	IgD	IgE
Mean serum concentration (mg ml^{-1})	10	2	1.2	0.03	0.0005
Subclasses	γ1–4	α1–2	μ1–2	–	–
Complement fixation	+ (IgG1 and 3)	–	++	–	–
Selective placental transfer	+	–	–	–	–

four-chain unit, is much smaller than IgM and diffuses more readily into extravascular spaces and tissues.

IgA is the predominant antibody secreted at most mucosal surfaces and into body fluids, where it occurs mostly in a dimeric or trimeric form. In these situations, mucosal plasma cells produce IgA which is taken up by epithelial cells which add a further molecule, known as secretory component. This facilitates Ig secretion at the luminal surface and protects IgA from degradation by proteases or acidic pH within the gastrointestinal lumen. IgD is found on the surface of immature B cells, but is present in only very low amounts in serum where its function is unknown. It is present in surprisingly high relative

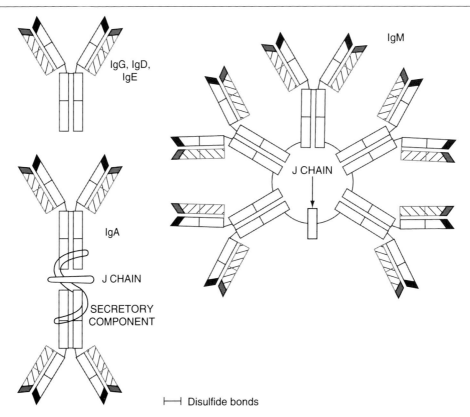

Fig. 1.6.2 *Basic structure of immunoglobulin classes. Refer to Fig. 1.6.1 on Page 61 for key.*

amounts in breast milk. IgE is involved in the immune response to certain parasites, but is better known for its role in allergy. Allergens bind to specific IgE engaged to specific IgE-Fc receptors on mast cells, leading to degranulation, release of vasoactive mediators and attendant adverse anaphylactic reactions in allergic (atopic) individuals.

B lymphocyte differentiation and function

B cells are the lymphocytes responsible for Ig production. They arise during fetal life from stem cells in the bone marrow (Fig. 1.6.3) where, independently of antigen, each developing B cell clone undergoes genetic rearrangement of the genes encoding Ig heavy and light chains to generate a unique, clonally distributed, IgM molecule expressed on the B cell surface.[1,2,4] The tremendous diversity of the antibody repertoire is generated by means of 'combinatorial' and 'junctional' diversity. Separate single heavy chain variable, diversity and joining gene segments are randomly selected from large pools of each of these genes and permanently rearranged in the B cell DNA (Fig. 1.6.4).[4] Additional diversity is acquired by imprecise joining of gene segments and addition of random nucleotides at the points of genetic recombination. A similar mechanism occurs for either κ or λ light chain genes, but these lack the so-called diversity gene segments. In this way, functional B

cells, expressing unique clonally distributed IgM receptors, are generated without prior contact with antigen. These cells also co-express cell surface IgD molecules having the same heavy chain variable domain, and thus antigenic specificity, as the surface IgM.

B cell antibody responses to most protein antigens are dependent upon the presence of T lymphocytes. When stimulated by specific antigen, previously unstimulated (naive) B cells undergo clonal expansion and differentiation in the presence of T cell help (i.e. soluble T cell-derived factors) to generate plasma cells secreting only antibody of binding specificity identical with the surface IgM receptor. However, the secreted IgM lacks a heavy chain C-terminal domain which, in cell surface IgM, is responsible for its plasma membrane attachment and interaction with an invariant B cell receptor molecular complex involved in signal transduction into the cell (Fig. 1.6.1).[5] Later in the primary immune response, many of the B cells stimulated in this way undergo Ig class switching, whereby IgG, IgA or IgE is produced bearing the same variable region and thus antigenic specificity as the original IgM. Cell surface IgG+ memory cells are also generated at this stage. As well as switching from IgM to other Ig classes, the antibody response undergoes affinity maturation by the introduction of point mutations within the Ig hypervariable region gene segments. Those B cells whose cell surface Ig receptors, by chance mutation, are now of higher affinity for antigen than the original B cell clones are

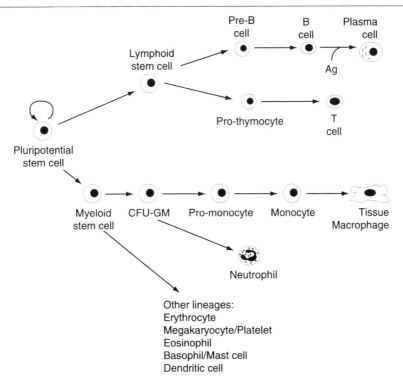

Fig. 1.6.3 *Hematopoiesis of cells of the immune system. This takes place largely within bone marrow, with the exception of the later stages of T cell maturation which take place within the thymus. CFU-GM, colony-forming unit, granulocyte/macrophage.*

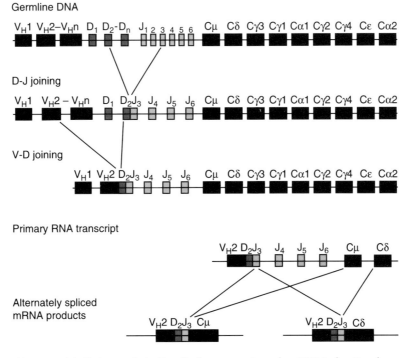

Fig. 1.6.4 *Generation of immunoglobulin heavy chain diversity from genomic nuclear DNA to functional messenger RNA.*

preferentially expanded, leading to a higher affinity antibody response. Thus, towards the end of a primary immune response, IgG[+] memory B cells are generated whose cell surface Ig molecules have a higher average affinity than those on naive B cells. Following secondary challenge with the same antigen, it is these memory B cells that are able to mount a more rapid and higher affinity secondary response in which IgG antibody will predominate.

Monoclonal antibodies

A monoclonal antibody (mAb) is the product of a single B cell clone that has been selected and immortalized *in vitro*.[1] Each mAb will have a unique specificity for a single antigenic site on the molecule against which it was originally raised. Being monospecific as well as relatively cheap and easy to produce in theoretically unlimited amounts, mAbs have many advantages over polyclonal antisera; they are now used extensively for research and diagnostic purposes, as well as for passive immunotherapy or immunodiagnosis *in vivo*. Examples include: monitoring of lymphocyte subsets by flow cytometry; immunoassays for a wide range of antigens and antigen subtypes in patient sera; immunohistochemical localization of antigens in tissue sections and tumor localization and treatment *in vivo*.[2]

However, as most mAbs are of mouse origin, their administration to patients normally results in induction of an immune response against mouse Ig, leading to rapid mAb elimination. This can be subverted by genetically engineering an antibody in which only the antigen-binding site is derived from the original mouse mAb whereas the remainder of the antibody molecule is of human origin. This minimizes the likelihood of the mAb being immunogenic in patients.

The role of HLA in antigen processing and presentation to T lymphocytes

Unlike B cells, T cells recognize only cellularly 'processed' antigenic peptides presented in association with cell surface molecules that are products of a group of genes in the major histocompatibility complex (MHC) on the short arm of chromosome 6; these glycoproteins are called human leucocyte antigens (HLA). The HLA cell surface glycoproteins are the major genetically characterized tissue antigens that define an individual's 'tissue type' and against which immune rejection responses to transplanted organs or tissues are directed. Of more fundamental importance is that T cells can only recognize antigens when bound as small peptides into a molecular complex with cell surface HLA molecules.[1,2,6] This is mediated by the clonally distributed T cell antigen receptor (TCR) that is broadly analogous to the B cell antigen receptor (i.e. Ig).

There are two main subpopulations of mature T cells, distinguished by mutually exclusive expression of the cell surface proteins CD4 and CD8 (Table 1.6.2).[1,2] CD4[+] ('helper') T cells recognize foreign antigenic peptides only in association with class II HLA molecules on the surface of 'antigen-presenting cells' (i.e. class II HLA-positive cells: macrophages, dendritic cells, B cells and certain epithelia), whereas CD8[+] (cytotoxic and regulatory) T cells recognize peptides only when presented in association with class I HLA molecules, which are expressed on most nucleated cells other than sperm and trophoblast.

Class I HLA molecules consist of a three-domain heavy (α) chain in association with an invariant β_2-microglobulin chain (Fig. 1.6.5).[1,2] The α chains exist as the products of three separate gene loci, HLA-A, -B and -C (Table 1.6.3), each of which are highly polymorphic and co-dominantly expressed. Thus, at each locus, each separate maternally and

Table 1.6.2 Cell surface antigen expression and function of human lymphocyte subpopulations

Lymphocyte subpopulation	Cell surface phenotype (CD number)											Predominant function	% of total PBL*
	2	3	4	5	8	16	19	20	56	57	Ig		
B cells	–	–	–	(+)	–	–	+	+	–	–	+	Antibody production	3–20
CD4[+] T cells	+	+	+	+	–	–	–	–	–	–	–	Cell-mediated immunity; B cell help	30–45
CD8[+] T cells	+	+	–	+	+	–	–	–	–	–	–	Cytotoxicity	20–30
NK cells	+	–	–	–	(+)	+	–	–	+	+	–	Antiviral; antitumor?	0–15

*Relative proportions of lymphocyte subsets in both lymphoid and non-lymphoid tissues will differ from those in peripheral blood leucocytes (PBL).

Table 1.6.3 Genetic polymorphisms (variants) at the class I and II HLA loci

Locus	HLA-A	HLA-B	HLA-C	HLA-DR	HLA-DQ	HLA-DP
No. of alleles	50	97	34	106	41	67

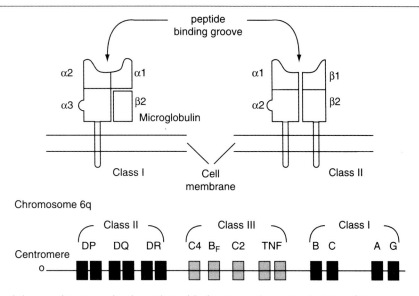

Fig 1.6.5 *Structure of class I and II HLA molecules and simplified HLA gene locus map (not to scale).*

paternally inherited 'tissue type' (sequence variation within each HLA molecule that is genetically inherited) is equally expressed. There are also three co-dominantly expressed forms of class II HLA: HLA-DP, -DQ and -DR, all of which are also polymorphic (Table 1.6.3) and consist of a hetero-dimeric pair of two-domain chains, α and β (Fig. 1.6.5). The role of the CD4 and CD8 molecules on the surface of T cells is to stabilize the interaction between TCR and HLA plus antigenic peptide by engaging an invariant part of class II and class I MHC molecules, respectively.

The fundamental feature of HLA molecules is the peptide-binding groove located between the α_1 and α_2 domains of class I and the α_1 and β_1 domains of class II HLA (Fig. 1.6.6).[1,6] The function of this site in class I and class II HLA molecules is to bind antigenic peptides and present them to either CD8+ or CD4+ T cells, respectively. In the case of class I HLA, peptides largely derived from the proteolytic breakdown of endogenously synthesized proteins (e.g. self-pro-

teins or intracellular viral proteins) become associated with class I HLA α-chain and β_2-microglobulin during assembly in the endoplasmic reticulum. In normal cells, only self-proteins will be present and peptides from these are inserted into the peptide-binding groove; these do not stimulate a T cell response as all 'autoreactive' T cells have been deleted during thymic development or inactivated during differentiation (Fig. 1.6.3).[7] When a cell is virally infected, viral peptides (i.e. non-self peptides) can also become inserted into the class I HLA peptide-binding groove and this complex of HLA and antigenic peptide is then transported to the cell surface where it serves as a recognition structure for specific CD8+ cytotoxic T lymphocytes (CTL).[1,6] This will lead to lysis of the virally infected cells, preventing release of further infective virus particles.

In the case of class II HLA, mostly exogenous foreign antigens are taken up by antigen-presenting cells (macrophages, dendritic cells or B cells) via phagocytosis or

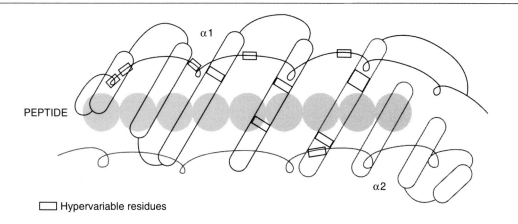

☐ Hypervariable residues

Fig 1.6.6 *Structure of the class I HLA peptide-binding groove.*

endocytosis and degraded into short peptides in the acidic protease-rich lysosomal compartment. In contrast to class I HLA, newly synthesized class II HLA molecules are associated with a protein known as invariant chain, which prevents peptides derived from endogenously synthesized proteins from being directly inserted into the peptide-binding groove.[8] In the acidic environment of the lysosome, invariant chain is degraded and dissociated, only then allowing largely exogenously derived peptides to be associated with class II HLA molecules. The class II HLA–peptide complexes are then transported to the cell surface to be presented to CD4⁺ T cells.

The peptide-binding groove of class I HLA will accommodate peptides of between 8 and 11 amino acids in length,[6] whereas that of class II HLA is more open-ended and may bind peptides of 12–24 amino acids in length, which would protrude from either end of the groove. Most genetic polymorphisms of HLA (sequence variations between individuals; Table 1.6.4) are localized in or around the groove region (Fig. 1.6.6) and hence products of different alleles (genetically inherited structurally distinct variations of the same gene) bind structurally distinct peptides. For each HLA allele studied, there are two or more consensus or 'anchor' amino acid residues, normally at either end of the peptide, which are the same in most peptides bound. Thus, individuals of different HLA types may respond well or poorly to any one antigenic protein, according to which peptides can be bound efficiently by their particular HLA molecules, whereas relative responses to another antigenic protein may show the opposite pattern. This is the basis for the genetic variation in immune responses that is the essence of protection of the species to a new pathogen.

T cell recognition and function

The specific antigen receptor on the surface of most T cells (T cell receptor; TCR) consists of a covalently associated αβ TCR heterodimeric protein together with an invariant CD3 protein molecular complex (γ, δ, ε and ζ chains; Fig. 1.6.7),[4] the role of the latter being in signal transduction. The αβ

Table 1.6.4 Human cellular expression and function of CD molecules mentioned in the text. The molecule(s) to which they bind (ligand) are also tabulated. Data are from reference 10.

CD number	Expressed by	Ligand	Function
CD2	T cells, NK cells	CD58	Cell–cell interaction; signal transduction
CD3 (+TCR)	T cells	HLA + antigenic peptide	Signal transduction
CD4	T cells, Mφ	Class II HLA	T cell accessory molecule; HIV receptor
CD8	T and NK cell subsets	Class I HLA	T cell accessory molecule
CD11a	Leucocytes	CD54	Cell adhesion (with CD18)
CD16	NK cells, Mφ, PMN	IgG	FcγRIII; opsonization, ADCC
CD18	Leucocytes	CD54	Cell adhesion (with CD11)
CD25	T,B,NK cells, Mφ	IL-2	IL-2 receptor α chain; cell proliferation
CD28	T cells	CD80	T cell co-stimulation
CD46	Many cell types	C3b, C4b	Complement regulation
CD55	Many cell types	C3 convertase	Complement regulation
CD56	NK cells	CD56?	Adhesion?; NCAM isoform
CD58	Many cell types	CD2	Cell–cell interaction
CD59	Many cell types	C8, C9	Complement regulation
CD80	B cells, dendritic cells	CD28	T cell co-stimulation
CD122	T and NK cells	IL-2	IL-2 receptor β chain; cell proliferation

ADCC, antibody-dependent cellular cytotoxicity; FcγR, receptor for the Fc portion of IgG; Mφ, macrophages; PMN, polymorphonuclear leucocytes.

Peptide antigen-HLA binding site

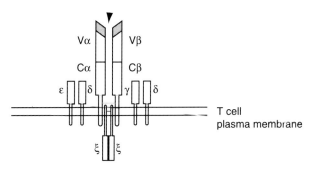

Components of the CD3 molecular complex

Fig 1.6.7 *Structure of the T cell antigen receptor complex.*

TCR resembles a Fab fragment of an Ig molecule in possessing variable, diversity, joining and constant gene segments. The TCR repertoire for antigen is generated during maturation of T cells in passage through the fetal thymus and occurs by unique rearrangements of TCR α and β gene segments within each developing clone of T cells, in a similar way to the generation of the Ig repertoire in B cells.[4] T cells potentially reactive with foreign peptide together with 'self' HLA are selected in the thymus, whereas any T cells reactive with 'self' peptides and 'self' HLA are triggered to die.[7] Unlike Ig, the TCR is found only in a cell-associated form and is not secreted. Also, the generation of a secondary T cell response is based solely upon expansion of clones with receptors of pre-existing specificities and there is no mechanism of affinity maturation as commonly found in B cell responses.

CD4+ T cells recognize processed antigenic peptide presented to them in association with class II HLA molecules on antigen-presenting cells (Fig. 1.6.8).[1,2] During a primary response, macrophages and dendritic cells both take up exogenous protein antigens and break them down to small peptides. In a secondary response, B cells are also important antigen-presenting cells, as they express class II HLA molecules and their surface Ig facilitates endocytosis of specific antigen. CD4+ T cells whose TCRs are specific for antigenic peptide plus self class II HLA are activated and induced to expand clonally. They can then provide help for antigen-specific B cells[9] and are also capable of activating macrophages to bring about enhanced killing of phagocytosed intracellular bacteria, e.g. *Listeria, Mycobacteria*, via a mechanism which has been termed delayed-type hypersensitivity (DTH).

The TCR is the antigen-specific ligand on the T cell surface, but other molecular interactions are also important in mediating full T cell activation by facilitating cell–cell adhesion (Fig. 1.6.9). For example, leucocyte function antigen-1 (LFA-1; CD11a/18), a member of the integrin family of molecules, interacts with intercellular adhesion molecules (CD54) on antigen-presenting cells or target cells (Table 1.6.4).[10] CD2 interacts with LFA-3 (CD58) and CD28 interacts with CD80 on antigen-presenting cells; the absence of the latter co-stimulatory interaction can lead to T cell anergy, or unresponsiveness.[1]

Following initial recognition of a peptide from an antigenic molecule in association with class I HLA on antigen-presenting cells (Fig. 1.6.8), naive CD8+ T cells need to undergo clonal proliferation and differentiation in order to generate a functional T cell cytotoxic (CTL) response.[1] CD4+ T cells specific for a different determinant of the same antigenic molecule are thought to participate as helper cells by providing a particular soluble 'communicator' between

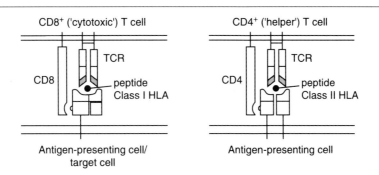

Fig 1.6.8 *Antigen recognition by CD4+ and CD8+ T cells.*

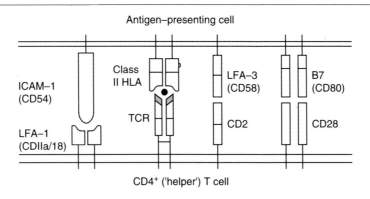

Fig 1.6.9 *Other molecular interactions involved in CD4+ T cell activation. ICAM, intercellular adhesion molecule; LFA, leucocyte function antigen.*

leucocytes called interleukin-2 (IL-2; see next section), the essential growth factor for CD8$^+$ T cells. In the case of viral antigens, mature CD8$^+$ CTL are able to kill autologous target cells infected with that virus. This is brought about by a type of programmed cell death known as apoptosis. CTL possess cytoplasmic granules containing a pore-forming protein known as perforin, together with several serine proteases known as granzymes. These are secreted locally at the point of contact between the effector T cell and the virus-infected target cell. Perforin inserts into the target cell membrane and in the presence of Ca^{2+} ions polymerizes to form membrane 'holes' which allow entry of other granule contents.[11] This permits activation of an endogenous nuclease, resulting in degradation of nuclear DNA into small fragments.

Cytokines in T cell responses

Cytokines are soluble molecular mediators which mostly act locally and are responsible for many of the cellular collaborations taking place during development of the immune response.[12] Many cytokines act on several cell types and show considerable overlap of function (Table 1.6.5). This reflects the variety of cell types that may express specific cell surface receptors that will bind a particular cytokine and promote an intracellular signal. For example, interleukin-1 (IL-1) has several pro-inflammatory functions but can also induce CD4$^+$ T cells to produce IL-2 and express IL-2 receptors. IL-1 (previously known as T cell activation factor) acts therefore as an antigen-non-specific co-stimulatory 'second'

signal for CD4$^+$ T cells whose TCRs have engaged specific antigenic peptide–HLA complex on antigen-presenting cells. IL-2 itself (previously known as T cell growth factor) is secreted by activated T cells and is an essential growth factor for both CD4$^+$ and CD8$^+$ T cells. IL-4, IL-5 and IL-6 are B cell growth and differentiation factors produced by B cells and mediating B cell–T cell collaboration. IL-10 (originally known as cytokine synthesis inhibitory factor) is produced by macrophages and T cells and is a down-regulator of immune responses.[1] Interferon-γ (IFN-γ) is produced mainly by T cells and has a variety of actions, including enhancement of cellular HLA expression and activation of macrophage functions. Another pro-inflammatory cytokine with a range of different functions is tumor necrosis factor-α (TNF-α), which is produced by macrophages and T cells and acts by stimulating the function of a range of different cell types including certain T cells.

Cytokines and the function of CD4$^+$ T cell subsets

Activated CD4$^+$ T cells are capable of providing help for activation of three distinct cell types: macrophages, CD8$^+$ T cells and B cells. These distinct functions necessarily require the participation of different cytokines, which has led to the characterization of two CD4$^+$ T cell subsets, based on differential production of cytokines, namely T$_H$1 and T$_H$2 cells (Table 1.6.6).[13]

Newly activated T cells produce a range of T cell cytokines and are termed T$_H$0 cells; it is only following pro-

Table 1.6.5 Cytokines and cells which produce and respond to them

Cytokine	Predominant cellular source	Predominant target cells
IL-1*	Macrophages, other cells	T cells, B cells, fibroblasts, other cells
IL-2	T cells, NK cells	T, B and NK cells
IL-4	T cells	B cells, T cells
IL-5	T cells	B cells, eosinophils
IL-6*	T cells, macrophages, fibroblasts	B cells, other cells
IL-10*	Macrophages, T cells	T cells, macrophages
IL-12	T cells, NK cells	T cells, NK cells
IFN-γ*	T cells, NK cells	Macrophages, other cells
TNF-α	Macrophages, T cells	Many cell types
GM-CSF	T cells, other cells	Hematopoietic stem cells, myeloid cells
G-CSF	Macrophages, fibroblasts, endothelial cells	Hematopoietic stem cells, polymorphs
M-CSF	Macrophages, fibroblasts, endothelial cells	Hematopoietic stem cells, macrophages
TGF-β*	Macrophages	Many cell types

*Also has other pro- or anti-inflammatory actions.

Table 1.6.6 Functions of activated CD4$^+$ T cell subsets

Subset	T$_H$1	T$_H$2
Helper cells for:	Macrophages; CD8$^+$ T cells	B cells
Cytokines produced	IL-2, IL-12, IFN-γ TNFα	IL-4, IL-5, IL-6 IL-10, TNFα
Regulatory functions	IFN-γ inhibits T$_H$2 cells	IL-4 and IL-10 inhibit T$_H$1 cells

longed antigenic stimulation that these are able to differentiate into T_H1 or T_H2 cells.[13] In T_H1 subset responses, activated CD4$^+$ T cells produce IL-2 which acts as an autocrine growth factor (i.e. stimulates growth of the same cells which produce IL-2) and also stimulates proliferation of other CD4$^+$ and CD8$^+$ T cells. IFN-γ and TNFα are also produced, which are up-regulators of HLA expression leading to enhanced T cell reactivity. IFN-γ can also activate macrophages to kill intracellular bacteria and can inhibit T_H2 cell function (Table 1.6.6). In T_H2 subset responses, IL-4, -5, -6 and -10 are preferentially produced (Table 1.6.6). IL-4, -5 and -6 are B cell growth and differentiation factors, and IL-4 and IL-10 can inhibit T_H1 function.

In this way, T_H1 cells are predominantly helper cells for macrophage and CTL-mediated responses, while T_H2 cells are mainly helper cells for antibody production by B cells. These two types of T cell response are mutually inhibitory, but the exact factors governing the balance between these CD4$^+$ T cell subsets are not known. An example of preferential activation of T_H1 or T_H2 subsets is the two extreme forms of leprosy. In the tubercular form, T_H1 cells predominate and a cell-mediated response is found which normally results in elimination of the mycobacteria. In the lepromatous form, mainly a T_H2 response is found, with a good antibody response but poor bacterial elimination.

Gamma-delta T cells

A small subset of T cells express an alternative $\gamma\delta$ heterodimeric form of the TCR, rather than the common $\alpha\beta$ form, which also exists on the cell surface in association with the CD3 molecular complex. These $\gamma\delta$ T cells are mainly CD4$^-$CD8$^-$ and it is unclear whether, by analogy with $\alpha\beta$ T cells, they normally recognize antigen in association with HLA molecules. $\gamma\delta$ T cells can respond to certain bacterial antigens and to so-called heat shock proteins, molecules produced by normal cells as a result of stress.[14] They can also mediate HLA-non-restricted cytotoxic function, that is killing of target cells independently of their expression of HLA molecules, following activation by IL-2 in a manner comparable to that of natural killer (NK) cells (see next section). In some mammals, $\gamma\delta$ T cells are greatly enriched in epithelial tissues such as gut and skin but this is not generally the case in humans. Their role is most likely to be elimination of stressed or damaged cells, including virus-infected or potentially malignant cells, and recognition of the most frequently encountered infectious agents.

The innate cellular immune response

As well as possessing Fc receptors for IgG, which facilitate phagocytosis of opsonized (antibody-coated) bacteria, macrophages have receptors for the activated complement component C3b produced on their surface following complement activation by the classical pathway (i.e. by IgM or IgG-containing immune complexes of antibody and antigen). Certain bacteria directly activate the alternative pathway of complement, which also leads to production of the activated component C3b and hence enhanced opsonization via the specific C3b receptor on macrophages in an antibody-independent fashion.[1,2] In addition, macrophages can also bind and internalize bacteria via receptors that interact with the polysaccharide component of bacterial cell walls.

Natural killer (NK) cells are large granular lymphocytes which are not of T or B cell lineage and do not express cell surface TCR or Ig. These cells also lack cell surface expression of CD3, but do express other cell lineage markers such as CD16 (Fc receptor for IgG) and CD56 (Table 1.6.4).[15] They recognize and kill certain hematopoietic tumors and virus-infected target cells *in vitro* in an HLA-non-restricted fashion and without prior exposure to or recognition of a specific antigen. Their cytotoxic function is enhanced following activation with IL-2 or IFN-γ and they also mediate antibody-dependent cellular cytotoxicity via Fc receptors (CD16; Table 1.6.4) in the presence of IgG antibody to target cell antigens. NK cells primarily recognize target cells with reduced HLA expression.[16] They kill their target cells via an apoptotic mechanism similar to that of CTL, mediated by perforin and granzymes.[11] Their main function is thought to be a rapid but relatively nonspecific response to virus infection by direct killing of infected cells and production of cytokines. More controversially, they may play a role in immune surveillance against the development or metastatic spread of certain tumours and in preventing inappropriate hematopoiesis outside of the bone marrow.

Development of the immune response
in vivo

On entering the body, foreign antigenic molecules are rapidly sequestered by and broken down within antigen-presenting cells in secondary lymphoid tissues. These comprise the spleen, lymph nodes and mucosal-associated lymphoid tissues (MALT). The latter can be subdivided into bronchial (BALT), gastrointestinal (GALT), urogenital and other tissues. Antigen entering the circulation is retained within the spleen, whereas antigen entering tissues drains via afferent lymphatics to regional lymph nodes. In the case of skin, local antigen-presenting cells (Langerhans cells) bind and process antigen and then migrate via the afferent lymph to draining lymph nodes where they persist for long periods as 'interdigitating' dendritic cells. These are bone marrow-derived cells (Fig. 1.6.3) and are responsible for presenting antigens to T cells,[17] whereas 'follicular dendritic cells' are not bone marrow-derived, occupy a different ultrastructural location within spleen and lymph nodes and instead present antigens to B cells.

B and T lymphocytes routinely traffic through spleen and lymph nodes, entering the latter in afferent lymph or from the circulation via specialized high endothelial venules.[1] They return to the circulation via efferent lymphatics and the thoracic duct. By retaining antigen on dendritic cells fixed within lymphoid tissues through which lymphocytes are constantly recirculating, the chances of antigen-specific lymphocytes meeting their specific antigen are maximized. Secondary follicles develop as a result of local proliferation of antigen-specific B and T cells and activated cells can then recirculate systemically to eliminate microorganisms or infected cells in tissues.

Foreign antigenic molecules entering the body via mucosal surfaces are retained within the BALT (tonsils, adenoids) or GALT (Peyer's patches) where a local immune response is generated. Lymphocytes from mucosal tissues also recirculate, but have the capacity to home to their tissue of origin. Intraepithelial lymphocytes are mainly CD8$^+$ T cells and, in the case of GALT, may also play a part in suppressing the immune response to dietary antigens. IgA is the main antibody at mucosal sites where it is secreted as a dimer or trimer after being specifically transported across mucosal epithelia by addition of secretory component,[2] which also enhances the stability of IgA in mucosal secretions.

Clinical aspects of the immune response

Immune dysfunction can lead to a variety of pathological consequences.[2] In autoimmune diseases, such as insulin-dependent diabetes mellitus, certain arthropathies and multiple sclerosis, cellular responses against self-antigens are thought to be involved in mediating tissue damage. Many such diseases show a strong association with particular HLA alleles, lending further support to the participation of the immune system in their etiology. In other autoimmune diseases, such as systemic lupus erythematosus (SLE) and myasthenia gravis, autoantibodies against cell nuclear constituents or the acetylcholine receptor, respectively, are involved in mediating tissue damage either by deposition of antigen–antibody immune complexes or by direct action on target tissue autoantigens.

Another way in which the immune response can be inappropriately activated is in allergy in which otherwise harmless substances, such as pollen, house dust mite antigens or nickel, trigger a strong IgE-mediated allergic response in sensitized individuals. Conversely, there is a group of diseases in which the immune system is compromised, leading to immunodeficiency.[2] This can be a result of a naturally occurring defect in the development of T cells, such as ataxia telangiectasia, or of both T and B cells, as in severe combined immunodeficiency. More frequently, in diseases such as common variable immunodefi-

ciency and selective IgA deficiency, the ability of B cells to produce normal amounts of antibody is compromised. Alternatively, infection with viruses such as human immunodeficiency virus (HIV), or therapeutic immuno-suppression in transplant or autoimmune patients, may also lead to immunodeficiency. Increased susceptibility to opportunistic infections and certain malignancies are common features in these instances.

A consequence of T cells recognizing foreign antigenic peptides in association with self-HLA molecules is that allogeneic HLA molecules themselves can resemble altered peptide-bound self HLA molecules. The resultant high frequency of alloreactive T cells can thus potently and adversely affect allograft survival in organ transplant patients or can lead to graft-versus-host disease in bone marrow transplantation. In pregnancy, the generation of a potentially harmful maternal immune response against the genetically dissimilar fetus must be avoided and the mechanisms by which this is achieved will be discussed in Chapter 3.3.

FUTURE PERSPECTIVES

It is clear that the next decade will be filled with attempts to introduce antigen-specific immunotherapy in both autoimmune diseases and transplantation (to suppress immune responses) as well as in cancer (to enhance or induce immune responses). Underlying any such therapeutic developments will be the better definition of clinically relevant tumor, transplantation and autoantigens. In a similar manner, specific immunomodulation will be tested whereby tolerance may be induced to allergens in infancy in order to reduce the incidence of allergic diseases.

Cytokines (e.g. IL-2 or IFN-γ) have been assessed as therapeutic drugs over recent years, but this avenue of clinical research is not yet exhausted. Biologically relevant combinations of cytokines have yet to be tested, as also have combinations of certain cytokines together with chemotherapeutic drugs or vaccine preparations, for example, cytokines that may particularly divert the immune response towards a T_H1 or T_H2 response, or a mucosal antibody response. Indeed, it is becoming increasingly appreciated that there is an urgent need to improve targeted mucosal vaccines, not least in respect of improved host defence to HIV at mucosal surfaces[18].

SUMMARY

- The immune system can respond to a very wide range of antigenic specificities, corresponding largely to external ('non-self') microbial agents, while failing to respond to normal tissue (self) antigens.
- The innate and adaptive immune responses complement each other in timing and degree of

specificity. The adaptive immune response (immunoglobulins, B and T lymphocytes) has an increased and more rapidly induced secondary response, i.e. memory, whereas innate host defence mechanisms (NK cells, macrophages, complement) do not.

- Antibodies recognize intact microorganisms

and facilitate their removal by direct lysis or by phagocytic cells. The primary immune response is predominantly IgM, while secondary responses predominantly involve IgG. IgA is the main antibody secreted at mucosal surfaces. Complement can enhance elimination of infectious agents in an antibody-dependent or -independent fashion.

T cells do not recognize intact soluble antigens but, instead, exclusively recognize only small antigenic peptides bound in association with cell surface HLA molecules (histocompatibility molecules that have genetically defined 'tissue type' differences between individuals).

Class I HLA molecules are expressed on nearly all nucleated cell types and normally bind peptides derived from endogenously-synthesized proteins. Class II HLA molecules are expressed predominantly on antigen-presenting cells (macrophages, dendritic cells, B cells) and normally bind peptides derived from exogenously synthesized antigens.

CD4$^+$ T cells selectively recognize foreign antigenic peptides in association with self class II HLA molecules and are helper cells for antibody responses and for activation of CD8$^+$ T cells as well as macrophages.

CD8$^+$ T cells selectively recognize foreign antigenic peptides in association with self class I HLA molecules and are the precursors of cytotoxic T cells.

T cells develop in the thymus, where autoreactive T cells are deleted and only those potentially reactive with self-HLA in association with foreign antigenic peptides are positively selected. B cells develop within the bone marrow and lymphoid tissues and are subject to a less rigorous process of elimination of autoreactive cells.

Cytokines are soluble molecular mediators released locally during an immune response and play an essential part in facilitating cell–cell collaborations.

Two main types of immune dysfunction can occur; in immunodeficiency, reduced immune responsiveness leads to an increased incidence of infection. Inappropriate immune responses to non-infective or self-antigens can lead to allergy or autoimmunity, respectively.

REFERENCES

1. Janeway CA, Travers P. *The Immune System in Health and Disease*. Oxford: Blackwell, 1994: 576pp.
2. Stites DP, Terr AI, Parslow TG (eds). *Basic and Clinical Immunology*, 8th edn. East Norwalk: Appleton & Lange, 1994: 870pp.
3. Lambris JD. The multifactorial role of C3, the third component of complement. *Immunol Today* 1988 **9**: 387–393.
4. Owen MJ, Lamb JR. *Immune Recognition*. Oxford: IRL Press, 1988: 73pp.
5. Reth M. Antigen receptors on B cells. *Annu Rev Immunol* 1992 **10**: 97–121.
6. Elliott T, Smith M, Driscoll P, McMichael A. Peptide selection by class I molecules of the major histocompatibility complex. *Curr Biol* 1993 **3**: 854–865.
7. von Boehmer H, Teh HS, Kisielow P. The thymus selects the useful, neglects the useless and destroys the harmful. *Immunol Today* 1989 **10**: 57–61.
8. Germain RN, Margulies DH. The biochemistry and cell biology of antigen processing and presentation. *Annu Rev Immunol* 1993 **11**: 403–450.
9. Parker DC. T cell-dependent B-cell activation. *Annu Rev Immunol* 1993 **11**: 331–360.
10. Barclay AN, Birkeland ML, Brown MH *et al. Leucocyte Antigen Facts Book*. London: Academic Press, 1992, 424pp.
11. Podack ER, Hengartner H, Lichtenheld MG. A central role of perforin in cytolysis. *Annu Rev Immunol* 1991 **9**: 129–157.
12. Hamblin AS. *Lymphokines*, Oxford: IRL Press. 1988: 71pp.
13. Mosmann TR, Coffman RL. T$_H$1 and T$_H$2 cells: different patterns of lymphokine secretion lead to different functional properties. *Annu Rev Immunol* 1989 **7**: 145–173.
14. Born W, Happ MP, Dallas A *et al.* Recognition of heat shock proteins and δ cell function. *Immunol Today* 1990 **11**: 40–43.
15. Robertson MJ, Ritz J. Biological and clinical relevance of human natural killer cells. *Blood* 1990 **76**: 2421–2438.
17. Steinman RM. The dendritic cell system and its role in immunogenicity. *Annu Rev Immunol* 1991 **9**: 271–296.
18. Bioca S, Cattaneo A. Intracellular immunization: antibody targeting to subcellular compartments. *Trends Cell Biol* 1995 **5**: 248–252.

1.7

Chromosomes

CM Gosden, M Robertson and C Davidson

INTRODUCTION

Chromosomes are important in life as they carry all the genes (which specify every cellular function) contiguously along them, each different chromosome forming a 'linkage group' of genes. For a human being, having 46 chromosomes is the norm; certain variants of this are possible without severe phenotypic consequences (for example, having two chromosomes joined together in a Robertsonian translocation). However, having too many or too few chromosomes usually has serious clinical consequences. Having the normal number of chromosomes is termed euploidy; aneuploidy refers to abnormalities of number such as trisomies, monosomies or abnormalities of whole sets of chromosomes as in triploidy or tetraploidy. For example, where there is an extra chromosome 21, this results in trisomy 21 or Down's syndrome. For most chromosomes, loss of a whole chromosome, monosomy, is usually lethal. There is one exception, monosomy X where although there is considerable lethality *in utero*, about 30% survive with 45,X Turner's syndrome.

Sometimes, parts of chromosomes, rather than whole chromosomes may be involved in deletions or duplications (partial monosomy or trisomy). In other cases, chromosomal segments may be lost or gained as a result of translocations, inversions or other rearrangements. Monosomy or trisomy (or partial monosomy or trisomy) can result in phenotypic consequences varying from minor to major depending on the chromosome or chromosomal region involved in the imbalance. Genes carried by the chromosomes determine sex; functional testes do not develop in the absence of a Y chromosome in man (or the essential Y sex determining genes or sequences). Just as Y chromosome sequences are important in determining maleness (and the presence of male gonads), so the presence of two X chromosomes (at least in ovarian tissue) is important for giving functional oocytes. In Turner's syndrome (45,X) where one of the X chromosomes has been lost, several million oocytes are present in the fetal ovaries at 20 weeks' ges-

tation, but these become atretic before birth so that effectively the menopause is reached before puberty.

Chromosomal abnormalities occur frequently and may have serious clinical consequences. This is because chromosomes exert important influences during development; fetuses with trisomy 13, 18 and 21 usually have major developmental defects such as cardiac, renal and brain anomalies. Trisomy 21 and other chromosomal syndromes are a major cause of physical and mental handicap with 1 in 150 newborns having a major chromosomal abnormality. Even if there are the right number of chromosomes, failing to have the genes arranged in the usual order (for example by having a chromosomal translocation) can lead to problems such as recurrent miscarriage. Many chromosomal abnormalities are so severe these cause infertility for those who are carriers and many of the unbalanced rearrangements or mutant abnormalities arising in the conceptus are lethal in early life. This selection is at its greatest during fetal life; about 50% of all human conceptions have major chromosomal disorders; a further 5% with major chromosomal abnormalities die *in utero* or at birth as stillbirths or neonatal deaths.[1] Of the survivors of this intrauterine and perinatal lethality, approximately 0.5% of newborns have major chromosomal disorders, the majority of which are clinically significant and cause long-term mental and physical handicap among survivors.

The purpose of this chapter is to consider the importance of chromosomes in reproductive medicine and interrelate the clinical aspects of cytogenetics with the underlying scientific mechanisms. There are many ways in which chromosomes are important: during development, during the reproductive years for their importance in determining genotype, phenotype, whether or not germ cells form, the constitution of germ cells and errors in their formation which give rise to aneuploid progeny and even the age at which the menopause occurs. There are numerous texts which explain chromosomal structure, nomenclature, methodology and details of mitosis and meiosis in full detail[2-8] and the reader should refer to these if further amplification is required.

CURRENT CONCEPTS

Causes of abnormalities and malformations

Chromosomal abnormalities

Chromosomal abnormalities are a major cause of morbidity and mortality in humans, being present in miscarriages, stillbirths and neonatal deaths. One in 150 livebirths have a major chromosome abnormality and at least 60% of these are clinically significant, leading to problems such as mental handicap, physical handicap or infertility. Recognition of the fact that there are 'new' conditions such as fragile X syndrome and the chromosomal instability syndromes has led to the recognition that there are no longer clear lines of demarcation between cytogenetics and Mendelian (single gene) defects and there really is a continuum of Mendelian cytogenetics.

Methods for study of possible genetic/cytogenetic abnormalities are changing rapidly with the advent of molecular genetics and molecular cytogenetics. These rapid expansions of knowledge are relevant to an understanding of the molecular pathology in reproductive medicine and for the new diagnostic potential from recent research findings. In this chapter we will try to give an overview of those aspects of chromosome studies which are important in reproductive medicine and delineate the extent of interaction of chromosomal abnormalities with single gene and multifactorial conditions. In order to help the reader and avoid overlap and duplication with the following chapter on genetic abnormalities, we have tried to make effective separations of the subject matter in the two chapters which we will try to illustrate and indicate briefly.

Cytogenetic conditions involve abnormalities of chromosomal number or structure, usually discernible by studying metaphase or pro-metaphase chromosomal preparations at the light microscope level. Some small chromosomal deletions or duplications are difficult to detect even by detailed microscopic examination using high resolution chromosomal banding (800 band level)[5] but the advent of the new chromosome-specific genetic probes utilizing chromosomal *in situ* hybdridization has made identification even of the smallest chromosomal abnormalities possible.

Single gene, multifactorial and teratogenic conditions

Single gene defects differ from chromosomal abnormalities in scale, as they involve mutations within a single gene whereas chromosomal abnormalities involve whole chromosomes or major chromosomal regions involving a number of genes on a contiguous chromosomal segment. The single gene abnormalities may be very small, involving only a single base change, or there may be larger deletions or alterations within a single gene and the actual change affects the mode of inheritance (see Chapter 1.8). Multifactorial conditions are considered to be due to a number of different genes with an environmental compo-

nent, e.g. neural tube defects where there is a genetic predisposition such as that in Celtic populations with some abnormality of folate in early pregnancy, at the time of neural tube closure. Cleft lip and palate (when not associated with specific genetic or chromosomal syndromes) is often thought to be multifactorial. Teratogens may sometimes produce phenotypic effects very similar to certain genetic syndromes, and it may take the demonstration of specific infection to try and establish causes. Teratogens include infectious agents such as rubella, toxoplasmosis, cytomegalovirus, parvovirus, syphilis; drugs such as warfarin, antiepileptics, many others and environmental agents such as ionizing radiation.

A brief guide to the essentials of chromosomology

Humans usually have 46 chromosomes. There are 23 pairs of chromosomes; 22 pairs called autosomes are numbered in order of size from 1 to 22; the remaining pair are called the sex chromosomes, because they detemine the sex of the individual; females have two X chromosomes but males have a dissimilar pair of an X and smaller Y chromosome. Normal females thus have a 46,XX karyotype and males a 46,XY karyotype. In 1956 two groups established that the diploid chromosome number in man was 46 not 48. In 1959, Lejeune reported an extra chromosome in Down's syndrome and this was rapidly followed by the discovery of human sex chromosome aberrations (in which there were extra or missing X and Y chromosomes) and translocation Down's syndrome (in which affected individuals had only 46 chromosomes instead of the expected 47, but had effectively three copies of chromosome 21 but with one of these translocated onto another chromosome, most usually chromosome 14 or 22).

One of the reasons that chromosome studies had been so difficult, and chromosome preparations so poor, was that there are few spontaneously dividing cells in human tissues which yield good, well-spread chromosomal preparations. Much of the early work had been done on bone marrow preparations but it is obviously a major problem to have to take a bone marrow biopsy in order to be able to study someone's chromosomes. The solution to the problem emerged when it was discovered that peripheral blood lymphocytes (which do not normally divide) could be stimulated to do so by mitogens such as phytohemagglutinin (derived from kidney beans), pokeweed mitogen or Epstein–Barr virus.[9]

The introduction of a short-term lymphocyte culture method in 1960 made it possible to do chromosome studies, just by taking a blood sample and culturing it under the appropriate conditions on patients with mental and physical handicap, recurrent miscarriage, infertility and with leukemia and related disorders. This led to descriptions of trisomy 13 (Patau's syndrome[10]), trisomy 18 (Edwards syndrome[11]), and the Philadelphia 9;22 translocation chromosome in chronic myeloid leukemia. Since then, advances have established the importance of molecular cytogenetics in fetal medicine, recurrent abortion, stillbirth and neonatal death, physical and mental handicap, infertility and oncology.

Modern banding techniques allow the identification of each of the 23 pairs.[12] Each chromosome has a narrow 'waist' or centromere (the site of attachment of the spindle fibers for mitosis) and the overall morphology of the chromosome is described according to the position of the centromere. Each chromosome has a long and a short arm; the short arm of each chromosome is called the p arm (from the French *petit*) and the long arm is called the q arm.

In the female the X chromosome is much larger than the Y chromosome and contains many more genes; in order to compensate for this genetic imbalance, one of the X chromosomes is inactivated during development in every cell in female mammals as a method of dosage compensation (Lyon hypothesis[13]). In the female, the inactivated X chromosome exists as a late replicating X which is seen as a sex chromatin or Barr body. In the male, the long (q) arm of the Y chromosome can be identified after quinacrine staining by brilliant fluorescence of the distal two-thirds of the long arm; this can be seen in interphase cells as the Y body. This fluorescent portion of the long arm of the Y chromosome and a number of other chromosomal regions such as the pericentromeric heterochromatin (C-band) regions of chromosomes 3, 4, 5 and centromeres and short arms of the acrocentric chromosomes 13, 14, 15, 21, 22 may vary in both size and intensity of fluorescence.[14] This is because these chromosomal regions contain multiple copies of short repeat sequences and the number of copies may vary between individuals. This leads to the phenomenon of chromosomal heteromorphisms; these are normal variants in the karyotype which can be traced in a pedigree from parent to offspring as chromosomal variants are transmitted as normal Mendelian characateristics. More sophisticated methods for cytogenetic sexing are now available using chromosome and gene-specific probes for the X and Y chromosome and segments of interest.[15] These can be demonstrated after *in situ* hybdridization of chromosomal probes by using fluoresecent tags to X or Y chromosomes (fluorescence *in situ* hybridization or FISH).[16] This is a very useful method as it can be used on interphase nuclei, rather than having to use dividing cells which is necessary for conventional chromosome studies.[17]

Normal and abnormal chromosomes; how chromosome abnormalities arise: non-disjunctional and other errors leading to trisomies and polyploidy

When germ cells (eggs and sperm) are formed, there is a need to have a reduction division or meiosis, otherwise chromosome numbers would double at each generation (46 chromosomes from each parent would give 92 chromosomes and so on). Meiotic divisions (which have complex names) essentially consist of a process in which the two chromosomes of each pair meet up, exchange genetic material in order to generate genetic diversity (a process termed 'crossing over') and then the two homologs sepa-

rate to form two daughter cells each with 23 chromosomes and this is immediately followed by a second division so that there are actually four cells produced as a result of this. There are, however, differences between males and females both in timing and other subtle processes (such as the formation of polar bodies in the female). Errors may arise during meiosis so that chromosomes fail to separate, so that the germ cells formed have too many, or too few chromosomes, or parts of chromosomes go missing, and this process is called non-disjunction.

Etiology of chromosome abnormalities: aneuploidy

The most common cause of monosomy, trisomy or triploidy is non-disjunction occurring during meiosis in a parent, so that there is failure of the relevant chromosome pair to separate. The egg or sperm then contains 22 or 24 instead of 23 chromosomes (or even at the most extreme the entire set of chromosomes fail to disjoin giving rise to a diploid egg or sperm). After fertilization by a normal gamete, the zygote has 45, 47 or even 69 chromosomes. Monosomy is lethal for autosomal anomalies but for some sex chromosome abnormalities both products may give rise to viable zygotes, e.g. 47,XXY and 45,X.

In about 80% of cases of autosomal trisomy, non-disjunction occurs in the formation of the oocyte (usually at the first meiotic division). Maternal errors leading to certain chromosomal abnormalities thus appear to be more common than paternal errors and this becomes increasingly common with advancing maternal age. All autosomal trisomies, some sex chromosome aneuploidies such as 47,XXX and 47,XXY and other abnormalities such as supernumerary marker chromosomes all show a predominantly maternal origin and the frequency rises with advancing maternal age.[18] 47,XYY obviously originates as a paternal meiotic error (as a second meiotic division non-disjunctional event) and, as would be expected, does not show any maternal age effect.

Non-disjunction in the father is not related to paternal age[18,19] although, because of the relationship which tends to exist between the ages of the parents (older women tend to have older partners), there can appear to be a correlation between paternal age and chromosomal abnormalities. In 60% of cases of Turner's syndrome it is the paternal X which is lost,[20,21] but this is because many cases of Turner's syndrome are due to an error of division in the early zygote rather than to a meiotic error in a parent and also to the fact that survival in Turner's syndrome is greater if the conceptus retains a maternal X chromosome. The incidence of Turner's syndrome is inversely related to maternal age, probably because younger mothers provide a better uterine environment for fetal survival. The majority of autosomal trisomies are lethal and result in failure of implantation or early spontaneous abortion. Only three autosomal trisomies are compatible with survival to birth: trisomy 13, trisomy 18 and trisomy 21 and only the latter of these, involving one of the smallest chromosomes, is found in surviving children and adults.

Unless a parent has a translocation or rearrangement which results in a chromosome abnormality in the child, there is usually a low risk of recurrence for a couple who have had a chromosomally abnormal child, fetus or abortus (this is in the order of 1–2% for mothers under 35 years).[22-24] The majority of disorders which exhibit Mendelian inheritance (autosomal dominant, autosomal recessive or X-linked diseases), as would be expected, show no recognizable chromosome abnormality, nor do the multifactorial conditions such as neural tube defects or isolated (non-syndromal) cleft lip and palate.

Many different factors including environmental mutagens and teratogens such as ionizing radiation,[25] and a variety of other agents such as anesthetic gases, alcohol and other substances have been implicated in chromosomal non-disjunction leading to aneuploidy.[26-28] Many of these reports have been controversial; for example, studies ascribing a significant effect on non-disjunction of low-doses of ionizing radiation are almost equal in number with those reporting no effect. Molecular studies of the chromosomes which fail to disjoin at meiosis suggests that there is reduced recombination in these chromosomes.[29]

Etiology of constitutional abnormalities: rearrangements and mosaicism

It is relatively easy to envisage non-disjunction involving whole chromosomes, but rather harder to picture more complex chromosomal errors occurring at meiosis or during early embryonic divisions. It is beyond the scope of this chapter to describe the complexities of the mechanisms involved since the texts on cytogenetics cover this in detail; the essence is that there are five major types:

1. **Mutant** – resulting from errors at meiosis in the formation of germ cells from a parent. This includes *de novo* chromosomal rearrangements such as translocations or inversions. Risks are given by Warburton,[30] and Buhler.[31]
2. **Unbalanced forms of a parental rearrangement or translocation**, e.g. translocation Down's syndrome, where a parent is a carrier of the translocation and the fetus inherits an unbalanced form; similarly for inversions and other rearrangements. Risks for different translocations have been described by Daniel *et al.*[23]
3. **Mosaics**, with two different cell lines resulting from a post-zygotic error in the early blastocyst or embryo.[32,33]
4. **Microdeletion/duplication or contiguous gene syndromes**, e.g. WAGR (Wilm's tumor, aniridia and gonadoblastoma) due to small deletions on the short arm of chromosome 11 at 11p13 or Beckwith syndrome (exomphalos, macroglossia) due to duplication of 11p15.
5. **Other, with chromosomal manifestations of single gene defects** including fragile X syndrome which should really be classified as an X-linked gene disorder, and chromosomal breakage syndromes such as Bloom's syndrome, Fanconi's pancytopenia and ataxia telangiectasia (which are inherited as autosomal recessive conditions and covered under the chapter on genetic abnormalities).

Specific chromosome abnormalities

Autosomal aneuploidy

Trisomy 21 (Down's syndrome or mongolism)

Incidence is 1 in 660 newborns. This syndrome was first reported by Down in 1886.[34] The principal features are mental handicap, general hypotonia, protruding tongue, brachycephaly with relatively flattened occiput, mild microcephaly with upslanting palpebral fissures, short hard palate, small nose with low nasal bridge, inner epicanthic folds, speckling of iris, macroglossia, short metacarpals and phalanges, clinodactyly, single palmar crease, distal position of axial triradius, ulnar loops on digits, wide sandal gap between first and second toes. Cardiac abnormalities occur in 40% of cases (ASD, VSD, PDA).

Males have hypogonadism and are infertile but females are fertile with a 50% risk of having a child with trisomy 21. Survival curves and causes of death for those with Down's syndrome are important in giving long-term prognoses.[35] Some cases involve mosaicism, which is the presence of more than one cell line in the same conceptus (compared with chimerism which involves cell lines from different conceptuses). The severity of the phenotype in mosaic cases tends to reflect the proportion of abnormal/normal cells as the presence of a normal cell line dilutes the abnormal phenotypic effects of the abnormal cell line.

Trisomy 18 (Edwards' syndrome)

Incidence is 1 in 3500 newborns. More than 130 different abnormalities have been described in this syndrome, but the principal features usually include growth deficiency, prominent occiput, low-set malformed ears, micrognathia, clenched hands, dermal arches, omphalocele, cardiac anomalies (VSD, ASD, PDA), urogenital anomalies including horseshoe kidney and diaphragmatic hernia. Long-term survival has been reported.[36] Warkany *et al.*[37] have described the abnormalities in autosomal trisomy syndromes.

Trisomy 13 (Patau's syndrome)

Incidence is 1 in 5000 births. Abnormalities include holoprosencephaly, microcephaly, cleft lip and palate, polydactyly, cardiac anomalies, omphalocele, heterotopic pancreas and spleen, polycystic kidney, hydronephrosis. Median survival is about 6 months, but extended survival has been described.[38,39]

Other trisomies

Trisomies for most of the human chromosomes have been described in abortuses, but few of these are compatible with survival except in mosaic form. Among surviving individuals with mosaic trisomies are mosaic trisomy 8,[40] mosaic trisomy 9[41] and trisomy 22 which is associated with the cat-eye syndrome.[42]

Partial trisomies and monosomies

For most of the trisomies, there are critical regions of the chromosome which give rise to the characteristic phenotype.[43] Thus even partial trisomies may have phenotypic effects similar to that of total trisomy, such as that of partial trisomy 22 and cat-eye syndrome. For other partial trisomies and monosomies there are characteristic patterns depending on the exact region which is duplicated or deleted and the genes it contains. The tip of the short arm of chromosome 4 (4p) may be duplicated to give partial trisomy 4p syndrome[44] or deleted to give the 4p- Wolf–Hischorn syndrome.[45] Deletions of the tip of chromosome 5 (5p-) give the characteristic 'cri du chat' syndrome.[46] There is now recognition of microdeletion syndromes such as Miller–Deiker lissencephaly syndrome due to a small interstitial deletion of chromosome 17 and aniridia/Wilm's tumor due to an interstitial deletion of chromosome 11p.[47]

Polyploidy

Triploidy

Triploidy can be 69,XXX or 69,XXY. This was first reported by Book et al. in 1960.[48] Triploidy is a common chromosome abnormality occurring in about 2% of all conceptions. The vast majority abort early in pregnancy (especially those with an XYY sex chromosome complement), with only 1 in 10,000 surviving to birth. In about 50% of cases there is hydatidiform change in the placenta; this occurs only in those triploid pregnancies where 46 of the 69 chromosomes are from the father (diandry). Triploidy arises from fertilization of an egg which has 46 chromosomes (due to failure to eject a polar body) by a sperm with a normal complement of 23 chromosomes, or to a diploid sperm (with 46 chromosomes) fertilizing a normal egg. In some cases there is dispermy, with two sperm fertilizing one egg. All result in embryos with 69 chromosomes. Most pregnancies with a triploid fetus have severe intrauterine growth retardation and multiple anomalies are present.[49,50]

Tetraploidy

Tetraploidy, 92,XXXX or 92,XXYY, is seen relatively frequently after cell culture, but not all tetraploid karyotypes have clinical significance. This is because culture conditions are often sufficient to permit chromosomal or nuclear division, but insufficient for the rate-limiting step of supplying precursor molecules to enable cytoplasmic and cell membrane division to occur as well. As a result, the chromosomes duplicate without cell division, leading to a state where the cells have effectively doubled the chromosome numbers from 46 to 92, giving tetraploidy. Thus, many cases of tetraploidy after culture are the result of culture artefact rather than non-disjunctional errors at meiosis or post-zygotic maldivisions.[32]

Sex chromosome aneuploidy

47,XXY Klinefelter syndrome

Incidence is about 1 in 600 newborn males. There is a tendency from childhood towards long lower limbs with low upper to lower segment ratio and relatively tall and slim stature, hypogonadism and hypogenitalism with low

testosterone values and infertility. Klinefelter et al.[51] first described the syndrome although the chromosomal aetiology was not recognized until 1960. Gynecomastia occurs in 40% of cases.

47,XYY

Incidence is 1 in 840 newborn males.[52] There is growth acceleration at puberty with tall stature, and temper tantrums in childhood. Most have normal fertility and the extra Y chromosome does not appear to be transmitted in the gametes of XYY males as it is lost during the process of spermatogenesis.

45,X Turner's syndrome

Incidence is 1 in 5000 newborns. This syndrome was first described by Turner in 1938.[53] Affected individuals have short stature, ovarian dysgenesis, congenital lymphedema, webbed neck, broad chest with widely spaced nipples, cubitus valgus, excess pigmented nevi, renal anomalies and cardiac abnormalities such as bicuspid aortic valve, coarctation of the aorta in 20% of patients. There is high lethality in utero. There are variants of Turner's syndrome such as those cases where there is mosaicism (usually involving a normal cell line which can either be female, so the karyotype is 45,X/46,XX or male 45,X/46,XY). In the latter case of 45,X/46,XY mosaicism, the phenotype may be either Turner female, intersex or male, depending on the relative proportions of 45,X and 46,XY cells.[54]

47,XXX

Incidence is 1 in 600 newborns. There are virtually no phenotypic manifestations of this karyotype except for mild learning disabilities with a characteristic IQ of between 75 and 85 in the majority of cases and a few cases showing more severe handicap and some with psychiatric illness. Most individuals have normal fertility. More extreme numbers of X chromosomes may occur, for example 49,XXXXX where the phenotypic effects are more severe.[55]

Chromosomal rearrangements

Chromosome abnormalities with major phenotypic effects can occur even when there are no abnormalities of chromosome number. These abnormalities include:

1. **Translocations**, reciprocal and Robertsonian.
2. **Inversions;** these include pericentric, which include the centromere, and paracentric, in which there is simply an inverted segment in one chromosome arm.
3. **Deletions** (including ring chromosomes) which usually result in partial monosomies.[56]
4. **Insertions or duplications:** these have been mentioned in the partial trisomies.

Reciprocal translocations

These involve the transfer of a segment of one chromosome to another; usually there is a reciprocal exchange. If there is no loss or gain of genetic material and the chromosomal material is merely rearranged, this usually causes no phenotypic abnormalities and is described as a balanced form of the translocation. At meiosis in a carrier of a balanced translocation however, abnormal chromosomal pairing and subsequent separation of the chromosomes may result in a gamete with chromosomal imbalance for the chromosomal segments involved, leading to partial monosomy and trisomy. Sometimes when a translocation occurs *de novo*, although it may appear to be apparently balanced at the cytological level, if the chromosomal breakpoints have occurred in a gene crucial for development or function, there may be phenotypic effects, the most frequent of which is mental handicap.

Robertsonian translocations, including translocation Down's syndrome

Robertsonian translocations are one of the most frequent chromosomal abnormalities seen in man. In a Robertsonian translocation, two acrocentric chromosomes which normally exist separately in most individuals are fused together at the centromeres. There are virtually no phenotypic effects of this provided that no chromosomal or genetic material is lost from the long arms of either chromosome during the fusion process. The main effects occur when the chromosomes of a Robertsonian translocation pair at meiosis as errors during this process occur more frequently than in normal individuals. The major consequences are thus sub- or infertility and the chances of having children with the unbalanced forms of the translocation.

The frequency of carriers of the balanced form of a 13/14 Robertsonian fusion (this is the most common form) is about 1 in 600 newborns. The frequency of 14/21 and 21/22 translocations (which are involved in translocation Down's syndrome) is much lower than that of 13/14 translocations at about 1 in 2500. These translocations are usually inherited in a familial manner from a parent, although a proportion occur *de novo*. About 1–3% of cases of Down's syndrome are due to translocation Down's. Carriers of Robertsonian translocations have 45 chromosomes instead of 46. They are usually phenotypically normal because all the essential chromosomal material is present. A female carrier of a Robertsonian translocation of the type involved in translocation Down's syndrome (which involves chromosome 21 and another acrocentric chromosome, usually chromosome 14) would have a karyotype 45,XX,-14 -21,+t(14q21q). This person would usually be phenotypically normal.[57] There are, however, differences in the risks for male and female carriers of Robertsonian translocations. For 14/21 translocations, female carriers have a 12–15% risk of having a child with translocation Down's syndrome whereas males have only a 1–3% risk of having an affected child because of the differences in behavior of the translocation chromosome in male and female meiosis. Male carriers, however, have a higher risk of infertility. Other chromosomal translocations may affect male and female fertility differently.

The highest risk of having an affected child is for people who have a homologous Robertsonian fusion, for example, that between two chromosomes 21 (21/21 translocation). These translocations are rare, since all must occur *de novo* as the only progeny will be those with translocation trisomy 21, or monosomy 21 (which is lethal). At meiosis in a 21/21 translocation carrier, the only gametes that can be made are thus with nullisomy 21 which is lethal or those with the 21/21 translocation which after fertilization with a normal egg or sperm carrying a normal chromosome 21 results in trisomy 21. There is thus a 100% risk, i.e. all the children of a carrier will have trisomy 21.

Inversions

An inversion involves two chromosomal breaks and then reinsertion of the chromosomal segment after rotating through 180 degrees. There are two types of inversion, the first called paracentric inversions result from two breaks in the same chromosome arm. The morphology of the chromosome does not change and even if crossing over occurs within the inverted segment, the chances of unbalanced offsping are very low. In contrast, pericentric inversions occur as a result of breaks occurring in two different arms of the same chromosome so that the centromere is included in the segment which is inverted. At meiosis there is a risk of a cross-over event occurring which could produce an unbalanced form of the inversion with duplication of part of the chromosome and deletion of other segments. The major risks are thus those for pericentric inversions where the risks of partial trisomy/monosomy differ for each chromosome and for the different breakpoints. Specific risks can be assessed from papers providing detail for each of the chromosomal breakpoints and types of interchange.[23,58]

FUTURE PERSPECTIVES

Interphase karyotyping, *in situ* hybridization, FISH and PCR *in situ* hybridization

One of the most important advances has been in the the ability to 'karyotype' non-dividing interphase cells, using new techniques such as chromosome painting with chromosome-specific probes and fluorescent *in situ* hybridization (FISH). This has enabled studies not previously possible such as studies of gonadal cells, gametes and brain cells. It also enables a rapid 'molecular karyotype' to be obtained within a few hours of taking the sample, which will be of value for rapid karyotyping in prenatal diagnosis.

Chromosomal mapping, microdissection libraries chromosome-specific and gene probes

The Human Genome Project which has, as its objective, mapping all the human genes to specific chromosomal loci, defining their interrelationships as linkage maps, cloning the genes and defining their function, has proved to be much more controversial than was originally foreseen. The ultimate aim of the genome project was to map major disease genes. However, fears about the eugenic aspects of any genetic mapping project have resulted in much public debate and some vocal opposition to gene mapping because of possible misuse of the information[59]. Two further complications have arisen; the costs have escalated and available resources diminished. Of great concern too has been the fact that there have been attempts (in many cases by commercial interests) to patent genes or genetic sequences, which would have serious financial implications for diagnostic testing. Despite these problems, chromosomal mapping of disease genes, the use of translocation breakpoint mapping and cloning strategies and the development of chromosome specific probes have revolutionized chromosomal diagnosis in all fields, dysmorphology, pedatrics, in solid tumors and hematological malignancies, mental and physical handicap, in infertility, and in prenatal diagnosis.

Clinical and family studies which are complementary to molecular genetic analysis are helping to refine the phenotype and to establish patterns of inheritance. Cytogenetic disorders have always been complex and refractory to genetic analysis because the majority occur as new mutations because of a meiotic error in a parent. Even for familial disorders, there may be differences between male and female carriers; for example for both reciprocal translocations and familial supernumerary marker chromosomes, male carriers may be infertile with severe oligospermia whereas female carriers of the same translocation may be fertile but more prone to miscarriage. The combination of scientific and clinical disciplines as molecular cytogenetics and reproductive medicine offers new prospects for diagnosis, prognosis and therapy.

SUMMARY

- The normal diploid number of human chromosomes is 46; abnormalities of number or structure are usually associated with clinical consequences and many of these have effects on fertility, reproductive failure or cause mental or physical handicap.
- Chromosomes can be visualized and counted most easily at metaphase of cell division. Dividing cells are thus needed for full karyotyping. These can be obtained by culturing cells from peripheral blood, skin, amniotic fluid or products of conception.
- New techniques such as FISH (fluorescent *in situ* hybridization) allow the number of chromosomes to be evaluated using chromosome-specific probes in non-dividing interphase cells.
- Each human chromosome has a characteristic pattern when chromosome banding techniques are used; high resolution chromosomal banding allows even small rearrangements such as small deletions, inversions or translocations (which may be of clinical significance) to be recognized.
- Even small chromosomal deletions can have serious phenotypic consequences and chromosomal syndromes are now associated with these microdeletions such as Prader–Willi syndrome on 15q, Miller–Dieker on chromosome 17, aniridia/Wilm's tumor on chromosome 11p and DiGeorge syndrome on 22q.
- The vast majority of constitutional chromosomal abnormalities arise as errors during meiosis (non-disjunctional errors) in the formation of eggs or sperm in a parent; about 5% occur as errors during an early cell division in the developing embryo.
- There is an increase in the proportion of babies with chromosomal abnormalities with advancing maternal age. As mothers over 35 years have less than 5% of the babies born, despite the increased risks for older mothers, the majority of babies with mutant chromosomal abnormalities are born to younger mothers with no previously identifiable risk factors.
- Acquired chromosomal abnormalities (in contrast to constitutional abnormalities arising at conception or as early mitotic errors in the embryo) are important in cancer, where specific chromosomal translocations or amplifications involve oncogenes and tumor suppressor genes and lead to inappropriate stimulation of cell division or uncontrolled cellular growth.
- Recurrence risks for constitutional chromosomal abnormalities after having an affected child depend on the type of chromosomal abnormality and whether the abnormality is mutant (i.e. has occurred *de novo*) or is familial. Risks for chromosomally normal parents who have had a child with a mutant abnormality are approximately 1% but also depend on the maternal age risks.
- For parents carrying a translocation these depend on the type of translocation, the chromosomal breakpoints and for Robertsonian translocations the sex of the parent carrying the translocation. For example a female carrier of a

Robertsonian t(14q;21q) translocation has about a 15% risk of having a child with translocation Down's syndrome whereas for a male carrier the risks are less than 3%. In the case of reciprocal translocations both parents usually have similar risks but these are translocation dependent and vary from about 15% up to about 30%.

REFERENCES

1. Hook EB, Topol BB, Cross PK. The natural history of cytogenetically abnormal fetuses detected at midtrimester amniocentesis which are not terminated electively: new data and estimates of the excess and relative risk of fetal death associated with 47, +21 and some other abnormal karyotypes. *Am J Hum Genet* 1989 **45**: 855–861.
2. Bergsma DS. *Birth Defects Atlas and Compendium*, 3rd edn. Baltimore: Williams and Wilkins, 1985.
3. de Grouchy J, Turleau C. *Clinical Atlas of Human Chromosomes*. New York: John Wiley, 1984.
4. ISCN. An International System for Human Cytogenetic Nomenclature 1978. *Birth Defects Orginal Articles Series* 1978 **14**(8).
5. ISCN. An International System for Human Cytogenetic Nomenclature – high resolution banding 1981. *Birth Defects Original Article Series* 1981 **17**(5).
6. Lindsten J. *The Nature and Origin of X Chromosome Aberration in Turner's Syndrome*. Stockholm: 1963 Almquist and Wikseel.
7. Rooney DE, Czepulkowski BH. *Human Cytogenetics A Practical Approach*. Oxford, New York, Tokyo: Oxford University Press, 1992.
8. Schinzel A. *Catalogue of Unbalanced Chromosome Aberrations in Man*. New York: Walter de Gruyter, 1984.
9. Gosden CM, Davidson C, Robertson M. Culture of human lymphocytes for cytogenetic analysis. In Rooney D, Czelplekowski B (eds) *Practical Human Cytogenetics*. Oxford: IRL Press 1992: 31–54.
10. Patau K. Multiple congenital anomaly caused by an extra chromosome. *Lancet* 1960: 790.
11. Edwards JH. A new trisomic syndrome. *Lancet* 1960 **i**: 787.
12. Caspersson T, Tomakka G, Zech Ll. 24 fluorescence patterns of human metaphase chromosomes: distinguishing characters and variability. *Hereditas* 1971 **67**: 89.
13. Lyon ME. Gene action in the X-chromosome of the mouse (*Mus musculus* L). *Nature* 1961 **190**: 372–373.
14. Bobrow M, Pearson PL, Pike MC, El Alfi OS. Length variation in the quinacrine binding segment of human Y chromosomes of different sizes. *Cytogenetics* 1971 **10**: 190.
15. Magenis RE, Casanova M, Fellous M, Olson S, Sheehy R. Further cytologic evidence for Xp–Yp translocation in XX males using *in situ* hybridisation with Y derived probe. *Hum Genet* **75**: 228–233.
16. Trask BJ. Fluorescence *in situ* hybridisation application in cytogenetics and gene mapping. *Trends Genet* 1991 7: 149–154.
17. Van de Kaa CA, Nelson KAM, Ramaekers FCS, Voojis PG, Hopman AHN. Interphase cytogenetics in paraffin sections of routinely processed hydatidiform moles and hydropic abortions. *J Pathol* 1991 **165**: 281–287.
18. Ferguson-Smith MA, Yates JRW. Maternal age specific rates for chromosome aberrations and factors influencing them: report of the collaborative European study on 52, 965 amniocenteses. *Prenat Diagn* 1984 4: 5–44.
19. Miller OJ, Mittwoch U, Penrose LS. Spermatogenesis in man with special reference to aneuploidy. *Heredity* 1960 14: 456.
20. Hassold TJ, Benham F, Leppert M. Cytogenetic and molecular analysis of sex-chromosome monosomy. *Am J Hum Genet* 1988 **42**: 534–551.
21. Cockwell A, Mackenzie M, Yoings S, Jacobs P. A cytogenetic study of 45, X fetuses and their parents. *J Med Genet* 1991 **28**: 151–155.
22. Berr C, Borghi E, Rethore MO, Lejeune J, Alperovitch A. Risk of Down syndrome in relatives of trisomy 21 children. A case control study. *Ann Genet* 1990 **33**: 137–140.
23. Daniel A, Hook EB, Wulf G. Risks of unbalanced progeny at amniocentesis to carriers of chromosome rearrangements: data from United States and Canadian Laboratories. *Am J Med Genet* 1989 **31**: 14–53.
24. Hassold TJ, Jacobs PA. Trisomy in man. *Annu Rev Genet* 1984 **18**: 69–97.
25. BEIR report. *The Effects on Populations of Low Levels of Ionising Radiation*. Committee on the Biological Effects of Ionising Radiation. Washington DC: National Academy Press, 1980.
26. Mikkelsen M, Poulsen H, Grinsted J, Lange A. Non-disjunction in trisomy 21: study of chromosomal heteromorphisms in 110 families. *Ann Hum Genet* 1980 **44**: 17–28.
27. Mikkelsen M, Poulsen H, Tommerup N. Genetic risk factors in human trisomy 21. In Hassold TJ, Epstein CJ (eds) *Progress in Clinical and Biological Research, Molecular and Cytogenetic Studies of Non-disjunction*, Vol. 311. New York: Alan R Liss 1989: 183–197.
28. Cohen EN, Belville JW, Brown BW. Anaesthesia, pregnancy and miscarriage: a study of operating room nurses and anesthetists. *Anesthesiology* 1971 **35**: 343.
29. Warren AC, Chakravati A, Wong C. Evidence for reduced recombination on the non-disjoined chromosomes 21 in Down's syndrome. *Science* 1987 **237**: 652–654.
30. Warburton D. Outcome of cases of *de novo* structural rearrangements diagnosed at amniocentesis. *Prenat Diagn* 1984 **4**: 69–80.
31. Buhler EM. Cat eye syndrome, a partial trisomy 22. *Humangenetik* 1972 **15**: 150.
32. Gosden CM. Prenatal diagnosis of chromosome anomalies. In Lilford RJ (ed.) *Prenatal Diagnosis of Fetal Abnormalities*. London, Boston, Sydney, Toronto: Butterworths 1990: 104–164.
33. Kohn G, Tayai T, Atkins TE, Mellman W. Mosaic mongolism. 1. Clinical correlations. *J Paediatr* 1970 **76**: 874.
34. Down JLH. Observations on an ethnic classification of Idiots. *Clinical Lecture Reports. London Hospital* 1886 **3**: 259.
35. Bell JA, Pearn JH, Firman D. Childhood deaths in Down's syndrome. Survival curves and causes of death from a total population study in Queensland Australia 1976–1985. *J Med Genet* 1989 **26**: 764–768.
36. Eaton FP, Kontras SB, Sommer A, Wehe RA. Long term survival in trisomy 18. New chromosomal and malformation syndromes. *Birth Defects* 1975 **11**: 327.
37. Warkany J, Passarge E, Smith LB. Congenital malformations in autosomal trisomy syndromes. *Am J Dis Child* 1966 **112**: 502.
38. Cowan JM. Trisomy 13 and extended survival. *J Med Genet* 1973 **16**: 155.
39. Goldstein H, Neilsen KG. Rates and survival of individuals with trisomy 13 and 18. Data form a 10 years period in Denmark. *Clin Genet* 1988 **34**: 266–272.
40. Berry AC. Mosaicism and the trisomy 8 syndrome. *Clin Genet* 1978 **14**: 105.
41. Haslam RHA. Trisomy 9 mosaicism and mutiple congenital abnormalities. *J. Med Genet* 1973 **10**: 180.
42. Cervenka J, Hansen CA, Francoisi, RA, Gorlin RJ. Trisomy 22 with 'cateye' anomaly. *J. Med Genet* 1977 **14**, 288.

43. Korenberg JR, Kawashima H, Pulst SM. Molecular definition of a region of chromosome 21 that causes features of the Down syndrome phenotype. *Am J Hum Genet* 1990 47: 236–246.

44. Gonzalez CH. The trisomy 4p syndrome Case report and a review. *Am J Med Genet* 1977 **1**: 137.

45. Wolf U, Reinwein H. Klinische und cytogenetische Differentiadiagnose der Defidienzen an den kurzen Armen der Bchromosomen. *Z Kinderheilkd* 1967 **98**: 235.

46. Lejeune J. Trois cas de deletion partielle du bras court du chromosome 5. *CR Acad Sci (D) Paris* 1963 **257**: 3098.

47. Riccardi VM. Chromosomal imbalance in the aniridia–Wilm's tumour association: 11p interstitial deletion. *Paediatrics* 1978 **61**: 604.

48. Book JA, Santesson B. Malformation syndrome in man associated with triploidy (69 chromosomes). *Lancet* 1960 **i**: 858.

49. Gosden CM, Wright MO, Paterson WG, Grant KA. Clinical details, cytogenetic studies and cellular physiology of a 69,XXX fetus with comments on the biological effect of triploidy in man. *J Med Genet* 1976 **13**: 371–380.

50. Nicolaides KH, Gosden CM, Snijders RJM. Ultrasonographically detectable markers of fetal chromosomal defects. In Nelson JP, Chambers SE (eds) *Obstetric Ultrasound 1*. Oxford: Oxford Medical Publications Oxford University Press, 1993: 41–48.

51. Klinefelter HF, Reifenstein EC, Albright F. Syndrome characterised by gynaecomastia, aspermatogenesis with aleydigism, and increased secretion of follicle stimulating hormone. *J Clin Endocrinol Metab* 1942 **2**: 615.

52. Sandberg AA. XYY human male. *Lancet* 1961 **ii**: 488.

53. Turner HH. A syndrome of infantilism, congenetal webbed neck and cubitus valgus. *Endocrinology* 1938 **23**: 566.

54. Dewhurst J. Fertility in 47, XXX and 45, X patients. *J Med Genet* 1978 **15**: 132.

55. Carpenter DG. The penta X (49, XXXXX) syndrome: danger of confusing phenotype with mongolism *Am J Dis Child* 1979 **133**: 330.

56. Taylor AI. Dq- Dr and retinoblastoma. *Humangenetik* 1970 **10**: 209.

57. Bonthron DT, Smith SJL, Fantes J, Gosden CM. De-novo microdeletion on an inherited robertsonian translocation chromosome – a cause for dysmorphism in the apparently balanced translocation carrier. *Am J Hum Genet* 1993 **53**(3): 629–637.

58. Groupe de Cytogeneticiens Francais. Pericentric inversions in man. A French collaborative study. *Ann Genet* 1986 **29**: 129–168.

59. Masood E *et al.* Gene tests: who benefits from risk? *Nature* 1996 **379**: 389–392.

Genetic Inheritance

DT Bonthron

INTRODUCTION

The massive amount of information currently being accumulated on the molecular basis for inherited (single gene) disease is only readily accessible through computer technology. This chapter cannot deal with specific disorders in depth, but outlines the major principles underlying genetic inheritance, emphasizing the practical consequences where possible. Precise classification of diseases in pathogenetic terms is of prime importance in genetics. The most widely used source for this purpose is McKusick's catalog *Mendelian Inheritance in Man* (MIM),[1] or its online computererized version OMIM. I have emphasized the need for standardization of terminology by attaching the appropriate MIM number to each genetic disorder mentioned in the text.

CURRENT CONCEPTS

Dominant inheritance

In clinical genetics, the term dominant is generally used to imply that a disease results from mutation of one allele at a particular gene locus. The affected individual therefore has one normal and one mutated gene, and the equal probability of transmission of either of these to offspring yields the classical 50% risk of inheriting the disease and the typical pattern of vertical transmission within families, within which many individuals may be affected.

New mutations

For most autosomal dominant disorders, new mutations are fairly frequently observed. Some conditions, such as Apert syndrome (acrocephalosyndactyly type IV, MIM 101200) have such severe effects that they are seldom passed on, and nearly all cases therefore result from new mutation. In some disorders, such as achondroplasia (MIM 100800), the 80% or so of cases which result from new mutation are easily distinguished from the inherited cases, since the phenotype is so easily recognized. For neurofibromatosis type 1 (NF1; MIM 162200), one of the commonest dominant disorders, about 50% of cases result from new mutation. However, in this condition, since affected individuals are often asymptomatic, proper examination of the parents of a case is necessary to distinguish inherited cases from new mutations.

Incomplete penetrance

Incomplete penetrance describes the failure of some individuals who carry a mutation to manifest any features of the disease. For an autosomal dominant disorder, this may result in apparent skipping of generations. This feature of some genetic disorders complicates the assessment of recurrence risks. For example, tuberous sclerosis (MIM 191100) may present dramatically in infancy with infantile spasms and then severe developmental delay. Parents carrying a TSC mutation however may be asymptomatic, and indeed it is possible for them to have no phenotypic features at all. Others may have small depigmented patches visible under UV light as the only clue to the fact that they are carrying a mutation. The distinction is critical, since in the latter case the recurrence risk for TSC is 50%, whereas for a clear new mutation (as in achondroplasia) the recurrence risk is extremely small.

For some dominant inherited disorders, late onset is the rule. This means that the apparent penetrance of the condition is age dependent, leading to two major areas of concern for genetic counseling. First, it may not be possible to be certain whether a patient at risk for such a disease is indeed carrying the mutation on clinical grounds alone. Even specific investigation may fail to resolve the issue; for example in autosomal dominant polycystic kidney disease (MIM 173900) a normal ultrasound scan at age 16 will still leave an appreciable risk that the condition will become apparent later in life. Secondly, presymptomatic testing may be requested, which can provide certainty as to the eventual development of the disease, but without offering any therapeutic options.

Variable expressivity

Variable expressivity is a phenomenon which ultimately is only distinguished from incomplete penetrance by semantics. It is variability in the type or severity of manifestations of a mutation. Thus one individual with NF1 may have only café au lait patches and axillary freckling, while his sibling also suffers from scoliosis and learning difficulties. Minor manifestations of some conditions need to be carefully sought by examination of asymptomatic relatives.

Anticipation is a term used to indicate increasing severity of a disease in succeeding generations of a family. For some conditions, notably myotonic dystrophy (MIM 160900), this is a real and common observation, and a molecular explanation in the form of transmission of unstable mutations (see below) is available.[2] However, for other conditions with variable expressivity, apparent anticipation may sometimes simply reflect bias in the way that families are ascertained; presentation tends to be through individuals who are severely affected at an early age, and mildly affected parents are only then brought to attention through deliberate study of the family.

Gonadal mosaicism

If a mutation or chromosome aberration occurs in a cell during embryonic development, the final result will be an individual who is a mosaic for normal and mutant cells. Whether that individual displays any phenotypic features depends on the extent and distribution of the cells containing the mutation. If the mutated cells contribute to the developing gonad, then even in the absence of any physical manifestation of the mutation, there is a risk that the mutation will be transmitted to the gametes, giving rise to a (non-mosaic) offspring with the disease associated with that mutation. Though gonadal mosaicism for chromosome abnormalities is sometimes seen, this phenomenon is most important in the context of autosomal dominant and X-linked recessive diseases.[3] A well-studied example concerns mutations of the type I collagen genes (α1 or α2 chain; COL1A1 or COL1A2).[4] These occur in heterozygous form in most cases of osteogenesis imperfecta (OI). This group of brittle bone diseases usually displays dominant inheritance (vertical transmission), in keeping with the molecular observation of a mutation of one allele only. The severest types of osteogenesis imperfecta, though (type II; multiple intrauterine fractures, perinatal death) have been believed to be recessive, on the grounds of recurrences in siblings, with apparently normal parents. Despite this, molecular analysis suggests that most type II cases, like the milder OI types, have a single (dominant) mutation of one allele only. Sibling recurrences are best explained by gonadal mosaicism for the mutation, in one or other parent. In a few cases this has been directly proven by analysis of the father's sperm.

The possibility of gonadal mosaicism means that even for a fully penetrant autosomal dominant disorder, whenever there appears to have been a new mutation (parents appear normal), the recurrence risk is likely to be higher than the general population risk. The absolute magnitude of this risk may still be very low, though it is seldom possible to quantify it accurately.

The mechanism of dominance

Most human diseases displaying vertical transmission are not truly dominant in the Mendelian sense; this would imply that homozygosity for a mutation has an effect indistinguishable from that of heterozygosity. In most 'dominant' disorders, the effect of homozygosity is unknown, but in a few cases it is known to result in a much more severe phenotype than that seen when only one allele is mutated. For example, the homozygous affected offspring of two achondroplastic parents has a much more severe lethal short-limbed dwarfism. True Mendelian dominance may, however, be seen in Huntington's disease (HD) (MIM 143100); in occasional families with this condition pedigree studies have demonstrated homozygosity for the mutation in individuals with typical HD.

Also, for some dominant disorders the effect of the mutation is not null (not equivalent to simple loss of function). Considering again achondroplasia, which results from a specific $Gly^{380} \rightarrow Arg$ mutation of the fibroblast growth factor receptor 3 (FGFR3) gene, the phenotype of achondroplasia is not seen in patients with chromosomal deletions of 4p16, the region containing FGFR3. Thus the codon 380 substitution must cause a very specific alteration in the biochemical properties of the fibroblast growth factor receptor 3 protein. Various such specific biochemical effects of heterozygosity for a non-null mutation can be envisaged.[5]

Autosomal recessive inheritance

A mutation is recessive if it only results in disease when in the homozygous state. For an autosomal gene both parents are expected to be heterozygous for the mutation (carriers), giving the sibling recurrence risk of 1 in 4. The risk for other family members (outside the immediate sibship) is small unless (a) there are consanguineous partnerships or (b) the general population carrier frequency is high. The latter can be calculated if the approximate frequency of the disease state is known; carrier frequency $\approx 2 \times \sqrt{}$ (disease frequency). For rare recessive disorders, parental consanguinity is increased in frequency, but the significance attached to an individual example of parental consanguinity is likely to be less in populations where inbreeding is relatively common.

Many autosomal recessive diseases show marked regional and racial variability in frequency and molecular pathology. In some cases this results from a 'founder effect', whereby a single mutation persists in a small geographically or reproductively isolated population for many generations. An example is aspartylglucosaminuria (MIM

208400) in the Finnish population (frequency about 1 in 3600, due to a 1 in 30 carrier rate for the mutation $Cys^{163} \rightarrow Ser$).[6,7] This disorder is very rare in other populations.

In outbred populations, though, most recessive diseases show allelic heterogeneity, with any of a large number of possible mutations being seen to inactivate the gene. In this situation, many patients are not true homozygotes but 'compound heterozygotes', with a different mutation being present in each of the two homologous genes. Different combinations of mutations can result in disease of varying severity if some mutations are not completely 'null', for example if they only result in partial deficiency of an enzyme. This may allow some attempt at correlating molecular pathology with clinical severity, particularly in metabolic disorders, for which the enzyme deficiency can usually be measured more or less precisely. Individual mutations are usually referred to using the single letter amino acid code and the residue number; thus C163S represents the aspartylglucosaminuria mutation referred to above.

Allelic heterogeneity in most recessive diseases greatly complicates the task of DNA analysis. It is rarely feasible for a clinical laboratory to search for a large number of mutations, since in general each mutation requires a separate assay. This means that if no biochemical method for carrier testing or prenatal diagnosis is available, then it is necessary to rely on analyzing the family by use of linked DNA polymorphisms (see below and Fig. 1.8.1). There are exceptions to this, in the form of a few disorders where one mutation predominates in a particular racial group. For example, in Anglo-Saxon populations some 85% of mutations causing hereditary fructose intolerance (hepatic

aldolase B deficiency, MIM 229600) are A149P,[8] and 89% of alleles causing MCAD (medium chain acyl CoA dehydrogenase) deficiency (MIM 201450) have a point mutation causing the substitution K304E.[9] This makes a search for these specific mutations worthwhile. However, it should be apparent that failure to find one of these mutations cannot be used to exclude the diagnosis. This general consideration limits the accuracy of population screening for carriers of common autosomal recessive disorders, in particular, in the UK, for cystic fibrosis (CF). In Scotland the five commonest mutations causing CF are: ΔF508 (73%), G551D (6.5%), G542X (3.5%) and R117H (1%).[10] Even together, these mutations only account for 84% of all CF alleles, and failure to find any of them still leaves a risk of about 1 in 160 of being a carrier. Nonetheless, because of the recessive inheritance of the condition, if a couple both screen negative for these mutations, the chance that both still carry unknown CF mutations is reduced to 1 in 26 000, and the predicted frequency of CF in the screened group's offspring to less than 1 in 100 000, compared to 1 in 2300 in the unscreened population. Population screening for carriers of recessive diseases can thus be effective even if the technology does not allow 100% detection rates.

X-linked inheritance

The cardinal feature which distinguishes X-linked from autosomal inheritance is that father to son transmission cannot occur in the former. On the other hand, *all* daughters of a male carrying an X-linked mutation will inherit the mutation from their father.

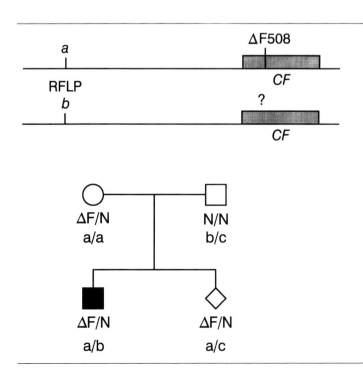

Fig. 1.8.1 *A simple example to show how both mutation analysis and linkage analysis (or 'indirect gene tracking') may be used to allow prenatal diagnosis of a genetic disorder which shows allelic heterogeneity. In the top part of the figure are shown both copies of the chromosomal region including the cystic fibrosis (CF) gene, in an affected child. A ΔF508 mutation has been found on one CF allele, but the other mutation is unknown (?). A nearby DNA sequence shows polymorphism, and the affected boy is heterozygous for two alleles a and b. Since the b allele of the polymorphism will be passed on together with the CF gene bearing the unknown mutation, it can be used to follow that mutation within this family only. This is shown in the small pedigree below. The ΔF508 mutation can be seen to have come from the patient's mother (along with the a allele of the polymorphism). Correspondingly, the b allele has come from the father along with the unknown mutation. The fetus being analysed at prenatal diagnosis can be seen to have inherited the opposite paternal allele c of the polymorphism. It is therefore highly likely that it has inherited the normal paternal CF gene, and is predicted to be a carrier. The accuracy of this type of analysis is limited by the chance of recombination between the polymorphic marker and the CF gene.*

X Inactivation

In the early female embryo, inactivation of one of the two X chromosomes occurs in every cell. The inactivation of maternal or paternal X appears to occur at random in each cell. However, the choice of inactivated X, once made, is then stably transmitted to all that cell's descendants. X inactivation occurs at an early enough stage of development that the number of cells involved is small. As a result, random variation may allow deviation from the expected 50:50 proportion of cells inactivating the maternal or paternal X. This effect may be more marked if an individual tissue is considered, which may derive from a very small number of progenitor cells at the time of X inactivation. The mature female is thus a mosaic of cells expressing either paternal or maternal X, with a 50:50 ratio expected, but with substantial deviation from this ratio possible. This has important implications for carrier testing in X-linked diseases (see below).

X-linked dominant inheritance

So-called X-linked dominant disorders are manifested in heterozygous females, and therefore may display vertical transmission from mother to daughter. As for autosomal dominant disorders, though, these mutations are not usually truly dominant in the Mendelian sense; hemizygous males are usually more severely affected, often lethally. An example of such a disorder is orofaciodigital syndrome type I (MIM 311200). Affected females have hamartomatous malformations of tongue and often brain, midline pseudo-cleft of the upper lip, hyperplastic oral frenulae, digital anomalies and cystic renal disease. Affected males have lethal malformations and do not survive to term. A similar situation is seen in the neurocutaneous disorder, incontinentia pigmenti (MIM 308310).

X-linked recessive disorders

In contrast to the small group of X-linked dominant conditions, the much commoner situation of a recessive mutation in a gene on the X chromosome results in a disorder affecting only hemizygous males. This group includes important conditions such as hemophilia A and B (MIM 306700 and 306900), Duchenne muscular dystrophy (MIM 310200), and glucose-6-phosphate dehydrogenase (G6PD) deficiency (MIM 305900), as well as two or three hundred other rarer diseases.

Lethal X-linked recessive genes are maintained in a population through ongoing new mutation. If male and female new mutation rates are equal, it can be calculated that one third of isolated cases of such disorders result from new mutations. For disorders which are not always reproductively lethal in the affected male (such as hemophilia), the proportion of new mutations is smaller.[11]

For the clinical geneticist, distinguishing new mutations from inherited cases is of prime importance. Results of classical biochemical assays, such as the factor VIII activity and antigen level in hemophilia, or the serum creatine kinase in Duchenne muscular dystrophy, may correctly identify carriers if results are clearly abnormal, but cannot alone exclude carrier status, since normal values may be seen in a proportion of obligate carriers. This results from the stochastic nature of X inactivation, which may be skewed by chance in favor of activity of the normal X. The normal and carrier ranges for a parameter such as creatine kinase therefore overlap significantly (Fig. 1.8.2).

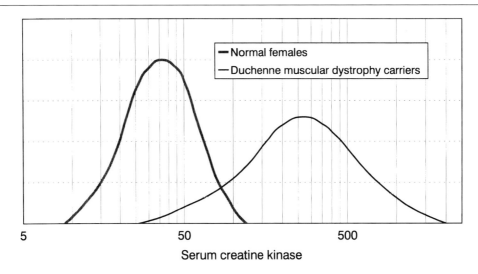

Fig. 1.8.2 *Hypothetical distributions of levels of a parameter such as creatine kinase in obligate carriers of Duchenne muscular dystrophy. The X axis is logarithmic. Some carriers by chance inactivate predominantly their affected X chromosome. They therefore have CK values in the normal range, hence the overlap with the non-carrier distribution. Some will by chance inactivate predominantly the normal X, giving high CK values. This variable pattern of X inactivation gives rise to the much broader distribution of CK values in the carrier than the normal population. Similar considerations apply to other measurable quantities such as the factor VIIIc level in hemophilia.*

The clonal nature of X-inactivation results in the female carrier of a null mutation in an X-linked gene having two populations of cells, those expressing the normal and those expressing the abnormal mutation. It is possible (though in clinical practice unusual) to exploit this fact for carrier testing, by analyzing clonal populations derived from a single cell. For example, carriers of iduronidate sulfate sulfatase (IDS) deficiency (Hunter syndrome; MIM 309900) can be identified by IDS assay on colonies, each cloned from a single skin fibroblast; such colonies have either normal or deficient IDS activity, depending on which X was inactivated in the cell from which they originated. The same principle of clonal analysis allows reasonably accurate testing by IDS assay of individual hair-roots from the suspected carrier of Hunter syndrome.[12]

In female carriers of some X-linked recessive conditions (e.g. Wiskott–Aldrich syndrome, MIM 301000[13]) a skewed pattern of X-inactivation in some tissues is seen more often than expected by chance. This may result from selection against cells (in this case lymphocytes) which have inactivated the normal X (Fig. 1.8.3). When such a pattern is documented (by studies of DNA methylation on the inactivated X), it may serve as a useful indicator of carrier status in that disorder .[13]

By far the most powerful general method of assessing carrier status in most families is by DNA analysis. This may be based either on direct detection of mutations, or more generally, by linkage study (gene tracking) of the wider family. Most of the significant X-linked disorders have now been mapped, allowing in the majority of cases the use of tightly linked microsatellite polymorphisms for carrier testing and prenatal diagnosis. This approach depends on there being enough pedigree information available to allow assignment of phase between the polymorphism and the disease gene (see below). However, phase can often be established from analysis of normal males in a family, even if the affected index case is not available.

Genomic imprinting

It is known from studies of mouse embryos containing two haploid genomes derived from one parent (gynogenetic or androgenetic) that specific abnormalities of development result, despite the presence of a normal diploid number of chromosomes. This suggests that paternal and maternal genomes are not equivalent, but undergo specific modifications during gametogenesis (imprinting) which specify the functions of some genes in a parental sex-specific way.[14, 15] In man, the effects of genomic imprinting can be revealed at the level of the whole chromosome by the occasional occurrence of uniparental disomy. This describes the situation in which both copies of one chromosome are derived from the same parent, perhaps by non-disjunction followed by post-zygotic loss of the chromosome from the other parent. In some cases (e.g. maternal uniparental disomy for chromosome 22) this is without effect, perhaps suggesting that no indispensible imprinted genes are present on that chromosome.[16] In other cases, reproducible patterns of abnormality result, the best known of which is the Prader–Willi syndrome (MIM 176270), which can

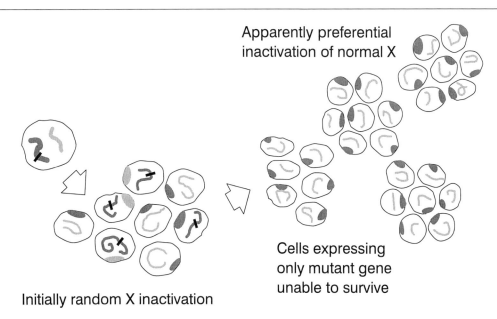

Apparently preferential inactivation of normal X

Cells expressing only mutant gene unable to survive

Initially random X inactivation

Fig. 1.8.3 *So-called 'non-random' X inactivation developing in a female carrier of an X-linked recessive disorder as a result of selection against cells expressing the mutation. Initially, inactivation (shown in the cartoon as condensation to a Barr body) of the mutated X (dark grey) and the normal X (light grey) occurs in early embryogenesis, at random. This leads to two populations of descendent cells, one expressing the normal gene and one the mutant gene. If the gene product in question is required for cell viability, the second of these populations will be selected against, leaving only the cells which have inactivated the mutant X. Since an inactivated X chromosome becomes heavily methylated, analysis in the DNA laboratory of polymorphisms and methylation on the X chromosome can detect this skewed X inactivation pattern, which may serve as a marker of the carrier state in some disorders.*

result from maternal uniparental disomy of chromosome 15.[17] Paternal uniparental disomy of the same chromosome gives an entirely different phenotype, Angelman syndrome (MIM 234400;[18]). Since each of these syndromes can also be produced by a microdeletion of a critical region of 15q (on a paternal chromosome in the case of Prader–Willi, maternal for Angelman), loss of function of, respectively, either the paternal or maternal copy of only one or a very few genes would appear to underlie the phenotype. This again suggests that the number of imprinted genes (and certainly the number of imprinted regions) is probably rather small, since if many dispersed genes were subject to imprinting, uniparental disomy of the whole of the chromosome would be expected to have diverse other effects. Similarly, if there were hundreds of imprinted genes, uniparental disomy for a whole chromosome such as 22 would be very unlikely to be without adverse outcome.

The physiological importance of genomic imprinting is uncertain, but one hypothesis holds that its evolution could be driven by the differing selective pressures on maternal and paternal genomes.[19] This idea derives in part from the fact that one important fetal growth-regulating gene (insulin-like growth factor II, *IGF2*) is expressed only from the paternal genome during development.[20-22] Thus paternal uniparental disomy for the region 11p13 (containing *IGF2*) results in fetal overgrowth as a result of *IGF2* over-expression. This can at least partly account for the phenotype in Beckwith syndrome (macrosomia, organomegaly, exomphalos and other features).[23] Whereas increased fetal size may favor transmission of the paternal genome, by improving neonatal survival in some environments, it is clearly in contrast in the mother's evolutionary interests to *restrict* fetal growth, so as to maximize her own chances of surviving delivery and producing further offspring. These different selective pressures could perhaps drive evolution of a genetic mechanism by which maternal and paternal genomes have opposing influences on fetal growth.

Unstable DNA

Dispersed around the human genome are many regions of DNA characterized by simple repetitive sequences. Among these are trinucleotide repeats such as $(CAG)_n$ and $(CGG)_n$. Although often within introns, such repetitive elements may also be found within the exons of genes (such as *FMR1*, the fragile X syndrome gene, and *DMK*, the protein kinase gene involved in myotonic dystrophy, MIM 160900) and even within the coding region (e.g. of the androgen receptor, and of the IT15 ('huntingtin') gene involved in Huntington's disease. Most such repetitive sequences display polymorphic variability in repeat number; for example in *FMR1* the CGG repeat number in normal individuals may be anything from 6 to 46. These variants are usually stably transmitted from parent to child. However, if a certain size limit is exceeded (different for each individual repeat), size instability during vertical transmission begins to be observable, with a change in repeat number (often an increase) on passing from parent to child. There may be a sex bias in the likelihood of repeat size changing. For example in Huntington's disease repeat

expansion is more likely to occur when a father transmits a large repeat to a child than when a mother with a repeat of the same size passes it on. Conversely, in fragile X syndrome, large changes in repeat size are seen only when the mother is the transmitting parent. Southern blotting is very effective at detecting the large size changes associated with fragile X mutation (Fig. 1.8.4).

The mechanism by which instability develops probably differs in different disorders. Although the parental sex-specificity would seem to suggest a meiotic event (since male and female meiosis are so different) for the fragile X CGG repeat (the best studied case) the evidence points towards expansion from premutation to full mutation occurring postzygotically, during a particular temporal window of early embryonic development.[24] This observation suggests that there must be an additional parent-specific modification of the chromosome (a type of imprinting) which makes paternal and maternal X distinguishable during early embryogenesis, and makes only the latter susceptible to *FMR1* CGG repeat instability. For some other disorders, including Huntington's disease and SCA1 (see below), repeat instability probably develops in meiosis, since somatic variation is not seen in the tissues of affected individuals, whereas expansion is seen on direct analysis of sperm DNA, so that affected males produce sperm carrying a range of different repeat sizes.[25]

Fragile X syndrome (MIM 309550)

The CGG repeat lies within the untranslated region of exon 1 of the *FMR1* gene.[26] The normal size range (no instability) is 6–46 repeats. Instability on maternal transmission is observed with increasing frequency within the range 50–200 repeats, with the sigmoidal curve closely approaching 100% probability above 90–95 repeats.[27,28] However, within this range (the so-called premutation) there are no phenotypic effects, even on males, who will transmit such premutations to all their daughters, usually without change in size. Thus, as in classical X-linked genetics, all daughters of a male with a premutation are carriers themselves, and may have affected children. However, their fathers are in this case 'normal transmitting males', whose existence in fragile X pedigrees was appreciated but not understood for many years prior to the identification of the fragile X mutation.[29] The risk of expansion from premutation to full mutation depends not just on repeat length, but on sequence variation (presence of AGG triplets) within the CGG repeat.[30] Long arrays of CGG repeats uninterrupted by AGG triplets confer the highest risk. This principle also applies to instability of the *SCA1* repeat (see below).[31]

The functional effect of a full fragile X mutation is transcriptional silencing of *FMR1* on that chromosome, associated with abnormal DNA methylation around the first exon. Neither methylation nor silencing of *FMR1* occurs in the presence of a premutation.[32] The fact that loss of *FMR1* function is the key event is shown by rare patients who have a fragile X phenotype without CGG repeat expansion, but instead have deletions or point mutations of *FMR1*.[33,34]

Three other cytogenetic fragile sites (*FRAXE*, *FRAXF* and *FRA16A*) also result from expansion of CGG repeat sequences.

(a)

(b)

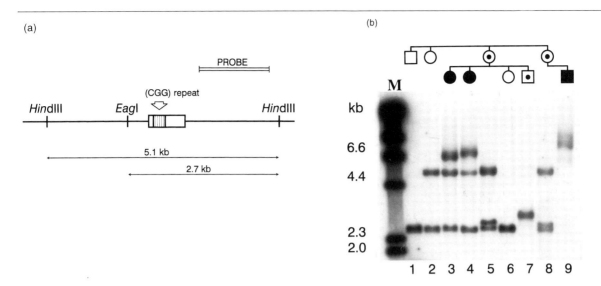

Fig. 1.8.4 *Southern blotting to detect the transmission of fragile X within a family. (a) shows the positions of the restriction sites ana-lyzed. DNA is cut with a combination of HindIII and EagI. On the X chromosome of a normal male this generates a 2.7 kb fragment. On an inactivated X chromosome in a normal female, methylation prevents cleavage by the methylation-sensitive enzyme EagI, thus gen-erating a 5.1 kb fragment. Normal females (lane 2 of (b)) thus have a 2.7 kb and a 5.1 kb band. Expansion of the CGG repeat into the premutation range causes a small increase in size of the fragments (lanes 5, 7, 8) but has no effect on methylation. Expansion to full mutation is accompanied not only by large increase in size, but also by methylation of the mutated X (in male or female) and by smear-ing as a result of somatic variation in repeat size. Thus no unmethylated fragments corresponding to full mutations are seen in either males or females. The blot shows a family in which two sisters (lanes 5 and 8) are both premutation carriers (small increase in band size, clearly seen in the unmethylated fragments). Expansion to full mutation has occurred in the two daughters (lanes 3 and 4) as shown by the large methylated fragments in addition to the normal fragment corresponding to their unaffected X. In the son in lane 7, slight expansion of the premutation has occurred, but it has remained in the (unmethylated) premutation range. This boy is a 'normal trans-mitting male'. The son of the second sister (lane 9) is affected, with a full mutation. M=marker lane. (Courtesy of Lisa Strain, Human Genetics Unit, University of Edinburgh.)*

Other disorders

Myotonic dystrophy (MIM 160900)

Expansion of a CAG trinucleotide repeat in the 3′ untrans-lated region of a protein kinase gene on chromosome 19q is seen in patients with myotonic dystrophy.[35] The repeat expands on transmission by both male and female, and its size correlates with disease severity, with the largest repeats seen in congenitally affected individuals. Small expansions are seen in mildly affected or asymptomatic gene carriers. Progressive expansion with succeeding generations under-lies the frequent observation of 'anticipation' (see above) in families with myotonic dystrophy.[2] There are sex differ-ences in the expansion probability on transmission of myotonic dystrophy mutations,[36] but as yet no completely satisfying explanation for the almost exclusive maternal inheritance of the congenital form of the disease.

Huntington's disease (HD; MIM 143100)

A CAG repeat within the coding region of the IT15 or 'huntingtin' gene is expanded in patients with HD.[37] In striking contrast to fragile X, the cut-off between normal range (6–34 repeats) and affected individuals is very fine, with the smallest mutation seen in the Edinburgh series

being 36 repeats[38] (Fig. 1.8.5). This clearly reflects differ-ences in disease mechanism; as mentioned above, HD expansions may be true dominant mutations; deletion of the HD gene in patients with Wolf–Hirschorn syndrome (del[4p]) does not cause HD. There is some correlation between mutation size and disease severity, with the largest mutations tending to be associated with early onset or juve-nile HD.[39] The mutations are only moderately unstable, with changes of one or two repeats being commonest. Larger jumps (up to 10 or 12 repeats) are occasionally seen, usually on transmission from an affected father. This may explain the paternal inheritance of juvenile HD.

Spinocerebellar ataxia type 1 (olivopontocerebellar degeneration; SCA1; MIM 164400)

This dominantly inherited disorder results from CAG repeat expansion in an HLA-linked gene on chromosome 6p. There is strong negative correlation between the size of the mutation and the age of onset and severity of the dis-ease,[40] an effect also seen in DRPLA and Machado–Joseph disease (see below).

Dentatorubropallidoluysian atrophy (DRPLA; MIM 125370)

Another neurodegenerative disease originally described in

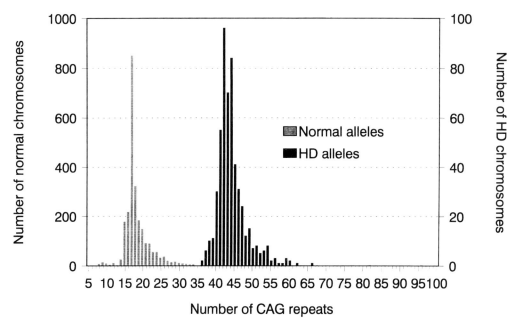

Fig. 1.8.5 *The Huntington's disease mutation. The x axis shows the number of CAG repeats in the HD gene and the y axis the number of individual alleles with each repeat size. Two populations are shown, normal individuals (light grey) and individuals with HD (dark grey), for whom only the affected allele has been scored. Normal HD genes have 8–34 repeats. Remarkably, there is a very fine line between normal and affected, with 36 repeats being the smallest seen in an affected individual. However, there is no overlap between normal and affected. Data from Scottish populations, analyzed in Edinburgh (courtesy of Jon Warner and Lilias Barron, Human Genetics Unit, University of Edinburgh).*

Japanese families and felt to be very rare, this condition results from expansion of a CAG repeat in a gene on chromosome 12p.[41] Preliminary results suggest that expansion of this repeat (which encodes a polyglutamine stretch) may be discovered in some patients with other diagnostic labels, and its true frequency is as yet unknown.

Machado–Joseph disease (MIM 109150)

This is a form of spinocerebellar ataxia whose frequency again appears greater than originally thought. It too results from a CAG repeat expansion causing enlargement of a polyglutamine sequence, within a protein of unknown function, for which the gene is on chromosome 14q.[42]

Kennedy's disease (spinal and bulbar muscular atrophy, partial androgen resistance)

A polyglutamine stretch encoded by a CAG repeat in exon 1 of the androgen receptor gene on Xq11-q12 is normally 17–26 amino acids long. Patients with Kennedy's disease have about double the usual number of CAG repeats. The alteration of androgen receptor structure results in a subtle degree of androgen resistance (late onset gynecomastia, impotence, infertility) and in some way also degeneration of spinal and bulbar motor neurones.[43]

It is striking that all of the unstable DNA disorders thus far described primarily affect the nervous system. From the brief descriptions above, it is clear that more than one biochemical mechanism (e.g. transcriptional effects vs. altered protein structure) is involved, but the emergence of a more detailed picture, particularly of the role of polyglutamine tracts in neural proteins, is awaited with interest.

Genetic diagnosis by linkage (gene tracking)

It is fortunately not necessary to identify the mutation causing a disease in order to perform DNA based diagnostic testing. The genome is rich in DNA segments which display polymorphic variation. Although always present at the same position on a particular chromosome, these sequences show some degree of variability when a number of individual allelic chromosomes are compared. The commonest and in practical use the most valuable type of polymorphism is known as a microsatellite. It consists of a short array of repeated simple sequences, most commonly based on a CA dinucleotide (i.e. CACACACACACA...), but sometimes on a tri- or tetranucleotide monomer. Microsatellites are widely dispersed in the genome, and vary in length (number of repeats) between individuals and between the two chromosomal homologues carried by one person. Since (with occasional exceptions; see unstable DNA above) the different length variants (or *alleles*) are stably inherited, they can be used to follow the inheritance of that particular chromosomal segment through a family. A microsatellite polymorphism close to or within a disease gene can similarly be used to follow the inheritance of the mutation (the precise nature of which may be unknown) *within that family.* Enough information must be assembled from the family to allow the determination of which microsatellite allele marks the presence of the mutation; this is known as *phase determination.* This information is usually most easily obtained from the affected individual(s), and the lack of key family studies (e.g. due to failure to store material from a deceased individual) can render the study difficult or impossible. It is important to appreciate that the same microsatellite allele may also occur on a chromosome not carrying a mutation, and similarly in a different family a mutation may occur on a chromosome carrying a different allele of the polymorphism. The polymorphism is simply an indirect indicator of the inheritance of the region containing the mutation of interest, within one family. Two simple examples of linkage analysis for an X-linked disorder are shown in Fig. 1.8.6.

The accuracy of linkage studies is limited by the occurrence of recombination, the exchange of DNA between homologous chromosomes which occurs during meiosis. Recombination between the gene of interest and the marker being used for tracking it will result in an error of interpretation if its occurrence is not appreciated (Fig. 1.8.7). This risk can be minimized by use of markers very close to or within the gene of interest, or by the general approach of using flanking markers, one on each side of the gene. In the latter case, recombination between marker and gene will then be detected as a recombination between the two flanking markers.

Less amenable to technical solutions is the problem of genetic (or *locus*) heterogeneity. This refers to a situation in which the same phenotype may be produced by mutations of two or more different genes. In order to perform diagnosis by genetic linkage, the involvement of a particular gene must be assumed, and since the mutation itself is not characterized, this assumption is not verified by the labora-tory study. Incorrect conclusions will be drawn if the disease in the family under study turns out to result from mutation of a different gene. An example of this situation is tuberous sclerosis, which can result from mutation in a gene on chromosome 16p (TSC2; MIM 191092), whereas in other families a gene on chromosome 9q appears to be responsible (TSC1; MIM 191100). Similarly, adult polycystic kidney disease (MIM 173900) results in 85–90% of cases from mutation in a gene on 16p, but another gene, on chromosome 4q (*PKD2*; MIM 173910) is involved in a minority of families with a clinically indistinguishable disease.

FUTURE PERSPECTIVES

Large-scale mapping and sequencing projects underway will eventually provide complete structural information on the human genome. Automation of various molecular genetic techniques is becoming more and more common, and the amount of published DNA sequence has grown almost exponentially (300 million bp as of April 1995). More efficient methods for scanning for mutations are also awaited, perhaps based on technologies derived from the microprocessor industry, which allow immobilization of matrices of oligonucleotides of defined sequence on small 'DNA chips'.[44] The hope is that such advances may allow facile detection of mutations for all patients with genetic disease, even where there is great allelic heterogeneity.

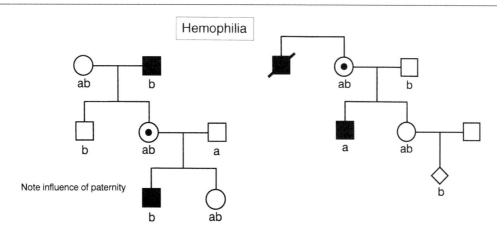

Hemophilia

Note influence of paternity

Fig. 1.8.6 *Use of polymorphism close to the factor VIII gene to study inheritance of a hemophilia A mutation in two families. In the first family ('phase known') the affected father has passed on his hemophilia mutation along with a b allele of the polymorphism, to his oblig-ate carrier daughter. Therefore the phase (see text) is certain; the carrier daughter's a allele is on her normal chromosome, the b on the X carrying the mutation. She has passed the b and the mutation both to her affected son, and to her daughter, who is therefore predicted to be a carrier. However, note the following. (1) We have to deduce that the carrier mother passed b to her daughter from the fact that her husband is a and the daughter is ab. If the paternity were not as indicated (i.e. if the girl's true biological father were b) this deduction would be erroneous. (2) Recombination could have occurred between the RFLP and the mutation, in the meiosis producing the carrier woman's daughter. This again would cause an error in diagnosis. In the second family, the phase between RFLP and mutation has to be deduced from the fact that the carrier mother passed a to her affected son along with the mutation. This however could have been the result of meiotic recombination between the maternal X chromosomes, so that the true phase might be b on the mother's mutated X, a on the normal X. There is then a further possibility for recombination in the meiosis producing the second child, whose carrier status is in question in this situation. The accuracy of the carrier test using this DNA marker is therefore less in the second pedigree compared to the first.*

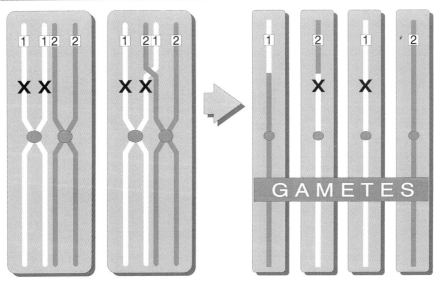

Fig. 1.8.7 *Meiotic recombination as a source of error in linkage analysis. Imagine the individual in question is affected by a dominant genetic disease, the mutation being shown as a cross on one of the chromosomal homologs at meiosis. A polymorphism (shown with alleles 1 and 2) is to be used to follow the mutation. If during meiosis, crossing over occurs as shown between the marker polymorphism and the disease-causing mutation, recombinant gametes will be produced in which the phase relationship between marker and mutation has been reversed, leading to an error of diagnosis.*

Currently the molecular basis of many inherited disorders (mostly the rare single gene defects) remains unknown, yet there are thousands of such disorders, and molecular analysis of each is required for accurate diagnosis, prenatal testing and design of therapeutic research. The genome project will facilitate a rapid change in this situation over the next ten years, by which time I expect rather few of the disorders listed in MIM to be 'unknown' in molecular terms. The majority of the 100 000 or so genes expressed in human tissues will also have been cloned and sequenced by that time[45].

Many of the commoner non-Mendelian disorders have a genetic basis, but space has prevented detailed discussion of this area. Two important groups may be considered: multifactorial diseases where an inborn genetic component(s) contributes to susceptibility to the disorder, and neoplasia. The unraveling of multifactorial predisposition to genetic disease is a complex area (for ischemic heart disease as an example see reference 46). Not only may several genes be involved, but different genes may confer susceptibility in different groups of patients with the same clinical disorder. An example of this situation is type 2 diabetes, a predominantly genetic group of conditions where the genes contributing to

impaired glucose tolerance and insulin resistance are undoubtedly different in different groups of patients.

The bulk of cancer is not inherited, yet myriad different mutations of growth regulatory genes have been found to underlie neoplasia, in all kinds of tumor.[47] The acquisition of mutations by somatic cells during the lifetime of the individual may be viewed as inevitable. The effects of some of these mutations to change growth regulation, causing clonal selection and stepwise acquisition of further mutations, represents another kind of 'polygenic' disorder, though this is somatic cell genetics rather than Mendelian genetics. Germline factors, however, can contribute in important ways to the likelihood of cancer developing. The recent demonstration that familial colon cancer can result from mutations of genes whose normal function is to repair postreplication DNA synthesis errors[48] underscores the fact that successful organisms have evolved efficient mechanisms for protecting themselves against somatic mutation and its neoplastic consequences. The complexity of the many possible genetic factors contributing towards the individual risk of neoplasia, however, means that within the next few years assessment of such risks will remain feasible only in a few families.

SUMMARY

An individual with a dominantly inherited condition has one normal and one mutated gene, with an equal probability of transmission of either of these to offspring.

New mutations are frequently observed for most autosomal dominant conditions.
Incomplete penetrance describes the failure of some individuals who carry such a mutation

to manifest any features of the disease.

A mutation is recessive if it only results in disease when in the homozygous state.

The cardinal feature of X-linked inheritance is that father to son transmission cannot occur.

In the early female embryo, inactivation of one of the two X chromosomes occurs in each cell – apparently at random.

Some genes function differently according to whether they are derived from the father or from the mother (imprinting). In man, the effects of genomic imprinting may be revealed by the occurrence of uniparental disomy.

Several inherited neurological conditions are characterized by the presence of expanded trinucleotide repeats, associated with DNA instability.

REFERENCES

1. McKusick VA. *Mendelian Inheritance in Man*, 11th edn. Baltimore: Johns Hopkins University Press, 1994.
2. Harper PS, Harley HG, Reardon W, Shaw DJ. Anticipation in myotonic dystrophy: new light on an old problem. *Am J Hum Genet* 1992 **51**: 10–16.
3. Bakker E, Veenema H, Den Dunnen JT, van Broeckhoven C, Grootscholten PM, Bonten EJ, van Ommen GJ, Pearson PL. Germinal mosaicism increases the recurrence risk for 'new' Duchenne muscular dystrophy mutations. *J Med Genet* 1989 **26**: 553–559.
4. Byers PH, Tsipouras P, Bonadio JF, Starman BJ, Schwartz RC. Perinatal lethal osteogenesis imperfecta (OI type II): a biochemically heterogeneous disorder usually due to new mutations in the genes for type I collagen. *Am J Hum Genet* 1988 **42**: 237–248.
5. Wilkie AOM. The molecular basis of genetic dominance. *J Med Genet* 1994 **31**: 89–98.
6. Mononen T, Mononen I, Matilainen R, Airaksinen E. High prevalence of aspartylglycosaminuria among school-age children in eastern Finland. *Hum Genet* 1991 **87**: 266–268.
7. Ikonen E, Aula P, Gron K, Tollersrud O, Halila R, Manninen T, Syvanen A-C, Peltonen L. Spectrum of mutations in aspartylglucosaminuria. *Proc Natl Acad Sci USA* 1991 **88**: 11222–11226.
8. Cross NCP, Cox TM. Molecular analysis of aldolase B genes in the diagnosis of hereditary fructose intolerance in the United Kingdom. *Q J Med* 1989 **3**: 1015–1020.
9. Matsubara Y, Narisawa K, Tada K. Medium chain acyl CoA dehydrogenase deficiency: molecular aspects. *Eur J Pediatr* 1992 **151**: 154–159.
10. Shrimpton AE, McIntosh I, Brock DJH. The incidence of different cystic fibrosis mutations in the Scottish population: effects on prenatal diagnosis and genetic counselling. *J Med Genet* 1991 **28**: 317–321.
11. Young ID. *Introduction to Risk Calculation in Genetic Counselling*. Oxford: Oxford University Press, 1991.
12. Nwokoro N, Neufeld EF. Detection of Hunter heterozygotes by enzymatic analysis of hair roots. *Am J Hum Genet* 1979 **31**: 42–49.
13. Fearon ER, Kohn DB, Winkelstein JA, Vogelstein B, Blaese RM. Carrier detection in the Wiskott–Aldrich syndrome. *Blood* 1988 **72**: 1735–1739.
14. Surani MA, Barton SC, Norris ML. Development of reconstituted mouse eggs suggests imprinting of the genome during gametogenesis. *Nature* 1984 **308**: 548–550.
15. McGrath J, Solter D. Completion of mouse embryogenesis requires both the maternal and paternal genomes. *Cell* 1984 **37**: 179–183.
16. Palmer CG, Schwartz S, Hodes ME. Transmission of a balanced homologous t(22q;22q) translocation from mother to normal daughter. *Clin Genet* 1980 **17**: 418–422.
17. Mascari MJ, Gottlieb W, Rogan PK *et al.* The frequency of uniparental disomy in Prader–Willi syndrome: implications for molecular diagnosis. *N Engl J Med* 1992 **326**: 1599–1607.
18. Malcolm S, Clayton-Smith J, Nichols M, Robb S, Webb T, Armour JA, Jeffreys AJ, Pembrey ME. Uniparental paternal disomy in Angelman's syndrome. *Lancet* 1991 **337**: 694–697.
19. Haig D. Genetic conflicts in human pregnancy. *Q Rev Biol* 1993 **68**: 495–532.
20. DeChiara TM, Robertson EJ, Efstratiadis A. Parental imprinting of the mouse insulin-like growth factor II gene. *Cell* 1991 **64**: 849–859.
21. Giannoukakis N, Deal C, Paquette J, Goodyer CG, Polychronakos C. Parental genomic imprinting of the human IGF2 gene. *Nature Genet* 1993 **4**: 98–101.
22. Ohlsson R, Nyström A, Pfeifer-Ohlsson S, Töhönen V, Hedbrog F, Schofield P, Flam F, Ekström TJ. IGF2 is parentally imprinted during human embryogenesis and in the Beckwith–Wiedemann syndrome. *Nature Genet* 1993 **4**: 94–97.
23. Henry I, Bonaiti-Pellié C, Chehensse V, Beldjord C, Schwartz C, Utermann G, Junien C. Uniparental paternal disomy in a genetic cancer-predisposing syndrome. *Nature* 1991 **351**: 665–667.
24. Wöhrle D, Hennig I, Vogel W, Steinbach P. Mitotic instability of fragile X mutations in differentiated cells indicates early post-conceptional trinucleotide repeat expansion. *Nature Genet* 1993 **4**: 140–146.
25. MacDonald ME, Barnes G, Srinidhi J *et al.* Gametic but not somatic instability of CAG repeat length in Huntington's disease. *J Med Genet* 1993 **30**: 982–986.
26. Verkerk AJMH, Pieretti M, Sutcliffe JS *et al.* Identification of a gene (*FMR-1*) containing a CGG repeat coincident with a breakpoint cluster region exhibiting length variation in fragile X syndrome. *Cell* 1991 **65**: 905–914.
27. Oberlé I, Rousseau F, Heitz D *et al.* Instability of a 550-base pair DNA segment and abnormal methylation in fragile X syndrome. *Science* 1991 **252**: 1097–1102.
28. Fu Y-H, Kuhl DPA, Pizzuti A *et al.* Variation of the CGG repeat at the fragile X site results in genetic instability: resolution of the Sherman paradox. *Cell* 1991 **67**: 1047–1058.
29. Yu S, Mulley J, Loesch D *et al.* Fragile-X syndrome: unique genetics of the heritable unstable element. *Am J Hum Genet* 1992 **50**: 968–980.
30. Eichler EE, Holden JJA, Popovich BW *et al.* Length of uninterrupted CGG repeats determines instability in the *FMR1* gene. *Nature Genet* **8**: 88–94.
31. Chung M, Ranum LPW, Duvick LA, Servadio A, Zoghbi HY, Orr HT. Evidence for a mechanism predisposing to intergenerational CAG repeat instability in spinocerebellar ataxia type I. *Nature Genet* 1993 **5**: 254–258.
32. Rousseau F, Heitz D, Biancalana V *et al.* Direct diagnosis by DNA analysis of the fragile X syndrome of mental retardation. *N Engl J Med* 1991 **325**: 1673–1681.
33. Gedeon AK, Baker E, Robinson H *et al.* Fragile X syndrome without CCG amplification has an *FMR1* deletion. *Nature Genet* 1992 **1**: 341–344.
34. De Boulle K, Verkerk AJMH, Reyniers E *et al.* A point mutation in the *FMR-1* gene associated with fragile X mental retardation. *Nature Genet* 1993 **3**: 31–35.
35. Brook JD. *et al.* Molecular basis of myotonic dystrophy: expansion of a trinucleotide (CTG) repeat at the 3′ end of a transcript encoding a protein kinase family member. *Cell* 1992 **68**: 799–808.

36. Lavedan C, Hofman-Radvanyi H, Shelbourne P *et al.* Myotonic dystrophy: size- and sex-dependent dynamics of CTG meiotic instability, and somatic mosaicism. *Am J Hum Genet* 1993 **52**: 875–883.

37. Huntington's Disease Collaborative Research Group. A novel gene containing a trinucleotide repeat that is expanded and unstable on Huntington's disease chromosomes. *Cell* 1993 **72**: 971–983.

38. Barron LH, Warner JP, Porteous M, Holloway S, Simpson S, Davidson R, Brock DJH. A study of the Huntington's disease associated trinucleotide repeat in the Scottish population. *J Med Genet* 1993 **30**: 1003–1007.

39. Snell RG, MacMillan JC, Cheadle JP *et al.* Relationship between trinucleotide repeat expansion and phenotypic variation in Huntington's disease. *Nature Genet* 1993 **4**: 393–397.

40. Orr HT, Chung M, Banfi S *et al.* Expansion of an unstable trinucleotide CAG repeat in spinocerebellar ataxia type I. *Nature Genet* 1993 **4**: 221–226.

41. Nagafuchi S, Yanagisawa H, Sato K *et al.* Dentatorubral and pallidoluysian atrophy expansion of an unstable CAG trinucleotide on chromosome 12p. *Nature Genet* 1994 **6**: 14–18.

42. Kawaguchi Y, Okamoto T, Taniwaki M *et al.* CAG expansions in a novel gene for Machado-Joseph disease at chromosome 14q32.1. *Nature Genet* 1994 **8**: 221–227.

43. La Spada AR, Wilson EM, Lubahn DB, Harding AE, Fishbeck KH. Androgen receptor gene mutations in X-linked spinal and bulbar muscular atrophy. *Nature* 1991 **352**: 77–79.

44. Pease AC, Solas D, Sullivan EJ, Cronin MT, Holmes CP, Fodor SP. Light-generated oligonucleotide arrays for rapid DNA sequence analysis. *Proc Natl Acad Sci USA* 1994 **91**: 5022–5026.

45. The Genome Directory. *Nature* 1995 **377** (suppl): 1–379.

46. Humphries SE, Dunning A, Xu CF, Peacock R, Talmud P, Hamsten A. DNA polymorphism studies. Approaches to elucidating multifactorial ischaemic heart disease: the apo B gene as an example. *Ann Med* 1992 **24**: 349–356.

47. Hodgson SV, Maher ER. *A Practical Guide to Human Cancer Genetics*, 1st edn. Cambridge: Cambridge University Press, 1993.

48. Karran P, Bignami M. DNA damage tolerance, mismatch repair and genome instability. *Bioessays* 1994 **16**: 833–839.

Molecular Techniques

PA Robinson and M Wells

INTRODUCTION

The rapid advance in molecular research and diagnosis over recent years has arisen because of the combination of both novel and established techniques. These include: (a) cleavage of DNA at defined sites by restriction enzymes and the application to the identification of genomic DNA polymorphisms (restriction fragment length polymorphisms, RFLPs), (b) the ability to clone and express fragments of DNA of up to 2 Mbp in size in both prokaryotic and eukaryotic cells, (c) the ability to amplify any short segment of DNA (< 30 kbp) providing DNA sequence information is available in flanking regions using the polymerase chain reaction, (d) *in situ* hybridization to identify sites of gene transcription in tissue sections or fluorescence *in situ* hybridization (FISH) to identify chromosomal localization of genes, and (e) the identification of repetitive elements (e.g. microsatellites) in the human genome that occur at regular intervals throughout the genome.[1-4]

A discussion of these techniques will form the basis of this chapter and will be discussed in more detail below. Certain fundamental facts such as the structure of chromosomes, the structure and function of DNA, the transcription into single-stranded messenger RNA (mRNA) and the synthesis of proteins will not be reiterated here. It should be remembered that the orientation of the two strands in double-stranded DNA is antiparallel, which means that when bound together in a helix one reads 5′ to 3′ and the other 3′ to 5′ (see Chapter 1.1).

CURRENT CONCEPTS

Restriction fragment length polymorphisms

Polymorphisms in the human genome may be due to natural variation in the population or the result of either an inherited or somatic mutation. These polymorphisms may be identified in certain instances by the loss or gain of a restriction enzyme motif.

Restriction enzymes are proteins that cleave DNA at specific recognition sequences. The length of the DNA segment that comprises the restriction site can be variable. For example, the restriction enzyme *Not1* has an eight base pair recognition motif, GCGGCCGC, whereas the recognition motif of *Eco*R1 is only six base pairs, GAATTC, and of *Hae*III is four base pairs, GGCC. As expected by statistical chance, *Hae*III will cut DNA at a greater frequency than either *Eco*R1 or *Not1*. Similarly, *Eco*R1 will be expected to cut DNA at a greater frequency than *Not1*.

In order to detect polymorphisms, DNA is digested by one or more restriction enzymes and the DNA separated by size by agarose gel electrophoresis. DNA migrates through the gel at a rate inversely proportional to its molecular size. Smaller DNA fragments will therefore travel further than larger molecules. The lack of restriction site in a segment of DNA will be reflected by the presence of a single band in the place of two smaller bands. DNA in the gel can be visualized and photographed in the gel by staining with ethidium bromide. This stain intercalates into the double-stranded DNA and fluoresces under ultraviolet light. When a complex mixture of DNA is being investigated and the segment of DNA of interest constitutes only a fraction of the total DNA it is not possible using ethidium bromide staining to identify a shift in size that is the result of a polymorphism. The technique of Southern blotting is employed.

Southern blotting (Fig. 1.9.1)

Southern blotting relies on the recognition of a particular segment of DNA in a complex mixture by binding its complementary sequence that is labeled with an easily identified probe, e.g. radioactivity. DNA is transferred from the agarose gel to a solid support such as nitrocellulose or a charged nylon membrane. The use of nylon membranes

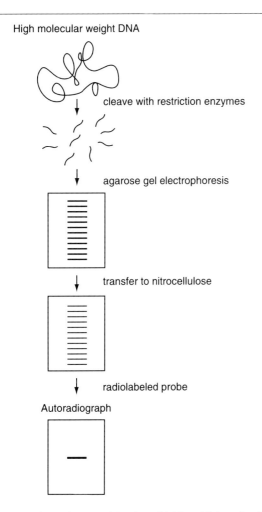

High molecular weight DNA

cleave with restriction enzymes

agarose gel electrophoresis

transfer to nitrocellulose

radiolabeled probe

Autoradiograph

Fig. 1.9.1 *The technique of Southern blotting. High-molecular-weight DNA is cleaved with one or more restriction enzymes. The resulting smaller molecules are separated according to size by agarose gel electrophoresis. The gel is laid on a nitrocellulose membrane and through the capillary action of a high salt solution, the DNA fragments are transferred to the membrane to which they bind electrostatically. Baking or treatment by ultraviolet light results in permanent fixing to the membrane. The 'Southern blot' is then exposed to a radioactively labeled probe which only hybridizes to specific restriction fragments. These can be localized subsequently using autoradiography.*

ture but also on other physical characteristics of the solution such as ion concentration and pH. Inter-strand bonding is promoted by increasing the salt concentration in the hybridization mixture. The presence of mis-matched base pairs in the double-stranded DNA will result in an instability of the product with respect to the perfectly matched alternative. The mis-matching will result in a lowering of the melting temperature under high stringency wash conditions. Therefore, by manipulating the temperature and salt concentration of the hybridization solution, i.e. by altering the stringency of the solution, it is possible to selectively cause the dissociation of mis-matched pairs compared to perfectly matched pairs.

Labeled DNA complementary to the region of DNA of interest will bind to this DNA sequence on the Southern blot. Methods of labeling DNA include radiolabeling, fluorescent labelling, enzyme labeling (alkaline phosphatase or peroxidase) and biotin labeling. DNA for labeling can be of any size, from small oligonucleotides, to complementary or copy DNA (cDNA) of a few hundred to a few thousand base pairs to genomic DNA megabases in size.

DNA cloning

In order to generate large quantities of DNA for techniques such as DNA labeling, sequencing, mutation and expression studies, fragments of DNA can be cloned into a variety of vectors.[5] The choice of vector/host system will depend on a number of different factors. These include: (a) the efficiency of the cloning procedure, (b) size of DNA to be cloned, (c) the need to generate RNA transcripts and protein corresponding to the cloned insert, (d) the necessity of generating post-translational modifications – the use of prokaryotic versus eukaryotic systems, (e) generation of single-stranded DNA for sequencing and DNA mutation, (f) the requirement for directional cloning, and (g) removal of intronic sequences.

Many different systems are now available. Furthermore, over the past decade they have become much more adaptable to include as many of the above requirements as possible in one vector. Vectors are available that are capable of being replicated in both eukaryotic and prokaryotic cells (shuttle vectors). The most adaptable such as the lambda ZAP Express™ vector (Stratagene), fulfill this requirement as well as many of those described above. Phagemids may be excised from these bacteriophage vectors *in vivo* and therefore remove the necessity for subcloning of the insert. One major drawback with these vectors is that the size of the DNA fragment to be cloned is generally less than 10 kbp. In order to clone larger fragments, cosmid (10–40 kbp) or yeast artificial chromosomes (100–2000 kbp) can be employed. Although the flexibility of these latter two vector systems is much more restricted, they replicate faithfully the cloned insert which is often genomic DNA.

If the material to be cloned is double-stranded (ds) DNA then the first step of the procedure is to digest it with restriction enzymes such as *Eco*R1 or *Bam*H1, that will generate ends that are compatible with those of a similarly digested vector. In contrast, the DNA may be digested

has generally superseded the use of nitrocellulose because of their higher nucleic acid binding capacity and greater mechanical strength. The hydrogen bonds between the two DNA strands attached to the membrane are broken by treatment with sodium hydroxide. Northern blotting refers to the same procedure except that RNA is transferred from the agarose gel to the solid support (see Chapter 1.1).

The presence of a specific fragment of DNA is determined using the technique of hybridization. Complementary single strands of DNA will reform double-stranded DNA (re-anneal) after denaturation under conditions of high stringency. The conditions under which the two strands dissociate is not only dependent on tempera-

with two different restriction enzymes. In this way the DNA can be 'directionally cloned'. Cohesive ends may also be generated using different restriction enzymes that generate the same overhang. For example digestion of genomic DNA with *Bgl* II (*A*GATC*T*) and *Bam*H1 (*G*GATC*C*) will both generate overhangs of GATC. However, cloning the Bgl II DNA fragments into a BamH1 digested vector will not re-create either the *Bam* H1 or the *Bgl* II restriction site. Similarly, dsDNA can be cut with restriction enzymes that generate blunt ends. These fragments can then be cloned into vector DNA that has been cut with the same or different restriction enzymes that also generate blunt-ended DNA. It should be noted, however, that the efficiency of cloning blunt-ended fragments is much less than cloning of cohesive ends. Further minor differences in approach include the use of partial digests. For example, the digestion with the restriction endonuclease *Sau*3A for differing periods of time is often used to generate a genomic DNA library. DNA is then size selected by agarose gel electrophoresis and cloned into a vector with compatible ends, e.g. *Bam*H1 digested vector.

If messenger RNA (mRNA) is the starting material for the cloning procedure then a number of steps have to be performed to generate clonable ds DNA. The first step, which is generally considered to be the most critical, is to reverse transcribe polyadenylated mRNA into single-stranded DNA. mRNA makes up approximately 1–5% of the total RNA population, the majority (approximately 90%) is ribosomal (r) RNA. The use of purified mRNA for this procedure is no longer necessary as the second generation of reverse transcriptases that are now available are not as sensitive to inhibition by impurities such as ribosomal RNA, e.g. murine Moloney leukemia virus reverse transcriptase.[5] These reverse transcriptases require a primer to initiate the reverse transcription. Generally the primer is constructed from a stretch of thymidine bases (oligo(dT)$_n$, $n=12–18$ residues)) such that it will prime from the polyadenylated tail of the mRNA. At the 5′ end of this primer a sequence of bases is often chemically attached that when turned into dsDNA will generate a restriction endonuclease site. These primers are often known as primer-adaptors. The presence of this site facilitates directional cloning into the vector of choice. dsDNA is generated from the single-stranded (ss) DNA–mRNA duplex using a combination of Rnase H and DNA polymerase 1. Rnase H has a specificity for RNA bound to DNA and generates a series of small oligonucleotide primers still bound to the ssDNA. These primers serve to initiate second-strand synthesis by the DNA polymerase 1. After generating blunt-ended DNA using a brief incubation with T4 DNA polymerase, DNA linkers are attached to each end of the dsDNA. These linkers are dsDNA molecules of small size (8–12 bp) designed to include a restriction enzyme site. Attaching them to the ends of the dsDNA attaches a restriction endonuclease site. The linkered DNA is then digested with a combination of restriction endonucleases. They correspond to the restriction site of the added linker and to the site located at the 5′ end of the primer-adaptor used for first strand synthesis. Internal restriction endonuclease sites may be protected by methylation prior

to linker ligation. After size fractionation of the cDNA, which also removes excess linkers, dscDNA is cloned into the vector of choice.

An alternative to the second-strand synthesis procedure described above, is to generate dscDNA from the reverse transcribed ss cDNA using the polymerase chain reaction (see below). This approach is particularly useful when the quantities of RNA are limited. The reverse transcribed mRNA strand is removed by alkaline hydrolysis. A string of deoxyguanosine residues is then added at the 3′ end of the sscDNA using terminal transferase. Two polymerase chain reaction (PCR) primers complementary to the sequences located at the 5′ (oligo(dT) primer-adaptor) and 3′ (oligo(dG)) ends of the ssDNA are then employed in a standard PCR reaction. Care must be taken with this procedure first to size fractionate the cDNA prior to amplification as PCR preferentially amplifies smaller products and secondly to increase the length of the extension time used in the PCR reaction to take into account the larger ss cDNA moieties present in the complex mixture.

These procedures can be used to clone a single DNA fragment or to generate a 'library' of different DNA fragments.

Polymerase chain reaction (PCR) (Fig. 1.9.2)

DNA or RNA identification in solution

This Nobel Prize winning technique, first described in 1985, has had a dramatic effect on the development of

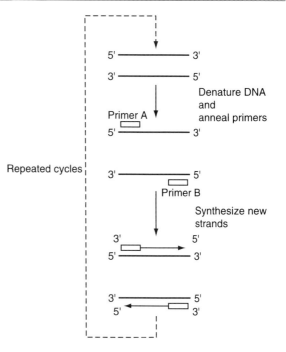

Fig. 1.9.2 *Schematic diagram of the polymerase chain reaction (see text for details).*

molecular biology and its applicability to the routine diagnostic laboratory.[6,7] The technique permits the analysis of DNA or RNA from any source and is potentially capable of amplifying DNA from a single cell.

In the diagnostic laboratory, the detection of very small amounts of DNA in clinical samples is of particular importance with regard to infections such as HPV and HIV. Because PCR is so sensitive, meticulous laboratory technique is essential to avoid contamination by previously amplified DNA. Furthermore, great care must be taken not to over-interpret a positive result. A positive reaction indicates the presence of DNA not its location. For example, the presence of virus in a sample does not indicate its cellular location; it may be bound non-specifically to a cell surface and not located intracellularly. The location of the virus would be confirmed by a technique such as *in situ* hybridization (see below).

For most diagnostic PCR procedures, DNA fragments of less than 1000 bp in size are amplified, although it is possible to amplify DNA of up to 10 kbp using standard procedures. Using modifications of the enzyme mixes and reaction conditions of standard PCR, DNA up to 30 kbp in size can be amplified. This procedure is known as long PCR.

One of the major attractions of PCR besides its sensitivity is its technical simplicity and the possibility of amplifying many samples simultaneously. A small proportion of DNA is placed in a tube. Two oligonucleotide primers are added at a molar concentration in vast excess to the DNA sequences that are to be amplified. These primers have DNA sequences that are complementary to sequences that flank the region of DNA to be amplified. A thermostable DNA polymerase (e.g. Taq polymerase) is added and the mixture is briefly heated (0.5–1.0 min) to the melting temperature of DNA, approximately 95°C, at which temperature DNA dissociates into its constituent single strands. The solution is then rapidly cooled to a temperature approximately 5°C below the melting temperature of the oligonucleotide primer(s)–DNA complex. At this temperature the oligonucleotides anneal to DNA where the complementary sequence is found. The temperature of the reaction is then increased to approximately 72°C, the optimum reaction temperature of the polymerase. The oligonucleotides now act as primers for the DNA polymerase which then attaches new deoxynucleotide bases to the 3′ end of the primers that are complementary to those in the strand being replicated. The cycle is repeated, with the amount of DNA doubling each time. After multiple rounds of amplification, the predominant double-stranded DNA species in the sample corresponds to a fragment whose two ends are defined by the 5′ ends of the two primer oligonucleotides. Normally 20–40 cycles are performed in automated thermocycling devices producing a 10^5–10^6 amplification of target DNA within a few hours. Amplified products of known length can be rapidly fractionated according to molecular weight by agarose or acrylamide gel electrophoresis and subsequent staining with ethidium bromide. There is no requirement for radioactive probes or blotting techniques to detect the product although they can be employed to confirm the specificity of the amplification procedure (Fig. 1.9.3).

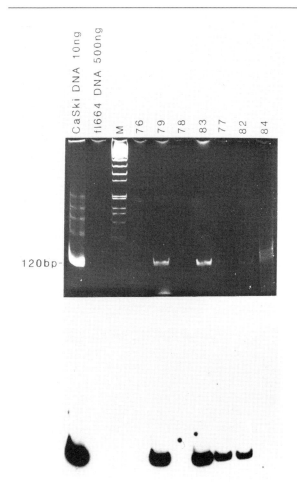

Fig. 1.9.3 *Amplification of DNA isolated from paraffin-wax-embedded cervical tissue with HPV 16-specific oligonucleotide primers. Upper panel: polyacrylamide gel electrophoresis and ethidium bromide staining of products of the polymerase chain reaction on DNA isolated from CaSki cells (HPV 16 positive cervical carcinoma cell line) fetal liver (f1664-negative control) and paraffin-wax-embedded cervical carcinomas (samples 76,79,78, 83,77,82,84). M = DNA size markers. Lower panel: Southern blot of amplified polymerase chain reaction products from the gel, confirming specificity for HPV 16 DNA. Amplified products from gel were electroblotted on to Hybond-N+ membrane (Amersham) and hybridized with an oligonucleotide probe of 40 nucleotides end-labeled with ^{32}P and taken from the region between the two HPV 16 E6 region primers. (Reproduced with permission of the Editor, J Clin Pathol).*

The specificity of the PCR reaction is determined by the sequence of the oligonucleotide primers. The degree of mis-matching that can be tolerated may be increased or decreased by changing the temperature of the reaction and/or the magnesium ion concentration. The remainder of the buffer constituents such as ion concentration must remain constant to preserve enzyme activity. Preliminary experiments are generally performed to establish optimum conditions.

In many instances, confirmation of the presence of specific gene transcripts (i.e. specific mRNA populations) is required, rather than the presence of genomic DNA containing the gene. The oligonucleotide primers can be designed in such a way as to amplify RNA selectively rather than genomic DNA. This is generally achieved by making use of the property that DNA contains introns. These introns are spliced from the mature RNA transcript. Therefore, by designing the primers to cross these intronic splice sites selective amplification is achieved. Amplification of contaminating DNA in the RNA preparations would result in a longer product than would be expected from the RNA sequence. To amplify RNA transcripts by reverse transcription PCR (RT-PCR), a preliminary step in which RNA is converted into single-stranded DNA using a reverse transcriptase (RNA-dependent DNA polymerase) is performed (see above). Murine Moloney leukemia virus reverse transcriptase is often the choice of enzyme for this step because of the reasons stated above and because of its superior stability compared to other reverse transcriptases such as avian myeloblastosis reverse transcriptase. Standard PCR is then employed to amplify the single-stranded cDNA molecules.

A technique that is gaining in its popularity is the 'differential display reverse transcription PCR', (DDRT-PCR).[8,9] This procedure is based on the RNA fingerprinting technique of Liang and Pardee[10] and generates an RNA fingerprint or RNA transcription profile of the RNA population under study. The procedure can be automated and has the major advantage over others such as subtractive hybridization[11] that transcriptional levels of large numbers of mRNA populations can be compared simultaneously and the levels of the majority of polyadenylated RNA moieties are investigated. Differentially expressed genes of interest can be rapidly cloned for further analysis.

There are two essential steps to DDRT-PCR. First, twelve separate reverse transcription reactions are performed using a series of anchored oligo (dT) primers based upon the general sequence oligo (dT).N_1.N_2.N_1 can be any deoxynucleotide base except thymidine whereas N_2 can be any deoxynucleotide. Any anchor primer should result, therefore, in the reverse transcription of, on average, one twelfth of the polyadenylated RNA population. The PCR step is performed using an arbitrary 5′ primer of ten base pairs and the anchor primer that was used for the reverse transcription step. The 26 decamers described by Bauer et al.[8] should result in the amplification of the majority of polyadenylated RNA species. The procedure can be performed in the presence of radiolabeled nucleotide, e.g.[32]P, ^{33}P, ^{35}S or a fluorescent marker can be tagged to the primer for automated analysis. The use of different fluorescent primers for the analysis of different RNA populations permits direct comparison of products in the same lane of a sequencing gel. The PCR procedure is performed at low temperature, 40–42°C, because of the small size of the primers. In order to drive the amplification of a specific target sequence, the six nucleotide bases at the 3′ end of the primer must be complementary to the target.[8] Reaction products from different RNA samples are either run in adjacent lanes of a non-denaturing polyacrylamide gel which is then autoradiographed or analyzed on an automated sequencer. Differentially expressed RNAs are indicated by increased/decreased band intensities. The portion of gel containing DNA bands of interest can then be isolated, PCR amplified and cloned. The number of samples run together is only limited by the number that can be included on the polyacrylamide gel or stored in an ABI sequencer database.

Genetic analysis of genomic DNA isolated from tissue

Cells in histological sections can be selected for DNA amplification by painting them with black ink. The sections can then be irradiated with ultraviolet light which will result in degradation of all DNA except in the areas protected by black ink. Loss of heterozygosity studies (see Chapter 4.5) can then be carried out by DNA extraction and amplification using appropriate primer sequences and the PCR.[12,13]

Mutational analysis

PCR is often used to identify a specific mutation or polymorphism in a gene that causes a given inherited disease in a patient or for analysis of genes in which mutations are suspected but the precise location of the mutation is not known, e.g. mutations in the p53 gene. In both instances DNA of interest is amplified by PCR. The detection of the mutation can be assessed in a number of different ways.

1. The design of the PCR oligonucleotide primers so that only mutated genes are amplified (ARMS, amplification refractory mutation system).[14] One of the PCR oligonucleotide primers is designed such that the nucleotide base at its 3′ end complements the expected mutated nucleotide base. Standard PCR conditions are then employed. Only mutated product is amplified.

2. PCR is performed such that the oligonucleotide PCR primers flank the mutation site. The DNA is then amplified. The mutation can then be identified by either sequencing the amplified product or, if the mutation causes the loss or generation of a restriction endonuclease site, the amplified product can be digested using the appropriate restriction enzyme. The former approach in particular depends on the level of the mutated DNA being present at a level that approximates the level of non-mutated DNA.

3. Single-stranded conformational polymorphism (SSCP) analysis is based on the principle that amplified wild-type and mutant DNA assume different three dimensional conformations when denatured into single strands (Fig. 1.9.4). The single-stranded wild-type and mutant DNA will then demonstrate differential migration in a non-denaturing polyacrylamide gel when electrophoresed side by side. PCR products with altered migration patterns can then be analyzed by DNA sequencing to determine the exact nature of the alteration. SSCP analysis is simple and relatively sensitive and multiple samples may be examined simultaneously. SSCP analysis detects 70–90% of mutations in PCR products of 400 base pairs or less but does not localize them within the fragment[15] (Fig. 1.9.5).

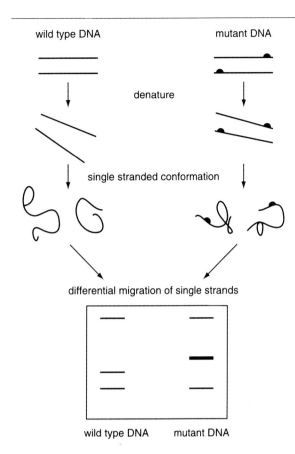

Fig. 1.9.4 *Single-stranded conformational polymorphisms (see text for details).*

In situ hybridization techniques

In situ hybridization has the advantage over techniques such as PCR in that the intracellular location of gene transcription or the cell population where gene transcription is taking place can be identified. It is not as sensitive as PCR, however, and is technically more demanding to perform. The technique may be applied to paraffin-embedded tissue sections, cytological preparations or metaphase spreads of chromosomes.[4]

Paraffin-embedded tissue sections

With labeled probes

Sections under study are hybridized with specific labeled probes and washed using conditions of stringency similar to those employed for Southern or Northern blots. Various precautions have to be taken to avoid sections lifting from glass slides such as the use of aminopropyltriethoxysilane to attach sections firmly to the glass slide prior to processing. Furthermore, sections often have to be treated with enzymes such as proteinase K or pepsin to expose the DNA/RNA for hybridization. The conditions such as enzyme concentration and temperature have to be determined experimentally and tend to be different for different tissues.

DNA or RNA probes may be employed and can either be non-isotopically or isotopically labeled. Probes to DNA viruses are constructed with whole viral DNA or restriction enzyme fragments of specific viral sequences. In non-isotopic *in situ* hybridization (NISH) the most popular methods for generating labeled probes are to label with either biotin (Fig. 1.9.6) or digoxigenin. These methods

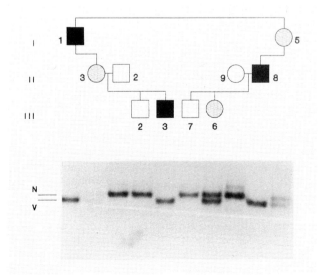

Fig. 1.9.5 *Mutational analysis of an X-linked trait through three generations of a family using SSCP. DNA, extracted from a salivary mouth wash, from individual family members was PCR amplified to give a 370 bp radiolabeled product. PCR amplified products were then analyzed by non-denaturing polyacrylamide gel electrophoresis. Filled squares, affected males; open squares, unaffected males; shaded circles, heterozygote females; open circles, unaffected females. N, amplified product from the normal gene; V, amplified product from mutant gene. Photograph kindly provided by Dr N Lench, Department of Molecular Medicine, University of Leeds, Leeds.*

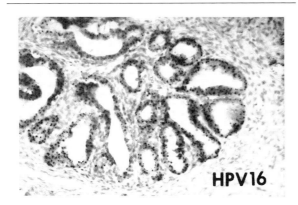

Fig. 1.9.6 In situ *hybridization for human papillomavirus type 16 in a case of cervical adenocarcinoma* in situ. *(Reproduced with permission of the Editor,* Int J Gynecol Pathol.)

have the advantages over isotopic labeling of being non-hazardous, rapid and employ simple detection techniques. After hybridization and washing, a protein blocking step is generally included to block non-specific protein binding sites. A primary antibody directed against the label is then added and the sections incubated for a predetermined time. This antibody is then washed off and a secondary antibody added and the incubation and washing procedure repeated. The primary or secondary antibody is labeled with a detection molecule which is visualized by a standard detection system, e.g. horseradish peroxidase or alkaline phosphatase. More recently viral probes have been produced synthetically. These oligonucleotides, containing complementary sequences to DNA or RNA viruses, can be easily labeled and used as probes but their use in conjunction with non-isotopic detection systems is limited. This is due to a lack of sensitivity, resulting from the lower amount of label available on these short sequences.

Primed in situ *labeling (PRINS)*

In this technique unlabeled DNA probes are hybridized to target sequences as described above. These probes are then extended by DNA polymerases in the presence of labeled deoxynucleotides. These deoxynucleotides can be labeled either isotopically or non-isotopically. This procedure has a major advantage that non-specific sticking of the probe does not result in a high background.

In situ PCR

DNA extraction and PCR preclude histological correlation with molecular biological findings and *in situ* hybridization is relatively insensitive with a detection threshold of approximately 20 copies per cell. *In situ* PCR (ISPCR) is a new molecular technique with potential to combine the high sensitivity of PCR with the precise topographical localization provided by *in situ* hybridization.[16] It can be problematical to perform. It appears to work best for single cell preparations compared to archival tissue.

In this procedure the cells or tissue are incubated in

PCR reaction mixture and PCR performed *in situ*. The amplified product is trapped by the cellular matrix. Amplified product is then identified by either including labeled deoxynucleotides during the PCR reaction (direct detection) or detection of *in situ* amplified products using oligonucleotide probes. Much care has to be taken with this approach to guarantee specificity. Diffusion artefact is a significant problem with ISPCR applied to tissue sections potentially leading to false positive results. If DNA has been fragmented during processing there is a significant possibility that deoxynucleotides will be incorporated into repairing this DNA during the amplification rounds of PCR. This will therefore increase the non-specific background. A few rounds of PCR in the absence of labeled deoxynucleotide may reduce this problem.

Although this procedure has the potential to yield significantly more information about the cellular location of DNA of interest such as viral DNA, that may be present in very small quantities, problems associated with developing the system to ensure its specificity probably preclude its routine application at the present time.

Fluorescent *in situ* hybridization (FISH)

FISH combines the specificity of molecular genetics with traditional cytogenetics. It is being widely incorporated into the clinical setting due to its speed, high resolution and reproducibility and the simple microscopy required for analysis. It is a technique whereby a biotin or digoxigenin-labeled nucleic acid probe is hybridized either to metaphase chromosomes or to cells.[17-19] The probes used are generally DNA. Increasingly labeled yeast artificial chromosomes (YACs) are being employed as the DNA to be labeled because their size (approximately 100–2000 kbp) enables them to be used to map chromosomal translocations. A map of the human genome has been constructed using YACs.[20] Visualization of hybridized probes by fluorescence microscopy is achieved using a fluorochrome such as fluorescein which is conjugated to avidin. This is then used to bind to hybridized probe labeled with biotin or biotinylated anti-digoxigenin (Fig. 1.9.7).

Various types of probes are commercially available that address different applications of the technology. Types of FISH probes include: chromosome-specific repetitive probes, whole chromosome painting probes or locus-specific probes.[19-21] Some applications of FISH include the following:

1. identification of marker chromosomes;
2. characterization of chromosomal rearrangements;
3. study of confined placental mosaicism;
4. rapid assessment of ploidy and major trisomies.

Furthermore, two-color probe combinations can be used for the determination of numerical chromosomal abnormalities and gene amplification. Results can be analyzed microscopically or by flow cytometry and areas showing focal chromosomal aberrations can be correlated with histological appearances.[22]

(a)

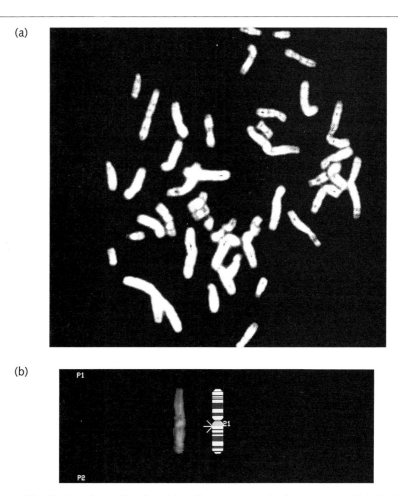

(b)

Fig. 1.9.7 *Chromosomal localization of a small proline-rich and involucrin gene to chromosome 1q21.3. Biotinylated probe was prepared from a YAC of 400 kbp that contains both the involucrin and a small proline-rich gene. (a) Fluorescence* in situ *hybridization (FISH) of metaphase spreads of human lymphoblastoid cells was then performed using this biotinylated probe.[19,21] The yellow signals (see Plate 5) indicate hybridization at this point. (b) YAC labeled chromosome 1 aligned with corresponding chromosome 1 G-banding ideogram. Photographs kindly provided by Mr J Leek and Professor A Markham, Department of Molecular Medicine, University of Leeds, Leeds.*

Molecular cytogenetic analysis

Comparative genomic hybridization

Most molecular techniques are highly focused; they target one specific gene or chromosome region at a time and leave the majority of the genome unexamined. The recently described technique of comparative genomic hybridization allows comparison of DNA from malignant and normal cells so that entire genomes can be examined and regions of gain or loss of DNA identified.[23]

Biotinylated tumor DNA and digoxigenin-labeled normal genomic reference DNA are simultaneously hybridized to normal metaphase spreads. Hybridization of tumor DNA can be detected with green-fluorescing fluorescein isothiocyanate (FITC)-avidin, and the reference DNA with red-fluorescing rhodamine antidigoxigenin. The fluorescence signals can then be quantitatively analyzed by means of a digital image analysis system. Changes in the green-to-red ratio will reflect differences in the relative amounts of tumor and reference DNA bound at a given chromosomal locus.

DNA fingerprinting

Very little difference is often observed in transcribed gene structures between individuals and where differences are observed they are usually correlated with the presence of disease. In contrast, however, there is a far greater variation in non-transcribed DNA. Distributed throughout the genome of any individual are many simple tandem repeat sequences of a short sequence of DNA. They are referred to as 'minisatellites' or when composed of smaller sequences 'microsatellites'. The number of these tandem repeats in one individual is often different from other individual members of a population. Unique patterns due to different lengths of these sequences are present in each individual's genome. In DNA fingerprinting, a probe is constructed which detects these minisatellite regions by ligating together several copies of the core repeat sequence. Genomic DNA is digested with various restriction endonucleases and are separated by electrophoresis and Southern blotted. The blot is then hybridized to a probe which detects the central core of the repeating unit. The resulting autoradiograph will show a large number of bands. Any individual will have inherited half of the bands from each parent, but the degree of polymorphism is so high that it appears that the banding pattern for each individual is unique.

More recently, probes have been introduced which detect unique sequences that are very highly polymorphic. These are also based on variable numbers of tandem repeat sequences (VNTR) but may be specific for an individual chromosome. These probes are easier to read since each individual will usually have only two bands rather than the large number seen with the original probes.[2,24]

Chromosome deletion identified using microsatellite analysis

Microsatellite repeat units consist of repeats (typically 15–30 repeats) of small segments of DNA, two, three or four base pairs in size, that appear to be evenly distributed throughout the human genome. It has been estimated that they occur on average once every 100 000 base pairs. As the number of repeats in the population often varies, the number of repeats in maternal and paternal chromosomes are also often different. The size of PCR amplified products from this segment of DNA from the maternal or paternal chromosomes will be different. Therefore, a deletion of chromosomal DNA from either can be identified. This type of analysis is often used to identify loss of chromosomes in tumor tissue. A comparison of DNA extracted from the tumor with that from the normal tissue (e.g. from blood) will indicate loss of chromosomal DNA if the appropriate microsatellite markers are employed.

FUTURE PERSPECTIVES

We have described above how recent advances in molecular biological techniques have enabled identification of genetic abnormalities associated with both inherited disease and malignant change. Their employment also permits identification of both bacteria and virus present in biological samples at very low titers. These powerful techniques are generally sensitive, specific and technically easy to perform. Moreover, they only require the collection of small samples obtained from either invasive techniques, such as the collection of blood samples, or non-invasive procedures such as retrieval of cells from a mouth rinse.

The employment of this technology presents, therefore, the possibility of routinely and rapidly screening whole populations to identify those individuals at risk of developing one of a multitude of diseases. Furthermore, their employment may be used for earlier diagnosis of the onset of disease processes such as cancer; these technologies permit the detection of mutated cells even when they represent only a small percentage of the total number of cells present. Early screening would present the obvious benefit of earlier clinical management for affected individuals.

SUMMARY

- Restriction enzymes cleave DNA at specific recognition sites. The distance that resulting fragments (when subject to agarose gel electrophoresis) will travel along the gel is dependent on their size; small fragments travel further than larger molecules.
- Southern blotting involves the transfer of DNA from an agarose gel to a nylon membrane.
- Northern blotting involves the transfer of RNA from an agarose gel to a nylon membrane.
- Identity of a specific DNA sequence of interest is by hybridization of a known labeled complementary DNA sequence.
- Large quantities of DNA can be produced by cloning the required fragments in a vector (e.g. cosmid or yeast artificial chromosomes).
- If messenger RNA (mRNA) is the starting material for cloning then there must be reverse transcription of polyadenylated mRNA into single-stranded DNA.
- Because it is so sensitive the polymerase chain reaction (PCR) requires meticulous laboratory technique to avoid contamination.
- A number of PCR-based techniques including single-stranded conformational polymorphism (SSCP) analysis can be used to detect mutations in DNA.
- *In situ* hybridization allows the topographical localization of DNA or RNA within tissues by either isotopic or non-isotopic methods. The latter includes fluorescent *in situ* hybridization (FISH).
- Microsatellite analysis involves the detection and comparison of short sequences of non-transcribed DNA which have unique patterns in each individual.

REFERENCES

1. Arends MJ, Bird CC. Recombinant DNA technology and its diagnostic applications. *Histopathology* 1992 **21**: 303–313.
2. Bennett P, Moore G. *Molecular Biology for Obstetricians and Gynaecologists*, Oxford: Blackwell Scientific Publications, 1992: 174pp.
3. Herrington CS, McGee J O'D. *Diagnostic Molecular Pathology. A Practical Approach*, Vols I and II. Oxford: IRL Press, 1992.
4. Wilkinson DG. *In Situ Hybridisation: A Practical Approach*. Oxford: Oxford University Press, 1992.
5. Robinson PA, Marley JJ, McGarva J. Construction of cDNA libraries from impure preparations of mRNA using Rnase-H free Moloney murine leukemia virus reverse transcriptase. *Meth Mol Cell Biol* 1992 **3**: 118–127.
6. Templeton NS. The polymerase chain reaction. History methods and applications. *Diagn Mol Pathol* 1992 **1**: 58–72.
7. Wright PA, Wynford-Thomas D. The polymerase chain reaction: miracle or mirage? A critical review of its uses and limitations in diagnosis and research. *J Pathol* 1990 **162**: 99–117.
8. Bauer D, Muller H, Reich J, Riedel H, Ahrenkiel V, Warthoe P, Strauss M. Identification of differentially expressed mRNA species by an improved display technique (DDRT-PCR). *Nucleic Acids Res* 1993 **21**: 4272–4280.
9. Zimmermann JW, Schultz RM. Analysis of gene expression in the preimplantation mouse embryo: use of mRNA differential display. *Proc Natl Acad Sci* 1994 **91**, 5456–5460.
10. Liang P, Pardee AB. Differential display of eukaryotic messenger-RNA by means of the polymerase chain reaction. *Science* 1992 **257**, 967–971.
11. Sive HL, St John T. A simple subtractive hybridisation technique employing photoactivatable biotin and phenol extraction. *Nucleic Acids Res* 1988 **16**, 10,937.
12. Shibata D, Hawes D, Li Z-H, Hernandez AM, Spruck CH, Nichols PW. Specific genetic analysis of microscopic tissue after selective ultraviolet radiation fractionation and the polymerase chain reaction. *Am J Pathol* 1992 **141**: 539–543.
13. Zheng J, Wan M, Zweizig S, Velicescu M, Yu MC, Dubeau L. Histologically benign or low-grade malignant tumours adjacent to high-grade ovarian carcinomas contain molecular characteristics of high-grade carcinomas. *Cancer Res* 1993 **53**: 4138–4142.
14. Newton CR, Graham A. Analysis of known mutations. In PCR: Oxford: IOS Scientific Publishers Ltd, 1994: 99–112.
15. Grompe M. The rapid detection of unknown mutations in nucleic acids. *Nature Genet* 1993 **5**: 111–117.
16. Nuovo G. PCR *in situ* hybridisation. *Protocols and Applications*, New York: Raven Press, 1992: 264pp.
17. Van de Kaa CA, Hanselaar AGJM, Hopman AHN *et al.* DNA cytometric and interphase cytogenetic analysis of paraffin-embedded hydatidiform moles and hydropic abortions. *J Pathol* 1993 **170**: 229–238.
18. Van Lijnschoten G, Albrechts J, Vallinga M *et al.* Fluorescence *in situ* hybridization on paraffin-embedded material as a means for retrospective chromosome analysis. *Hum Genet* 1994 **94**: 518–522.
19. Jalal, SM, Law, ME, Christensen, ER, Spurbeck, JL, Dewald, GW. Method for sequential staining of GTL-banded metaphases with fluorescent-labelled chromosome specific paint probes. *Am J Med Genet* 1993 **46**: 98–103.
20. Chumakov I *et al.* A YAC contig map of the human genome. *Nature* 1995 **377**(suppl): 175–297.
21. Landegent, JE, Dewal NJI, Dirk RW *et al.* Use of whole cosmid cloned genomic sequences for chromosomal localisation by non-radioactive *in situ* hybridisation. *Hum Genet* 1987 **77**: 336–370.
22. Persons DL, Hartmann LC, Herath JF *et al.* Interphase molecular cytogenetic analysis of epithelial ovarian carcinomas. *Am J Pathol* 1993 **142**: 733–741.
23. Kallionemi A, Kallionemi O-P, Sudar D *et al.* Comparative hybridization for molecular cytogenetic analysis of solid tumours. *Science* 1992 **258**: 818–821.
24. Gruis NA, Abeln ECA, Bardoel AFJ, Devileep, Franks RR, Cornelisse CJ. PCR-based microsatellite polymorphisms in the detection of loss of heterozygosity in fresh and archival tumour tissue. *Br J Cancer* 1993 **68**: 308–313.

Section 2

Development and Function of the Genital Tract

Gonadal Differentiation

C Yding Andersen and AG Byskov

INTRODUCTION

The gonads maintain the flow of genetic information and diversity from each generation to the next. To achieve this they produce: (a) haploid gametes with different genetic information, and (b) sex hormones that regulate reproductive function and sexual behavior. Thus the one function affects the genotype, whereas the other affects the phenotype of each new individual.

Genetic sex is determined at conception but morphological differences between the sexes do not become apparent until the gonads become sex-differentiated during fetal life. Gonadal differentiation ultimately influences the sexual development of the entire body – brain, bones and muscle, etc., as well as the reproductive tract. This chapter will survey current understanding of gonadal development and sexual differentiation, building on earlier knowledge that has been comprehensively reviewed elsewhere.[1–4]

CURRENT CONCEPTS

The primordial germ cells (PGCs)

The PGCs are the precursors of spermatozoa and oocytes. They are set aside as a germ-cell line early in life. When stained with alkaline phosphatase, PGCs can be identified about three weeks after fertilization in the human yolk sac outside the embryo proper, indicating their endodermic origin.[5] These cells can be traced back even further during development in mice, to the epiblast of the inner cell mass of the blastocyst.[6]

The PGCs migrate by ameboid movement to the gonadal anlagen. They travel from the developing hind gut through the dorsal mesentery into the celomic epithelium covering the gonadal ridges. When PGCs arrive at the gonadal ridges, they are termed 'oogonia' in the developing ovary and 'prespermatogonia' in the developing testis.

What determines the migratory route of PGCs is largely unknown, but chemotropic effects of growth factors, e.g. transforming growth factor-β (TGF-β), possibly in concert with other factors, seem to be important.[7] PGCs possess a unique glucoconjugate at the surface of the plasma membrane[8] that may play a role in the translocation of the PGC, by for instance following chemotactic signals or specific proteins like fibronectin along the migratory route. No specific function has been ascribed to the high level of alkaline phosphatase present in PGCs.

PGC numbers increase by mitosis during migration. In the 5-week-old human embryo, the number of migrating germ cells is between 700 and 1300.[5] Similar to other stem cells, PGC survival and proliferation depend on the Steel gene, which encodes for a pleiotropic growth factor, termed *stem cell factor* (SCF), *mast cell growth factor* (MGF, or *kit* ligand).[9] PGC fate is, however, likely to be determined by more than one factor – other candidates being *basic fibroblast growth factor* (bFGF) and *leukemia inhibitory factor* (LIF).[10]

Genetic determination of sex

Gonadal sex in mammals is determined by the sex chromosome constitution, established when the oocyte is fertilized by a spermatozoa carrying either an X or a Y chromosome. The presence of a Y chromosome dictates testicular formation and will result in the development of a phenotypic male. Indeed, no matter how many X chromosomes are present in the genome, the presence of a single Y chromosome will enforce the formation of testes and male development (as in the human 47, XXY, 48, XXXY and 48, XXYY). In the absence of a Y chromosome, ovaries will be formed and phenotypic female development will occur (as in the human 46, XX, 45, XO, 47, XXX).[11] Sex determination is thus equivalent to testis determination. However, two X chromosomes are usually essential for normal ovarian development, whereas the presence of two X chromosomes, as in the human male 47,XXY, impairs spermatogenesis.[12]

Sex-determining genes

In 1959, it was shown that the Y chromosome in mammals is essential for development as a male.[13] Researchers then began to hunt for 'the master sex-determining gene'. The sex-determining region was gradually located to ever smaller regions of the Y chromosome, until in 1991 a small fragment of DNA containing a single gene was shown to be the genetic determinant of 'maleness' (Fig. 2.1.1).

The sex-determining region was first located to the short arm of the Y chromosome and named *Tdy* (testis-determining genes on the Y). This result came from studies showing that abnormal Y chromosomes consisting of two long arms resulted in the failure of testicular formation and in the development of a female phenotype, whereas abnormal Y chromosomes consisting of two short arms resulted in normal male development.[14]

During the 1970s and 1980s, there was considerable interest in the theory that H-Y (histocompatible-Y) antigen encoded by the sex-determining gene might be responsible for testicular development. However, this concept was abandoned when it was found that male mice could develop lacking the H-Y antigen.[15] It was later shown that the gene encoding the H-Y antigen is located on the long arm of the Y chromosome.[16]

More detailed information came from studies of human XX males and XY females using modern DNA technology. The XX men were all males that had inherited a small fragment of the Y chromosome from their fathers, and the XY females had lost a crucial part of their Y chromosome: a 140 kb segment localized to the 1A2 region of the short arm of the Y chromosome.[17] This segment contained a gene, encoding a protein with many 'fingers' – loops of amino acids formed by zinc cation bridges, and was named *ZFY*.[17] However, *ZFY* proved not to be the master sex-

determining gene. *ZFY* was not expressed in somatic cells crucial to gonadal sex determination, and some XX males did not have *ZFY*. Instead, these XX males had a fragment of the Y chromosome very close to where the *ZFY* gene was located, in the neighboring 1A1 segment[18] (Fig. 2.1.1).

This small piece of the Y chromosome coded for a single gene: *SRY* (sex-determining region Y) in human beings, and *Sry* in mice. *SRY/Sry* encoded a protein with DNA-binding properties, indicating it to be a regulatory gene.[18,19] The gene was expressed in the somatic cells of the testis at around the time of gonadal differentiation in the mouse fetus. Final proof that *SRY/Sry* is the master sex-determining gene was obtained when the *Sry* gene on a 14 kb genomic DNA fragment was introduced into mouse embryos:[20] a number of the transgenic female mice showed testicular differentiation and subsequent male development.

It is believed that *SRY/Sry* acts as a type of 'on-off' switch. When *SRY/Sry* is active, a panel of genes is transcribed that leads to testicular development. Experiments by Koopman and co-workers showed that these genes are located on the X chromosome as well as on autosomal chromosomes.[20] If the switch is not turned on, another pathway of genes is transcribed to allow ovarian development.

Meiosis

Meiosis is the process of reduction division by which haploid gametes are produced from the diploid stem germ cells. Meiosis is unique to germ cells and includes two meiotic divisions (Fig. 2.1.2). The process begins with premeiotic DNA-synthesis, at which stage the germ cell is equipped with a DNA content of 4c-DNA and a chromosome number of 2n, both characteristic of a normal diploid cell before a mitotic division.[21,22]

During the first (reductional) meiotic division, the maternal and paternal genes are exchanged before homologous chromosomes separate into the daughter cells, which

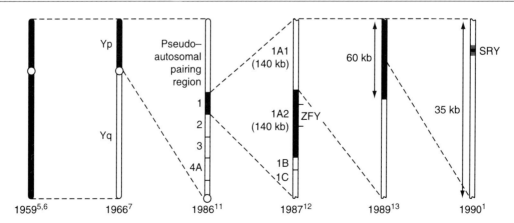

Fig. 2.1.1 *Location of the sex-determining region* (SRY) *on the Y chromosome. (From reference 79, with permission.)*

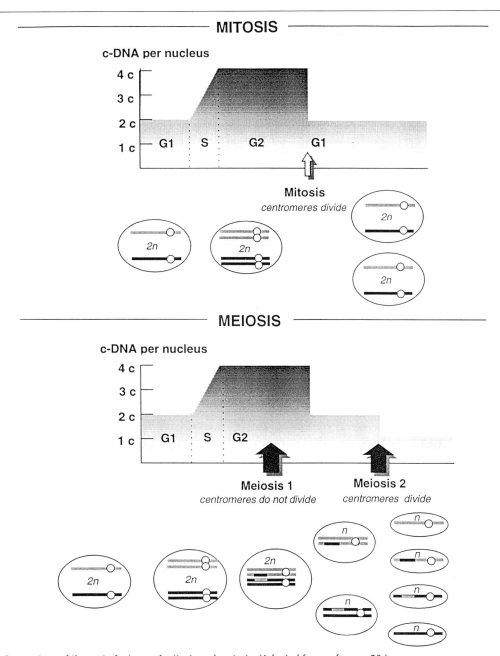

Fig. 2.1.2 *Comparison of the main features of mitosis and meiosis. (Adapted from reference 23.)*

therefore each contain 1n chromosomes and 2c-DNA. In contrast to mitosis, where the centromeres divide, the first meiotic division results in two daughter cells with different genetic constitutions. This is because crossing over occurs between sister chromatids and the centromeres do not divide. In the second meiotic division, which is not preceded by DNA-synthesis, the non-sister chromatids separate and segregate, resulting in the haploid gametes with 1n chromosomes and 1c-DNA. Due to the exchange of genetic material between non-sister chromatids in the first meiotic prophase, all four daughter cells are genetically different (Fig. 2.1.2).[23]

The first meiotic prophase consists of five consecutive stages: leptotene, zygotene, pachytene, diplotene and diakinesis. During the first three stages, the homologous chromosomes line up and increasingly condense. In the pachytene stage, the synaptonemal complex assembles. This consists of two dense parallel rod-like structures, the lateral elements, separated by a central, less dense element. The lateral elements arise from the condensed sister chromatids. When the synapsis between the chromosomes is complete, the chromatids are positioned for gene exchange, i.e. crossing over, visualized by the chiasmata.[24] Evidence is growing that the proper formation of the synaptonemal complex is crucial for ensuring proper segregation of the chromosomes in the first meiotic division.[25]

Meiosis in the female germ line

When the PGCs arrive at the developing ovary they are called oogonia. Oogonia continue to multiply by mitosis until meiosis begins. All oogonia enter meiosis early in life, often before birth,[26] and thereafter are termed oocytes. The process of meiosis is, however, arrested in the diplotene stage of the first meiotic prophase and does not resume until around the time of ovulation during adulthood (Fig. 2.1.3).

Germ cell destiny is determined once meiosis is initiated.

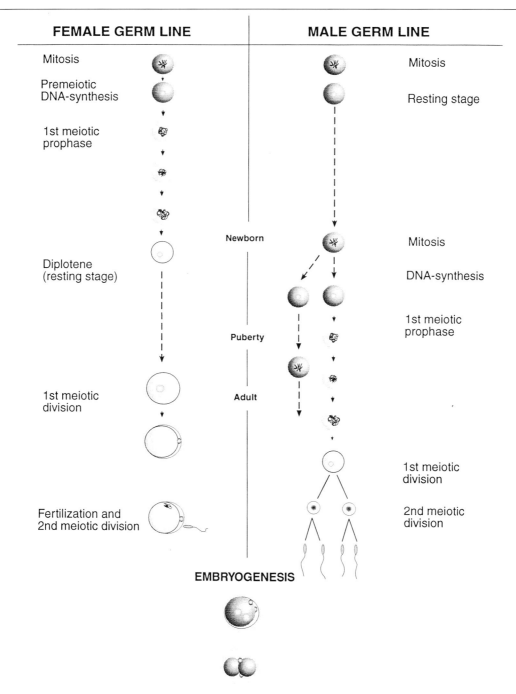

Fig. 2.1.3 *The life cycles of male and female mammalian germ cells. The germ cells of both sexes proliferate mitotically until shortly after sex-differentiation. All oogonia of the ovary enter the first meiotic prophase at early stages of development but are arrested in the diplotene stage (with 2n chromosomes and 4c-DNA). Meiosis of the oocyte is only resumed after puberty, at the time of ovulation. The spermatogonia of the testis form a stem cell population (with 2n chromosomes and 2c-DNA) that can divide mitotically and from which meiotic germ cells can be drawn throughout fertile life.*

A meiotic germ cell can either degenerate or complete meiosis but cannot return to mitotic proliferation. The female mammal therefore possesses a finite number of germ cells by the time all the oogonia have entered meiosis, whereupon oocyte number begins to decline and continues to do so throughout the fertile lifespan (Fig. 2.1.4).[27] In women, oocytes have vanished from the ovaries by around the onset of menopause, whereas the females of many other mammalian species remain fertile throughout life.[28]

The processes that control the switch from mitotis to meiosis, the maintenance of meiotic arrest at diplotene, and the resumption of meiosis in the mature oocyte are not well understood (see Chapter 2.4). Certain X-chromosome-linked genes, which are completely unmethylated and thereby active in the oogonia, may be important for the onset of meiosis.[29] Secretion of a meiosis-activating sterol (MAS), the chemical nature of which has recently been identified (Fig. 2.1.5),[30] may be the trigger for the ini-

tiation of meiosis early in life[31] as well as for the resumption of meiosis in the fertile period.[32] The arrest in diplotene, which occurs simultaneously with initiation of folliculogenesis, is still a mystery. At later stages of follicular development, locally produced purines, e.g. hypoxanthine and adenosine, may inhibit the resumption of meiosis.[33] Whether purines are responsible for meiotic arrest at the diplotene stage is not yet known.

Meiosis in the male germ line

When male PGCs settle in the developing testis they are termed prespermatogonia[34] (see Chapter 2.6). The confinement of prespermatogonia to a germ-cell compartment, i.e. the testicular cords, is crucial to their survival, just as it is for oocytes to be enclosed in follicles (see above).

Like oogonia, prespermatogonia divide mitotically for some time after arriving at the gonadal anlage but they cease

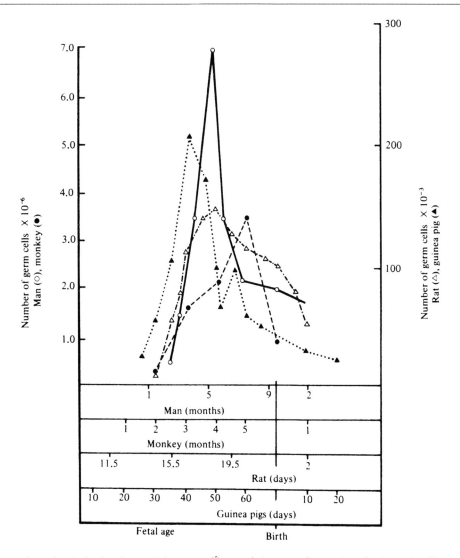

Fig. 2.1.4 *Germ cell number in fetal and neonatal ovaries of human beings, monkeys, rats and guinea pigs. (From reference 27, with permission.)*

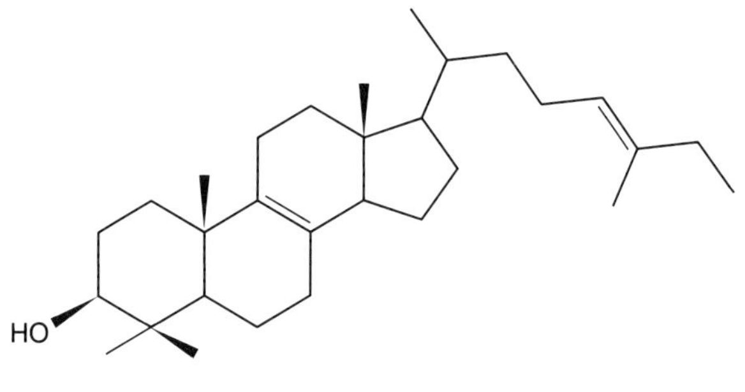

Fig. 2.1.5 *Chemical structure of meiosis-activating sterol (MAS).*[30]

to proliferate shortly after being enclosed in testicular cords.[35] A second wave of proliferation sets in some time before puberty, before meiosis is initiated[36] (Fig. 2.1.3). In contrast to oocytes, a stem-cell population of mitotically dividing male germ cells, spermatogonia, is maintained throughout fertile life, giving rise to continual spermatogenesis.[37] As in the female, mechanisms regulating mitotic arrest, resumption of proliferation and meiotic initiation are not well understood in the male (see below). Presumably, both endocrine and paracrine factors are important to these processes.

Pairing of X and Y chromosomes during meiosis

X and Y chromosomes pair to ensure appropriate segregation during meiosis.[38] However, in contrast to the two X chromosomes that are held together at the centromere, the X and Y chromosomes pair at a homologous region on the distal short arms of the two chromosomes: the so-called pseudoautosomal pairing region (Fig. 2.1.1). This ensures that two types of spermatozoa are formed during the second meiotic division – those that carry an X chromosome and those that carry a Y chromosome.

During the first meiotic division, crossing-over occurs between the X and Y chromosomes, as it does with other chromosomes.[38] Because *SRY/Sry* is located near the region of X–Y pairing, this gene is occasionally transferred to the X chromosome, causing sex reversal (see below). Sex-reversed individuals develop with testes, normal male Wolffian duct derivatives, and male external genitalia. However, such XX males are infertile without spermatogenesis.[39] The incidence of a 46, XX karyotype in phenotypic men is approximately 1:20 000.[40] This is comparable with the spontaneous frequency of X-linked disease such as hemophilia-A, which is approximately 1:5000 to 1:10 000.[41]

Formation of gonads and ducts: role of mesonephros

The gonads begin to form when germ cells arrive at the ventral cranial part of the mesonephros, the second fetal kidney anlage (Fig. 2.1.6).[42] Apart from germ cells and mesonephric cells, the gonad consists of mesenchymal and ingrowing cells from the celomic epithelium. In some

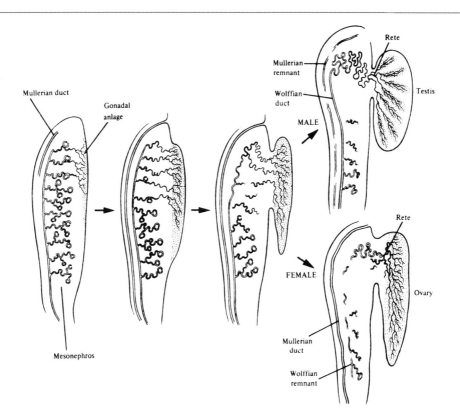

Fig. 2.1.6 *Transformation of genital duct system during the period when gonads pass from an undifferentiated state to recognizable testes and ovaries. (From reference 42, with permission of Cambridge University Press.)*

species, the mesonephros serves as a fetal excretory kidney, whereas in others it is rudimentary. Irrespective of its renal function, the mesonephros fulfills several other functions crucial to gonadal formation.

Wolffian ducts

In males, the excretory duct of the mesonephros – the Wolffian duct – differentiates in response to stimulation by testosterone to form the epididymis, the vas deferens and the upper part of the seminal vesicle. In females, the Wolffian duct degenerates during the early stages of ovarian differentiation due to the lack of stimulation by testosterone (see below).

Müllerian ducts

The Müllerian duct arises from celomic mesothelium in close association with the Wolffian duct. In females, the Müllerian duct becomes the oviduct, the uterus and the upper part of the vagina. In males, the Müllerian duct degenerates after testicular differentiation due to the local production of anti-Müllerian hormone (AMH), also known as Müllerian-inhibiting substance (MIS) or Müllerian inhibiting factor (MIF) (see below).

Mesonephric cells

The mesonephros itself donates cells to the developing gonad at the time of germ cell invasion.[43] Shortly thereafter, nerves and blood vessels invade the organ.[44] The mesonephros also influences the onset of meiosis, gonadal sex differentiation *in vitro* and sex-steroid production.[45]

Testis

In the testis, the ingrowth of mesonephric cells decreases or stops when sex differentiation occurs and the germ cells become enclosed in testicular cords. The testis itself rounds off and the connection to the mesonephros diminishes. From this point on, testicular growth mainly depends on the proliferation of those cells that already lie within the gonadal boundary.

Ovary

Mesonephric cells continue to migrate into the developing ovary for an extended period of time, depending on animal species. In some species (e.g. sheep and pig) a large part of the central area becomes occupied by mesonephric cells, whereas in others (e.g. mouse) the area occupied by mesonephric cells is small. The developing ovary does not round off like the testis, and in many species a broad connection to the regressing mesonephric tissue remains for a long time. In some species this connection becomes part of the gonadal endocrine tissue.

Differentiation of the ovary

Morphologically and endocrinologically, the ovary differentiates after the testis. However, histologically, the female gonad is potentially recognizable as an ovary if not simultaneously with the testis, then shortly thereafter. It is usually possible to recognize one of two characteristic patterns of ovarian differentiation based on the onset of meiosis in relation to the time at which morphological sex-differentiation occurs in males (i.e the stage of development at which testicular cords can be recognized). In some species (i.e. those with 'immediate meiosis'), the first female germ cells to enter meiosis do so shortly after morphological sex-differentiation occurs in males, whereas in others (i.e. those with 'delayed meiosis') there is a time lapse, known as the 'delay period', before meiosis begins.[46]

In species with 'immediate meiosis', the newly differentiated ovary is characteristically a homogeneous structure with little morphological compartmentalization. For example, in the mouse, the germ cells are closely packed in the cortex, which fills most of the ovary. In the human, which represents an intermediate meiotic pattern, a better defined peripheral cortex is seen (Fig. 2.1.7). The tissue in the center or basal area of the ovary, the medulla, contains far fewer germ cells.

In species with 'delayed meiosis' such as sheep and pig, a testis-like pattern of ovarian differentiation is seen during

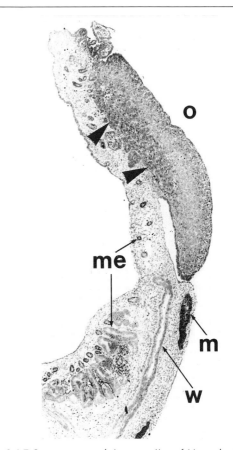

Fig. 2.1.7 *Ovary–mesonephric connection of 11-week-old human fetus. The ovary (**o**) is attached to the cranial part of mesonephros (arrowheads). Caudally, mesonephric tubules (**me**), Wolffian duct (**w**), and Müllerian duct (**m**) are seen. ×200. (From reference 4, with permission.)*

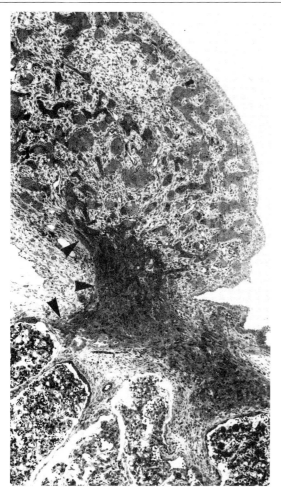

Fig. 2.1.8 *Part of ovary and mesonephros of 42-day-old pig fetus. Dense cell masses (arrowheads) of mesonephric origin connect germ cell cords of ovary with parietal layers of Bowman's capsules. ×200. (From reference 4, with permission.)*

the delay period. The ovary becomes clearly compartmentalized with germ cells enclosed in irregular cords (Fig. 2.1.8). It is often a characteristic of species with delayed meiosis that the cortex contains many germ cells within cords, while the the medulla is packed with rete cords and is almost devoid of germ cells.

Induction of meiosis in oogonia

The first oogonia to enter meiosis in the mammalian ovary are those located at the border between the cortex and the medulla. These will have been the first germ cells to make contact with invading mesonephric cells, fostering the idea that meiosis is initiated by MIS (see above), secreted by mesonephros-derived rete cells.[47] This has been confirmed by experiments showing that germ cells entering meiosis in the fetal mouse ovary secrete a substance which induces meiosis in fetal mouse testicular anlage.[48] MIS-activity was also found in adult testes and in follicular fluids from the ovaries of various species.[4] Recently, it was discovered that

MIS is a novel C_{29} sterol, now known as meiosis-activating sterol (MAS)[30] (Fig. 2.1.5), confirming earlier studies.[49]

Folliculogenesis

The diplotene oocyte depends for survival on its enclosure within a layer of granulosa cells. Once granulosa cells have surrounded the oocyte and enclosed themselves in a basement membrane, the follicle is formed.[50–52]

The first follicles are organized in the inner part of the ovarian cortex. Gradually folliculogenesis spreads towards the periphery (Fig. 2.1.9). Before the basement membrane is formed, granulosa cells often form contacts with cells of the medullary intraovarian rete cords (Fig. 2.1.9). Such granulosa–rete associations, which are seen in many mammalian species, suggest that rete cells might also supply follicles with granulosa cells. Various experiments support this idea. For example, when the ovarian primordium is separated from adherent mesonephric tissue, follicular formation is impaired or inhibited *in vitro*.[53] The ovarian surface epithelium may also give off cells to the granulosa cell layer, which, like rete cells, are often closely associated with peripherally situated oocytes. Thus, granulosa cells may originate at two different sites, although the influence of the ovarian surface epithelium seems less important than that of the rete cells with respect to early follicle formation.[43,53] In a study of XX/XY chimeras it was shown that both the granulosa cells and the celomic epithelium covering the gonad were predominantly XX.[54] Other cell types, e.g. mesenchymal cells, may also be enclosed in the granulosa cell compartment.

The centrally located follicles that are first to be formed are also first to show signs of growth. What triggers their growth is still unknown, but neither gonadotropins nor sex steroids seem to be responsible.[52] Gradually those follicles that are situated more distally also begin to grow. Only a small fraction of follicles that start to grow will ever reach the preovulatory stage. The vast majority degenerate, becoming atretic, and may do so at any developmental stage.[52] Thus, an ever-diminishing reserve of small, nongrowing follicles is kept in the distal part of the cortex.

Regardless of where granulosa cells originate, the characteristic pattern of follicular growth within the ovary implies that a growth-control gradient is established within the cortex by the time that oocytes reach the diplotene stage.[55] It has been suggested that those oocytes that first enter meiosis and first commence growth are also the first to ovulate, and vice versa: the 'first in-first out, last in-last out' theory.[56]

Mesonephric influences on ovarian development

The size and the excretory function of the mesonephros in female mammals have been correlated with onset of meiosis.[45] Species with a 'large' mesonephros tend to exhibit delayed meiosis (e.g. rabbit, pig and sheep), whereas meiosis is immediate in species with a smaller mesonephros (e.g. rat and mouse). In species with delayed meiosis, meiosis appears to begin when the renal excretory activity

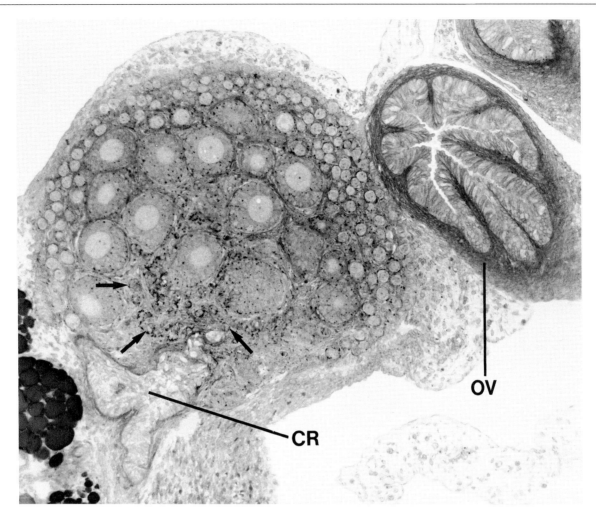

Fig. 2.1.9 *Developing ovary and oviduct (**OV**) from a 7-day-old immature mouse. Growing follicles are seen in the inner part and small non-growing follicles in the outer part of the ovary. Lipid droplets are present in intraovarian rete cords in the centre of the ovary (arrows).* **CR**, *connecting rete. ×400. (From reference 4, with permission.)*

of mesonephros ceases. It has been proposed that the mesonephric kidney function or perhaps its secretory products interfere with the onset of meiosis.[45] The mesonephros influences steroid production *in vitro* by the fetal and immature rabbit ovary.[57] In fetal life, steroid secretion is lowered by the mesonephros, but a few days after birth when meiosis has begun, the mesonephros stimulates estradiol production. At this stage the altered interaction between the ovary and the mesonephros could result in the secretion of MAS.

Hormone secretion by the fetal ovary

The human ovary – morphologically undifferentiated at the time that males develop testicular cords – is incapable of *de novo* synthesis of steroids until later stages of fetal life when follicles are formed.[58] However, the ovary acquires the ability to convert testosterone into estradiol almost simultaneously with the onset of testosterone production

by the testis, i.e. shortly after sex-differentiation.[59] The functional significance of this is unclear, given that the maternally derived estradiol concentration is so high. Possibly this aromatase system protects the female fetus from virilization.

The time of onset of *de novo* ovarian steroidogenesis is species-related. In species with immediate meiosis (e.g. rat and mouse) *de novo* synthesis of estradiol does not take place immediately after sexual differentiation, whereas it does so during the delay period in species with delayed meiosis, e.g. rabbit, sheep and cow. When meiosis is eventually initiated, estradiol synthesis temporarily ceases. Thus steroid synthesis and onset of meiosis seem to be inversely related.[4]

AMH is not expressed during fetal life in the female, permitting continuous growth of the Müllerian duct, ovarian differentiation and the subsequent development of the female reproductive tract (Figs. 2.1.6 and 2.1.10). AMH is, however, expressed later on in the granulosa cells of

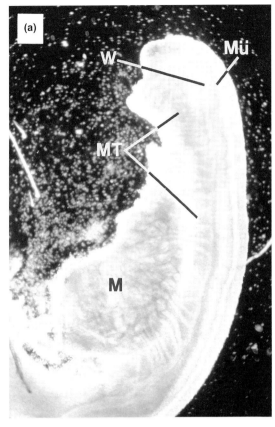
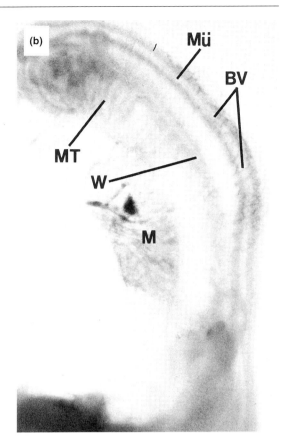

Fig. 2.1.10 *Whole mount preparations of cranial and middle parts of urogenital ducts and mesonephros of two human female fetuses from which gonads have been removed. (a) 9 weeks old. Mesonephros (M) is still prominent, with many tubules connecting to Wolffian duct (W). The Müllerian duct (Mü) is still rather thin. (b) 12 weeks old. Mesonephros is regressing and only cranially situated tubules (MT) connect to the Wolffian duct (W). Müllerian duct (Mü) is well developed, wrapped in a network of blood vessels (BV), and with a distinct lumen. (From reference 4, with permission.)*

growing ovarian follicles. The intrafollicular function of AMH and the mechanisms that regulates its expression remain unknown.[60]

Differentiation of the testis

Genetic sex is reflected in the dimorphism of the gonads, the first sign being the formation of the testicular cords. During this process two somatic cell lines differentiate, the Sertoli cells and the Leydig cells. The Sertoli cells aggregate with the germ cells to form solid cell cords. Outside the developing cords, the Leydig cells differentiate and become the main steroid producing cells of the testis (see Chapter 2.5). As the Sertoli cells aggregate to form the testicular cords, they envelop germ cells at the middle of the cords and separate themselves from their surroundings by a basement membrane.[61]

The testicular cords develop as a continuation of the mesonephros-derived rete testis, to form the permanent connection between the testis and the epididymis (Fig. 2.1.11). The rete connection becomes very narrow as the testis rounds off shortly after differentiation.

Sertoli cells are thought to originate mainly from the mesonephros-derived rete testis. Surface epithelial cells might also contribute to the formation of Sertoli cells, since connections between these two cell types exist at early stages of testicular differentiation.[62] Studies of chimeric mice indicate that only a few cells of the surface epithelium contribute to the Sertoli cells.[54] As testicular differentiation progresses, Sertoli cells undergo waves of proliferation and differentiation that equip them with the specialized properties necessary to support spermatogenesis[63] (see Chapter 2.6).

Prevention of meiosis in fetal male germ cells

When the prespermatogonia become enclosed in the testicular cords at the time of testicular differentiation, their rate of proliferation decreases and finally ceases after birth. This sequence of events is referred to as 'prespermatogenesis'.[64] In contrast, the proliferation rate of the Sertoli cells is high during the period when the prespermatogonia rest.[36] Thus, it is likely that different factors control the proliferation of germ cells and Sertoli cells. It has been proposed that a meiosis-preventing substance

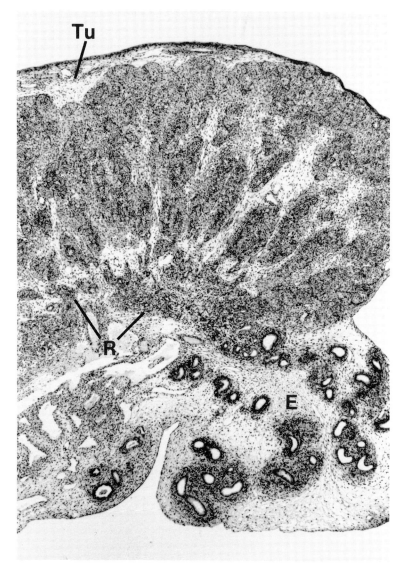

Fig. 2.1.11 *Part of the testis and epididymis (**E**) of a 21-week-old human fetus. The rete testis (**R**) connects testicular cords and epididymis. Tunica albuginea (**Tu**). ×350. (From reference 4, with permission.)*

(MPS) produced within the testicular cords prevents or counteracts MAS activity, resulting in the resting stage of prespermatogonia. A MAS/MPS balance may act in concert with testicular steroids to control meiosis.[46]

Mesonephric influences on testicular differentiation

In contrast to the female, there is no suggestion of a direct correlation between the size or function of the mesonephros and testicular differentiation. For example, in the rabbit, testicular differentiation takes place on around day 15 of fetal life, when the mesonephros is still a large, functional kidney.[45]

With the onset of meiosis in the mouse ovary, the mesonephros of the fetal male mouse exhibits meiosis-inducing activity. This 'feminizing' effect of the mesonephros is clearly seen when fetal mouse testicular anlage is cultured with its adherent mesonephric tissue. For a limited period around the time of testicular differentiation, the mesonephros inhibits testicular cord formation and meiosis is induced in male germ cells.[65] The rapid rounding off of the testis and the consequent diminished influence of the mesonephros (by now a developing epididymis) after sex differentiation may serve to prevent further 'feminization' of the testis by the mesonephros.

Hormone secretion by the fetal testis

The testis starts to produce hormones as soon as it differentiates. The classic experiments of Jost[66, 67] showed that the testis secretes two hormones essential to male development:

the male sex-steroid, testosterone, which virilizes the Wolffian duct derivatives, and AMH, which causes regression of the Müllerian duct (Fig. 2.1.10) (see below). In the absence of these two hormones a female phenotype develops.

Testosterone

Almost as soon as the testicular cords form, Leydig cells develop in the interstitial tissue of the testis. The Leydig cells are the primary androgen secreting cells, which start producing testosterone shortly after differentiation.[68] Testosterone is the main androgen secreted by the fetal and adult testis (see Chapter 2.5). In fetal life, testosterone maintains the growth and differentiation of the internal and external genitalia. Virilization of the Wolffian ducts, urogenital sinus and external genitalia fails to occur in individuals with genetic defects that result in either the failure of testosterone production or in the lack of responsiveness of target cells to testosterone.

Testosterone acts via androgen receptors located within target cell nuclei. Some cells convert testosterone into 5α-dihydrotestosterone (DHT), which binds to the androgen receptor with a higher affinity than testosterone.[69] Activated androgen–receptor complexes interact with regulatory regions of androgen responsive genes to stimulate or inhibit their transcription, as described in Chapter 1.4.

Testosterone is reduced to DHT by steroid 5α-reductase. This enzyme is almost undetectable in Wolffian duct derivatives until after sex differentiation but is expressed in the male urethra, prostate and external genitalia before virilization occurs.[70] This has prompted the idea that testosterone and DHT might play separate roles in male differentiation, with testosterone being responsible for the virilization of Wolffian derivatives and DHT being responsible for development of the male external genitalia.[71] However, since both androgens bind to the same receptor, it is not understood how these two androgens might perform separate functions in male differentiation.

In addition to governing the growth and differentiation of the male internal and external genitalia, testosterone is believed to be essential for priming the brain in the male direction at an early developmental stage.[72]

AMH

Anti-Müllerian hormone is a homodimeric (140 kDa) glycoprotein secreted by Sertoli cells that is a member of the TGF-β/activin family of growth/differentiation factors.[73] Its vital function in males is to suppress Müllerian duct development during fetal life. The mechanism through which AMH acts is not yet known. The putative AMH receptor is a member of the superfamily of transmembrane serine/threonine kinase receptors.[73]

The fetal Müllerian duct is only sensitive to AMH for a short time after sex-differentiation. Exposure to AMH before or after this critical period is ineffective. The female Müllerian duct will also degenerate *in vivo* and *in vitro* if exposed to AMH at this point.[74,75] However, AMH is not usually secreted in the female fetus.

The AMH-cDNAs for rat, mouse, cow and man have been cloned,[75] sharing an overall 75% homology. The genes show 95% homology at the C-terminal end, where it is believed that the putative receptor binding site is located. The AMH genes have all been mapped to autosomal chromosomes and the human AMH gene is located on the short arm of chromosome 19.

AMH may have functions other than to cause Müllerian duct regression. Although the fetal ovary does not produce AMH (see above), in adult ovaries granulosa cells lining the cavities of large antral follicle produce AMH.[60,76] Cumulus granulosa cells cease to produce AMH shortly before ovulation, which is when oocyte meiosis resumes, suggesting that AMH is an inhibitor of meiosis.[77] If the fetal ovary is exposed to AMH, morphological sex-reversal occurs, accompanied by a switch in the pattern of sex steroid synthesis from predominantly female (estradiol) to predominantly male (testosterone), highlighting the pivotal role of AMH in gonadal differentiation.[78]

FUTURE PERSPECTIVES

We now know that the *SRY/Sry* gene governs gonadal sex in mammals. The next step is to understand how *SRY/Sry* expression is regulated and how the encoded products in turn regulate expression of homeotic genes vital to gonadal development such as fushi tarazu factor 1 (Ftz-F1).[79]

A recent advance has been the discovery of a new class of gonadal C_{29} sterols, of which MAS is a member, that participate in the regulation of germ cell maturation.[30] MAS is implicated in the initiation and resumption of meiosis in both the male and female gonad. The impetus now is to identify the intragonadal source of MAS, to determine how its synthesis is regulated and to elucidate the mechanisms through which it acts.

We still know little about the paracrine factors that initiate follicular growth. Candidate paracrines are polypeptide growth/differentiation factors that are members of the TGF-β/activin family, which includes AMH.[80] Further research on the roles played by these factors and their receptors in gametogenesis should be rewarding. A question mark hangs over the effects of estrogens and estrogen-like compounds (xeno-estrogens) on gonadal development. Evidence is growing that inappropriate exposure to these substances during fetal life can damage gonadal function in adulthood, resulting in reduced fertility.[81,82] How estrogens exert such effects and how the fetus is protected from maternal estrogens are public health as well as basic science issues.

Finally, the formation of definitive sex glands involves coordinated phases of cellular proliferation, differentiation and death. Programmed cell-death (apoptosis) presumably occurs during, for example, Müllerian duct regression and follicular atresia in fetal gonads. Research on the apoptotic program in developing gonads may thus shed new light on the mechanisms through which production of spermatozoa and oocytes is sustained during adulthood.

SUMMARY

- Genetic sex is normally determined by the presence of either two X chromosomes in females or both an X and a Y chromosome in males. The Y chromosome encodes the gene *SRY*, the master sex-determining gene that regulates the development of maleness.

- Meiosis generates haploid gametes each having one unique set of chromosomes. In the female, the first part of meiosis is initiated in fetal life and only completed years later when the follicle undergoes ovulation. In the male, meiosis begins at puberty leaving a stem germ cell population from which meiotic cells can be recruited throughout fertile life.

- In the male, crossing-over between X and Y chromosomes during the first meiotic division is obligatory in order to obtain normal segregation.

- The mesonephros, the second kidney anlage, donates cells to the developing gonad and supports the development of the Wolffian duct in the male and the Müllerian duct in the female. The mesonephros also influences the initiation of meiosis, gonadal sex differentiation and sex-steroid production by the gonads.

- The initiation of meiosis in the female is regulated by a recently characterized C_{29} sterol, named MAS.

- Folliculogenesis begins during fetal life, consisting of the enclosure of the oocyte (at the diplotene stage of meiosis) by a few granulosa cells. Follicular growth begins first among follicles located centrally in the ovarian medulla, followed by follicles located distally in the ovarian cortex.

- As the testis differentiates, germ cells become enclosed in testis cords. The mechanism that inhibits meiotic progression until puberty is unknown; the influence of a meiosis preventing substance (MPS) has been proposed.

- Hormone production begins as the testis differentiates: Leydig cells produce testosterone and Sertoli cells produce AMH.

- Testosterone, the classic male sex steroid, is responsible for the virilization of the Wolffian duct. AMH, a homodimeric glycoprotein belonging to the TGF-β/activin family of regulatory factors, causes the regression of the Müllerian duct.

- Local actions of testosterone, AMH and related regulatory proteins are crucial to gonadal differentiation.

ACKNOWLEDGEMENT

We thank Mrs S. Peters for her careful revision of our English.

REFERENCES

1. Austin CR, Short RV (eds). *Reproduction in Mammals*, 2nd edn. New York: Cambridge University Press, 1992.
2. Lamming GE (ed.). *Marshall's Physiology of Reproduction*, 4th edn, Vol 1. New York: Churchill Livingstone, 1984.
3. George FW, Wilson JD. Sex determination and differentiation. In Knobil E, Neill JD (eds) *The Physiology of Reproduction*. New York: Raven Press, 1994: 3–28.
4. Byskov AG Hoyer PE. Embryology of mammalian gonads and ducts. In Knobil E, Neill JD (eds). *The Physiology of Reproduction*. New York: Raven Press, 1994: 487–540.
5. Witschi E. Migration of the germ cells of human embryos from the yolksac to the primitive gonadal fold. *Contrib Embryol* 1948 32: 67–80.
6. Ginsburg M, Snow MHL, McLaren A. Primordial germ cells in the mouse embryo during gastrulation. *Development* 1990 110: 521–528.
7. Godin I, Wylie CC. TGF-β inhibits proliferation and has a chemotropic effect on mouse primordial germ cells in culture. *Development* 1991 113: 1451–1457.
8. Fazel AR, Schulte BA, Spicer SS. Glycoconjugate unique to the migrating primordial germ cells differs with genera. *Anat Rec* 1990 228: 177–184.
9. Williams DE, de Vries P, Namen AE, Widmer MB, Lyman SD. The *Steel* factor. *Dev Biol* 1992 151: 368–376.
10. Resnik JL, Bixler LS, Cheng L, Donovan PJ. Long term proliferation of mouse primordial germ cells in culture. *Nature (London)* 1992 359: 550–551.
11. Polani PE. Sex chromosome anomalies in man. In Hamerton JL (ed.) *Chromosomes in Medicine. Little Club Clinics in Developmental Medicine*. London: National Spastic Society with William Heinemann Medical Books, 1962: 74–133.
12. Davis RM. Localisation of male determining factors in man: A thorough review of structural anomalies of the Y chromosome. *J Med Genet* 1981 18: 161–195.
13. Beatty RA. Genetic basis for the determination of sex. *Philos Trans R Soc Lond (Biol)* 1970 259: 3–13.
14. Jacobs PA, Ross A. Structural abnormalities of the Y chromosome in man. *Nature (London)* 1966 210: 353–354.
15. McLaren A. Chimeras and sexual differentiation. In LeDouarin N, McLaren A (eds) *Chimeras in Developmental Biology*. New York: Academic Press, 1984: 381–388.
16. Cantrell MA, Bogan JS, Simpson E *et al*. Deletion mapping of H–Y antigen to the long arm of the human Y chromosome. *Genomics* 1992 13: 1255–1260.
17. Page DC, Mosher R, Simpson EM *et al*. The sex-determining region of the human Y chromosome encodes a finger protein. *Cell* 1987 51: 1091–1104.
18. Sinclair AH, Berta P, Palmer M *et al*. A gene from the human sex-determining region encodes a protein with

homology to a conserved DNA-binding motif. *Nature (London)* 1990 **346**: 240–244.

19. McElreavey K, Vilain E, Cotinot C, Payen E, Fellous M. Control of sex determination in animals. *Eur J Biochem* 1993 **218**: 769–783.

20. Koopman P, Gubbay J, Vivian N, Goodfellow PN, Lovell-Badge R. Male development of chromosomally female mice transgenic for Sry. *Nature (London)* 1991 **351**: 117–121.

21. Goodenough V, Levine RP. *Genetics.* London: Rinehart, Winston, 1974.

22. Moens PB (ed.). *Meiosis.* London: Academic Press, 1987.

23. Susuki DT, Griffiths AJF, Miller JH, Lewontin RC. *An Introduction to Genetic Analysis.* New York: WH Freeman, 1989.

24. Roeder GS. Chromosome synapsis and genetic recombination: their role in meiotic segregation. *Trends Genet* 1990 **6**: 386–389.

25. Mahadevaiah SK, Lovell-Badge R, Burgoyne PS. Tdy-negative XY, XXY and XYY female mice: breeding data and synaptonemal complex analysis. *J Reprod Fertil* 1993 **97**: 151–160.

26. Peters H. Migration of gonocytes into the mammalian gonad and their differentiation. *Philos Trans R Soc Lond B Biol Sci* 1970 **9**: 91–101.

27. Baker TG. Oogenesis and ovarian development. In Balin H, Glasser S (eds) *Reproductive Biology.* Amsterdam: Excerpta Medica, 1972: 398–437.

28. Mossman HW, Duke KL. *Comparative Morphology of the Mammalian Ovary.* Wisconsin: The University Wisconsin Press, 1973.

29. Singer-Sam J, Goldstein L, Dai A, Gartler SM, Riggs AD. A potentially critical Hpa II site of the X chromosome-linked PGK1 gene is unmethylated prior to the onset of meiosis of human oogenic cells. *Proc Natl Acad Sci USA* 1992 **89**: 1413–1417.

30. Byskov AG, Yding Andersen C, Nordholm L, Thøgersen H, Guoliang X, Wassmann O, Andersen JV, Roed T. Chemical structure of novel meiosis activating steroids crucial to reproduction. *Nature* 1995 **374**: 559–562.

31. Byskov AG, Fenger M, Westergaard LG, Anderson CY. Forskolin and the meiosis inducing substance synergistically initiate meiosis in fetal male germ cells. *Mol Reprod Dev* 1993 **34**: 47–52.

32. Guoliang X, Byskov AG, Andersen CY. Cumulus cells secrete a meiosis inducing substance by stimulation with forskolin and dibutyric cyclic adenosine monophosphate. *Mol Reprod Dev* 1994 **39**: 17–24.

33. Downs SM. Purine control of mouse oocyte maturation: evidence that nonmetabolized hypoxanthine maintains meiotic arrest. *Mol Reprod Dev* 1993 **35**: 82–94.

34. Gondos B. Development and differentiation of the testis and male reproductive tract. In Steinberger A, Steinberger E (eds) *Testicular Development, Structure and Function.* New York: Raven Press, 1980: 3–20.

35. Hilscher W. T1-prospermatogonia (Primordial Spermatogonia of Rauh): the 'ameiotic' counter part of early oocytes. *Fortschr Androl* 1981 7: 21–32.

36. Vergouwen RPFA, Jacobs SGPM, Huiskamp R, Davids JAG, de Rooij DG. Proliferative activity of gonocytes, Sertoli cells and interstitial cells during testicular development in mice. *J Reprod Fertil* 1991 **93**: 233–243.

37. Leblond CP, Clermont Y. Definition of the stages of the cycle of the seminiferous epithelium in the rat. *Ann NY Acad Sci* 1952 **55**: 548–573.

38. Burgoyne PS, Mahadevaiah SK. Unpaired sex chromosomes and gametogenic failure. In Sumner AT, Chandley AF (eds) *Chromosomes Today*, Vol. 11. London: Chapman and Hall, 1993: 243–263.

39. Perez-Palacios G, Medina M, Ulla-Aguirre A *et al.* Gonadotropin dynamics in XX males. *J Clin Endocrinol Metab* 1981 **53**: 254–257.

40. de la Chapelle A. The etiology of maleness in XX men. *Hum Genet* 1981 **58**: 105–116.

41. Gitschier J, Wood WI, Goralka TM, Wion KL, Chen EY, Eaton DH, Vehar GA, Capon DJ, Lawn RM. Characterization of the human factor VIII gene. *Nature (London)* 1984 **312**: 326.

42. Byskov AG. Primordial germ cells and regulation of meiosis. In Austin CR, Short RV (eds) *Reproduction in Mammals*, 2nd edn. New York: Cambridge University Press, 1984: 1–16.

43. Byskov AG. Differentiation of mammalian embryonic gonad. *Physiol Rev* 1986 **66**: 71–117.

44. Pelliniemi LJ, Fröjdman, Paranko J. Embryological and prenatal development and function of the Sertoli cells. In Russell LD, Griswold MD (eds) *The Sertoli Cell.* Clearwater: Cache River, 1993: 87–113.

45. Grinsted J, Ügesen L. Mesonephric excretory function related to its influence on differentiation of fetal gonads. *Anat Rec* 1984 **210**: 551–556.

46. Byskov AG. Regulation of meiosis in mammals. *Biol Anim Biochim Biophys* 1979 **19**: 1251–1261.

47. Byskov AG. The role of the rete ovarii in meiosis and follicle formation in the cat, mink and ferret. *J Reprod Fertil* 1975 **45**: 201–209.

48. Byskov AG, Saxen L. Induction of meiosis in foetal mouse testis *in vitro. Dev Biol* 1976 **52**: 193–200.

49. Yding Andersen C, Byskov AG, Grinsted J. Partial purification of the meiosis-inducing substance (MIS). In Byskov AG, Peters H (eds) *The Development and Function of the Reproductive Organs.* Amsterdam: Exerpta Medica, 1981: ICS serie no. 559, 73–80.

50. Peters H, McNatty KP. *The Ovary.* London: Granada Publishing, 1980.

51. Hirshfield AN. Development of follicles in the mammalian ovary. *Int Rev Cytol* 1991 **124**: 43–101.

52. Greenwald GS, Roy SK. Follicular development and its control. In Knobil E, Neill JD (eds) *The Physiology of Reproduction.* New York: Raven Press, 1994: 629–724.

53. Byskov AG, Skakkebaek NE, Stafanger G, Peters H. Influence of ovarian surface epithelium and rete ovarii on follicle formation. *J Anat* 1977 **123**: 77–86.

54. Patek CE, Kerr JB, Gosden RG *et al.* Sex chimaerism, fertility and sex determination in the mouse. *Development* 1991 **113**: 311–325.

55. Byskov AG, Guoliang X, Høyer PE, Andersen CY. Early postnatal growth pattern of mouse oocytes is imprinted during fetal life. (submitted).

56. Hendersen SA, Edwards RG. Chiasma frequency and maternal age in mammals. *Nature (London)* 1968 **218**: 22–28.

57. Grinsted J, Byskov AG, Christensen IJ, Jensenius JC. Influence of the mesonephros on fetal and neonatal rabbit gonads. I. Sex-steroid release by the testis *in vitro. Acta Endocr (Copenhagen)* 1982 **99**: 272–280.

58. Reyes FI, Winter JSD, Faiman C. Studies on human sexual development. I. Fetal gonadal and adrenal sex steroids. *J Clin Endocrinol Metab* **37**: 74–78.

59. George FW, Wilson JD. Conversion of androgen to estrogen by the human fetal ovary. *J Clin Endocrinol Metab* 1978 **47**: 550–555.

60. Munsterberg A, Lovell-Badge R. Expression of the mouse anti-Müllerian hormone gene suggests a role in both male and female sexual differentiation. *Development* 1991 **113**: 613–624.

61. Magre S, Jost A. Sertoli cells and testicular differentiation in the rat fetus. *J Electron Microsc Tech* 1991 **19**: 172–188.

62. Wartenberg H, Kinsky I, Viebahn C, Schmolke C. Fine structural characteristics of testicular cord formation in the developing rabbit gonad. *J Electron Microsc Tech* 1991 **19**: 133–157.

63. Russel LD, Griswold MD. *The Sertoli cell.* Clearwater: Cache River Press, 1993.

64. Hilsher B, Hilsher W, Bülthoff-Ohnholz B, Krämer U, Birke A, Pelzer H, Gauss G. Kinetics of gametogenesis. I. Comparative histological and autoradiographic studies of

oocytes and transitional prospermatogonia during oogenesis and prespermatogenesis. *Cell Tissue Res* 1974 **154:** 443–470.

65. Byskov AG, Grinsted J. Feminizing effect of mesonephros on cultured differentiating mouse gonads and ducts. *Science* 1981 **212:** 817–818.

66. Jost A. Problems in fetal endocrinology: the gonadal and hypophyseal hormones. *Recent Prog Horm Res* 1953 **8:** 379–418.

67. Jost A. A new look at the mechanism controlling sexual differentiation in mammals. *Johns Hopkins Med J* 1972 **130:** 38–53.

68. Siiteri PK, Wilson JD. Testosterone formation and metabolism during male sexual differentiation in the human embryo. *J Clin Endocrinol Metab* 1974 **38:** 113–125.

69. George FW, Noble JF. Androgen receptors are similar in fetal and adult rabbits. *Endocrinology* 1984 **115:** 1451–1458.

70. Wilson JD, Griffin JE, George FW, Leshim M. The endocrine control of male phenotypic development. *Aust J Biol Sci* 1983 **36:** 101–128.

71. Wilson JD, Lasnitzki I. Dihydrotestosterone formation in fetal tissues of the rabbit and rat. *Endocrinology* 1971 **89:** 659–668.

72. McEwen DS. Gonadal steroids and brain development. *Biol Reprod* 1980 **22:** 43–48.

73. Cate RL, Wilson CA. Müllerian-Inhibiting Substance. In Gwatkin RBL (ed.) *Genes in Mammalian Reproduction.* New York: Wiley-Liss, 1993: 185–206.

74. Josso N, Picard J-Y. Anti-Müllerian hormone. *Physiol Rev* 1986 **66:** 1038–1090.

75. Taguchi O, Chunha GR, Lawrence WD, Robboy SJ. Timing and irreversibility of Müllerian duct inhibition in the embryonic reproductive tract of the human male. *Dev Biol* 1984 **106:** 394–398.

76. Ueno S, Kuroda T, MacLaughlin DT, Ragin RC, Manganaro TF, Donahoe PK. Mullerian inhibiting substance in the adult rat ovary during various stages of the estrous cycle. *Endocrinology* 1989 **125:** 1060–1066.

77. Takahashi M, Koide SS, Donahoe PK. Müllerian inhibiting substance as oocyte meiosis inhibitor. *Mol Cell Endocrinol* 1986 **47:** 225–234.

78. Vigier B, Forest MG, Eychenne B, Bezard J, Garrigou O, Robel P, Josso N. Anti-Müllerian hormone produces endocrine sex reversal of fetal ovaries. *Proc Natl Acad Sci USA* 1989 **86:** 3684–3688.

79. Luo X, Ikeda Y, Schlosser DA, Parker KL. Steroidogenic factor 1 is the essential transcript of the mouse *Ftz-F1* gene. *Mol Endocrinol* 1995 **9:** 1233–1239.

80. Matzuk, MM. Functional analysis of mammalian members of the transforming growth factor beta superfamily. *Trends Endocrinol Metab* 1995 **6:** 120–127.

81. Sharpe RM, Skakkebaek NE. Are oestrogens involved in falling sperm counts and disorders of the male reproductive tract? *Lancet* 1993 **341:** 1392–1395.

82. Editorial. Male reproductive health and environmental oestrogens. *Lancet* 1995 **345:** 933–934.

2.2

The Hypothalamo–Pituitary Axis

IJ Clarke

INTRODUCTION

Reproduction is controlled by the brain through a delicately designed network of gonadotropin-releasing hormone (GnRH) neurones that translate neural signals into endocrine messages by action on the pituitary gland. The synthesis and secretion of GnRH (also known as luteinizing hormone (LH) releasing hormone) is controlled by higher neural centres in the brain, allowing integration of a variety of influences (nutrition, stress etc). GnRH is secreted into the hypophysial portal blood system, that runs between the hypothalamus and the pituitary gland[1,2] (Fig. 2.2.1). The pituitary hormones that orchestrate gonadal function are the gonadotropins, LH and follicle stimulating hormone (FSH); these are synthesized in the gonadotropes in response to stimulation by GnRH. Prolactin, a pituitary hormone secreted from the lactotropes, may also act on the ovaries to stimulate the secretion of progesterone from the corpus luteum in some species, although not in human beings. The main role for prolactin, however, is in the stimulation of the onset of milk production in mothers after parturition.

The hypothalamo–pituitary axis is an anatomical and functional masterpiece, integrating neuronal, metabolic and hormonal factors to produce the patterns of circulating gonadotropins in peripheral plasma, which determine reproductive success or failure. This chapter surveys current understanding of the molecular and cellular processes through which this neuroendocrine system is controlled.

CURRENT CONCEPTS

The hypothalamo–pituitay axis is regulated at two main levels. At the 'higher level', GnRH neurones of the *hypothalamus* have an inherent mode of operation driven by afferent inputs from the central nervous system. Superimposed on this is the endocrine control of GnRH synthesis and secre-

tion, regulated by gonadal feedback mechanisms and GnRH itself. At the 'lower' level, the rate of synthesis and mode of secretion of FSH and LH by the gonadotropes in the *anterior pituitary gland* is dependent upon GnRH, modulated by gonadal endocrine feedback, paracrine mechanisms and various extrinsic factors. Prolactin secretion from the pituitary gland is also controlled by the hypothalamus but the regulation of its synthesis and secretion is less well understood. Each of these components of the neuroendocrine system will now be considered.

The GnRH neurones

Embryonic origins

The GnRH neurones arise from the olfactory placode.[3] From this embryonic origin they migrate to the basal forebrain in and around the preoptic area where they colonize the hypothalamus. The anosmic condition of Kallman's syndrome, in which gonadotropin secretion is absent, has an embryonic etiology, characterized by partial or total absence of GnRH neurones and infertility during adulthood.[4]

The final location of the GnRH neurones in the hypothalamus is site-dependent. Transgenic replacement of the GnRH gene in the hypogonadal (*hpg*) mouse[5] with a >33.5 kb deletion in the GnRH gene leads to expression of GnRH neurones exclusively in the hypothalamus.[6]

Migration of GnRH neurones from the olfactory placode has been demonstrated *in vitro*.[7] In cultured explants from fetal monkey placodes, GnRH cells visualized by immunostaining migrated out of the explants, led by 'pioneer' cells. The GnRH cells matured in culture, and released GnRH in response to K+ induced depolarization. *In vivo*, the GnRH expressing cells migrate along and within a scaffold created by nerve cell adhesion molecule (NCAM). The 'pioneer cells' are themselves NCAM positive, forming a cellular aggregate which links nasal tissue to the developing basal forebrain.[3]

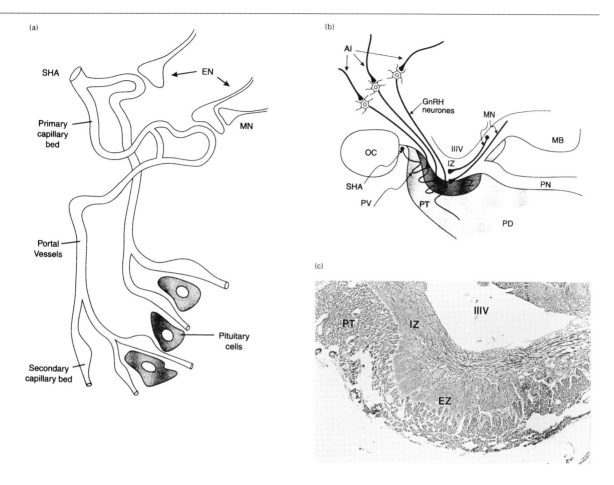

Fig. 2.2.1 *Anatomy of the hypothalamus–pituitary axis. (a) The hypophysial portal vessels connect a primary capillary bed in the median eminence to a secondary capillary bed in the anterior pituitary gland. The blood supply arises from the superior hypophysial artery* **(SHA)***. Effector neurones* **(EN)** *abut the capillaries to discharge, and release inhibiting factors. Presynaptic control of EN may occur by modulatory neurones* **(MN)***. (b) Sagittal view of the sheep hypothalamo–pituitary axis. GnRH neurones are found generally in the septal preoptic area with a greater population in the mediobasal hypothalamus of some primate species. The cells are regulated by afferent inputs from various brain regions. The GnRH neurones project to the external zone of the median eminence* **(EZ)** *to discharge into the primary capillary bed of the portal system.* **OC***, optic chiasma;* **IZ***, internal zone;* **IIIV***, third cerebral ventricle;* **PT***, pars distalis of the pituitary gland, which forms the outer layer of the infundibulum;* **PN***, pars nervosa;* **PD***, pars distalis. (c) Sagittal section of the sheep median eminence displaying the neurohemal zone where the effector neurones of the hypothalamus abut the primary capillary bed.*

The *in vitro* model mentioned above offers a potentially powerful way of studying the function of GnRH cells. GnRH cells in primary culture are probably more useful than GnRH cell lines derived from transgenic mice,[8] the properties of which may not be representative of normal GnRH cells.

Neuronal networks

There are relatively few GnRH neurones: approximately 2400 is the estimate for the adult rhesus monkey brain.[9] Using *in situ* hybridization, more GnRH cells have been detected in the human brain[10] with a wider distribution than previously seen by immunohistochemistry. Such a wide distribution of GnRH neurones raises the interesting question of how their activities are synchronized to produce bursts of firing required for pulsatile GnRH secretion (see below).

Some, but not all, GnRH cells appear to communicate with each other.[11] Some GnRH neurones have a glial ensheathment that may be modified for regulatory purposes.[12] Changes in neuronal morphology occur in response to treatment with steroids and stage of the estrous cycle,[13] however, their physiological significance has yet to be evaluated.

GnRH 'pulse generator'

The GnRH neuronal network controls pituitary gonadotropin release by periodic and pulsatile secretion of GnRH into the hypophysial portal circulation. There is a paucity of data on the electrophysiology of GnRH neurones, since they present such a diffuse target to investigate *in vivo*. However, electrical recordings from unidentified hypothalamic neuroendocrine cells suggest that they have inherent phasic firing patterns, which may constitute the underlying mechanism of pulsatile GnRH release.[14] Knobil and colleagues have identified a pattern of multi-unit electrical activity in the mediobasal hypothalamus that could provide the pulse generating mechanism for GnRH[15] (Fig. 2.2.2). However, the source of this phasic electrical activity is unknown.

The GnRH neuronal network may itself constitute, or be part of, the 'pulse-generator' system responsible for the control of pulsatile gonadotropin secretion. However, multi-unit electrical activity has also been described in species in which GnRH cells are sparse in the mediobasal hypothalamus, such as goat[16] and rat.[17]

Pulsatile secretion of LH – and by inference GnRH – can be inhibited by pharmacological intervention (e.g. adrenergic receptor blockade[18]) at the level of the GnRH cell bodies, suggesting that afferent inputs to the GnRH neurones are vital to the phasic nature of their activity.

GnRH biosynthesis

GnRH-associated peptide (GAP)

GnRH is synthesized as a prohormone that consists of a 23 amino acid signal peptide, the decapeptide sequence of GnRH and a 56 amino acid C-terminal extension that has been called GnRH-associated peptide or GAP.[19] The prohormone is detectable in the cell bodies, and the axons and terminals of the GnRH neurones. Pulses of GAP are detectable in hypophysial portal blood coincident with pulses of LH measured in the peripheral plasma of sheep, indicative of co-secretion with GnRH.[20] The early suggestion that GAP may be a prolactin-releasing factor[21] has not been substantiated.

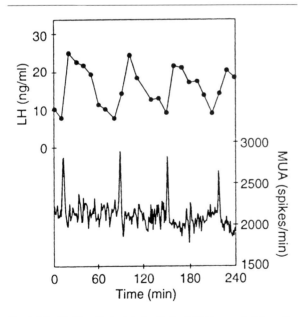

Fig. 2.2.2 *Multi-unit electrical activity (MUA) recorded from the mediobasal hypothalamus in an ovary-intact rhesus monkey on day 5 of the follicular phase of the menstrual cycle. Note the coincidence of each volley of MUA with a pulse of LH determined by radioimmunoassay in peripheral serum. (From reference 15, with permission.)*

Cyclic changes

The suggestion that cyclic changes in hypothalamic GnRH content reflect alterations in secretion have not been reliably substantiated. In sheep, there appears to be little change in the amount of GnRH in the median eminence throughout the estrous cycle, suggesting that the rate of GnRH biosynthesis is relatively constant.[22]

Studies of GnRH mRNA expression by *in situ* hybridization suggests that GnRH synthesis is regulated by steroids.[22] However, such data provide information on the abundance of mRNA only, and not peptide formation *per se*. GnRH mRNA levels increase after the onset of the LH surge in cyclic rats,[23] which could be in response to the depletion of GnRH stores during the preovulatory GnRH/LH surge. Effects of hyperprolactinemia, ageing, starvation and castration on the levels of mRNA for GnRH have also been reported.[24-26]

Since GnRH neurones do not contain steroid receptors,[27] effects of steroids on the synthesis of GnRH must be mediated via another neuronal system. GnRH mRNA levels were reduced when ovariectomized rats were treated with the α-adrenergic antagonist, prazosin,[28] suggesting that noradrenergic inputs to the GnRH cells may regulate GnRH expression. Other studies implicate neurosteroids such as γ-aminobutyric acid (GABA) and excitatory amino acids. Nitric oxide (NO) synthase is also present in brain and local production of NO has been postulated as a mediator of synchronized GnRH neuronal activity (see reference 29 for review).

Gonadotropin biosynthesis

The gonadotropins LH and FSH are heterodimeric polypeptides comprising a common α-subunit and a unique, structurally related β-subunit that confers biological specificity. They belong to a family of glycoproteins that includes thyroid-stimulating hormone (TSH) and placenta derived chorionic gonadotropin (HCG). Each gonadotropin subunit results from the post-translational maturation of independent precursor polypeptides that are encoded by different genes. The α and β chains are linked by disulfide bonds and the molecules are glycosylated. Free gonadotropin subunits have no known biological activities. The level of complexity in the structures of these molecules allows for substantial regulation in the biosynthetic pathway.[30] As a result, there are a number of gonadotropin isoforms with varying biological activities.[31,32]

GnRH receptor

The GnRH receptor is the crucial regulatory molecule that transduces the action of GnRH to stimulate gonadotropin synthesis and release. It is a member of the seven-transmembrane domain, G-protein coupled family of receptors (see Chapter 1.4) located in the gonadotrope plasma membrane. Occupation of the receptor by GnRH or a GnRH agonist triggers a rapid increase in intracellular calcium levels and activation of protein kinase C, both of which may lead to the exocytosis of secretory granules and enhanced biosynthesis of gonadotropin subunits.

The maintenance of both α- and β-subunit mRNA levels is reliant upon GnRH input. They decline rapidly after withdrawal of GnRH and are regulated by changes in the frequency and the amplitude of GnRH pulses.[33]

Negative feedback regulation

Gonadal hormones also directly regulate gonadotropin subunit gene expresion. Castration of animals of either sex results in an increase in gonadotropin mRNA levels (reviewed in reference 33), However, this could be secondary to increased secretion of GnRH and not to a reduction of steroid negative-feedback to the pituitary gland. Nilson *et al.*[34] showed that chronic administration of estradiol to ovariectomized ewes reduced the mRNA levels of α-subunit and LHβ by around 90%, but when ovariectomized ewes were subjected to hypothalamo–pituitary disconnection (removing GnRH input to the pituitary gland) and were then given hourly pulses of GnRH at a fixed dose, chronic estradiol treatment had no effect on the levels of mRNA for these subunits.[35] Similar estradiol treatment caused a profound suppression of GnRH secretion.[36] Thus the predominant negative feedback effect of estrogen on LH secretion is likely to be indirect, via an effect on GnRH secretion.

Androgens negatively regulate gonadotropin synthesis in the male. Gonadotropin mRNA levels increase after orchidectomy and return to normal after physiological androgen replacement.[37] Supraphysiological doses of testosterone selectively increase FSHβ mRNA levels,[38] apparently by prolonging mRNA half-life.[39]

Progesterone alone does not directly regulate gonadotropin mRNA levels or the secretion of gonadotropins by the pituitary gland.[40,41] However, progesterone may negatively regulate gonadotropin secretion when acting in concert with estrogen.[42]

Positive feedback regulation

In addition to the *chronic* negative-feedback action of estrogen on GnRH and gonadotropin secretion, estrogen also has an *acute* positive-feedback effect at the level of the brain and the pituitary gland. This positive feedback mechanism is primarily responsible for generating the preovulatory LH surge in females. The positive feedback effect of estrogen is exerted at the level of the hypothalamus to increase the secretion of GnRH, and at the level of the pituitary gland to increase the responsiveness of gonadotropes to GnRH.

Does the positive feedback action of estrogen at the level of the pituitary gland involve increased synthesis of LH and FSH? In rats, an increase in LHβ-subunit mRNA levels occurs before the LH surge,[43] with an increase in FSHβ mRNA levels after the surge.[44] During the follicular phase of the estrous cycle in ewes, there is a doubling in the level of α-subunit mRNA, a non-significant increase in LHβ mRNA and a fall in FSHβ mRNA.[45] Thus both sets of data show

divergent regulation of gonadotropin subunit mRNAs, with LHβ tending to be upregulated. However, even if the expression of LHβ mRNA is increased during the preovulatory period, such an increase does not appear to be mandatory for the generation of an LH surge by estrogen.[46,47]

Steady-state synthesis

Transcription of gonadotropin subunit genes is subject to negative feedback regulation by gonadal steroids and peptides. Regulatory domains have been identified on some subunit genes but details of their function are lacking. The regulation of the gonadotropin α-subunit has been studied in cultured cell lines but there is limited information on the regulation of β-subunit genes. Those immortalized cell lines described to date express α-subunit but not the β-subunits,[48] which is unfortunate since synthesis of β-subunits is rate-limiting in the synthesis of gonadotropins.

Regulation by inhibin

The control of FSH synthesis and secretion by peptidergic gonadal hormones deserves special mention. Inhibin and related peptides such as activin specifically regulate the secretion of FSH by direct actions at the level of the pituitary gland, *without any effect on the secretion of GnRH*.[49] The direct action of inhibin appears to be at the level of FSHβ mRNA. Within hours of administration of inhibin, a marked reduction occurs in the steady-state level of FSHβ mRNA with no effect on LHβ mRNA or α-subunit mRNA. This effect is only partially accounted for by a reduction in the transcription rate of the FSH gene.[50]

Inhibin appears to have a specific destabilizing action on FSHβ mRNA in the gonadotropes. FSHβ mRNA has a long 3′ untranslated region[30] containing a number of AUUUA repeat sequences that are believed to be involved in destabilizing the mRNA.[51] It is hypothesized that inhibin, or some induced factor, binds to the 3′ region of the message and effects or initiates its destruction. Deletion of all but 135 base pairs of the 3′-untranslated region of the FSHβ gene results in the expression of increased amounts of FSHβ mRNA in transfected COS cells,[51] confirming a regulatory function for this region of the gene.

Cyclic patterns of GnRH and gonadotropin secretion

Pulsatility

The development of a system in sheep for the simultaneous sampling from both the hypophysial portal vessels and the pituitary gland in the conscious animal has allowed simultaneous measurements of GnRH and gonadotropin secretion.[52]

Using this experimental approach it has been shown that short-lived pulses of GnRH produce correspondingly large pulses of LH secretion (Fig. 2.2.3). However, the pattern of FSH secretion in peripheral plasma is not rigidly pulsatile,[53] possibly due to the 'smoothing' effect of the long half-life of FSH compared to LH.

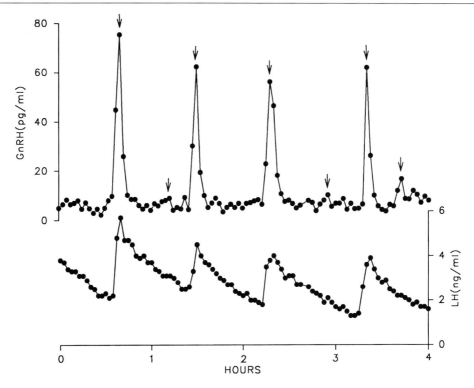

Fig. 2.2.3 *Relationship between hypothalamic GnRH secretion and pituitary LH secretion. Large, short-lived pulses of GnRH (upper panel) produce correspondingly large secretory episodes of LH secretion (lower panel). Smaller pulses not associated with discernible rises in the peripheral levels of LH may serve a role in maintaining the synthesis of the gonadotropins. (Reproduced from reference 60, with permission.)*

In addition to the major secretory episodes of GnRH, there appear to be a number of smaller pulses not associated with discernible rises in the peripheral levels of LH. These small pulses of GnRH may serve a role in maintaining the synthesis of the gonadotropins (see above).[54] Recently, sampling of blood from the cavernous sinus of the sheep has revealed small LH pulses measurable at the site of secretion from the pituitary gland that are not seen with sampling of the jugular vein (I.J. Clarke, unpublished data). These small pulses of LH are probably produced by the small GnRH pulses.

Cyclicity

The pattern of hypothalamic GnRH secretion in relation to pituitary LH secretion has been examined in considerable detail in sheep (Fig. 2.2.4). During the luteal phase of the estrous cycle, GnRH pulses are large and relatively infrequent, leading to a similar pattern of LH secretion.[55–58] In the follicular phase, the frequency of secretory episodes of both hormones increases.[55–58] This is probably due to the reduction in the plasma levels of progesterone upon regression of the corpus luteum, since progesterone has been shown to exert powerful inhibitory effects on the secretion of GnRH,[36] and somewhat lesser effects on the secretion of LH at the level of the pituitary gland.[41]

During the follicular phase of the cycle, the frequency of GnRH pulses increases slightly, and there is a progressive reduction in GnRH pulse amplitude. LH pulses also increase in frequency during the follicular phase of the cycle and there is also evidence for progressive reduction in LH pulse amplitude.[56–58]

The LH surge

Is the ovulation-inducing gonadotropin surge due to a rise in GnRH secretion, increased responsiveness of the gonadotropes to GnRH, or both? The original data of Sarkar *et al.*[59] first demonstrated an unambiguous and remarkable increase in the secretion of GnRH at the time of the pro-estrous rise in LH secretion in the rat. Subsequent data from conscious sheep showed a detectable rise in GnRH secretion at the time of the LH surge in some but not all animals.[55] More recent studies suggest that there is an unequivocal rise in GnRH secretion at this time but there is considerable variation between animals in the magnitude of the rise.[56] This leads to the proposition that initiation of the surge may be due to a variety of factors, and that more than one pattern of GnRH secretion can initiate it.

Rapid sampling of the portal blood suggests that the pre-ovulatory rise in GnRH secretion is generally brought about by a dramatic increase in the frequency of GnRH pulses.[60] Indirect measurement of the secretion of GnRH in the monkey by sampling cerebrospinal fluid from the infundibular recess of the third ventricle[61] or by push–pull perfusion of the median eminence[62] confirms that there is also a preovulatory GnRH surge in primates. This sheds

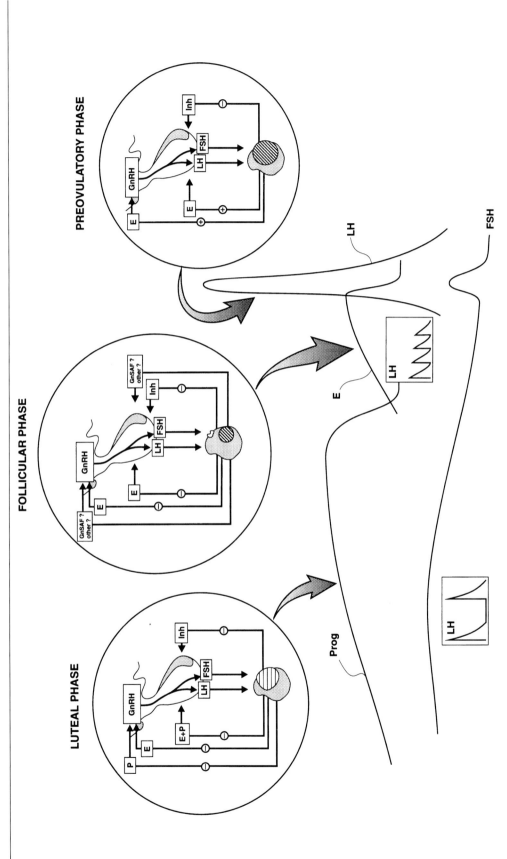

Fig. 2.2.4 Schematic illustration of dynamic changes in the hypothalamo–pituitary–ovarian axis during the ovine estrous cycle. During the luteal phase the frequency of GnRH pulses is reduced by the negative feedback action of estrogen (**E**) and progesterone (**P**). Both E and P can act in combination but not individually to limit LH responsiveness to GnRH. E and inhibin (**Inh**) negatively regulate FSH secretion. During the follicular phase the GnRH pulse frequency is increased due to the absence of P negative feedback. E limits GnRH pulse amplitude. LH responses to GnRH pulses may be limited by E and other feedback factors (such as gonadotropin surge attenuating factor (**GnSAF**)). Increased secretion of E and Inh provide more powerful inhibition of FSH secretion at this time than during the luteal phase of the cycle. In the preovulatory phase the negative feedback action of E is switched to a positive feedback effect. This is a transient, time-delayed response to rising E levels which having reached a threshold, cause a surge in GnRH secretion and enhanced responsiveness of the pituitary gonadotrope to GnRH. The mechanism involves a 'switch' from negative to positive feedback and is coordinated at the brain and pituitary level. A surge in FSH secretion also occurs.

light on the role of GnRH in gonadotropin surge onset that has been debated since the 1970s. Classic studies by Knobil and colleagues on monkeys bearing radiofrequency lesions of the arcuate nucleus (hence, preventing endogenous GnRH production) showed that when the pituitary gonadotropes were 'driven' by exogenously administered GnRH,[63] delivery of GnRH in hourly pulses at fixed dose was sufficient to initiate follicular development and ovulation. These results were interpreted as evidence that cyclic changes in the secretion of GnRH are not a prerequisite for the normal ovarian cycle. However, although it is clearly possible to drive the ovarian cycle in this way, it is not necessarily physiological.[61,62] Nevertheless, the experimental studies[63] on arcuate-lesioned monkeys have had important practical implications, leading to the development of pulsatile GnRH treatment to treat various forms of infertility in patients with hypothalamic insufficiency.[53]

Relationship between GnRH pulse frequency and LH pulse amplitude

A tight inverse relationship between the frequency of GnRH pulses and the amplitude of LH pulses has been demonstrated in GnRH-treated monkeys with radiofrequency lesions to the arcuate nucleus (see above)[64] and in hypothalamo–pituitary disconnected sheep.[65] The latter is a surgical preparation in which all neural inputs to the median eminence are removed but the vascular supply to the pituitary gland is preserved. In such models – and in the absence of steroidal feedback – the inverse relationship between the frequency of administered GnRH pulses and the amplitude of the LH pulses is well demonstrated.[65] Furthermore, the relationship can be accounted for by alterations in the size of the releasable pool of LH in the pituitary gland, such that a slower pulse rate appears to allow a greater build up of releasable LH.[66] It is important to note that generally not all of the LH in the gonadotropes is in a releasable state, presumably because biosynthesis is continual.

Negative feedback actions of gonadal hormones

Secretion of GnRH can be regarded as 'free-running' after gonadectomy. In this situation, the frequency of GnRH and LH pulses is around one per hour, reflecting the inherent activity of the 'pulse generator' mentioned above. Negative feedback effects operate in the male and throughout the luteal and follicular phases of the estrous/menstrual cycle in the female. Testosterone reduces the GnRH pulse frequency in the castrated male sheep.[67] In the female, progesterone acts as the major negative regulator of GnRH pulse frequency.[36] This explains the relatively low pulse frequency of GnRH and LH during the luteal phase of the menstrual cycle. Estradiol is also a negative regulator of GnRH secretion[36] and both ovarian steroids probably act in concert to regulate the secretion of GnRH during the luteal phase of the menstrual cycle (Fig. 2.2.4).

The reduction in circulating progesterone and estradiol levels upon regression of the corpus luteum explains changes in LH pulses that occur at the luteal-follicular transition phase of the estrous/menstrual cycle. GnRH pulses increase in frequency and decrease in amplitude at

this time, causing similar changes in the pattern of LH pulses. The reduction in LH pulse amplitude is further accentuated by the increase in GnRH pulse frequency (see above). In addition, there is negative feedback regulation at the level of the pituitary gland during the follicular phase. Some studies in sheep show a progressive reduction in the amplitude of LH pulses across the follicular phase of the estrous cycle,[68] which is most likely due to a negative feedback effect of estrogen secreted by the growing preovulatory follicles at this time.

Factors other than estrogen that exert negative feedback regulation of gonadotropin secretion during the follicular phase include inhibin[70,71] and possibly gonadotropin surge-attenuating factor (GnSAF).[69] Inhibin, acting in concert with estradiol, is an established negative feedback regulator of FSH secretion in the estrous cycles of rats and sheep. The contribution of inhibin to the control of FSH release during the human menstrual cycle is less clear (see Chapter 2.3). GnSAF, an uncharacterized protein secreted by ovarian follicles, may reduce pituitary responsiveness to GnRH (reviewed in reference 69). In combination with estradiol it might provide a negative feedback clamp on the secretion of LH at this time. However, purification of a biologically active protein and the development of specific assays for GnSAF are required before its physiological significance can be fully evaluated.

Positive feedback actions of gonadal hormones

The positive feedback actions of estrogen that trigger the preovulatory LH surge involve increased GnRH secretion (see above) and increased responsiveness to GnRH.[72] How does the switch from negative to positive feedback control occur? One contributory factor could be the increased number and/or affinity of the GnRH receptors during the follicular phase.[73] This increase, which occurs at a time during the cycle when LH secretion is still under negative feedback control, could help maximize the eventual *responsiveness* of the pituitary to the LH surge but cannot explain the *timing* of surge onset (Fig. 2.2.5). Estrogen causes an increase in the number of GnRH receptors long before increased responsiveness to GnRH is manifest.[74] The switch from negative to positive feedback control could be initiated by the GnRH surge but this seems unlikely in view of the evidence cited above that fixed rates of pulsatile GnRH administration to arcuate-lesioned animals are able to initiate an LH surge.[63]

The most probable cause of the switch from negative to positive feedback control lies at the level of the gonadotrope, brought about by the sudden rise in estradiol in the absence of progesterone (Fig. 2.2.5). Gonadotropin-containing secretory granules adjacent to the plasma membrane represent a readily releasable pool of hormone. Acute responses to estrogen by the gonadotrope include mobilization of LH stores into secretory granules that migrate to the cell periphery,[75] and altered second-messenger signaling – notably increased activation of protein kinase C.[76] Other second-messenger systems that may also be involved at this time have been less well studied.[76]

The self-priming action of GnRH is another factor that contributes to the positive feedback event. This may be

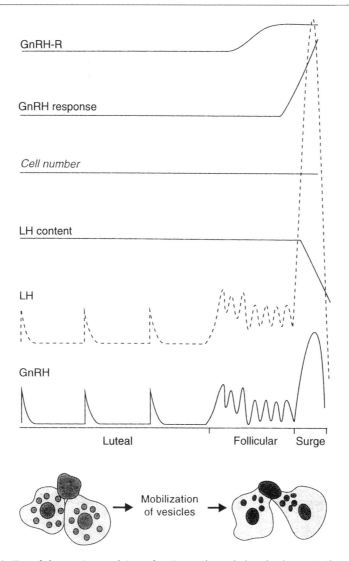

Fig. 2.2.5 *Schematic illustration of changes in gonadotrope function and morphology leading up to the preovulatory LH surge. Changes occur at the beginning of the follicular phase in response to the fall in plasma progesterone levels (luteal regression) and the rise in estrogen levels (preovulatory follicular development). GnRH-R, GnRH receptor number; GnRH response, responsiveness to GnRH; Cell number, gonadotrope number; LH, peripheral plasma LH level; GnRH, portal plasma GnRH level. The timing of maximum responsiveness to GnRH coincides with the preovulatory surge in GnRH secretion by the GnRH neurones.*

demonstrated by observing responses to the administration of two injections of GnRH within an hour or so of each other.[77] The self-priming action is greater during the preovulatory period and involves the upregulation of G-protein coupled second-messenger systems within the gonadotropes.[76]

Major changes in the number of GnRH receptors occur throughout the estrous cycle, as discussed above. The recent cloning of the GnRH receptor has allowed more fundamental studies of its regulation.[78] An interesting new finding is the existence of multiple GnRH mRNA transcripts that appear to be differentially regulated (IJ Clarke and RP Millar, unpublished observations). Studies to date suggest that the expression of the GnRH receptor gene is highly regulated, as is GnRH receptor number on the gonadotropes.[78]

Prolactin biosynthesis

In addition to its classic lactogenic role, prolactin can exert effects on gonadal function in some animal species. In women, it is an important factor in certain forms of hypogonadism and infertility associated with hyperprolactinemia. This chapter concludes with a brief examination of the mechanisms that regulate prolactin secretion by the anterior pituitary gland.

Negative regulation by dopamine

Lactotropes in the anterior pituitary gland synthesize, store and release prolactin by mechanisms that are common to all secretory cells (see Chapter 1.2). Prolactin secretion is under tonic inhibitory control by the hypothalamus, being elevated by the removal of neural input to the median eminence.[79] Studies in rats point to dopamine as the predominant negative regulator. Dopamine acts on specific receptors on lactotropes to inhibit the secretion of prolactin, providing the basis for widespread use of dopamine agonists to treat hyperprolactinemia and prolactinoma in women.

Although dopamine was not measurable in the portal blood of sheep,[80] norepinephrine (noradrenaline) – another amine that inhibits prolactin secretion – was. Dopamine may reach the lactotropes by way of short portal vessels that link the posterior and anterior lobes of the pituitary. Evidence for this comes from studies in which the selective removal of the posterior lobe led to elevation of prolactin secretion.[81,82]

Positive regulation by TRH

The most potent stimulator of prolactin secretion is thyrotropin-releasing hormone (TRH). TRH cannot, however, be regarded as a specific regulator of prolactin secretion, since it also stimulates the secretion of thyroid-stimulating hormone (TSH). Immunization against TRH did not compromise prolactin secretion in sheep[83] and only caused a minor delay in the pro-estrous prolactin surge in rats.[84] Furthermore, the pulsatile secretion of TRH into portal blood of sheep is not related to the secretion of prolactin.[85] A variety of other peptides have been implicated in the positive regulation of prolactin (see reference 2 for review). Acute release of prolactin is produced by lactation, stressors and various pharmacological manipulations, supporting the view that another physiological factor(s) exists that regulates prolactin release.[86] There is evidence for the production of a 'prolactin-releasing factor' by the posterior pituitary but its identity is as yet unknown.[87]

Another possible mechanism for stimulation of prolactin release is interruption of tonic inhibition by dopamine, as demonstrated experimentally in monkeys.[86] However, measurements of dopamine secretion into portal blood do not support the view that this is a physiological mechanism.

Positive regulation by estrogen

Estrogen is a potent stimulator of prolactin synthesis, via direct action at the pituitary level.[88] The prolactin gene contains an estrogen response element in the 5′ upstream region that allows for direct transcriptional control.[89] Accordingly, estrogen stimulates prolactin secretion in rats, causing a surge in secretion on the afternoon of pro-estrus.[90,91] The preovulatory rise in estrogen does not, however, evoke a rise in prolactin secretion in primates.[86]

Estrogen also reduces transcription of the tyrosine hydroxylase enzyme in the median eminence, thereby reducing dopamine turnover.[92–94] The inhibitory effect of estrogen on tyrosine hydroxylase is antagonized by progesterone.[95]

Diurnal rhythm

The combined effect of estrogen to increase prolactin synthesis and to suppress the inhibitory effect of dopamine is thought to explain the daily prolactin surge that occurs in estrogen-treated rats.[95]

Marked diurnal secretion of prolactin also occurs in humans, with an increase at night,[96] especially during the early hours of sleep.[97] Prolactin secretion is also stimulated by GnRH,[98] and LH and prolactin pulses coincide in some situations.[99] The mechanism through which this occurs is unclear. However, the effect of GnRH appears to be specific, since it can be blocked by a GnRH antagonist.[100]

FUTURE PERSPECTIVES

Factors that regulate the developmental biology and functioning of GnRH neurones should become more clearly understood in the next few years through the use of recently developed *in vitro* models. Cells produced from cultured explants appear to offer the most 'physiological' model for this purpose. Immortalized cell lines may also be useful,[8] but the question remains whether the functioning of transformed cells is relevant to normal cells.

The concept of a 'pulse generator' within the brain that in some way regulates GnRH pulse frequency has prevailed for over two decades. However, the 'pulse generator' may not exist as a discrete entity. The phasic nature of GnRH neuronal activity may simply represent modulation by various afferent inputs. Future research to resolve this issue is likely to depend on the use of pharmacological methods to manipulate GnRH cell function *in vitro* and *in vivo*. Techniques of brain dialysis, voltametry, microinjection and histochemistry should assist in this area.

Reproductive success depends on ovulation occurring timeously: i.e. when the oocyte is mature and the reproductive tract is ready to support fertilization and conception. It is therefore of fundamental and practical (clinical) importance to gain improved knowledge of the mechanisms through which ovarian steroidal (estrogen) and nonsteroidal (inhibin, GnSAF, etc.) factors differentially regulate FSH and LH secretion and trigger the ovulation-inducing gonadotropin surge.

The challenge with regard to prolactin is to identify the prolactin-releasing factor, which could open up new avenues for the medical treatment of disorders associated with hyperprolactinemias.

SUMMARY

- GnRH neurones originate embryologically in the olfactory placode and migrate into the hypothalamus.
- The GnRH decapetide is synthesized in GnRH neurones, processed from a pre-propeptide.
- Synthesis and secretion of GnRH is regulated by gonadal steroids. Estrogen has both positive and negative feedback effects.
- Pituitary gonadotropins, FSH and LH are heterodimeric glycoproteins, comprising a common α-subunit and a unique, structurally related, β-subunit that determines hormonal specificity.
- Genes encoding gonadotropin subunits are expressed in gonadotropes, regulated by GnRH. Gonadal steroids exert feedback control of the synthesis and secretion of FSH and LH. FSH is specifically regulated by inhibin.
- Secretion of LH and FSH by the anterior pituitary is governed by the frequency and amplitude of GnRH input from the hypothalamus.
- The secretion of LH is substantially affected by the negative and positive feedback actions of estrogen at the level of the pituitary gland.
- The secretion of prolactin secretion is under tonic inhibitory control by the hypothalamus. The major negative regulator of prolactin synthesis is most probably dopamine.
- Prolactin secretion is stimulated by TRH. However, there is circumstantial evidence that a more specific prolactin-releasing factor exists, possibly produced by the posterior lobe of the pituitary gland. Prolactin secretion is also stimulated by estrogen, acting at both hypothalamic and pituitary levels.
- Prolactin secretion may be stimulated by GnRH, and in certain circumstances LH and prolactin pulses coincide.

REFERENCES

1. Page RB. The pituitary portal system. In Ganten D, Pfaff D (eds) *Current Topics in Neuroendocrinology Morphology of Hypothalamus and its Connections*. Berlin: Springer-Verlag, 1986: 1–47.
2. Clarke IJ. Effector mechanisms of the hypothalamus that regulate the anterior pituitary gland. In Unsicker K (ed.) *The Autonomic Nervous System* Autonomic Endocrine Interactions, vol. 10. London: Harwood, 1996: 45–88.
3. Pfaff DW, Weesner GD, Schwanzel-Fukuda M. GnRH neurons during migration and in basal forebrain. In Bouchard P, Caraty A, Coelingh-Benink HJT, Pavlou SN (eds) *GnRH, GnRH Analogs, Gonadotropins and Gonadal Peptides*. London: Parthenon, 1993: 15–21.
4. Schwanzel-Fukuda M, Bick D, Pfaff DW. Luteinizing hormone-releasing hormone (LHRH)-expressing cells do not migrate normally in an inherited hypogonadal (Kallmann) syndrome. *Mol Brain Res* 1989 **6**: 311–326.
5. Mason AJ, Hayflick JS, Zoeller T, Scott Young III W, Phillips HS, Nikolics K, Seeburg PH. A deletion truncating the gonadotropin-releasing hormone gene is responsible for hypogonadism in the *hpg* mouse. *Science* 1986 **234**: 1366–1371.
6. Mason AJ, Pitts SL, Nikolics K, Szonyi E, Wilcox JN, Seeburg PH, Stewart TA. The hypogonadal mouse: reproductive functions restored by gene therapy. *Science* 1986 **234**: 1372–1378.
7. Terasawa E, Quanbeck CD, Schulz CA, Burich AJ, Luchansky LL, Claude PA. Primary cell culture system of luteinizing hormone releasing hormone neurons derived from embryonic olfactory placode in the rhesus monkey. *Endocrinology* 1993 **133**: 2379–2390.
8. Mellon PL, Windle JJ, Goldsmith P, Pedula C, Roberts J, Weiner RI. Immortalization of hypothalamic GnRH neurons by genetically targeted tumorigenesis. *Neuron* 1990 **5**: 1–10.
9. Marshall PE, Goldsmith PC. Neuroregulatory and neuroendocrine GnRH pathways in the hypothalamus and forebrain of the baboon. *Brain Res* 1980 **193**: 353–372.
10. Rance NE, Young WS, McMullen NT. Topography of neurons expressing luteinizing hormone-releasing hormone gene transcripts in the human hypothalamus and basal forebrain. *J Comp Neurol* 1991 **339**: 573–586.
11. Lehman MN, Karsch FJ, Robinson JE, Silverman A-J. Ultrastructure and synaptic organization of luteinizing hormone-releasing hormone (LHRH) neurons in the anestrous ewe. *J Comp Neurol* 1988 **273**: 447–457.
12. Witkin JW, Ferin M, Popilskis SJ, Silverman A-J. Effects of gonadal steroids on the ultrastructure of GnRH neurons in the rhesus monkey: synaptic input and glial apposition. *Endocrinology* 1991 **129**: 1083–1092.
13. Naftolin F, Leranth C, Garcia-Segura LM. Ultrastructural changes in hypothalamic cells during estrogen-induced gonadotrophin feedback. *Neuroprotocols* 1992 **1**: 16–26.
14. Andrew RP, Dudek FE. Burst discharge in mammalian neuroendocrine cells involves an intrinsic regenerative mechanism. *Science* 1983 **221**: 1050–1052.
15. O'Byrne KT, Chen MD, Nishihara M, Williams CL, Thalabard JC, Hotchkiss J, Knobil E. Ovarian control of gonadotropin hormone-releasing hormone pulse generator activity in the rhesus monkey: duration of the associated hypothalamic signal. *Neuroendocrinology* 1993 **57**: 588–592.
16. Mori Y, Nishihara M, Tarraka T, Shimizu T, Yamaguchi M, Takeuchi Y, Hoshino K. Chronic recording of electrophysiological manifestation of the hypothalamic gonadotropin-releasing hormone pulse generator activity in the goat. *Neuroendocrinology* 1991 **53**: 392–395.
17. Nishihara M, Sano A, Kimura F. Cessation of the electrical activity of gonadotropin-releasing hormone pulse generator during the steroid-induced surge of luteinizing hormone in the rat. *Neuroendocrinology* 1994 **59**: 513–519.
18. Barraclough CA, Wise PM. The role of catecholamines in the regulation of pituitary luteinizing hormone and follicle stimulating hormone secretion. *Endocr Rev* 1982 **3**: 91–119.

19. Seeburg PH, Adelman JP. Characterisation of cDNA for precursor of human luteinizing hormone releasing hormone. *Nature* 1984 311: 666–668.

20. Clarke IJ, Karsch FJ, Cummins JT, Seeburg PH, Nikolics PE. Secretion of GnRH associated peptide (GAP) into hypophyseal portal blood of ovariectomized ewes. *Biochem Biophys Res Commun* 1987 143: 665–672.

21. Nikolics K, Mason AJ, Szonyi E, Ramachandran J, Seeburg PH. A prolactin-inhibiting factor within the precursor for gonadotropin-releasing hormone. *Nature* 1985 316: 511–517.

22. Clarke IJ. GnRH synthesis, secretion and action and ovarian steroidal feedback. *Oxf Rev Reprod Biol* 1987 9: 54–95.

23. Park O-K, Gugneja S, Mayo KE. Gonadotropin-releasing hormone gene expression during the rat estrous cycle: effects of pentobarbital and ovarian steroids. *Endocrinology* 1990 127: 365–372.

24. Selmanoff M, Shu C, Petersen SL, Barraclough CA, Zoeller RT. Single cell levels of hypothalamic messenger ribonucleic acid encoding luteinizing hormone-releasing hormone in intact, castrated, and hyperprolactinemic male rats. *Endocrinology* 1991 128: 459–466.

25. Gruenewald DA, Matsumoto AM. Reduced gonadotropin-releasing hormone gene expression with fasting in the male rat brain. *Endocrinology* 1993 132: 480–482.

26. Zoeller RT, Seeburg PH, Young SW. *In situ* hyridization histochemistry for messenger ribonucleic acid (mRNA) encoding gonadotropin-releasing hormone (GnRH): effect of estrogen on cellular levels of GnRH mRNA in female rat brain. *Endocrinology* 1988 122: 2570–2577.

27. Watson RE Jr, Langub MC Jr, Landis JW. Further evidence that most luteinizing hormone-releasing hormone neurons are not directly estrogen-responsive: simultaneous localization of luteinizing hormone-releasing hormone and estrogen receptor immunoreactivity in the guinea-pig brain. *J Neuroendocrinol* 1993 4: 311–318.

28. Weesner GD, Bergen HT, Pfaff DW. Differential regulation of luteinizing hormone-releasing hormone and galanin messenger ribonucleic acid levels by alpha$_1$-adrenergic agents in the ovariectomized rat. *J Neuroendocrinol* 1993 5: 331–336.

29. Negro-Vilar A, Wetsel W, López F, Valenca M, Moretto M, Liposits Z, Merchenthaler I. Novel concepts in the physiology of the LHRH pulse generator. In Bouchard P, Caraty A, Coelingh-Benink HJT, Pavlou SN (eds) *GnRH, GnRH Analogs, Gonadotropins and Gonadal Peptides*. London: Parthenon, 1993: 39–51.

30. Gharib SD, Wierman ME, Shupnik MA, Chin WW. Molecular biology of the pituitary gonadotropins. *Endocr Rev* 1990 II: 177–199.

31. Stanton PG, Robertson DM, Burgon PG, Schmauk-White B, Hearn MTW. Isolation and physiochemical characterization of human follicle-stimulating hormone isoforms. *Endocrinology* 1992 130: 2820–2832.

32. Stanton PG, Pozvek G, Burgon PG, Robertson DM, Hearn MTW. Isolation and characterization of human LH isoforms. *J Endocrinol* 1993 138: 529–543.

33. Marshall JC, Dalkin AC, Haisenleder DJ, Paul SJ, Ortolano GA, Kelch RP. Gonadotropin-releasing hormone pulses: regulators of gonadotropin synthesis and ovulatory cycles. *Recent Prog Horm Res* 1991 47: 155–189.

34. Nilson JH, Nejedlik MT, Virgin JB, Crowder ME, Nett TM. Expression of subunit and luteinizing hormone genes in the ovine anterior pituitary. *J Biol Chem* 1983 258:12087–12091.

35. Mercer JE, Clements JA, Funder JW, Clarke IJ. LH-β mRNA levels are regulated primarily by GnRH and not by negative estrogen feedback on the pituitary. *Neuroendocrinology* 1988 47: 563–566.

36. Karsch FJ, Cummins JT, Thomas GB, Clarke IJ. Steroid feedback inhibition of pulsatile secretion of gonadotropin-releasing hormone in the ewe. *Biol Reprod* 1987 36: 1207–1218.

37. Papavasiliou SS, Zmeili S, Khoury S, Landefeld TD, Chin WW, Marshall JC. Gonadotropin-releasing hormone differentially regulates expression of the genes for luteinizing hormone and subunits in male rats. *Proc Natl Acad Sci USA* 1986 83: 4026–4029.

38. Wierman ME, Gharib SD, LaRovere JM, Badger TM, Chin WW. Selective failure of androgens to regulate follicle stimulating hormone messenger ribonucleic acid levels in the male rat. *Mol Endocrinol* 1988 2: 492–498.

39. Sander JP, Ortolano GA, Haisenleder DJ, Stewart JM, Shupnik MA, Marshall JC. Gonadotropin subunit messenger RNA concentrations after blockade of gonadotropin-releasing hormone action: testosterone selectively increases follicle-stimulating hormone subunit messenger RNA by posttranscriptional mechanisms. *Mol Endocrinol* 1990 4: 1943–1948.

40. Clarke IJ, Cummins JT. Direct pituitary effects of estrogen and progesterone on gonadotropin secretion in the ewe. *Neuroendocrinology* 1984, 39: 267–274.

41. Hamernik DL, Kim KE, Maurer RA, Nett TM. Progesterone does not affect the amount of mRNA for gonadotropins in the anterior pituitary gland of ovariectomized ewes. *Biol Reprod* 1987 37: 1225–1232.

42. Girmus RL, Wise ME. Progesterone directly inhibits pituitary luteinizing hormone secretion in an estradiol-dependent manner. *Biol Reprod* 1992 46: 710–714.

43. Zmeili SM, Papavasilou SS, Thorner MO, Evans WS, Marshall JC, Landefeld TD. Alpha and luteinizing hormone beta subunit messenger ribonucleic acids during the rat estrous cycle. *Endocrinology* 1986 119: 1867–1869.

44. Ortolano GA, Haisenleder DJ, Dalkin AC, Iliff-Sizemore SA, Landefeld TD, Maurer RA, Marshall JC. Follicle-stimulating hormone beta subunit messenger ribonucleic acid concentrations during the rat estrous cycle. *Endocrinology* 1988 123: 2149–2151.

45. Leung K, Kim KE, Maurer RA, Landefeld TD. Divergent changes in the concentrations of gonadotropin subunit messenger ribonucleic acid during the estrous cycle of sheep. *Mol Endocrinol* 1988 2: 272–276.

46. Mercer JE, Phillips DJ, Clarke IJ. Short-term regulation of gonadotropin subunit mRNA levels by estrogen: studies in the hypothalamo–pituitary intact and hypothalamo–pituitary disconnected ewe. *J Neuroendocrinol* 1993 5: 591–596.

47. Haisenleder DJ, Barkan AL, Papavasiliou S, Zmeili SM, Dee C, Jameel ML, Ortolano GA, El-Gewely MR, Marshall JC. LH subunit mRNA concentrations during LH surge in ovariectomized estradiol-replaced rats. *Am J Physiol* 1988 254: E99–E103.

48. Mellon PL, Wetsel WC, Windle JJ, Valencas MM, Goldsmith C, Whyte DB, Eraly SA, Negro-Vilar A, Weiner RI. Immortalized hypothalamic gonadotropin-releasing hormone neurons. In Ciba Foundation Symposium *Functional Anatomy of the Neuroendocrine Hypothalamus*. Chichester: Wiley, 1992: 104–126.

49. Clarke IJ, Findlay JK, Cummins JT, Ewens WJ. Effects of ovine follicular fluid on plasma LH and FSH in ovariectomized ewes; determination of the site of action of inhibin. *J Reprod Fertil* 1986 77: 575–585.

50. Clarke IJ, Rao A, Fallest PC, Shupnik MA. Transcription rate of the follicle stimulating hormone (FSH) beta subunit gene is reduced by inhibin in sheep but this does not fully explain the decrease in mRNA. *Mol Cell Endocrinol* 1993 91: 211–216.

51. Mountford PS, Brandon MR, Adams TE. Removal of 3′ untranslated sequences dramatically enhances transient expression of ovine follicle-stimulating hormone beta gene messenger ribonucleic acid. *J Neuroendocrinol* 1992 4: 655–658.

52. Clarke IJ, Cummins JT. The temporal relationship between gonadotropin-releasing hormone (GnRH) and luteinizing hormone (LH) secretion in ovariectomized ewes. *Endocrinology* 1982 111: 1737–1739.

53. Crowley WF, Filicori M, Spratt DI, Santoro NF. The physiology of gonadotropin-releasing hormone (GnRH) secretion in men and women. *Recent Prog Horm Res* 1985 **41**: 471–531.

54. Clarke IJ, Cummins JT, Burman KR, Doughton BW. Effects of constant infusion of GnRH in ovariectomized ewes: further evidence for differential control of LH and FSH secretion and the lack of a priming effect. *J Endocrinol* 1986 **111**: 43–49.

55. Clarke IJ, Thomas GB, Yao B, Cummins JT. GnRH secretion throughout the ovine estrous cycle. *Neuroendocrinology* 1987 **46**: 82–88.

56. Moenter SM, Caraty A, Locatelli A, Karsch FJ. Pattern of GnRH secretion leading up to ovulation in the ewe: existence of a preovulatory GnRH surge. *Endocrinology* 1991 **129**: 1175–1182.

57. Evans NP, Dahl GE, Glover BH, Karsch FJ. Central regulation of pulsatile gonadotropin releasing hormone (GnRH) by estradiol during the period leading up to the preovulatory GnRH surge in the ewe. *Endocrinology* 1994 **134**: 1806–1811.

58. Clarke IJ. Evidence that the switch from negative to positive feedback at the level of the pituitary gland is an important timing event for the onset of the preovulatory surge in luteinising hormone. *J Endocrinol* 1994 **145**: 271–282.

59. Sarkar DK, Chiappa SA, Fink G, Sherwood NM. Gonadotrophin-releasing hormone surge in pro-oestrous rats. *Nature (Lond)* 1976 **264**: 461–463.

60 Clarke IJ. Variable patterns of gonadotropin-releasing hormone secretion during the estrogen-induced luteinizing hormone surge in ovariectomized ewes. *Endocrinology* 1993 **133**: 1624–1632.

61. Xia L, van Vugt D, Alston EJ, Luckhaus J, Ferrin M. A surge of gonadotropin-releasing hormone accompanies the estradiol-induced gonadotropin surge in the rhesus monkey. *Endocrinology* 1992 **131**: 2812–2820.

62. Pau F K-Y, Berria M, Hess DL, Spies HG. Preovulatory gonadotropin-releasing hormone surge in ovarian-intact rhesus macaques. *Endocrinology* 1993 **133**: 1650–1656.

63. Knobil E. The neuroendocrine control of the menstrual cycle. *Recent Prog Horm Res* 1980 **36**: 53–88.

64. Wildt L, Häusler A, Marshall G, Hutchinson JS, Plant TM, Belchetz PE, Knobil E. Frequency and amplitude of gonadotropin-releasing hormone stimulation and gonadotropin secretion in the rhesus monkey. *Endocrinology* 1981 **109**: 376–385.

65. Clarke IJ, Cummings JT, Findlay JK, Burman KJ, Doughton BW. Effects on plasma luteinizing hormone and follicle stimulating hormone of varying the frequency and amplitude of gonadotropin-releasing hormone pulses in ovariectomized ewes with hypothalamo–pituitary disconnection. *Neuroendocrinology*, 1984 **39**: 214–221.

66. Clarke IJ, Cummins, JT. GnRH pulse frequency determines LH pulse amplitude by altering the amount of releasable LH in the pituitary gland. *J Reprod Fertil* 1985 **73**: 425–431.

67. Tilbrook AJ, de Kretser DM, Cummins JT, Clarke IJ. The negative feedback effect of testicular steroids on gonadotrophin secretion in the ram is due to reduced GnRH secretion and not a direct effect on the pituitary gland. *Endocrinology* 1991 **129**: 3080–3092.

68. Thomas GB, Martin GB, Ford JR, Moore PM, Campbell BK, Lindsay DR. Secretion of LH, FSH and oestradiol-17 during the follicular phase of the oestrous cycle in the ewe. *Aust J Biol Sci* 1988 **41**: 303–308.

69. Danforth DR, Cheng CY. The identification of gonadotrophin surge inhibiting factor and its role in the regulation of pituitary gonadotrophin secretion. *Hum Reprod* 1993 **8**: 117–122.

70. Findlay JK, Clarke IJ, Robertson DM. Inhibin concentrations in ovarian and jugular venous plasma and the concentrations in ovarian and jugular venous plasma and the relationship of inhibin with FSH and LH during the ovine estrous cycle. *Endocrinology* 1990 **126**: 528–535.

71. Martin GB, Price CA, Thiery J-C, Webb R. Interactions between inhibin, oestradiol and progesterone in the control of gonadotrophin secretion in the ewe. *J Reprod Fertil* 1988 **82**: 319–328.

72. Yen SSC, Lasley BL, Wang CF, Leblanc H, Siler TM. The operating characteristics of the hypothalamic–pituitary system during the menstrual cycle and observations of biological action of somatostatin. *Recent Prog Horm Res* 1975 **31**: 321–357.

73. Clayton RN, Catt KJ. Gonadotropin-releasing hormone receptors characterization, physiological regulation, and relationship to reproductive function. *Endocr Rev* 1981 **2**: 186–209.

74. Clarke IJ, Cummins JT, Crowder ME, Nett, TM. Pituitary receptors for GnRH in relation to changes in pituitary and plasma gonadotropins in ovariectomized hypothalamo–pituitary disconnected ewes II. A marked rise in receptor number during acute feedback effects of estradiol. *Biol Reprod* 1988 **39**: 349–354.

75. Childs GV. Functional ultrastructure of gonadotropes: a review. *Curr Top Neuroendocrinol* 1986 **7**: 49–97.

76. Hawes BE, Conn PM. Molecular mechanism of GnRH action: do G proteins and inositol phosphates have a role? In Bouchard P, Caraty A, Coelingh-Benink HJT, Pavlou SN (eds) *GnRH, GnRH Analogs, Gonadotropins and Gonadal Peptides*. London: Parthenon, 1993: 63–80.

77. Aiyer MS, Chiappa SA, Fink G. A priming effect of luteinizing hormone releasing factor on the pituitary gland in the female rat. *J Endocrinol* 1974 **62**: 573–588.

78. Davidson JS, Flanagan CA, Becker II, Illing N, Sealfon SC, Millar RP. Molecular function of the gonadotropin-releasing hormone receptor: insights from site-directed mutagenesis. *Mol Cell Endocrinol* (in press).

79. Thomas GB, Cummins JT, Cavanagh L, Clarke IJ. A transient elevation of prolactin secretion following hypothalamo-pituitary disconnection in the ewe during anoestrus and the breeding season. *J Endocrinol* 1986 **111**: 425–431.

80. Thomas GB, Cummins JT, Smythe GA, Gleeson RM, Dow RC, Fink G, Clarke IJ. Concentrations of dopamine and noradrenaline in hypophysial portal blood in the sheep and the rat. *J Endocrinol* 1989 **121**: 141–147.

81. Thomas GT, Cummins JT, Canny BJ, Rundle SE. Griffin N, Katsahambas S, Clarke I. The posterior pituitary regulates prolactin, but not adrenocorticotropin or gonadotropin secretion in the sheep. *Endocrinology* 1989 **125**: 2204–2211.

82. Peters LL, Hoefer MT, Ben-Jonathan N. The posterior pituitary; regulation of anterior pituitary prolactin secretion. *Science* 1981 **213**: 659–661.

83. Fraser HM, McNeilly AS. Effect of chronic immunoneutralization of thyrotropin-releasing hormone on the hypothalamic–pituitary–thyroid axis, prolactin, and reproductive function in the ewe. *Endocrinology* 1982 **111**: 1964–1973.

84. Horn AM, Fraser HM, Fink G. Effects of antiserum to thyrotropin-releasing hormone on the concentrations of plasma prolactin, thyrotrophin and LH in the pro-oestrous rat. *J Endocrinol* 1985 **104**: 205–209.

85. Thomas GB, Cummins JT, Yao B, Gordon K, Clarke IJ. The release of prolactin is independent of the secretion of thyrotropin-releasing hormone into hypophysial portal blood of sheep. *J Endocrinol* 1988 **117**: 115–122.

86. Frawley LS, Neill JD. Neuroendocrine regulation of prolactin secretion in primates. In Bhatnagar AS (ed.) *The Anterior Pituitary Gland*. New York: Raven Press, 1983: 253–268.

87. Liu J-W, Ben-Jonathan N. Prolactin-releasing activity of neurohypophyseal hormones: structure–function relationship. *Endocrinology* 1994 **134**: 114–118.

88. Frawley LS, Neill JD. Effect of estrogen on serum prolactin levels in rhesus monkeys after hypophyseal stalk transection. *Biol Reprod* 1980 **22**: 1089–1093.

89. Maurer RA, Notides AC. Identification of an estrogen responsive element from the 5′ flanking region of the rat prolactin gene. *Mol Cell Biol* 1987 **7**: 4247–4254.

90. Neill JD. Prolactin: its secretion and control. In Greep RO, Astwood EB, Knobil E, Sawyer WH, Geiger SR (eds) *Handbook of Physiology Section 7 Volume IV The Pituitary Gland and its Neuroendocrine Control Part 2*. Washington: American Physiological Society, 1974. 469–488.

91. Maurer RA. Estradiol regulates the transcription of the prolactin gene. *J Biol Chem* 1982 **257**: 2133–2136.

92. Pilotte NS, Burt DR, Barraclough CA. Ovarian steroids modulate the release of dopamine into hypophysial portal blood and the density of anterior pituitary [³H]Spiperone-binding sites in ovariectomized rats. *Endocrinology* 1984 **114**: 2306–2311.

93. Crowley WR. Effects of ovarian hormones on norepinephrine and dopamine turnover in individual hypothalamic and extrahypothalamic nuclei. *Neuroendocrinology* 1982 **34**: 381–386.

94. Pasqualini C, Leviel V, Guibert B, Faucon-Biguet N, Kerdelhue B. Inhibitory actions of acute estradiol treatment on the activity and quantity of tyrosine hydroxylase in the median eminence of ovariectomized rats. *J Neuroendocrinol* 1991 **3**: 575–580.

95. Arbogast LA, Voogt JL. Progesterone reverses the estradiol-induced decrease in tyrosine hydroxylase mRNA levels in the arcuate nucleus. *Neuroendocrinology* 1993 **58**: 501–510.

96. Tennekoon KH, Lenton EA. Early evening prolactin rise in women with regular cycles. *J Reprod Fertil* 1985 **73**: 523–527.

97. Rossmanith WG, Mortola JF, Yen SSC The effects of dopaminergic blockade on the sleep-associated changes in luteinizing hormone pulsatility in early follicular phase women. *Neuroendocrinology* 1988 **48**: 634–639.

98. Yen SSC, Hoff JD, Lasley BL, Casper RF, Sheehan K. Induction of prolactin release by LRF and LRF-agonist. *Life Sci* 1980 **26**: 1963–1967.

99. Cetel NS, Yen SSC. Concomitant pulsatile release of prolactin and luteinizing hormone in hypogonadal women. *J Clin Endocrinol Metab* 1983 **56**: 1313–1317.

100. Gambacciani M, Yen SSC, Rasmussen DD. GnRH stimulates *in vitro* release of ACTH, β-endorphin and prolactin from the rat pituitary. *Life Sci* 1988 **43**: 755–760.

The Ovary: Endocrine Function

AJ Zeleznik and SG Hillier

INTRODUCTION

The primary endocrine function of the ovaries is to secrete sex steroids – estradiol and progesterone – that are essential to prepare the reproductive tract for pregnancy (Fig. 2.3.1). The preovulatory (Graafian) follicle develops under the influence of the gonadotropins follicle-stimulating hormone (FSH) and luteinizing hormone (LH) during the first half of the menstrual cycle. During late preovulatory development, this follicle secretes estradiol as well as the polypeptide hormone inhibin. At mid-cycle, in response to the ovulation-inducing LH surge, the preovulatory follicle ruptures, releases the oocyte and is transformed into the corpus luteum, which secretes progesterone, estradiol and inhibin, regulated by LH (Fig. 2.3.1). If pregnancy does not occur, the corpus luteum undergoes regression (luteolysis), luteal hormone secretion ceases and a new menstrual

cycle begins. Thus the endocrine functions of the ovaries are intrinsically linked to follicular and luteal development. Here we summarize current concepts of the hormonal and cellular mechanisms that regulate these processes.

CURRENT CONCEPTS

Follicular development and estrogen synthesis

Around 400 follicles sequentially mature and ovulate during an average woman's reproductive lifetime. From birth to the menopause, the other ~99.98% of her follicles begin development but never complete it. Instead they default to atresia due to inadequate stimulation by FSH.[1] Follicular growth to the stage of antrum formation (~0.25 mm

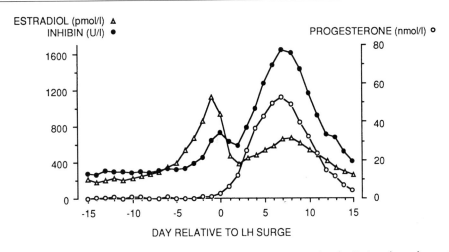

Fig. 2.3.1 *Serum levels of estradiol, progesterone and inhibin during the human menstrual cycle. (Data redrawn from reference 78, with permission).*

diameter) is independent of gonadotropic stimulation (Fig. 2.3.2a) (see Chapter 2.1). However, follicular antrum formation (Fig. 2.3.2b) and growth to the stage at which follicles are potentially able to begin preovulatory development (2–5 mm diameter) require stimulation by FSH (Fig. 2.3.2c). Before the onset of puberty, blood levels of FSH do not rise sufficiently to sustain development beyond this stage. Therefore all antral follicles that develop in juvenile ovaries eventually become atretic. After puberty, at the beginning of each menstrual cycle FSH levels rise beyond a critical 'threshold' level that is sufficient to stimulate several follicles to enter early preovulatory

stages of development. Due to increases in its responsiveness to FSH and LH, one of these follicles is eventually selected to ovulate while the others become atretic. At the mid-follicular phase, the dominant follicle reaches ≥10 mm in diameter and increasingly synthesizes estradiol. Tonic stimulation by FSH and LH, underpinned by local paracrine signaling, maintains estrogen secretion by the dominant follicle, which grows to ≥20 mm in diameter before it ovulates in response to the mid-cycle LH surge. The cellular mechanisms that underlie preovulatory follicular growth and estrogen secretion will now be considered in detail.

(a) Initiation of folliculogenesis

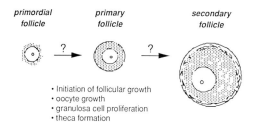

(b) Antrum formation

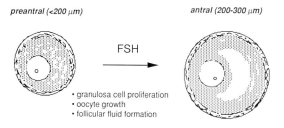

(c) Antral growth

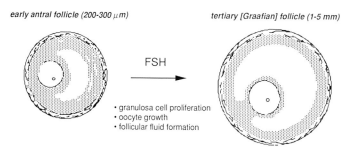

Fig. 2.3.2 *Early stages in ovarian folliculogenesis.* **(a)** *At birth the ovaries contain around two million follicles arrested at primordial stages of development. Throughout infancy, childhood and adolescence, continuing throughout the reproductive years, individual follicles exit the primordial pool and folliculogenesis begins independent of gonadotropic stimulation.* **(b)** *Granulosa cell proliferation, theca formation and oocyte growth during preantral stages of folliculogenesis also occur independently of gonadotropic stimulation. However, antrum formation requires tonic stimulation by FSH, facilitated by local steroidal and non-steroidal regulatory factors.* **(c)** *Small antral follicles grow to intermediate sizes (up to ~5 mm diameter) in response to tonic stimulation by FSH. Before adolescence, follicles do not normally progress beyond this stage because circulating plasma FSH levels are too low. Thus all follicles that begin to develop before the onset of cyclic (adult) levels of pituitary FSH secretion are destined to undergo atresia.*

Preantral and early antral follicular development

The growth of a primordial follicle to the large preantral stage in humans takes approximately 85 days, whereas the final maturation of the large preantral follicle to the preovulatory stage.takes approximately 14 days, representing the duration of the follicular phase (Fig. 2.3.3).[2] Thus a follicle that ovulates in one menstrual cycle will actually have begun to mature at least two cycles previously. Although the initiation of folliculogenesis occurs independently of gonadotropic stimulation antrum formation requires stimulation by FSH, beginning when follicles reach about 0.25 mm in diameter[3] (Fig. 2.3.2).

FSH stimulates granulosa cell division and the formation of glycosaminoglycans that are essential components of antral fluid.[4] Granulosa cells are the only cells in the female body known to possess FSH receptors, and binding of FSH to its receptor on the cell surface activates adenylyl cyclase and cyclic AMP-dependent protein kinase(s) (see Chapters 1.4 and 1.5), leading to altered expression of multiple genes crucial to cytoproliferation and differentiation.[5] Granulosa cell genes that are responsive to FSH include: aromatase (P450arom) the steroidogenic cytochrome P450 crucial to estrogen synthesis;[6] cholesterol side-chain cleavage (P450scc), rate-limiting in progesterone synthesis;[5] the LH receptor;[7] polypeptide 'growth factors' and binding-proteins such as insulin-like growth factors (IGFs) and IGFBPs;[8–10] proteolytic enzymes and inhibitors such as tissue plasminogen activator (TPA) and inhibitor (PAI) involved in follicular rupture;[11] regulatory peptides such as inhibin, activin and follistatin;[12] and subcellular factors involved in steroid hormone action such as 'heat-shock' proteins.[13]

The mitogenic action of FSH is facilitated by locally produced polypeptide growth factors, production and/or action of which may be modified by FSH.[14] Tonic stimulation by FSH is adequate to sustain the development of small antral follicles to intermediate sizes around 5 mm in diameter. Before adulthood, all follicles that survive to this stage become atretic. Any larger follicles that develop are likely to be cystic or degenerate.[15] When sufficiently high levels of FSH are reached during adulthood, follicles at such intermediate stages are rescued from atresia and preovulatory development begins.

Preovulatory follicular 'recruitment'

At the beginning of each menstrual cycle, pituitary secretion of FSH increases due to withdrawal of the negative feedback action of estradiol, progesterone and inhibin produced by the previous corpus luteum.[16–18] This intercyclic rise in plasma FSH level causes multiple antral follicles with diameters in the range 2–5 mm to enter preovulatory stages of development. Evidence from ovulation induction using exogenous FSH suggests that each follicle within this cohort has a 'threshold' requirement for FSH beyond which it must be stimulated by FSH if it is to be protected from atresia and continue to develop.[19,20] Small (10–30%) differences exist between individual follicles at this stage of

development with respect to the threshold amount of FSH required to initiate preovulatory development, which explains how one follicle is eventually selected to mature and ovulate as discussed below.

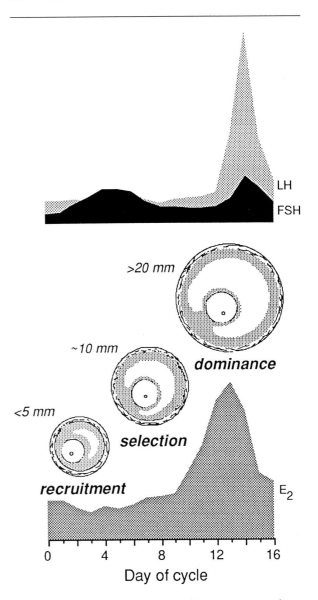

Fig. 2.3.3 *Gonadotropin-dependent stages in preovulatory follicular development. 'Recruitment': at the beginning of each adult menstrual cycle, plasma FSH levels rise sufficiently to stimulate proliferation and functional differentiation of granulosa cells in multiple follicles beween <5 mm and ~10 mm in diameter, including induction of LH receptors and aromatase activity. Tonic stimulation by LH maintains thecal androgen synthesis in these follicles. The next follicle that will ovulate emerges as the one that is most responsive to FSH (i.e. has the lowest FSH 'threshold'). 'Dominance': by the mid-follicular phase, the preovulatory (Graafian) follicle becomes recognizable as the largest (≥10 mm diameter) healthy follicle in either ovary, containing granulosa cells expressing LH receptors coupled to aromatase. Since this follicle is uniquely responsive to both FSH and LH, it continues to grow and secrete estradiol in the face of declining plasma levels of FSH. Development-dependent paracrine signals maintain the dominance of this follicle, amplifying its responsiveness to FSH and LH. Modified from reference 1.*

Preovulatory follicular 'selection'

Usually only one of the several follicles initially recruited to begin preovulatory development actually survives to secrete estrogen in the late follicular phase. The ability of this follicle most rapidly to begin estrogen synthesis is crucial to its survival as the dominant follicle.[20,21] As the plasma FSH level rises, P450arom, responsible for estrogen synthesis (see Fig. 2.3.4), is increasingly expressed in its granulosa cell layer. This activation of the aromatase system has been likened to an on/off switch that is thrown as the FSH threshold level is surpassed.[22]

Follicles with greatest sensitivity to FSH (i.e. having the lowest FSH thresholds) are recruited to progress beyond the early antral stage, and the first (presumably the most sensitive to FSH) begins to secrete estradiol.[23] FSH also stimulates granulosa cell inhibin synthesis.[12] Although both estradiol and inhibin have the potential to negatively

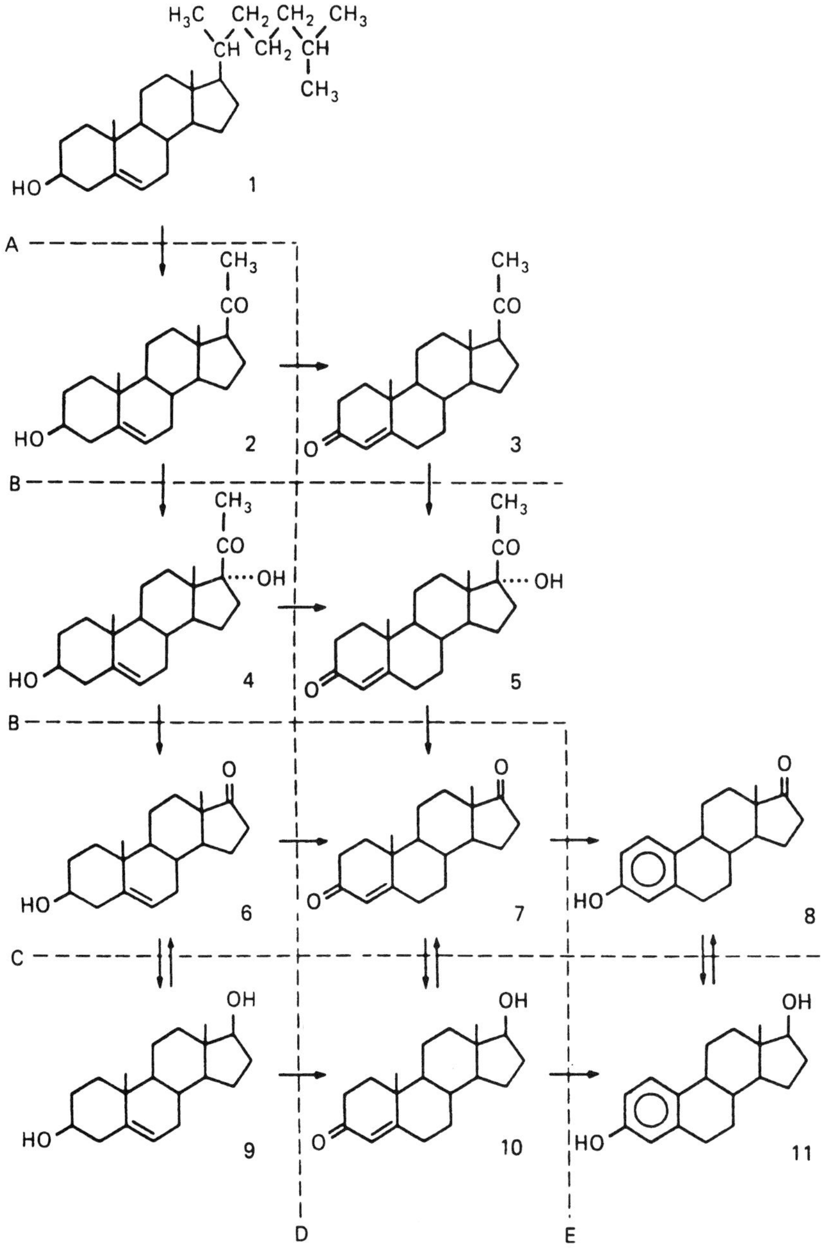

Fig. 2.3.4 *Pathways of ovarian steroid hormone synthesis. Enzymes: (A) cholesterol side-chain cleavage (P450scc); (B) 17-hydroxy-lase/C$_{17-20}$-lyase (P450c17); (C) 17β-hydroxysteroid dehydrogenase; (D) 3β-hydroxysteroid dehydrogenase/Δ^{5-4} isomerase; (E) aromatase (P450arom). Steroids: (1) cholesterol; (2) pregnenolone; (3) progesterone; (4) 17-hydroxypregnenolone; (5) 17-hydroxyprogesterone; (6) dehydroepiandrosterone; (7) androstenedione; (8) estrone; (9) androstenediol; (10) testosterone; (11) estradiol.*

regulate pituitary FSH secretion,[24] there is experimental evidence that estradiol is the primary regulator of FSH secretion during the follicular phase of human and non-human primate ovarian cycles.[23] Thus blood FSH levels fall to levels too low to sustain the development of other follicles within the cohort and they therefore become non-ovulatory and undergo atresia. As discussed in the next section, the maturing follicle continues to develop in the presence of diminishing FSH concentrations because, as a direct consequence of FSH stimulation, it undergoes maturation dependent changes which further increase its sensitivity to gonadotropins (i.e. its threshold further decreases).

The following development-related variables are likely to influence follicular sensitivity to FSH, hence giving rise to follicular selection.

FSH and LH receptor levels

From the law of mass action it would be predicted that increases in receptor numbers for FSH and LH should directly increase the sensitivity of the follicle to the prevailing gonadotropic milieu. In rats, the density of granulosa cell FSH receptors increases slightly during preovulatory follicular growth which could provide an advantage to developing follicles as plasma FSH concentrations fall.[25] In addition to changes in the density of FSH receptors on granulosa cells, a hallmark of FSH action on the maturing follicle is the induction of cell surface receptors for LH.[26] As both FSH and LH exert their actions, at least in part, via the stimulation of adenylyl cyclase and elevation of intracellular cyclic AMP concentrations, the presence of LH receptors on granulosa cells of the maturing follicle could protect it from the fall in FSH.[27] Because less mature follicles possess only FSH receptors, they would be highly susceptible to a fall in FSH concentrations while the selected follicle, as a result of the FSH-mediated increase in LH receptors, may survive the fall in FSH concentrations by developing the ability to respond to LH.

Vascularization

In addition to changes in the density of cell surface receptors for the gonadotropic hormones, a preferential delivery of gonadotropins to the maturing follicle could protect it from the fall in FSH. In rhesus monkeys, the density of capillaries that supply the selected follicle is at least three times greater than that of other less mature follicles and this increased density of capillaries results in preferential delivery of gonadotropin to the maturing follicle.[28] Observations that extracts of follicular cells or conditioned tissue culture media from granulosa cells stimulate endothelial cell growth suggest that the developing follicle may produce diffusible angiogenic factors that cause the selective vascularization of the follicle. In this regard, it has been demonstrated recently that mRNA for vascular endothelial growth factor (VEGF) is selectively expressed by the maturing follicle indicating that this protein could be responsible for the angiogenesis that accompanies follicular development.[29,30]

Paracrine and autocrine signaling

A variety of locally produced steroidal and non-steroidal factors have been shown to modify FSH action *in vitro*

and thus could serve a role in providing increased sensitivity of the maturing follicle to gonadotropins.[31] Many potential regulatory substances are known to be produced in antral follicles. Putative paracrine modulators of FSH action on granulosa cells are androgenic steroids and polypeptides such as transforming growth factors (TGF-α and TGF-β) produced by LH-stimulated thecal cells.[32] Conversely, FSH-stimulated granulosa cells produce steroidal (e.g. estradiol and progesterone) and non-steroidal (e.g. inhibin/activin and IGFs)[33,34] substances that may influence thecal responsiveness to LH. These and many other factors may also exert autocrine regulation within the cells that produce them. The potential relevance of paracrine regulation to selection of the preovulatory follicle will be discussed below.

Steroidogenic enzymes

The major biochemical pathways of steroid hormone synthesis in the ovaries are illustrated in Fig. 2.3.4.[35,36] Principal components of the steroidogenic machinery are: (a) proteins that participate in the acquisition of cholesterol, including lipoprotein receptors and enzymes involved in *de novo* cholesterol synthesis; (b) mixed-function oxidases that catalyze the cleavage of carbon side-chains from the sterol nucleus (P450scc and cytochrome P450c17 (17-hydroxylase/C_{17-20}-lyase)), introduce hydroxyl groups (cytochrome P450c17) and aromatize the A ring (cytochrome P450arom); (c) the oxidoreductases (or hydroxysteroid dehydrogenases) catalyze in some cases, reversibly, the oxidation or reduction of oxy functions at C-3, C-17 and C-20 (e.g. 3β-hydroxysteroid dehydrogenase, 17β-hydroxysteroid dehydrogenase and 20α-hydroxysteroid dehydrogenase); and (d) reductases, which irreversibly reduce the Δ^4 olefinic bond of the A ring of Δ^{4-3} keto steroids (e.g. 5α-reductase).

Mechanism of follicular estrogen synthesis

The onset of follicular estrogen secretion reflects a functional interplay between the two major steroidogenic cell types in the follicle – granulosa and thecal – regulated by FSH and LH. LH stimulates precursor androgen synthesis in the theca and FSH stimulates granulosa cell aromatase activity. Thus both cell types and both gonadotropins are crucial to estrogen synthesis (Fig. 2.3.5).[37,38]

Thecal androgen synthesis

Thecal cells minimally express P450arom (Fig. 2.3.6a) and are therefore unable to synthesize estrogens *de novo*.[39] However, thecal cells abundantly express P450c17[40] (Fig. 2.3.6b), the rate-limiting steroidogenic enzyme in androgen synthesis, which is positively regulated by LH.[41] The vascularized theca interna has direct access to blood-borne precursor cholesterol and thecal cells contain steroidogenic enzymes necessary to synthesize androgens from acetate and cholesterol. IGF-I and insulin receptors functionally coupled to androgen synthesis are also present on thecal cells,[42] and physiological concentrations of IGF-I, IGF-II and insulin augment basal and LH-stimulated thecal

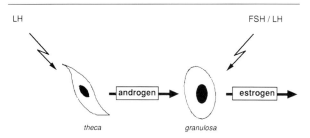

Fig. 2.3.5 *The '2-cell, 2-gonadotropin' model of follicular estra-diol biosynthesis. Androgen synthesis occurs in the theca interna regulated by LH, rate-limiting metabolism of C_{21} substrates to C_{19} androgens being catalyzed by 17-hydroxylase/C_{17-20}-lyase (P450c17). Aromatase (P450arom), the granulosa cell enzyme that converts C_{19} androgens (androstenedione and testosterone) to C_{18} estrogens (estrone and estradiol) is induced by FSH. FSH also induces granulosa cell LH receptors that are functionally coupled to aromatase. Thus, uniquely in the preovulatory follicle, both the synthesis of androgen (in thecal cells) and its aromatization to estradiol (in granulosa cells) are directly regulated by LH. (Based on reference 37.)*

androgen synthesis *in vitro*.[43] Thus circulating IGFs and insulin of hepatic origin as well as IGFs produced within the follicle have the potential to modulate LH-stimulated androgen synthesis *in vivo*.

The major androgen secreted by the human preovulatory follicle is androstenedione. During the follicular phase of the menstrual cycle, the ovary contributes about 30% of the total blood androstenedione and the adrenal accounts for the rest. Towards mid-cycle, the ovarian contribution rises to about 60% due to increased synthesis and secretion of the steroid by the LH-stimulated theca of the preovulatory follicle, reflecting its role as a precursor for estradiol.[44] The mechanism by which androgen synthesis is selectively upregulated in this follicle is likely to involve paracrine control,[31] as discussed below. It is noteworthy that one of the major causes of anovulatory infertility in women – polycystic ovarian syndrome – is associated with hyperthecosis and hyperandrogenism. The strong correlation between hyperandrogenism and hyperinsulinism in many of these patients further emphasizes the likely importance of insulin and IGFs in the regulation of thecal androgen synthesis.[43,45]

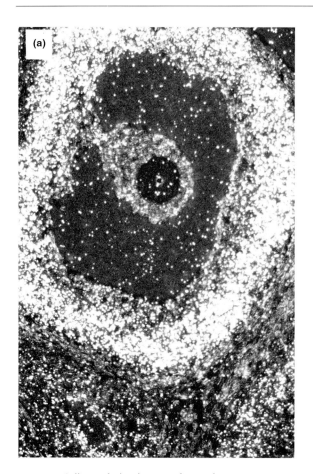

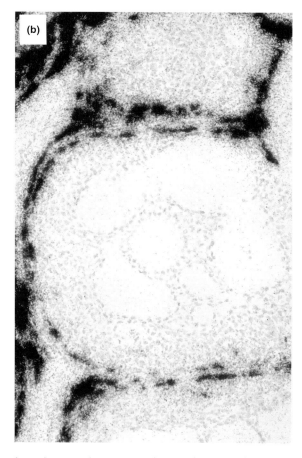

Fig. 2.3.6 *Cell-specific localization of steroidogenic enzymes necessary for androgen and estrogen synthesis in the rat Graafian follicle, revealed by* in situ *hybridization.* **(a)** *Selective localization of P450arom mRNA in granulosa cells[39] (dark-field view, ×70);* **(b)** *selective localization of P450c17 mRNA to thecal cells[59] (bright-field view, ×70).*

Androgen synthesis in the preovulatory follicle is temporarily suppressed at mid-cycle immediately following the onset of the ovulation inducing LH surge. This poorly understood effect seems to involve thecal 'desensitization' to the extreme elevation in the circulating LH level. Thecal 17-hydroxylase/C_{17-20}-lyase activity becomes suppressed at this time, possibly due to local inhibition by estradiol.[41]

Granulosa cell estrogen synthesis

Granulosa cells are unable to synthesize androgens *de novo* since they do not express P450c17 (Fig. 2.3.6b). They are, however, intrafollicular sites of androgen metabolism and express 17β-hydroxysteroid dehydrogenase (17β-HSD),[46] 3β-HSD,[47] as well as aromatase P450arom[39] (Fig. 2.3.6a). Each of these enzymatic activities is stimulated by FSH and increases during preovulatory follicular development. Granulosa cells also possess 5α-reductase activity[48] and undertake steroid conjugation,[49] but the control of these enzymes is poorly understood.

Within the preovulatory follicle, the avascular granulosa cell layer is exposed to high concentrations of aromatizable androgen that reach it by diffusion from the theca interna. More than 99.9% of this follicle's enzymatic capacity to aromatize androgen resides in its granulosa cell layer, based on measurements of aromatase activity in isolated granulosa and thecal cells[50] and on the localization of P450arom mRNA and protein by immunocytochemistry[51,52] and *in situ* hybridization.[39] Cells in the outer (mural) granulosa cell layer are presumed to be particularly active sites of aromatization, since they express more P450arom mRNA and LH receptors than do cells distal to the lamina basalis[39,53] (Fig. 2.3.6a). The thecal vasculature is so well developed in the preovulatory follicle that murally located granulosa cells are effectively in direct contact with adjacent blood vessels. They are therefore well placed to respond to changes in the circulating LH level, and the estrogen they produce can be discharged directly into the venous effluent of the preovulatory follicle.[29]

The ability of FSH to induce LH receptors functionally coupled to steroidogenesis in granulosa cells has implications for the maintenance of follicular dominance,[54] as outlined below. LH acts via its receptors on mature granulosa cells and thecal/interstitial cells to activate adenylyl cyclase signaling, which increases precursor-cholesterol uptake and sustains characteristically high steroidogenic enzyme activities.[55] Intracellular signal transmission via phosphoinositide hydrolysis and activation of the diacylglycerol/ protein kinase C pathway may also mediate LH action on luteal steroidogenesis (see Chapter 1.5).[56]

Maintenance of follicular 'dominance'

By the mid-follicular phase, the dominant follicle is recognizable as the largest healthy follicle in either ovary.[57] At this time, maintenance of its status as the dominant follicle becomes increasingly dependent on LH. As discussed above, LH receptors are constitutively present on thecal cells and develop on granulosa cells following stimulation by FSH. Thus the dominant follicle secretes increased amounts of androstenedione as well as estradiol in response

to stimulation by LH.[58] Paracrine signaling (granulosa on theca) is thought to contribute to the selective enhancement of LH-responsive androgen synthesis that occurs in this follicle.[31,50,59] *In vitro*, LH coordinately stimulates aromatase activity and inhibin synthesis in granulosa cells from the dominant follicle,[60] and inhibin potently enhances LH-stimulated thecal androgen synthesis.[31] Thus inhibin is likely to participate in the paracrine system that leads to enhanced secretion of estrogen by the dominant follicle (Fig. 2.3.7).

Ovulation

Ovulation is the central event in the ovarian cycle when the secondary oocyte is discharged on to the surface of the ovary and passes into the oviduct where it may be fertilized (see Chapter 2.4). It is also the terminal step in the growth and differentiation of the follicle, marking the onset of corpus luteum formation.

The LH surge

Ovulation is triggered by the mid-cycle LH surge, which is itself triggered by the sustained high circulating level of estradiol produced by the preovulatory follicle (see Chapter 2.2). Ovulation can also be induced by exogenous human chorionic gonadotropin (HCG), given as a surrogate LH after appropriate gonadotropic priming of the preovulatory follicle(s) with FSH.

Onset of progesterone production

At the granulosa cell level, immediate responses to the LH surge are inhibition of mitosis (i.e. cessation of follicular growth) and increased expression of P450scc,[27,61] the major steroidogenic enzyme necessary for progesterone synthesis.

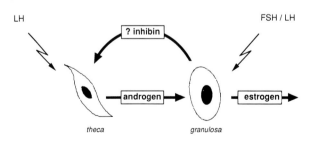

Fig 2.3.7 *Hypothetical regulatory function of inhibin in maintaining follicular 'dominance' during the late follicular phase of the human menstrual cycle. Granulosa cells in the preovulatory follicle respond to stimulation by FSH and LH with increased production of inhibin, paralleling the preovulatory increase in aromatase activity. Inhibin acts locally to promote LH/IGF-stimulated androgen synthesis in the theca interna. As inhibin production increases, a positive-feedback loop is created through which thecal androgen synthesis is amplified to sustain estrogen synthesis in the granulosa cell layer.[31]*

Estrogen synthesis declines due to inhibition of thecal 17-hydroxylase/C_{17-20}-lyase activity (see above) and the attendant lack of aromatase substrate.[62] Thus as ovulation approaches, the ovary increasingly secretes progesterone while estrogen secretion temporarily declines.

Follicular Rupture

The LH surge stimulates a proteolytic cascade within the preovulatory follicle, resulting in its rupture approximately 36 hours later. The biochemical basis of ovulation – which can be likened to an inflammatory response,[63] is the activation of diverse second-messenger systems in thecal and granulosa cells, leading to ovarian hyperemia and local increases in proteolytic enzyme activities that reduce the tensile strength of the apical region of the follicle wall.

At least three postreceptor signaling systems mediate the LH/HCG-induced cellular changes that bring about follicular rupture: cyclic AMP and cyclic AMP-dependent protein kinase A; phosphoinositide metabolism and calcium- dependent protein kinase C; and arachidonic acid metabolism to prostaglandins and leukotrienes[11,64] (see Chapter 1.5). The follicular response to LH/HCG includes increased production of prostaglandins, leukotrienes, cytokines, platelet-activating factor, PAF, kinins, PAs and matrix metalloproteinases (MMPs) such as collagenases, gelatinases and stromelysins (Fig. 2.3.8). Locally synthesized prostaglandins appear to be essential to follicular rupture, being primarily responsible for the increase in vascular permeability which sustains positive intrafollicular pressure during the period when follicular fluid begins to leak through the partially digested follicular wall. The gradual reduction in the tensile strength of the follicular wall eventually results in its complete rupture. The flow of follicular fluid and vascular transudate then carries the

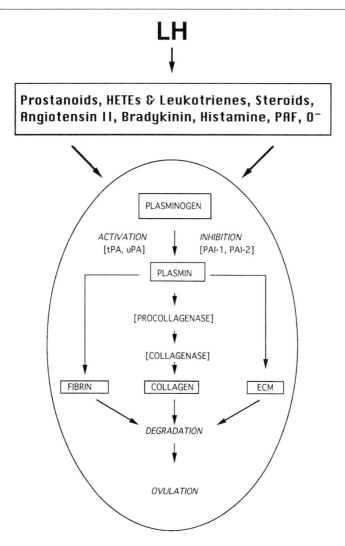

Fig. 2.3.8 *Biochemistry of follicular rupture. LH binds to its receptor on granulosa and thecal cells to activate multiple postreceptor signaling pathways in the Graafian follicle. This incites an 'inflammatory response'[63] involving multiple regulatory factors, some of which are listed in the rectangle. The subsequent proteolytic cascade causes breakdown of collagen, fibrin and extracellular matrix in the apical region of the follicle wall, leading to ovulation. (See references 11, 64 and 65 for further details).*

cumulus-enclosed oocyte out of the follicle on to the surface of the ovary.[11,64,65]

A local role for progesterone in ovulation?

Progesterone levels in follicular fluid rise markedly following the LH surge or injection of HCG and it is possible that the preovulatory increase in progesterone formation is essential to follicular rupture. In rats and pigs, LH/HCG stimulates transient expression of progesterone receptor mRNA in the granulosa cells of preovulatory follicles[66] and there is evidence for a specific local function for progesterone in ovulation in these species.[67,68] Human and monkey granulosa-lutein cells also contain progesterone receptors.[69,70] Incubation of pieces of human follicular wall with progesterone *in vitro* decreases the formation of collagen.[71] *In vivo*, such an effect of progesterone could accelerate the net loss of collagen fibers, thereby expediting follicular rupture.

A direct action of progesterone on the synthesis of a proteolytic enzyme(s) involved in follicular rupture was first suggested by the work of Rondell[72] who showed that treatment with progesterone *in vitro* specifically increases the distensibility of porcine preovulatory follicular strips. More recently, follicular steroids have been implicated in the regulation of PA synthesis and the activation of collagenase, thereby facilitating breakdown of the follicle wall.[73] Estradiol,[74] progestins and androgens[75] were shown to potentiate gonadotropin-induced elevation of PA activity in rat preovulatory follicles and granulosa cells, respectively. Moreover, inhibition of progesterone synthesis in the ovine ovary resulted in suppression of the preovulatory rise in collagenolysis, possibly mediated by a decrease in PA activity.[76]

Luteal development and luteolysis

The corpus luteum is pivotal to the control of the menstrual cycle.[77] Hormones secreted by the corpus luteum (progesterone, estrogen and inhibin) collectively exert negative feedback regulation of pituitary FSH secretion, thereby inhibiting preovulatory follicular development. Regression of the corpus luteum (luteolysis) is therefore necessary to terminate a non-fertile cycle so that a new menstrual cycle can begin. On the other hand, if conception occurs and pregnancy begins, prolongation of luteal function beyond its intrinsic 14–16 day lifespan is essential for the maintenance of pregnancy until the placenta develops sufficiently to carry the burden of progesterone secretion. The cellular and molecular processes underpinning luteal development and luteolysis will briefly be reviewed here.

Luteal Development

Luteinization of the follicle by LH is accompanied by neovascularization of the granulosa cell layer and breakdown of the blood–follicle barrier. The increased access of luteinizing granulosa cells to blood-borne precursor cholesterol allows high rates of progesterone secretion to commence. Plasma progesterone levels rise to a maximum in the mid-luteal phase when luteal progesterone secretion

peaks at a rate of ~25 mg (~80 μmol) progesterone per day. Luteal phase plasma levels of estradiol and inhibin follow the same pattern[78,79] (Fig. 2.3.1).

The luteotropic function of LH

LH plays an obligatory role in the control of luteal progesterone secretion,[80,81] exerting both acute and chronic effects on steroidogenesis, similar to its effects on androgen synthesis in the testis (see Chapter 2.5). A close temporal association exists between secretory bursts of LH and episodes of progesterone production by the corpus luteum.[82–84] The speed of the progesterone response to each pulse of LH implies an acute effect of LH on precursor cholesterol metabolism through existing steroidogenic pathways rather than increased production of steroidogenic enzymes *per se*. The precise mechanism through which intracellular cholesterol dynamics are regulated is unknown. It is thought to include the cyclic AMP-dependent mobilization of cholesterol to the inner mitochondrial membrane for conversion into pregnenolone by P450scc.[35]

LH exerts longer-term effects on luteal steroidogenesis through maintaining cellular levels of mRNAs encoding 3β-HSD and P450scc.[85,86] Paradoxically, as the corpus luteum matures and plasma progesterone levels rise, the capacity for luteal cells to biosynthesize progesterone declines[87] (Fig. 2.3.9). Cellular levels of 3β-HSD and

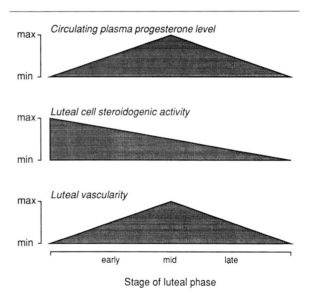

Fig. 2.3.9 *Relation between circulating plasma progesterone level, luteal cell steroidogenic activity, and the degree of vascularization of the corpus luteum throughout the luteal phase of the human menstrual cycle. As the blood progesterone level rises during the early luteal phase, the steroidogenic activity of luteal cells declines, as determined by measurement of cellular steroidogenic mRNA levels and production of progesterone by isolated luteal cells in vitro (see references 85–87). This paradox is probably explained by the development of the luteal vasculature, which increases throughout the first half of the luteal phase, thereby allowing luteal cells increased access to blood-borne substrates (e.g. LDL-associated cholesterol) necessary to sustain high rates of steroid synthesis. In the absence of pregnancy, all three parameters decline during the second half of the luteal phase due to the functional and morphological regression of the corpus luteum.*

P450scc mRNAs are also highest shortly after ovulation, declining progressively throughout the luteal phase.[85] This dissociation of luteal steroid secretion rate and biosynthetic potential may occur because the new corpus luteum is incompletely vascularized such that its access to precursor cholesterol in the form of blood-borne low-density lipoprotein (LDL) is restricted.[55] On the other hand, when the luteal vasculature becomes fully developed in the mid-luteal phase precursor cholesterol no longer rate-limits steroidogenesis. Thus the luteal progesterone secretion rate progressively increases during the early luteal phase in spite of an age-related decline in steroidogenic potential at the cellular level.

The luteal-phase plasma estradiol pattern mirrors progesterone in reaching a maximum in the mid-luteal phase when total luteal aromatase activity is declining.[87] Similar to granulosa cells in the preovulatory follicle, granulosa-lutein cells in the corpus luteum cannot undertake estradiol synthesis unless supplied with an aromatase substrate.[63] Theca-lutein cells are presumed to provide precursor androgen for aromatization by granulosa-lutein cells in an extension of the 'two-cell' type mechanism of estrogen synthesis that occurs in the preovulatory follicle (see earlier). High rates of C_{19} steroid synthesis in the theca depend on access to extracellular precursor cholesterol.[55] Presumably, therefore, androgen synthesis in theca-lutein cells, like progesterone synthesis in granulosa-lutein cells, benefits from the increased vascularization of the corpus luteum that occurs during the first week after ovulation.

Luteal regression

Although luteal function unequivocally depends on LH, changes in LH secretion *per se* do not seem to be responsible for luteal regression in non-fertile menstrual cycles. The major change in LH secretion during the luteal phase is a progesterone-mediated reduction in the frequency of pulsatile LH secretion by the pituitary gland, falling from approximately 1 pulse an hour during the early luteal phase to 1 pulse every 4–8 hours during the mid–late luteal phase.[83,84] However, this decline in LH pulse frequency cannot be the direct cause of luteal regression because setting the pulse frequency at 1 pulse per hour throughout the luteal phase does not prolong the life span of the corpus luteum.[88,89] Similarly, premature reduction of the LH pulse frequency to 1 pulse every 8 hours during the early luteal phase does not cause premature luteal regression.[90,91]

Currently, the best explanation for luteal regression is that the corpus luteum undergoes an age-related reduction in sensitivity to LH, such that progressively more intense stimulation by LH (i.e. a higher plasma LH level) is required to sustain luteal function. In other words, the corpus luteum may regress not because of reduced exposure to LH, but due to its ever-decreasing ability to respond to the low plasma levels of LH that prevail throughout the luteal phase.

At the cellular level, factors thought to be involved in the initiation of luteolysis include estrogen, oxytocin, prostaglandins and various polypeptide growth factors and cytokines.[92] However, any involvement of specific paracrine factors in luteolysis may be secondary to more general regulatory processes set in train when granulosa cells become terminally differentiated (i.e. luteinized) by the LH surge. This suggestion is borne out by evidence that programmed cell-death (apoptosis) is hormonally regulated in the ovaries,[93] being implicated in follicular atresia as well as regression of the corpus luteum.[94]

Luteal rescue by HCG

If conception occurs, trophoblastic cells in the implanting blastocyst secrete HCG. Stimulation of the corpus luteum by HCG delays its regression, serving to 'rescue' luteal progesterone secretion until the placenta is sufficiently developed to take over the role of progesterone synthesis.

Structurally and functionally, the HCG molecule is similar to LH and both interact with the same cell-surface receptor.[95,96] The question therefore arises how HCG, unlike LH, is able to prevent the corpus luteum from involuting. It is possible that HCG provides a more intense and sustained gonadotropic stimulus to the ageing corpus luteum, overriding its diminished responsiveness to the intermittent pulses of LH secreted by the pituitary gland. HCG becomes detectable in peripheral plasma within 8–10 days after fertilization and the plasma HCG level increases exponentially over the first trimester of pregnancy. The substantially longer half-life of HCG compared to LH would serve further to enhance the strength of HCG as a luteotropic signal.[97]

Recent evidence indicates that there may be a 'point of no return' at the mid-luteal phase, beyond which the corpus luteum can no longer be rescued by HCG.[98] The cellular mechanisms responsible for the loss of responsiveness to LH and HCG that occurs as the corpus luteum ages remain unknown. A better understanding of these mechanisms would be likely to provide valuable new insights into the causes of luteal phase dysfunction and early pregnancy loss.

FUTURE PERSPECTIVES

Current understanding of the roles of FSH and LH in the control of ovarian function are based on the use of more-or-less pure hormone preparations isolated from pituitary glands or urine. Neither hormone had been available completely free from contamination from the other until recently when FSH and LH produced by recombinant DNA technology became available for experimental use.[99] These materials are expected to provide new tools for exploring the cellular levels at which each gonadotropin acts within the preovulatory follicle and the corpus luteum.

A challenge for basic scientists is to unravel the cellular mechanisms through which FSH 'threshold' requirements are altered as follicles mature. A challenge to clinicians will be to exploit this knowledge to develop improved strategies for stimulating follicular development in anovulatory women. With the ability to administer pure FSH and LH independently, it should be possible to understand the precise roles of FSH and LH in regulating the final stages of follicular development, and to tailor individual therapy accordingly.[100] With respect to the corpus luteum, the availability of purified LH will provide an opportunity to develop dynamic tests of luteal function by administering exogenous LH.

Finally, a better understanding of the cellular and molecular mechanisms that regulate luteal function should provide us with the knowledge more effectively to target the corpus luteum for the development of novel forms of contraception.

SUMMARY

- Around 400 follicles sequentially mature and ovulate during an average woman's reproductive lifetime. Throughout birth to the menopause, the other ~99.98% of her follicles begin to develop but never mature. Instead, they default to atresia due to inadequate stimulation by FSH.
- The initiation of folliculogenesis and preantral follicular growth up to a diameter of 200–300 μm occur independently of cyclic changes in pituitary FSH secretion. Antral follicular development up to a diameter of 2–5 mm requires tonic stimulation by FSH, providing a constantly available population from which preovulatory follicles can be drawn.
- Recruitment of antral follicles to preovulatory stages of development requires appropriate stimulation by FSH beyond levels exceeding the threshold requirements of responding follicles, which are set by development-dependent changes in gonadotropin receptor numbers, thecal vascularization and paracrine/autocrine signaling.
- FSH induces granulosa cell proliferation and differentiation leading to the expression of LH receptors coupled to steroidogenic enzymes necessary for estrogen synthesis (cytochrome P450arom) by the preovulatory follicle and progesterone synthesis (cytochrome P450scc) by the corpus luteum.
- LH stimulates thecal cells to produce androgens (modulated by paracrine signaling emanating in granulosa cells) that are metabolized to estradiol in FSH-stimulated granulosa cells:

the 'two-cell, two-gonadotropin' mechanism of estrogen synthesis.
- The preovulatory follicle is 'selected' to ovulate, because it is the first follicle in the cohort (a) to acquire aromatase and LH receptors, and (b) to produce estrogen. Estrogen (and perhaps inhibin) produced by this follicle suppresses FSH concentrations below the threshold needs of other early antral follicles, and as a direct consequence, they become atretic. The maturing follicle is spared from the reduction in FSH because it progressively becomes more sensitive to FSH (and perhaps LH), as a direct result of its stimulation by FSH and autocrine and paracrine factors.
- The mid-cycle LH surge induces follicle rupture and terminates granulosa cell differentiation, leading to formation of the corpus luteum, which secretes progesterone, estradiol and inhibin throughout the luteal phase of the menstrual cycle.
- Hormone secretion by the corpus luteum is regulated by LH (HCG if pregnancy ensues).
- In the absence of pregnancy, luteal regression occurs in association with an age-related diminution in the responsiveness of the corpus luteum to LH. Luteolysis involves programmed cell death, possibly initiated during advanced stages of preovulatory development, regulated by FSH.
- The corpus luteum is rescued during early pregnancy due to the more intense gonadotropic signal generated by HCG secreted by the implanting blastocyst.

REFERENCES

1. Hillier SG. Hormonal control of folliculogenesis and luteinization. In Findlay JK (ed.) *Molecular Biology of the Female Reproductive System.* London: Academic Press, 1994: pp 1–37.
2. Gougeon A. Dynamics of follicular growth in the human: a model from preliminary results. *Hum Reprod* 1986 1: 81–87.
3. Aittomäki K, Lucena JLD, Pakarinen P *et al.* Mutation in the follicle-stimulating hormone receptor gene causes hereditary hypergonadotropic ovarian failure. *Cell* 1995 82: 959–968.

4. Hillier SG. Cellular basis of follicular endocrine function. In Hillier SG (ed.) *Ovarian Endocrinology.* Oxford: Blackwell Scientific Publications, 1991: 25–72.
5. Richards JS. Hormonal control of gene expression in the ovary. *Endocr Rev* 1994 15: 725–751.
6. Simpson ER, Mahendroo MS, Means GD *et al.* Aromatase cytochrome P450, the enzyme responsible for estrogen biosynthesis. *Endocr Rev* 1994 15: 342–355.
7. Segaloff DL, Ascoli M. The lutropin/chorionic gonadotrophin receptor...4 years later. *Endocr Rev* 1993 14: 1324–1347.
8. Giudice L. Insulin-like growth factors and ovarian follicular development. *Endocr Rev* 1992 13: 641–669.

9. Adashi E, Resnick CE, Hurwitz A, Ricciarelli E, Hernandez ER, Roberts CT, Leroith D, Rosenfeld R. Insulin-like growth factors: the ovarian connection. *Hum Reprod* 1991 **6**: 1213–1219.

10. Hernandez ER, Hurwitz A, Vera A, Pellicer A, Adashi E, LeRoith D, Roberts CTJr. Expression of the genes encoding the insulin-like growth factors and their receptors in the human ovary. *J Clin Endocrinol Metab* 1992 **74**: 419–425.

11. Tsafriri A, Dekel N. Molecular mechanisms in ovulation. In Findlay JK (ed.) *Molecular Biology of the Female Reproductive System.* London: Academic Press, 1994: 207–258.

12. Findlay JK. An update on the roles of inhibin, activin and follistatin as local regulators of folliculogenesis. *Biol Reprod* 1993 **48**: 15–23.

13. Ben-Ze'ev A, Amsterdam A. Regulation of heat shock protein synthesis by gonadotropins in cultured granulosa cells. *Endocrinology* 1989 **124**: 2584–2594.

14. Skinner MH, Parrott JA. Growth factor-mediated cell–cell interactions in the ovary. In Findlay JK (ed.) *Molecular Biology of the Female Reproductive System.* London: Academic Press, 1994: 67–82.

15. Peters H, Byskov AG, Grinsted J. The development of the ovary during childhood in health and disease. In Coutts JRT (ed.) *Funtional Morphology of the Human Ovary.* Lancaster: MTP Press, 1981: 26–34.

16. Baird DT, Bäckström T, McNeilly AS, Smith SK, Wathen CG. Effect of enucleation of the corpus luteum at different stages of the luteal phase of the human menstrual cycle on subsequent follicular development. *J Reprod Fertil* 1984 **70**: 615–624.

17. Goodman AL, Hodgen GD. The ovarian triad of the primate menstrual cycle. *Recent Prog Horm Res* 1983 **39**: 1–73.

18. Le Nestour E, Marraoui J, Lahlou N, Roger M, de Ziegler D, Bouchard P. Role of estradiol in the rise in follicle-stimulating hormone levels during the luteal–follicular transition. *J Clin Endocrinol Metab* 1993 **77**: 439–442.

19. Brown JB. Pituitary control of ovarian function – concepts derived from gonadotrophin therapy. *Aust NZ J Obstet Gynaecol* 1978 **18**: 46–54.

20. Goodman AL, Nixon WE, Johnson DK, Hodgen GD. Regulation of folliculogenesis in the cycling rhesus monkey; selection of the dominant follicle. *Endocrinology* 1977 **100**: 155–161.

21. Zeleznik AJ. Premature elevation of systemic estradiol reduces serum levels of follicle stimulating hormone and lengthens the follicular phase of the menstrual cycle in rhesus monkeys. *Endocrinology* 1981 **109**: 352–355.

22. Hillier SG. Regulation of follicular oestrogen biosynthesis: a survey of current concepts. *J Endocrinol* 1981 **89** (suppl): 3P–18P.

23. Zeleznik AJ, Kubik CJ. Ovarian responses in macaques to pulsatile infusion of follicle stimulating hormone and luteinizing hormone: increased sensitivity of the maturing follicle to FSH. *Endocrinology* 1986 **119**: 2025–2032.

24. Groome NP, O'Brien M, Illingworth P, Pai R, Mather J, Priddle J, McNeilly AS. Inhibin B is a major circulating form of inhibin in men and women. *Abstracts of the 77th Annual Meeting of the Endocrine Society, 1995.* Washington DC OR41-6, p 103.

25. LaPolt PS, Tilly JL, Aihara T, Nishimori K, Hsueh AJW. Gonadotropin-induced up-and down-regulation of ovarian follicle stimulating hormone receptor gene expression in immature rats: effects of pregnant mares serum gonadotropin, human chorionic gonadotropin and recombinant FSH. *Endocrinology* 1992 **130**: 1289–1295.

26. Zeleznik AJ, Midgley ARJr, Reichert LEJr. Granulosa cell maturation in the rat: increased binding of human chorionic gonadotropin following treatment with follicle stimulating hormone *in vivo. Endocrinology* 1974 **95**: 818–825.

27. Yong E, Baird DT, Hillier SG. Mediation of gonadotrophin-stimulated growth and differentiation of human granulosa cells by adenosine 3′,5′-monophosphate: one molecule, two messages. *Clin Endocrinol* 1992 **37**: 51–58.

28. Zeleznik AJ, Schuler HM, Reichert LEJr. Gonadotropin-binding sites in the rhesus monkey ovary: role of the vasculature in the selective distribution of human chorionic gonadotropin to the preovulatory follicle. *Endocrinology* 1981 **109**: 356–362.

29. Ravindranath N, Little-Ihrig LL, Phillips HS, Ferrara N, Zeleznik AJ. Vascular endothelial growth factor messenger ribonucleic acid expression in the primate ovary. *Endocrinology* 1992 **131**: 254–260.

30. Ferrara N, Houck K, Jakeman L, Leung DW. Molecular and biological properties of the vascular endothelial growth factor family of proteins. *Endocr Rev* 1994 **13**: 18–32.

31. Hillier SG. Paracrine control of follicular estrogen synthesis. *Semin Reprod Endocrinol* 1991 **9**: 332–340.

32. Magoffin DA, Erickson GF. Control systems of theca-interstitial cells. In Findlay JK (ed.) *Molecular Biology of the Female Reproductive System.* London: Academic Press, 1994: 39–66.

33. Park-Sarge OK, Mayo KE. Molecular biology of endocrine receptors in the ovary. In Findlay JK (ed.) *Molecular Biology of the Female Reproductive System.* London: Academic Press, 1994: 153–206.

34. Erickson GF, Nakatani A, Liu, XJ, Shimasaki S, Ling N. Role of insulin-like growth factors (IGF) and IGF binding proteins in folliculogenesis. In Findlay JK (ed.) *Molecular Biology of the Female Reproductive System.* London: Academic Press, 1994: 101–128.

35. Strauss JF, Miller WL. Molecular basis of ovarian steroid synthesis. In Hillier SG (ed.) *Ovarian Endocrinology.* Oxford: Blackwell Scientific Publications, 1991.

36. Hinshelwood MM, Demeter-Arlotto M, Means GD, Simpson ER. Expression of genes encoding steroidogenic enzymes in the ovary. In Findlay JK (ed.) *Molecular Biology of the Female Reproductive System.* London: Academic Press, 1994: 129–151.

37. Armstrong DT, Goff AK, Dorrington JH. In Midgley AR, Sadler WA (eds) *Ovarian Follicular Development and Function.* New York: Raven Press, 1979: 169–182.

38. Hillier SG, Whitelaw PF, Smyth CD. Follicular oestrogen synthesis: the 'two-cell, two-gonadotrophin' model revisited. *Mol Cell Endocrinol* 1994 **100**: 51–54.

39. Whitelaw PF, Smyth CD, Howles CM, Hillier SG. Cell-specific expression of aromatase and LH receptor mRNAs in rat ovary. *J Mol Endocrinol* 1992 **9**: 309–313.

40. Sasano H, Okamoto M, Mason JI, Simpson ER, Mendelson CR, Sasano N, Silverberg SG. Immunolocalization of aromatase, 17α-hydroxylase and side-chain cleavage cytochromes P-450 in the human ovary. *J Reprod Fertil* 1989 **85**: 163–169.

41. Erickson GF, Magoffin DA, Dyer CA, Hofeditz C. The ovarian androgen producing cells: a review of structure/function relationships. *Endocr Rev* 1985 **6**: 371–399.

42. Bergh C, Olsson JH, Hillensjö T. Effect of insulin-like growth factor I on steroidogenesis in cultured human granulosa cells. *Acta Endocrinol (Copenh)* 1991 **125**: 177–185.

43. Nahum R, Thong KJ, Hillier SG. Metabolic regulation of androgen production by human thecal cells *in vitro. Hum Reprod* 1995 **10**: 75–81.

44. Baird DT. Synthesis and secretion of steroid hormones by the ovary *in vivo.* In Zuckerman S, Weir BJ (eds) *The Ovary,* Vol. 3 2nd edn. London: Academic Press, 1977: 305–357.

45. Poretsky L. On the paradox of insulin-induced hyperandrogenism in insulin-resistant states. *Endocr Rev* 1991 **12**: 3–13.

46. Ghersevich S, Nokelainen P, Poutanen M, Orava M, Autio-Harmainen H, Rajaniemi H, Vihko R. Rat 17β-hydroxysteroid dehydrogenase type 1: primary structure and regulation of enzyme expression in rat ovary by diethylstilbestrol and gonadotropins *in vivo. Endocrinology* 1994 **135**: 1477–1487.

47. Teerds KJ, Dorrington JH. Immunohistochemical localization of 3β-hydroxysteroid dehydrogenase in the rat ovary during follicular development and atresia. *Biol Reprod* 1993 **49**: 989–996.

48. McNatty KP, Makris A, Reinhold VN, DeGrazia C, Osathanondh R, Ryan KJ. Metabolism of androstenedione by human ovarian tissue *in vitro* with particular reference to reductase and aromatase activity. *Steroids* 1979 **34**: 429–443.

49. Lischinsky A, Khali MW, Hobkirk R, Armsstrong DT. Formation of androgen conjugates by porcine granulosa cells. *J Steroid Biochem* 1983 **19**: 1435–1440.

50. Hillier SG, Reichert LEJr, van Hall EV. Control of preovulatory follicular estrogen biosynthesis in the human ovary. *J Clin Endocrinol Metab* 1981 **52**: 847–856.

51. Tamura T, Kitawaki J, Yamamoto T, Osawa Y, Kominami S, Takemori S, Okada H. Immunohistochemical localization of 17α-hydroxylase/C17-20 lyase and aromatase cytochrome P-450 in the human ovary during the menstrual cycle. *J Endocrinol* 1992 **135**: 589–595.

52. Fitzpatrick SL, Richards JS. Regulation of cytochrome P450 aromatase messenger ribonucleic acid and activity by steroids and gonadotropins in rat granulosa cells. *Endocrinology* 1991 **129**: 1452–1462.

53. Amsterdam AA, Koch Y, Lieberman ME, Lindner HR. Distribution of binding sites for human chorionic gonadotropin in the preovulatory follicle of the rat. *J Biol Chem* 1975 **67**: 894–900.

54. Zeleznik AJ, Hillier SG. The role of gonadotropins in the selection of the preovulatory follicle. *Clin Obstet Gynecol* 1984 **27**: 927–940.

55. Carr BR, MacDonald PC, Simpson ER. The role of lipoproteins in the regulation of progesterone secretion by the human corpus luteum. *Fertil Steril* 1982 **38**: 303–311.

56. Leung PCK, Steele GL. Intracellular signaling in the gonads. *Endocr Rev* 1993 **13**: 476–498.

57. Gougeon A, Lefévre B. Evolution of the largest healthy and atretic follicles during the human menstrual cycle. *J Reprod Fertil* 1983 **69**: 497–502.

58. McNatty KP, Baird DT, Bolton A, Chambers P, Corker CS, McLean H. Concentration of oestrogens and androgens in human ovarian venous plasma and follicular fluid throughout the menstrual cycle. *J Endocrinol* 1976 **71**: 77–85.

59. Smyth CD, Miró F, Whitelaw PF, Howles CM, Hillier SG. Ovarian thecal/interstitial androgen synthesis is enhanced by a follicle-stimulating hormone-stimulated mechanism. *Endocrinology* 1993 **133**: 1532–1538.

60. Hillier SG, Wickings EJ, Illingworth PI, Yong EL, Reichert LEJr, Baird DT, McNeilly AS. Control of immunoreactive inhibin production by human granulosa cells. *Clin Endocrinol* 1991 **35**: 71–78.

61. Yong EL, Hillier SG, Turner M, Baird DT, Ng SC, Bongso A, Ratnam SS. Differential regulation of cholesterol side-chain cleavage (P450scc) and aromatase (P450arom) enzyme mRNA expression by gonadotrophins and cyclic AMP in human granulosa cells. *J Mol Endocrinol* 1994 **12**: 239–249.

62. Hillier SG, Wickings EJ. Cellular aspects of corpus luteum function. In Jeffcoate SL (ed.) *The Luteal Phase*. London: Wiley, 1985: 1–23.

63. Espey LL. Ovulation as an inflamatory process – a hypothesis. *Biol Reprod* 1980 **22**: 73–106.

64. Brannström M, Janson PO. The biochemistry of ovulation. In Hillier SG (ed.) *Ovarian Endocrinology*. London: Blackwell Scientific Publications, 1991: 132–166.

65. Adashi EY, Kokia E, Hurwitz A. Potential relevance of cytokines to ovarian physiology. In Findlay JK (ed.) *Molecular Biology of the Female Reproductive System*. London: Academic Press, 1994: 83–99.

66. Park-Sarge O-K, Mayo KE. Regulation of the progesterone receptor gene by gonadotropins and cyclic adenosine 3′,5′-monophosphate in rat granulosa cells. *Endocrinology* 1994 **134**: 709–718.

67. Mori T, Suzuki A, Nishimura T, Kambegawa A. Inhibition of ovulation in immature rats by antiprogesterone antiserum. *J Endocrinol* 1977 **73**: 185–186.

68. Natraj U, Richards JS. Hormonal regulation, localization and functional activity of the progesterone receptor in granulosa cells of rat preovulatory follicles. *Endocrinology* 1993 **133**: 761–769.

69. Chaffkin LM, Luciano AA, Peluso JJ. The role of progesterone in regulating human granulosa cell proliferation and differentiation *in vitro*. *J Clin Endocrinol Metab* 1993 **76**: 696–700.

70. Duffy DM, Hess DL, Stouffer RL. Acute administration of a 3β-hydroxysteroid dehydrogenase inhibitor to rhesus monkeys at the midluteal phase of the menstrual cycle: evidence for possible autocrine regulation of the primate corpus luteum by progesterone. *J Clin Endocrinol Metab* 1994 **79**: 1587–1594.

71. Tjugum J, Dennefors B, Nortström A. Influence of progesterone, androstenedione and oestradiol-17β on the incorporation of [³H]proline in the human follicular wall. *Acta Endocrinol (Copenh)* 1984 **105**: 552–557.

72. Rondell P. Role of steroid synthesis in the process of ovulation. *Biol Reprod* 1970 **2**: 64–89.

73. Ohno Y, Mori T. Correlation between progesterone and plasminogen activator in rat ovaries during the ovulatory process. *Acta Obst Gynaecol Jpn* 1985 **37**: 247–256.

74. Reich R, Tsafriri A, Mechanic GL. The involvement of collagenolysis in ovulation in the rat. *Endocrinology* 1985 **116**: 522–527.

75. Ny T, Bjersing L, Hsueh AJW, Loskutoff DJ. Cultured granulosa cells produce two plasminogen activators and an antiactivator, each regulated differently by gonadotropins. *Endocrinology* 1985 **116**: 1666–1668.

76. Murdoch WJ, Peterson TA, Van Kirk EA, Vincent DL, Inskeep EK. Interactive roles of progesterone, prostaglandins and collagenase in the ovulatory mechanism of the ewe. *Biol Reprod* 1986 **35**: 1187–1194.

77. Baird DT, Baker TG, McNatty KP, Neal P. Relationship between the secretion of the corpus luteum and the length of the follicular phase of the ovarian cycle. *J Reprod Fertil* 1975 **45**: 611–619.

78. McLachlan RI, Robertson DM, Healy DL, Burger HG, de Kretser DM. Circulating immunoreactive inhibin levels during the normal menstrual cycle. *J Clin Endocrinol Metab* 1987 **65**: 954–961.

79. Muttukrishna S, Fowler PA, Groome NP, Mitchell GG, Robertson WR, Knight PG. Serum concentrations of dimeric inhibin during the spontaneous human menstrual cycle and after treatment with exogenous gonadotrophin. *Hum Reprod* 1994 **9**: 1634–1642.

80. Hutchison JS, Zeleznik AJ. The rhesus monkey corpus luteum is dependent on pituitary gonadotropin secretion throughout the luteal phase of the menstrual cycle. *Endocrinology* 1984 **115**: 1780–1786.

81. Fraser HM, Abbott M, Laird NC, McNeilly AS, Nestor JJJr, Vickery BH. Effects of an LH releasing hormone antagonist on the secretion of LH, FSH, prolactin and ovarian steroids at different stages of the luteal phase in the stumptailed macaque (*Macaca arctoides*). *J Endocrinol* 1986 **111**: 83–90.

82. Mais V, Kazer RR, Cetel NS, Rivier J, Vale W, Yen SS. The dependency of folliculogenesis and corpus luteum function on pulsatile gonadotropin secretion in cycling women using a gonadotropin-releasing hormone antagonist as a probe. *J Clin Endocrinol Metab* 1986 **62**: 1250–1255.

83. Ellinwood WE, Norman RL, Spies HG. Changing frequency of pulsatile luteinizing hormone and progesterone secretion during the luteal phase of the menstrual cycle of rhesus monkeys. *Biol Reprod* 1984 **31**: 714–722.

84. Filicori M, Butler JP, Crowley WFJr. Neuroendocrine regulation of the corpus luteum in the human. Evidence for pulsatile progesterone secretion. *J Clin Invest* 1984 **73**: 1638–1647.

85. Bassett SG, Little-Ihrig LL, Mason JI, Zeleznik AJ. Expression of messenger ribonucleic acids that encode for 3β-hydroxysteroid dehydrogenase and cholesterol side-chain cleavage enzymes throughout the luteal phase of the macaque menstrual cycle. *J Clin Endocrinol Metab* 1991 **72**: 362–366.

86. Ravindranath N, Little-Ihrig L, Benyo DF, Zeleznik AJ. Role of luteinizing hormone in the expression of cholesterol side-chain cleavage cytochrome P450 and 3β-hydroxy-steroid dehydrogenase, Δ^{5-4} isomerase messenger ribonucleic acids in the primate corpus luteum. *Endocrinology* 1992 **131**: 2065–2070.

87. Fisch B, Margara RA, Wintston RM, Hillier SG. Cellular basis of luteal steroidogenesis in the human ovary. *J Endocrinol* 1989 **122**: 303–311.

88. Knobil E, Plant TM, Wildt L, Belchetz PE, Marshall G. Control of the rhesus monkey menstrual cycle: permissive role of hypothalamic gonadotropin releasing hormone. *Science* 1980 **207**: 1371–1373.

89. Leyendecker G, Wildt L, Hansmann M. Pregnancies following chronic intermittent (pulsatile) administration of GnRH by means of a portable pump ('Zyklomat') – a new approach to infertility in hypothalamic amenorrhea. *J Clin Endocrinol Metab* 1980 **51**: 1214–1216.

90. Hutchison JS, Nelson PB, Zeleznik AJ. Effects of different gonadotropin pulse frequencies on corpus luteum function during the menstrual cycle of rhesus monkeys. *Endocrinology* 1986 **119**: 1964–1971.

91. Zelinski-Wooten MB, Hutchison JS, Chandrasekher YA, Wolf DP, Stouffer RL. Administration of human luteinizing hormone (hLH) to macaques after follicular development: further titration of the LH surge requirements for ovulatory changes in primate follicles. *J Clin Endocrinol Metab* 1992 **75**: 502–507.

92. Braden TD, Belfiore CJ, Niswender GD. Hormonal control of luteal function. In Findlay JK (ed.) *Molecular Biology of the Female Reproductive System.* London: Academic Press, 1994: 259–287.

93. Hsueh AJW, Billig H, Tsafriri A. Ovarian follicular atresia: a hormonally controlled apoptotic process. *Endocr Rev* 1994 **15**: 707–724.

94. Zeleznik AJ, Ihrig LL, Bassett SG. Developmental expression of Ca⁺⁺/Mg⁺⁺ sensitive endonuclease activity in rat granulosa and luteal cells. *Endocrinology* 1989 **125**: 2218–2220.

95. Lapthorn AJ, Harris DC, Littlejohn A, Lustbader JW, Canfield RE, Machin KJ, Morgan FJ, Isaacs NW. Crystal structure of human chorionic gonadotropin. *Nature (London)* 1994 **369**: 455.

96. Cameron JL, Stouffer RL. Gonadotropin receptors of the primate corpus luteum. I. Characterization of ^{125}I-labeled human luteinizing hormone and human chorionic gonadotropin binding to luteal membranes from the rhesus monkey. *Endocrinology* 1982 **110**: 2059–2067.

97. Monfort SL, Hess DL, Hendrickx AG, Lasley BL. Absence of regular pulsatile gonadotropin secretion during implantion in the rhesus macaque. *Endocrinology* 1989 **125**: 1766–1773.

98. Baird DD, Weinberg CR, Wilcox AJ, McConnaughey DR, Musey PI, Collins DC. Hormonal profiles of natural conception cycles ending in early, unrecognized pregnancy loss. *J Clin Endocrinol Metab* 1991 **72**: 793–800.

99. Hillier SG. Current concepts of the roles of follicle stimulating hormone and luteinizing hormone in folliculogenesis. *Hum Reprod* 1994 **9**: 188–191.

100. Filicori M, Flamigni C. (eds) *Ovulation Induction: Basic Science and Clinical Advances.* Amsterdam: Excerpta Medica International Congress Series 1046, 1994: 395pp.

The Ovary: Oogenesis

JJ Eppig

INTRODUCTION

The discoverers of mammalian ovarian follicles, even Regnier de Graaf himself, thought that the entire ovarian follicle might constitute the oocyte itself.[1] Although it was shown almost 150 years later that the oocyte actually resides within the ovarian follicle, we now appreciate that the follicular granulosa cells and the oocyte are actually a structural and functional unit and that, in non-atretic follicles, the egg is divorced from most of the somatic cells only by ovulation. Complex interactions between the two cell types are essential for the normal development and function of both. This chapter will describe these interactions and the coordination of the development of the follicle and the oocyte. The product of these interactions and oocyte-autonomous developmental programs is an egg competent to undergo fertilization and embryogenesis.

CURRENT CONCEPTS

Formation of primordial follicles

Oocytes originate at an extragonadal site (Fig. 2.4.1). Primordial germ cells probably originate in the embryonic ectoderm but abandon the embryo for temporary residence in the extraembryonic mesoderm during gastrulation. They appear as clusters of alkaline phosphatase-positive cells in this extraembryonic site before they begin their migration back into the embryo and their sojourn to the genital ridge.[2] The expression of two gene loci in the mouse, the *dominant spotting* (*W*) and *steel* (*Sl*) loci, is essential for the survival of the primordial germ cells during their journey to the genital ridge.[3,4] Mutations at these loci greatly reduce the number of germ cells found in the primitive gonad. The *W* locus codes for the receptor c-kit and the *Sl* locus codes for the specific ligand of this recep-

tor. The ligand is known by various names including kit ligand (KL), stem cell factor (SCF) or mast cell growth factor (MGF). *W* is expressed by the primordial germ cells and, later, by the oocytes while *Sl* is expressed by the cells of the germ cell environment.[5-7] KL might function later in germ cell development by promoting oocyte growth and maturation.[8] Factors from the primitive gonad probably attract the migrating primordial germ cells,[9] though some go astray and undergo limited development at extragonadal sites.[10]

After the primordial germ cells arrive at the primitive ovary, they are called oogonia. Oogonia proliferate by mitotic division in the primitive ovary until they enter meiosis and become oocytes. The number of female germ cells never increases from this time.

Granulosa cells, which are vital for the development of oocytes, also arise at an extragonadal site. They probably derive from the chords of the rete ovarii, which originate from the mesonephric tubules.[11,12] The oocytes and the presumptive granulosa cells become associated in the developing ovary (Fig. 2.4.1) and, with the participation of the ovarian mesenchymal cells, assemble to form the primordial follicle enclosed by a basal lamina.[12] (Further details of the origin of oocytes and early events in folliculogenesis are given in Chapter 2.1.)

Oocyte growth

Upon the initiation of follicular development, oocytes embark on a period of dramatic growth in which they enlarge from 15–20 μm to sometimes more than 100 μm in diameter, depending upon the species. Granulosa cells communicate with the oocyte throughout follicular development via membrane specializations known as gap junctions.[13,14] These channels allow the exchange of low-molecular weight molecules including those known to participate in cellular signaling mechanisms and nutrition. This network of gap junctions unites the granulosa cells with the oocyte as a structural and functional syncytium and is essential for oocyte growth.[15] The rate of oocyte growth directly correlates with the number of granulosa cells coupled to it.[16] The necessity of somatic cell participation in oocyte growth probably reflects qualitative and quantitative deficiencies in the nutrient transport capabilities of the oocyte plasma membrane, metabolic deficiencies in the oocyte, and the need for regulatory signals from the somatic cells.

Formation of the zona pellucida

The most obvious change in the structure of the growing oocyte, besides the dramatic increase in size, is the formation of the zona pellucida, which is the extracellular coat of the oocyte. Glycoprotein components of the zona pellucida function during fertilization to mediate sperm binding, induce the acrosome reaction and promote sperm

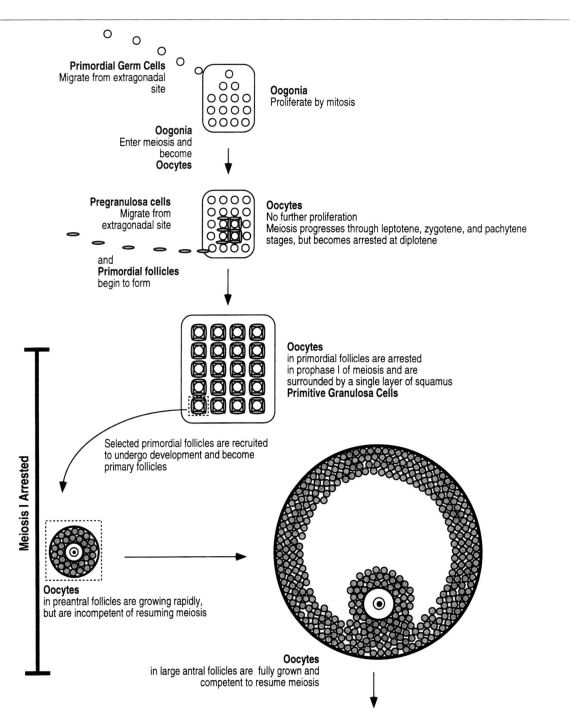

Fig. 2.4.1 *See caption opposite.*

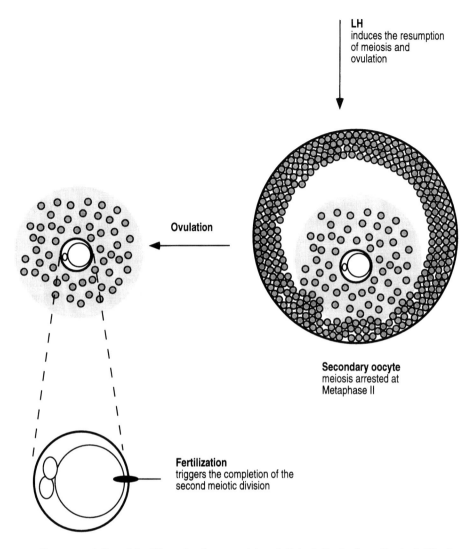

LH
induces the resumption
of meiosis and
ovulation

Ovulation

Secondary oocyte
meiosis arrested at
Metaphase II

Fertilization
triggers the completion of the
second meiotic division

Fig. 2.4.1 *Diagrammatic representation of the life-cycle of a preovulatory follicle: follicular formation to fertilization.*

penetration and, after modification by the contents of the egg's cortical granules, prevent multiple sperm entry into the egg.[17,18] The expression of zona pellucida (*Zp*) genes in the mouse is oocyte specific and developmentally controlled,[18,19] though in the rabbit some evidence suggests that both the oocyte and the adjacent granulosa cells produce a component of the zona pellucida.[20] The synthesis of zona pellucida glycoproteins is detected shortly after the initiation of oocyte growth and is completed by the time the oocyte reaches full size. Although zona pellucida mRNAs are detected mainly in immature oocytes beginning shortly after the initiation of oocyte growth,[18,19] the highly sensitive polymerase chain reaction (PCR) has detected small numbers of ZP2 transcripts, and transcripts of a factor that might regulate the transcription of the *Zp-2* gene, at the time the oocytes enter the dictyate (arrested diplotene) stage of meiosis during late fetal life.[21]

Meiosis in oocytes

Meiosis is a specialized process of cell division that occurs in germ cells. It occurs in two parts. The first part is characterized by the pairing of homologous chromosomes, which allows the exchange of genetic material between the homologous pairs, followed by segregation of the homologs into the daughter cells. This reduces the number of chromosomes from the diploid (2n) to the haploid (n) number. The second part resembles a mitotic division in the sense that sister chromatids segregate into the daughter cells. Mitosis and the second meiotic division differ in the number of chromosomes that segregate; mitosis usually involves the diploid number of chromosomes whereas the meiosis II involves the haploid number. Unlike meiotic divisions of spermatogenesis, the daughter cells of meiotic divisions of oocytes are unequal in size; one daughter cell is relatively small and is called a polar body. Thus the majority of the cytoplasmic components of the oocyte are conserved for use during early embryogenesis. Meiosis is necessary during both oogenesis and spermatogenesis to maintain a constant number of chromosomes from one generation to the next. Another major difference between meiosis during spermatogenesis and oogenesis is that meiosis in the male is continuous but is discontinuous in the female (Fig. 2.4.1). Meiosis in oocytes becomes arrested during prophase of the first meiotic division and remains in this arrested state for long periods depending upon the species. In some species, such as humans, this arrest can last as long as 50 to 60 years. This arrested diplotene stage of meiotic prophase is called the dictyate stage. Meiosis does not resume in the oocytes of non-atretic follicles until after the preovulatory surge of gonadotropins. Meiosis in mammalian oocytes normally becomes arrested for yet a second time at metaphase II and resumes again only after fertilization. Meiosis II also resumes after experimentally induced parthenogenesis or after spontaneous parthenogenesis, which occurs only rarely in mammals.

Nuclear and cytoplasmic maturation of oocytes

Nuclear maturation refers to the resumption of meiosis and the progression of meiosis to its next natural arresting point, metaphase II. The most obvious morphological manifestation of the resumption of meiosis is the disappearance of the oocyte's nucleolus and nuclear (germinal vesicle) envelope. This is called germinal vesicle breakdown, or GVB. Cytoplasmic maturation refers to the processes that prepare the egg for activation, formation of pronuclei, and preimplantation development.

Nuclear maturation

Meiotic cell divisions appear to be driven by the same, or similar, molecules that drive mitotic cell division. The best characterized participants in driving the G_2 to M phase transition in these divisions are cyclin B and p34^{cdc2} (also known as Cdc2, see Chapter 1.3). As illustrated in Fig. 2.4.2, these two molecules become associated and then the p34^{cdc2} is dephosphorylated at critical loci and becomes an active serine/threonine kinase often referred to as maturation (or M-phase) promoting factor (MPF): (see reference 22 for review). The product of the *cdc25* locus likely carries out the dephosphorylation of the p34^{cdc2} kinase.[23,24] The initiation of nuclear maturation and condensation of metaphase I chromosomes requires active MPF and entry into anaphase I correlates with the inactivation of MPF. Proteolytic degradation of the cyclin component of MPF probably causes the inactivation of MPF and drives entry into anaphase.[25] With no real interphase, a second increase in MPF activity causes entry of the oocytes into metaphase II where they await fertilization to instigate another round of cyclin degradation and entry into anaphase.

Meiotic arrest

The classic experiments of Pincus and Enzmann[26] demonstrated that oocytes undergo gonadotropin-independent (spontaneous) nuclear maturation when released from large antral follicles and cultured. However, oocytes isolated from preantral follicles cultured under similar conditions do not.[27,28] That the oocytes from the antral follicles resume meiosis when liberated from the mass of follicular somatic cells demonstrates that these oocytes contain all of the cell cycle regulatory molecules necessary to drive the initiation of nuclear maturation. Moreover, it follows that the somatic cells of antral follicles function to prevent the

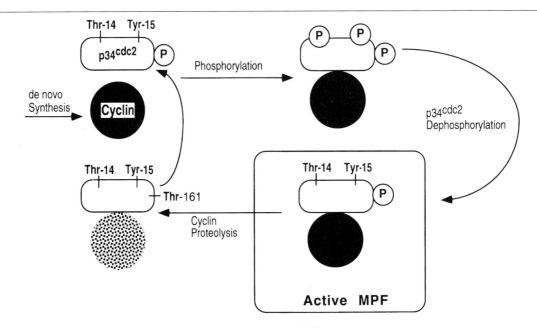

Fig. 2.4.2 *Pathway for the production of maturation promoting factor (MPF).*

oocyte from undergoing nuclear maturation inappropriately. In contrast, the oocytes of preantral follicles are fundamentally different from those in antral follicles since they do not undergo nuclear maturation after liberation from their follicles probably because these oocytes lack one or more of the critical molecules that drive the cell cycle. Thus, there are key differences in the mechanism for maintenance of meiotic arrest in preantral and antral follicles. Arrest in preantral follicles probably results from deficiencies within the oocyte in the molecules necessary to drive the resumption of meiosis while granulosa cells sustain the meiotic arrest of resumption-competent oocytes in antral follicles.

How do the granulosa cells of antral follicles maintain meiotic arrest? Although many of the earlier studies on the maintenance of meiotic arrest focused on substances present in follicular fluid, this fluid is not necessary for meiotic arrest. Rather, the critical substances are probably transmitted intracellularly to the oocyte from the mural granulosa cells through the cumulus granulosa cells. Contact of the oocyte–cumulus cell complex with the follicle wall, in the absence of follicular fluid, maintains meiotic arrest. Detachment of the complex from the wall induces GVB.[29,30] Gap junctions are probably the avenue for the communication of molecules that regulate the reinitiation of meiosis.[31,32]

Purines and their derivatives are potent inhibitors of GVB. Several lines of evidence indicate that cyclic adenosine monophosphate (cAMP) participates in the maintenance of meiotic arrest: (see references 33 and 34 for reviews). For example, membrane-permeable analogs of cAMP maintain meiotic arrest; the oocytes of laboratory rodents are more sensitive to these compounds than primate oocytes. Preventing the normal decrease in the amount of cAMP preceding GVB in oocytes of rodents with cAMP phosphodiesterase inhibitors such as 3-isobutyl-1-methylxanthine (IBMX) prevents GVB. Finally, microinjecting an inhibitor of the catalytic subunit of PK-A into IBMX-arrested oocytes induces GVB demonstrating that the phosphorylation of proteins via the PK-A pathway mediates the action of cAMP in the maintenance of meiotic arrest *in vitro*. The granulosa cells probably maintain meiosis-inhibiting levels of cAMP in the oocyte by transferring cAMP to the oocytes, by regulating the production and hydrolysis of cAMP within the oocytes, or most probably by a combination of both mechanisms.

Two other purines, hypoxanthine and adenosine, also participate in the maintenance of meiotic arrest, both promoting elevated cAMP levels in the oocyte. Hypoxanthine, a naturally occurring cAMP-phosphodiesterase inhibitor, directly suppresses cAMP degradation in oocytes.[35] Adenosine probably acts in concert with hypoxanthine by stimulating adenylate cyclase and by serving as a substrate for cAMP production.[36,37] Thus, adenosine promotes the generation of cAMP, and hypoxanthine prevents its degradation.

Finally, guanyl compounds play a clear and vital role in the maintenance of meiotic arrest. Guanosine is the most potent of all of the purines in suppressing the resumption

of meiosis *in vitro*[38] and, most importantly, inhibitors of inosine monophosphate dehydrogenase, a key enzyme in the formation of guanosine monophosphate, induce the resumption of meiosis by GVB-competent oocytes *in vivo*.[39]

Competence to resume meiosis

As described above, growing oocytes in preantral follicles do not spontaneously resume meiosis upon isolation from their follicles and culture. These oocytes are incompetent to resume meiosis probably because they are deficient in the amounts or configuration of one or more molecules critical to drive entry into M-phase. Incompetent oocytes display characteristics of cells at the G_2 phase of the cell cycle while oocytes acquiring competence begin to display characteristics typical of the G_2/M border such as chromatin condensation, microtubule reorganization, and phosphorylated centrosomes.[40] As oocytes near completion of their growth phase they become competent to undergo spontaneous GVB *in vitro* but they acquire competence to complete nuclear maturation and progress to metaphase II only after further development at the germinal vesicle stage. Thus, oocytes acquire competence to complete nuclear maturation in at least two sequential steps. The first probably involves the appropriate production and activation of MPF, which drives entry into M-phase as manifested by GVB and condensation of chromosomes to a prometaphase configuration, and the second involves the inactivation of MPF, which correlates with entry into anaphase.

The participation of both oocyte-autonomous and somatic cell-dependent processes is necessary for the acquisition of competence to undergo the first step. GVB-incompetent oocytes become partially competent *in vitro* by an oocyte-autonomous developmental program.[41,42] However, external signals provided by companion somatic cells participate in the process of acquiring competence to undergo GVB. These signals are probably universal promoters of cell cycle progression since they are produced by fibroblasts in culture as well as granulosa cells. In addition, cAMP, which promotes the proliferation of primordial germ cells[43] and maintains meiotic arrest in fully grown GVB-competent oocytes (see above), also participates in the acquisition of GVB-competence by growing oocytes.[42] Thus, cAMP participates in the regulation of the cell cycle at several critical stages in the development of the female gamete.

The processes that drive entry of oocytes into anaphase I have not been studied in detail, particularly in mammalian oocytes, although it is known that decreased MPF activity is correlated with anaphase in all mammalian oocytes studied. A mutant form of cyclin B, which is proteolysis-resistant, prevents the inactivation of MPF and exit from M-phase in frog embryonic cells.[25] Likewise, the injection of this 'indestructible' form of cyclin B into frog oocytes arrests maturation at the onset of anaphase I.[44] These results indicate that the destruction of cyclin B by proteolytic degradation at metaphase I is critical for the inactivation of MPF and driving entry into anaphase I. Perhaps mammalian oocytes that are competent to undergo GVB but that become arrested at metaphase I do not possess the proteases necessary for cyclin B degradation or the molecules necessary to activate or target the proteases and maturation consequently does not proceed beyond metaphase I. Nevertheless, insemination of metaphase I-arrested oocytes induces the completion of meiosis I and the production of a polar body. Thus, although oocytes that have acquired competence to undergo GVB, but not to progress beyond metaphase I, do not initially possess a functional system to drive entry into anaphase I, they may develop this system later during cytoplasmic maturation and it may remain dormant unless initiated by anaphase II-triggering mechanisms. On the other hand, the triggers for entry into anaphase II may be sufficient to launch entry into anaphase I even if the anaphase I and anaphase II triggers are not the same. If so, this implies that anaphase II-initiating mechanisms can develop in oocytes incapable of producing the systems sufficient to drive normal entry into anaphase I.

Gonadotropin-induced nuclear maturation

The preovulatory surge of gonadotropins induces the resumption of meiosis *in vivo*. Gap junctional communication within the ovarian follicle is probably involved in the resumption process, but its role is not clearly defined. Some investigators have proposed that the reduction in gap junctional communication between the oocyte–cumulus cell complex and the membrana granulosa reduces the flow of meiosis-arresting substances to the oocyte and thus causes the resumption of meiosis.[32,45] Others have postulated that gonadotropins induce the generation of a positive maturation-inducing signal within the granulosa cells and that the transmission of this signal to the oocyte actu-

ally requires patent gap junctional communication.[31,46] The nature of this signal has not been resolved, but it has been hypothesized that it might be either calcium (Ca^{2+}) or a Ca^{2+}-releasing factor such as inositol 1,4,5-trisphosphate (IP_3).[34,47] In this model (Fig. 2.4.3), the preovulatory surge of luteinizing hormone (LH) induces a rise in the level of Ca^{2+}, IP_3, or both in the mural granulosa cells, which, unlike the oocytes themselves, express LH-receptors. The Ca^{2+}/IP_3 is then passed through the cumulus cells to the oocyte, via the gap junctions, where the Ca^{2+}/IP_3 either overcomes the meiosis-arresting action of cAMP or promotes cAMP hydrolysis and maturation ensues. There are experimental observations reviewed by Eppig[34] and Homa *et al.*[47] that both support and dispute this hypothetical model.

Cytoplasmic maturation

Cytoplasmic maturation refers to the processes that prepare the egg for activation, formation of pronuclei, and preimplantation development. Early studies of spontaneous nuclear maturation of mammalian oocytes in culture implied that cytoplasmic maturation does not occur spontaneously since these oocytes failed to undergo fertilization and embryo development, but oocytes that underwent gonadotropin-induced maturation within intact follicles did.[48] These early failures were probably due to inadequate culture conditions since there has now been successful fertilization and development after *in vitro* maturation of oocyte–cumulus cell complexes isolated from many species[49] including humans.[50] Similarly to nuclear maturation, competence to undergo cytoplasmic maturation is

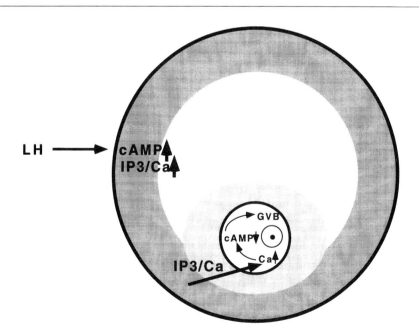

Fig. 2.4.3 *Hypothetical model for the possible participation of calcium in LH-induced oocyte maturation. The preovulatory surge of LH induces a rise in the level of Ca^{2+}, IP_3, or both in the mural granulosa cells. Ca^{2+}/IP_3 is then passed through the cumulus cells to the oocyte, via the gap junctions, where the Ca^{2+}/IP_3 either overcomes the meiosis-arresting action of cAMP or promotes cAMP hydrolysis and maturation ensues. Reproduced from reference 34, with permission.*

acquired in sequential steps by GV-stage oocytes; mouse oocytes first become competent to undergo cleavage to the 2-cell stage after insemination and, after further development at the GV-stage, they become competent to complete the 2-cell stage to blastocyst transition. In general, higher proportions of oocytes isolated from larger antral follicles are competent to develop to the blastocyst stage than oocytes from smaller follicles.[49,51] This is not due simply to a higher proportion of the oocytes that are competent to complete nuclear maturation to metaphase II after isolation from the larger follicles; a higher proportion of oocytes that matured to metaphase II after isolation from large follicles completed the 2-cell stage to blastocyst transition than oocytes that matured to metaphase II after isolation from small antral follicles.[52] Thus, even though oocytes may be competent to complete nuclear maturation, they can still be deficient in cytoplasmic maturation. These oocytes require further differentiation at the GV-stage to produce eggs containing maternal factors essential for development of embryos beyond the time of zygotic gene activation at the 2-cell stage.

Nuclear and cytoplasmic maturation usually occur in approximate synchrony since pronuclear formation fails unless sperm penetration of the oocyte occurs shortly before, or at the time of, the emission of the first polar body.[53] Nevertheless, oocytes incompetent to complete nuclear maturation can undergo at least some aspects of cytoplasmic maturation. Oocytes arrested at metaphase I of nuclear maturation can undergo (a) fertilization, pronuclear formation and preimplantation development, and (b) activation after treatment with Ca^{2+} ionophore.[52] Since cytoplasmic maturation of mouse oocytes occurs despite metaphase I arrest, the molecules required to regulate both the initiation and completion of cytoplasmic maturation are obviously present in oocytes that have not developed the cell cycle regulators required for the completion of meiosis I. Thus, oocytes can acquire competence to undergo cytoplasmic maturation independently of competence to complete nuclear maturation.

Cytoplasmic maturation obviously entails many changes that are necessary to prepare for fertilization, egg activation and preimplantation development. The following discussion details some of these changes.

Roles of inositol lipids and calcium

Sperm binding/fusion promotes a Ca^{2+}-dependent series of events leading to egg activation. The release of Ca^{2+} from intracellular stores occurs via an IP_3-dependent signal transduction mechanism. Persuasive evidence for this mechanism comes from studies showing that microinjection of antibodies to IP_3 prevents the generation of Ca^{2+} oscillations after insemination.[54] IP_3 is probably generated in response to the binding of sperm to G-protein-linked receptors on the oocyte surface since activators of G proteins, such as GTPγS, promote some, but not all, events of egg activation.[55] The oocyte's capacity to release intracellular stores of Ca^{2+} in response to microinjection of IP_3 is relatively low during the early stages of maturation, but reaches maximum sensitivity about the time that nuclear maturation has progressed to metaphase II.[56] Thus this

aspect of cytoplasmic maturation, which is essential for egg activation and pronuclear formation, normally coincides with nuclear maturation.

Protein synthesis

The pattern of proteins synthesized by oocytes during maturation undergoes both quantitative and qualitative changes until meiosis becomes arrested again at metaphase II.[57-59] Some of these changes are probably related to the regulation of nuclear maturation. Other changes, however, are probably directly concerned with processes associated with cytoplasmic maturation. Inhibition of protein synthesis during certain critical stages in maturation of pig oocytes, although having little effect on the decondensation of the sperm nucleus, dramatically impaired the transformation of the sperm nucleus to a male pronucleus.[60] Oocyte mRNA that will be translated during oocyte maturation is stored in a stable, dormant form until after GVB.[61] One of these transcripts studied in detail codes for tissue plasminogen activator (tPA). Although the function of tPA in oocytes is not known, it is used as a model to study the regulation of translation during oocyte maturation. Beginning about 3 h after GVB, the tPA mRNA undergoes progressive polyadenylation followed by translation and then degradation.[62] Destruction of a critical region of the 3′ untranslated sequence of tPA mRNA, using antisense RNA, prevents polyadenylation, translation and subsequent degradation.[62] This region, plus the 3′-processing signal AAUAAA, are essential for initiating polyadenylation, which is both necessary and sufficient for translation during oocyte maturation.[62]

Glutathione production

A male pronucleus does not form after sperm penetration of immature oocytes.[63] A critical step in the formation of a male pronucleus is the decondensation of the sperm nucleus. This process probably requires the reduction of the disulfide bonds of protamine so that factors within the oocyte can extract or degrade the protamine and replace it with somatic histones.[63] The reducing agent glutathione probably plays a key role in this process.[64,65] The concentration of glutathione increases during oocyte maturation and inhibition of the synthesis of this reducing agent suppresses male pronuclear formation.[64,65] Thus, the production of glutathione is a critical part of cytoplasmic maturation. The failure to provide culture conditions adequate for the production of necessary concentrations of glutathione[66] may explain, in part, the inability of earlier investigators to produce *in vitro* matured oocytes that can form a male pronucleus.[48]

Competence to release cortical granules

The development of competence to release cortical granules is a critical component of cytoplasmic maturation. If an egg is penetrated by more than one spermatozoon, the diploid number of chromosomes in the zygote will not be maintained and the embryo will degenerate. Oocytes, therefore, establish mechanisms to prevent the entry of more than one spermatozoon (see Chapter 2.10). Foremost among these mechanisms is the release of cortical granules whose contents proteolytically alter the structure of components of the zona pellucida in a way that prevents sperm penetration. The fusion or penetration of a single spermatozoon into the egg triggers the release of the cortical granules thereby blocking multiple sperm penetrations (polyspermy).[67] There is a high incidence of polyspermy when oocytes are inseminated before they complete maturation.[68] This is one reason that immature human oocytes, removed from follicles before ovulation, are subjected to continued maturation *in vitro* before *in vitro* fertilization (IVF).[69] The exocytosis of cortical granules is a Ca^{2+}-dependent process;[70] the Ca^{2+} is probably released from smooth membrane vesicles located in the egg's cortical region.[71] Ca^{2+} ionophore, therefore, induces release of the granules from mature oocytes: (see reference 67 for review). The density of the cortical vesicles, which potentially store calcium, is relatively sparse in GV-stage oocytes compared to mature oocytes[71] and the exocytosis of cortical granules in response to Ca^{2+} ionophore increases dramatically with the progression of maturation.[72]

Relationship between cytoplasmic and nuclear maturation

Maturation-associated changes in the pattern of protein synthesis are similar during the spontaneous maturation of either nucleated or enucleated mammalian oocytes.[73,74] Thus, at least some aspects of cytoplasmic maturation are under cytoplasmic control. Nevertheless, contents of the GV that mix with the cytoplasm following GVB may be required for complete cytoplasmic maturation. For example, the formation of a male pronucleus requires mixing of the contents of the GV with the cytoplasm.[75] In addition, the maturation-specific deadenylation of mRNAs in frog oocytes requires an activity derived from the GV and does not occur in anucleate fragments.[76] Thus, the initial event of nuclear maturation, GVB, is probably essential for activating cytoplasmic maturation even though the oocyte's developmental program for acquiring competence to complete cytoplasmic maturation does not appear to be linked to the acquisition of competence to complete nuclear maturation. Nuclear and cytoplasmic maturation would be normally coordinated by this mechanism requiring the mixing of the GV contents with the cytoplasm at the time of GVB, but cytoplasmic maturation can still occur without coordinated completion of nuclear maturation.[52]

The oocyte and granulosa cell function

Initial attempts to assess the role of the oocyte in follicular development were made by Nalbandov.[77] After excising the oocyte from pig and rabbit follicles *in situ*, he reported luteinization of the remaining granulosa cells and concluded that factors produced by oocytes prevent untimely luteinization. Although these studies were questioned,[78] recent studies have shown that communication between granulosa cells and oocytes is clearly bidirectional (Fig. 2.4.4).

Cumulus-expansion enabling factor(s)

Just before ovulation, gonadotropins stimulate cumulus cells to produce and secrete hyaluronic acid that disperses

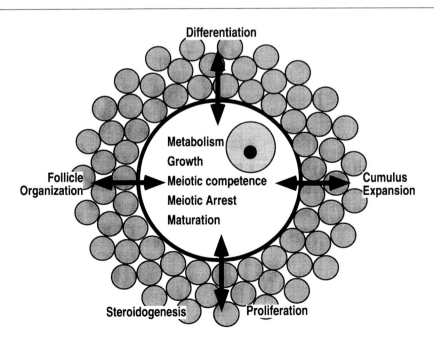

Fig. 2.4.4 *Diagramatic representation of granulosa cell-dependent processes in oocytes and oocyte-dependent processes in granulosa cells.*

the cumulus cells and embeds them in a mucus-like matrix; a process called cumulus expansion or mucification.[79–81] Cumulus expansion requires the synthesis and secretion of hyaluronic acid, a non-sulfated glycosaminoglycan, by the cumulus cells. LH stimulates cumulus expansion *in vivo*, and in intact large antral follicles *in vitro*, but FSH is required to stimulate the expansion of cumuli oophori of isolated oocyte–cumulus cell complexes *in vitro*.[80,82] When cumulus cells are removed from mouse oocytes and cultured as dispersed cells, however, they fail to produce hyaluronic acid when stimulated with FSH.[83] Likewise, the cumuli oophori of isolated complexes do not undergo expansion after removing the oocyte by microsurgery.[84,85] Nevertheless, medium conditioned by oocytes enables the cumulus cells to respond to FSH by synthesizing hyaluronic acid and undergoing expansion.[83,84] Thus, oocytes produce a paracrine factor(s) essential for cumulus expansion. Both the enabling factor(s) and FSH must be present at the same time for expansion to occur; neither this factor nor gonadotropin alone can stimulate cumulus expansion. The secretion of cumulus expansion enabling factor is developmentally regulated; significant secretion of the enabling factor by mouse oocytes coincides with the acquisition of competence to resume meiosis.[86] Oocyte competence to secrete the factor is probably promoted by paracrine factors from follicular somatic cells.[87]

Interestingly, pig oocytes secrete cumulus expansion enabling factor that functions in mouse cumuli oophori, but do not seem to need it for their own cumuli oophori to undergo expansion.[88] This conservation of the factor itself suggests that it may have other functions in the ovarian follicle. Alternatively, it is possible that the pig cumuli oophori actually do require the enabling factor for expansion, but the factor functions earlier in follicular development and the cumulus cells are able to 'remember' the action.

Granulosa cell proliferation factor(s)

Mouse oocytes produce one or more factors that stimulate the proliferation of granulosa cells derived from either the relative undifferentiated granulosa cells of preantral follicles or the more differentiated cumulus cells of antral follicles *in vitro*.[89] This supports earlier observations that cell division occurs more frequently in the population of granulosa cells nearest to the oocyte than in the more distal cells.[90,91]

Granulosa cell steroidogenesis factor(s)

Mouse oocytes secrete a factor(s) that inhibits the production of progesterone by cumulus cells.[92] Since spontaneous luteinization is characterized by the production of progesterone,[93] these studies support the classic observations of Nalbandov that oocytes suppress spontaneous luteinization of granulosa cells.[77]

Follicular organizing factor(s)

In the male, seminiferous tubules form in the absence of germ cells, but in the female, follicles do not form in the absence of oocytes.[94] Oocytes are therefore critical for the development and function of follicles even from the very earliest stages of follicle formation. Oocytectomized preantral follicles lose their three-dimensional organization and flatten on the culture surface, but paracrine factors secreted by oocytes restore three-dimensional organization to the oocytectomized follicles.[86,89]

FUTURE PERSPECTIVES

Exciting progress is being made in the identification of cell-cycle regulatory factors using yeast genetics and oocytes of lower vertebrates. This knowledge will be applied to resolve the mechanisms that govern nuclear maturation of mammalian oocytes. Genetic variants of oocyte maturation will be extremely useful in this effort.[95] It will be important to identify not only the molecules that orchestrate the initiation and completion of nuclear maturation but also the maternal factors produced during oocyte development that enable the oocyte to undergo fertilization and embryogenesis. An exciting new strategy to identify these factors is to use the cytoplasmic polyadenylation elements that drive maturation-specific translation to isolate previously unidentified maternal mRNAs. The function of these transcripts could then be resolved through the use of microinjected antisense oligonucleotides to selectively cleave the transcripts and subsequently observe effects on oocyte maturation and early embryogenesis.[96]

Methods are available to assess oocyte and somatic cell development and function *in vitro*.[97–100] The development and function of both the granulosa cells and oocytes in mammalian ovarian follicles require bidirectional communication and it is essential to understand which processes are regulated by intercellular communication and the nature of the signals. The influence of the oocyte on the function of the somatic cells certainly adds a new layer of complexity to an already complicated cellular system involving autocrine, paracrine and endocrine factors. Nevertheless, since oocytes probably play a critical role throughout follicular development in the organization, proliferation, differentiation and function of the granulosa cells, studies of follicular development that ignore this fact risk difficulties in interpretation. Identification of the components of the bidirectional control processes will certainly promote novel approaches to resolving the fundamental mechanisms of ovarian development, function and dysfunction, and contribute to analyzing fertility problems in zoological, agricultural and clinical fields.

SUMMARY

- Oocytes arise as primordial germ cells at an extragonadal site and migrate to the primitive gonad.
- In the female, there is no further increase in the number of germ cells after the initiation of meiosis, which usually occurs during fetal life.
- Meiosis in oocytes is not continuous, it becomes arrested at prophase of the first meiotic division and can remain in this stage for many years, depending on the species.
- Throughout most of oocyte growth, oocytes are incompetent to resume meiosis because of deficiencies in molecules that drive the entry into M-phase, but after they become competent to resume meiosis, meiotic arrest is sustained by the oocyte's companion somatic cells.
- Cyclic AMP is an important component of the meiosis-arresting system and purines such as hypoxanthine, adenosine and guanosine sustain meiotic arrest by maintaining elevated levels of cAMP in the oocyte.
- The resumption of meiosis is induced *in vivo* by the preovulatory surge of gonadotropins.
- Nuclear maturation of the oocyte refers to the reinitiation of meiosis and progression to metaphase II. It is driven by an initial increase in the activity of MPF, a complex of $p34^{cdc2}$ kinase and cyclin B but a decrease in MPF activity is associated with entry into anaphase. Metaphase II arrest is sustained by high MPF activity until fertilization.
- Cytoplasmic maturation refers to the processes that prepare the egg for activation, formation of pronuclei, and preimplantation development.
- Competence to undergo cytoplasmic maturation is acquired by GV-stage oocytes independently of competence to complete nuclear maturation.
- Oocytes play a critical role throughout follicular development in the organization, proliferation, differentiation and function of the granulosa cells.

ACKNOWLEDGEMENTS

I am very grateful to Drs Franck Chesnel, Ales Hampl and Larry Mobraaten for critically reading this manuscript and for their helpful suggestions. Research on oocyte development in my laboratory is supported by grants HD-20575, HD-23839 and HD-21970 from the National Institutes of Child Health and Human Development of the National Institutes of Health.

REFERENCES

1. Short RV. The discovery of the ovaries. In Zuckerman S, Weir BJ (ed.) *The Ovary*, 1. *General Aspects*. New York: Academic Press, 1977: 1–39.
2. McLaren A. Development of primordial germ cells in the mouse. *Andrologia* 1992 **24**: 243–247.
3. Dolci S, Williams DE, Ernst MK, Resnick JL, Brannan CI, Lock LF *et al*. Requirement for mast cell growth factor for primordial germ cell survival in culture. *Nature* 1991 **352**: 809–811.
4. Matsui Y, Toksoz D, Nishikawa S, Nishikawa S-I, Williams D, Zsebo K *et al*. Effects of Steel factor and leukemia inhibitory factor on murine primordial germ cells in culture. *Nature* 1991 **353**: 750–752.
5. Keshet E, Lyman SD, Williams DE, Anderson DM, Jenkins NA, Copeland NG *et al*. Embryonic RNA expression patterns of the c-*kit* receptor and its cognate ligand suggest multiple functional roles in mouse development. *Embo J* 1991 **10**: 2425–2435.
6. Manova K, Nocka K, Besmer P, Bachvarova RF. Gonadal expression of c-*kit* encoded at the *W* locus of the mouse. *Development* 1990 **110**: 1057–1069.
7. Motro B, Van Der Kooy D, Rossant J, Reith A, Bernstein A. Contiguous patterns of c-*kit* and steel expression: analysis of mutations at the *W* loci and *Sl* loci. *Development* 1991 **113**: 1207.
8. Manova K, Huang EJ, Angeles M, DeLeon V, Sanchez S, Pronovost SM *et al*. The expression pattern of the c-*kit* ligand in gonads of mice supports a role for the c-*kit* receptor in oocyte growth and in proliferation of spermatogonia. *Dev Biol* 1993 **157**: 85–99.
9. Godin I, Wylie C, Heasman J. Genital ridges exert long-range effects on mouse primordial germ cell numbers and direction of migration in culture. *Development* 1990 **108**: 357–363.
10. Zamboni L, Upadhyay S. Germ cell differentiation in mouse adrenal glands. *J Exp Zool* 1983 **228**: 173–193.
11. Byskov AG. The role of the rete ovarii in meiosis and follicle formation in the cat, mink and ferret. *J Reprod Fertil* 1975 **45**: 201–209.
12. Rajah R, Glaser EM, Hirshfield AN. The changing architecture of the neonatal rat ovary during histogenesis. *Dev Dynam* 1992 **194**: 177–192.
13. Albertini DF, Anderson E. The appearance and structure of the intercellular connections during the ontogeny of the rabbit ovarian follicle with special reference to gap junctions. *J Cell Biol* 1974 **63**: 234–250.
14. Gilula NB, Epstein ML, Beers WH. Cell-to-cell communication and ovulation. A study of the cumulus–oocyte complex. *J Cell Biol* 1978 **78**: 58–75.
15. Eppig JJ. Mouse oocyte development *in vitro* with various culture systems. *Dev Biol* 1977 **60**: 371–388.
16. Brower PT, Schultz RM. Intercellular communication between granulosa cells and mouse oocytes: existence and possible nutritional role during oocyte growth. *Dev Biol* 1982 **90**: 144–153.
17. Bleil JD. Sperm receptors of mammalian eggs. In

Wassarman PM (ed.) *Elements of Mammalian Fertilization.* I. *Basic Concepts.* Boca Raton: CRC Press, 1991: 133–151.

18. Dean J. Biology of mammalian fertilization: role of the zona pellucida. *J Clin Invest* 1992 **89**: 1055–1059.

19. Kinloch RA, Lira SA, Mortillo S, Schickler M, Roller RJ, Wassarman PM. Regulation of expression of *mZP3*, the sperm receptor gene, during mouse development. In Bernfield M (ed.) *Molecular Basis of Morphogenesis.* New York: Wiley-Liss, 1993: 19–33.

20. Lee VH, Dunbar BS. Developmental expression of the rabbit 55-kDa zona pellucida protein and messenger RNA in ovarian follicles. *Dev Biol* 1993 **155**: 371-382.

21. Millar SE, Lader ES, Dean J. ZAP-1 DNA binding activity is first detected at the onset of zona pellucida gene expression in embryonic mouse oocytes. *Dev Biol* 1993 **158**: 410–413.

22. Norbury C, Nurse P. Animal cell cycles and their control. *Annu Rev Biochem* 1992 **61**: 441–470.

23. Gautier J, Solomon MJ, Booher RN, Bazan JF, Kirschner MW. Cdc25 is a specific tyrosine phosphatase that directly activates p34cdc2. *Cell* 1991 **67**: 197–211.

24. Gabrielli BG, Lee MS, Walker DH, Piwnica-Worms H, Maller JL. Cdc25 regulates the phosphorylation and activity of the *Xenopus* cdk2 protein kinase complex. *J Biol Chem* 1992 **267**: 18040–18046.

25. Murray AW, Solomon MJ, Kirschner MW. The role of cyclin synthesis and degradation in the control of maturation promoting factor activity. *Nature* 1989 **339**: 280–286.

26. Pincus G, Enzmann EV. The comparative behavior of mammalian eggs *in vivo* and *in vitro*. I. The activation of ovarian eggs. *J Exp Med* 1935 **62**: 655–675.

27. Erickson GF, Sorensen RA. *In vitro* maturation of mouse oocytes isolated from late, middle, and pre-antral Graafian follicles. *J Exp Zool* 1974 **190**: 123–127.

28. Sorensen RA, Wassarman PM. Relationship between growth and meiotic maturation of the mouse oocyte. *Dev Biol* 1976 **50**: 531–536.

29. Leibfried L, First NL. Follicular control of meiosis in the porcine oocyte. *Biol Reprod* 1980 **23**: 705–709.

30. Racowsky C, Baldwin KV. *In vitro* and *in vivo* studies reveal that hamster oocyte meiotic arrest is maintained only transiently by follicular fluid, but persistently by membrana/cumulus granulosa cell contact. *Dev Biol* 1989 **134**: 297–306.

31. Fagbohun CF, Downs SM. Metabolic coupling and ligand-stimulated meiotic maturation in the mouse oocyte–cumulus cell complex. *Biol Reprod* 1991 **45**: 851–859.

32. Wert SE, Larsen WJ. Preendocytotic alterations in cumulus cell gap junctions precede meiotic resumption in the rat cumulus–oocyte complex. *Tissue Cell* 1990 **22**: 827–851.

33. Schultz RM. Meiotic maturation of mammalian oocytes. In Wassarman PM (ed.) *Elements of Mammalian Fertilization.* Vol. I. *Basic Concepts.* Boston: CRC Press 1991: 77–104.

34. Eppig JJ. Regulation of mammalian oocyte maturation. In Adashi EY, Leung PCK (eds) *The Ovary.* New York: Raven Press, 1993: 185–208.

35. Downs SM. Purine control of mouse oocyte maturation: evidence that nonmetabolized hypoxanthine maintains meiotic arrest. *Mol Reprod Dev* 1993 **35**: 82–94.

36. Eppig JJ, Ward-Bailey PF, Coleman DL. Hypoxanthine and adenosine in murine ovarian follicular fluid: concentrations and activity in maintaining oocyte meiotic arrest. *Biol Reprod* 1985 **33**: 1041–1049.

37. Salustri A, Petrungaro S, Conti M, Siracusa G. Adenosine potentiates forskolin-induced delay of meiotic resumption by mouse denuded oocytes: evidence for an oocyte surface site of adenosine action. *Gamete Res* 1988 **21**: 157–168.

38. Downs SM, Coleman DL, Ward-Bailey PF, Eppig JJ. Hypoxanthine is the principal inhibitor of murine oocyte maturation in a low molecular weight fraction of porcine follicular fluid. *Proc Natl Acad Sci* 1985 **82**: 454–458.

39. Downs SM, Eppig JJ. Induction of mouse oocyte maturation *in vivo* by perturbants of purine metabolism. *Biol Reprod* 1987 **36**: 431–437.

40. Wickramasinghe D, Albertini DF. Cell cycle control during mammalian oogenesis. *Curr Top Dev Biol* 1993 **28**: 125–153.

41. Canipari R, Palombi F, Riminucci M, Mangia F. Early programming of maturation competence in mouse oogenesis. *Dev Biol* 1984 **102**: 519–524.

42. Chesnel F, Wigglesworth K, Eppig JJ. Acquisition of meiotic competence by denuded mouse oocytes: participation of somatic-cell products and cAMP. *Dev Biol* 1994 **161**:285–295.

43. De Felici M, Dolchi S, Pesce M. Proliferation of mouse primordial germ cells *in vitro*: a key role for cAMP. *Dev Biol* 1993 **157**: 277–280.

44. Huchon D, Rime H, Jessus C, Ozon R. Control of metaphase I formation in *Xenopus* oocyte: effects of an indestructible cyclin B and of protein synthesis. *Biol Cell* 1993 **77**: 133–141.

45. Dekel N. Spatial relationship of follicular cells in the control of meiosis. In Haseltine FP, First NL (eds) *Progress in Clinical and Biological Research. Meiotic Inhibition: Molecular Control of Meiosis.* New York: Alan R. Liss, 1988: 87–101.

46. Downs SM, Daniel SAJ, Eppig JJ. Induction of maturation in cumulus cell-enclosed mouse oocytes by follicle-stimulating hormone and epidermal growth factor: evidence for a positive stimulus of somatic cell origin. *J Exp Zool* 1988 **245**: 86–96.

47. Homa ST, Carroll J, Swann K. The role of calcium in mammalian oocyte maturation and egg activation. *Hum Reprod* 1993 **8**: 1274–1281.

48. Thibault C. Are follicular maturation and oocyte maturation independent processes? *J Reprod Fertil* 1977 **51**: 1–15.

49. Eppig JJ. Establishment of competence for preimplantation embryogenesis during oogenesis in mice. In Bavister B (ed.) *Preimplantation Embryo Development.* New York: Springer Verlag, 1993: 43–53.

50. Cha KY, Choi DH, Koo JJ, Han SY, Ko JJ, Yoon TK. Pregnancy after *in vitro* fertilization of human follicular oocytes collected from nonstimulated cycles, their culture *in vitro* and their transfer in a donor oocyte program. *Fertil Steril* 1991 **55**: 109–113.

51. Pavlok A, Lucas-Hahn A, Niemann H. Fertilization and developmental competence of bovine oocytes derived from different categories of antral follicles. *Mol Reprod Dev* 1992 **31**: 63–67.

52. Eppig JJ, Schultz RM, O'Brien M, Chesnel F. Relationship between the developmental programs controlling nuclear and cytoplasmic maturation of mouse oocytes. *Dev Biol* 1994 **164**: 1–9.

53. Iwamatsu T, Chang MC. Sperm penetration *in vitro* of mouse oocytes at various times during maturation. *J Reprod Fertil* 1972 **31**: 237–247.

54. Miyazaki S, Yuzaki M, Nakada K, Shirakawa H, Nakanishi S, Nakade S *et al.* Block of Ca²⁺ wave and Ca²⁺ oscillation by antibody to the inositol 1,4,5-trisphosphate receptor in fertilized hamster eggs. *Science* 1992 **257**: 251–255.

55. Kurasawa S, Schultz RM, Kopf GS. Egg-induced modifications of the zona pellucida of mouse eggs: effects of microinjected inositol 1,4,5-trisphosphate. *Dev Biol* 1989 **133**: 295–304.

56. Fujiwara T, Nakada K, Shirakawa H, Miyazaki S. Development of inositol trisphosphate-induced calcium release mechanism during maturation of hamster oocytes. *Dev Biol* 1993 **156**: 69–79.

57. Moor RM, Gandolfi F. Molecular and cellular changes associated with maturation and early development of sheep eggs. *J Reprod Fertil Suppl* 1987 **34**: 55–69.

58. Schultz RM, Wassarman PM. Specific changes in the pattern of protein synthesis during meiotic maturation of mammalian oocytes *in vitro*. *Proc Natl Acad Sci USA* 1977 **74**: 538–541.

59. Kastrop PMM, Bevers MM, Destree OHJ, Kruip TAM. Changes in protein synthesis and phosphorylation patterns

during bovine oocyte maturation *in vitro*. *J Reprod Fertil* 1990 **90**: 305–310.

60. Ding JC, Moor RM, Foxcroft GR. Effects of protein synthesis on maturation, sperm penetration, and pronuclear development in porcine oocytes. *Mol Reprod Dev* 1992 **33**: 59–66.

61. Bachvarova R. Gene expression during oogenesis and oocyte development in mammals. In Browder LW (ed.) *Developmental Biology. A Comprehensive Synthesis, 1. Oogenesis.* New York: Plenum Press, 1985: 453–524.

62. O'Connell ML, Huarte J, Belin D, Vassalli J-D, Strickland S. Translation control in oocytes: a critical role for the poly(A) tail of maternal mRNAs. In Bavister BD (ed.) *Preimplantation Embryo Development.* New York: Springer-Verlag, 1993: 38–42.

63. Perreault SD. Regulation of sperm nuclear reactivation during fertilization. In Bavister BD, Cummins J, Roldan ERS (eds) *Fertilization in Mammals.* Norwell: Serono Symposia, 1990: 285–296.

64. Perreault SD, Barbee RR, Slott VL. Importance of glutathione in the acquisition and maintenance of sperm nuclear decondensation activity in maturing hamster oocytes. *Dev Biol* 1988 **125**: 181–186.

65. Yoshida M. Role of glutathione in the maturation and fertilization of pig oocytes *in vitro*. *Mol Reprod Dev* 1993 **35**: 76–81.

66. Yoshida M, Ishigaki K, Nagai T, Chikyu M, Pursel VG. Glutathione concentration during maturation and after fertilization in pig oocytes: relevance to the ability of oocytes to form male pronucleus. *Biol Reprod* 1993 **49**: 89–94.

67. Cherr GN, Ducibella T. Activation of the mammalian egg: cortical granule distribution, exocytosis, and the block to polyspermy. In Bavister BD, Cummins J, Roldan ERS (eds) *Fertilization in Mammals.* Norwell: Serono Symposia, 1990: 309–330.

68. Iwamatsu T, Chang MC. Factors involved in the fertilization of mouse eggs *in vitro*. *J Reprod Fertil* 1971 **26**: 197–208.

69. Trounson AO, Mohr LR, Wood C, Leeton JF. Effect of delayed insemination on *in-vitro* fertilization, culture and transfer of human embryos. *J Reprod Fertil* 1982 **64**: 285–294.

70. Ducibella T, Kurasawa S, Duffy P, Kopf GS, Schultz RM. Regulation of the polyspermy block in the mouse egg: maturation-dependent differences in cortical granule exocytosis and zona pellucida modifications induced by inositol 1,4,5-trisphosphate and an activator of protein kinase C. *Biol Reprod* 1993 **48**: 1251–1257.

71. Ducibella T, Rangarajan S, Anderson E. The development of mouse oocyte cortical reaction competence is accompanied by major changes in cortical vesicles and not cortical granule depth. *Dev Biol* 1988 **130**: 789–792.

72. Ducibella T, Kurasawa S, Rangarajan S, Kopf GS, Schultz RM. Precocious loss of cortical granules during mouse oocyte meiotic maturation and correlation with an egg-induced modification of the zona pellucida. *Dev Biol* 1990 **137**: 46–55.

73. Schultz RM, Letourneau GE, Wassarman PM. Meiotic maturation of mouse oocytes *in vitro*: protein synthesis in nucleate and anucleate oocyte fragments. *J Cell Sci* 1978 **30**: 251–264.

74. Sun FZ, Moor RM. Nuclear-cytoplasmic interactions during ovine oocyte maturation. *Development* 1991 **111**: 171–180.

75. Borsuk E. Anucleate fragments of parthenogenetic eggs and of maturing oocytes contain complementary factors required for development of a male pronucleus. *Mol Reprod Dev* 1991 **29**: 150–156.

76. Varnum SM, Hurney CA, Wormington WM. Maturation-specific deadenylation in *Xenopus* oocytes requires nuclear and cytoplasmic factors. *Dev Biol* 1992 **153**: 283–290.

77. Nalbandov AV. Interactions between oocytes and follicular

cells. In Biggers JD, Schuetz AW (eds) *Oogenesis.* Baltimore: University Park Press, 1972: 513–522.

78. Channing CP, Tsafriri A. Lack of an inhibitory influence of oocytes upon luteinization of porcine granulosa cells in culture. *J Reprod Fertil* 1977 **50**: 103–105.

79. Dekel N, Kraicer PF. Induction *in vitro* of mucification of rat cumulus oophorus by gonadotropins and adenosine 3′,5′-monophosphate. *Endocrinology* 1978 **102**: 1797–1802.

80. Eppig JJ. FSH stimulates hyaluronic acid synthesis by oocyte-cumulus cell complexes from mouse preovulatory follicles. *Nature* 1979 **281**: 483–484.

81. Salustri A, Yanagishita M, Hascall VC. Synthesis and accumulation of hyaluronic acid and proteoglycans in the mouse cumulus cell–oocyte complex during follicle-stimulating hormone-induced mucification. *J Biol Chem* 1989 **264**: 13840–13847.

82. Eppig JJ. Regulation of cumulus oophorus expansion by gonadotropins *in vivo* and *in vitro*. *Biol Reprod* 1980 **23**: 545–552.

83. Salustri A, Yanagishita M, Hascall VC. Mouse oocytes regulate hyaluronic acid synthesis and mucification by FSH-stimulated cumulus cells. *Dev Biol* 1990 **138**: 26–32.

84. Buccione R, Vanderhyden BC, Caron PJ, Eppig JJ. FSH-induced expansion of the mouse cumulus oophorus *in vitro* is dependent upon a specific factor(s) secreted by the oocyte. *Dev Biol* 1990 **138**: 16–25.

85. Eppig JJ. Oocyte-somatic cell communication in the ovarian follicles of mammals. *Sem Dev Biol* 1994 **5**: 51–59.

86. Vanderhyden BC, Caron PJ, Buccione R, Eppig JJ. Developmental pattern of the secretion of cumulus-expansion enabling factor by mouse oocytes and the role of oocytes in promoting granulosa cell differentiation. *Dev Biol* 1990 **140**: 307–317.

87. Eppig JJ, Wigglesworth K, Chesnel F. Secretion of cumulus expansion enabling factor by mouse oocytes: relationship to oocyte growth and competence to resume meiosis. *Dev Biol* 1993 **158**: 400–409.

88. Vanderhyden BC. Species differences in the regulation of cumulus expansion by an oocyte-secreted factor(s). *J Reprod Fertil* 1993 **98**: 219–227.

89. Vanderhyden BC, Telfer EE, Eppig JJ. Mouse oocytes promote proliferation of granulosa cells from preantral and antral follicles *in vitro*. *Biol Reprod* 1992 **46**: 1196–1204.

90. Bullough WS. The method of growth of the follicle and corpus luteum in the mouse ovary. *J Endocrinol* 1942 **3**: 150–156.

91. Hirshfield AN. Patterns of [³H] thymidine incorporation differ in immature rats and mature, cycling rats. *Biol Reprod* 1986 **34**: 229–235.

92. Vanderhyden BC, Cohen JN, Morley P. Mouse oocytes regulate granulosa cell steroidogenesis. *Endocrinology* 1993 **133**: 423–426.

93. Channing CP. Effect of stage of the estrous cycle and gonadotropins upon luteinization of porcine granulosa cells in culture. *Endocrinology* 1970 **87**: 156–164.

94. Coulombre JL, Russell ES. Analysis of the pleiotropism at the W-locus in the mouse. The effects of W and Wv substitution upon postnatal development of germ cells. *J Exp Zool* 1954 **126**: 277–295.

95. Eppig JJ, Wigglesworth K. Atypical maturation of oocytes of strain I/LnJ mice. *Human Reprod* 1994 **9**: 1136–1142.

96. Sallés FJ, Darrow AL, O'Connell ML, Strickland S. Isolation of novel murine maternal mRNAs regulated by cytoplasmic polyadenylation. *Genes Dev* 1992 **6**: 1202–1212.

97. Eppig JJ, Schroeder AC. Capacity of mouse oocytes from preantral follicles to undergo embryogenesis and development to live young after growth, maturation and fertilization *in vitro*. *Biol Reprod* 1989 **41**: 268–276.

98. Eppig JJ. Mammalian oocyte development *in vivo* and *in vitro*. In Wassarman PM (ed.) *Elements of Mammalian*

Fertilization 1. *Basic Concepts.* Boca Raton: CRC Press, 1991: 57–76.

99. Nayudu PL, Osborn SM. Factors influencing the rate of preantral and antral growth of mouse ovarian follicles *in vitro. J Reprod Fertil* 1992 **95**: 349–362.

100. Boland NI, Humpherson PG, Leese HJ, Gosden RG. Pattern of lactate production and steroidogenesis during growth and maturation of mouse ovarian follicles *in vitro. Biol Reprod* 1993 **48**: 798–806.

2.5

The Testis: Endocrine Function

ID Morris

INTRODUCTION

Male fertility totally depends on the endocrine and paracrine functions of androgens produced by the testes. Until recently the testis was generally considered to be a relatively simple endocrine gland, androgen secretion being driven primarily by pituitary luteinizing hormone (LH) and spermatogenesis by follicle-stimulating hormone (FSH). Homeostatic regulation occurred by simple negative feedback signals – testosterone produced by Leydig cells and inhibin produced by Sertoli cells (Fig. 2.5.1). Since testicular endocrine pathologies are relatively rare and access to normal testicular tissue for experimental purposes is uncommon, new insight into the physiology of the testis has been slow to develop. However, intricacies in the control of testicular endocrine secretion are now becoming apparent, largely due to new experimental approaches based on rapid developments in molecular biology. These advances reveal that the endocrinology of the testis is at least as complex as any other endocrine gland. This chapter summarizes our current understanding of the central role of testicular hormones in reproduction, as an important prerequisite for the investigation of disorders in male fertility.

CURRENT CONCEPTS

Leydig cells and androgen secretion

The androgen-producing cells of the testis are the Leydig cells, so named after Franz Leydig who described the testicular intertubular tissue in 1850.[1] Leydig also noticed the paucity of these cells relative to other cells in the testicular parenchyma. In men, Leydig cells constitute less than 1% of the total testicular mass. However, their scarcity belies their importance to reproduction as the exclusive cellular sites of androgen synthesis.

Interstitial tissue

Leydig cells are located in the spaces between the seminiferous tubules (Fig. 2.5.2). They are therefore ideally placed to provide the high concentrations of androgen necessary for spermatogenesis, which are many times higher than the testosterone concentration present in plasma.[2] The Leydig cell represents about 75% of the interstitial cell population, the majority of the remainder comprising macrophages, fibroblasts, lymphocytes, mast cells and the endothelial cells of the blood vessels.

Leydig cell ultrastructure

The Leydig cell is polyhedral in shape and has a distinctive ultrastructure.[3,4] The nuclear heterochromatin is distributed in a thin irregular layer around the nuclear membrane. In the adult testis, mitosis is extremely rare. The Leydig cell is considered to be terminally differentiated although Leydig cell tumors do rarely occur.[5] Mitochondria and smooth endoplasmic reticulum are extremely abundant as would be expected of a secretory cell. The rough endoplasmic reticulum and dense granules are not prominent, since the Leydig cell does not store protein hormones.

Leydig cell ontogeny

Leydig cells have been shown to originate from at least two sources. The first is through differentiation from mesenchymal precursors stimulated by locally produced growth factors; the second is via the division of Leydig cells themselves under the influence of LH, testosterone,[6] and possibly FSH.[7] LH also appears to be important to the growth of Leydig cells in men, since a mutation in the LH β-subunit gene that decreases binding of LH to the LH receptor is associated with hypogonadism and absence of Leydig cells.[8]

The adult testicular Leydig cell population is more or less static. In the rat, Leydig cell turnover has been estimated to be 240 days, i.e. longer than most rats live![9] However, experiments have shown if all Leydig cells are destroyed by

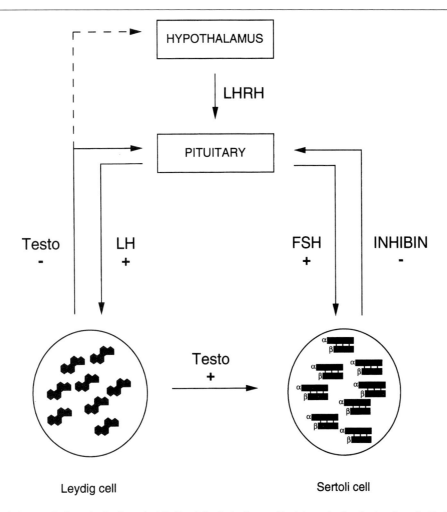

Fig. 2.5.1 *The hypothalamo–pituitary–testicular axis. LH stimulates testosterone (Testo) production by Leydig cells. Testosterone exerts negative feedback regulation of LH and FSH production by the pituitary gland and paracrine regulation of Sertoli cell function. FSH and androgen stimulate inhibin production by Sertoli cells. Inhibin selectively suppresses FSH production, but the relative contributions of inhibin and testosterone to negative feedback regulation of FSH secretion are controversial.*

treatment with a cytotoxin, a new Leydig cell population regenerates within weeks.[10] Regeneration requires the action of testicular growth factors to establish a precursor population, presumably by mitosis, which then differentiate into androgen–secreting Leydig cells in response to stimulation by LH.[7] Thus the testis has the potential to act quickly to maintain the Leydig cell population and hence the circulating androgen levels that are essential to male fertility. It is not however known if this mechanism is activated under normal physiological conditions.

Androgens

Androgens are C_{19} steroids (Fig. 2.5.3) characterized by their ability to stimulate and maintain the development of secondary sexual tissues through binding to specific, high-affinity androgen receptors located within target cells[11] (see Chapter 1.4). Testosterone is the major testicular androgen. In men, 95% of the testosterone circulating in blood

originates from Leydig cells. Only 20% of circulating di-hydrotestosterone (DHT) is of testicular origin – the rest arises from the peripheral conversion of testosterone and dehydroepiandrosterone (DHEA). Only 10% of serum DHEA and even less androstenedione (2%) originates from the Leydig cell, since these androgens are secreted in greater amounts by the adrenal gland.

Binding to plasma proteins

Most (>98%) secreted androgen circulates in blood bound to proteins. Binding occurs in approximately equal amounts to albumin and sex hormone-binding globulin (SHBG).[12] Serum albumin binds steroids non-specifically with low affinity but high capacity. SHBG, a homodimeric protein secreted by the liver, binds androgens and estrogens with high affinity but limited capacity.[13] Collectively, the steroid-binding properties of albumin and SHBG determine the proportion of androgen that circulates 'free', and hence in a biologically active form.

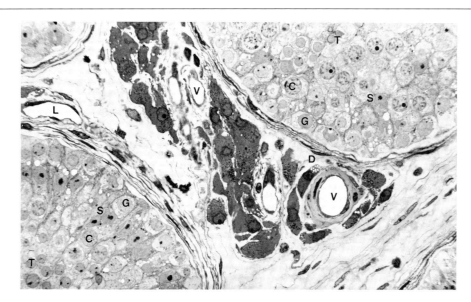

Fig. 2.5.2 *The histological appearance of the adult human testis (×530). The intertubular space contains the darkly staining androgen-secreting Leydig cells, some containing lipid droplets (**D**). The Leydig cells aggregate around the capillary vessels (**V**). Much of the inter-tubular space is filled with loose connective tissue in which the lymphatic vessels (**L**) can be seen. The germ cells almost fill the seminiferous tubules, the stem cell spermatogonia (**G**), which lie around the perimeter of the tubule, divide to give rise to spermatocytes (**C**) which differentiate into spermatids (**T**) and eventually spermatozoa. The Sertoli cells, which secrete inhibin and related peptides, envelop all the germ cells and can be identified by their characteristic irregular nuclei (**S**) in the cellular layer above the spermatogonia. (Micrograph kindly provided by Professor J Kerr, Monash University, Australia.)*

ANDROGENS

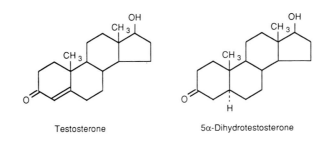

INHIBINS AND ACTIVINS

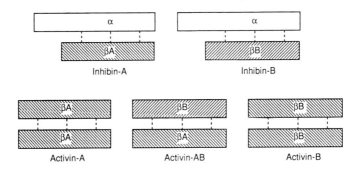

Fig. 2.5.3 *The major testicular hormones. Androgens are low molecular-weight C_{19} steroids of which testosterone and 5α-dihydrotestos-terone are the most potent. Inhibins and activins are large, water-soluble, glycoproteins with molecular weights of 20 000–50 000. Inhibins are heterodimeric proteins, comprising a common α-subunit in association with β_A (inhibin-A) or β_B (inhibin-B) subunits. Activins are homodimeric: β_A,β_A (activin-A) or β_A,β_B (activin-AB). Theoretically, the β_B,β_B (activin-B) form also exists but has not been isolated.*

Secretory dynamics

Testicular androgen secretion is a dynamically regulated process that depends on the rapid production and metabolism of intermediates in C_{19} steroid synthesis. Leydig cells undertake increased secretion of testosterone within minutes of stimulation by LH, reflecting *de novo* steroid synthesis.[14,15] This dynamic property is readily seen in the pulsatile nature of androgen secretion, with serum androgen levels being closely correlated with serum LH levels, which themselves reflect the pulsatile secretion of luteinizing hormone releasing hormone (LHRH) by the hypothalamus[16,17] (see Chapter 2.2).

Steroidogenic pathways

Androgen biosynthesis depends on an adequate supply of precursor cholesterol, which is catabolized to C_{19} androgens via C_{21} progestogen intermediates (Figs. 2.5.4 and 2.5.5).

Cholesterol synthesized within the cell from acetate is an important, but not exclusive, substrate for testicular androgen biosynthesis. Cholesterol taken up in association with high-density lipoproteins (HDL) via HDL receptors in the cell surface membrane[18] is the other major source. It is not known if the relative contribution of intra- and extracellular cholesterol to androgen synthesis alters with changes in

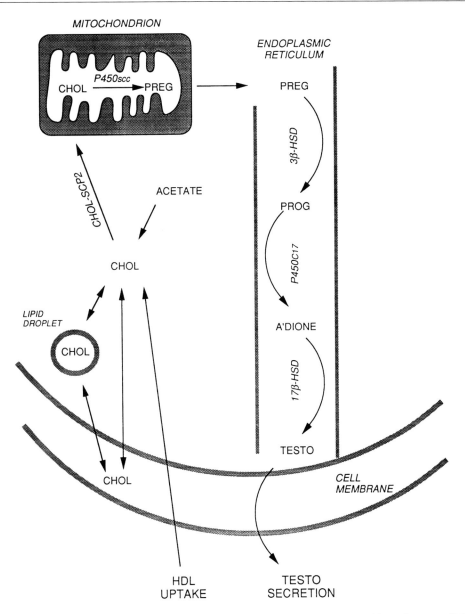

Fig. 2.5.4 *Organization of the steroidogenic pathway in Leydig cells. Cholesterol (CHOL) imported from the extracellular fluid via the high-density lipoprotein (HDL) receptor or synthesized de novo is transported into mitochondria as a complex with SCP-2. The conversion of cholesterol into pregnenolone (PREG) is carried out by the cytochrome P450scc within the mitochondrial membrane. Pregnenolone is then converted into progesterone (PROG) and testosterone (TESTO) by steroidogenic enzymes in microsomes. The rate-limiting steps in androgen synthesis are transport of cholesterol to the mitochondria and the conversion of cholesterol into pregnenolone.*

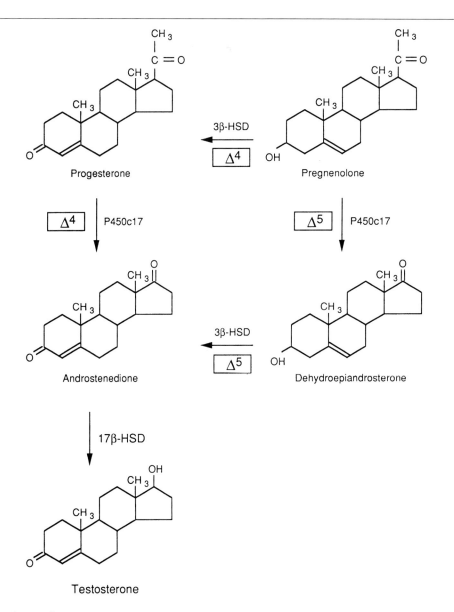

Fig. 2.5.5 *The 'Δ^4' and 'Δ^5' pathways of androgen biosynthesis. Pregnenolone and dehydroepiandrosterone are both potential 3β-HSD substrates, whereas pregnenolone and progesterone are both potential P450c17 substrates. Both routes of androgen synthesis operate in the human testis.*

the androgen secretion rate. Under situations of low androgen secretion, cholesterol is esterified and stored in microscopic lipid droplets, which are particularly numerous in the prepubertal testis. When cholesterol is needed for steroidogenesis, LH stimulates the hydrolysis of esterified cholesterol to produce free cholesterol, which is translocated by sterol carrier-protein 2 (SCP-2)[15] to the mitochondria (Fig. 2.5.4). The recently discovered 'steroidogenic acute regulatory protein' (STAR) is also involved in this process.[19]

Androgen synthesis within Leydig cells is highly regionalized due to the specific localization of the major steroidogenic enzymes in different organelles of the cell.[14] The process begins when cholesterol is delivered by SCP-2 to the inner mitochondrial membrane, which is where the

steroidogenic cyctochrome P450 *cholesterol side-chain cleavage enzyme* (P450scc/CYP11A) is found. Prolonged stimulation of the testis by LH upregulates P450scc gene expression.[20] However, the delivery of cholesterol to the inner mitochondrial membrane by SCP-2 is thought to be the rate-limiting step in steroidogenesis, unless cholesterol is provided in excess, in which case the conversion of cholesterol into pregnenolone by P450scc becomes limiting.[15] P450scc removes the isocapraldehyde side chain of cholesterol to produce pregnenolone. All subsequent steps in androgen synthesis take place within the lipophilic membranes of the endoplasmic reticulum (microsome), where pregnenolone presumably arrives by diffusion. The first microsomal steroidogenic reaction is catalyzed by *3β-hydroxysteroid dehydrogenase/Δ^{5-4} isomerase* (3β-HSD), which converts pregnenolone into progesterone. The presence of the 3β-HSD enzyme protein is often used as a histochemical Leydig cell marker because of its relatively high abundance in these cells. The next microsomal reaction is another steroidogenic cytochrome P450 *17α-hydroxylase/ C$_{17-20}$-lyase* (P450c17/CYP17) which removes the progestogenic C-21 side chain at the D ring of progesterone to produce androstenedione, a weak androgen that is not secreted in significant amounts by the testis. Finally, another microsomal non-P450 enzyme *17β-hydroxysteroid dehydrogenase* converts androstenedione into testosterone, which is then drawn down a concentration gradient into the extracellular fluid from where it subsequently enters the blood (Fig. 2.5.4).

The 'Δ^4' steroidogenic pathway (pregnenolone–progesterone–androstenedione–testosterone) is the major route of androgen synthesis in the rat testis. P450c17 can also convert pregnenolone into dehydroepiandrosterone (DHEA), which can then be converted into androstenedione by 3β-HSD. This reaction sequence (pregnenolone–DHEA–androstenedione–testosterone) is the 'Δ^5' pathway. Both the Δ^4 and Δ^5 pathways of androgen synthesis operate in man (Fig. 2.5.5). Testicular cells also contain low levels of aromatase (see Chapter 2.3), which is why the testis also produces small amounts of estrogen.

Regulation of androgen secretion

Role of LH

LH is the primary endocrine regulator of testicular androgen synthesis, acting via cell-surface receptors for LH that are located on Leydig cells [21] (see Chapter 1.4). Binding of LH to the LH receptor activates the binding of GTP to the Gs (stimulatory) protein, which interacts with adenylyl cyclase to promote the generation of cyclic AMP from ATP. Cyclic AMP then stimulates protein kinase A to phosphorylate various proteins that can increase steroidogenesis through enhancing steroidogenic enzyme activity or stimulating the synthesis of new enzyme proteins (see Chapter 1.5). A rare form of precocious puberty, testotoxicosis, in which testicular androgen production is raised in the absence of LH stimulation, is due to the constitutive activation of adenylyl cyclase because of a point mutation in the Gs subunit leading to changes in GTP binding.[22]

Although cyclic AMP plays a major role in mediating LH action on androgen secretion, maximal steroidogenesis in response to LH-stimulation is reached when only about 1% of LH receptors are occupied by LH, i.e. before cellular cyclic AMP levels begin to rise. This discrepancy is resolved if only cyclic AMP bound to protein kinase is taken into account, which corresponds more closely to LH-receptor occupancy than the total intracellular cyclic AMP level.[21,23]

Testicular androgen synthesis is inhibited when excessively large doses of LH or HCG are administered. This is due to ligand-induced desensitization, in which coupling between the LH receptor and the Gs subunit is disrupted and the receptor becomes internalized. Although membrane and G-protein-related mechanisms account for some

of this inhibitory effect, changes in the transcription of the LH receptor gene may also play a role. Thus, testicular LH receptor mRNA levels decline after a desensitizing dose of HCG, leading to loss of receptor protein.[21,24]

There is experimental evidence for the involvement of other intracellular messengers in LH action, although their roles may be less central than cyclic AMP. Increases in cellular calcium liberated from intracellular stores by inositol triphosphate or by the opening of calcium channels in the cell membrane increase steroidogenesis. Calmodulin and chloride channels may also be involved, as may be arachidonic acid metabolites such as prostaglandins and leukotrienes,[14,21] consistent with the emerging concept that receptors are linked to multiple transduction systems (see Chapter 1.5).[25]

Physiological regulation

LH-stimulated testosterone produced by Leydig cells causes negative feedback regulation of the synthesis and release of LH by the anterior pituitary gland. This is the major physiological mechanism through which androgenic homeostasis is maintained (Fig. 2.5.1). Stress, resulting in raised plasma glucocorticoid levels, also causes decreased testicular androgen secretion and has been associated with impotence and infertility.[26,27] This may be explained at least in part by a negative feedback effect of glucocorticoids on pituitary LH secretion.[28] However, a direct effect of glucocorticoids on steroidogenesis is also possible, as implied by the presence of glucocorticoid receptors in Leydig cells.[29,30] A microsomal 11β-hydroxysteroid dehydrogenase (11β-HSD) isoenzyme present in Leydig cells[31] is believed to protect these cells from the deleterious effects of pathologically high glucocorticoid levels by reduction to biologically inactive 11β-hydroxy metabolites (i.e. cortisol→cortisone (man) or corticosterone→11-dehydrocorticosterone (rat)) similar to the mechanism proposed to operate in the kidney.[32]

Developmental aspects

Leydig cell androgen secretion is activated during two developmental phases: *in utero* at the time of sexual differentiation of the fetus beginning about the 12th week of human gestation, and at puberty in the early teenage years of boys.[33]

Leydig cells begin to secrete testosterone in the 8-week old fetus, increasing to a maximum around 11–12 weeks of gestation. Thereafter secretion declines as the negative feedback axis becomes established.[33,34] Fetal testicular androgen secretion is driven by HCG, which enters the fetal circulation from the placenta. The high steroidogenic capacity of fetal Leydig cells could be related to unique features of the fetal LH receptor system. In the neonatal rat high levels of LH or HCG do not down-regulate the LH receptor and androgen secretion is not inhibited. The Gi (inhibitory) subunit is not functional in fetal Leydig cells. Thus a lack of intracellular negative feedback could increase the capacity of the fetal Leydig cell to secrete androgen.[35]

Testosterone secretion persists for up to six months after birth in boys. However, the testis is effectively quiescent during childhood, since gonadotropin levels are too low to stimulate Leydig cell development. Leydig cells become noticeable in the testis when puberty is initiated by the rising LH and FSH levels that occur at around 10 years of age (see Chapter 2.8). Nocturnal and diurnal androgen secretion then commences as the testes begin to enlarge and spermatogenesis begins in response to stimulation by FSH and androgen.

The Sertoli cell and inhibin secretion

Sertoli cells, the testicular homologs of ovarian granulosa cells, are embedded within the germinal epithelium of the seminiferous tubule, where they serve functions vital to the control of spermatogenesis (see Chapter 2.6). The primary endocrine function of the Sertoli cells is to secrete inhibin, which participates in the negative feedback regulation of pituitary FSH release (Fig. 2.5.1). Sertoli cell function is subject to endocrine regulation by FSH and paracrine regulation by the androgen produced in LH-stimulated Leydig cells through mechanisms that will be briefly reviewed here.

The seminiferous tubule

There are two types of somatic cell in the seminiferous tubules: the Sertoli cells and the peritubular myoid or smooth muscle-like cells. In addition there are five types of germ cells: spermatogonia, primary and secondary spermatocytes, spermatids and spermatozoa (see Chapter 2.6). Sertoli cells make up 37% of the cellular complement of the germinal epithelium in the human testis,[36] reflecting the elaborate way in which they envelop the germ cells.

The Sertoli cells form specialized tight junctions between themselves to compartmentalize the epithelium so that spermatogonia and early spermatocytes lie outside and the remaining germ cell inside the testis–tubule barrier. This barrier acts to maintain the specialized environment within the tubule conducive to spermatogenesis, as well as to exclude potentially damaging agents such as antibodies and toxins.[37]

Sertoli cell ultrastructure

The intracellular organelles of Sertoli cells are not particularly remarkable. Surprisingly, given that they secrete proteins such as inhibin and androgen-binding protein (ABP), the rough endoplasmic reticulum and secretory granules are sparse, suggesting protein secretion is not the primary role of the Sertoli cell.[38]

Similar to Leydig cells, the Sertoli cells in the adult testis do not divide. However, they proliferate rapidly in fetal and immature testes. The initial wave of proliferation appears to be under the control of local growth factors, since Sertoli cells do not possess FSH receptors at this time. Once FSH receptors appear, Sertoli cells proliferate under the influence of FSH.[39] During proliferation, the specialized tight junctions that characterize fully differentiated Sertoli cells are not present. However, when proliferation ceases at about around the time of puberty, the Sertoli cells become interconnected and the testis–tubule barrier is

established. The size of the adult testis and the amount of spermatozoa it produces are directly related to Sertoli cell number, which is why interference with FSH secretion has damaging consequences for fertility.[40]

Inhibins and activins

McCullagh[41] first recognized that the testis produces a nonsteroidal substance capable of exerting negative feedback regulation of pituitary FSH secretion in 1932.[41] This substance, which he named inhibin, is also produced in the ovary (see Chapter 2.3), whence it was eventually isolated and purified.[42–46]

Mature inhibin is an ~32 kDa heterodimeric glycoprotein composed of a common α-subunit and one of two β-subunits, $β_A$ (inhibin-A) and $β_B$ (inhibin-B). Activins are homodimeric forms of inhibin β-subunits capable of stimulating pituitary FSH secretion: activin-A ($β_A,β_A$), activin-AB ($β_A,β_B$) and activin-B ($β_B,β_B$) (Fig. 2.5.3). The three inhibin/activin subunits are encoded by separate genes, and biologically active recombinant forms of both inhibin and activin have been expressed in mammalian kidney cells.[42–46]

A high degree of structural homology exists between the inhibins/activins and other members of a growth/differentiation superfamily that are synthesized from precursors of high molecular weight and whose expression occurs in embryologic, fetal and adult tissues across a wide range of animal phyla. Members of this gene family include transforming growth factor-β (TGF-β), anti-Müllerian hormone/Müllerian duct inhibiting substance (AMH/MIS; causes Müllerian duct regression in males), decapentaplegic gene complex (DPP-C; active during insect embryogenesis), and the encoded product of *vg1* (a mesoderm-inducing factor in frog embryos). Activin is itself implicated as a regulatory factor in several fundamental processes including erythropoiesis, nerve cell survival, mesoderm induction in amphibian embryos and gonadal cell proliferation.[43,47–49] Thus this family of genes is highly conserved and is likely to be involved in the fundamental control of cell growth and differentiation.

Spermatogenesis is the obvious focus of paracrine inhibin/activin action in the testis (see Chapter 2.6). *In vitro* and *in vivo* experiments suggest that activin stimulates the proliferation of spermatogonia whereas inhibin is inhibitory.[50] Targeted gene deletion of the murine inhibin α-subunit, which knocks out inhibin production, results in gonadal sex cord-stroll tumors after puberty, indicating that the inhibin α-subunit is a tumor suppresser.[51] Current research is attempting to unravel the paracrine and autocrine functions that inhibins and activins undoubtedly play in the regulation of testicular function. More is known about the role of the inhibins in the endocrine control of pituitary gonadotropin secretion, which will now be discussed.

Control of inhibin/activin gene expression

Sertoli cells express mRNAs encoding both the inhibin α- and β-subunits, and both inhibin and activin have been purified from conditioned media from Sertoli cells.[44,52] The isolation and characterization of the genes for the inhibin subunits has allowed investigations into the factors that control their expression in Sertoli cells (Fig. 2.5.6). The inhibin α-subunit promoter region lacks TATA and CATT boxes at the transcription site but contains regulatory sites which may be responsive to cyclic AMP, glucocorticoid and estrogen.[53] The inhibin/activin β-subunit genes are less tightly regulated and have characteristics similar to 'housekeeping' genes.[54] FSH acting via intracellular cyclic AMP regulates the secretion of the inhibin α-subunit, but not the β-subunits in Sertoli cell cultures. Similarly, hypophysectomy causes a reduction in testicular inhibin α-subunit levels, which can be restored by treatment with FSH whereas the $β_B$-subunit is unaffected.[55,56] This suggests that the relative availability of the α-subunit determines whether inhibin or activin is secreted.[57]

The Sertoli cell was once considered the exclusive source of testicular inhibin production. However, in situ hybridization studies have located all three inhibin/activin subunit mRNAs in the Leydig cells of immature rat testes, and α-subunit mRNA has been found in the Leydig cells of the adult rat testis.[52] In vitro production of immunoreactive inhibin by immature Leydig cells has also been reported.[58]

Sertoli-germ cell interaction

The secretion of inhibin by Sertoli cells is dependent upon interactions with germ cells. Secretion occurs from both the apical and basal aspects of the Sertoli cell, such that inhibin and activin are found in both the intratubular and interstitial fluids. Germ cells influence the direction of inhibin secretion, their absence promoting secretion from the base of the Sertoli cell into the interstitial lymph.[59]

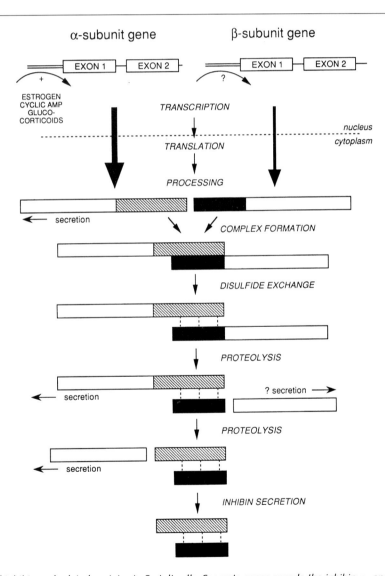

Fig. 2.5.6 *Synthesis of inhibin and related proteins in Sertoli cells. Separate genes encode the inhibin α- and β-subunits. The inhibin α-subunit gene is expressed in greatest abundance, being regulated by FSH, estrogens and glucocorticoids. The greater availability of the α-subunit presumably dictates that α,β (inhibin) heterodimers are formed in preference to β,β (activin) homodimers. Assembly proceeds with the formation of disulfide bridges and glycosylation. The pre-pro-proteins are cleaved by proteolysis to form inhibin dimers, which are secreted and not stored.*

Regulation of inhibin secretion

The spermatogenic epithelium regresses after hypophysectomy, highlighting the dependence of Sertoli cells on FSH. However, replacement therapy with FSH alone does not quantitatively restore spermatogenesis, since androgen is also required. Thus, in as much as LH stimulates androgen synthesis (see above), Sertoli cell function also depends on LH.[60,61]

Role of FSH and androgen

FSH receptors are present in the testis located exclusively on Sertoli cells. In the adult rat, FSH receptors are limited to the basal aspect of Sertoli cells, outside the testis–tubule barrier. FSH receptor density and inhibin secretion by these cells are closely correlated.[62]

Stimulation of Sertoli cell inhibin secretion by FSH is mainly via the cyclic AMP second messenger system, involving cyclic AMP-dependent protein kinases. FSH also induces a rapid Ca^{2+} influx into Sertoli cells not mediated by G proteins.[63] Phosphatidylinositol metabolism is not stimulated by FSH but there is evidence for the involvement of phospholipase A_2 activity and eicosanoid generation.[64]

Androgen receptors appear to be located exclusively in Sertoli cells within the spermatogenic epithelium. However, androgen receptors are also present at high concentrations in peritubular cells and Leydig cells. Androgen receptors are less abundant in Sertoli cells of the immature testis and begin to appear after the adult complement of Sertoli cells is reached at about the time that spermatogenesis is established.[65,66] The ligand bound by the Sertoli cell androgen receptor may be DHT (Fig. 2.5.2), since Sertoli cells contain significant amounts of 5α-reductase.[67]

FSH may modulate the responsiveness of Sertoli cells to androgen, since androgen receptor mRNA and protein concentrations increase in Sertoli cells cultured with FSH.[68] Interactions between FSH and androgen appear to be additive and there is no clear evidence that androgens exert a significant influence on the FSH signaling pathways. Independent stimulatory effects of androgen on Sertoli cell secretion of inhibin *in vitro* have not been observed, making it difficult to explain the role of androgen in the stimulation of inhibin secretion by LH *in vivo*. However, as mentioned above, peritubular and Leydig cells also contain androgen receptors and the poor response of isolated Sertoli cells to androgen could be due to the disruption of essential cell–cell interactions involving these other testicular cell types.

Negative feedback function of inhibin

The original hypothesis that inhibin negatively regulates pituitary FSH secretion has been confirmed many times.[69] However, androgen also suppresses FSH secretion, and there is continuing debate about the relative importance of androgen and inhibin to this feedback process.

The relationship between testicular inhibin production and plasma FSH levels has been difficult to evaluate experimentally because the inhibin assays available to date usually have not distinguished between free inhibin α-subunit and the biologically active, dimeric forms of inhibin. In studies of men with testicular disorders in which spermato-genesis was abnormal and serum FSH levels were raised, no changes in serum immunoreactive inhibin values were observed.[70,71] However, where there was a high degree of testicular damage due to X-irradiation, serum inhibin and FSH levels were inversely related.[72] Presently, both inhibin and androgen must be assumed to contribute to the homeostatic regulation of FSH secretion.

Leydig cells are also potential sources of testicular inhibin secretion (see above). Increases in serum immunoreactive inhibin levels have been observed in both rats and men after the administration of LH or HCG.[73,74] In hypogonadal men, inhibin levels are only restored to normal by combined treatment with FSH and HCG. Moreover, inhibin is detectable in the serum of men with Klinefelter's syndrome, in which the Sertoli cells are absent or severely damaged. Thus both LH(HCG)-stimulated Leydig cells and FSH-stimulated Sertoli cells could contribute to testicular inhibin secretion.[75,76] However, experimental destruction of Leydig cells in rats does not cause significant changes in serum inhibin levels, suggesting that inhibin of Leydig cell origin is likely to be of little physiological relevance to the regulation of gonadotropin release.[76]

FUTURE PERSPECTIVES

Testicular paracrine control

In addition to classic endocrine functions, androgen[2] and inhibin[52] serve local regulatory functions within the testis. Untold numbers of other steroidal and non-steroidal factors also participate in the testicular paracrine system, and future advances in our understanding of testicular function will depend on research directed at this level of control.[24,77–79]

Reproductive toxicology

Sperm counts in fertile men appear to have fallen over the past fifty years, during which environmental pollution has increased.[80] Certain environmental pollutants that possess estrogenic activities are believed to be deleterious to the testis.[81] Research is needed to understand the impact of such substances on adult testicular endocrine function.

Intracellular signaling

Progress towards understanding the molecular events underlying FSH and LH action on testicular cells illustrates the complexity of the receptor and postreceptor mechanisms involved. The seven-transmembrane domain, G-protein coupled receptor family to which the FSH and LH receptors belong show remarkable diversity in ligand specificity. What roles might other members of this family of ubiquitous signaling molecules play in testicular pathophysiology?

Gonadotropin receptor variants

The genes encoding LH and FSH receptors contain multiple exons, and variable transcription leads to complex patterns of gene splice variants.[82] The presence of multiple gonadotropin receptor mRNAs in testicular cells raises the possibility that variant gonadotropin receptor subtypes exist. A challenge for the future is to identify them and determine their functions.

Inhibins and activins

Although much has been learnt about the endocrine and paracrine functions of testicular inhibin, many questions remain unanswered – notably: 'What is the true contribution of inhibin to the negative feedback regulation of FSH secretion?' A major limitation has been the lack of specificity of the inhibin immunoassays used in most clinical and experimental studies to date. New assays, specific for individual molecular forms of inhibin and activin circulating in plasma, are currently under development to resolve these issues.[83]

SUMMARY

- The major hormones secreted by the testis are testosterone and inhibin.
- Leydig cells synthesize testosterone, regulated by LH (HCG in the fetus). Sertoli cells synthesize inhibin, regulated by FSH and androgens.
- Gonadotropins stimulate testicular hormone synthesis via G-protein-coupled receptors located on Leydig cells (LH receptor) and Sertoli cells (FSH receptor).
- Cyclic AMP is the major intracellular mediator of gonadotropin action on both Leydig cells and Sertoli cells.
- Testicular androgen synthesis is activated by maternal HCG during fetal and neonatal life. After birth, androgen secretion declines and remains low until puberty, when testosterone secretion recommences in response to increased stimulation by LH.
- Testosterone is biosynthesized from cholesterol, obtained from blood-borne HDL or synthesized from acetate *de novo*. Precursor cholesterol is converted into testosterone in four enzymic steps catalyzed by P450scc, P450c17, 3β-HSD and 17β-HSD.
- Testosterone is secreted in a pulsatile manner in response to pulsatile LH release by the pituitary gland. Circulating testosterone acts via androgen receptors located in target cells to stimulate secondary sexual characteristics and exert negative feedback regulation of LH secretion.
- Inhibin exerts negative feedback regulation of FSH secretion before puberty. However, androgen also negatively regulates FSH, and both inhibin and testosterone participate in the homeostatic control of circulating plasma FSH levels during adulthood.
- Genes encoding inhibin/activin subunits are expressed mainly in Sertoli cells regulated by FSH. Expression of the α-inhibin subunit relative to β-inhibin/activin subunit(s) determines whether mainly inhibin or activin is produced.
- Testicular androgens and inhibins/activins play paracrine and autocrine roles crucial to the regulation of spermatogenesis by FSH and LH.

REFERENCES

1. Ober WB, Sciagura C. Leydig, Sertoli and Reinke: three anatomists who were on the ball. *Pathol Annu* 1981 **16**: 1–13.
2. Sharpe RM. Testosterone and spermatogensis. *J Endocrinol* 1987 **113**: 1–3.
3. Mori H. Ultrastructure and sterological analysis of Leydig cells. In Motta P (ed.) *Ultrastructure of Endocrine Cells and Tissues*. The Hague: Martinus Nijhoff, 1984: 225–237.
4. De Kretser DM, Kerr JB. The cytology of the testis. In Knobil E, Neill JD (eds) *The Physiology of Reproduction,* 2nd edn. New York: Raven Press, 1994: 1177–1290.
5. Bertram KA, Bratloff B, Hodges GF, Davidson H. Treatment of malignant Leydig cell tumor. *Cancer* 1991 **68**: 2324–2329.
6. Shan L-X, Hardy DO, Catterall JF, Hardy MP. Effects of luteinizing hormone (LH) and androgen on steady state levels of messenger ribonucluic acid for LH receptors, androgen receptors, and steroidogenic enzymes in rat Leydig cell progenitors *in vivo. Endocrinology* 1995 **136**: 1686–1693.
7. Teerds KJ, de Rooij DG, Rommerts FFG, van der Tweel F, Wensing CJG. Turnover time of Leydig cells and other interstitial cells in testes of adult rats. *Arch Androl* 1989 **23**: 105–111.
8. Weiss J, Axelrod L, Whitcomb RW, Harris DE, Crowley WF, Jameson JK. Hypogonadism caused by a single amino acid substitution in the β-subunit of luteinizing hormone. *N Engl J Med* 1992 **326**: 179–183.
9. Teerds KJ, Veldhuizen MB, Rommerts FFG, de Rooij DG, Dorrington JH. Proliferation and differentiation of testicular interstial cells: aspects of Leydig cell development in the (pre)pubertal and adult testis. In Verhoeven G, Habenicht UF (eds) *Molecular and Cellular Endocrinology of the Testis*. Berlin: Springer-Verlag, 1994: 37–65.
10. Morris ID, Philips DM, Bardin CW. Ethylene dimenthane sulphonate destroys Leydig cells in the rat testis. *Endocrinology* 1986 **118**: 709–719.
11. Zhou ZX, Wong CI, Sar M, Wilson EM. The androgen receptor: an overview. *Recent Prog Horm Res* 1994 **49**: 249–274.
12. Rosner W. Plasma steroid-binding proteins. *Endocrinol Metab Clin Nrth Am* 1991 **4**: 697–720.
13. Hammond GL. Sex hormone-binding globulin. In Parker MG (ed.) *Steroid Hormone Action: Frontiers in Molecular Biology*. Oxford: IRL Press, 1993: 1–25.

14. Hall PF. Testicular steroid synthesis: organisation and regulation. In Knobil E, Neill JD (eds) *The Physiology of Reproduction,* Vol. 1. New York: Raven Press, 1994: 1335–1362.

15. Stocco DM, Clarke BJ. Regulation of the acute production of steroids in steroidogenic cells. In Verhoeven G, Habenicht UF (eds) *Molecular and Cellular Endocrinology of the Testis.* Berlin: Springer Verlag, 1994: 367–98.

16. Reyes-Fuentes A, Veldhuis JD. Neuroendocrine physiology of the male gonadal axis. *Endocrinol Metab Clin North Am* 1993 **22:** 93–124.

17. Plant TM, Dubey AK. Evidence from the rhesus monkey (*Macaca mulatta*) for the view that negative feedback control of luteinizing hormone secretion by the testis is mediated by a deceleration of hypothalamic gonadotropin-releasing hormone pulse frequency. *Endocrinology* 1984 **115:** 2145–2153.

18. Brown MS, Goldstein JL. A receptor-mediated pathway for cholesterol homeostasis. *Science* 1988 **232:** 34–47.

19. Clark BJ, Wells J, King SR, Stocco DM. The purification, cloning, and expression of a novel luteinizing hormone-induced mitochondrial protein in MA-10 mouse Leydig tumor cells. Characterization of the steroidogenic acute regulatory protein (StAR). *J Biol Chem* 1994 **269:** 28314–28322.

20. Hanukoglu I. Steroidogenic enzymes: structure function, and role in the regulation of steroid hormone biosynthesis. *J Steroid Biochem Mol Biol* 1992 **43:** 779–804.

21. Cooke BA, Choi MC, Dirami G, Lopez-Ruiz MP, West AP. Control of steroidogenesis in Leydig cells. *J Steroid Biochem Mol Biol* 1992 **43:** 445–449.

22. Liri T, Herzmark P, Nakamoto J M, van Dop C, Bourne HR. Rapid GDP release from G-s alpha in patients with gain and loss of endocrine function. *Nature (London)* 1994 **371:** 164–168.

23. Dufau ML, Tsuruhara T, Horner KA, Podesta E, Katt KJ. Intermediate role of cyclic adenosine-3′:5′-monophosphate and protein kinase during gonadotrophin induced steroidogenesis in testicular cells. *Proc Natl Acad Sci USA* 1997 **74:** 3419–3423.

24. Saez JM. Leydig cells: endocrine, paracrine, and autocrine regulation. *Endocr Rev* 1994 **15:** 574–615.

25. Thompson EB. Comment: single receptors, dual second messengers. *Mol Endocrinol* 1992 **6:** 501.

26. Cumming DC, Quigley ME, Yen SS. Acute suppression of circulating testosterone levels by cotisol in men. *J Clin Endocrinol Metab* 1983 **57:** 671–673.

27. Dong Q, Hawker F, McWilliam D, Bangah M, Burger HG, Handlesman DJ. Circulating immunoreactive inhibin and testosterone levels in men with critical illness. *Clin Endocrinol (Oxf)* 1992 **36:** 399–404.

28. Michael AE, Cooke BA. A working hypothesis for the regulation of steroidogenesis and germ cell development in the gonads by glucocorticoids and 11β-hydroxysteroid dehydrogenase (11βHSD). *Mol Cell Endocrinol* 1994 **100:** 55–63.

29. Li J. Effect of cortisol on testosterone production by immature pig Leydig cells. *J Steroid Biochem Mol Biol* 1991 **38:** 205–212.

30. Trzeciak WH, LeHoux JG, Waterman MR, Simpson ER. Dexamethasone inhibits corticotropin-induced accumulation of CYP11A and CYP17 messenger RNAs in bovine adrenocortical cells. *Mol Endocrinol* 1993 **7:** 206–213.

31. Monder C, Miroff Y, Marandici A, Hardy MP. 11β-hydroxysteroid dehydrogenase alleviates glucocorticoid-mediated inhibition of steroidogenesis in rat Leydig cells. *Endocrinology* 1994 **134:** 1199–1204.

32. Seckl JR. 11β-hydroxysteroid dehydrogenase isoforms and their implications for blood pressure regulation. *Eur J Clin Invest* 1993 **23:** 589–601.

33. Reyes FI, Winter JSD, Faiman C. Endocrinology of the fetal testis. In Burger H, de Kretser DM (eds) *The Testis,* 2nd edn. New York: Raven Press, 1989: 119–142.

34. Rabinovici J, Jaffe RB. Development and regulation of growth and differentiated function in human and subhuman primate fetal gonads. *Endocr Rev* 1990 **11:** 532–557.

35. Huhtaneimi I. Fetal testis – a very special endocrine organ. *Eur J Endocrinol* 1994 **130:** 25–31.

36. Russell LD, Ren HP, Sinha-Hikim I, Schulze W, Sinha-Hikim AP. A comparative study in twelve mammalian species of volume densities, volumes, and numerical densities of selected testicular components, emphasing those related to the Sertoli cell. *Am J Anat* 1990 **188:** 21–30.

37. Dym M, Fawcett DW. The blood–testis barrier in the rat and the physiological compartmentalisation of the seminiferous epithelium. *Biol Reprod* 1970 **3:** 308–326.

38. Russell LD. Form dimensions and cytology of mammalian Sertoli cells. In Russell LD, Griswold MD (eds) *The Sertoli Cell.* Clearwater: Cache River Press, 1993: 1–37.

39. Orth JM. Cell biology of testicular development in the fetus and neonate. In Desjardins C, Ewing LL (eds) *Cell and Molecular Biology of the Testis.* New York: Oxford University Press, 1993: 3–42.

40. Heckert L, Griswold MD. The changing functions of follicle stimulating hormone in the testes of prenatal, newborn, immature, and adult rats. In Hunzicker-Dunn M, Schwartz NB (eds) *Follicle-Stimulating Hormone: Regulation of Secretion and Molecular Mechanisms of Action.* New York: Springer-Verlag, 1992: 237–245.

41. McCullagh DR. The dual endocrine activity of the testis. *Science* 1932 **76:** 19.

42. de Jong FH, Grootenhuis AJ, Klaij IA, van Beurden WMO. Inhibin and related proteins: localisation, regulation and effects. In Porter JC, Jezova D (eds) *Circulating Regulatory Factors and Neuroendocrine Function.* New York: Plenum Press, 1990: 271–293.

43. Vale W, Hsueh A, Rivier C, Yu J. The inhibin/activin family of hormones and growth factors. In Sporn MA, Roberts AB (eds) *Peptide Growth Factors and their Receptors. Handbook of Experimental Pharmacology.* New York: Springer-Verlag, 1990: 211–248.

44. Robertson DM, McLachlan RI, Burger HG, de Kretser DM. Inhibin and inhibin related proteins in the male. In Burger HG, de Kretser DM (eds) *The Testis.* New York: Raven Press, 1989: 231–254.

45. Robertson DM, Risbridger GP, de Kretser DM. The physiology of testicular inhibin and related proteins. *Balliéres Clin Endocrinol Metab* 1992 **6:** 355–372.

46. Robertson DM, Risbridger GP, de Kretser DM. Inhibin and inhibin related proteins. In Desjardins C, Ewing LL (eds) *Cell and Molecular Biology of the Testis.* New York: Oxford University Press, 1993: 220–237.

47. Tiedemann H, Lottspeich F, Davids M, Knochel S, Hoppe P, Tiedemann H. The vegetalizing factor. A member of the evolutionarily highly conserved activin family. *FEBS Lett* 1992 **300:** 123–126.

48. Wei WH, Gustafson ML, Hirobe S, Donahoe PK. Developmental expression of four novel serine/threonine kinase receptors homologous to the activin/transforming growth factor-beta type II receptor family. *Dev Dynam* 1993 **196:** 133–142.

49. Mathews LS. Activin receptors and cellular signaling by the receptor serine kinase family. *Endocr Rev* 1994 **15:** 310–325.

50. Moore A, Krummen LA, Mather JP. Inhibins, activins, their binding proteins and receptors: interactions underlying paracrine activity in the testis. *Mol Cell Endocrinol* 1994 **100:** 81–86.

51. Shikone T, Matzuk MM, Perlas E, Finegold MJ, Lewis KA, Vale W, Bradley A, Hseuh AJW. Characterisation of gonadal sex cord-stromal tumor cell lines from inhibin-alpha and p-53 deficient mice: the role of activin as an autocrine growth factor. *Mol Endocrinol* 1994 **8:** 983–995.

52. Mather JP, Woodruff TK, Krummen LA. Paracrine regulation of reproductive function by inhibin and activin. *Proc Soc Exp Biol Med* 1992 **201:** 1–15.

53. Su JG, Hseuh AJW. Characterisation of mouse inhibin-α gene and its promoter. *Biochem Biophys Res Commun* 1992 **186:** 293–300.

54. Mason AJ, Berkemier LM, Schmenlzer CH, Schwall RH. Activin-B: precursor sequences, genomic structure and *in vitro* activities. *Mol Endocrinol* 1989 **3:** 1352–1358.

55. Krummen LA, Toppari J, Kim WH, Morelos BS, Ahmed N, Swerdloff RS, Ling N Shimaski S, Esch F, Bhasin S. Regulation of testicular inhibin subunit messenger ribonucleic acid levels *in vivo*: effects of hypophysectomy and selective follicle stimulating hormone replacement. *Endocrinology* 1989 **125:** 1630–1637.

56. Feng ZM, Li YP, Chen CLC. Analysis of the 5′-flanking regions of rat inhibin α- and β-B subunit genes suggest two different regulatory mechanisms. *Mol Endocrinol* 1989 **3:** 1914–1925.

57. Klaij IA, Toebosch AMW, Themmen APN, Shimaski S, de Jong FH, Grootegoed JA. Regulation of inhibin alpha and beta subunit mRNA levels in rat Sertoli cells. *Mol Cell Endocrinol* 1990 **68:** 45–52.

58. Simpson BJB, Risbridger GP, Hedger MP, De Kretser DM. The role of calcium in luteinizing hormone/chorionic gonadotrophin stimulation of Leydig cell immunoreactive inhibin secretion *in vitro*. *Mol Cell Endocrinol* 1991 **44:** 937–944.

59. Maddocks S, Kerr JB, Allenby G, Sharpe RM. Evaluation of the role of germ cells in regulating the route of secretion of immunoactive inhibin from the rat testis. *J Endocrinol* 1992 **132:** 439–448.

60. Matsumoto AM, Bremner WJ. Endocrinology of the hypothalamic–pituitary–testicular axis with particular reference to the hormonal control of spermatogenesis. *Balliéres Clin Endocrinol Metab* 1987 **1:** 71–87.

61. Weinbauer G, Neischlag E. Hormonal control of spermatogenesis. In de Kretser DM (ed.) *Molecular Biology of the Male Reproductive System*. London: Academic Press, 1993: 99–142.

62. Parvinen M. Cyclic function of Sertoli cells. In Russell LD, Griswold MD (eds) *The Sertoli Cell*. Clearwater: Cache River Press, 1993: 331–348.

63. Monaco L, Adamo S, Stefanini M, Conti M. Signal transduction in the Sertoli cell: serum modification of the response to FSH. *J Steroid Biochem* 1989 **32:** 129–134.

64. Jannini EA, Ulisse S, Cecconi S, Cironi L, Colonna R, D'Armiento M, Santoni A, Cifone G. Follicle-stimulating hormone-induced phospholipase A₂ activity and eicosanoid generation in rat Sertoli cells. *Biol Reprod* 1994 **51:** 140–145.

65. Sanborn BM, Caston LA, Chang C, Liao S, Speller R, Porter ID, Ku CY. Regulation of androgen receptor mRNA in rat Sertoli and peritubular cells. *Biol Reprod* 1991 **45:** 634–641.

66. Sar M, Hall SH, Wilson EM, French FS. Androgen regulation of the Sertoli cell. In Russell LD, Griswold MD (eds) *The Sertoli Cell*. Clearwater: Cache River Press, 1993: 331–348.

67. Dorrington JH, Fritz IB. Androgen synthesis and metabolism by preparations from the seminiferous tubule of the rat testis. In French FS, Hansson V, Ritzen EM, Nayfeh SH (eds) *Hormonal Regulation of Spermatogenesis*. New York: Plenum, 1975: 37–52.

68. Jegou B. The Sertoli cell. *Balliéres Clin Endocrinol Metab* 1992 **6:** 273–311.

69. Medhamurthy R, Abbeyawardene SA, Culler MD, Negro-Vilar A, Plant TM. Immunoneutralization of circulating inhibin in the hypophysiotropically clamped male rhesus monkey (*Mucaca mulatta*) results in a selective hypersecretion of follicle-stimulating hormone. *Endocrinology* 1990 **126:** 2116–2124.

70. De Kretser DM, McLachlan RI, Robertson DM, Burger HG. Serum inhibin levels in normal men and men with testicular disorders. *J Endocrinol* 1989 **120:** 517–523.

71. Tsatoulis A, Shalet SM, Robertson WR, Morris ID, Burger HG, de Kretser DM. Plasma inhibin levels in men with chemotherapy induced severe damage to the seminiferous epithelium. *Clin Endocrinol (Oxford)* 1988 **29:** 659–665.

72. Tsatsoulis A, Shalet SM, Morris ID, de Kretser DM. Immunoreactive inhibin as a marker of Sertoli cell function following cytotoxic damage to the human testis. *Horm Res* 1990 **34:** 254–259.

73. Drummond AE, Risbridger GP, de Kretser DM. The involvement of Leydig cells in the regulation of inhibin secretion by the testis. *Endocrinology* 1989 **125:** 510–515.

74. Burger HG, Tiu SC, Bangah ML, de Kretser DM. Human chorionic gonadotrophin raises serum inhibin levels in men with hypogonadotropic hypogonadism. *Reprod Fertil Dev* 1990 **2:** 137–144.

75. McLachlan RI, Matsumoto AM, de Kretser DM, Burger HG, Bremner WJ. Follicle-stimulating hormone is required for quantitatively normal inhibin secretion in men. *J Clin Endocrinol Metab* 1988 **82:** 1–5.

76. Maddocks S, Sharpe RM. Assessment of the contribution of the Leydig cells to the secretion of inhibin by the rat testis. *Mol Cell Endocrinol* 1989 **67:** 113–118.

77. Skinner MK. Cell–cell interactions in the testis. *Endocr Rev* 1991 **12:** 45–72.

78. Jegou B, Sharpe RM. Paracrine mechanisms in testicular control. In de Kretser DM (ed.) *Molecular Biology of the Male Reproductive System*. London: Academic Press, 1993: 271–310.

79. Spiteri-Grech J, Nieschlag E. Paracrine factors relevant to the regulation of spermatogenesis – a review. *J Reprod Fertil* 1993 **98:** 1–14.

80. Auger J, Kunst JM, Czyglik F, Jouannet P. Decline in semen quality among fertile men in Paris during the past 20 years. *N Engl J Med* 1995 **332:** 281–285.

81. Editorial. Male reproductive health and environmental oestrogens. *Lancet* 1995 **345:** 933–934.

82. Themmen APN, Kraaij R, Grootegoed JA. Regulation of gonadotropin receptor gene expression. *Mol Cell Endocrinol* 1994 **100:** 15–19.

83. Groome NP, Illingworth PJ, O'Brien M, Priddle J, Weaver K, McNeilly AS. Quantification of inhibin pro-αC-containing forms in human serum by a new ultrasensitive two-site enzyme-linked immunosorbent assay. *J Clin Endocrinol Metab* 1995 **80:** 2923–2926.

2.6

The Testis: Spermatogenesis

JA Grootegoed

INTRODUCTION

A man's testes produce as many as 2×10^{12} spermatozoa in a lifetime. The process of spermatogenesis requires testicular differentiation (see Chapter 2.1) and reaches fruition during puberty, with the release of the first mature spermatozoa into the lumen of the seminiferous tubule.[1-5] Within the spermatogenic epithelium, the process is sustained by extensive interactions between Sertoli cells and germ cells, that are subject to endocrine control by follicle-stimulating hormone (FSH) and paracrine control by local factors that include the androgens produced by LH-stimulated Leydig cells (see Chapter 2.5). Gene expression in germ cells and the cellular and molecular mechanisms that underpin Sertoli–germ cell interaction – rapidly expanding fields of research[6-12] – form the focus of this chapter.

CURRENT CONCEPTS

Spermatogenesis

The spermatogenic epithelium

The spermatogenic cells are embedded in Sertoli cells (Fig. 2.6.1), which require stimulation by FSH and testosterone to develop into the mature cells that can support spermatogenesis[13,14] (see Chapter 2.5). Interactions with the basement membrane of the tubules and other testicular cell types influence Sertoli cell function.[15] Peptide growth/differentiation factors, produced locally by different testicular cell types – including Sertoli cells themselves – participate in the regulatory network that controls Sertoli cell function, and hence spermatogenesis (see later).[16,17]

Spermatogenesis itself comprises the mitotic divisions of spermatogonia, followed by the meiotic prophase and the meiotic divisions of spermatocytes, the transformation of round spermatids into spermatozoa (spermiogenesis), and

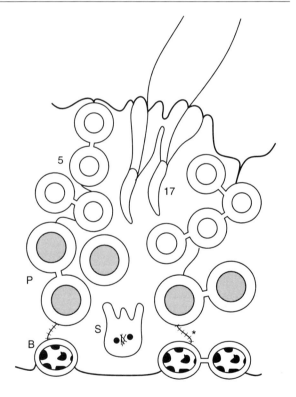

Fig. 2.6.1 *Cell–cell interactions in the spermatogenic epithelium. The diagram shows a Sertoli cell interacting with different germinal cell types at stage V of the spermatogenic cycle (see Fig. 2.6.2). The type B spermatogonia are in the basal compartment, separated from the more advanced germ cell types in the adluminal compartment by tight junctions on all sides in between neighboring Sertoli cells (indicated with asterisk): the 'Sertoli cell barrier', or 'blood–testis barrier'). At stage VIII of the spermatogenic cycle, preleptotene spermatocytes start to migrate through the Sertoli cell barrier.* **S**, *Sertoli cell nucleus;* **B**, *B spermatogonia;* **P**, *pachytene spermatocytes;* **5**, *step 5 spermatids;* **17**, *step 17 spermatids.*

events leading to the release of spermatids into the tubule lumen (spermiation).[18–22] Fig. 2.6.2 illustrates the different phases of spermatogenesis, and the 14 stages of the spermatogenic cycle, as they occur in the rat testis.

Spermatogonia

The 'spermatogonial' phase involves mitotic proliferation of 'type A', 'intermediate' and 'type B' spermatogonia. Type A spermatogonia can be classified into four increasingly differentiated subtypes (A1 to A4) that are continually being generated from undifferentiated type A spermatogonia throughout adult life.

Meiosis

Type A spermatogonia pass through the intermediate stage to become type B spermatogonia, which undergo mitotic division to form preleptotene spermatocytes. Preleptotene spermatocytes perform DNA replication for the last time during spermatogenesis, resulting in diploid 4C-DNA spermatocytes (see Chapter 2.1) which become leptotene,

zygotene, pachytene and diplotene primary spermatocytes. At the end of this lengthy prophase, the primary spermatocytes undergo the first meiotic division resulting in haploid secondary spermatocytes. The second meiotic division gives rise to the haploid round spermatids. Four haploid 1C-DNA spermatids are formed from one diploid 4C-DNA primary spermatocyte.

Spermiogenesis

The development of spermatids (also referred to as spermiogenesis) involves phases of acrosome development (*steps 1–7*), nuclear elongation and condensation (*steps 8–15*), and cytoplasma reduction (*steps 16–19*). Finally, spermatids are released from the spermatogenic epithelium (*spermiation*) (Fig. 2.6.2).

The spermatogenic cycle

Sperm formation does not occur randomly within the spermatogenic tubules. Certain germinal cell types only occur in characteristic associations with one another. In the rat,

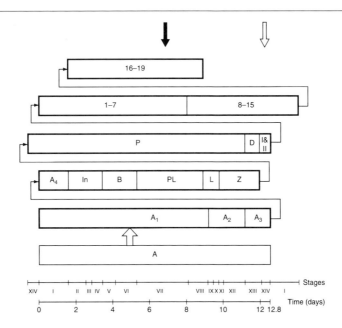

Fig. 2.6.2 *The different phases of spermatogenesis, and the 14 stages of one spermatogenic cycle, as they occur in the Wistar rat. The spermatogonial phase involves mitotic proliferation of types A, intermediate, and B spermatogonia (**A, In, B**). The differentiating types A_1 to A_4 spermatogonia are continually being generated from undifferentiated type A spermatogonia throughout adult life. At the beginning of the meiotic phase, preleptotene spermatocytes (formed after mitotic division of type B spermatogonia) perform DNA replication for the last time during spermatogenesis, resulting in 4C-DNA diploid cells. The preleptotene spermatocytes (**PL**) develop into leptotene (**L**), zygotene (**Z**), pachytene (**P**), and diplotene (**D**) primary spermatocytes. At the end of this lengthy prophase, the primary spermatocytes undergo the first meiotic division (**I**) resulting in haploid secondary spermatocytes. The second meiotic division (**II**) gives rise to the haploid round spermatids. Four 1C-DNA haploid spermatids are formed from one diploid primary spermatocyte. The development of spermatids (also referred to as spermiogenesis) involves phases of acrosome development (steps 1–7), nuclear elongation and condensation (steps 8–15), and cytoplasm reduction (steps 16–19). Finally, the spermatids are released from the spermatogenic epithelium (spermiation). See text for further details. From the figure it can be inferred that the development of, for example, preleptotene spermatocytes into spermatids that are ready to be released from the spermatogenic epithelium, takes three consecutive spermatogenic cycles (3×12.8 days in the Wistar rat). At a given point of time, a definable Sertoli cell at, for example, stage VII of the spermatogenic cycle interacts simultaneously with type A_1 spermatogonia, preleptotene and mid-pachytene spermatocytes, and round (step 7) and elongated (step 19) spermatids (solid arrow). At a later point of time, for example 6 days later at stage XIV of the spermatogenic cycle, the same Sertoli cell will interact with type A_3 spermatogonia, early pachytene spermatocytes, the meiotic divisions, and step 14 spermatids (in the phase of nuclear condensation) (open arrow).*

14 such associations give rise to *stages I–XIV* of the spermatogenic cycle (Fig. 2.6.2). In a random tubular cross-section, any one – but only one – association (stage) will be present. However, in time, each Sertoli cell supports every germ cell association in a cyclic manner and the same cell associations recur every 12.8 days. The stages of the spermatogenic cycle are present sequentially along the spermatogenic tubule, giving rise to the spermatogenic wave.

In the human testis *stages I–VI* of the spermatogenic cycle are organized along the tubule in a helical pattern, so that multiple stages can be observed in one tubular cross-section.[14,18,21]

Gene expression during spermatogenesis

Spermatogenesis involves development-related differential expression of genes encoding regulatory proteins, structural proteins, enzymes, and cell surface proteins. Regulatory genes include proto-oncogenes, that encode nuclear transcription factors, various protein kinases, and other regulatory proteins.[7,8,11,12] In addition, there are thought to be a number of germ cell-specific gene regulatory proteins, including proteins that regulate mRNA stability and translation (see later). Since the post-meiotic transformation of spermatids into spermatozoa is an unique process, many of the sperm structural proteins, enzymes, and cell surface proteins are encoded by genes that are expressed exclusively in the developing male germ cells.

A number of genes involved in spermatogenesis are located on the Y chromosome, which also encodes the testis determining factor *SRY*[4,23] (see Chapter 2.1). An example is the so-called *'azoospermia' factor (AZF)* locus, which maps to interval 6 of the human Y chromosome long arm. Microdeletions in interval 6, hence loss of *AZF*, result in male infertility.[24,25] Testis determination occurs normally in men lacking *AZF* but they show azoospermia or oligospermia. Candidate *AZF* genes have been identified, which show testis-specific expression and encode proteins with RNA-binding protein homology, suggesting a role in RNA processing or translational control during spermatogenesis.[25]

The sex body

The 'sex body' is formed during the meiotic prophase in early primary spermatocytes when the XY chromosome bivalent condenses[26,27] (Fig. 2.6.3). Unlike autosomal chromosome bivalents, X and Y chromosomes of the sex body show little, if any, transcriptional activity[28] (Fig. 2.6.3). The exact meaning of this is unclear. However, certain X chromosome ploidies in men are known to give rise to dysregulation of spermatogenesis and to infertility,[33] e.g. Klinefelter's syndrome (47,XXY). Thus there may be genes on the X chromosome, expression of which is detrimental to meiosis in male germ cells. On the other hand, transcriptional inactivation of the X chromosome in spermatocytes might be related to the chromosome pairing events of meiosis.[27] In meiotic oocytes, both X chromosomes are transcriptionally active.[27]

A number of genes on the X and Y chromosomes are

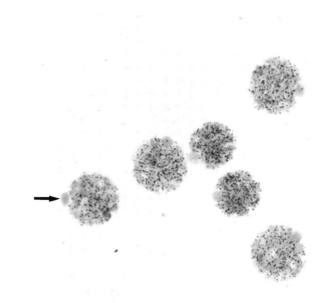

Fig. 2.6.3 *RNA synthesis in pachytene spermatocytes. Radioautogram of Giemsa-stained nuclei of isolated rat pachytene spermatocytes that were incubated for 2 h in the presence of 5-[³H]uridine.[29,30] The grains over the nucleus represent RNA synthesis. The arrow points to the condensed XY chromosome bivalent (the 'sex body'), that shows little, if any, transcriptional activity.[28] Following the meiotic divisions, the sex chromosomes are divided over two haploid sister cells, and are more actively transcribed.[26,27,31,32]*

transcribed in spermatids, once meiotic divisions are completed. All of the genes on the Y chromosome that have been characterized to date are transcribed in spermatids, whereas transcription of the X chromosome seems to be much more selective.[11,31,32]

Cytoplasmic bridges

Both the X and Y chromosomes may encode proteins important to spermiogenesis and/or sperm function. However, meiosis gives rise to haploid spermatids containing only an X or a Y chromosome. This may explain why 'cytoplasmic bridges' exist between developing germ cells so that exchange of X and Y chromosomal gene products can occur. Throughout the spermatogonial stages of spermatogenesis, germ cells do not complete cytoplasmic division during mitosis and meiosis, and remain connected to one another by cytoplasmic bridges. These cytoplasmic bridges persist until the very end of spermatogenesis.[18,34] There is experimental evidence that gene products can be transported in between spermatids sharing a common cytoplasm, which implies that the cells are functionally diploid.[35,36] This does not exclude other functions for the cytoplasmic bridges, such as sharing of autosomal gene products, and synchronization of the development of the interconnected germ cells.

Gene 'switching'

During X chromosome inactivation in primary spermatocytes, various genes on the X chromosome that encode proteins essential for sperm development and function are not expressed, alternative genes located on autosomal chromosomes are therefore brought into play.

Spermatozoa have high energy demands and require an active glycolytic pathway. Phosphoglycerate kinase (PGK) is an enzyme, catalyzing an essential step in glycolysis, that spermatozoa do not contain. All somatic cells that perform glycolysis use the PGK-1 isoform, encoded by *Pgk-1* on the X chromosome. However, because of X chromosome inactivation the *Pgk-1* gene is silent during the meiotic prophase in sperm. Absence of PGK-1 is compensated by the expression of autosomal *Pgk-2* that encodes another PGK isoform, PGK-2.[37,38] The *Pgk-2* gene is a so-called 'processed' gene, that lacks introns.[39,40] It may have originated from mature mRNA encoded by *Pgk-1* that has been re-inserted into the DNA at another chromosomal site through viral intervention at some point in evolution. Usually, such intron-less genes become mutated and lose their function, but in sperm it has not mutated and is of vital importance for the provision of energy requirements.

The pyruvate dehydrogenase (PDH) E1α-subunit in spermatocytes and spermatids is also encoded by a processed autosomal gene, which compensates for the absence of the isotypic subunit encoded by the X chromosome in somatic cells.[41,42]

Spermatids and spermatozoa make use of alternative autosomally encoded gene products not only to compensate for inactivated genes on the X chromosomes. Several autosomal genes that encode 'house-keeping' proteins also

become silent during spermatogenesis, and are substituted for by the sperm-specific expression of alternative autosomal genes. Examples include glyceraldehyde 3-phosphate dehydrogenase, lactate dehydrogenase subunits, and cytochrome *c*.[43–46] Sperm-specific variants of these proteins are expressed in spermatogenic cells but in no other cell type[43,44,47] (Table 2.6.1).

It is noteworthy that each of the above proteins forms part of the energy-yielding machinery of spermatozoa. Possibly spermatogenic cells and spermatozoa require these specific isoenzymes and other isotypic proteins to sustain their unique metabolic requirements. The metabolic machinery is structurally reorganized during spermatogenesis and distinguishes itself from that found in somatic cell types.[47] Glycolytic enzymes in spermatozoa may be complexed together, perhaps in association with the mitochondrial sheath in the middle piece, forming a highly active glycolytic and ATP-generating unit.[47]

Table 2.6.1 Spermatogenic cells make use of specific isoenzymes

Isoform expressed in somatic cells		Isoform expressed in germ cells
PGK-1	→	PGK-2
PDH E1α (X)	→	PDH E1α (A)
GAPD	→	GAPD-s
LDH-A/B	→	LDH-C
Cytochrome c	→	Cytochrome c$_T$

During spermatogenesis, particularly during the lengthy meiotic prophase, several genes become transcriptionally inactive. There appears to be a developmental switch, from the use of the protein products of 'somatic' genes (expressed in many somatic cell types) to the use of protein products that are encoded by 'sperm-specific' genes (expressed exclusively in spermatogenic cells). The genes *Pgk-1* and *Pdh E1α (X)* are on the X chromosome, and the other gene products are encoded by autosomal genes. LDH-C4 is also referred to as LDH-X, but the gene encoding the C subunit is not located on the X chromosome. The genes *Pgk-2* and *Pdh E1α (A)* lack introns (processed genes).

Abbreviations: PGK, Phosphoglycerate kinase; PDH E1α, Pyruvate dehydrogenase E1α subunit; GAPD, Glyceraldehyde 3-phosphate dehydrogenase; LDH-A/B/C, Lactate dehydrogenase subunits A, B and C (references 37 to 46).

Translational control of gene expression

Mechanisms controlling mRNA stability and translation play an important role during spermatogenesis. Translational control has been observed for several mRNAs in spermatocytes and spermatids. This includes PGK-2 mRNA (see above), which although present in pachytene spermatocytes is not translated until the spermatids develops.[38]

Sperm-specific structural proteins such as protamines are also expressed subject to translational control. Protamine genes (two genes in humans) are transcribed in elongating spermatids, giving rise to stable mRNAs that are not translated until several days later in condensing spermatids.[9,36,48,49]

Non-functional gene expression?

Not all genes transcribed in spermatogenic cells seem to be functional.[6] For example, the *Sry* gene, which encodes a DNA-binding protein (see Chapter 2.1) and is transcribed during the period of testis determination in the male embryo, is also expressed in spermatids. However, the major *Sry* mRNA species in spermatids appears to be circular and hence unlikely to be translatable.[50]

The proto-oncogene *Wnt-1* is another example of a non-functional gene expressed during spermatogenesis. The encoded protein is involved in cell-to-cell communication during embryonic development[51] and is expressed in the neural tube of mid-gestational mouse embryos (see Chapter 3.1). *Wnt-1* mRNA is also found in elongated spermatids[52] but does not seem to be an absolute requirement for fertility in male mice.[51,53]

Thus the overall transcription machinery in male germ cells may be influenced by the general process of chromatin reorganization during meiotic and postmeiotic development.[48] This reorganization, which includes the replacement of nuclear histones by transition proteins and subsequently by protamines, may lead to the inadvertent transcription of genes not essential to spermatogenesis.

An autonomous genetic program?

The time taken for spermatogonia to develop into spermatozoa is species-specific: in man it is 10 weeks. The duration of spermatogenesis is not markedly influenced by the principal endocrine regulators of spermatogenesis, FSH and testosterone.[13,14] However, if stimulation of Sertoli cells by these hormones is interrupted, massive degeneration of germ cells occurs, most obviously in the more mature cells.[30,54]

Although Sertoli cells undoubtedly support the survival of the germ cells (see below) and 'fine-tune' their development, the germ cells appear to have much autonomy. This likelihood is strengthened by observations on the development of isolated germ cells from a non-mammalian species, the frog *Xenopus laevis*, which can pass through the meiotic prophase, the meiotic divisions, and the early steps of spermiogenesis, in an incubation system that does not include Sertoli cells.[55]

Sertoli cell–germ cell interactions

Germ cells not only program their own meiotic and morphological development but also participate, both structurally and functionally,[18,20] in interactions with Sertoli cells that ensure that spermatogenesis and spermiation once initiated are sustained throughout adulthood.

Sertoli cell maturation

The maximum number of germ cells per testis, and hence testis size and sperm output, is determined by Sertoli cell number. In the human testis, a single Sertoli cell can support four round spermatids (and four elongating spermatids).[14] The testicular Sertoli cell complement is established when the replication of these cells becomes arrested at puberty.[14]

Sertoli cells mature morphologically[5] and functionally as they cease to proliferate. Biochemical markers of Sertoli cell maturation include decreased expression of aromatase activity (cytochrome P450arom) and anti-Müllerian hormone (AMH), and altered expression of various other genes.[56–58] Certain features of Sertoli cell maturation occur in the absence of germ cells,[59] but full functional maturation of Sertoli cells requires ongoing spermatogenesis.

Sertoli–cell barrier

The Sertoli–cell barrier (also known as the 'blood–testis' barrier) is created by the tight junctions between neighboring Sertoli cells that are established during sexual maturation. This is when spermatogenesis is initiated and the first spermatocytes give rise to spermatids.[18] Passage of spermatocytes in early meiotic prophase across the Sertoli cell barrier occurs from then onwards (Fig. 2.6.1). Germ cells from the mitotically proliferating region move into the adluminal compartment of the spermatogenic epithelium, where meiotic and postmeiotic development is completed in close association with the Sertoli cells.

Germ cells require support by Sertoli cells

Sertoli cells and germ cells have very different biochemical properties.[47,60,61] Metabolically, Sertoli cells show remarkable flexibility and can carry out diverse transformations at high rates, whereas spermatocytes and spermatids are more metabolically constrained and specialized. For example, isolated pachytene spermatocytes and round spermatids require exogenous pyruvate or lactate for ATP production, apparently because glycolysis is rate-limited by the availability of energy substrates[47] (Fig. 2.6.4). However, even in the presence of pyruvate and lactate, isolated spermatocytes and spermatids from mammalian species cannot survive in culture for more than several days. Germ cell survival and differentiation to the round spermatid stage in culture requires direct contact with Sertoli cells.[63–65] Possible support mechanisms include the intercellular transport of lactate, amino acids and glutathione, and iron via Sertoli cell transferrin.[47,60,66,67] In addition to transferrin, Sertoli cells produce and secrete a number of other serum proteins in relatively high quantities into the adluminal compartment of the tubule.[58] Thus, spermatocytes and spermatids are not deprived of essential serum proteins otherwise excluded by the Sertoli–cell barrier.

Ectoplasmic specializations

Sertoli cells engage in a variety of specialized contacts among themselves and developing germ cells. Structures known as ectoplasmic specializations (ES) are found at basal Sertoli–Sertoli cell junctions, but also near pachytene spermatocytes and to a greater extent near elongating spermatids (Fig. 2.6.5). ES are composed of actin filament bundles, positioned close to the plasma membrane in

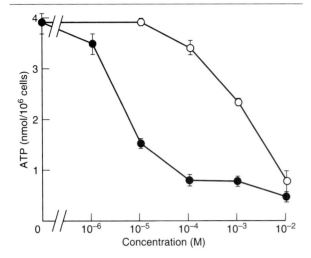

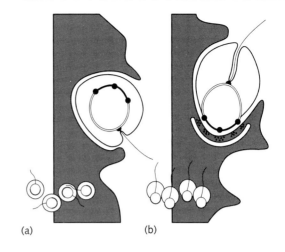

(a)   (b)

Fig. 2.6.4 *Effects of glucose and fructose on the ATP content of isolated rat spermatids. Round spermatids were isolated in the absence of glucose, but in the presence of L-lactate. Subsequently, the cells were incubated for 30 min (at 32°C) in the presence of glucose (closed circles) or fructose (open circles), but in the absence of L-lactate. The figure shows that glucose and fructose exert a strong negative effect on the cellular ATP level. The glucose/fructose-induced ATP dephosphorylation can be prevented by the addition of pyruvate or L-lactate to the incubation medium (resulting in a cellular ATP content of 6–8 nmol/10⁶ cells). The effect of glucose/fructose is explained by a rate-limitation of glycolysis in spermatids, presumably at the level of glyceraldehyde 3-phosphate dehydrogenase and phosphoglycerate kinase, resulting in accumulation of phosphorylated intermediates (such as fructose 1,6-bisphosphate) and thereby in a negative net ATP yield of glycolysis. (From reference 62.)*

Fig. 2.6.5 *Attachment of spermatids to Sertoli cells. When the nucleus, covered by the acrosome, moves towards the cell surface of the spermatids during mid-spermiogenesis, ectoplasmic specializations (ES) appear in the cytoplasm of Sertoli cells in apposition to the plasma membrane covering the acrosome.[20] This points to an as yet unknown mechanism for Sertoli cell–germ cell signaling. The ES is probably involved in attachment of the spermatid to the Sertoli cell, allowing for proper head-tail orientation of the spermatids, and remains apposed to the spermatid heads until spermiation. This schematic drawing reflects stage VII **(a)** and stage VIII **(b)** of the rat spermatogenic cycle. (Based on references 20 and 21.)*

association with a cistern of the endoplasmic reticulum.[18,20] Elongating spermatids adhere firmly to Sertoli cells. A mantle of ES is positioned around the area of contact with the spermatid head, and may serve as a site of attachment. Cell surface molecules such as cell adhesion molecules (CAMs) and integrins may play an important role in this attachment.[65,68]

In round spermatids, the growing acrosome points in different directions. As soon as the acrosome and the nucleus move to an eccentric position, marking the onset of spermatid elongation, all acrosomes point towards the basement membrane of the tubule, with ES in Sertoli cells holding the spermatids in position (Fig. 2.6.5). In the rat, this more fixed orientation of the elongating spermatids is established at *stage VIII* of the spermatogenic cycle.[20,21] At this stage, there is also transport of a new cohort of early primary spermatocytes across the Sertoli cell barrier, and the Sertoli cells are involved in the final steps of spermiogenesis and spermiation.[18,19]

During these final stages of spermatogenesis, which take about 3–4 days (*stages VII* and *VIII* in the rat), the cytoplasmic volume of spermatids becomes markedly reduced[20,69] (Fig. 2.6.6). This removal of cytoplasm from spermatids is probably facilitated by so-called 'tubulobulbar' complexes. This structure is composed of the cytoplasmic projections of spermatids that protrude into

Sertoli cells to form bulbous dilatations.[19] Most of the residual cytoplasm is pulled off (residual bodies) and phagocytosed by the Sertoli cells, when the spermatids (now called spermatozoa) are released from the Sertoli cells into the tubule lumen.[18]

Cyclic changes in Sertoli cell function

The high and complex workload of Sertoli cells during spermatid development and spermiation causes pronounced changes in the Sertoli cell cytoarchitecture and corresponding changes in the pattern of Sertoli cell gene expression.[70] Changes in Sertoli cell morphology and biochemistry show a cyclic pattern, mirroring the spermatogenic cycle.[70–72] An example of a functional change is the production of plasminogen activator, which peaks at *stages VII* and *VIII* of the spermatogenic cycle.[73] Plasminogen activator enzyme is involved in tissue restructuring and cell migration at these stages of spermatogenesis.

Another protein product of Sertoli cells, cyclic protein 2 (CP-2), is secreted maximally at *stages VI* and *VII* of the cycle.[74] CP-2 is the proenzyme form of cathepsin-L, a cysteine protease that may degrade adhesion molecules that bind spermatids to Sertoli cells, in preparation for spermiation.[75] There is experimental evidence that the expression of CP-2 is controlled by the presence of elongated spermatids.[76]

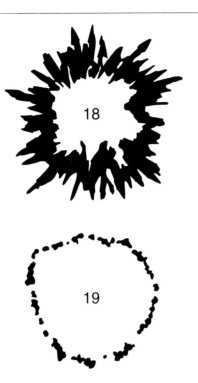

Fig. 2.6.6 *The reduction in cytoplasmic volume of spermatids that occurs shortly before spermiation. Extensive loss of cytoplasm from elongated spermatids at stages VII and VIII of the spermatogenic cycle in the rat, as illustrated by this line drawing showing the circumference of the cytoplasm of step 18 (**18**) and step 19 (**19**) spermatids in tubular cross-sections. Approximately 70% of the cytoplasm from the head region of the spermatids is eliminated in the period before sperm release. Sertoli cells play an active role in this process. (Based on references 20 and 69.)*

Certain changes in Sertoli function may occur in response to physical interactions with germ cells or as a response to the phagocytosis of residual bodies at the time of spermiation.[18,71] However, other mechanisms of intercellular signaling within the spermatogenic epithelium may involve the local production of growth/differentiation factors, which will now be discussed.

Paracrine signaling

Intercellular signaling underpinning the endocrine regulation of spermatogenesis by FSH and androgen involves many known (and unknown) peptide growth/differentiation factors and cytokines and their receptors, including stem cell factor (SCF) and kit,[77-81] insulin-like growth factor I (IGF-I), nerve growth factor (NGF), epidermal growth factor (EGF), basic fibroblast growth factor (bFGF/FGF-4), interleukins,[16,17] transforming growth factors α and β (TGF-α and TGF-β) and other members of the TGF-β family of growth/differentiation factors such as activin, inhibin and AMH.[57,82-84] The relative importance of individual factors is uncertain but collectively they create a vital paracrine/autocrine regulatory network.

The transgenic approach has been used to investigate the role of the α-inhibin gene (encoding the α-subunit of the het-

erodimeric inhibin molecule (see Chapter 2.5) in spermatogenesis).[86] In mice with both copies of the α-inhibin gene deleted, spermatogenesis was initially active, but from 5–7 weeks of age spermatogenesis regressed due to the formation and enlargement of Sertoli cell tumors. These observations indicate a role for α-inhibin in the control of Sertoli cell proliferation, rather than a direct role in spermatogenesis.

On the other hand, the inhibin/activin β,β-subunit homodimer, activin (see Chapter 2.5) is implicated in the control of spermatogonial proliferation.[82] Activin receptor mRNA is present in spermatocytes and spermatids (Fig. 2.6.7)

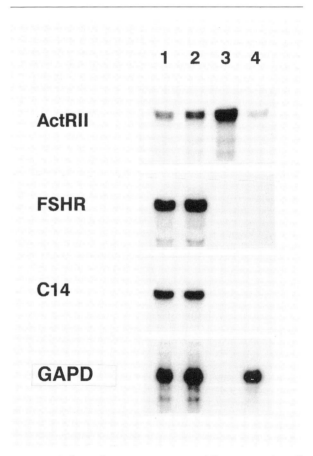

Fig. 2.6.7 *Cell-specific gene expression in different testicular cell types. RNase protection assays on Sertoli cells from immature 3-week-old rats (**Lane 1**), Sertoli cells from adult rats (**Lane 2**), round spermatids (**Lane 3**), and a cell preparation enriched in peritubular cells (**Lane 4**). FSH receptor mRNA (**FSHR**) is found in both immature and mature Sertoli cells. Similarly, Sertoli cells from immature and adult rats express mRNA encoding a novel member (C14) of the transmembrane serine/threonine kinase receptor family, members of which bind TGF-β and related peptide growth/differentiation factors.[83] **C14** represents the putative receptor for AMH (AMI IR).[89,90] C14 and FSHR mRNAs are not expressed by round spermatids or peritubular cells. However, round spermatids do express mRNA encoding another member of the serine/threonine kinase receptor family, namely the activin type II receptor (**ActRII**). Sertoli cells also express ActRII. **GAPD** represents mRNA encoding the glycolytic enzyme glyceraldehyde 3-phosphate dehydrogenase, which was used as a control to show the presence of intact mRNA in all samples. Note that spermatids are different from somatic cells in that they do not express the same GAPD gene, as discussed in the text and Table 2.6.1. (From reference 89.)*

and binding of radiolabeled activin to spermatids has been demonstrated *in vitro*.[87,88] Sertoli cells express β_B-subunit mRNA[82] but 'knock-out' mutation of this β_B-subunit gene does not result in male infertility in mice.[91] This leaves open the possibility that the related activin/inhibin β_A-subunit may compensate for the loss of the β_B-subunit.

Germ cells lack receptors for the principal regulators of spermatogenesis, FSH and testosterone, but express genes encoding other receptors, such as activin and SCF receptors (see above), and, surprisingly, even a member of the olfactory receptor family.[92,93] Spermatocytes and spermatids also express proteins that could take part in signal transduction pathways, including a number of proto-oncogene products.[7,8,12,76–81]

Sperm-specific forms of adenylyl cyclase and cyclic AMP phosphodiesterase have been found in germ cells.[94–96] Moreover, the cyclic AMP-responsive element modulator (CREM) gene that encodes both activators and repressors of cyclic AMP-induced transcription – generated through alternative splicing (see Chapter 1.5) – is also expressed in the spermatogenic epithelium under the control of FSH.[97–100] However, it is not known which Sertoli cell factors modulate cyclic AMP levels in spermatogenic cells. Beginning in spermatocytes, there is an increased level of CREM activator mRNA (transcript stabilization). This mRNA is translated in spermatids (translational control), resulting in a 'developmental switch' in CREM function, from transcriptional repression to activation.[99] Thus, CREM may have a particular role in the regulation of haploid gene expression. An FSH-induced signal transmitted from Sertoli cells to spermatids is believed to bring about the aforementioned switch in CREM function.[97,100] The nature of this FSH-induced signal is not yet known, but the data point to a possible mechanism for 'fine-tuning' of gene expression in germ cells by Sertoli cells.

Cell surface proteins may also play a role both during spermatogenesis and in sperm function. A possible example for a protein with such a dual function, is the integral membrane protein PH-30.[101] This protein is composed of two subunits, α and β, synthesized as larger precursors and then processed to mature forms during spermatogenesis. The subunits are multifunctional, containing metalloprotease and disintegrin domains, and a potential fusion peptide.[102] At the cell surface of spermatogenic cells, the metalloprotease activity of PH-30 might be active in facilitating migration of the germ cells within the spermatogenic epithelium. Disintegrins are ligands that bind to the integrin class of cell surface adhesion proteins. As indicated above, integrins are present at sites of attachment of spermatids to Sertoli cells, and PH-30, being an integral membrane protein of spermatids, might therefore participate in this attachment. With respect to the function of processed PH-30 on spermatozoa, a disintegrin domain and a potential fusion peptide in the mature subunits may be necessary for the binding and fusion of sperm and egg plasma membranes.[101–103]

Spermatids become spermatozoa!

Certain genes and signal transduction components expressed in spermatids that may have no role during spermatogenesis *per se* could nevertheless be involved in mature sperm function. After all, ejaculated spermatozoa need to be able to respond to extracellular signals that regulate their motility and equip them to engage in the various steps involved in fertilization of the egg[104,105] (see Chapter 2.10).

FUTURE PERSPECTIVES

Progress in our understanding of the control of spermatogenesis is likely to occur through further improvements in the cell culture systems being used, continued application of the ever-increasing power of molecular biology, and targeted gene deletion in mice (see also Chapter 3.1). Such approaches should provide more information on the regulation of gene expression in Sertoli cells and germ cells, and permit the elucidation of pathways of signal transfer between the two cell types.

It will remain important to try to establish a firm link between our experimental knowledge of cells and genes, and the clinical questions concerning male fertility and infertility. Our ignorance regarding several aspects of spermatogenesis is perhaps best illustrated by the fact that we still do not have a straightforward explanation for the phenomenon that spermatogenesis cannot occur when the testis is at body temperature (cryptorchidism).[106]

The net result of proper Sertoli cell function and Sertoli cell–germ cell communication concerns not only the quantity, but also the quality of sperm produced. Disturbance of the intricate spermiation process may result in the production of spermatozoa with an excess amount of cytoplasm, showing biochemical defects. Several studies indicate a correlation between biochemical defects in spermatozoa and their fertilizing capacity.[107,108] Thus, it will be important to study the relationship between Sertoli cell function and sperm quality, in trying to define causes of male infertility. Such research may yield useful parameters of Sertoli cell function and sperm quality. This may improve the diagnosis and treatment of 'idiopathic' infertility.

Finally, an important goal of research on spermatogenesis should be to develop methods for male contraception.[109] Such methods might be based, conventionally, on the hormonal manipulation of spermatogenesis.[110] On the other hand, there is a challenge to exploit the unique features of Sertoli cell–germ cell biology to define specific molecular targets for non-hormonal methods of disrupting sperm development or function.[111]

SUMMARY

- The principal regulators of spermatogenesis, FSH and testosterone, act on Sertoli cells. In the absence of these hormones, Sertoli cells fail to support spermatogenesis.
- Testicular growth/differentiation factors participate in a regulatory network that controls Sertoli cell development, and maintenance of the functions of the mature cell.
- Developing germ cells exert feedback effects on Sertoli cells, possibly mediated through effects on Sertoli cell structure or involving other pathways of cell-to-cell signaling.
- Sertoli cells probably control proliferation and survival of spermatogonia, and support development of spermatocytes and spermatids.
- Supporting activities of Sertoli cells include the creation of a conditioned micro-environment, as well as direct and intricate structural/mechanical Sertoli cell germ cell interactions.
- Gene expression in spermatogenic cells is geared towards transformation of the cells into highly specialized spermatozoa. This gene expression proceeds according to a defined pattern with a precise temporal control.
- Notable aspects of gene expression in spermatocytes and spermatids are:
  - (a) Germ cell-specific expression of genes encoding isoenzymes/isotypes of gene products that are expressed in somatic cell types (switching);
  - (b) Germ cell-specific expression of genes encoding structural proteins, metabolic enzymes, and cell surface proteins, that are unique to developing germ cells/spermatozoa;
  - (c) Transcription of genes which might be non-functional with respect to spermatogenesis;
  - (d) Translational control, and sharing of gene products between haploid spermatids.
- Relatively little is known about the specific gene-regulatory proteins involved in the control of gene expression in the spermatogenic cells. Such control occurs both at the level of gene transcription and at the level of mRNA stability and translation. It seems possible that Sertoli-to-germ cell signaling exerts fine-tuning of the activity of gene-regulatory proteins in the germ cells.
- Sperm quality is determined not only by gene expression in the spermatogenic cells, but also by proper functioning of Sertoli cells, e.g. Sertoli cell malfunction during spermiation may lead to the release of spermatozoa with excess cytoplasm, causing biochemical/functional defects.
- Improved knowledge of spermatogenesis is essential to obtain useful methods for the analysis and treatment of male infertility, and to define possible targets for non-hormonal male contraception.

REFERENCES

1. Koopman P, Gubbay J, Vivian N, Goodfellow P, Lovell-Badge R. Male development of chromosomally female mice transgenic for *Sry*. *Nature* 1991 **351**: 117–121.
2. McLaren A. The making of male mice. *Nature* 1991 **351**: 96.
3. Bogan JS, Page DC. Ovary? Testis? – A mammalian dilemma. *Cell* 1994 **76**: 603–607.
4. Harley VR. Genetic control of testis determination. In Kretser D de (ed.) *Molecular Biology of the Male Reproductive System*. San Diego: Academic Press, 1993: 1–20.
5. Gondos B, Berndtson WE. Postnatal and pubertal development of Sertoli cells. In Russell LD, Griswold MD (eds) *The Sertoli Cell*. Clearwater FL: Cache River Press, 1993: 115–154.
6. Willison K, Ashworth A. Mammalian spermatogenic gene expression. *Trends Genet* 1987 **3**: 351–355.
7. Propst F, Rosenberg MP, Vande Woude G. Proto-oncogene expression in germ cell development. *Trends Genet* 1988 **4**: 183–187.
8. Grootegoed JA. Proto-oncogenes and spermatogenesis. *Int J Androl* 1989 **12**: 251–253.
9. Hecht NB. Regulation of 'haploid expressed genes' in male germ cells. *J Reprod Fertil* 1990 **88**: 679–693.
10. Erickson RP. Post-meiotic gene expression. *Trends Genet* 1990 **6**: 264–269.
11. Eddy EM, Welch JE, O'Brien DA. Gene expression during spermatogenesis. In Kretser D de (ed.) *Molecular Biology of the Male Reproductive System*. San Diego: Academic Press, 1993: 181–232. .
12. Winer MA, Wolgemuth DJ. Patterns of expression and potential functions of proto-oncogenes during mammalian spermatogenesis. In Kretser D de (ed.) *Molecular Biology of the Male Reproductive System*. San Diego: Academic Press, 1993: 143–179.
13. Weinbauer GF, Nieschlag E. Hormonal control of spermatogenesis. In Kretser D de (ed.) *Molecular Biology of the Male Reproductive System*. San Diego: Academic Press, 1993: 99–142.
14. Sharpe RM. Regulation of spermatogenesis. In Knobil E, Neill JD (eds) *The Physiology of Reproduction*. New York: Raven Press, 1994: 1363–1434.
15. Dym M. Basement membrane regulation of Sertoli cells. *Endocr Rev* 1994 **15**: 102–115.
16. Skinner MK. Cell–cell interactions in the testis. *Endocrine Rev* 1991 **12**: 45–77.
17. Robertson DM, Risbridger GP, Hedger M, McLachlan RI.

Growth factors in the control of testicular function. In Kretser D de (ed.) *Molecular Biology of the Male Reproductive System.* San Diego: Academic Press, 1993: 411–438.

18. Kretser DM de, Kerr JB. The cytology of the testis. In Knobil E, Neill JD (eds) *The Physiology of Reproduction*, 2nd edn. New York: Raven Press, 1994: 1177–1290.
19. Russell LD. Role of Sertoli cells in spermiation. In Russell LD, Griswold MD (eds) *The Sertoli Cell.* Clearwater FL: Cache River Press, 1993: 269–303.
20. Russell LD. Morphological and functional evidence for Sertoli–germ cell relationships. In Russell LD, Griswold MD (eds) *The Sertoli Cell.* Clearwater FL: Cache River Press, 1993: 365–390.
21. Russell LD, Ettlin RA, Sinha Hikim AP, Clegg ED. *Histological and Histopathological Evaluation of the Testis.* Clearwater FL: Cache River Press, 1990: 286pp.
22. Clermont Y. Kinetics of spermatogenesis in mammals: seminiferous epithelium cycle and spermatogonial renewal. *Physiol Rev* 1972 52: 198–236.
23. Burgoyne PS, Mahadevaiah SK, Sutcliffe MJ, Palmer SJ. Fertility in mice requires X–Y pairing and a Y-chromosomal 'spermiogenesis' gene mapping to the long arm. *Cell* 1992 71: 391–398.
24. Ma K, Inglis JD, Sharkey A *et al*. A Y chromosome gene family with RNA-binding protein homology: candidates for the azoospermia factor AZF controlling human spermatogenesis. *Cell* 1993 75: 1287–1295.
25. Chandley AC, Cooke HJ. Human male fertility: Y-linked genes and spermatogenesis. *Hum Mol Genet* 1994 3: 1449–1452.
26. Handel MA, Hunt PA, Kot MC, Park C, Shannon M. Role of sex chromosomes in the control of male germ-cell differentiation. *Ann NY Acad Sci* 1991 637: 64–73.
27. Handel MA, Hunt PA. Sex-chromosome pairing and activity during mammalian meiosis. *BioEssays* 1992 14: 817–822.
28. Monesi V. Differential rate of ribonucleic acid synthesis in the autosomes and sex chromosomes during male meiosis in the mouse. *Chromosoma (Berl)* 1965 17: 11–21.
29. Grootegoed JA, Grollé-Hey AH, Rommerts FFG, Molen HJ van der. Ribonucleic acid synthesis *in vitro* in primary spermatocytes isolated from rat testis. *Biochem J* 1977 168: 23–31.
30. Grootegoed JA, Meerkerk LM van, Rommerts FFG, Molen HJ van der. Effect of hypophysectomy on ribonucleic acid synthesis in primary spermatocytes isolated from rat testis. *Int J Androl* 1979 2: 330–342.
31. Hendriksen PJM, Hoogerbrugge JW, Themmen APN, Koken MHM, Hoeijmakers JHJ, Oostra BA, Lende T van der, Grootegoed JA. Post-meiotic transcription of X and Y chromosomal genes during spermatogenesis in the mouse. *Dev Biol* 1995 170: 730–733.
32. Shannon M, Handel MA. Expression of the *Hprt* gene during spermatogenesis: implications for sex-chromosome inactivation. *Biol Reprod* 1993 49: 770-778.
33. Lifschytz E, Lindsley DL. The role of X chromosome inactivation during spermatogenesis. *Proc Natl Acad Sci USA* 1972 69: 182–186.
34. Dym M, Fawcett DW. Further observations on the numbers of spermatogonia, spermatocytes, and spermatids connected by intercellular bridges in the mammalian testis. *Biol Reprod* 1971 4: 195–215.
35. Braun RE, Behringer RR, Peschon JJ, Brinster RL, Palmiter RD. Genetically haploid spermatids are phenotypically diploid. *Nature* 1989 337: 373–376.
36. Caldwell KA, Handel MA. Protamine transcript sharing among post-meiotic spermatids. *Proc Natl Acad Sci USA* 1991 88: 2407–2411.
37. VandeBerg JL, Cooper DW, Close PJ. Testis specific phosphoglycerate kinase B in mouse. *J Exp Zool* 1976 198: 231–240.
38. Gold B, Fujimoto H, Kramer JM, Erickson RP, Hecht NB. Haploid accumulation and translational control of phosphoglycerate kinase-2 messenger RNA during mouse spermatogenesis. *Dev Biol* 1983 98: 392–399.
39. McCarrey JR, Thomas K. Human testis-specific PGK gene lacks introns and possesses characteristics of a processed gene. *Nature* 1987 326: 501–505.
40. Boer PH, Adra CN, Lau YF, McBurney MW. The testis-specific phosphoglycerate kinase gene *pgk-2* is a recruited retroposon. *Mol Cell Biol* 1987 7: 3107–3112.
41. Dahl H-HM, Brown RM, Hutchison WM, Maragos C, Brown GK. A testis-specific form of the human pyruvate dehydrogenase E1a subunit is coded for by an intronless gene on chromosome 4. *Genomics* 1990 8: 225–232.
42. Iannello RC, Dahl H-HM. Transcriptional expression of a testis-specific variant of the mouse pyruvate dehydrogenase E1a subunit. *Biol Reprod* 1992 47: 48–58.
43. Mori C, Welch JE, Sakai Y, Eddy EM. *In situ* localization of spermatogenic cell-specific glyceraldehyde 3-phosphate dehydrogenase (Gapd-s) messenger ribonucleic acid in mice. *Biol Reprod* 1992 46: 859–868.
44. Welch JE, Schatte EC, O'Brien DA, Eddy EM. Expression of a glyceraldehyde 3-phosphate dehydrogenase gene specific to mouse spermatogenic cells. *Biol Reprod* 1992 46: 869–878.
45. Millan JL, Driscoll CE, LeVan KM, Goldberg E. Epitopes of human testis-specific lactate dehydrogenase deduced from a cDNA sequence. *Proc Natl Acad Sci USA* 1987 84: 5311–5315.
46. Virbasius JV, Scarpulla RC. Structure and expression of rodent genes encoding the testis-specific cytochrome-C. *J Biol Chem* 1988 263: 6791–6796.
47. Grootegoed JA, Boer PJ den. Energy metabolism of spermatids: a review. In Hamilton DW, Waites GM (eds) *Cellular and Molecular Events in Spermiogenesis.* Cambridge: Cambridge University Press, 1989: 193–216.
48. Meistrich ML. Nuclear morphogenesis during spermiogenesis. In Kretser D de (ed.) *Molecular Biology of the Male Reproductive System.* San Diego: Academic Press, 1993: 67–97.
49. Eddy EM, O'Brien DA. The spermatozoon. In Knobil E, Neill JD (eds) *The Physiology of Reproduction.* 2nd edn, New York: Raven Press, 1994: 29–77.
50. Capel B, Swain A, Nicolis S *et al*. Circular transcripts of the testis-determining gene *Sry* in adult mouse testis. *Cell* 1993 73: 1019–1030.
51. Nusse R, Varmus HM. *Wnt* genes. *Cell* 1992 69: 1073–1087.
52. Shackleford GM, Varmus HE. Expression of the proto-oncogene Wnt-1 is restricted to postmeiotic male germ cells and the neural tube of mid-gestational embryos. *Cell* 1987 50: 89–95.
53. Erickson RP, Lai L-W, Grimes J. Creating a conditional mutation of *Wnt-1* by antisense transgenesis provides evidence that *Wnt-1* is not essential for spermatogenesis. *Dev Genet* 1993 14: 274–281.
54. Russell LD, Clermont Y. Degeneration of germ cells in normal, hypophysectomized and hormone treated hypophysectomized rats. *Anat Rec* 1977 187: 347–366.
55. Risley MS. Spermatogenic cell differentiation *in vitro*. *Gamete Res* 1983 4: 331–346.
56. Dorrington JH, Armstrong DT. Effects of FSH on gonadal functions. *Recent Prog Horm Res* 1979 35: 301–342.
57. Josso N, Cate RL, Picard J-Y *et al*. Anti-müllerian hormone: the Jost factor. *Recent Prog Horm Res* 1993 48: 1–59.
58. Bardin CW, Cheng CY, Mustow NA, Gunsalus GL. The Sertoli cell. In Knobil E, Neill JD (eds) *The Physiology of Reproduction*, 2nd edn. New York: Raven Press, 1994: 1291–1333.
59. Means AR, Fakunding JL, Huckins C, Tindall DJ, Vitale R. Follicle-stimulating hormone, the Sertoli cell, and spermatogenesis. *Recent Prog Horm Res* 1976 32: 477–527.
60. Grootegoed JA, Jansen R, Molen HJ van der. Intercellular pathway of leucine catabolism in rat spermatogenic epithelium. *Biochem J* 1985 226: 889–892.

61. Griswold MD. Unique aspects of the biochemistry and metabolism of Sertoli cells. In Russell LD, Griswold MD (eds) *The Sertoli Cell*. Clearwater FL: Cache River Press, 1993: 485–492.

62. Grootegoed JA, Jansen R, Molen HJ van der. Effect of glucose on ATP dephosphorylation in rat spermatids. *J Reprod Fertil* 1986 77: 99–107.

63. Toebosch AMW, Brussée R, Verkerk A, Grootegoed JA. Quantitative evaluation of the maintenance and development of spermatocytes and round spermatids in cultured tubule fragments from immature rat testis. *Int J Androl* 1989 12: 360–374.

64. Rassoulzadegan M, Paquis-Flucklinger V, Bertino B *et al*. Transmeiotic differentiation of male germ cells in culture. *Cell* 1993 75: 997–1006.

65. Kierszenbaum AL. Mammalian spermatogenesis *in vivo* and *in vitro*: a partnership of spermatogenic and somatic cell lineages. *Endocr Rev* 1994 15: 116–134.

66. Boer PJ den, Mackenbach P, Grootegoed JA. Glutathione metabolism in cultured Sertoli cells and spermatogenic cells from hamsters. *J Reprod Fertil* 1989 87: 391–400.

67. Sylvester SR, Griswold MD. Molecular biology of iron transport in the testis. In Kretser D (ed.) *Molecular Biology of the Male Reproductive System*. San Diego: Academic Press, 1993: 311–326.

68. Palombi F, Salanova M, Tarone G, Farini D, Stefanini M. Distribution of β1 integrin subunit in rat seminiferous epithelium. *Biol Reprod* 1992 47: 1173–1182.

69. Russell LD. Spermatid–Sertoli tubulobulbar complexes as devices for elimination of cytoplasm from the head region of late spermatids of the rat. *Anat Rec* 1979 194: 233–246.

70. Jégou B. The Sertoli–germ cell communication network in mammals. *Int Rev Cytol* 1993 147: 25–96.

71. Vogl AW, Pfeiffer DC, Redenbach DM, Grove BD. Sertoli cell cytoskeleton. In Russell LD, Griswold MD (eds) *The Sertoli Cell*. Clearwater FL: Cache River Press, 1993: 39–86.

72. Parvinen M. Cyclic function of Sertoli cells. In Russell LD, Griswold MD (eds) *The Sertoli Cell*. Clearwater FL: Cache River Press, 1993: 331–347.

73. Fritz IB, Tung PS, Ailenberg M. Proteases and antiproteases in the seminiferous tubule. In Russell LD, Griswold MD (eds) *The Sertoli Cell*. Clearwater FL: Cache River Press, 1993: 217–235.

74. Wright WW, Parvinen M, Musto NA *et al*. Identification of stage-specific proteins synthesized by rat seminiferous tubules. *Biol Reprod* 1983 29: 257–270.

75. Erickson-Lawrence M, Zabludoff SD, Wright WW. Cyclic protein-2, a secretory product of rat Sertoli cells, is the proenzyme form of cathepsin L. *Mol Endocrinol* 1991 5: 1789–1798.

76. Maguire SM, Millar MR, Sharpe RM, Saunders PTK. Stage-dependent expression of mRNA for cyclic protein 2 during spermatogenesis is modulated by elongate spermatids. *Mol Cell Endocrinol* 1993 94: 79–88.

77. Fleischman RA. From white spots to stem cells: the role of the Kit receptor in mammalian development. *Trends Genet* 1993 9: 285–290.

78. Raff MC. Social controls on cell survival and cell death. *Nature* 1992 356: 397–400.

79. Yoshinaga K, Nishikawa S, Ogawa M *et al*. Role of c-kit in mouse spermatogenesis: identification of spermatogonia as a specific site of c-kit expression and function. *Development* 1991 113: 689–699.

80. Tajima Y, Onoue H, Kitamura Y, Nishimune Y. Biologically active *c-kit* ligand growth factor is produced by mouse Sertoli cells and is defective in *Sl/d* mutant mice. *Development* 1991 113: 1031–1035.

81. Rossi P, Dolci S, Albanesi C *et al*. Follicle-stimulating hormone induction of Steel factor (SLF) mRNA in mouse Sertoli cells and stimulation of DNA synthesis in spermatogonia by soluble SLF. *Dev Biol* 1993 155: 68–74.

82. Vale W, Bilezikjian LM, Rivier C. Reproductive and other roles of inhibins and activins. In Knobil E, Neil JD (eds) *The Physiology of Reproduction*, 2nd edn. New York: Raven Press, 1994: 1861–1878.

83. Massagué J, Attisano L, Wrana JL. The TGF-β family and its composite receptors. *Trends Cell Biol* 1994 4: 172–178.

84. Lee MM, Donahoe PK. Müllerian inhibiting substance: a gonadal hormone with multiple functions. *Endocr Rev* 1993 14: 152–164.

85. Capecchi MR. Targeted gene replacement. *Sci Am* 1994 **March**: 34–41.

86. Matzuk MM, Finegold MJ, Su J-GJ, Hsueh AJW, Bradley A. α-Inhibin is a tumour-suppressor gene with gonadal specificity in mice. *Nature* 1992 360: 313–319.

87. Winter JP de, Themmen APN, Hoogerbrugge JW *et al*. Activin receptor mRNA expression in rat testicular cell types. *Mol Cell Endocrinol* 1992 83: R1–R8.

88. Krummen LA, Moore A, Woodruff TK *et al*. Localization of inhibin and activin binding sites in the testis during development by *in situ* ligand binding. *Biol Reprod* 1994 50: 734–744.

89. Baarends WM, Helmond MJL van, Post M *et al*. A novel member of the transmembrane serine/threonine kinase receptor family is specifically expressed in the gonads and in mesenchymal cells adjacent to the Müllerian duct. *Development* 1994 120: 189–197.

90. Grootegoed JA, Baarends WM, Themmen APN. Welcome to the family: the anti-Müllerian hormone receptor. *Mol Cell Endocrinol* 1994 100: 29–34.

91. Vassalli A, Matzuk MM, Gardner HAR, Lee K-F, Jaenisch R. Activin/inhibin βB subunit gene disruption leads to defects in eyelid development and female reproduction. *Genes Dev* 1994 8: 414–427.

92. Parmentier M, Libert F, Schurmans S *et al*. Expression of members of the putative olfactory receptor gene family in mammalian germ cells. *Nature* 1992 355: 453–455.

93. Vanderhaeghen P, Schurmans S, Vassart G, Parmentier M. Olfactory receptors are displayed on dog mature sperm cells. *J Cell Biol* 1993 123: 1441–1452.

94. Adamo S, Conti M, Geremia R, Monesi V. Particulate and soluble adenylate cyclase activities of mouse male germ cells. *Biochem Biophys Res Commun* 1980 97: 607–613.

95. Gordeladze JO, Hansson V. Purification and kinetic properties of the soluble Mn^{2+}-dependent adenylyl cyclase of the rat testis. *Mol Cell Endocrinol* 1981 23: 125–136.

96. Welch JE, Swinnen JV, O'Brien DA, Eddy EM, Conti M. Unique adenosine 3′,5′ cyclic monophosphate phosphodiesterase messenger ribonucleic acids in rat spermatogenic cells: evidence for differential gene expression during spermatogenesis. *Biol Reprod* 1992 46: 1027–1033.

97. Delmas V, Sassone-Corsi P. The key role of CREM in the cAMP signaling pathway in the testis. *Mol Cell Endocrinol* 1994 100: 121–124.

98. Foulkes NS, Sassone-Corsi P. More is better: activators and repressors from the same gene. *Cell* 1992 68: 411–414.

99. Foulkes NS, Mellström B, Benusiglio E, Sassone-Corsi P. Developmental switch of CREM function during spermatogenesis: from antagonist to activator. *Nature* 1992 355: 80–84.

100. Foulkes NS, Schlotter F, Pévet P, Sassone-Corsi P. Pituitary hormone FSH directs the CREM functional switch during spermatogenesis. *Nature* 1993 362: 264–267.

101. Blobel CP, Wolfsberg TG, Turck CW, Myles DG, Primakoff P, White JM. A potential fusion peptide and an integrin ligand domain in a protein active in sperm–egg fusion. *Nature* 1992 356: 248–252.

102. Wolfsberg TG, Bazan JF, Blobel CP *et al*. The precursor region of a protein active in sperm–egg fusion contains a metalloprotease and a disintegrin domain: structural, functional, and evolutionary implications. *Proc Natl Acad Sci USA* 1993 90: 10783–10787.

103. Myles DG. Molecular mechanisms of sperm–egg membrane binding and fusion in mammals. *Dev Biol* 1993 158: 35–45.

104. Hardy DM, Garbers DL. Molecular basis of signalling in spermatozoa. Kretser D de (ed.) *Molecular Biology of the Male Reproductive System.* San Diego: Academic Press, 1993: 233–270.

105. Yanagimachi R. Mammalian fertilization. In Knobil E, Neill JD (eds) *The Physiology of Reproduction,* 2nd edn. New York: Raven Press, 1994: 189–317.

106. Kandeel FR, Swerdloff RS. Role of temperature in regulation of spermatogenesis and the use of heating as a method for contraception. *Fert Steril* 1988 **49**: 1–23.

107. Huszar G, Vigue L, Corrales M. Sperm creatine kinase activity in fertile and infertile oligospermic men. *J Androl* 1990 **11**: 40–46.

108. Aitken RJ, Irvine DS, Wu FC. Prospective analysis of sperm–oocyte fusion and reactive oxygen species generation as criteria for the diagnosis of infertility. *Am J Obstet Gynecol* 1991 **164**: 542–551.

109. Waites GMH. Male fertility regulation: the challenges for the year 2000. *Br Med Bull* 1993 **49**: 210–221.

110. World Health Organisation Task Force on Methods for the Regulation of Male Fertility. Contraceptive efficacy of testosterone-induced azoospermia in normal men. *Lancet* 1990 **ii**: 955–959.

111. Hamilton DW, Waites GMH (eds). Cellular and molecular events in spermiogenesis. Cambridge: Cambridge University Press, 1990: 334 pp.

2.7

Uterus and Tubes

HOD Critchley

INTRODUCTION

The uterus and Fallopian tubes are of fundamental importance to reproduction. The uterus develops as a muscular expansion of the Müllerian duct (see Chapter 2.1), which nourishes the early embryo and accommodates the growth and differentiation of the developing fetus (Fig. 2.7.1).[1] The Fallopian tubes – also Müllerian derivatives – conduct the egg from the ovary to the uterus and spermatozoa from uterus to the distal part of the tube where they fertilize the egg.

The three major functional components of the uterus are its glandular lining membrane (endometrium) that nourishes the early embryo, the smooth muscle of the uterine body (myometrium), which greatly increases in

amount during pregnancy and whose contraction ultimately expels the fetus and placenta, and the cervix – the cylindrical lower part of the uterus opening to the vagina, containing numerous glands that supply mucus to the vagina.

Functionally, the most important tasks of the endometrium are implantation and regeneration and in order to assure appropriate maturation and receptivity each month, the endometrium must be able to be discarded and regenerate quickly in the absence of a conceptus.[2] The endometrium is thus distinctive in both form and function.[3]

The myometrium undergoes spontaneous rhythmic contractions that vary with stage of menstrual cycle and stage of pregnancy. Ultimately, at the end of pregnancy, myometrial contractions occur that enable labor and

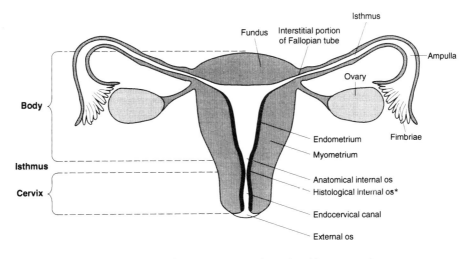

Fig. 2.7.1 *Coronal section of uterus and Fallopian tubes.*

delivery to take place. In contrast to the myometrium of the body of the uterus, the normal cervix is a collagenous structure with smooth muscle fibers accounting for only 10–15% of its tissue composition.[4] Hence the cervix has the capacity to undergo profound tissue remodeling during pregnancy and labor, and rapidly to return to its former state thereafter. The important functions of the cervix are to allow migration and transport of spermatozoa through the cervical canal, to act as a barrier to retain the conceptus, and, at an appropriate time, to open and permit the conceptus to be expelled from the uterus.[5]

The Fallopian tubes have several roles but their main function is in the process of natural conception. Gamete transport, maturation, fertilization, and early embryo development and transport all take place within the fallopian tube.[6] The Fallopian tubes also provide nutrition in the earliest stages of development and provide a defence against infection.[7]

This chapter surveys current knowledge of the regulation of uterine and tubular function, emphasizing the roles of ovarian steroids and local control mechanisms.

CURRENT CONCEPTS

Steroidal regulation

Uterus

Progesterone is essential for the establishment and maintenance of pregnancy in all mammalian species.[8] The first half of the menstrual cycle, the follicular phase, is estrogen dominated; and the second half of the cycle, the luteal phase is progesterone dominated.[9,10] Progesterone secretion

by the corpus luteum converts an estrogen primed proliferative endometrium into a secretory one, which is receptive to the blastocyst. The blastocyst interacts with secretory endometrium during implantation and, on coming into contact with stromal cells, decidual transformation occurs. In the absence of pregnancy, stromal differentiation into decidual tissue still occurs largely under the influence of ovarian hormones. When the corpus luteum regresses and progesterone levels fall, the endometrium (largely decidua) breaks down and menses occurs. Although the exact mechanisms of endometrial regeneration, implantation, and menstruation are unknown, several lines of evidence suggest that the interplay between the endocrine and immune systems, i.e. interaction between steroid hormones, leucocytes, cytokines and locally produced growth factors, are crucial to the maintenance of normal uterine function.

Conventional steroid receptor assays depend on the measurement of specific binding of a labeled steroid (ligand) to receptors in homogenized tissue extracts, e.g. the 'dextran-coated charcoal' (DCC) ligand-binding assay. Although such techniques permit quantification of receptors, the process of homogenization disrupts tissue architecture and precludes identification of the cellular site(s) within the tissue where receptors are located. Estrogen receptor (ER) and progesterone receptor (PR) levels in human uterus measured using a DCC assay are illustrated in Fig. 2.7.2.[11] A rise in ER content is observed throughout the proliferative phase, paralleled by a delayed rise in PR content. During the secretory phase, both ER and PR contents return to low levels.[11]

Over recent years, with the availability of specific monoclonal antibodies to ER and PR, histochemical techniques have been employed to determine receptor distribution, both within cells and between coexistent cell types in the same tissue.[11] ER and PR distribution in the non-pregnant

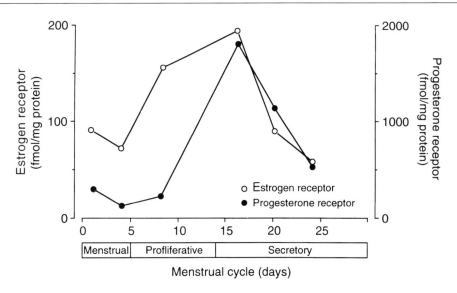

Fig. 2.7.2 *Relationship of uterine ER and PR concentration to stage of the menstrual cycle using a DCC ligand-binding assay (fmol/mg protein). (Reproduced from reference 11, with permission of the Endocrine Society.)*

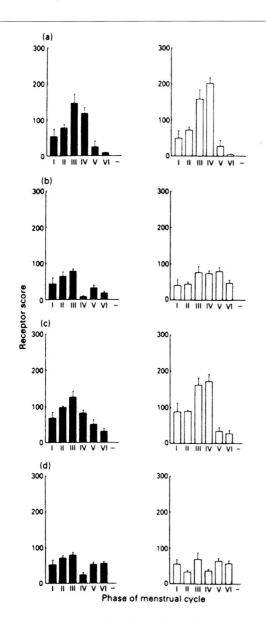

Fig. 2.7.3 *Immunocytochemical ER (closed bars) and PR (open bars) scores (mean+/- SEM, n=5) in* (**a**) *glandular epithelium functionalis,* (**b**) *stroma functionalis,* (**c**) *glandular epithelium basalis and* (**d**) *stroma basalis during the menstrual cycle phases I–VI (I–III = menstruation, early, late proliferative; IV–VI = early, mid, late secretory). (Reproduced from reference 13, with permission.)*

human uterus has now been well described in a number of immunohistochemical studies[11-14] (Table 2.7.1, Fig. 2.7.3).

The PR is induced by estradiol at the transcriptional level, and down-regulated by its own ligand, progesterone, at the transcriptional and post-transcriptional levels.[15] Both ER and PR are localized within the nuclei of target cells.[11] Figs. 2.7.4–2.7.7 illustrate nuclear immunolocalization of ER and PR in late proliferative phase endometrium (Figs. 2.7.4 and 2.7.5) and secretory-phase endometrium (Figs. 2.7.6 and 2.7.7). Recent immunohistochemical data[16] have shown that administration of the antigestogen RU486 in the early luteal phase blocks the progesterone-induced down-regulation of PR (and ER) in non-pregnant human endometrium.

In contrast to the changes reported for ER and PR over the menstrual cycle, no changes in glandular or stromal androgen receptor expression have been reported.[17,18]

The documented changes in ER and PR are consistent with the various physiological functions of the uterus, these being endometrial regeneration, implantation, menstruation, myometrial contractility and the role played by the Fallopian tubes in conception (see later).

Endometrial regeneration and repair

Angiogenesis – growth of new blood vessels – rarely occurs in normal adult tissues. A notable exception is the female reproductive tract.[19] In the female, regular angiogenic activity occurs during endometrial repair and proliferation, development of the endometrial spiral arterioles and placentation.[20] Rogers *et al.*[20] described three episodes of angiogenesis in endometrium during the primate menstrual cycle. Postmenstrual repair occurs in the early proliferative phase[20,21] and further angiogenesis and repair continues during the mid-proliferative phase under the influence of estrogen.[19,22] Growth of coiled arterioles takes place in the secretory phase under the influence of progesterone.[19,22,23] Thus the immunohistochemical evidence for presence of ER in proliferative phase endometrium is consistent with the regenerative role of its ligand, estrogen, at this stage of the cycle. Clarke and Sutherland[24] reviewed the complex effects of progestins on endometrial stromal cells. Significant stromal proliferation is observed during the proliferative phase, which declines shortly after ovulation. Thereafter, there is a second wave of proliferation, presumably in response to progesterone. Immunohistochemical studies

Table 2.7.1 Summary of sex steroid receptor localization in the uterus and Fallopian tubes (as determined by immunohistochemistry)[13,41]

	Uterus						Fallopian tube			
	Endometrium				Myometrium		Medial epithelium		Fimbrial epithelium	
	ER	PR	ER	PR	ER	PR	ER	PR	ER	PR
	Glands	Glands	Stroma	Stroma						
Follicular phase	+↑	+↑	+↑	+↑ Persist	+↑	+↑ Persist	+↑/−↑	+↑ Persist	+↑	Patchy
Luteal phase	−↓	−↓	−↓	+	−↓	+	−↓ (Late LP)	+/−	+/−	Patchy

Abbreviations: ER, Estrogen receptor; PR, Progesterone receptor; ↑ Increases; ↓ Decreases; + Marked; +/− Low/moderate; − Low/absent.

have provided evidence for the presence of PR late in the cycle and support a role for progesterone action in the stroma at this time.[11] An example of such progestin action might be a role, either direct or indirect, in the growth of spiral arterioles. (See Chapter 2.9 for further details of angiogenesis and menstruation.)

Implantation

Almost every structural component of the endometrium (glands, stroma, blood vessels) is involved in the preparation for implantation, and normal nidation requires a delicate balance between the prevailing steroid environment and essential tissue components. Hormonal control of the

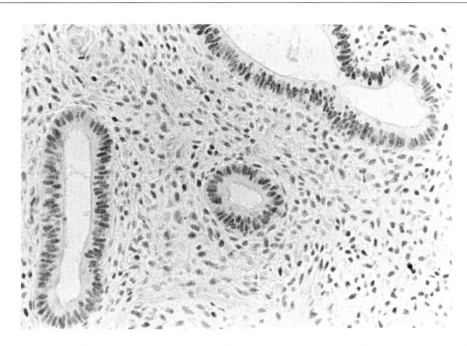

Fig. 2.7.4 *Photomicrograph of ER immunostaining in late proliferative phase endometrium. Glandular and stromal ER expression is maximal.*

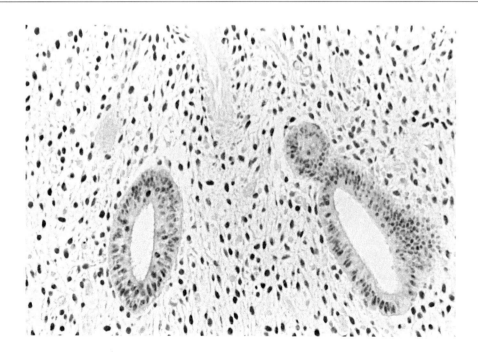

Figure 2.7.5 *Photomicrograph illustrating maximal PR immunoreactivity (both glandular and stromal) in late proliferative phase endometrium.*

endometrium is mediated by estradiol and progesterone acting via the cognate receptors in target cell-types. The intense ER and PR immunoreactivity observed in the late proliferative and early secretory phases, i.e. peri-ovulation, is correlated with increased estradiol secretion. The decrease of ER and PR from the glandular compartment of the endometrium during the mid- and late luteal phases reflect down-regulation of the receptors by progesterone. Observations in anovulatory women (all endometrial tissue displayed positive glandular ER and PR immunoreactivity) confirmed this concept.[12,25] Thus patterns of sex steroid immunoreactivity may be useful for assessing endometrial maturation; that is, increases in sex steroid receptors reflect the actions of estradiol and decreases in receptors in the

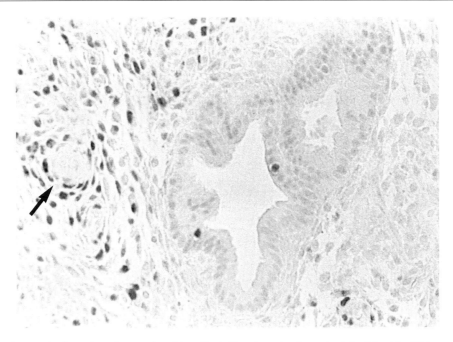

Fig. 2.7.6 *Photomicrograph of secretory phase endometrium illustrating stromal cells moderately stained for PR in contrast to epithelial gland cells which show no or very weak immunostaining. Note the positive immunoreactivity (arrow) in close association with blood vessels.*

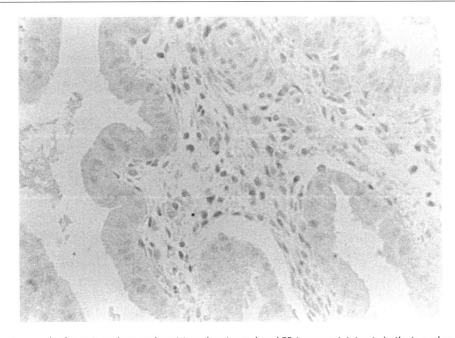

Fig.2.7.7 *Photomicrograph of secretory phase endometrium showing reduced ER immunostaining in both stromal and glandular cells.*

glands are an index of the cumulative action of progesterone during the luteal phase.[12,25] Moreover, the perivascular location of ER and PR[25,26] is consistent with the modulation of physiological uterine vascular changes by sex steroids. Estradiol at physiological concentrations has been shown to decrease vascular resistance in uterine arteries.[27]

If conception occurs and pregnancy proceeds, PR expression remains fairly constant throughout pregnancy (4–38 weeks) and PR are widely expressed in stromal cells and in blood vessel walls.[28,29] ER expression is initially weak and then undetectable. During early pregnancy, ER expression is restricted to scattered stromal cells and a few cells within the walls of spiral arteries. Both PR and ER are absent from the glandular epithelium. Such observations support a role for progesterone in stromal decidualization. Significant PR down-regulation by progesterone during pregnancy only occurs in epithelial cells. Absent or low endometrial ER expression is consistent with the down-regulation by steroid hormones of ER mRNA or receptor protein levels. Increase in ER in human decidua after administration of an antigestogen suggests that the main cause of low ER levels is progesterone secretion.[28,30]

Menstruation

Sex steroid hormones are important in the regulation of normal uterine function, including the normal uterine bleeding – menstruation – that occurs with the demise of the corpus luteum. The menstrual phase of the cycle is associated with rising levels of ER and PR in the glands and an increase of ER in the stromal tissue (Fig. 2.7.3). Stromal cells of the endometrium show only minor fluctuations in PR over the phases of the cycle (Fig. 2.7.3).[13] The effects of estrogen or progesterone upon the vascular epithelium or smooth muscle may be direct or indirect. ER and PR have been reported in non-pregnant uterine vascular smooth muscle, but not in endothelium.[25,26] Vascular tissue exists to serve the needs of the stromal and epithelial compartments, thus sex steroid receptors located in smooth muscle cells may respond to signals sent by the stroma and epithelium.[31] Certain lymphoid cells in human endometrium express steroid receptors (ER),[32] and the uterine cell population of hemopoietic lineage produces cytokines which may act as mediators of uterine function (see later). This endocrine–immune interaction and the further interplay of other local mediators no doubt have crucial roles in the control of normal menstruation (see Chapter 2.9).

Myometrial function

In non-pregnant uterine smooth muscle cells of the myometrium, ER expression is maximum in the mid- to late proliferative phase and declines sharply in the early secretory phase.[11,13] An increase in ER immunoreactivity has been reported in the mid- and late secretory phases.[13] Following an increase in PR immunoreactivity in the proliferative phase, there is no significant change in smooth muscle cells over the menstrual cycle. This observation is in keeping with the suggestion that progesterone inhibits the contractility of the myometrium in early pregnancy.[11,13] No regional variations in steroid receptor distribution in myometrium have been reported.[13]

Coordinated contractions of the myometrium are necessary for the normal progression of parturition, and complex endocrine and paracrine regulatory mechanisms activate uterine motility when gestation is complete.[33] The contractility of the non-pregnant human uterus is also hormonally regulated, being related to circulating concentrations of sex steroids throughout the menstrual cycle.[34]

Myometrial smooth muscle cells are both ER and PR positive in early pregnancy. In late pregnancy, PR immunoreactivity persists and less than 1% of cells show positive ER immunoreactivity. In early pregnancy uterine activity is decreased and the response to oxytocin is suppressed due to a blocking effect of luteal progesterone.[34] Swahn and Bygdeman[34] were able to demonstrate increased uterine activity following 24–36 hours of antiprogestin treatment and these data suggested that the effect of progesterone on uterine contractility was mediated through the progesterone receptor system. Prostanoids may also increase myometrial contractility.[35] It should be remembered that decidua is a rich source of prostaglandins (PGs) and cytokines, is well vascularized and lies adjacent to the myometrium.[35]

The sequence of contraction and relaxation of the myometrium is dependent on underlying cyclic electrical activity within the membranes of smooth muscle cells. The observation of gap junctions appearing between myometrial cells during the onset and progression of labor has contributed greatly to understanding the mechanisms controlling this process. Excellent detailed reviews are available concerning the anatomy and electrophysiology of the myometrium.[33,36]

Cervix

In the ectocervix, basal and parabasal cells of squamous epithelium moderately stain for ER in the proliferative phase. ER expression is more evident in the parabasal and intermediate cell layers in the secretory phase. Superficial cell layers remain unstained for ER.[13,37] PR expression is absent or weak in squamous epithelium throughout the menstrual cycle.[13] In the endocervix epithelial cells showed ER immunoreactivity throughout the cycle[13,37] and PR expression is maximum in the late proliferative phase. Both ER and PR are constant and moderately expressed in cervical stromal and smooth muscle cells over the menstrual cycle.[13]

Fallopian tube

Both the structure and function of the Fallopian tubes are influenced by estrogen and progesterone. The Fallopian tubes are paired organs, 7–14 cm long enclosed in the mesosalpingeal borders of the broad ligaments. The well-described regions of the Fallopian tube are the fimbria, ampulla, ampullary-isthmic region, isthmus and uterotubal junction (Fig. 2.7.1). The isthmus is considered to act as a sperm reservoir and fertilization takes place in the ampullary region. The Fallopian tube itself consists of an outer myosalpinx responsible for tubal contraction and an inner endosalpinx which creates the luminal environment.[7]

The tubal epithelium is essentially composed of two cell types: ciliated and non-ciliated secretory cells (Fig. 2.7.8). Ciliated epithelium predominates in the fimbrial region and non-ciliated secretory cells in the isthmic portions of the tubes.[7] Turnover of tubal epithelium is low when compared to endometrial regeneration. There are, however, well established hormone-regulated morphological changes in the tubal epithelium in relation to the ovarian cycle.[38,39] Ciliogenesis in the Fallopian tube is estrogen dependent and takes place during the proliferative phase;[39] the process is antagonized by progesterone. Mature differentiated cells are seen at mid-cycle, under the influence of estrogen.[39] Mitosis is uncommon in the adult fallopian tube (in contrast to endometrium) at any stage of the menstrual cycle, so there is little change in cell number. Maximal height and ciliation of the luminal epithelium is apparent in the late follicular phase with evidence of atrophy and deciliation at the end of the luteal phase. Progestins increase the number of non-ciliated relative to ciliated cells.

(a)

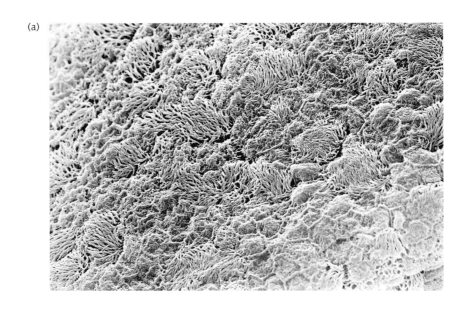

(b)

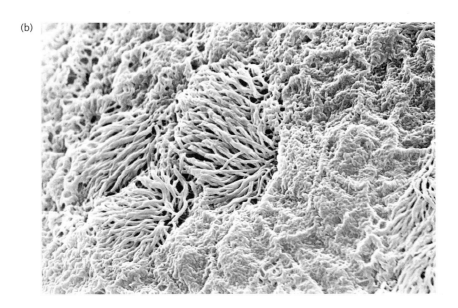

Fig. 2.7.8 *Secretory-phase (day 23 of cycle) tubal epithelium demonstrating both ciliated and non-ciliated secretory cells (scanning electron microscope, Leica-Cambridge Steroscan 360). Note the greater numbers of non-ciliated cells at this stage of cycle due to the influence of progesterone. (*a*) x1675, (*b*) x4250.*

The non-ciliated secretory cells show marked cyclic changes, especially in the isthmic region (see Fig. 2.7.8). At mid-cycle (estrogen peak) serous granules are evident in the apical cytoplasm. With increasing ovarian progesterone production, secretory activity ceases.[39]

The pattern of sex steroid receptor (ER and PR) distribution is broadly consistent with the morphological changes in tubal epithelium just described (Table 2.7.1). Ciliated tubal epithelium has been reported to contain more ER than secretory cells in the tubal lumen and were noted to be most intense in the follicular phase.[40] A very recent report[41] has provided a detailed description of both ER and PR in Fallopian tube. The fimbrial region displayed a different pattern of ER immunoreactivity from the rest of the tube, i.e. strong staining in the early and mid-follicular phase. This was coincident with the formation of new cilia formation in this region. Elsewhere in the fallopian tube, low to moderate ER immunoreactivity was observed in the epithelium of the isthmus and mid-ampulla in the follicular and early luteal phases. ER expression declined in the late luteal phase. PR immunoreactivity was marked along the length of the Fallopian tube epithelium during most of the ovarian cycle except for a slight decline in the late luteal phase. Patchy expression was reported in the fimbrial epithelium.

Attention has been drawn to the differential control of PR in the endometrium and tubal epithelium.[41] PR immunoreactivity falls in the glandular endometrium in the luteal phase, whereas in tubal epithelium moderate staining persists. The exception is the fimbrial region, the behavior of which appears to be a 'mirror image' of the remainder of the tube.

Estrogen stimulates the production of oviductal fluid.[42] Secretion is maximal at mid-cycle (coincident with the estradiol peak). Protein concentration is, however, inversely related to estrogen levels. The secretory function of the fallopian tube would appear to be hormonally regulated. Moderate ER immunoreactivity in tubal epithelium and stroma has been reported[41] in the isthmic region in the follicular and early luteal phase and mid-cycle in the ampullary region.

A number of uterine and tubal secretions are hormonally regulated. The two best characterized are placental protein 14 (PP14) and insulin-like growth factor-binding protein-1 (IGFBP-1).[43,44] PP14 is synthesized in the glandular compartment of the endometrium during the later luteal phase. Synthesis of PP14 is under the influence of progesterone. Progesterone also increases IGFBP-1 synthesis from decidualized endometrial stromal cells.[44] PP14 mRNA is most abundant in the late secretory phase. IGFBP-1 mRNA is maximal earlier in the secretory phase.[43] Interestingly, in contrast to the endometrium, both PP14 and IGFBP-1 mRNAs are only present in low abundance in the Fallopian tubes and these two mRNAs are synthesized in the same cell type of fallopian tube, i.e. the epithelium.[43] This is another illustration that different local mechanisms regulate gene expression in the endometrium and Fallopian tube despite the common mesonephric origin of these tissues. The functional roles of these proteins remain unknown but paracrine actions have been suggested.[44]

The extent to which locally produced mediators, such as growth factors[45] are involved in the effects of estrogen and progesterone on the tubal epithelium is unknown (see below).

Local regulation

Although reproductive events are primarily dependent upon the endocrine actions of sex steroids and other hormones, some of the hormonal effects may involve local mediators, such as growth factors, cytokines and prostaglandins.

Growth factors and cytokines

Growth factors are peptides or polypeptides that interact with cell membrane receptors and usually promote mitogenesis or differentiation. Cytokines are proteins which modulate various cellular functions. The complex interactions of the network of uterine cells, i.e. epithelial, stromal, endothelial, and cells of hemopoietic origin (lymphoid, macrophage, neutrophil) which are responsible for endometrial proliferation and differentiation, and menstrual shedding, require a well-developed assembly of intercellular communication signals.[10,46] Many of the events in human endometrium, such as menstrual shedding and abortion in early pregnancy, resemble inflammatory and regenerative processes. There is increasing evidence for the involvement of pro-inflammatory cytokines in normal uterine function, and several excellent reviews exist in the literature.[10,46,47] Sex steroids may influence cytokine production/action in various ways, including: altered expression of cytokine protein at transcriptional or post-transcriptional levels, altered expression of cytokine receptors, or altered cellular response (e.g. through affecting post-receptor signaling within the target cell).[46]

A more detailed review of current knowledge of likely local mediators of uterine function, i.e. interleukins (IL-1, IL-6, IL-8), tumor necrosis factor, interferons, growth factors (transforming growth factors α, β; epidermal growth factor; IGFs and IGFBPs) is provided in Chapter 2.9. Table 2.7.2 summarizes the localization of these mediators within the uterus. The list is by no means exhaustive and reference should be made to more detailed publications concerning cytokine expression in human endometrium.[10,31,46-48]

Prostaglandins

This comment on local mediators would be incomplete if mention was not made of another very important group of modulators of uterine function, the prostaglandins (PGs). There is good evidence that progesterone modulates PG activity in decidua.[56,57] PGs are likely to be involved with the modulation of blood vessel tone and the transmigration of leucocytes. The activity of the main PG metabolizing enzyme prostaglandin dehydrogenase (PGDH) is stimulated by progesterone; PGDH is increased in the

Table 2.7.2 Presence and location of mediators of uterine function

Mediator	Stroma	Epithelium	Perivascular
Cytokines			
IL-1 (10,50)	+	+	+
IL-1 receptor (10,50)	+	+	+
IL-6 (10,46,49)	+	+	−
IL-8 (51)	−	−	+
IF-γ receptor (10,46)	−	+	−
TNF-α (10,52)	+	+	−
IGFBP-1 (46)	+	−	−
Growth factors			
EGF (10,53)	+	+	+
EGF receptor (10,46)	+	+	+
TGF-β (10,54)	+	+	−
FGF (10,55)	−	+	−
Prostaglandins			
PGE (57)		+	+
PGF$_{2\alpha}$(77)		+	
Sex steroids			
ER (11,13,25)	+	+	+
PR (11,13,25)	+	+	+

luteal phase[58]. Furthermore, progesterone suppresses PG production in secretory endometrium.[59] Administration of an antigestogen (Mifepristone, RU486), simulating progesterone withdrawal, resulted in an increase in PGE$_2$ due to a reduction in PG metabolism.[56,57] Particularly striking was the elevation of PGE in small blood vessels.

Many of the local mediators noted above are likely to interact in some way with the leucocyte populations present within the uterus. The leucocyte populations may be stimulated or inhibited by these local mediators, as well as being a source of production. It is therefore necessary to summarize current knowledge concerning these important components of the normal uterine milieu.

Leucocyte profiles

The local tissue response to withdrawal of progesterone resulting in menstruation shows many features characteristic of an inflammatory response. Immediately prior to spontaneous menstrual bleeding there is release of PGs, a breakdown of blood vessel walls and an abundance of leucocytes in the endometrium. The number and type of leucocytes in human endometrium and decidua varies during the menstrual cycle, with implantation and throughout pregnancy. This suggests a measure of endocrine and local (paracrine) control of leucocyte infiltration and replication in this tissue.[60]

Leucocytes contain small membrane-bound intracellular organelles containing hydrolytic enzymes, called lysosomes.[61] Common lysosomal enzymes include phospholipase A$_2$ (involved in PG metabolism) and plasminogen activator.

The profile of leucocytes in non-pregnant human endometrial stroma is formed primarily by macrophages and lymphocytes. Withdrawal of ovarian progesterone in the sheep produces an influx of polymorphonuclear (PMN) leucocytes.[62] Consequently there is a marked

increase in lysosomal activity both immediately prior to and at the beginning of menstruation.

Data concerning neutrophil subpopulations in human endometrium and early decidua are scarce and there are no data on the mechanism of recruitment. The crucial importance of endometrial and decidual lymphocyte populations is recognized and thus it is necessary to include a resume of current knowledge regarding the role of this leucocyte subpopulation. A population of phenotypically unusual lymphocytes (CD56+,CD16−,CD3−) has been described which increase in the late luteal phase and aggregate in the vicinity of glands and spiral arteries.[63,64] It has yet to be clearly established whether increases in this subpopulation of lymphocytes are a consequence of *in situ* proliferation or alternatively arise from *de novo* peripheral migration from the circulation.[65-68] Following a significant increase in decidual CD56+ lymphocytes in the first trimester of pregnancy, there is a decline in the third trimester.[69] The role of CD56+ lymphocytes, which comprise 70% of first trimester decidual leucocytes, is uncertain. The missing self hypothesis suggests that they interact with non-classical Class I MHC antigen (HLA-G) expressed on extravillous trophoblast but are cytolytic for cells not expressing this antigen. By such a selective action, they might regulate the implantation process.[64]

Polymorphonuclear (PMN) leucocytes can synthesize and release a range of immunoregulatory cytokines and thus initiate and amplify cellular and humoral immune responses. Activated macrophages also produce a wide range of cytokines (including IL-1 and TNF-α) and prostaglandins.[69] Reports concerning the distribution and numbers of macrophages across the menstrual cycle are not consistent. Bulmer *et al.*[70] have described the presence of macrophages in both the stratum basalis and functionalis throughout the menstrual cycle, but did not observe any fluctuation over the cycle and conclude that the recruitment of macrophages is not under hormonal control. On the other hand, Kamat and Isaacson[71] reported a premenstrual increase in the endometrial macrophage population. Furthermore, Klentzeris *et al.*[66] reported that macrophages constitute 30% of the endometrial leucocyte population with an increase in numbers in the latter part of the cycle (LH+10 to LH+13). Macrophages are the most prominent population in decidual stroma of basal decidua,[69] and may be important during embryo–maternal interactions in the peri-implantation period.[72] An excellent review by Hunt[48] has described the role of macrophages within the utero-placental unit.

Prolactin

Extrapituitary prolactin is synthesized and released from endometrial decidua and the identification of prolactin mRNA in decidua has reinforced the view that decidual prolactin is a functional molecule of endometrial origin.[73,74] Only decidualized cells are involved in the biosynthesis of prolactin.[74] Endometrial stromal cells decidualize under the influence of progesterone. The stimulation of prolactin secretion from endometrial cells by progesterone is dose-dependent. There is *in vivo* evidence that decidual prolactin production in early pregnancy occurs as a consequence of decidualization induced by progesterone.[75]

Prolactin synthesis and secretion have also been identified in myometrium and cytokines appear to be involved in the regulation of both synthesis and secretion of prolactin from this reproductive tissue.[76] A paracrine immunomodulatory role for prolactin has been proposed.[73,74]

FUTURE PERSPECTIVES

Improved knowledge of the interplay between sex steroids and cytokines in the control of human endometrial (and decidual) function can be anticipated, hand-in-hand with continuing advances in our understanding of endocrine–immune interactions in the control of reproductive processes.

Further research on the molecular and cellular bases of implantation should be particularly rewarding, since unraveling the local regulatory networks within the uterus could ultimately assist in the identification of new and more acceptable methods of contraception.

Finally, it is apparent that the same local mediators and regulatory systems influence cyclic changes in uterine function throughout the reproductive cycle. Understanding how these mechanisms affect implantation and menstruation could point to new therapeutic options for the management of menstrual disorders and certain complications of early pregnancy.

SUMMARY

- The network of uterine cells – epithelial, stromal, endothelial – and cells of hemopoietic origin (lymphoid, macrophage, neutrophil) that are responsible for endometrial proliferation and differentiation, implantation and menstrual shedding, makes use of a well-developed assemblage of intercellular signal factors (cytokines, growth factors, etc.).
- Estradiol up-regulates and progesterone down-regulates the uterine ER. Administration of an antigestogen in the early luteal phase blocks the progesterone-induced down-regulation of sex steroid receptors in non-pregnant human endometrium.
- Changes in sex steroid receptor distribution during the cycle are consistent with known physiological roles of the uterus: endometrial regeneration, implantation, menstruation, myometrial contractility and normal tubal function (see Table 2.7.1).
- Withdrawal of progesterone elicits a uterine response with features that are characteristic of an inflammatory response: release of PGs, breakdown of blood vessel walls and an abundance of leucocytes in endometrium.

- Pro-inflammatory cytokines are involved in the maintenance of normal uterine function.
- Progesterone modulates PG activity in endometrium and decidua.
- The number and type of leucocytes in human endometrium and decidua vary with the menstrual cycle, at the time of implantation and during pregnancy. This suggests that both endocrine and paracrine mechanisms control leucocyte migration *to* and replication *within* this tissue.
- Prolactin is synthesized and released from endometrial decidua. The localization of prolactin mRNA to the decidua reinforces the view that decidual prolactin is a functional molecule of endometrial origin.
- The contractility of both the non-pregnant and pregnant human uterus are hormonally regulated; changes in uterine contractility during the menstrual cycle are related to circulating sex steroid concentrations.
- The Fallopian tube is related structurally and functionally to the uterus. Dynamic changes in tubular epithelial structure and function also occur in response to cyclic changes in ovarian steroids.

ACKNOWLEDGEMENTS

I am most grateful to Mr C Gilpin, Biological Sciences Electron Microscope Unit, University of Manchester for providing the illustrations of fallopian tube. Thanks are also due to Mr Tom McFetters and Mr Ted Pinner for assistance with the photomicrographs and to Mrs Vicky Watters for secretarial support.

REFERENCES

1. Healy DL, Hodgen GD. The endocrinology of human endometrium. *Obstet Gynecol Surv* 1983 **38**: 509–530.
2. Carson SA. A summary of normal female reproductive physiology. In Alexander NJ, d'Areangues C (eds) *Steroid Hormones and Uterine Bleeding*. Washington: AAAS Press, 1992.
3. Buckley CH, Fox H. The anatomy and histology of the

endometrium. In Gottlieb LS, Neville AM, Walker F (eds) *Biopsy Pathology of the Endometrium. Biopsy Pathology Series*, Vol. 14. London: Chapman & Hall Medical, 1989: 11–29.

4. Rorie DK, Newton M. Histologic and chemical studies of smooth muscle in the human cervix and uterus. *Am J Obstet Gynecol* 1967 **99**: 466–469.

5. Danforth DN. The morphology of the human cervix. *Clin Obstet Gynecol* 1983 **26**: 7–13.

6. Maguiness SD, Djahanbakhch O, Grudzinskas JG. Assessment of the fallopian tube. *Obstet Gynecol Surv* 1992 **47**: 587–603.

7. Leese HJ, Dickens CJ. Tubal physiology and function. In Templeton AA, Drife JO (eds) *Infertility*. Berlin, Heidelberg: Springer-Verlag, 1992: 157–168.

8. Rothchild I. Role of progesterone in initiating and maintaining pregnancy. In Bardin CW, Milgrom E, Mauvais-Jarvis P (eds) *Progesterone and Progestins*. New York: Raven Press, 1983: 219–229.

9. Noyes RW, Hertig AT, Rock J. Dating the endometrial biopsy. *Fertil Steril* 1950 **1**: 3–25.

10. Giudice LC. Growth factors and growth modulators in human uterine endometrium: their potential relevance to reproductive medicine. *Fertil Steril* 1994 **61**: 1–17.

11. Lessey BA, Killam AP, Metzger DA, Haney AF, Greene GL, McCarty KS. Immunohistochemical analysis of human uterine estrogen and progesterone receptors throughout the menstrual cycle. *J Clin Endocrinol Metab* 1988 **67**: 334–340.

12. Garcia E, Bouchard P, DeBrux J *et al.* Use of immunocytochemistry of progesterone and estrogen receptors for endometrial dating. *J Clin Endocrinol Metab* 1988 **67**: 80–87.

13. Snijders MPML, de Goeij AFPM, Debets-Te Baerts MJC, Rousch MJM, Koudstaal J, Bosman FT. Immunocytochemical analysis of oestrogen receptors and progesterone receptors in the human uterus throughout the menstrual cycle and after the menopause. *J Reprod Fertil* 1992 **94**: 363–371.

14. Critchley HOD, Bailey DA, Au CL, Affandi B, Rogers PAW. Immunohistochemical sex steroid receptor distribution in endometrium from long-term subdermal levonorgestrel users and during the normal menstrual cycle. *Hum Reprod* 1993 **8**: 1632–1639.

15. Chaucherau A, Savouret J-F, Milgrom E. Control of biosynthesis and post-transcriptional modification of progesterone receptor. *Biol Reprod* 1992 **46**: 174–177.

16. Maentausta O, Svalander P, Danielsson KG, Bygdeman M, Vihko R. The effects of an antiprogestin, Mifepristone, and an antiestrogen, Tamoxifen, on endometrial 17β-hydroxysteroid dehydrogenase and progestin and estrogen receptors during the luteal phase of the menstrual cycle: an immunohistochemical study. *J Clin Endocrinol Metab* 1993 **77**: 913–918.

17. Tamaya T, Murakami T, Okada H. Concentrations of steroid receptors in normal human endometrium in relation to the day of the menstrual cycle. *Acta Obstet Gynecol Scand* 1986 **65**: 195–198.

18. Horie K, Takakura K, Imai K, Liao S, Mori T. Immunohistochemical localisation of androgen receptor in the human endometrium, decidua, placenta and pathological conditions of the endometrium. *Hum Reprod* 1992 **7**: 1461–1466.

19. Goodger (Macpherson) AM, Rogers PAW. Endometrial endothelial cell proliferation during the menstrual cycle. *Hum Reprod* 1994 **9**: 399–405.

20. Rogers PAW, Abberton KM, Susil B. Endothelial cell migratory signal produced by human endometrium during the menstrual cycle. *Hum Reprod* 1992 **7**: 1061–1066.

21. Markee JE. Menstruation in intraocular endometrial transplants in the rhesus monkey. *Contrib Embryol Carnegie Inst* 1940 **177**: 219–308.

22. Ferenczy A, Bertrand G, Gelfand MM. Proliferation kinetics of human endometrium during the normal menstrual cycle. *Am J Obstet Gynecol* 1979 **133**: 859–867.

23. Kaiserman-Abramof IR, Padykula HA. Angiogenesis in the postovulatory primate endometrium: the coiled arteriolar system. *Anat Rec* 1989 **224**: 479–489.

24. Clarke CL, Sutherland RL. Progestin regulation of cellular proliferation. *Endocr Rev* 1990 **11**: 266–301.

25. Bouchard P, Marraoui J, Massai MR *et al.* Immunocytochemical localisation of oestradiol and progesterone receptors in human endometrium: a tool to assess endometrial maturation. *Bailliere's Clin Obstet and Gynaecol* 1991 **5**: 107–115.

26. Perrot-Applanat M, Groyer-Picard MT, Garcia E *et al.* Immunocytochemical demonstration of estrogen and progesterone receptors in muscle cells of uterine arteries in rabbits and humans. *Endocrinology* 1988 **123**: 1511–1519.

27. de Ziegler D, Bessis R, Frydman R. Vascular resistance of uterine arteries: physiological effects of estradiol and progesterone. *Fertil Steril* 1991 **55**: 775–779.

28. Perrot-Applanat M, Deng M, Fernandez H, Lelaider C, Meduri G, Bouchard P. Immunohistochemical localisation of oestradiol and progesterone receptors in human uterus throughout pregnancy: expression in endometrial blood vessels. *J Clin Endocrinol Metab* 1994 **78**: 216–224.

29. Wang J-D, Fu Y, Shi W-L *et al.* Immunohistochemical localisation of progesterone receptor in human decidua of early pregnancy. *Hum Reprod* 1992 **7**: 123–127.

30. Shi W-L, Wang J-D, Fu Y, Xu L-K, Zhu P-D. The effect of RU486 on progesterone receptor in villous and extravillous trophoblast. *Hum Reprod* 1993 **8**: 953–958.

31. Clark DA. Cytokines and uterine bleeding. In Alexander NJ, d'Arcangues C (eds) *Steroid Hormones and Uterine Bleeding*. Washington: AAAS Press, 1992: 263–275.

32. Tabibzadeh SS, Satyaswaroop PG. Sex steroid receptors in lymphoid cells of human endometrium. *Am J Clin Pathol* 1989 **91**: 656–663.

33. Garfield RE, Blennerhassett MG, Miller SM. Control of myometrial contractility: Role and regulation of gap junctions. *Oxford Rev Reprod Biol* 1988 **10**: 436–490.

34. Swahn ML, Bygdeman M. The effect of the antiprogestin RU486 on uterine contractility and sensitivity to prostaglandin and oxytocin. *Br J Obstet Gynaecol* 1988 **95**: 126–134.

35. Kelly RW. Pregnancy maintenance and parturition; the role of prostaglandin in manipulating the immune and inflammatory response. *Endocr Rev* 1994 **15**: 684–706.

36. Garfield RE, Yallampalli C. Control of myometrial contractility and labor. In Chwalisz K, Garfield RE (eds) *Basic Mechanisms Controlling Term and Preterm Birth*. Ernst Schering Research Foundation Workshop 7. Berlin, Heidelberg, New York: Springer-Verlag, 1994.

37. Press MF, Nousek-Goebl NA, Bur M, Greene GL. Estrogen receptor localisation in the female genital tract. *Am J Pathol* 1986 **123**: 280–292.

38. Verhage HG, Bareither ML, Jaffe RC, Akbar M. Cyclic changes in ciliation, secretion and cell height of the oviductal epithelium in women. *Am J Anat* 1979 **156**: 505–522.

39. Jansen RPS. Endocrine response in the Fallopian tube. *Endocr Rev* 1984 **5**: 525–551.

40. Land JA, Arends JW. Immunohistochemical analysis of estrogen and progesterone receptors in fallopian tubes during ectopic pregnancy. *Fertil Steril* 1992 **59**: 335–337.

41. Amso NN, Crow J, Shaw RW. Comparative immunohistochemical study of oestrogen and progesterone receptors in the fallopian tube and uterus at different stages of the menstrual cycle and the menopause. *Hum Reprod* 1994 **9**: 1027-1037.

42. Lippes J, Kasner J, Alfonso LA, Dacalos ED, Lucero R. Human oviductal fluids proteins. *Fertil Steril* 1981 **36**: 623–629.

43. Julkunen M, Koistinen R, Suikkari AM, Seppälä M, Jänne OA. Identification by hybridisation histochemistry of human endometrial cells expressing mRNAs encoding a uterine β-lactoglobulin homologue and insulin-like growth factor-binding protein-1. *Mol Endocrinol* 1990 **4**: 700–707.

44. Seppälä M, Koistinen R., Rutanen EM. Uterine endocrinology and paraendocrinology: insulin-like growth factor binding protein-1 and placental protein 14 revisited. *Hum Reprod* 1994 **9**: Suppl 2: 96–106.

45. Giudice LC, Dsupin BA, Irwin JC, Eckert RL. Identification of insulin-like growth factor binding proteins in human oviduct. *Fertil Steril* 1992 **57**: 294–301.

46. Tabibzadeh, S. Human endometrium: an active site of cytokine production and action. *Endocr Rev* 1991 **12**: 272–290.

47. Clark D, Cytokines, decidua, and early pregnancy. *Oxf Rev Reprod Biol* 1993 **15**: 83–111.

48. Hunt JS. Cytokine networks in the utero-placental unit: macrophages as pivotal regulatory cells. *J Reprod Immunol* 1989 **16**: 1–17.

49. Tabibzadeh S, Sun XZ. Cytokine expression in human endometrium throughout the menstrual cycle. *Hum Reprod* 1992 **7**: 1214–1221.

50. Simon C, Piquette GN, Frances A, Polan ML. Localisation of interleukin-1 type receptor and interleukin-1β in human endometrium throughout the menstrual cycle. *J Clin Endocrinol Metab* 1993 **77**: 549–555.

51. Critchley HOD, Kelly RW, Kooy J. Perivascular expression of chemokine interleukin-8 in human endometrium: a preliminary report. *Hum Reprod* 1994 **9**: 1406–1409.

52. Hunt JS, Chien H-L, Hu X-L, Tabibzadeh SS. Tumor necrosis factor-α messenger ribonucleic acid and protein in human endometrium. *Biol Reprod* 1992 **47**: 141–147.

53. Haining RE, Cameron IT, van Papendorf C *et al.* Epidermal growth factor in human endometrium: proliferative effects in culture and immunocytochemical localisation in normal and endometriotic tissues. *Hum Reprod* 1991 **6**: 1200–1205.

54. Murphy LJ, Gong Y, Murphy LC. Growth factors in normal and malignant uterine tissue. *Ann NY Acad Sci* 1991 **622**: 383–401.

55. Cordon-Cardo C, Vlodavsky I, Haimovitz-Friedman A, Hicklin D, Fuks Z. Expression of basic fibroblast growth factor in normal human tissues. *Lab Invest* 1990 **63**: 832–840.

56. Cheng L, Kelly RW, Thong KJ, Hume R, Baird DT. The effect of mifepristone (RU486) on prostaglandin dehydrogenase in decidual and chorionic tissue in early pregnancy. *Hum Reprod* 1993 **8**: 705–709.

57. Cheng L, Kelly RW, Thong KJ, Hume R, Baird DT. The effect of mifepristone (RU486) on the immunohistochemical distribution of prostaglandin E and its metabolite in decidual and chorionic tissue in early pregnancy. *J Clin Endocrinol Metab* 1993 **77**: 873–877.

58. Casey ML, Hemsell DL, Johnston JM, MacDonald PC. NAD dependent 15-hydroxyprostaglandin dehydrogenase activity in human endometrium. *Prostaglandins* 1980 **19**: 115–122.

59. Abel MH, Baird DT. The effect of 17β estradiol and progesterone on prostaglandin production by human endometrium maintained in organ culture. *Endocrinology* 1980 **106**: 1599–1606.

60. Lea RG, Clark DA. Macrophages and migratory cells in endometrium relevant to implantation. *Bailliere's Clin Obstet Gynaecol* 1991 **5**: 25–59.

61. Wang IYS, Fraser IS. Lysosomes: an important mediator in the female reproductive tract. *Obstet Gynecol Surv* 1989 **45**: 18–33.

62. Staples LD, Heap RB, Wooding FBP, King GJ. Migration of leukocytes into the uterus after acute removal of ovarian progesterone during early pregnancy in the sheep. *Placenta* 1983 **4**: 339–350.

63. Bulmer JN, Longfellow M, Ritson A. Leukocytes and resident blood cells in endometrium. *Ann NY Acad Sci* 1991 **622**: 57–68.

64. King A, Loke YW. Uterine large granular lymphocytes: a possible role in embryonic implantation? *Am J Obstet Gynecol* 1990 **162**: 308–310.

65. Tabibzadeh S. Proliferative activity of lymphoid cells in human endometrium throughout the menstrual cycle. *J Clin Endocrinol Metab* 1990 **70**: 437–443.

66. Klentzeris LD, Bulmer JN, Warren A, Morrison L, Li T-C, Cooke ID. Endometrial lymphoid tissue in the timed endometrial biopsy: Morphometric and immunohistochemical aspects. *Am J Obstet Gynecol.* 1992 **167**: 667–674.

67. Marzusch K, Ruck P, Geiselhart A *et al.* Distribution of cell adhesion molecules on CD56⁺⁺,CD3⁻,CD16⁻ large granular lymphocytes and endothelial cells in first-trimester human decidua. *Hum Reprod* 1993 **8**: 1203–1208.

68. Rees MCP, Heryet AR, Bicknell R. Immunohistochemical properties of the endothelial cells in the human uterus during the menstrual cycle. *Hum Reprod* 1993 **8**: 1173–1178.

69. Haller H, Radillo O, Rukavina D *et al.* An immunohistochemical study of leucocytes in human endometrium, first and third trimester basal decidua. *J Reprod Immunol* 1993 **23**: 41–49.

70. Bulmer JN, Lunny DP, Hagin SV. Immunohistochemical characterisation of stromal leucocytes in nonpregnant human endometrium. *Am J Reprod Immunol Microbiol* 1988 **17**: 83–90.

71. Kamat BR, Isaacson PG. The immunocytochemical distribution of leukocytic subpopulations in human endometrium. *Am J Pathol* 1987 **127**: 66–73.

72. Tachi C, Tachi S. Macrophages and implantation. In Yoshinaga K (ed.) Nidation. *Ann NY Acad Sci* 1986 **476**: 158–182.

73. Healy DL, Salamonsen L, Moon J, Cameron IT, Findlay JK. Human endometrial prolactin. In D'Arcangues C, Fraser IS, Newton JR, Odlind V (eds) *Contraception and Mechanisms of Endometrial Bleeding.* Cambridge: Cambridge University Press, 1990: 213–221.

74. Wu W-X, Brooks J, Millar MR *et al.* Localisation of the sites of synthesis and action of prolactin by immunocytochemistry and *in-situ* hydridisation within the human utero-placental unit. *J Mol Endocrinol* 1991 **7**: 241–247.

75. Wu W-X, Glasier A, Norman J, Kelly RW, Baird DT, McNeilly AS. The effects of the antiprogestin mifepristone, *in vivo*, and progesterone, *in vitro*, on prolactin production by the human decidua in early pregnancy. *Hum Reprod* 1990 **5**: 627–631.

76. Bonhoff A, Gellersen B. Modulation of prolactin secretion in human myometrium by cytokines. *Eur J Obstet Gynecol Reprod Biol* 1994 **54**: 55–62.

77. Rees MCP, Parry DM, Anderson ABM, Turnbull AC. Immunohisto-chemical localisation of cyclo-oxygenase in the human uterus. *Prostaglandins* 1982 **23**: 207–214.

2.8

Puberty

K Oerter Klein and GB Cutler Jr

INTRODUCTION

Puberty is the series of physiological and chemical events that leads to the development of secondary sex characteristics, growth spurt, psychological changes, and fertility. This process increases the activity of the hypothalamic–pituitary–gonadal axis so that the gonads are stimulated to produce adult levels of sex steroids. 'Puberty is the final stage of two decades of reproductive development and maturation.'[1] Understanding puberty, its initiation and its progression, is a necessary background to understanding the end result of puberty – a fully mature adult.

CURRENT CONCEPTS

Development

The hypothalamic–pituitary–gonadal axis becomes functional during fetal development, continues during early infancy, is inhibited during childhood, and is reactivated at the time of puberty.

Fetal

The morphogenesis of the hypothalamic–pituitary unit is complete by mid-gestation, but functional maturation is not complete until after birth. By 14 weeks' gestation all the hypothalamic nuclei are present.[2] By 14.5 weeks the hypothalamic–pituitary portal system is intact (see Chapter 2.2). Luteinizing hormone releasing hormone (LHRH) is present by 8 weeks gestation. This development is independent of the maternal hypothalamic–pituitary unit. Maternal LHRH and gonadotropins are not transferred across the placenta. Luteinizing hormone (LH) and follicle-stimulating hormone (FSH) reach peak levels

at mid-gestation and then decrease to low levels by term (Fig. 2.8.1). The female fetus has higher FSH levels than does the male.[3] The inhibition of LH and FSH secretion in late gestation appears to be the result of negative feedback by high levels of estrogen and progesterone in the fetal circulation.

Plasma levels of progesterone rise progressively during fetal life with no apparent sex difference. In contrast, 17α-hydroxyprogesterone levels are higher in cord blood of girls than boys. Levels fall rapidly after birth in both sexes. In boys, levels rise until the second month of life and then fall to prepubertal levels by seven months of age. In girls, levels do not start to decrease until one to four months of age and do so more slowly. Between one and two years, 17α-hydroxyprogesterone levels are the lowest and there is no sex difference.

Fetal levels of estrone and estradiol rise progressively throughout gestation in both boys and girls.[4] Estrone and estradiol fall rapidly during the first five days of life. Estrone levels remain low throughout infancy and childhood. Estradiol levels increase during the first two months in boys, and the first four to twelve months in girls. There is wide variation in estradiol levels from children with low levels early in life to children with high levels persisting up to two years.[5]

Testosterone secretion begins early in gestation and reaches a peak at 10 to 18 weeks.

Prolactin is secreted by the fetal pituitary such that by the third fetal month levels are in the adult normal range. Cord prolactin levels are usually greater than those in maternal blood. Plasma levels remain elevated during the first day of postnatal life and then fall rapidly over the next seven days. Prolactin levels continue to fall over the next two to three months until they reach prepubertal levels.[6]

Infancy

During the first few days to one week after birth, the concentration of human chorionic gonadotropin (hCG) and placenta steroids fall.[7,8] This fall is followed by an increase

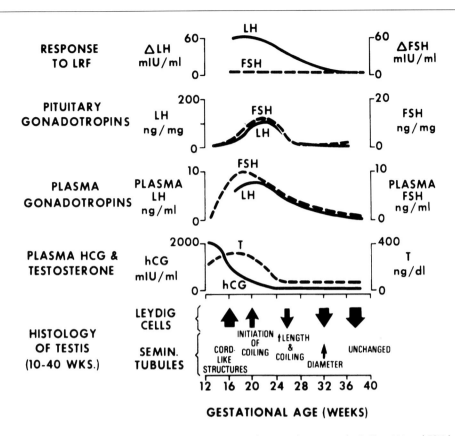

Fig. 2.8.1 *Comparison of the pattern of change of serum testosterone, hCG, and serum and pituitary LH and FSH levels in the human male fetus during gestation in relation to the morphological changes in fetal testis. The top graph illustrates the regression curve for the increment between a baseline plasma LH and FSH level and the 15-min response to administration of LHRH to the male fetus plotted as a function of gestational age. (Modified from reference 70.)*

in plasma LH and FSH. FSH rises to a peak at 3 months in both boys and girls, but reaches a much higher peak in girls and remains elevated longer, up to two years. LH levels increase in both sexes by the second week of life and remain elevated during the first 4–6 months of life in both boys and girls. Maximal levels of LH are observed in girls by the third month and then decrease by the end of the first year of life. In boys, LH levels are highest between one to four months and then decrease during the first year.

LH and FSH are secreted in a pulsatile pattern during infancy, childhood and puberty.[9] The amplitude and frequency of FSH pulses are greater in girls, and the amplitude and frequency of LH pulses are greater in boys (Fig. 2.8.2). The nocturnal augmentation of secretion described in the prepubertal and pubertal period has not been described in infancy.

The pituitary is responsive to LHRH stimulation immediately after birth, but more so after the third day of life. The response is primarily LH predominant in boys and FSH predominant in girls. FSH levels are 8 to 10 times higher in girls than in boys.[10] The FSH response to LHRH is higher during the first six months of life than at any time thereafter. After six months the response decreases gradually over the next two years.

Plasma testosterone levels in boys increase to a peak at 6–15 weeks and then decrease to low levels by 6 months. In girls, testosterone levels decrease in the first week of life and remain low. Estradiol levels in girls are elevated during the first 6–12 months after birth. There is wide variability among girls and estradiol levels may remain elevated up to two years.

Prepubertal period

The inhibitory stage preceding puberty lasts from late infancy through most of childhood. It is characterized by relatively high FSH levels in relation to LH levels, and a low pituitary responsiveness to LHRH. There is only a slight increase in gonadotropins in agonadal children.

Pulsatility and nocturnal augmentation of gonadotropin secretion were previously thought to occur only after the onset of puberty. With the increased use of sensitive and specific radioimmunoassays, pulsatile gonadotropin secretion was observed during prepuberty as well as puberty.[11,12]

Pubertal period

The pattern of gonadotropin secretion during puberty is controlled both by LHRH secretion and by feedback inhibition from sex steroids. FSH appears to be more

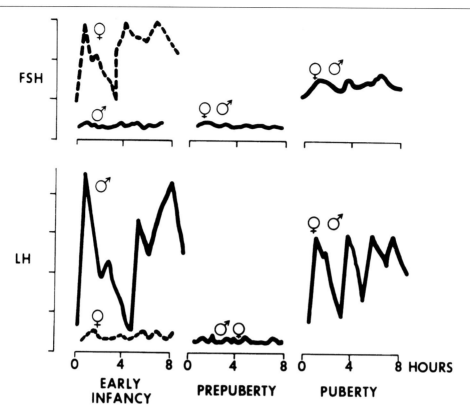

Fig. 2.8.2 *The change in the pattern of pulsatile FSH and LH secretion. (Data from reference 9.)*

influenced by sex steroid feedback, and LH more dependent on LHRH pulses.[13,14]

LH, FSH, testosterone, and testicular volume all rise continuously with age once puberty starts. Estradiol remains undetectable with most currently available radioimmunoassays (RIAs) until the end of puberty. Prolactin levels are stable throughout puberty in boys, but increase until after menarche in girls.

The pulsatility of LHRH has been studied indirectly by measuring LH and FSH pulsatility. During puberty the LHRH pulse amplitude is higher than it was prepubertally. Puberty represents an augmentation of gonadotropin release rather than an initiation of gonadotropin release. In prepubertal children, a pubertal pattern of gonadotropin secretion can be induced by pulsatile administration of LHRH.[15]

Boyar *et al.* first described the nocturnal augmentation of gonadotropin secretion in early and mid-puberty.[16] Daytime pulses were detected by late puberty. Oerter *et al.* described increasing mean LH and FSH levels with increasing pubertal stage as well as nocturnal augmentation during stages 1 to 4 of puberty in girls and boys (Figs. 2.8.3 and 2.8.4).[17] They also showed that the LHRH-stimulated peak LH to peak FSH ratio was greater in boys than girls during pubertal stages 1–3.[17]

Adrenarche

The increase in sex steroids results from two independent processes, gonadarche and adrenarche. Adrenarche is a maturational change in adrenal function that causes increased adrenal secretion of androgens and estrogens. Adrenarche precedes gonadarche by several years. Adrenarche causes an increase in the adrenal secretion of dehydroepiandrosterone (DHA), DHA sulfate (DHAS), androstenediol, androstenedione, testosterone, estrone, pregnenolone and 17-hydroxypregnenolone. DHA and DHAS are derived almost entirely from the adrenal gland, whereas the other steroids come from both adrenals and gonads. Mean plasma DHEA increases steadily from age 5 to 20 in boys and girls. Estrone follows a similar pattern in boys suggesting that it originates primarily from the adrenal. Androstenedione increases more rapidly once puberty starts, because of its derivation from both adrenal and gonadal sources. Adrenarche is no longer thought to play a role in the control of the onset of puberty.

The adrenal androgens cause pubic hair and axillary hair development. There is also a small effect of androgens on growth and bone maturation.

Adrenarche and gonadarche are both part of normal puberty, but they appear to be independent processes, as one can occur without the other in pathological states.

The mechanism of onset of adrenarche is unknown. Estrogen, cortisol, LH, prolactin, growth hormone, pro-opiomelanocortin-derived peptides, pituitary adrenal androgen-stimulating hormone, or genetic programming of the adrenal gland have all been proposed as mechanisms to initiate adrenarche.[18]

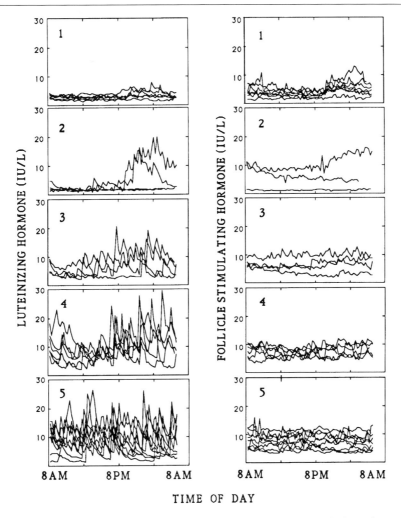

Fig. 2.8.3 *LH and FSH profiles for girls over 24 hours. Girls in each pubertal stage are graphed together to convey the overall temporal pattern of gonadotropin secretion. (From reference 17, with permission.)*

Theories on the onset of puberty

The control of the onset of puberty is not yet well understood. Several hypotheses are presented here. The timing of the onset of puberty is related more to bone age than to chronological age.

LHRH neurons receive synaptic contacts from several neurotransmitter systems including noradrenergic, dopaminergic, γ-aminobutryric acid (GABA)ergic and opioid neurons. Whether all these synaptic connections are needed for puberty is not known. The morphology of the LHRH neurons does change during development.

Knobil and colleagues studied the GnRH pulse generator using techniques of multiunit electrical activity (MUA). They placed electrodes in the medial basal hypothalamus. MUA was coincident with the initiation of LH pulses in the periphery.[19]

Gonadostat

A clock-driven rhythm is characterized as a regularly occurring event with a predictable repeat time. A clock can run at various speeds and can be reset. The biological rhythms described for gonadotropins include circadian rhythms and ultradian rhythms. A constant source of light blocks the circadian rhythm of LH secretion in the rat, but does not interfere with the pulsatility of LH.[20]

Central inhibitor

The CNS is widely believed to exercise the only major restraint on the onset of puberty. The neuroendocrine control of puberty is mediated by the hypothalamic GnRH neurons, which act as an endogenous pulse generator. This pulse generator functions at a low level of activity in the

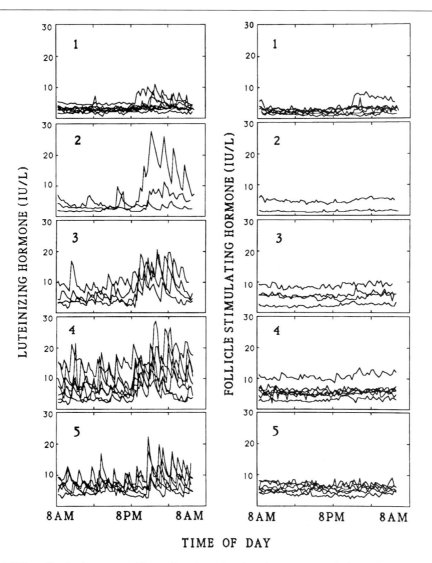

Fig. 2.8.4 *LH and FSH profiles for boys over 24 hours. Boys in each pubertal stage are graphed together to convey the overall temporal pattern of gonadotropin secretion. (From reference 17, with permission.)*

prepubertal child. At puberty this oscillator is hypothesized to be reactivated or disinhibited.

LHRH acts via plasma membrane receptors to stimulate LH release. Regulation of the receptors occurs via changes in the rate of secretion of LHRH. The gonadotropins are secreted from the pituitary in response to pulses of LHRH, whereas a continuous infusion of LHRH inhibits gonadotropin secretion. Estrogen also feeds back on the pituitary to inhibit gonadotropin release.[10]

Negative feedback

The negative feedback ('gonadostat') hypothesis proposes that the hypothalamic–pituitary unit is exquisitely sensitive to suppression by low levels of sex steroids in the prepubertal period. As sex steroid receptors in the hypothalamus and pituitary mature, this inhibition decreases. Evidence for this hypothesis is found in the syndromes of gonadal dysgenesis in which gonadotropin levels increase at the

expected age of puberty (Fig. 2.8.5) and the gonadotropin response to LHRH stimulation is augmented.[21]

Intrinsic inhibition

Evidence for an intrinsic inhibition in contrast to a sex-steroid dependent negative feedback mechanism lies in the fact that agonadal children have low levels of gonadotropins during the childhood years after the initially elevated levels during infancy.

Inhibition of the hypothalamic–pituitary unit is lost in some CNS lesions, which has been hypothesized to result from the destruction of inhibitory neural pathways.

A combination of negative feedback and intrinsic inhibition may exist (Fig. 2.8.6). Grumbach *et al.*[22] propose that the negative feedback mechanism is dominant during the first 2 to 3 years of life and that intrinsic inhibition is dominant from that point through the prepubertal period. After pubertal onset, the intrinsic inhibition has been

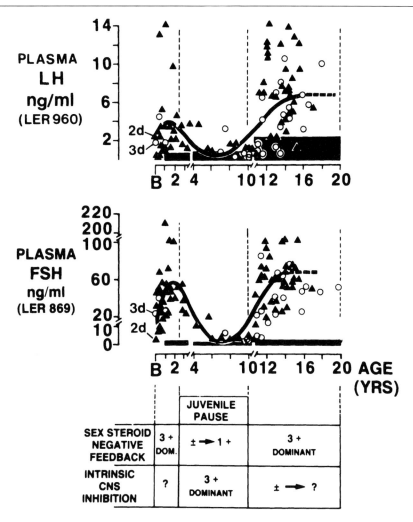

Fig. 2.8.5 *Interaction of the negative feedback mechanism and the putative intrinsic CNS inhibitory mechanism in restraining puberty as extrapolated from the pattern of change in the concentrations of FSH and LH in agonadal infants, children, and adolescents. Triangles designate patients with 45,X karyotype; circles indicate patients with X chromosome mosaicism or structural abnormalities. (Modified from reference 22, with permission.)*

removed and the negative feedback system is again in place to regulate adult sex steroid levels.

Cell bodies elaborating LHRH are located in the mediobasal hypothalamus (see Chapter 2.2). The major group of these neurons projects to neurovascular junctions in the median eminence and supplies the peptide to the pituitary. A minor group of neurons projects to the telencephalon and the mid-brain where LHRH has been shown to evoke postsynaptic potentials and participate in the regulation of sex behavior.[23] Noradrenergic neurons have been shown in close proximity to LHRH cell bodies. A dense population of GABA-containing interneurons has been shown to innervate LHRH cell bodies and establish connections with the noradrenergic fibers.[24,25] A few dopaminergic nerve terminals are also believed to innervate the GnRH neurons, but most dopamine-containing fibers interact with LHRH fibers in the median eminence. β-endorphin-containing fibers connect the arcuate nucleus with LHRH fibers in the median eminence and, to a lesser

extent, with LHRH neurons located in the arcuate nucleus and the preoptic area.[26]

'Immortalized' mouse LHRH neurons have been found to release LHRH in a pulsatile fashion only after they are allowed to form cell–cell interconnections, suggesting that LHRH neurons *in vivo* form a discrete network that is capable of pulsatile LHRH release.[27]

LHRH neurons also receive input from corticotropin-releasing factor (CRF)-containing fibers from the paraventricular nucleus. The turnover rate of noradrenalin correlates with circulating LH levels, whereas the turnover of GABA decreases as gonadotropin secretion increases.[28]

Dopamine, GABA, and opiate peptides have been shown to inhibit LH pulsatility. GABA, dopamine, and β-endorphin neurons have also shown the ability to express receptors for steroid hormones, which is consistent with the hypothesis that they play a role in controlling pulsatility of LHRH neurons.

Opioids have been observed to suppress the frequency

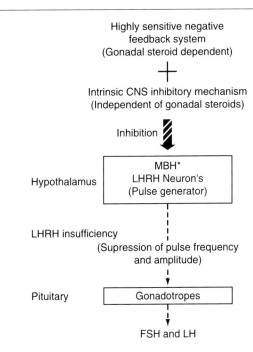

Fig. 2.8.6 *Postulated dual mechanism of restraint of puberty involving gonadal steroid-dependent and gonadal steroid-independent processes. MBH, medical basal hypothalamus. (Modified from reference 22, with permission.)*

and amplitude of LH pulsatile secretion *in vitro* and *in vivo* by a direct action on opiate receptors on LHRH neurons.[29] Studies of the effect of naloxone, an opioid receptor blocker, on prepubertal gonadotropin secretion showed no effect in five children studied.[30]

Melatonin from the pineal gland has been studied as a candidate for the inhibitor of the LHRH pulse generator. This hypothesis is considered unlikely after several studies of pinealectomies in animals,[31] melatonin levels in prepubertal and pubertal children,[32,33] and the discovery that precocious puberty from tumors in the pineal region is mediated by hCG production by the tumors.

Ojeda *et al.*[34] have studied the possibility that pubertal onset is determined by the activation of neurotransmitter systems. One system involves excitatory amino acids that exert their effects via specific receptors. A class of these receptors binds selectively the analog of aspartic acid, *N*-methyl-D-aspartic acid (NMDA). Ojeda *et al.* administered NMDA to rats prior to puberty and observed an increase in LH secretion and an earlier onset of puberty.[34] They also showed that an antagonist of NMDA blocked LH secretion and delayed the onset of puberty in rats.

Nerve growth factor (NGF) is expressed in the developing hypothalamus. The direct effects of NGF are not known. Epidermal growth factor (EGF) and transforming growth factor-α (TGF-α) stimulate LHRH secretion from median eminence fragments *in vitro*.

Nutrition

The age of menarche is affected by nutrition, weight, exercise, stress, high altitude, and other factors (see Chapter 2.9).[35,36]

The age of menarche has decreased at a rate of two to three months per decade between 1950 and 1980. It has been suggested that this is secondary to improved nutrition and life style.[37,38] Conditions that lead to weight loss, such as anorexia, tend to delay or interrupt puberty. The onset of menarche is correlated not only with weight but with percentage of body fat.[39] In women with anorexia nervosa, LH and FSH secretion is low, suggesting a central mechanism for control of their menses.[40] In contrast, moderate obesity is associated with earlier menarche, but pathological obesity is associated with delayed menarche.[41]

A large energy expenditure may delay puberty. The amount of delay appears to be related to the amount of exercise prior to menarche. The combination of nutritional restriction and increased exercise compounds the delay, as is seen in ballet dancers. Whereas athletic performance is better in sexually immature girls, the superior athletes among boys tend to be more advanced in puberty.[42]

Chronic illness, such as uremia, regional enteritis, ulcerative colitis, congenital heart disease, cystic fibrosis and diabetes, can delay pubertal maturation.

The effect of stress on pubertal onset is difficult to study objectively. Personality profiles have shown that ammenorrhea occurs more often in stressed athletes.[43]

The mechanisms for delayed pubertal progression in each of the above situations are unknown. Hormonal changes, however, are similar among the different conditions associated with delayed puberty: glucose and insulin decrease, whereas glucagon, growth hormone, prolactin, cortisol, β-endorphin, and catecholamines increase. T4 does not change but T3 decreases and reverse T3 increases. TSH decreases with food restriction and increases with exercise. Gonadotropin secretion is decreased for age.

Effects of puberty

The normal sequence of pubertal changes in girls is breast budding between 8 and 13 years (Fig 2.8.7), onset of pubic hair several months later, peak growth velocity between 9.5 and 14.5 years, and menarche between 10 and 16.5 years. Other physical changes include adult body odor, acne, oily skin, and vaginal discharge. The average occurrence of ovulation is ten months after menarche.

The normal sequence of pubertal changes in boys is the onset of testicular growth between 9.5 and 13.5 years, the onset of pubic hair, penile growth between 10.5 and 14.5 years (Fig. 2.8.8), and peak growth velocity between 10.5 and 17.5 years. Other physical changes include adult body odor, acne, oily skin, deep voice, erections, increased muscle strength and development of facial and body hair.

Growth

Prepubertal growth velocity is nearly identical in both sexes.[44] Growth is most rapid in the fetus and in early

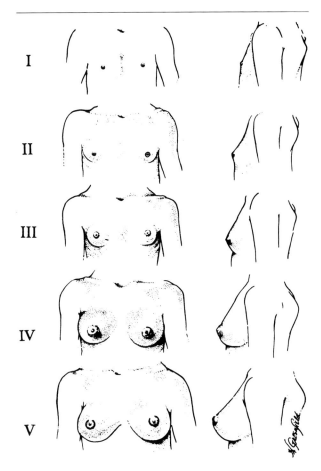

I

II

III

IV

V

Fig. 2.8.7 *Stages of breast development according to Tanner. Stage I, prepubertal; no breast tissue. Stage II, breast bud with diameter no greater than areola. Stage III, further enlargement of breast to greater than areola. Stage IV, projection of areola and papilla to form secondary mound. Stage V, fully mature breast; projection of papilla only. (Redrawn from reference 71.)*

infancy, decreases quickly over the first two years of life, then declines slowly to its lowest growth velocity just prior to the onset of the pubertal growth spurt. The pubertal growth spurt is earlier and slightly smaller in girls compared to boys.

The greater adult height in men than in women is attributable to the greater peak velocity at puberty in boys and the delayed epiphyseal fusion in boys.

There is no growth spurt in the absence of sex steroids. The onset of the growth spurt corresponds to the onset of gonadarche rather than adrenarche, suggesting that it is the gonadal sex steroids rather than the adrenal steroids that are stimulating growth.

Evidence for links between sex steroids and GH

Linear growth is most rapid *in utero* and immediately after birth. Growth rate quickly declines during the first two years of life and then increases again at puberty.[45,46] The timing and magnitude of the pubertal growth spurt is different for girls and boys, with an average peak growth

velocity of 9.4 ± 2.4 cm/year at 13.5 years in boys, and an average peak growth velocity of 8.3 ± 2.1 cm/year at 11.5 years in girls. Growth hormone (GH) and sex steroids are both changing during puberty and both influence growth during that period. Boys on GH therapy were reported to have a decreased growth velocity during puberty when their growth hormone was discontinued.[47] In GH-deficient hypogonadal boys, both testosterone replacement and GH replacement are necessary for normal pubertal growth velocities.[48] Low-dose estrogen increases growth in pre-pubertal boys.[49]

Mean 24-hour GH levels increase during puberty in both girls and boys with the highest levels at mid-puberty. The increase begins before the onset of breast budding in girls and slightly later in boys.[50]

In boys, mean 24-hour GH levels are highest in late puberty.[51] The pubertal growth spurt corresponds to the changes in GH concentration. Insulin-like growth factor-1 (IGF-1) levels follow the same pattern of increase during late puberty. Androgen[52,53] and estrogen[54] have been shown to stimulate GH release.

IGF-1 levels rise during puberty and decline in adulthood in association with the pubertal growth spurt.[55–57] Administration of testosterone or estradiol to hypogonadal children increases IGF-1 to pubertal levels.[58] It has been suggested that IGF binding protein-1 (IGFBP-1) may also play a role in the initiation of puberty.[59]

Optimal growth is only possible if both sex steroids and GH are present. Aynsley-Green *et al.*[60] studied five groups of boys to resolve the influences of testosterone and GH. One group had isolated gonadotropin deficiency; a second group had congenital anorchia or absence of testes; the third had gonadotropin deficiency and GH deficiency, and were treated with GH; the fourth had gonadotropin deficiency and GH deficiency, and were not treated with GH; and the fifth group were normal. All groups except the control group were treated with testosterone to initiate puberty. The growth spurt was greatest in the isolated gonadotropin deficiency and the anorchia groups. The growth spurt was modest in the GH-treated group and very slight in the GH-deficient group.

Other hormones

Testosterone and estradiol are reversibly bound to testosterone-binding globulin (TeBG) (also known as sex-hormone binding globulin (SHBG); see Chapter 2.5). TeBG levels are similar in girls and boys before puberty. TeBG levels decrease as puberty progresses. This decrease is smaller in girls than in boys.

Inhibin is produced by the Sertoli cells of the testes and the granulosa cells of the ovary. Inhibin exerts a negative feedback on the secretion of FSH from the pituitary. FSH in turn stimulates production of inhibin (see Chapters 2.3 and 2.5).

Anti-Müllerian hormone (AMH) is produced by the Sertoli cells of the fetal testis and by the granulosa cells of the fetal ovary (see Chapter 2.1). Levels are high in newborn boys, rise soon after birth, decrease by age 10, and decrease further during puberty. Newborn girls have

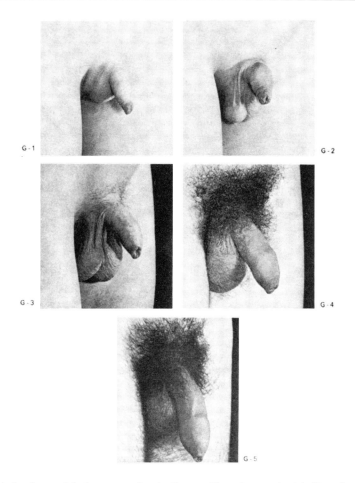

Fig. 2.8.8 *Stages of genital development in boys according to Tanner. Stage 1, prepubertal. Stage 2, scrotum and testicles have enlarged; scrotum is reddened and textured; sparse pubic hair. Stage 3, further enlargement of testicles; growth of penis; pubic hair crosses midline. Stage 4, continued enlargement of testicles and penis with darkening of scrotum and extension of pubic hair. Stage 5, fully mature; pubic hair extends to thighs. (From reference 71.)*

undetectable levels which may increase slightly at puberty.[61]

Fasting insulin levels increase two- to threefold with peak height velocity, and insulin secretion after a glucose load increases, suggesting insulin resistance.[62]

Testosterone increases serum low-density lipoprotein (LDL) cholesterol and decreases high-density lipoprotein (HDL) cholesterol concentrations.[63]

Acquisition of reproductive competence

Primordial follicles appear during the fourth month of fetal development and continue to be formed until about six months postnatally.[64] After that time, no new follicles are formed.[65] At the time of puberty, growth of the follicle resumes and the follicle undergoes characteristic changes (see Chapters 2.1 and 2.4). There is evidence in animals and humans for anovulatory cycles that begin before the onset of ovulation.[66,67]

The onset of spermatogenesis and a rise in testosterone production occurs at the time of puberty. Before puberty the germ cells in the testes are prespermatogonia. Spermatogenesis is signaled by the development and maturation of spermatogonia from a series of mitotic divisions. The onset is related to the sharp rise in testosterone production. The onset is also associated with the maturation of Sertoli cells and the formation of the blood–testes barrier (see Chapter 2.6). A rise of FSH levels correlates with the maturation of Sertoli cells. The mechanism by which FSH acts on Sertoli cells is not yet understood.

The Leydig cells also hypertrophy at puberty. These changes are associated with the sharp rise in testosterone production. The first recognizable change associated with early pubertal testicular development is a rise in FSH. This eventually leads to changes in the Sertoli cells described above. Subsequently, there is a rise in LH and the changes in Leydig cells and the rise in testosterone follows (see Chapter 2.5). Spermatogonia then begin to appear. Spermaturia and the first conscious ejaculation occur between 12 and 14 years.

Behavioral changes

Infants go through a phase of heightened concern with their genitalia often accompanied by masturbation efforts. This phase does not last long and the child goes into a latency period which lasts 6 to 7 years before the onset of puberty. The relationship between these behavioral changes and the hormonal changes in infancy and puberty has not been studied longitudinally.

The relationship of psychopathology to puberty has been looked at by Weiner and Del Gaudio.[68] Neurosis showed a female preponderance throughout puberty. Personality disorders showed a male preponderance until age 15 years. Attempted suicide increases abruptly in females by age 14 years. The evidence linking the physical and hormonal changes of puberty to the increased rate of depression in female adults compared to male adults, in contrast to the equivalent rates of depression between prepubertal girls and boys has been reviewed.[16]

Uniform crime reports indicate a peak of behaviors such as arson and vandalism at age 13–14 years, whereas assaults, robbery, murder, and sex offenses peak at 17–18 years. The frequency of all these crimes decreases thereafter except for assault, murder and sex offenses which remain high into the 20s.

FUTURE PERSPECTIVES

LHRH regulation The future is sure to hold advances in understanding of the LHRH neurons and their regulation at the cellular and physiological levels. Important avenues of research include the mechanisms governing the differentiation of LHRH neurons in the olfactory placode, their migration to the hypothalamus, and their cell surface receptors and mechanisms of signal transduction. An unanswered fundamental question is what molecular differences distinguish the pubertal from the prepubertal LHRH neuron.

Estrogen levels New assays are being developed to measure levels of estradiol substantially lower than those which can currently be detected by conventional radioimmunoassay. This will be of great help in understanding gonadal changes in the prepubertal and pubertal periods, and in evaluating disorders of puberty.

Factors that influence pubertal onset and progression The control of the onset of puberty is not yet understood. The relationship between LHRH regulation, bone growth, and changes in other hormones and growth factors continues to be studied. Further study of abnormalities of puberty will continue to lead to greater understanding of the mechanism of normal puberty.

SUMMARY

- Puberty is the series of physiological and hormonal events that leads to the development of secondary sex characteristics, the pubertal growth spurt, adolescent psychological changes, and fertility.
- The hypothalamic–pituitary–gonadal axis becomes functional during fetal development, is activated during early infancy, is inhibited during childhood, and is reactivated at the time of puberty.
- LH and FSH are secreted in a pulsatile pattern in infancy as well as childhood and puberty. Nocturnal augmentation of gonadotropin secretion occurs in both the prepubertal and pubertal periods. At the completion of puberty gonadotropin secretion is nearly the same during the day and night.
- The mechanisms controling the onset of puberty are not known. Theories include the release from a central inhibitor and a developmental decrease of sex steroid negative feedback. There is a wide range in the normal time of onset and rate of progression through puberty.

- Nutritional status affects the timing and progression of normal puberty.
- Puberty is accompanied by a pubertal growth spurt. This increase in growth velocity is greater in boys and occurs earlier in girls. The spurt is initiated by gonadal sex steroids and requires the presence of growth hormone.
- Adrenarche is a maturational change in adrenal function that causes increased adrenal secretion of androgens and estrogens. Adrenarche precedes gonadarche by several years.
- Adrenarche and gonadarche are both part of normal puberty, but they appear to be independent processes, as one can occur without the other in pathological states.
- Fundamental areas of current research include the mechanisms of the differentiation, migration, and signal transduction of the LHRH neuron.
- An unresolved issue is whether puberty can be explained entirely by different regulatory inputs to the LHRH neurons, or whether the LHRH neurons themselves undergo fundamental changes in their electrophysiological properties, such as by the expression of new ion channels.

REFERENCES

1. Forest MG. Pituitary gonadotropin and sex steroid secretion during the first two years of life. In Grumbach MM, Sizonenko PC, Aubert ML (eds) *Control of the Onset of Puberty II.* Baltimore: Williams and Wilkins, 1990: 451–478.
2. Thliveris JA, Currie RW. Observations on the hypothalamic-hypophyseal portal vasculature in the developing human fetus. *Am J Anat* 1980 157: 441–444.
3. Grumbach MM, Kaplan SL. Ontogenesis of growth hormone, insulin, prolactin, and gonadotropin secretion in the human foetus. In Cross KW, Nathanielsz PW (eds) *Fetal and Neonatal Physiology.* Cambridge: Cambridge University Press, 1973: 462–487.
4. Reyes FI, Borditsky RS, Winter JSD, Faiman C. Studies on human sexual development. II. Fetal and maternal serum gonadotropin and sex steroid concentrations. *J Clin Endocrinol Metab* 1974 38: 612–617.
5. Winter JSD, Faiman C, Hobson WC, Prasad Av, Reves FI. Pituitary–gonadal relations in infancy 2. Patterns of serum gonadal steroid concentrations in man from birth to two years of age. *J Clin Endocrinol Metab* 1976 42: 679–686.
6. Aubert MIL, Sizonenko PC, Kaplan SL *et al.* The ontogenesis of human prolactin from fetal life to puberty. In: Crosignani PG, Robyn C (eds) *Prolactin and Human Reproduction.* New York: Academic Press, 1977: 9–20.
7. Winter JSD, Faiman C, Hobson WC, Prasad Av, Reves FI. Pituitary–gonadal relations in infancy 1. Patterns of serum gonadotropin concentrations from birth to four years of age in man and chimpanzee. *J Clin Endocrinol Metab* 1975 40: 515–554.
8. Forest MG, Sizonenko PC, Cathiard AM, Bertrand J. Hypophysogonadal function in infants during the first year of life. I. Evidence for testicular activity in early infancy. *J Clin Invest* 1974 53: 819–828.
9. Waldhauser F, Weissenbacher G, Frisch H, Prich Z. Pulsatile secretory pattern of gonadotropins in infants. *Pediatr Res* 1980 15: 77.
10. Garnier PE, Chaussain JL, Biner E, Schlumberger A, Job JC. Effect of synthetic luteinizing hormone-releasing hormone on the release of gonadotropins in children and adolescents. VI. Relations to age, sex, and puberty. *Acta Endocrinol (Copenh)* 1974 77: 422–434.
11. Kulin HE, Moore RG Jr, Santner SJ Jr. Circadian rhythms in gonadotropin excretion in prepubertal and pubertal children. *J Clin Endocrinol Metab* 1976 42: 770–773.
12. Jakacki RI, Kelch RP, Sauder SE, Lloyd JS, Hopwood NJ, Marshall JC. Pulsatile secretion of luteinizing hormone in children. *J Clin Endocrinol Metab* 1982 55: 453–458.
13. Marshall JC, Case GD, Valk TW, Corley KP, Sauder SE, Kelch RP. Selective inhibition of follicle-stimulating hormone secretion by estradiol. Mechanism for modulation of gonadotropin responses to low dose pulses of gonadotropin-releasing hormone. *J Clin Invest* 1983 71: 248–257.
14. Goji K. Twenty-four hour concentration profiles of gonadotropin and estradiol (E2) in prepubertal and early pubertal girls: the diurnal rise of E2 is opposite the nocturnal rise of gonadotropin. *J Clin Encocrinol Metab* 1993 77: 1629–1635.
15. Corley KP, Valk TW, Kelch RP, Marshall JC. Estimation of GnRH pulse amplitude during pubertal development. *Pediatr Res* 1981 15: 157–162.
16. Boyar RM, Wu RH, Roffwarg H, Kapen S, Weitzman ED, Hellman L, Finkelstein JW. Human puberty: 24-hour estradiol in pubertal girls. *J Clin Endocrinol Metab* 1976 43: 1418–1421.
17. Oerter KE, Uriarte MM, Rose SR, Barnes KM, Cutler GB Jr. Gonadotropin secretory dynamics during puberty in normal girls and boys. *J Clin Endocrinol Metab* 1990 71: 1251–1258.
18. Cutler GB Jr, Schiebinger RJ, Albertson BD *et al.* The adrenarche (human and animal). In Grumbach MM, Sizonenko PC, Aubert ML (eds) *Control of the Onset of Puberty II.* Baltimore: Williams and Wilkins, 1990: 506–533.
19. Knobil E, Hotchkiss J. In Knobil E, Neill JD (eds) *The Physiology of Reproduction.* New York: Raven Press 1988: 1971–1994.
20. Watts AG, Fink G. Constant light blocks diurnal but not pulsatile release of luteinizing hormone in the ovariectomized rat. *J Endocrinol* 1981 89: 111–116.
21. Conte FA, Grumbach MM, Kaplan SL. A diphasic pattern of gonadotropin secretion in patients with the syndrome of gonadal dysgenesis. *J Clin Endocrinol Metab* 1980 40: 670–674.
22. Grumbach MM, Kaplan SL. The neuroendocrinology of human puberty: an ontogenetic perspective. In Grumbach MM, Sizonenko PC, Aubert ML (eds) *Control of the Onset of Puberty.* Baltimore: Williams and Wilkins, 1990: 1–68.
23. Pfaff DW. Luteinizing hormone-releasing factor potentiates lordosis behavior in hypophysectomized ovariectomized female rats. *Science* 1973 182: 1148–1149.
24. Leranth C, Maclusky N, Salamoto H, Shanabrough M, Naftolin F. Glutamic acid decarboxylase-containing axons synapse on LHRH neurons in the rat medial preoptic area. *Neuorendocrinology* 1985 40: 536–539.
25. Flugge G, Oertel W, Wuttke W. Evidence for estrogen-receptive GABAergic neurons in the preoptic/anterior hypothalamic area of the rat brain. *Neuorendocrinology* 1986 43: 1–5.
26. Swanson LW, Sawchenko PE, Rivier J, Vale W, Organization of ovine corticotropin-releasing factor immunoreactive cells and fibers in the rat brain: an immunohistochemical study. *Neuroendocrinology* 1983 36: 165–186.
27. Martinez de la Escalera G, Choi AL, Weiner RI. Generation and synchronization of gonadotropin-releasing hormone (GnRH) pulses: intrinsic properties of the GT1-1 GnRH neuronal cell line. *Proc Natl Acad Sci USA* 1992 89: 1852–1855.
28. Fuchs E, Mansky T, Stock K, Vijayan E, Wuttke W. Involvement of catecholamines and glutamate in GABAergic mechanism regulatory to luteinizing hormone and prolactin secretion. *Neuroendocrinology* 1984 38: 484–489.
29. Wilkes MM, Yen SS. Augmentation by naloxone of efflux of LRF from superused medial basal hypothalamus. *Life Sciences* 1981 28: 2355–2359.
30. Sauder SE, Case GD, Hopwood NJ, Kelch RP, Marshall JC. The effects of opiate antagonism on gonadotropin secretion in children and in women with hypothalamic amenorrhea. *Pediatr Res* 1984 18: 322–328.
31. Reiter RJ. The pineal and its hormones in the control of reproduction in mammals. *Endocr Rev* 1980 1: 109–131.
32. Lang U, Lenko HL, Bradtke J, Delavy B, Aubert ML, Sizonenko PC. Melatonin, pineal gland, and puberty. In Grumbach MM, Sizonenko PC, Aubert ML (eds) *Control of the Onset of Puberty II.* Baltimore: Williams and Wilkins, 1990: Chapter 13.
33. Cavallo A. Melatonin and human puberty: current perspectives (review). *J Pineal Res* 1993 15: 115–121.
34. Ojeda SR, Urbanski HF. Puberty in the rat. In Knobil E, Neill JD (eds) *The Physiology of Reproduction.* New York: Raven Press, 1988.
35. Warren MP. The effects of exercise on pubertal progression and reproductive function in girls. *J Clin Endocrinol Metab* 1980 51: 1150–1157.
36. Warren MO. Anorexia nervosa. In Sciarra JJ (ed.) *Gynecology and Obstetrics.* Hagerstown, MD: Harper and Row, 1981.
37. Tanner JM. Trend towards earlier menarche in London, Oslo, Copenhagen, the Netherlands and Hungary. *Nature* 1973 243: 95–96.

38. Bullough VL. Age at menarche: a misunderstanding. *Science* 1981 **213**: 365–366.

39. Frisch RE. Influences on the age of menarche. *Lancet* 1973 **i**: 1077.

40. Marshall JC, Kelch RP. Low dose pulsatile gonadotropin releasing hormone in anorexia nervosa: a model of human pubertal development. *J Clin Endocrinol Metab* 1979 **49**: 712–719.

41. Hartz AJ, Barboriak PN, Wong A. The association of obesity with infertility and related menstrual abnormalities in women. *Int J Obes* 1979 **3**: 57–73.

42. Cumming DC, Wheeler GC. Exercise-associated changes in reproduction: A problem common to women and men. In Frisch RE (ed.) *Adipose Tissue and Reproduction.* Berne: Karger, 1990: 125–135.

43. Schwartz DM, Thompson MG, Johnson CL. Anorexia nervosa and bulimia: the socio-cultural context. *Int J Eat Dis* 1982 **1**: 20–36.

44. Prader A. Normal growth and disorders of growth in children and adolescents (author's translation) [in German]. *Klin Wochensch* 1981 **59**: 977–984.

45. Tanner JM, Davies PW. Clinical longitudinal standards for height and height velocity for North American Children. *J Pediatr* 1985 **107**: 317.

46. Tanner JM, Whitehouse RH, Takaishi M. Standards from birth to maturity for height, weight, height velocity and weight velocity: British children. 1965 Part II. *Arch Dis Child* 1966 **41**: 613.

47. Tanner JM, Whitehouse RH, Hughes PCR *et al.* Relative importance of growth hormone and sex steroids for the growth at puberty of trunk length, limb length, and muscle width in growth-hormone deficient children. *J Pediatr* 1976 **89**: 1000.

48. Aynsley-Green A, Zachmann M, Prader A. Interrelation of the therapeutic effects of growth hormone and testosterone on growth in hypopituitarism. *J Pediatr* 1976 **89**: 992.

49. Caruso-Nicoletti M, Cassorla F, Skerda M *et al.* Short term, low dose estradiol accelerates ulnar growth in boys. *J Clin Endocrinol Metab* 1985 **61**: 896.

50. Rose SR, Municchi G, Barnes KM, Kamp GA, Uriarte MM, Ross JL, Cassorla F, Cutler GB Jr. Spontaneous growth hormone secretion increases during puberty in normal girls and boys. *J Clin Endocrinol Metab* 1991 **73**: 428–435.

51. Martha PM Jr, Gorman KM, Blizzard RM, Rogol AD, Veldhuis JD. Endogenous growth hormone secretion and clearance rates in normal boys, as determined by deconvolution analysis: relationship to age, pubertal status, and body mass. *J Clin Endocrinol Metab* 1992 **74**: 336–344.

52. Martin LG, Grossman MS, Connor TB *et al.* Effect of androgen on growth hormone secretion and growth in boys with short stature. *Acta Endocrinol (Copenh)* 1979 **91**: 201.

53. Mauras LG, Blizzard Rm, Link K *et al.* Augmentation of growth hormone secretion during puberty: evidence for a pulse amplitude-modulated phenomenon. *J Clin Endocrinol Metab* 1987 **64**: 596.

54. Moll GW Jr, Rosenfield RL, Fang VS. Administration of low-dose estrogen rapidly and directly stimulates growth hormone production. *Am J Dis Child* 1986 **140**: 124.

55. Cara JF, Rosenfield RL, Furlanetto RW. A longitudinal study of the relationship of plasma somatomedin-C concentration to the pubertal growth spurt. *Am J Dis Child* 1987 **141**: 562.

56. Luna AM, Wilson DM, Wibbelsman CJ *et al.* Somatomedins at adolescence: a cross-sectional study of the effect of puberty on plasma insulin-like growth factor I and II levels. *J Clin Endocrinol Metab* 1983 **57**: 268.

57. Rosenfield RL, Furlanetto R, Bock D. Relationship of Somatomedin-C concentrations to pubertal changes. *J Pediatr* 1983 **103**: 723.

58. Rosenfield RL, Furlanetto R. Physiologic testosterone or estradiol induction of puberty increases plasma somatomedin-C. *J Pediatr* 1985 **3**: 415.

59. Jenkins PJ, Grossman A. The control of the gonadotropin releasing hormone pulse generator in relation to opiod and nutritional cues. *Hum Reprod* 1993 **2**: 154–161.

60. Aynsley-Green A, Zachmann M, Prader A. Interrelation of the therapeutic effects of growth hormone and testosterone on growth in hypopituitarism. *J Pediatr* 1976 **89**: 992–999.

61. Hudson PL, Dougas I, Donahoe PK *et al.* An immunoassay to detect human mullerian inhibiting substance in males and females during normal development. *J Clin Endocrinol Metab* 1990 **70**: 16–22.

62. Hindmarsh PC, DiSilvio L, Pringle PJ *et al.* Changes in serum insulin concentration during puberty and their relationship to growth hormone. *Clin Endocrinol* 1988 **28**: 381–388.

63. Kirkland RT, Keenan BS, Probstfield JL *et al.* Decrease in plasma high-density lipoprotein cholesterol levels at puberty in boys with delayed adolescence. Correlation with plasma testosterone levels. *J Am Med Assoc* 1987 **257**: 502–507.

64. Rabinovici J. The differential effects of FSH and LH on the human ovary. *Baillieres Clin Obstet Gynaecol* 1993 **7**: 263–281.

65. Peters H, Byskov AG, Grinsted J. Follicular growth in fetal and prepubertal ovaries of humans and other primates. *J Clin Endocrinol Metab* 1978 **7**: 469–485.

66. Hansen JW, Hoffman HJ. Urinary gonadotropin cycles in prepubertal girls. *Pediatr Res* 1979 **13**: 379.

67. Hoffman HJ. Time series methods for detecting monthly gonadotropin cycles in pubescent girls. *Biometrics* 1978 (Sept): 532–533.

68. Weiner IB, del Gaudio AC. Psychopathology in adolescence. An epidemiological study. In Chess S, Thomas A (eds) *Annual Progress in Child Psychiatry and Child Development.* New York: Brunner/Mazel, 1977: 471–488.

69. Angold A, Worthman CW. Puberty onset of gender differences in rates of depression: a developmental, epidemiologic and neuroendocrine perspective. *J Affective Disord* 1993 **29**: 145–158.

70. Kaplan SL, Grumbach MM. Pituitary and placental gonadotrophins and sex steroids in the human and subhuman primate fetus. *Clin Endocrinol Metab* 1978 **7**: 487–511.

71. Van Wieringen JD, Wafelbakker F, Verbrugge HP *et al.* Growth diagrams 1965 Nertherlands: Second National Survey on 0–24 year olds. Netherlands Institute for Preventative Medicine TNO. Gröningen: Wolters-Noordhoff, 1971.

2.9

Menstruation

IT Cameron, G Irvine and JE Norman

INTRODUCTION

Menstruation can be defined as the shedding of the superficial layers of the endometrium following the withdrawal of ovarian steroids. The process is associated with a variable degree of blood loss, and in the human usually lasts for up to six days.

Before the availability of effective contraception and sterilization, women experienced episodes of pregnancy and lactational amenorrhea interspersed with the occasional ovulatory menstrual cycle.[1] The regular 28 day menstrual cycle is considered normal, and as a result

menstruation will occur on some 400 occasions during a woman's reproductive lifetime (Fig. 2.9.1).

The process of menstruation itself does not occur widely throughout the animal kingdom, but is confined to humans, non-human primates, and two non-primate species, the elephant shrew (*Elephantus myuras jamesoni*) and the bat (*Glossophaga sorcinina* and *Carollia* spp.).[2-4] Menstruation may be the inevitable consequence of the way in which the mechanism of implantation has evolved in these species.[5] Although in some mammals, such as the pig, implantation merely involves close apposition between the embryo and the luminal epithelium of the endometrium, in women the blastocyst actively invades the

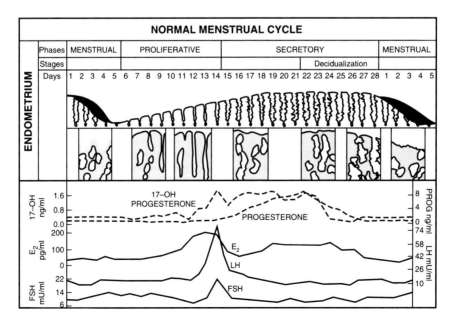

Fig. 2.9.1 *Temporal relationship between endometrial and hormonal changes during the menstrual cycle. (Adapted and redrawn from reference 106.)*

uterus, with extravillous trophoblast extending through the endometrium towards the myometrium. In menstruating species, implantation is preceded by decidualization, whereby endometrial stromal cells undergo hormone-dependent proliferation and differentiation following the influence of progesterone on an estrogen-primed endometrium in the late luteal phase of the cycle. Should pregnancy not occur and progesterone concentrations decline, the decidualized cells die and menstruation follows.

This chapter examines the major cellular and molecular mechanisms that underpin the process of menstruation in women.

CURRENT CONCEPTS

The endometrial 'cycle'

It is appropriate to summarize the morphological events seen in the endometrium before considering the mechanisms which are thought to play a role in the control of menstruation itself. Endometrial histology has been extensively documented.[6] The well-described cyclic changes are known to be regulated by ovarian steroids, and are illustrated in Figs 2.9.1 and 2.9.2.

Estradiol plays a major role in the follicular phase, leading to repair of the glandular, stromal and vascular elements of the endometrium (Fig. 2.9.2a,b). By the late follicular phase the endometrial glands are short, straight and narrow, and the stroma is compact (Fig. 2.9.2c). After ovulation, the endometrium is exposed to increasing concentrations of progesterone from the corpus luteum. In the early luteal phase the endometrial glands elongate and coil, and their lumina fill with glycogen-rich secretions (Fig. 2.9.2d,e). By the late luteal phase these changes become accentuated, and the glands assume a 'saw-tooth' appearance (Fig. 2.9.2f). The stromal compartment becomes progressively more edematous due to fluid accumulation in the extracellular matrix. Three distinct layers can be identified: the superficial zona compacta, the intermediate zona spongiosa and the zona basalis. The compacta and spongiosa make up the 'functional' endometrium which is shed during menstruation (Fig. 2.9.2g–i).

The cyclic changes in the epithelial and stromal compartments are paralleled by simultaneous events in the endometrial vasculature. The spiral arterioles which are destined to provide the maternal side of the interface between the placental blood supply and the uterus, regrow from remaining vascular fragments in the basal endometrium into markedly coiled end-arterioles, each supplying 4–7 mm^2 of the endometrial surface.[7] These arterioles feed a network of superficial capillaries which in turn drain into superficial venous lakes and larger veins towards the endometrial–myometrial junction.

Recent work has described the ultrastructure of endometrial remodeling and regeneration.[8] With the exception of the epithelium lining glandular stumps, most of the endometrial surface epithelium was desquamated

within 24 h of the onset of bleeding, and open-ended blood vessel segments were seen, devoid of platelet–fibrin clots. Within a further 24–48 h, new endometrial epithelial growth was detected, originating from the retained glandular stumps. On cycle day 4, most of the interglandular endometrial surface had been replaced by new epithelium, and by day 5–6 the endometrium had been completely re-epithelialized, following which stromal tissue began to grow.[8] These studies illustrate the three main mechanisms that are required to control menstrual bleeding. First, there is a need for a potent vasoconstrictor to check blood loss from the damaged vessels. Next, although there should be an associated deposition of platelet–fibrin plugs,[9] there is an even greater requirement for an active fibrinolytic system to prevent clot organization with subsequent scarring and intrauterine adhesion formation, which would constitute a distinct evolutionary disadvantage. Finally, the bleeding will be controlled definitively by the repair of both the endometrial surface and the blood vessels themselves.

Decidualization

The process of decidualization is integral to the mechanism of menstruation. Decidualization is the hormone-dependent transient formation of decidual tissue which encompasses cellular proliferation, differentiation and death, and which is seen in species in which the trophoblast invades the uterine stroma to reach the maternal blood vessels.[10] The process is characterized by the differentiation of stromal fibroblasts into decidual cells, which in turn leads to modification of the extracellular matrix, alterations in cellular secretory function and recruitment of precursor granulated lymphocytes in readiness for implantation. Though removal of steroid hormone support from decidualized endometrium results in menstruation, it appears that cell death is programmed once decidualization has been induced,[10] and that menstruation itself is an inevitable consequence unless appropriate signals are received from an implanting embryo.[11]

Mechanism of endometrial hemostasis

The physiology of the hemostatic mechanism has been studied extensively. In the periphery, blood vessel damage reveals subendothelial collagen. This is followed by the cascade of platelet accumulation, fibrin deposition, and platelet degranulation and interdigitation to form the primary hemostatic plug within 3 min of injury. Over the next few hours, the plug is transformed by cellular lysis and further fibrin deposition to form a secondary plug composed of fibrin and empty platelet remnants.[12]

Hemostatic events in the menstruating uterus are markedly different.[13] Detailed studies were performed on the uteri of women who underwent hysterectomy within 72 h of the onset of menses. In the earliest specimens, stromal disintegration and vessel lesions were seen in the absence of platelet adhesion. Following this, blood

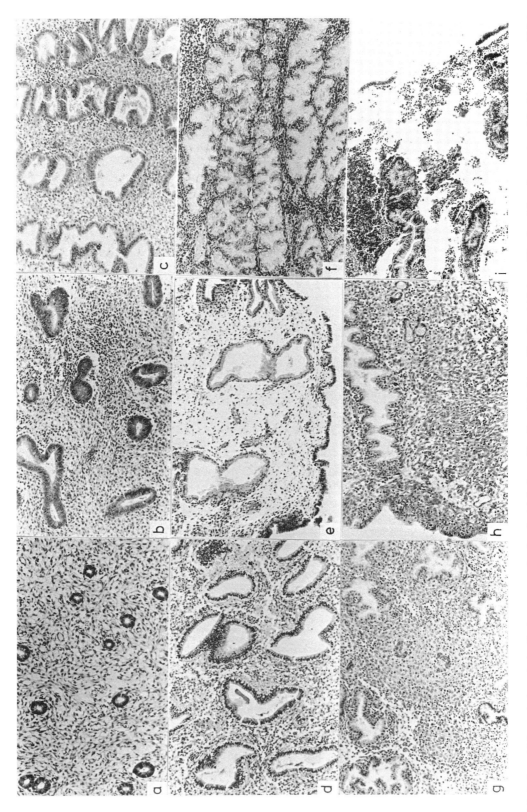

Fig. 2.9.2 *Endometrial morphology during the human menstrual cycle.* **(a)** *Early proliferative,* **(b)** *mid-proliferative,* **(c)** *late proliferative,* **(d)** *early secretory,* **(e)** *mid-secretory,* **(f)** *late secretory ('saw-tooth' glands),* **(g)** *late secretory (pre-decidual change around arterioles),* **(h)** *pre-menstrual,* **(i)** *menstrual. (Reproduced with permission from reference 106.)*

Table 2.9.1 Paracrine and autocrine factors in the initiation and control of menstruation: agents known or thought to play a role in the hemostatic and repair process within the endometrium

Event	Mediator	Result
Initiation of bleeding		
Endometrial regression	Collapse of ECM	Shear stress, release of growth factors.
Vasoconstriction	$PGF_{2\alpha}$, ET-1	Ischemia, release of reactive oxygen species.
Control of bleeding		
Hemostasis	PGs	Vasoconstriction, dilatation, proliferation.
	Fibrinolysis	Prevention of intrauterine adhesions.
	PAF	Paracrine/vasoactive actions.
	ETs	Vasoconstriction, paracrine actions, mitogenesis.
Myometrial contraction	ADH, OT	Vasoconstriction.
	his, heparin	Paracrine/vasoactive actions, reduced endometrial blood flow.
Repair		
Epithelium	*Cytokines:*	
	IL, TNF, IFN	Immune response, inflammation, repair.
	Growth factors:	
	TGF-α, TGF-β, EGF, IGF	Paracrine actions, repair.
Vessels	*Angiogenic growth factors:*	
	aFGF, bFGF, VEGF	Angiogenesis.

ECM, extracellular matrix; PG, prostaglandin; ET, endothelin; PAF, platelet-activating factor; ADH, vasopressin; OT, oxytocin; his, histamine; IL, interleukin; TNF, tumor necrosis factor; IFN, interferon; TGF, transforming growth factor; EGF, epidermal growth factor; IGF, insulin-like growth factor; FGF, fibroblast growth factor; VEGF, vascular endothelial growth factor.

extravasation was a prominent feature in the functional endometrium, and damaged blood vessels were sealed by intravascular thrombi consisting of various amounts of platelets and fibrin. By 20 h after the onset of bleeding, most of the functional endometrium had been shed, and subsequent hemostasis appeared to be achieved not by the deposition of stable platelet-fibrin plugs, but by vasoconstriction.[14]

Impaired platelet plug formation might be expected in the presence of potent inhibitors of platelet adhesion and aggregation in the endometrium. Prostacyclin (prostaglandin I_2), a potent inhibitor of platelet aggregation,[15] is produced by the endometrium and myometrium.[16–18] Furthermore, recent work using a rat model has shown that the uterus is also a major source of nitric oxide,[19] a ubiquitous vasodilator and powerful inhibitor of platelet aggregation.[20]

Evaluation of the mechanisms underlying the process of menstruation requires an understanding of three main events, namely the initiation of bleeding and endometrial shedding, the control and cessation of bleeding and endometrial shedding, and the subsequent repair process. Each of these events will be considered in turn, together with those mediators thought to play a key role (Table 2.9.1).

Local regulation of menstruation

Initiation of bleeding

The studies by Markee, assessing endometrial explants in the anterior eye chamber of the rhesus monkey, showed that the earliest changes prior to the onset of menstrual bleeding were regression of the endometrium and intense vasoconstriction of the spiral arterioles.[7] Vasodilatation and tissue breakdown followed. That these early premenstrual events could be reproduced by withdrawing exogenous estradiol and progesterone suggested that the falling concentration of circulating ovarian steroids following luteolysis was a main determinant of the onset of menstruation. Although the precise mechanism by which changes in ovarian steroids result in menstrual bleeding remains to be determined, recent data suggest that the steroids act through intermediate paracrine or autocrine factors within the endometrium itself.[21]

Regression of the functional endometrium may be the result of collapse of the extracellular matrix due to loss of progesterone. A number of events would be predicted to follow. For example, regression would lead to distortion of the tightly coiled spiral arterioles causing shear stress, which in turn would lead to tissue damage either directly or via the release of potent vasoactive peptides such as endothelin-1 from the vascular endothelium (see below). Alterations of the structure of the extracellular matrix would also lead to the release of growth factors which are stored within it, and which are thought to play an important role in endometrial repair.[22]

Whatever the mechanism of regression and vasoconstriction, the subsequent ischemia and tissue damage will initiate the release of a host of mediators including reactive oxygen species, which will result in leukocyte infiltration, abnormal arachidonic acid metabolism and disrupted mitochondrial function, and will lead to menstruation proper.[23]

Control and cessation of bleeding

Prostaglandins

Extensive data have accumulated supporting a role for the prostaglandins (PGs) in the pathogenesis of menorrhagia. Most work has concentrated on direct actions of the prostaglandins on the uterine vasculature.[24-26]

The main endometrial products of the arachidonic acid cascade are PGE_2 and $PGF_{2\alpha}$.[27] Endometrial PG concentrations are low in the proliferative phase, and increase in the second half of the cycle.[28,29] One effect of progesterone is to promote the storage of arachidonic acid which is released as steroid concentrations fall after luteolysis, resulting in PG formation at the time of menstruation itself. The endometrium also synthesizes smaller amounts of PGD_2,[30] and the vasodilator prostacyclin, measured as its metabolite 6 oxo-$PGF_{1\alpha}$.[16,17,31] The major PG in myometrium is prostacyclin (PGI_2).[18] Although the production rate per gram of tissue is similar to that of the endometrium, the large muscle mass of the myometrium makes prostacyclin the main PG product of the uterus as a whole.

It has already been suggested that the local production of prostacyclin might contribute to the impaired platelet-plug formation seen during menstruation. When the functional endometrium has been shed, PGE_2 and $PGF_{2\alpha}$ are thought to control the degree of bleeding from the remaining spiral arteriolar fragments by vasodilatation and vasoconstriction, respectively; indeed in the endometrium of women with menorrhagia the balance between PGE_2 and $PGF_{2\alpha}$ is tilted in favor of the vasodilator PGE_2.[30]

The precise nature of the vasoconstrictor responsible for endometrial hemostasis is not known. Although $PGF_{2\alpha}$ has been implicated, it is a weak vasoconstrictor in comparison with the potent vasodilatory properties of prostacyclin, and pharmacological concentrations are required to contract small branches of human uterine artery *in vitro*.[32] Furthermore, in a canine *in vitro* model, physiological concentrations of $PGF_{2\alpha}$ caused not vasoconstriction, but vasodilatation of the uterine artery by stimulating the release of prostacyclin from vascular smooth muscle.[33]

An alternative mechanism whereby the PGs may be involved in endometrial hemostasis is by inducing myometrial contraction, for the anatomy of the uterine vascular bed is such that the entire endometrial blood supply reaches its destination by traversing the myometrial smooth muscle. That menstruation is accompanied by contractions of the myometrium has been documented in detail.[27,34]

Platelet-activating factor

Platelet-activating factor (PAF) is a D-glycerol derivative formed from alkyl-acyl-glycerol-3-phosphocholine by the action of phospholipase A_2 and acetyl transferase.[35] Increasing evidence has shown that PAF may be an important local mediator in the maternal recognition of pregnancy, but it might also play a role in the paracrine control of the uterine vascular bed in the non-pregnant cycle. Platelet-activating factor stimulated the release of PGE_2, but not $PGF_{2\alpha}$ from separated human endometrial glandular cells from secretory endometrium.[36,37] Other work showed an inhibitory effect of PAF on $PGF_{2\alpha}$ release from cell cultures of glandular and stromal cells from luteal phase endometrium.[38] Since PGE_2 stimulated PAF release in stromal cell cultures in the presence of progesterone,[38] a mechanism was envisaged whereby positive feedback of PGE_2 production could occur. In turn, PGE_2 could either act on vascular smooth muscle and myometrium, or having angiogenic properties, could contribute to the vascular repair process.[39] Being a vasoconstrictor,[40] and stimulating platelet aggregation,[41] PAF itself is also likely to make a direct contribution to menstrual hemostasis.

Endothelins

The endothelins are a family of three vasoactive peptides, endothelin-1, endothelin-2 and endothelin-3, which act by binding to at least two distinct receptor subtypes, ET_A and ET_B (see reference 42 for review). Initially described as products of vascular endothelium, the endothelins are now known to be released from a variety of epithelial cell types. Endothelin-1, which has been described as the most potent vasoconstrictor yet discovered, is a powerful constrictor of small vessels in the human uterus.[32,43,44] Endothelin-like immunoreactivity has been localized to human uterine glandular epithelium,[45-47] and was released into the supernatant after endometrial tissue culture.[48,49] An action for the endothelins in the uterus was further suggested by the demonstration of specific binding sites for iodinated endothelins on myometrium and on endometrial vascular smooth muscle and glandular epithelium.[50] These studies were supported by the demonstration of mRNA for endothelin-1, endothelin-2 and endothelin-3 and the receptors ET_A and ET_B in human endometrium.[51]

Endothelin-1 is thought to mediate vasoconstriction by binding to the ET_A receptor, whereas activation of the ET_B receptor may lead to the release of vasodilators including prostacyclin and nitric oxide.[52] As endothelin peptide appears to be present in endometrium throughout the cycle, the differential distribution of ET_A and ET_B receptors might provide a mechanism to modify the physiological action of the endothelins.

It is not known whether the endothelins are involved in the initiation of menstruation, but the release of endothelin-1 from vascular endothelium following the potent stimulus of shear stress at the time of premenstrual endometrial regression would provide a strong candidate for the vasoconstrictor described by Markee.[7] Furthermore, once the endometrium begins to break down, disruption of glandular epithelium would lead to the release of stored endothelins which could gain access to the smooth muscle of the spiral arterioles to effect a potent and long-lasting vasoconstriction. Increased endothelin activity at the time of menstruation might also come about as a result of the inhibition of endothelin metabolism. The endothelins are degraded by the metalloendopeptidase enkephalinase.[53] Enkephalinase activity in human endometrium was greatest in the mid-luteal phase, and fell in concert with the premenstrual decline in circulating progesterone,[54] revealing at least indirectly, that endometrial endothelin activity is under ovarian steroid control.

Fibrinolysis

Fibrinolysis within the uterine cavity is a necessary consequence of activation of the coagulation cascade during menstruation, to prevent clot formation with subsequent organization and the development of intrauterine adhesions. Endometrial tissue explants release two types of plasminogen activator *in vitro*: tissue-type and urokinase-type. Estradiol stimulates urokinase plasminogen activator, whereas progesterone not only reduces the secretion of both types of activator, but also increases the release of plasminogen activator inhibitor.[55] In addition to the activation of the fibrinolytic system by the coagulation cascade itself, and plasminogen release as a result of endometrial disintegration, falling progesterone concentrations after luteolysis may provide a further stimulus for plasminogen formation.

That fibrinolysis plays an important role in the control of uterine bleeding is illustrated by the fact that endometrial fibrinolysis is excessive in women with menorrhagia.[56] In addition, the widely documented increase in menstrual blood loss experienced by women after insertion of inert or copper-containing intrauterine contraceptive devices has been attributed in part to a local effect of the device on endometrial fibrinolysis.[57,58] Whereas uterine plasminogen activator activity was highest in the endometrium surrounding intrauterine devices,[59] suppression of both tissue and urokinase plasminogen activator by the combined contraceptive pill could contribute to the reduced blood loss seen in women receiving these agents.[60]

Other vasoactive agents

A variety of other agents might contribute to the control and cessation of menstrual bleeding. Arginine vasopressin and oxytocin have potent direct vasoconstrictor actions on small branches of human uterine artery *in vitro*,[61] and the demonstration that mRNA for oxytocin is present in rat endometrium suggests a possible physiological role.[62]

The innervation of the uterine artery and myometrium is also likely to be instrumental in the mechanism of menstrual hemostasis. In addition to adrenergic and cholinergic pathways, the smooth muscle of the human uterine artery has been shown to contain fibers exhibiting vasoactive intestinal peptide-, histidine-, methionine- and neuropeptide-Y-like immunoreactivity.[61]

Mast cell-derived histamine and heparin are powerful effectors of the local hemostatic response. In the uterus, most mast cells are located in the myometrium, adjacent to capillaries and small venules.[56] Histamine concentrations in endometrium are greatest in the late luteal phase.[56] Besides a direct action to contract large blood vessels, dilate small arterioles and capillaries and increase capillary permeability, histamine may contribute to the hemostatic mechanism by stimulating the release of tissue plasminogen activator and Factor VIII.[63,64] A contribution of locally produced heparin to the control of menstrual blood loss was suggested by the observation that heparin-like activity was increased in uterine fluid collected from women with menorrhagia.[65] Alternatively, heparin might aid the cessation of menstrual bleeding by permitting the release of growth factors from the extracellular matrix to promote endometrial regeneration.[22]

Repair and angiogenesis

The eventual cessation of menstrual bleeding depends on repair of the endometrium and its vasculature, initiated from the remaining glandular epithelium, vascular endothelium and stroma of its basal layer. If the basal endometrium is removed, as is the case after complete endometrial resection, normal regeneration of the functional endometrium fails to occur. Local agents which may play a fundamental role in endometrial regeneration include cytokines, peptide growth factors and angiogenic growth factors.

Cytokines

The cytokines comprise a diverse group of proteins which regulate a variety of cellular functions. Cytokines usually act in autocrine or paracrine fashion, and are seldom present in serum. They are important mediators of immune and inflammatory responses, and of the reparative response to injury, and as cytokines influence vasoconstriction, hemostatic platelet-plug formation, mitogenesis and angiogenesis, they are likely to play a key role in the mechanism of menstruation. Interleukins, tumor necrosis factor and interferons are outlined here (see reference 66 for review).

The **interleukins** may contribute to the control of menstruation by modulating cellular proliferation, inducing the release of other cytokines and activating stromal T cells.[67] Messenger RNA for interleukin-1α, interleukin-1β, and interleukin-receptor antagonist has been demonstrated in human endometrium throughout the menstrual cycle using the polymerase chain reaction (PCR),[67] whereas the less sensitive method of Northern analysis showed interleukin-1β in the secretory phase only,[68] coincident with the peak concentration of interleukin-1 in serum.[69] A role for interleukin-1 in the uterus was supported by the demonstration of binding sites for the cytokine on endometrial epithelial and stromal cells.[70,71] Other members of the interleukin family found in the uterus include interleukin-6 and interleukin-8.[72]

Tumor necrosis factor (TNF)-α, or cachectin has also been detected in endometrium. This peptide exerts a variety of effects including stimulation of the inflammatory response, stimulation and inhibition of growth, modulation of the immune response, angiogenesis and cytotoxicity.[78] Using immunocytochemistry, the cytokine was localized to endometrial glandular epithelial cells in mid- and late luteal phases, whereas immunoreactivity in stromal cells was seen throughout the cycle. Subsequent studies detected mRNA for TNF-α in endometrium throughout the menstrual cycle using PCR.[71]

The **interferons** (IFNs), IFN-α, IFN-β and IFN-γ, make up a family of regulatory peptides with anti-viral and immunoregulatory activities, which plays an important role in the control of cell growth and differentiation. A potential source of IFN-γ in the uterus is the lymphoid aggregates adjacent to the glands of the basal endometrium.[75] Interferon-γ inhibits proliferation of human endometrial cells *in vitro*, and receptors for the cytokine have been demonstrated on human endometrial cells throughout the menstrual cycle.[75,76]

Growth factors

Transforming growth factors (TGFs) are peptide growth factors with diverse paracrine actions. Although TGF-α and TGF-β are similarly named, they represent distinct families of peptides with different structures and actions.[77,78]

TGF-α binds to the same receptor as epidermal growth factor (EGF) to exert its biological action. In human endometrium, TGF-α has been localized to stromal cells in the proliferative phase of the cycle. The distribution was different in the secretory phase, when TGF-α-like immunoreactivity was localized to glandular and luminal epithelium, with moderate to intense staining around spiral arterioles.[79] The presence of TGF-α in close proximity to endometrial blood vessels in the luteal phase might suggest a role either in the development of the placental vasculature following implantation, or in the repair process following menstruation.

The TGF-β group, which currently comprises a family of three distinct isoforms, plays a crucial part in the regulation of epithelial homeostasis and epithelial–mesenchymal interactions.[80] Of specific relevance to the mechanism of menstruation, TGF-β is expressed after vascular insult and is involved in the repair of damaged epithelium in a variety of human tissues.[81] In addition, it promotes gland formation, and is both chemotactic and angiogenic.[82] Messenger RNA for TGF-β has been demonstrated in human endometrium,[68] whereas in early pregnancy TGF-β-like immunoreactivity was localized to the decidual extracellular matrix, syncytiotrophoblast and extracellular matrix within chorionic villi.[83] As TGF-β inhibits growth in a variety of epithelial cell types and interferes with the mitogenic actions of other peptide growth factors including EGF, TGF-α and platelet-derived growth factor,[78] TGF-β itself may be central in regulating the control of endometrial repair.

Regeneration and repair of the endometrium involves estrogen-induced cellular proliferation. Increasing evidence indicates that this process is mediated by **epidermal growth factor** (EGF). This growth factor, first isolated from the submaxillary glands of adult male mice, is a potent stimulator of proliferation in various cell types, including epithelial cells.[84,85] Furthermore, that EGF can replace the effects of estradiol on the growth and differentiation of the genital tract in ovrectomized rodents provides compelling evidence for the physiological role of the peptide.[86]

Epidermal growth factor appears to be produced by human endometrium. Radioimmunoassay demonstrated EGF-like immunoreactivity with the greatest concentration in homogenates of late proliferative endometrium.[87] Messenger RNA for EGF was detected using PCR amplification, and EGF-like immunoreactivity has been localized to glands and stroma throughout the menstrual cycle.[88,89] The demonstration of specific binding sites for iodinated

EGF in human endometrium lends further support to the hypothesis that the peptide is involved in endometrial proliferation.[90,91]

The **insulin-like growth factors** (IGFs), like EGF, are widely distributed. They bind to specific binding proteins (IGFBPs), release from which provides a mechanism to control their bioavailability. Animal studies suggested that IGF-1 may increase uterine DNA synthesis *in vitro*.[93] In the human, IGFBP-1 (placental protein 12, PP12, see reference 93 for review) has been identified as a major secretory product of decidualized endometrium. Whether IGFs play a part in the mechanism of menstruation is not known, however IGFBP-1 mRNA and peptide have been localized to stromal cells in late secretory endometrium,[94,95] suggesting the facilitation of IGF bioavailability at the onset of menstruation.

Angiogenic growth factors

Angiogenesis, the formation of new capillaries from existing blood vessels, is a basic requirement for the regeneration of the endometrium following menstruation. The process involves degradation of the basement membrane around pre-existing blood vessels, endothelial cell migration and proliferation, structural re-organization to form a lumen and functional maturation.[96,97] Several members of the heparin-binding family of growth factors influence this important process, including fibroblast growth factors (FGFs) and vascular endothelial growth factor (VEGF), as described below.

Fibroblast growth factors (FGFs) exist in two molecular forms: acidic FGF and basic FGF. Both forms bind to the same receptor to exert their biological actions, though basic FGF is 10 to 100 times more potent than its acidic counterpart.[97] In endometrium, FGF has been localized to glandular epithelium,[98] and has been shown to be mitogenic for endometrial stromal cells in culture.[99] Fibroblast growth factors are not secreted but are stored, either within the cell, or in the extracellular matrix.[22] Whichever is the case, cellular and extracellular matrix destruction at the time of menstruation would be expected to release bioavailable FGF to participate in the endometrial vascular repair process.

Vascular endothelial growth factor (VEGF) is a potent angiogenic growth factor which is a highly specific mitogen for endothelial cells.[100] In contrast to the FGFs, VEGF can be a secretory product. Messenger RNA for VEGF has been detected in normal endometrium and myometrium, and in endometrial carcinoma cell lines.[101] Using *in situ* hybridization, expression of mRNA for VEGF was localized to stroma and glands in proliferative endometrium, with increased glandular and diminished stromal staining in the secretory phase. In menstrual tissue, there was intense hybridization in glands and in necrotic groups of cells thought to be macrophages.[101]

Control of VEGF expression was investigated by Northern analysis, which showed that VEGF mRNA was increased in endometrial carcinoma cell lines pretreated with estradiol.[101] The authors suggested at least two mechanisms controlling VEGF production in endometrium. First, estradiol appeared to increase VEGF production. As estradiol levels rise in the follicular phase, an increase in VEGF would promote blood vessel formation, thus providing the regenerating endometrium with a blood supply and repairing those vessels damaged during menstruation. Secondly, the increased expression of VEGF mRNA in menstrual endometrium might be triggered by hypoxia,[102] indicating that hypoxic conditions at the onset of and during menstruation might stimulate the release of this potent angiogenic factor to initiate the repair process.

FUTURE PERSPECTIVES

The mechanism whereby ovarian steroid withdrawal initiates the process of menstruation is thought to involve the activation or inhibition of a host of paracrine and autocrine mediators from the epithelial, stromal and vascular com-partments of the endometrium (Fig. 2.9.3). A detailed understanding of the ways in which estradiol and progesterone influence these local mediators is of paramount importance, and is the focus of continuing research.

Menstruation might be viewed as the inevitable consequence of failure of fertilization. Similarly, those factors which play a role in the initiation and control of menstrual bleeding and the subsequent repair process are also likely to be involved in the establishment and maintenance of pregnancy.[103] A better understanding of these factors should lead to improved treatments for women with menorrhagia and greater insight into the cause of irregular bleeding with exogenous contraceptive steroids or hormone replacement therapy. In addition, such understanding will also provide a model to elucidate the local mechanisms responsible for implantation, placentation and subsequent growth *in utero*, which in turn might have far-reaching implications for the development of cardiovascular and respiratory disease in adult life.[104]

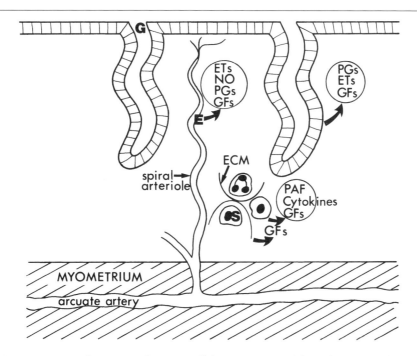

Fig. 2.9.3 *Paracrine interactions in endometrium. The major cellular components of the endometrium, glandular epithelium, stroma and vascular endothelium, synthesize a wide range of locally acting factors which are thought to play a fundamental role in the initiation and maintenance of menstrual bleeding, and the subsequent repair process. G, gland; S, stroma; E, endothelium; ECM, extracellular matrix; ET, endothelin; GF, growth factor; NO, nitric oxide; PAF, platelet activating factor; PG, prostaglandin.*

SUMMARY

- Menstruation is the shedding of the superficial layers of the endometrium following the withdrawal of ovarian steroids.
- The process occurs in humans, other primates, the elephant shrew and the bat, and is the consequence of the way in which implantation has evolved in these species.

- The first events prior to the onset of bleeding are endometrial regression and vasoconstriction of the spiral arterioles.
- Once the functional endometrium is shed, hemostasis is achieved almost exclusively by vasoconstriction of remaining arteriolar fragments.

- The degree of menstrual blood loss is determined in part by the balance between the vasoconstrictor $PGF_{2\alpha}$ and the vasodilator PGE_2.
- Endothelin-1 may be a potent vasoconstrictor in human endometrium.
- Endometrium possesses an active fibrinolytic system: fibrinolysis is greatest in the endometrium of women with menorrhagia.
- Cytokines, which coordinate immune and inflammatory responses, and the reparative response to injury, are abundant in endometrium.
- The proliferative effects of estradiol on endometrium are mediated by locally released peptide growth factors.
- Angiogenic growth factors may play a fundamental role in the repair and regeneration of the endometrial vascular bed.

ACKNOWLEDGEMENTS

We thank Mrs Kay Byrne for secretarial help, and the Medical Illustration Department of the Yorkhill NHS Trust.

REFERENCES

1. Short RV. The evolution of human reproduction. *Proc R Soc Lond* 1976 **195**: 3–24.
2. Van der Horst CJ, Gilman J. The menstruation cycle in *Elephantulus myuras jamesoni* – family Macroscelididae. *South Afr J Med Sci* 1941 **6**: 27–47.
3. Hamlett GW. Uterine bleeding in a bat (*Glossophaga sorcina*). *Anat Rec* 1934 **60**: 9–17.
4. Rasweiler IV JJ, de Bonilla H. Menstruation in short-tailed fruit bats (*Carollia* spp.). *J Reprod Fertil* 1992 **95**: 231–248.
5. Finn CA. Why do women and some other primates menstruate? *Perspect Biol Med* 1987 **30**: 566–574.
6. Noyes RW, Hertig AT, Rock J. Dating the endometrial biopsy. *Fertil Steril* 1952 **1**: 3–25.
7. Markee JE. Menstruation in intraocular endometrial transplants in the rhesus monkey. *Contrib Embryol* 1940 **28**: 219–308.
8. Ludwig H, Metzger H, Frauli M. Endometrium: tissue remodelling and regeneration. In D'Arcangues C, Fraser IS, Newton JR, Odlind V (eds) *Contraception and Mechanisms of Endometrial Bleeding*. Cambridge: Cambridge University Press, 1990: 441–466.
9. Van Eijkeren MA, Christiaens GCML, Gueze JJ, Haspels AA, Sixma JJ. Morphology of menstrual hemostasis in essential menorrhagia. *Lab Invest* 1991 **64**: 284–294.
10. Bell SC. Decidualization and relevance to menstruation. In D'Arcangues C, Fraser IS, Newton JR, Odlind V (eds) *Contraception and Mechanisms of Endometrial Bleeding*. Cambridge: Cambridge University Press, 1990: 187–212.
11. Findlay JK, Rees MCP. Factors controlling menstrual blood volume. In D'Arcangues C, Fraser IS, Newton JR, Odlind V (eds) *Contraception and Mechanisms of Endometrial Bleeding*. Cambridge: Cambridge University Press, 1990: 138.
12. Sixma JJ, Wester J. The hemostatic plug. *Semin Hematol* 1977 **14**: 265–269.
13. Christiaens GCML, Sixma JJ, Haspels AA. Hemostasis in menstrual endometrium: a review. *Obstet Gynecol Surv* 1982 **37**: 281–303.
14. Christiaens GCML, Sixma JJ, Haspels AA. Morphology of haemostasis in menstrual endometrium. *Br J Obstet Gynecol* 1980 **87**: 425–439.
15. Gryglewski RJ, Bunting S, Moncada S, Flower RJ, Vane JR. Arterial walls are protected against deposition of platelet thrombi by a substance (prostaglandin X) which they make from prostaglandin endoperoxides. *Prostaglandins* 1976 **12**: 685–713.
16. Kelly RW, Lumsden MA, Abel MH, Baird DT. The relationship between menstrual blood loss and prostaglandin production in the human: evidence for increased availability of arachidonic acid in women suffering from menorrhagia. *Prostaglandins Leukot Med* 1984 **16**: 69–78.
17. Rees MCP, Anderson ABM, Demers LM, Turnbull AC. Endometrial and myometrial prostaglandin release during the menstrual cycle in relation to menstrual blood loss. *J Clin Endocrinol Metab* 1984 **58**: 813–818.
18. Abel MH, Kelly RW. Differential production of prostaglandins within the human uterus. *Prostaglandins* 1979 **18**: 821–828.
19. Yallampalli C, Izumi H, Byam-Smith M, Garfield RE. An L-arginine-nitric oxide–cyclic guanosine monophosphate system exists in the uterus and inhibits contractility during pregnancy. *Am J Obstet Gynecol* 1994 **170**: 175–185.
20. Lowenstein C, Snyder SH. Nitric oxide: a novel biologic messenger. *Cell* 1992 **70**: 705–707.
21. Findlay JK, Salamonsen LA. Paracrine regulation of implantation and uterine function. *Bailliere's Clinical Obstet Gynaecol* 1991 **5**: 117–131.
22. Ruoslahti E, Yamaguchi Y. Proteoglycans as modulators of growth factor activities. *Cell* 1991 **64**: 867–869.
23. Rice-Evans C, Cooke B. Oxygen radicals, bleeding and tissue injury. In D'Arcangues C, Fraser IS, Newton JR, Odlind V (eds) *Contraception and Mechanisms of Endometrial Bleeding*. Cambridge: Cambridge University Press, 1990: 411–430.
24. Hagenfeldt K. The role of prostaglandins and allied substances in uterine haemostatis. *Contraception* 1987 **36**: 23–35.
25. Bell SC, Smith SK. The endometrium as a paracrine organ. In Chamberlain G (ed.) *Contemporary Obstetrics and Gynaecology*. London: Butterworth, 1988: 273–298.
26. Cameron IT. Prostaglandins and menstruation. In Drife JO, Calder AA. (eds) *Prostaglandins and the Uterus. 24th RCOG Study Group*. London: Springer Verlag, 1992: 17–32.
27. Pickles VR, Hall WJ, Best FA, Smith GN. Prostaglandins in endometrium and menstrual fluid from normal and dysmenorrhoeic subjects. *J Obstet Gynaecol Br Cmmwlth* 1965 **72**: 185–192.
28. Downie J, Poyser NL, Wunderlich M. Levels of prostaglandins in human endometrium during the normal menstrual cycle. *J Physiol* 1974 **236**: 464-472.
29. Maathius JB, Kelly RW. Concentrations of prostaglandins $F_{2\alpha}$ and E_2 in the endometrium throughout the human menstrual cycle, after the administration of clomiphene or an estrogen–progesterone pill, and in early pregnancy. *J Endocrinol* 1978 **77**: 361–371.
30. Smith SK, Abel MH, Kelly RW, Baird DT. Prostaglandin synthesis in the endometrium of women with ovular dysfunctional uterine bleeding. *Br J Obstet Gynaecol* 1981 **88**: 434–442.
31. Cameron IT, Leask R, Kelly RW, Baird DT. Endometrial

prostaglandins in women with abnormal menstrual bleeding. *Prostaglandins Leukot Med* 1987 **29**: 249–257.

32. Ekstrom P, Alm P, Akerlund M. Differences in vasomotor responses between main stem and smaller branches of the human uterine artery. *Acta Obstet Gynaecol Scand* 1991 **70**: 429–433.

33. Kimura T, Yoshida Y, Toda N. Mechanisms of relaxation induced by prostaglandins in isolated canine uterine arteries. *Am J Obstet Gynecol* 1992 **167**: 1409–1416.

34. Novak E, Reynolds BR. The cause of primary dysmenorrhea with special reference to hormonal factors. *JAMA* 1932 **99**: 1466–1472.

35. Braquet P, Touqui L, Shen TY, Vargarfig BB. Perspectives in platelet-activating factor research. *Pharmacol Rev* 1987 **39**: 97–145.

36. Smith SK, Kelly RW. Effect of platelet-activating factor on the release of $PGF_{2\alpha}$ and PGE_2 by separated cells of human endometrium. *J Reprod Fertil* 1988 **82**: 271–276.

37. Ahmed A, Smith SK. Platelet-activating factor stimulates phospholipase C activity in human endometrium. *J Cell Physiol* 1992 **152**: 207–214.

38. Alecozay AA, Harper MJK, Schenken RS, Hanahan DJ. Paracrine interactions between platelet-activating factor and prostaglandins in hormonally-treated human luteal phase endometrium *in vitro. J Reprod Fertil* 1991 **91**: 301–312.

39. Ben Ezra D. Neovasculogenic ability of prostaglandins, growth factors and synthetic chemoattractants. *Am J Ophthalmol* 1978 **86**: 455–461.

40. Bjork J, Smedegard G. Acute microvascular effects of PAF-acether, as studied by intravital microscopy. *Eur J Pharmacol* 1983 **96**: 87–94.

41. Pinckard RN, Farr RS, Hanahan DJ. Physicochemical and functional identity of rabbit platelet-activating factor (PAF) released *in vivo* during IgE anaphylaxis with PAF released *in vitro* from IgE sensitized basophils. *J Immunol* 1979 **123**: 1847–1857.

42. Cameron IT, Davenport AP. Endothelins in reproduction. *Rep Med Rev* 1992 **1**: 99–113.

43. Fried G, Samuelson U. Endothelin and neuropeptide Y are vasoconstrictors in human uterine blood vessels. *Am J Obstet Gynecol* 1991 **164**: 1330–1336.

44. Svane D, Larsson B, Andersson KE, Forman A. Endothelin-1: immunocytochemistry, localization of binding sites, and contractile effects in human uteroplacental smooth muscle. *Am J Obstet Gynecol* 1993 **168**: 233–241.

45. Cameron IT, Davenport AP, van Papendorp CL *et al.* Endothelin-like immunoreactivity in human endometrium. *J Reprod Fertil* 1992 **95**: 623–628.

46. Cameron IT, Plumpton C, Champeney R, van Papendorp CL, Ashby MJ, Davenport AP. Identification of endothelin-1, endothelin-2 and endothelin-3 in human endometrium. *J Reprod Fertil* 1993 **97**: 251–255.

47. Salamonsen LA, Butt AR, Macpherson AM, Rogers PAW, Findlay JK. Immunolocalization of the vasoconstrictor endothelin in human endometrium during the menstrual cycle and umbilical cord at birth. *Am J Obstet Gynecol* 1992 **167**: 163–167.

48. Economos K, MacDonald PC, Casey ML. Endothelin-1 gene expression and protein biosynthesis in human endometrium: potential modulator of endometrial blood flow. *J Clin Endocrinol Metab* 1992 **74**: 14–19.

49. Marsh MM, Hampton AL, Riley SC, Findlay JK, Salamonsen LA. Production and characterization of endothelin released by human endometrial epithelial cells in culture. *J Clin Endocrinol Metab* 1994 **79**: 1625–1631.

50. Davenport AP, Cameron IT, Smith SK, Brown MJ. Binding sites for iodinated endothelin-1, endothelin-2 and endothelin-3 demonstrated on human uterine glandular epithelial cells by quantitative high-resolution autoradiography. *J Endocrinol* 1991 **129**: 149–154.

51. O'Reilly G, Charnock-Jones DS, Davenport AP, Cameron IT, Smith SK. Presence of mRNA for endothelin-1, endothelin-2 and endothelin-3 in human endometrium,

and a change in the ratio of ET_A and ET_B receptor subtype across the menstrual cycle. *J Clin Endocrinol Metab* 1992 **75**: 1545–1549.

52. Takayanagi R, Kitazumi K, Takasaki C *et al.* Presence of non-selective type of endothelin receptor on vascular endothelium and its linkage to vasodilatation. *FEBS Lett* 1991 **282**: 103–106.

53. Vijayaraghavan J, Scicli AG, Carretero OA, Slaughter C, Moomaw C, Hersh LB. The hydrolysis of endothelins by neutral endopeptidase 24.11 (enkephalinase). *J Biol Chem* 1990 **265**: 14150–14155.

54. Casey ML, Smith JW, Nagai K, Hersh LB, MacDonald PC. Progesterone-regulated cyclic modulation of membrane metalloendopeptidase (enkephalinase) in human endometrium. *J Biol Chem* 1991 **266**: 23041–23047.

55. Casslen B, Andersson A, Nilsson IM, Astedt B. Hormonal regulation of the release of plasminogen activators and of a specific activator inhibitor from endometrial tissue in culture (42360). *Proc Soc Exp Biol Med* 1986 **182**: 419–424.

56. Hourihan HM, Sheppard BL, Brosens IA. Endometrial hemostasis. In D'Arcangues C, Fraser IS, Newton JR, Odlind V (eds) *Contraception and Mechanisms of Endometrial Bleeding.* Cambridge: Cambridge University Press, 1990: 95–116.

57. Andrade ATL, Orchard EP. Quantitative studies on menstrual blood loss in IUD users. *Contraception* 1987 **36**: 129–144.

58. Toppozada M. Treatment of increased menstrual blood loss in IUD users. *Contraception* 1987 **36**: 145–157.

59. Shaw ST, Macauley LK, Sun NC, Tanaka MS, Roche PC. Changes of plasminogen activator in human uterine tissue induced by intrauterine contraceptive devices. *Contraception* 1983 **27**: 131–140.

60. Casslen B, Astedt B. Reduced plasminogen activator content of the endometrium in oral contraceptive users. *Contraception* 1983 **28**: 181–188.

61. Akerlund M. Function of endometrial blood vessels. In D'Arcangues C, Fraser IS, Newton JR, Odlind V (eds) *Contraception and Mechanisms of Endometrial Bleeding.* Cambridge: Cambridge University Press, 1990: 81–94.

62. Lefebvre DL, Giaid A, Bennett H, Lariviere R, Zingg HH. Oytocin gene expression in rat uterus. *Science* 1992 **256**: 1553–1555.

63. Hamilton KK, Sims PJ. Changes in cytosolic Ca^{2+} associated with von Willebrand factor release in human endothelial cells exposed to histamine. Study of microcarrier cell monolayers using the fluorescent probe indo-1. *J Clin Invest* 1987 **79**: 600–608.

64. Hanss M, Collen D. Secretion of tissue-type plasminogen activator and plasminogen activator inhibitor by cultured human endothelial cells: modulation by thrombin, endotoxin and histamine. *J Lab Clin Med* 1987 **109**: 97–104.

65. Foley ME, Griffin BD, Zuzel M *et al.* Heparin-like activity in uterine fluid. *Br Med J* 1978 **2**: 322–324.

66. Tabibzadeh SS. Human endometrium: an active site of cytokine production and action. *Endocr Rev* 1981 **12**: 272–290.

67. Tabibzadeh SS, Sun XY. Cytokine expression in human endometrium throughout the menstrual cycle. *Hum Reprod* 1992 **7**: 1214–1221.

68. Kauma A, Matt D, Strom S, Eierman D, Turner T. Interleukin-1β, human leukocyte antigen HLA-DRα and transforming growth factor β expression in endometrium, placenta and placental membranes. *Am J Obstet Gynecol* 1990 **163**: 1430–1437.

69. Cannon JG, Dinarello CA. Increased plasma interleukin-1 activity in women after ovulation. *Science* 1985 **227**: 1247–1249.

70. Tabibzadeh SS, Kafka KL, Satyaswaroop PG, Kilian PL. Interleukin-1 regulation of human endometrial function: presence of IL-1 receptor correlates with IL-1-stimulated prostaglandin E_2 production. *J Clin Endocrinol Metab* 1990 **70**: 1000–1006.

71. Tabibzadeh SS. Cytokine regulation of human endometrial function. *Ann NY Acad Sci* 1991 **622**: 89–98.

72. Critchley HOD, Kelly RW, Kooy J. Perivascular location of chemokine interleukin-8 in human endometrium: a preliminary report. *Hum Reprod* 1994 **9**: 1406–1409.

73. Arai K-I, Lee F, Miyajiima A, Miatake S, Arai N, Yokota T. Cytokines: coordination of immune and inflammatory responses. *Annu Rev Biochem* 1990 **59**: 783–793.

74. Tabibzadeh SS. Ubiquitous expression of TNFα1 cachectin immunoreactivity in human endometrium. *Am J Reprod Immunol* 1991 **26**: 1–4.

75. Tabibzadeh SS, Satyaswaroop PG, Rao PN. Antiproliferative effect of interferon γ in human endometrial epithelial cells *in vitro*: potential local growth modulatory role in endometrium. *J Clin Endocrinol Metab* 1988 **67**: 131–138.

76. Tabibzadeh SS. Evidence of T-cell activation and potential cytokine action in human endometrium. *J Clin Endocrinol Metab* 1990 **71**: 645–649.

77. De Larco JE, Todaro GJ. Growth factors from murine sarcoma virus-transformed cells. *Proc Natl Acad Sci USA* 1978 **75**: 4001–4005.

78. Roberts AB, Sporn MB. Transforming growth factor β. *Adv Cancer Res* 1988 **51**: 107–145.

79. Horowitz GM, Scott RT, Drews MR, Mavot D, Hofmann GE. Immunohistochemical localization of transforming growth factor α in human endometrium, decidua, and trophoblast. *J Clin Endocrinol Metab* 1993 **76**: 786–792.

80. Akhurst RJ, Fitzpatrick DR, Fowlis DJ, Gatherer D, Millan FA, Slager H. The role of TGF-βs in mammalian development and neoplasia. *Mol Reprod Dev* 1992 **32**: 127–135.

81. Casscells W, Bazoberry F, Speir E *et al.* Transforming growth factor-β1 in normal heart and in myocardial infarction. *Ann NY Acad Sci* 1990 **593**: 148–160.

82. Sporn MB, Roberts AB. The transforming growth factor-βs: past, present and future. *Ann NY Acad Sci* 1990 **593**: 1–6.

83. Graham CH, Lysiak JJ, McCrae KR, Lala PK. Localization of transforming growth factor β at the human fetal–maternal interface: role in trophoblast growth and differentiation. *Biol Reprod* 1992 **46**: 561–572.

84. Cohen S. Isolation of a mouse submaxillary gland protein accelerating incisor eruption and eyelid opening in the newborn animal. *J Biol Chem* 1962 **237**: 1455–1462.

85. Carpenter G, Cohen S. Epidermal growth factor. *Annu Rev Biochem* 1979 **48**: 193–216.

86. Nelson KG, Takahashi T, Bossert NL, Walmer DK, McLachlan JA. Epidermal growth factor replaces estrogen in the stimulation of female genital tract growth and differentiation. *Proc Natl Acad Sci USA* 1991 **88**: 21–25.

87. Ishihara S, Tatetani Y, Mizuno M. Epidermal growth factor-like immunoreactivity in human endometrium. *Asia Oceania J Obstet Gynaecol* 1990 **16**: 165–168.

88. Haining REB, Cameron IT, van Papendorp CL *et al.* Epidermal growth factor in human endometrium: proliferative effects in culture and immunocytochemical localization in normal and endometriotic tissues. *Hum Reprod* 1991 **6**: 1200–1205.

89. Haining REB, Schofield JP, Jones DSC, Rajput-Williams J, Smith SK. Identification of mRNA for epidermal growth factor and transforming growth factor α present in low

copy number in human endometrium and decidua using reverse transcriptase-polymerase chain reaction. *J Mol Endocrinol* 1991 **6**: 207–214.

90. Chegini N, Rao CV, Wakim N, Sanfilippo J. Binding of ^{125}I-epidermal growth factor in human uterus. *Cell Tissue Res* 1986 **246**: 543–548.

91. Berchuck A, Soisson A.P, Olt G J *et al.* Epidermal growth factor receptor expression in normal and malignant endometrium. *Am J Obstet Gynecol* 1989 **161**: 1247–1252.

92. Ghahary A, Chakrabarti S, Murphy LJ. Localization of the sites of synthesis and action of insulin-like growth factor-1 in the rat uterus. *Mol Endocrinol* 1990 **4**: 191–195.

93. Fay TN, Grudzinskas JG. Human endometrial peptides: a review of their potential role in implantation and placentation. *Hum Reprod* 1991 **6**: 1311–1326.

94. Waites GT, James RFL, Bell SC. Immunohistochemical localization of the human endometrial secretory protein pregnancy-associated endometrial α-1-globulin, an insulin-like growth factor binding protein, during the menstrual cycle. *J Clin Endocrinol Metab* 1988 **67**: 1100–1104.

95. Julkunen M, Koistinen R, Suikkari AM, Seppala M, Janne OA. Identification by hybridization histochemistry of human endometrial cells expressing mRNAs encoding a uterine β-lactoglobulin homologue and insulin-like growth factor-binding protein-1. *Mol Endocrinol* 1990 **4**: 700–707.

96. Folkman J, Klagsbrun M. Angiogenic factors. *Science* 1987 **253**: 442–447.

97. Bohlen P. Angiogenic factors. In D'Arcangues C, Fraser IS, Newton JR, Odlind V (eds) *Contraception and Mechanisms of Endometrial Bleeding*. Cambridge: Cambridge University Press, 1990: 467–489.

98. Cordon-Caro C, Vlodavsky I, Haimovitz-friedman A, Hicklin D, Fuks Z. Expression of basic fibroblast growth factor in normal human tissues. *Lab Invest* 1990 **63**: 832–840.

99. Irwin JC, Utian WH, Eckert RL. Sex steroids and growth factors differentially regulate the growth and differentiation of cultured human endometrial stromal cells. *Endocrinology* 1991 **129**: 2385–2392.

100. Ferrarra N, Houck K, Jakman L, Leung DW. Molecular and biological properties of the vascular endothelial growth factor family of proteins. *Endocr Rev* 1992 **13**, 18–32.

101. Charnock-Jones DS, Sharkey AM, Rajput-Williams J *et al.* Identification and localization of alternately spliced mRNAs for vascular endothelial growth factor in human uterus and estrogen regulation in endometrial carcinoma cell lines. *Biol Reprod* 1993 **48**: 1120-1128.

102. Shweiki D, Itin A, Soffer D, Keshet E. Vascular endothelial growth factor induced by hypoxia may mediate hypoxia-initiated angiogenesis. *Nature* 1992 **359**: 843–845.

103. Tabibzadeh S, Babaknia A. The signals and molecular pathways involved in implantation, a symbiotic interaction between blastocyst and endometrium involving adhesion and tissue invasion. *Mol Hum Reprod* 1, *Hum Reprod* 1995 **10**: 1579–1602.

104. Barker DJP (ed.) Fetal and infant origins of adult disease. London: British Medical Journal, 1992: 343pp.

105. Healy DL, Cameron IT. Clinical physiology of the endometrium. In Riddick DH (ed.) *Reproductive Physiology in Clinical Practice*. New York: Thieme Medical Publishers.

Fertilization and Early Embryogenesis

RJ Aitken

INTRODUCTION

Fertilization is the process by which the haploid male and female gametes unite to create a unique individual that is genetically distinct from either of its parents. The cell biology of fertilization and early embryonic development has excited the interest of research scientists interested in fundamental mechanisms of cellular control, because this process can occur *in vitro* and is, therefore, accessible. From a clinical perspective, this stage of the reproductive cycle is of interest because failures of fertilization and early embryonic development make a significant contribution to the etiology of human infertility. Our basic understanding of the biological mechanisms regulating these events led directly to the introduction of the *in vitro* fertilization (IVF) technology[1] that has come to dominate the management of patients attending infertility clinics. Moreover, these early stages of development are strategically important because they represent suitable targets for contraceptive intervention, particularly the development of contraceptive vaccines that aim to block either the fertilization of the oocyte or the implantation of the early human embryo. In order to create a platform from which to appreciate the clinical significance of the most recent advances in gamete and developmental biology, this chapter sets out the scientific essentials of this field with emphasis on those aspects of some relevance to clinical practice.

CURRENT CONCEPTS

Sperm transport

The passage of sperm from the site at which they are deposited in the vagina to the proximal region of the Fallopian tube where fertilization occurs depends on a dynamic sequence of changes in the biochemistry and morphology of sperm, which will now be discussed.

Semen liquefaction

In a vast majority of mammals, including man, the spermatozoa are deposited in the anterior fornix of the vagina. Shortly after insemination the seminal plasma coagulates, possibly to enhance the retention of the semen in the vaginal canal, and subsequently takes about 30 min to liquefy. This liquefaction process is thought to involve the action of proteolytic enzymes derived from the prostate gland.[2,3] Normal liquefaction of the semen is essential if the spermatozoa are to leave the seminal compartment and penetrate the cervix. Even in the context of IVF therapy, the recovery of sufficient functional spermatozoa to conduct IVF may be heavily influenced by the normality of semen liquefaction. If this does not occur then treatment of the semen with proteases such as bromelin or chymotrypsin may be necessary, although the influence of these reagents on the subsequent fertilizing potential of the spermatozoa is unknown.[4]

Sperm movement

Following deposition of the semen and liquefaction of the seminal plasma, the spermatozoa have the task of penetrating the cervical mucus. This process is biologically and clinically important and is almost entirely dependent on the propulsive forces generated by the beating of the sperm tail. For spermatozoa attempting to penetrate the cervical mucus interface, it is essential that they exhibit a progressive, linear pattern of movement associated with high frequency, symmetrical flagellar waves of moderate amplitude, that propel the spermatozoa forward at speeds in excess of 25 μm s^{-1}. The correlation between sperm movement and cervical mucus penetration is so strong that around 70% of the information generated by a cervical mucus penetration assay can be gleaned from a detailed analysis of sperm movement using computer-aided sperm analysis.[5]

Anti-sperm antibodies

In addition to the movement characteristics of the spermatozoa, another factor that can have a profound effect on

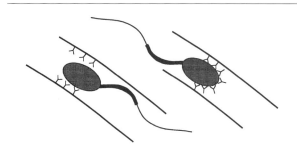

Fig. 2.10.1 *Sperm progress through cervical mucus may be impaired by the presence of antibodies, particularly IgA, on the surface of the spermatozoon or in the cervical mucus. An interaction between the Fc portion of the antibody and cervical mucin tethers the spermatozoa to the latter and initiates the expression of a characteristic 'shaking phenomenon'.*

cervical mucus penetration is the presence of anti-sperm antibodies on either the surface of the spermatozoa or in the cervical mucus (Fig. 2.10.1). This is particularly true of IgA class antibodies, the Fc portion of which possesses a binding affinity for cervical mucin.[6] As a consequence of this interaction, the spermatozoa become tethered to the cervical mucin chains and develop a spectacular pattern of movement, termed the 'shaking phenomenon' by its discoverer, Jan Kremer,[7] as the spermatozoa struggle to set themselves free.

Formation of the isthmic sperm store

Once the spermatozoa have colonized the cervical mucus they may remain viable in this location for many days, while they initiate the process of capacitation. The competence of human spermatozoa to invade the cervical mucus and establish a viable sperm store, is one of the most important properties assessed in the postcoital test. This test, though much maligned, has been shown to have significant prognostic value when performed in a carefully standardized manner.[8]

Following penetration of the cervical mucus, the spermatozoa swim along the the longitudinal microstructure of the mucus glycoproteins to reach the surface of the secretory epithelium. From this position, the spermatozoa progress along the folds and grooves of the cervical epithelium until they ultimately reach the uterus. During the preovulatory period the uterine cavity is filled with fluid and the spermatozoa become rapidly dispersed throughout this space owing to the muscular movements of the uterine wall. From the uterine cavity, the spermatozoa penetrate the isthmic regions of the Fallopian tube and in certain species, such as the sheep and cow, establish a sperm store in this location.[9] Similar isthmic stores of spermatozoa have also been observed in rodents and it is possible that this is a universal feature of sperm transport in mammals, although as far as primates are concerned this suggestion is entirely speculative.

Although located in the isthmic store, the spermatozoa appear to attach firmly to the oviducal epithelium and their

motility is suppressed. In this state, the spermatozoa can remain viable, in readiness for fertilization, for many days.[10,11] Even *in vitro*, it has recently been shown that human spermatozoa can remain viable for 48 h when co-cultured with human oviducal epithelia.[12] The preservation of the spermatozoa under these circumstances could not be accomplished by conditioned media from cultures of oviducal cells or the presence of cells of non-oviducal origin. Even in the presence of oviducal epithelia, the maintenance of sperm viability did not involve attachment of the spermatozoa to the epithelium. Thus, whatever the nature of the factors produced by the oviduct that promote sperm survival, they must be actively secreted by the epithelium and exhibit a relatively short half-life.

Hyperactivation

Once ovulation has occurred, the spermatozoa are released from their isthmic store and progress towards the ampulla of the Fallopian tubes, where fertilization occurs. The factors responsible for inducing the sudden discharge of the spermatozoa from the isthmic epithelium are unknown. It is possible that a key factor in initiating the escape of spermatozoa from the isthmic store is the onset of 'hyperactivated' motility.[13,14] This pattern of movement has been observed in most mammalian species and appears to be a common feature of sperm capacitation. It is characterized by large amplitude, asymmetrical thrashings of the sperm tail that normally cause the sperm head to describe a characteristic figure-of-eight trajectory, known as the 'star-spin' pattern of hyperactivated movement. The intracellular factors responsible for the induction of hyperactivated movement have still to be resolved in detail, although the important roles of calcium and cyclic AMP have already been recognized.[14] In principle, both of these second messengers could be generated by follicular fluid released into the oviducal lumen following ovulation. Thus, follicular fluid is known to induce sperm hyperactivation and contains: (a) phosphodiesterase inhibitors, such as hypoxanthine, that would raise the intracellular concentration of cyclic AMP, and (b) progesterone, a steroid that induces rapid calcium transients in human spermatozoa.[15–17]

Sperm capacitation

As spermatozoa ascend the female reproductive tract they are said to undergo a physiological transformation resulting in the attainment of a state of 'capacitation'. The biological concept of capacitation dates back to experiments conducted more than 40 years ago demonstrating that freshly ejaculated or epididymal spermatozoa were unable to fertilize ova *in vivo*, whereas spermatozoa that have resided in the oviducts of donor animals for 4–8 h were able to do so.[14] The conclusion of these experiments was that before fertilization can take place, the spermatozoa must be *capacitated* in the female tract for a number of hours to gain the ability to respond to the cell recognition signals generated when male and female gametes make contact.

Roles of calcium and cyclic AMP

Analysis of the mechanisms involved in sperm capacitation became possible when it was discovered that the spermatozoa of certain species could be readily capacitated *in vitro*. Careful dissection of the events associated with capacitation in the golden hamster, suggested that this process involves a gradual increase in the levels of intracellular calcium which, in turn, enhance the intracellular generation of cyclic AMP.[18] In response to the high intracellular levels of cyclic AMP and calcium, the spermatozoa adopt a hyperactivated pattern of movement and become primed to undergo the acrosome reaction. In addition to these changes in second messenger status, the sperm plasma membrane also increases in fluidity during capacitation, in part due to the loss, or relocation, of cholesterol.[19] In this primed state, with calcium and cyclic AMP levels raised and the sperm plasma membrane in a fluid state, the spermatozoa are said to be 'capacitated' and in response to an appropriate stimulus, such as the zona glycoprotein ZP3, will admit a second influx of calcium over the acrosomal region of the cell and rapidly complete the acrosome reaction.[14]

Clinically, attempts have been made to promote the capacitation of human spermatozoa in the context of *in vitro* fertilization therapy for male factor infertility. The most widely used strategy in this context is the use of reagents, such as pentoxyfylline[20] or 2-deoxyadenosine[21] to elevate the intracellular levels of cyclic AMP. Such reagents certainly render the spermatozoa extremely sensitive to changes in intracellular calcium levels[22] and stimulate a moderate rise in the incidence of hyperactivated movement. There are also recent data suggesting that addition of this reagent can enhance the success of IVF treatment for male factor infertility,[23] although there is some controversy in this area. Clearly, if the spermatozoa are not cyclic AMP deficient, then reagents designed to elevate the level of this second messenger will not be of therapeutic value. Unfortunately, clinical trials do not appear to have been conducted in which the use of phosphodiesterase inhibitors has been examined in relation to defined pathologies involving deficiencies in the cyclic AMP-generating system.

Decapacitation factors

In addition to the changes in membrane fluidity, cyclic AMP and calcium referred to above, the attainment of a capacitated state also appears to involve alterations in several other aspects of sperm biochemistry and structure. One recurring theme in the literature, is that capacitation involves the removal of coating materials from the sperm surface[14] including so-called 'decapacitation factors'.[24-26] The general concept behind such decapacitation factors is that they are deposited on the sperm surface from epididymal and/or seminal plasma and play a key role in suppressing the capacitation of the spermatozoa until these cells have embarked on their migration through the female reproductive tract. During the transport of the spermatozoa to the site of fertilization, these decapacitation factor(s) are removed from the sperm surface, thereby allowing the spermatozoa to initiate the cascade of biochemical changes that culminate in a state of capacitation. An essential feature of this hypothesis is that the changes induced by the removal of the decapacitation factor(s) are reversible. Thus, capacitated cells can be decapacitated once more by adding seminal plasma or even conditioned medium in which spermatozoa have previously been incubated.[14]

The chemistry of the decapacitation factors, and their mechanism of action, have yet to be resolved. They appear to block one or more of the major events associated with capacitation, including the progressive increases in intracellular calcium levels and membrane fluidity. The cholesterol present in seminal plasma could, for example, induce a reversible stabilization of the sperm plasma membrane in such a way as to account for the decapacitating activity of this material. In addition, seminal plasma contains calmodulin-like proteins[27] that are thought to stimulate the $Ca^{2+} Mg^{2+}$-ATPase activity in the sperm plasma membrane and, in this way, prevent the gradual increase in intracellular calcium levels that promote the capacitation process.

In association with the removal of decapacitation factors from the sperm surface during capacitation, the antigenic structure of the sperm plasma membrane becomes extensively modified. Such changes may involve the removal or masking of sperm surface proteins or their processing by proteases or glycosidases. Monoclonal antibodies[14,28] and lectins[14,29,30] have been used to map such changes during capacitation but, as yet, the functional significance of the modifications observed is poorly understood.

Intramembranous particles

One set of changes that does appear to be of functional relevance involves alterations in the distribution of intramembranous particles within the sperm plasma membrane.[31,32] As spermatozoa capacitate, patches of plasma membrane develop that are free of intramembranous particles and contain little if any sterols, such as cholesterol. These particle-free domains are thought to be particularly fusogenic and to play an important role in facilitating the subsequent fusion of the plasma and outer acrosomal membranes during acrosomal exocytosis.[14,33]

In summary, capacitation is a biological phenomenon that results in the spermatozoa acquiring a capacity to respond to the activating stimuli presented by the cumulus–oocyte complex. It involves a number of biochemical changes in the spermatozoa, the most important of which involve increases in intracellular calcium and cyclic AMP, as well as an enhancement of membrane fluidity. Structurally, the pattern of surface antigen expression is modified and particle-free fusogenic domains are created in the sperm plasma membrane. In terms of behavior, the only outward sign that a spermatozoon has capacitated is the onset of the hyperactivated pattern of motility. These changes are reversible and are thought to be largely brought about by the release of decapacitation factors from the sperm surface. Since the latter appears to be a passive process, it can be appreciated that capacitation is not a tightly synchronized phenomenon either within or between ejaculates. This inherent heterogeneity creates considerable difficulties in the analysis of the molecular mechanisms that control this process. Nevertheless, this same heterogeneity in the rates at which individual human spermatozoa capacitate may be biologically important, in extending the period of time over which a sperm population remains competent to fertilize the ovum.

Interaction with the cumulus mass

In concert with the completion of capacitation and the appearance of hyperactivated motility, the spermatozoa break away from the epithelial lining of the isthmus of the Fallopian tube and head towards the oocyte. Although some authors have suggested that the cumulus–oocyte complex may generate chemotactic factors to assist the spermatozoa in locating the ovum,[34] this evidence is not convincing.[14] The initial contact between the male and female gametes in the ampulla of the Fallopian tube is probably a chance event, brought about by the hyperactivated movement of the spermatozoa and the active contractile activity displayed by the oviduct, around the time of ovulation.

Role of cumulus extracellular matrix

The primary recognition event that initiates the cascade of interactions comprising the fertilization process involves the sperm plasma membrane and the surface of the cumulus mass (Fig 2.10.2). The latter comprises cumulus cells embedded in an extracellular matrix that is particularly rich in hyaluronic acid. Data from animal experiments suggest that only capacitated spermatozoa with intact acrosomes are able to penetrate the cumulus mass.[14] This association may reflect the importance of the hyperactivated motility displayed by capacitated mammalian spermatozoa in achieving physical penetration of the cumulus matrix. Since sea urchin, frog and rooster spermatozoa will penetrate the hamster cumulus mass, it seems likely that mechanical forces do play a major role in achieving cumulus penetration.[14,35] It is even possible that the motility of mammalian spermatozoa is altered by the hyaluronic acid present in the cumulus matrix in order to improve the chances of penetration. Spermatozoa from a wide variety of species possess a hyaluronic binding protein on the plasma membrane and incubation of human spermatozoa in synthetic hyaluronic acid polymers enhances sperm motility.[36,37] Moreover, there are data to suggest that the hyaluronidase-digested cumulus mass can influence the movement of capacitated human spermatozoa in order to induce a more progressive, linear pattern of motility.[38]

In addition to the active movement of the spermatozoa, it is possible that cumulus penetration is facilitated by hyaluronidase associated with the sperm surface.[14] It has recently been noted that bee venom hyaluronidase exhibits some sequence homology with PH-20, a guinea-pig protein involved in sperm-zona recognition.[39] This observation raises the intriguing possibility that spermatozoa may possess dual purpose molecules on their surface that

mediate both cumulus penetration and sperm binding to the zona pellucida.

Sperm binding to the zona pellucida

Once the spermatozoa have negotiated a path through the cumulus mass, they make contact with the surface of the zona pellucida (Fig. 2.10.2). This is an acellular structure that is secreted around the oocyte during folliculogenesis. In addition to a general protective function, the zona pellucida also acts as a cell-specific recognition site for spermatozoa and represents the location at which they undergo the acrosome reaction. The biochemistry of the zona pellucida has been thoroughly investigated over the past decade and we now have quite a detailed understanding of the molecular composition of this structure.

Zona proteins

The mammalian zona pellucida comprises three major glycoprotein species (ZP 1–3) which, in the mouse, are arranged such that interconnecting filaments of heterodimers of ZP2 (M_r=120 000) and ZP3 (M_r=83 000) are held together by dimers of ZP1 (M_r=200 000) to give an open, porous, matrix.[40,41] These proteins are heavily glycosylated and possess both N-linked and O-linked oligosaccharide side chains that are linked to the polypeptide backbone by asparagine and serine/threonine residues, respectively.

The most closely studied zona glycoprotein is ZP3, since it is this molecule that, in the mouse at least, plays a key role in sperm recognition and the induction of the acrosome reaction. Molecular characterization of ZP3 has revealed the existence of considerable homology between species. In general, this protein is approximately 424 amino acids long and is particularly rich in serine and threonine residues, which are potential sites of O-linked glycosylation. There is also a proline rich region in the centre of ZP3 which may explain why the molecule possesses very few α-helices. An additional conserved feature is the number and location of cysteine residues: the human, marmoset, mouse and hamster ZP3 sequences all possessing 15 cysteine residues at identical sites.[42] This would suggest that intramolecular disulfide bonds place important architectural constraints on the molecule, which may be essential to its biological function. Despite the similarity in the amino acid sequences, there are considerable differences in relative molecular mass within this family of ZP3 glycoproteins (human ZP3 M_r=57 000–73 000, mouse M_r=83 000, hamster M_r=56 000) presumably due to differences in glycosylation.

ZP3 carbohydrates

The O-linked carbohydrate side chains on ZP3 are thought to play a key role in the biological activity of this molecule. If these oligosaccharides are removed and purified they retain the properties of a sperm receptor and, at nanomolar concentration, are able to block sperm–zona interaction in

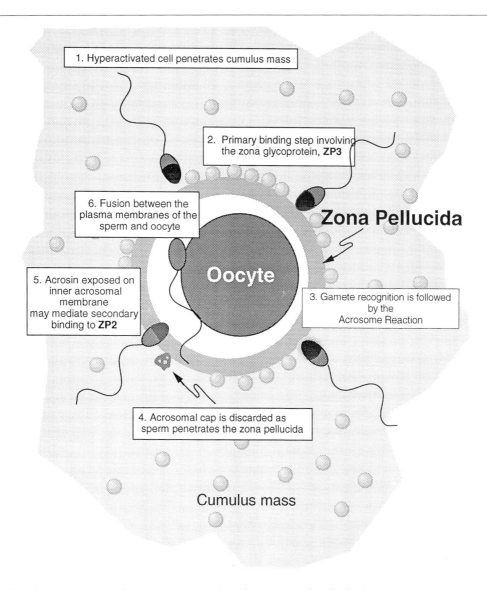

1. Hyperactivated cell penetrates cumulus mass

2. Primary binding step involving the zona glycoprotein, **ZP3**

6. Fusion between the plasma membranes of the sperm and oocyte

Zona Pellucida

Oocyte

5. Acrosin exposed on inner acrosomal membrane may mediate secondary binding to **ZP2**

3. Gamete recognition is followed by the Acrosome Reaction

4. Acrosomal cap is discarded as sperm penetrates the zona pellucida

Cumulus mass

Fig. 2.10.2 *Schematic representation of sperm–ovum interaction during mammalian fertilization.*

a competition assay.[40] However, the purified oligosaccharides lose their ability to induce the acrosome reaction, emphasizing the importance of the polypeptide backbone in mediating this effect through the cross-linking of zona binding sites on the sperm surface.[40,43] The composition and structural configuration of these *O*-linked carbohydrate side chains is the subject of ongoing research and studies in the pig have revealed the presence of a series of (sialated) sulfated oligosaccharides with a linear (*N*-acetyl-lactosamine) backbone.[44] In the mouse, a galactose residue located at the non-reducing terminus has been shown to be essential for sperm binding.[45] Removal of the galactose by digestion with α-galactosidase, or oxidation of its C-6 hydroxyl to an aldehyde group, can lead to a complete loss of sperm receptor activity. An alternative model involving a sperm surface β-1,4-galactosyl transferase, that behaves like a lectin by binding to a specific glycoside substrate of ZP3, has also been reported.[46]

Engineering an anti-zona vaccine

Molecular characterization of ZP3, and its complementary receptor on the surface of the spermatozoon, is of considerable importance to the development of contraceptive vaccines that suppress fertility by blocking fertilization. Studies in animal models, including primates, demonstrate that the long-term suppression of fertility through the induction of immunity against the zona pellucida is a feasible objective, although certain vaccine formulations have been observed to disrupt normal ovarian function. Engineering vaccines that retain the contraceptive effect but do not induce ovarian pathology is an objective that has been successfully achieved, using the mouse as an animal model. In light of these results, the prospects for developing a safe, effective vaccine targeting the zona pellucida seem, for the present at least, to be excellent.[47]

Acrosome reaction

As a consequence of the binding of spermatozoa to ZP3, these cells are induced to undergo a secretory event known as the acrosome reaction (Fig. 2.10.3). This process involves the focal fusion of the plasma membrane and outer acrosomal membrane, to create a fenestrated structure over the surface of the acrosome, the purpose of which is to effect the release of the most soluble components of the acrosomal vesicle. This initial fusion of acrosomal and plasma membranes appears to take place on the surface of the zona pellucida. The vigorous motility of the spermatozoa is then thought to drive the sperm head down through the zona matrix towards the perivitelline space (Fig. 2.10.2). The acrosomal membranes are left at the surface of the zona pellucida so that during penetration the spermatozoon possesses, on its apical surface, the slowly dispersing constituents of the acrosomal vesicle (Fig. 2.10.2).

Acrosin

One of these constituents, a protease known as acrosin, is thought to facilitate zona penetration by: (a) dissolving the zona matrix in advance of the penetrating spermatozoon, and (b) maintaining intimate contact with the zona pellucida by virtue of an affinity for a second zona glycoprotein, ZP2.[48] This interaction between the acrosome-reacted cell and ZP2 is referred to as the *secondary phase of sperm–zona interaction.*

Acrosin is generated from a precursor molecule, proacrosin, during the acrosome reaction, through modifications to both the N-terminal and C-terminal ends of the

protein.[49–51] The nature of the binding site for proacrosin/acrosin on ZP2 is not known although the results of competition studies utilizing a variety of polysaccharides indicate that the presence of sulfate ester groups on the zona glycoproteins mediate interactions with basic residues on proacrosin/acrosin and that the density and location of sulfate groups along the polymer backbone are key determinants of biological activity.[52] Thus, acrosin is an extremely important molecule in mediating the secondary phase of sperm–zona interaction, achieving both the binding of spermatozoa to the zona pellucida and the proteolytic cleavage of the zona matrix during sperm penetration. These processes are accomplished using a bind-and-cut mechanism that utilizes the diverse biochemical properties expressed by different regions of the same, intricate molecule.

The acrosome reaction as a diagnostic test

Because the constituents of the acrosomal vesicle, such as acrosin, are required during zona penetration, it follows that, *in vivo*, the outer plasma and acrosomal membranes must be dispersed more rapidly than the acrosomal contents. This sequence of events also occurs when the acrosome reaction is induced biochemically using, for example, calcium ionophores. These observations are of relevance in the design of diagnostic tests with which to assess the competence of human spermatozoa to undergo the acrosome reaction, since they have a direct bearing on the nature of the probes that may be used to monitor this event. Thus fluorescent labels that target the outer acrosomal membrane (such as *Arachis hypogaea* lectin) are dispersed early in the acrosome reaction and are much more sensitive probes of the acrosome reaction than reagents (such as *Pisum sativum* lectin) that target the acrosomal contents;[53] Fig. 2.10.4).

Sperm–oocyte fusion

During the course of the acrosome reaction, a discrete band of plasma membrane around the equatorial segment of the sperm head suddenly acquires the capacity to recognize and fuse with the vitelline membrane of the oocyte (Fig. 2.10.3). Until the acrosome reaction has occurred, spermatozoa have no capacity to interact with the oocyte whatsoever. Sperm–oocyte fusion is clearly an important aspect of sperm function to monitor for diagnostic purposes and, to this end, a bioassay for this phenomenon has been developed, based on the unusual capacity of zona-free hamster oocytes to fuse with acrosome reacted spermatozoa from a wide variety of species including man.[54] In the absence of a zona pellucida, the spontaneous rates of acrosome reaction and sperm oocyte fusion observed with this bioassay are low. A variety of different strategies have therefore been developed to induce the activation of the spermatozoa artificially. The divalent cation ionophore, A23187, is probably the most widely used reagent in this context and the rates of sperm–oocyte fusion obtained with this compound have been shown to exhibit excellent

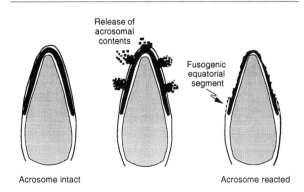

Release of acrosomal contents

Fusogenic equatorial segment

Acrosome intact

Acrosome reacted

Fig. 2.10.3 *Schematic representation of the acrosome reaction. As a consequence of this process, enzymes are released in the acrosomal contents that facilitate zona penetration and a discrete band of plasma membrane around the equatorial region of the sperm head suddenly acquires the capacity to recognize and fuse with the oocyte.*

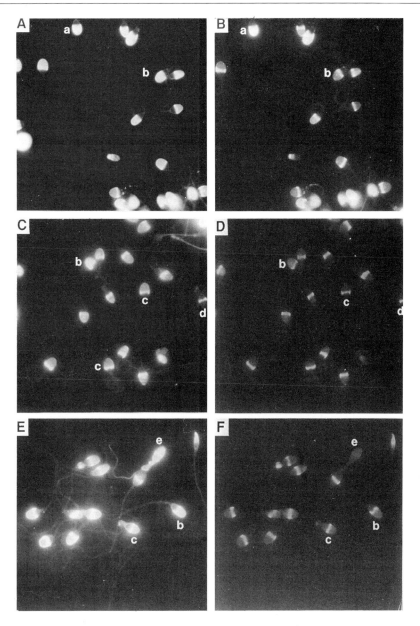

Fig. 2.10.4 *Differences in the staining patterns observed with lectins derived from* Arachis hypogaea *and* Pisum sativum *using a double labeling technique.*[53] *The panels designated* **A**, **C** *and* **E** *were stained with fluorescein-labeled P.* sativum *lectin whereas* **B**, **D** *and* **F** *were stained with rhodamine-labeled A.* hypogaea. *Within these panels it is possible to identify the following staining patterns:* (**a**) *acrosome intact spermatozoa that are uniformly labeled over the acrosomal region with both lectins;* (**b**) *spermatozoa that still appear to be acrosome intact when stained with P.* sativum *lectin and yet display dissipation of the A.* hypogaea *labeling, indicating the initiation of the acrosome reaction;* (**c**) *spermatozoa in which the acrosomal contents appear to be dispersing, as indicated by a the reduction in P.* sativum *staining, whereas the labeling pattern observed with A.* hypogaea *is confined to the equatorial segment. In such cells the acrosomal membranes have been lost although elements from the acrosomal vesicle are still present.* (**d**) *Spermatozoa in which the labeling of the spermatozoa is confined to the equatorial segment with both lectins and in which both the acrosomal contents and membranes have dispersed; and* (**e**) *morphologically abnormal spermatozoa characterized by an intense staining with P.* sativum *but lacking the target sites for A.* hypogaea (x600).

correlations with the fertilizing potential of human spermatozoa *in vivo* and *in vitro*.[55–57]

Role of sperm movement

Although the acrosome reaction is a prerequisite for sperm–oocyte fusion, bioassays of these two phenomena are not tightly correlated. The reason for this is that sperm–oocyte fusion is highly dependent on the movement characteristics of the spermatozoa whereas the histochemical detection of the acrosome is not tightly linked with sperm motility. Spermatozoa that are weakly motile, but viable, will still give positive acrosome reactions following exposure to ionophore. These observations emphasize that bioassays of the acrosome reaction and sperm–oocyte fusion are not synonymous but give slightly different diagnostic information. Specifically, whenever the acrosome reaction is used as a diagnostic test it should be coupled to an analysis of the movement characteristics of the spermatozoa, in order to give a balanced view of the functional competence of these cells.[58]

Fusion molecules

The way in which the acrosome reaction confers upon the sperm plasma membrane the capacity to recognize and fuse with the vitelline membrane of the oocyte is still not fully understood. Despite numerous attempts nobody has yet succeeded in making an acrosome intact spermatozoon, fusogenic. It is likely that proteolytic enzymes released during the acrosome reaction are responsible for inducing the processing of precursor fusion molecules located in the equatorial region of the sperm head.[14] In the case of human spermatozoa a variety of complement factors have been implicated in the fusion process including CD46, C3 and C1q.[59-61]

In the guinea pig, a protein known as PH-30 is thought to be involved in mediating sperm–oocyte fusion.[62] This molecule consists of two subunits that are tightly coupled and behave as a single integral membrane protein. One subunit, the α, is specialized for membrane fusion and contains domains that appear to be similar to viral fusion proteins. It therefore appears as if nature's masterpieces of gene transfer technology, viral infection and fertilization, have come to depend on similar molecules to achieve the process of fusion. In order for the α-subunit of PH-30 to mediate sperm–oocyte fusion, the plasma membranes of the male and female gametes must be brought into close apposition. This is the function of the second subunit of PH-30, the β, which contains an integrin binding domain which is thought to interact with integrins of the surface of the oocyte, to mediate the juxtaposition of male and female gametes. How this fascinating molecule becomes processed during the acrosome reaction in order to express its fusogenic properties, is currently unknown.

Egg activation

Following sperm–oocyte fusion, the egg becomes activated and initiates the cascade of events that culminate in the initiation of embryonic differentiation. The most obvious expressions of egg activation are the release of the cortical granules, the resumption of meiosis, and the formation of male and female pronuclei.[14] Biochemically, the first responses of the oocyte to fertilization are the generation of a series of periodic membrane hyperpolarizations and calcium transients after fusion has occurred. The oscillatory pattern of calcium elevations observed following sperm–oocyte fusion is thought to play an important role in programming normal embryonic development.

Cortical granule release

The release of the cortical granules during egg activation is a key component of the oocyte's strategy to prevent polyspermy and appears to be induced by the calcium transients observed at the moment of sperm–oocyte fusion.[14] The cortical granules prevent polyspermy by inducing changes in the zona pellucida in terms of the penetrability of this structure and its affinity for spermatozoa. These changes appear to involve the proteolytic cleavage of zona glycoproteins which, in the mouse, comprise the proteolytic cleavage of ZP2 (120 kDa) to form a new molecule ZP2$_f$ (90 kDa).[63] Simultaneously, ZP3 becomes dysfunctional, possibly as a result of modifications to the O-linked oligosaccharide side chains by glycosidases released by the cortical granules.[64] In addition to these changes, it is also possible that hardening of the zona pellucida due to the cross-linking of tyrosine residues under the influence of cortical granule peroxidase activity, contributes to the prevention of polyspermy.[65]

The 'vitelline block'

In addition to the changes in the zona pellucida that block polyspermy, the vitelline membrane of the oocyte also becomes resistant to fusion with additional spermatozoa, after the first fusion event has occurred. The mechanisms by which this refractory state develops are currently unresolved. Nevertheless the so called 'vitelline block' is an extremely important component of the block to polyspermy and in some species, such as the rabbit, constitutes the major means by which multiple fertilizations are prevented. In other species, such as the human, the combination of a fast 'vitelline block' and slower 'zona block' is used to prevent polyspermy. In the context of assisted conception, polyspermy can prove a problem when immature ova are inseminated and the cortical granules have not fully completed their migration to the undersurface of the plasma membrane.[66] In light of this factor, it is common practice to preincubate ova aspirated from ovarian follicles for several hours before the addition of the spermatozoa. In this way, the oocyte has time to arrange its defenses before the first spermatozoon arrives at the surface of the vitelline membrane.

Pronuclear formation and cleavage

Following fusion with the oocyte, the sperm nucleus decondenses and initiates the formation of a male pronucleus. The recent introduction of ICSI (Intra Cytoplasmic Sperm Injection) (see Chapter 2.11) as a therapeutic technique for treating severe male factor infertility has placed great emphasis on the mechanisms by which nuclear decondensation is brought about, since approximately half of the oocytes treated in this manner fail to fertilize.[67,68] The mechanisms by which sperm nucleus decondensation is achieved involve the breakdown of the nuclear envelope, reduction of the S–S bonds in the nuclear protamines and replacement of the protamines by histones.[14]

Sperm nucleus decondensation will occur in the oocyte regardless of whether the the egg has been activated or not. However, the transformation of this nuclear material into a male pronucleus is dependent on the activation of the oocyte and the concomitant formation of the female pronucleus. DNA synthesis within the male and female pronuclei begins synchronously several hours (12 h in the human) after sperm–oocyte fusion and is accompanied by the movement of these structures to the center of the oocyte. The pronuclear membranes then break down and the process of syngamy occurs whereby the two sets of chromosomes unite and organize themselves for the first cleavage division, that heralds the beginning of embryonic development.

FUTURE PERSPECTIVES

The advent of new techniques in cell and molecular biology is likely to have a major impact on our understanding of the cellular mechanisms that control fertilization and early embryonic development. In the wake of this knowledge we should witness significant advances in our capacity to diagnose and treat human infertility and develop novel forms of contraception. In terms of diagnostics, the recent production of biologically active recombinant human ZP3[69] should revolutionize the development of sperm function bioassays, by replacing the ionophores in current use with a much more biologically relevant agonist. The availability of this reagent will also facilitate fundamental studies on the cascade of events that occur downstream of receptor activation in the human spermatozoon. In the light of this knowledge, we should then be able to go back into the patient population and determine the biochemical basis for defective sperm function. This information should, in turn, shed light on the etiology of male infertility the cause of which is, at the present time, largely unknown.

Information on the cell biology of defective sperm function should also facilitate the development of rational strategies for the treatment of the infertile male. At present the only hope for most male infertility cases is ICSI. In the future, it is probable that the micromanipulation technology that underpins the ICSI procedure, will permeate through to the less specialized clinical centers and become a recognized routine technique for the treatment of infertile men. The extension of this technique to cover the intracytoplasmic injection of spermatids as well as spermatozoa has already been achieved in animals and human pregnancies have been obtained with this technique for certain cases of spermatogenic arrest.[70] In the longer term, the treatment of the patient rather than his spermatozoa should be the goal. However, attaining this objective is entirely dependent on improvements in our understanding of the fundamental pathophysiology of male infertility.

In terms of contraception, a deeper understanding of the cellular mechanisms involved in fertilization is likely to have its greatest impact on the development of contraceptive vaccines. The latter offer the prospect of prolonged, safe protection against pregnancy by interfering with specific molecules involved in fertilization and early development. The fact that clinical conditions exist in which men and women appear to suffer from long-term infertility due to the presence of anti-sperm antibodies, in the absence of any discernible side-effects, suggests that this objective is achievable. Substantial progress has already been made on the development of contraceptive vaccines based on the zona glycoprotein, ZP3, and parallel work on sperm surface antigens is at last beginning to yield results.[71]

SUMMARY

- Colonization of the female reproductive tract is heavily dependent on the capacity of human spermatozoa to penetrate the cervix. This function is, in turn, reliant on the expression of linear, progressive patterns of movement.
- In many animal species the spermatozoa are stored in the isthmic region of the Fallopian tube in readiness for fertilization. Whether isthmic sperm stores occur in primates is unknown.
- As the spermatozoa ascend the female reproductive tract they undergo a process of capacitation, involving increases in intracellular cyclic AMP and calcium and enhanced membrane fluidity.
- The biological expression of these capacitation-dependent changes in sperm biochemistry is the onset of hyperactivated motility.
- As a consequence of capacitation, the spermatozoa are able to penetrate the cumulus mass and make contact with the surface of the zona pellucida.
- Capacitated spermatozoa respond to a glycoprotein constituent of the zona pellucida (ZP3) by undergoing a secretory event known as the acrosome reaction.
- As a consequence of the acrosome reaction, the spermatozoa acquire the capacity to penetrate the zona pellucida. A protease exposed on the surface of the spermatozoa after the acrosome reaction, acrosin, is thought to effect the cleavage of the zona matrix and mediate the secondary binding of the acrosome reacted cell to the zona pellucida.
- As a consequence of the acrosome reaction, the spermatozoon also acquires the capacity to recognize and fuse with the vitelline membrane of the oocyte via a process that appears to have homologies with the fusion of a virus to its host cell.

- Sperm–oocyte fusion is followed by nuclear decondensation and, in concert with the activation of the oocyte, pronucleus formation and syngamy.
- Analyses of the molecular mechanisms underlying these events during fertilization and early embryonic development will contribute to the clinical resolution of male infertility and the development of new forms of fertility control that target the process of conception.

REFERENCES

1. Steptoe PC, Edwards RG. Birth after re-implantation of a human embryo. *Lancet* 1978 ii: 366.
2. Boonsaeng V. Molecular structure of human seminal coagulum: the role of proteolysis. *Andrologia* 1986 **18**: 252–258.
3. Mandal A, Bhattacharyya AK. Isolation of the predominant coagulum protein of human semen before liquefaction. *Hum Reprod* 1994 **9**: 320–324.
4. World Health Organization. WHO Laboratory Manual for the Examination of Human Semen and Semen–Cervical Mucus Interaction. Cambridge: Cambridge University Press, 1992.
5. Aitken RJ, Bowie H, Buckingham D, Harkiss D, Richardson DW, West KM. Sperm penetration into a hyaluronic acid polymer as a means of monitoring functional competence. *J Androl* 1992 **13**: 44–54.
6. Kremer J, Jager S, Kuiken J, van Slochteren-Draaisma T. Recent advances in diagnosis and treatment of infertility due to antisperm antibodies. In Cohen J, Hendry WF (eds) *Spermatozoa, Antibodies and Infertility*. Oxford: Blackwell, 1978: 117–128.
7. Kremer J, Jager S. The sperm cervical mucus contact test: a preliminary report. *Fertil Steril* 1976 **27**: 335–340.
8. Hull MGR, Savage PE, Bromham DR. Prognostic value of the postcoital test: prospective study based on time specific conception rates. *Br J Obstet Gynaecol* 1982 **89**: 299–305.
9. Hunter RHF. *Physiology and Technology of Reproduction in Female Domestic Animals*. New York: Academic Press, 1980: 250.
10. Smith TT, Yanagimachi R. The viability of hamster spermatozoa stored in the isthmus of the oviduct: the importance of sperm-epithelium contact for sperm survival. *Biol Reprod* 1990 **42**: 450–457.
11. Overstreet JW. Transport of gametes in the reproductive tract of the female mammal. In Hartmann JF (ed.) *Mechanisms Controlling Animal Fertilization*. New York: Academic Press, 1983: 499–543.
12. Kervancioglu ME, Djahanbakhch O, Aitken RJ. Epithelial cell co-culture and the induction of sperm capacitation. *Fertil Steril* 1994 **61**: 1103–1108.
13. Yanagimachi R. *In vitro* capacitation of hamster spermatozoa by follicular fluid. *J Reprod Fertil* 1969 **18**: 275–286.
14. Yanagimachi R. Mammalian fertilization. In Knobil E, Neill JD (eds) *The Physiology of Reproduction, 2nd edn*. New York: Raven Press, 1994: 189–317.
15. Eppig JJ, Downs SM, Schroeder AC. Perspectives of mammalian oocyte maturation *in vitro* and practical applications. In Testart J, Frydman R (eds) *Human in Vitro Fertilization: INSERM Symposium No 24*. Amsterdam: Elsevier, 1985: 33–44.
16. Blackmore PF, Beebe SJ, Danforth DR, Alexander N. Progesterone and 17-hydroxyprogesterone: novel stimulators of calcium influx in human sperm. *J Biol Chem* 1990 **265**: 1376–1380.
17. Kay VJ, Coutts JRT, Robertson L. Pentoxyfylline stimulates hyperactivation in human spermatozoa. *Hum Reprod* 1993 **8**: 727–731.
18. White D, Aitken, RJ. Relationship between calcium, cyclic AMP, ATP and intracellular pH and the capacity of hamster spermatozoa to express hyperactivated motility. *Gamete Res* 1989 **22**: 163–177.
19. Langlais J, Roberts KD. A molecular membrane model of sperm capacitation and the acrosome reaction of mammalian spermatozoa. *Gamete Res* 1985 **12**: 183–224.
20. Yovich JM, Edirisinghe WR, Cummins JM, Yovich JL. Influence of pentoxyfylline in severe male factor infertility. *Fertil Steril* 1990 **53**: 715–722.
21. Aitken RJ, Mattei A, Irvine S. Paradoxical stimulation of human sperm-motility by 2-deoxyadenosine. *J Reprod Fertil* 1986 **78**: 515–527.
22. Carver-Ward JA, Jaroudi KA, Einspenner M,Parhar RS, Al-Sedairy ST, Sheth KV. Pentoxyfylline potentiates ionophore (A23187) mediated acrosome reaction in human sperm: flow cytometric analysis using CD46 antibody. *Hum Reprod* 1994 **9**: 71–76.
23. Tesarik J, Thebault A, Testart J. Effect of pentoxyfylline on sperm movement characteristics in normospermic and asthenozoospermic specimens. *Hum Reprod* 1992 **7**: 1257–1263.
24. Fraser LR, Harrison RAP, Herod JE. Characterization of a decapacitation factor associated with epididymal mouse spermatozoa. *J Reprod Fertil* 1990 **89**: 135–148.
25. Miller DJ, Ax RL. Carbohydrates and fertilization in animals. *Mol Reprod Dev* 1990 **26**: 184–198.
26. Oliphant G. Removal of sperm-bound seminal plasma components as a prerequisite to induction of the rabbit acrosome reaction. *Fertil Steril* 1976 **27**: 28–38.
27. Bradley MP, Forrester IT. Human and ram seminal plasma both contain a calcium-dependent regulator protein, calsemin. *J Androl* 1982 **3**: 289-296.
28. Okabe M, Takada K, Adachi T, Kohama Y, Miura T, Aonuma S. Inconsistent reactivity of an anti-sperm monoclonal antibody and its relationship to sperm capacitation. *J Reprod Immunol* 1986 **9**: 67–70.
29. Koehler JK. The mammalian sperm surface: studies with specific labelling techniques. *Int Rev Cytol* 1978 **54**: 73–108.
30. Ahuja KK. Lectin-coated agarose beads in the investigation of sperm capacitation in the hamster. *Dev Biol* 1984 **104**: 131–142.
31. Friend DS, Rudolf I. Acrosomal disruption in sperm. *J Cell Biol* 1974 **63**: 466–478.
32. Suzuki F, Yanagimachi R. Changes in the distribution of intra membranous particles and filipin-reactive membrane sterols during *in vitro* capacitation of golden hamster spermatozoa. *Gamete Res* 1989 **23**: 335–347.
33. Bearer EL, Friend DS. Modifications of anionic lipid domains preceding membrane fusion in guinea pig sperm. *J Cell Biol* 1982 **92**: 604–615.
34. Aitken RJ. Do sperm find eggs attractive? *Nature* 1991 **351**: 19–20.
35. Talbot P, Di Carlantonio G, Zao P, Penkala J, Haimo LT. Motile cells lacking hyaluronidase can penetrate the hamster oocyte cumulus complex. *Dev Biol* 1985 **108**: 387–398.
36. Huszar G, Willetts M, Corrales M. Hyaluronic acid (Sperm Select) improves retention of sperm motility and velocity in normospermic and oligospermic specimens. *Fertil Steril* 1990 **54**: 1127–1134.
37. Ranganathan S, Ganguly AT, Datta K. Evidence for presence of hyaluronan binding protein on spermatozoa and its possible involvement in sperm function. *Mol Reprod Dev* **38**: 69–76.
38. Tesarik J, Oltras CM, Testart J. Effect of the human

cumulus oophorus on movement characteristics of human capacitated spermatozoa. *J Reprod Fertil* 1990 **88**: 665–675.

39. Gmachi M, Gunther K. Bee venom hyaluronidase is homologous to a membrane protein of mammalian sperm. *Proc Natl Acad Sci USA* 1993 **90**: 3569–3573.

40. Wassarman PM. Profile of a sperm receptor. *Development* 1990 **108**: 1–17.

41. Greve JM, Wassarman PM. Mouse extracellular coat is a matrix of interconnected filaments possessing a structural repeat. *J Mol Biol* 1985 **81**: 253–264.

42. Thillai Koothan P, van Duin M, Aitken RJ. Cloning, sequencing and oocyte-specific expression of the marmoset sperm receptor protein, ZP3. *Zygote* 1993 **1**: 93–101.

43. Leyton L, Saling P. Evidence that aggregation of mouse sperm receptors by ZP3 triggers the acrosome reaction. *J Cell Biol* 1989 **108**: 2163–2168.

44. Hokke CH, Damm JBL, Penninkhof B, Aitken RJ, Kamerling JP, Vliegenthart JFG. Structure of the O-linked carbohydrate chains of porcine zona pellucida glycoproteins. *Eur J Biochem* 1994 **221**: 491–512.

45. Bleil JD, Wasarman PM. Galactose at the nonreducing terminus of O-linked oligosaccharides of mouse egg zona pellucida glycoprotein ZP3 is essential for the glycoprotein's sperm receptor activity. *Proc Natl Acad Sci USA* 1988 **85**: 6778–6782.

46. Miller DJ, Macek MB, Shur BD. Complementarity between sperm surface β-1,4-galactosyltransferase and egg coat ZP3 mediates sperm–egg binding. *Nature* 1992 **357**: 589–593.

47. Paterson M, Aitken RJ. Development of a vaccine based on zona pellucida antigens. *Curr Opin Immunol* 1990 **5**: 743–747.

48. Töpfer-Petersen E, Henschen A. Acrosin shows zona and fucose binding, novel properties for a serine proteinase. *FEBS Lett* 1987 **226**: 38–42.

49. Fock-Nuzel R, Lottspeich F, Henschen A, Muller-Esterl W. Boar acrosin is a two-chain molecule. Isolation and primary structure of the light chain; homology with the pro-part of other serine proteinases. *Eur J Biochem* 1984 **141**: 441–446.

50. Cechova D, Topfer-Petersen E, Henschen A. Boar proacrosin is a single chain molecule which has the N-terminus of the acrosin A-chain (light chain). *FEBS Lett* 1988 **241**: 136–140.

51. Baba T, Kashiwabara S, Watanabe K, Itoh H, Michikawa Y, Kimura K, Takada M, Fukamizu A, Arai Y. Activation and maturation mechanisms of boar acrosin zymogen based on deduced primary structure. *J Biol Chem* 1989 **264**: 11920–11927.

52. Jones, R. Identification and functions of mammalian sperm–egg recognition molecules during fertilization. *J Reprod Fertil* 1990 **42**: 89–105.

53. Aitken RJ, Brindle JP. Comparison of probes targeting constituents of the outer acrosomal membrane and acrosomal vesicle for their ability to detect the acrosome reaction in human spermatozoa. *Hum Reprod* 1993 **8**: 1663–1669.

54. Yanagimachi R, Yanagimachi H, Rogers BJ. The use of zona free animal ova as a test system for the assessment of the fertilizing capacity of human spermatozoa. *Biol Reprod* 1976 **15**: 471–476.

55. Aitken RJ, Irvine DS, Wu FC. Prospective analysis of sperm–oocyte fusion and reactive oxygen species generation as criteria for the diagnosis of infertility. *Am J Obstet Gynecol* 1991 **164**: 542–551.

56. Aitken RJ, Ross A, Hargreave T, Richardson DW, Best FSM. Analysis of human sperm function following exposure to the ionophore A23187. Comparison of normospermic and oligozoospermic men. *J Androl* 1984 **5**: 321–329.

57. Aitken RJ, Thatcher S, Glasier AF, Clarkson JS, Wu FCW, Baird DT. Relative ability of modified versions of the hamster oocyte penetration test, incorporating hyperosmotic medium or the ionophore A23187, to predict IVF outcome. *Hum Reprod* 1987 **2**: 227–231.

58. Aitken RJ, Buckingham D, Harkiss D. Analysis of the extent to which sperm movement can predict the results of ionophore-enhanced functional assays of the acrosome reaction and sperm–oocyte fusion. *Hum Reprod* 1994 **9**: 1867–1874.

59. Anderson DJ, Abbot AF, Jack RM. The role of complement component C3b and its receptors in sperm–oocyte interaction. *Proc Natl Acad Sci USA* 1993 **90**: 10051–10055.

60. Okabe M, Matzno S, Nagira T, Mimura T, Kawai Y, Mayumi T. A human sperm antigen possibly involved in binding and/or fusion with zona-free hamster eggs. *Fertil Steril* 1990 **54**: 1211–1126.

61. Fusi F, Bronson RA, Hong Y, Ghebrehiwei B. Complement component C1q and its receptor are involved in the interaction of human sperm with zona free hamster eggs. *Mol Reprod Dev* 1991 **29**: 180–188.

62. Primakoff P, Hyatt H, Tredick-Kline J. Identification and purification of a sperm surface protein with a potential role in sperm–egg membrane fusion. *J Cell Biol* 1987 **104**: 141–149.

63. Moller CC, Wassarman PM. Characterization of a proteinase that cleaves zona pellucida glycoprotein ZP2 following activation of mouse eggs. *Dev Biol* 1989 **132**: 103–112.

64. Wassarman PM. The biology and chemistry of fertilization *Science* 1987 **235**: 553–560.

65. Schmell ED, Gulyas BJ. Ovoperoxidase activity in ionophore treated mouse eggs. II. Evidence for the enzyme's role in hardening the zona pellucida. *Gamete Res* 1980 **3**: 279–290.

66. Sathananthan AH, Trounson AO. The human pronuclear ovum: fine structure of monospermic and polyspermic fertilization *in vitro*. *Gamete Res* 1985 **12**: 385–398.

67. Van Steirteghem AC, Liu J, Joris H, Nagy Z, Janssenswillen C, Tournaye H, Derde M-P, Van Assche E, Devroey P. Higher success rate by intracytoplasmic sperm injection than by subzonal insemination. Report of a second series of 300 consecutive cycles. *Hum Reprod* 1993 **8**: 1055–1060.

68. Van Steirteghem AC, Nagy Z, Joris H, Liu J, Staessen, Smitz J, Wisanto A, Devroey P. High fertilization and implantation rates after intracytoplasmic injection. *Hum Reprod* 1993 **8**: 1061–1066.

69. Van Duin M, Polman JEM, De Breet ITM, van Ginneken K. Bunschoten H, Grootenhuis A, Brindle J, Aitken RJ. Production, purification and biological activity of recombinant human zona pellucida protein, ZP3. *Biol Reprod* 1994 **51**, 607–617.

70. Aitken RJ, Irvine DS. Fertilization without sperm. *Nature* 1996 **379**: 493–495.

71. Aitken RJ, Paterson M, Thillai Koothan P. Contraceptive vaccines. *Br Med Bull* 1993 **49**: 88–99.

2.11

Assisted Reproduction

A Van Steirteghem, I Liebaers and P Devroey

INTRODUCTION

The birth of Louise Brown in July, 1978, following *in vitro* fertilization and embryo transfer (IVF/ET: Table 2.11.1) was a landmark in the treatment of infertility.[1] Initially developed to treat women who were unable to conceive because of tubal infertility, IVF/ET has since been extended to treat many other indications including unexplained infertility and endometriosis (Fig. 2.11.1), as well as infertility in couples where there is a problem with the male partner's sperm (Fig. 2.11.2). Worldwide, hundreds of thousands of children have been born to IVF and related procedures such as gamete and zygote intrafallopian transfer (GIFT and ZIFT) (Table 2.11.1). In the UK alone, in 1992[2] there were 18 224 IVF treatment cycles carried out, resulting in 3080 clinical pregnancies and 2318 live births.

Despite these impressive advances, it is still the general experience that standard IVF fails in certain couples, especially in those with severe male-factor infertility where sperm numbers are too low and/or sperm function is defective. To treat these cases it has been necessary to develop assisted fertilization procedures that circumvent the barriers to fertilization *in vitro*: partial zona dissection (PZD), subzonal insemination (SUZI) and intra cytoplasmic sperm injection (ICSI) (Table 2.11.1). This chapter surveys the current status of assisted reproduction technology,

emphasizing conventional IVF/ET and the newer techniques of assisted fertilization that have recently been introduced into clinical practice.

CURRENT CONCEPTS

In vitro fertilization

IVF is a well-established treatment for certain types of infertility.[3,4] GIFT and ZIFT are variations on IVF/ET that are only appropriate if tubal function is normal. The various stages in a cycle of IVF treatment consist of: (a) patient selection, (b) ovarian stimulation, (c) oocyte retrieval, (d) semen preparation, (e) insemination, (f) assessment of fertilization, (g) embryo cleavage, (h) embryo replacement, (i) cryopreservation of excess embryos, and (j) detection of pregnancy. Each of these stages will now be summarized (Fig. 2.11.3).

Table 2.11.1 Common assisted reproduction techniques

Acronym	Definition
IVF/ET	*In vitro* fertilization and embryo transfer
GIFT	Gamete intra-Fallopian transfer
ZIFT	Zygote intra-Fallopian transfer
DI	Donor insemination
PZD	Partial zona dissection
SUZI	Subzonal sperm injection
ICSI	Intracytoplasmic sperm injection
MESA	Micro-epididymal sperm aspiration

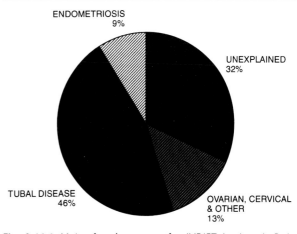

Fig. 2.11.1 *Major female reasons for IVF/ET treatment. Data from the Third Annual Report of the Human Fertilization and Embryology Authority (HFEA).*[2]

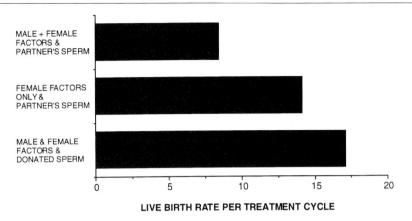

Fig. 2.11.2 *IVF live-birth rates according to male factor and donated or partner's sperm (excluding frozen embryo transfers, unstimulated cycles, donated eggs and embryos). Data from the Third Annual Report of the HFEA.*[2]

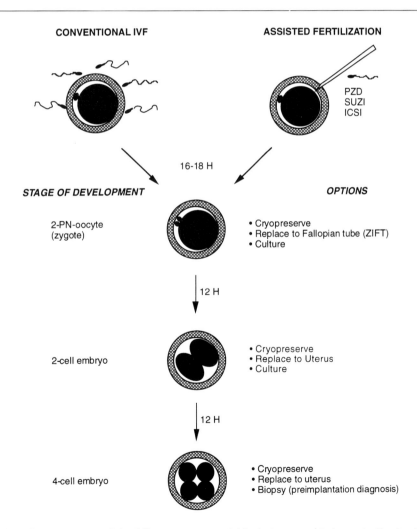

Fig. 2.11.3 *Flow-sheet illustrating some of the different options available during an assisted reproduction treatment cycle.*

Patient selection

The various indications for IVF treatment include tubal disease, andrological infertility, endometriosis, immunological and idiopathic infertility. It is not uncommon for several causes of infertility to be present in one couple. IVF can also be applied in infertile couples requiring oocyte donation. This involves two distinct groups of patients: (1) females without gonadal function due to gonadal dysgenesis, premature menopause (which may occur spontaneously, or after surgical castration or castration induced by chemo- or radiotherapy) or resistant-ovary syndrome, and (2) women with functional ovaries but who do not wish to use their own oocytes to become pregnant because of the risk of transmitting chromosomal abnormalities to the offspring (e.g. if there is a history of autosomal dominant disease or X-linked disease, or when both partners are carriers of an autosomal recessive disease).[5,6]

Ovarian stimulation

The aim of ovarian stimulation is to bring about the development of multiple mature follicles so that multiple oocytes can be harvested to maximize the likelihood of successful IVF treatment. Currently the most frequently used protocol of controlled ovarian stimulation combines treatment with a gonadotropin-releasing hormone agonist (GnRHa) and human menopausal gonadotropin (HMG).[7] HMG is a urinary preparation containing roughly equal amounts of follicle-stimulating hormone (FSH) and luteinizing hormone (LH). GnRHa is given to bring about desensitization of the pituitary gonadotropes to endogenous GnRH so that ovarian stimulation can be exerted by administering HMG.[8-10] When several follicles have sufficiently matured, based on their size (≥17 mm diameter, as assessed by ovarian ultrasound scanning) and measurement of serum estradiol concentration (≥3.7 nmol/l) ovulation can be induced by administering human chorionic gonadotropin (HCG). Since this regimen suppresses pituitary LH secretion, the subsequent luteal phase must be 'supported' by giving low-dose HCG to stimulate luteal progesterone production or by administering exogenous progesterone directly.[11,12]

Oocyte retrieval

The purpose of this step is safely and quickly to aspirate as many mature oocytes as possible from the patient's ovaries. In the early days of IVF, oocyte retrieval was carried out by laparoscopy under general anesthesia, which required the availability of a fully staffed operating theatre and usually an overnight stay in hospital. Nowadays, egg collection is usually performed by transvaginal ultrasound-guided follicular puncture under local anesthesia. This makes IVF more practicable and convenient, since it can be carried out on an outpatient basis.

Immediately after the contents of each follicle have been aspirated, the cumulus–oocyte complex is identified and transferred into culture medium for incubation at 37°C until it is inseminated, usually 4–6 h later.

The culture medium

Many different culture media can be used for IVF. Most are bicarbonate-buffered, containing a protein supplement (patient serum, cord blood serum, human or bovine serum albumin).[13-19] Incubation is at 37°C, usually in an atmosphere of 5% O_2, 5% CO_2 and 90% N_2. *In vitro* culture can be done in open test tubes or culture dishes if large (≥0.5 ml) volumes of medium are used, or in small droplets (e.g. 25 μl) of medium covered by lightweight paraffin oil.

Semen preparation

Motile spermatozoa must be separated from seminal fluid and allowed to capacitate before they can be used for conventional IVF (see Chapter 2.10). Semen produced by masturbation is allowed to liquefy before being diluted with culture medium and centrifuged to sediment the spermatozoa. One of two procedures is then commonly employed to isolate motile sperm from the centrifuged sperm pellet:

1. *'Swim-up'* In this type of protocol[20-21] fresh medium is overlayed onto the sperm pellet. Upon incubation at 37°C, the most motile sperm 'swim up' into the medium above, away from immotile sperm and debris in the centrifuged pellet.
2. *Density-gradient centrifugation* is more popular where the motile sperm content of the initial ejaculate is low. In this protocol the centrifuged sperm pellet is resuspended in medium and centrifuged through a two- or three-layer discontinuous Percoll™ gradient.[22-26] A typical 'three-layer' gradient comprises 90%–70%–50% Percoll (vol/vol) as a discontinuous gradient in culture medium, whereas a 'two-layer' system would comprise 95% and 47.5% Percoll. Motile sperm sediment to the bottom of the tube upon centrifugation.

Motile sperm separated by either technique are harvested, washed by centrifugation, resuspended in culture medium and kept at 37°C until insemination.

Insemination

Capacitated spermatozoa are added to cumulus-enclosed oocytes a few hours after oocyte retrieval, by which time most oocytes are expected to be at the metaphase-II stage of development ready for fertilization (see Chapter 2.4). The number of spermatozoa added to each oocyte usually varies between 100 000 and 200 000 spermatozoa/ml culture medium. In the authors' laboratory, gamete and embryo culture are carried out in 25 μl microdrops of medium covered by lightweight paraffin oil. The number of spermatozoa added to each oocyte varies between 2000 and 5000 spermatozoa, corresponding to a concentration of 80 000–200 000 sperm cells/ml of medium. The higher number of spermatozoa is used for couples with male-factor infertility.

Assessment of fertilization

About 16–18 h after the spermatozoa have been added, cumulus cells are removed from each oocyte by gentle pipetting using finely drawn glass pipettes with diameters between 200 and 300 μm. The denuded oocytes are then transferred to fresh culture medium and examined microscopically (×200 magnification) for the presence of pronuclei and polar bodies (Fig. 2.11.4). Normal fertilization is indicated by the presence of two distinct pronuclei and usually also two polar bodies. If only one pronucleus is present, a second observation is made out 3–4 h later. In our experience, approximately 25% of inseminated oocytes that show only one pronucleus will develop the second within this time.[27] Around 5% of inseminated oocytes will only ever develop one pronucleus, whereas another 5% develop more than two (i.e. become polyspermic).

Embryo cleavage

Fertilized oocytes are usually re-examined after a further 24 h incubation (i.e. ~42 h postinsemination) to confirm that embryonic cleavage has occurred and assess embryo 'quality' (Fig. 2.11.4). The assessment is based on the extent of anucleate fragments present in the cleaving embryos. A typical embryo scoring system is as follows. 'Excellent' (type A) embryos are those without anucleate fragments, 'good' (type B) have 1–20% of their volume filled with anucleate fragments, 'fair' (type C) have 21–50% anucleate fragments, and 'poor' (type D) have more than 50% fragmentation.[28–32] It must be emphasized that assignment of a good morphological score to an individual embryo is no guarantee that it is chromosomally 'normal'.[33]

Preimplantation diagnosis of genetic disease

At the 4-cell stage of development or beyond, it is possible to remove one of the blastomeres by micromanipulation for genetic analysis. It is estimated that 21 000 children are born each year in the UK with a significant genetic defect such as cystic fibrosis, hemophilia, Huntington's chorea and many others.[2] Preimplantation diagnosis of certain genetic defects can now be carried out on a single blastomere to determine whether defective genes are present. It is then possible to transfer to the woman only those embryos which are unaffected. The first single gene defect to be tackled in this way was cystic fibrosis.[34] Subsequently the approach has been extended to Lesch–Nyan's disease, Tay–Sachs disease and Duchenne's muscular dystrophy. In principle, any single gene defect might eventually be tackled in this way.[35]

Embryo replacement

After embryonic cleavage has been established, several embryos are selected for transcervical transfer to the uterus. The replacement of cleaved embryos of sufficient morphological quality (i.e. types A–C) is usually carried out 44–48 h after insemination when they should be at the 2–4 cell stage (Fig. 2.11.3). The pregnancy rate after IVF increases with the number of embryos replaced. However, the multiple pregnancy rate also increases with the number of

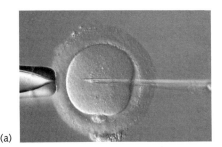

(a)

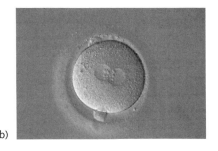

(b)

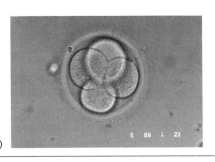

(c)

Fig. 2.11.4. Assisted fertilization and early human embryogenesis: **(a)** metaphase II oocyte undergoing ICSI; **(b)** a 2-PN (i.e. normally fertilized) oocyte; **(c)** 'type A' 4-cell embryo. Magnification ×330 (approx.) (see Plate 3).

embryos replaced, therefore the number of embryos replaced at any one time is generally restricted to a maximum of three. In younger women who are more likely to become pregnant it is even advisable to restrict this number to two. This avoids the occurrence of triplet pregnancies without influencing the pregnancy rate.[28,36]

GIFT and ZIFT

In the GIFT procedure, oocytes and sperm are collected as for IVF/ET but then both sets of gametes are combined and immediately transferred to the Fallopian tube so that fertilization can occur *in vivo* (Fig. 2.11.4). A limited number of cumulus–oocyte complexes (usually no more than three, see above) is placed into the fimbrial end of the Fallopian tube together with 100 000–200 000 motile spermatozoa.[37] ZIFT is another IVF/ET variant in which uncleaved, fertilized oocytes (zygotes) are placed into the Fallopian tube on the first day after oocyte retrieval. Alternatively, cleaved embryos are replaced to the Fallopian tube in a similar manner once embryonic cleavage has begun.[38–41] Most replacements of zygotes and embryos to the Fallopian tube involve laparoscopy and general anesthesia, although tubal replacement can also be carried out through the uterus.

Embryo freezing

Not all of the multiple embryos produced in any one IVF cycle can always be replaced to the patient in that cycle because of the risk of high-order multiple pregnancy. It is, therefore, common practice to cryopreserve (freeze-store) excess embryos for future use. If the replacement of fresh embryos does not lead to pregnancy, the patient can receive thawed embryos in a later cycle. Similarly, successfully treated patients wishing repeat treatment(s) in the future can make use of their freeze-stored embryos, thus making IVF treatment more efficient and cost-effective.

Factors that influence the success of embryo cryopreservation include: (a) the cryopreservation protocol (i.e. the cryoprotectant used and rates of freezing and thawing), (b) the morphological quality of the embryos and their stage of development at the time of freezing, (c) the degree of damage suffered by the embryos during freezing or thawing, (d) the ovarian stimulation protocol leading up to egg collection, (e) the management of the cycle in which thawed embryos are replaced, (f) the timing of embryo replacement, and (g) the number of embryos replaced.[42,43] In most experienced centers, implantation rates using freeze–thawed embryos are comparable with implantation rates using fresh embryos.

Establishment of pregnancy

Within 10–12 days of insemination, implantation of embryos replaced to the uterus can be detected by an increase in serum HCG levels. Trophoblastic cells in the blastocysts secrete HCG, levels of which in plasma increase exponentially during the first trimester of pregnancy. In a viable pregnancy, HCG levels double approximately every 1.3 days. Marked deviations from this normal pattern of increase are consistent with an abnormal pregnancy such as ectopic implantation, blighted ovum or an impending miscarriage.

The diagnosis of a clinical pregnancy depends on visualization by ultrasound of a gestational sac containing a viable fetus (i.e.with a detectable heartbeat) located within the uterine cavity.

IVF audit

IVF has become a widely applied and generally successful treatment, and live birth rates have generally increased over recent years (Fig. 2.11.5). However, IVF outcomes vary greatly with the age of the patient and the cause of infertility under treatment. The likelihood of achieving pregnancy and live birth decrease with age where a woman uses her own eggs. Her age is less significant if she receives donor eggs or embryos. A high proportion of IVF treatments involving a female factor also involve a male factor.[44,45] Recent statistics from the UK[2] show that where the partner's sperm was used and there is a male factor, the live birth rate is 8.4% per treatment cycle compared with 17.1% where donor sperm was used. For those with no male factor the live birth rate was 14.1 % (Fig. 2.11.2).

Highest live birth rates following conventional IVF are found among women having IVF with donated embryos or donor sperm, suggesting that many couples treated with IVF have a male factor problem as well as a female factor.[2]

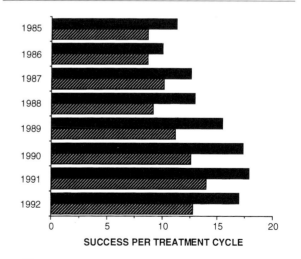

Fig. 2.11.5 *IVF success rates in the UK since 1985. Data from the Third Annual Report of the HFEA.[2]*

Assisted fertilization

Gamete micromanipulation

In the last five years, several procedures of assisted fertilization based on the micromanipulation of eggs and sperm have been applied to couples with severe male-factor infertility who cannot be helped by conventional IVF. The strategy has been to reduce or remove the barrier to fertilization *in vitro* by disrupting the zona pellucida, thus allowing sperm direct access to the perivitelline space of the oocyte. The first such technique was PZD (Fig. 2.11.6a), in which a small slit is made in the zona to allow sperm to pass through to the oolemma. The results of PZD were generally found to be unsatisfactory, being associated with erratic but generally low fertilization rates.[46,47] The next technique to gain sway was SUZI, in which several (between 3 and 20) motile spermatozoa are injected through the zona pellucida into the perivitelline space (Fig. 2.11.6b). The monosper-

mic fertilization rate using SUZI was still low at about 20% of all metaphase-II oocytes injected.[46,48–52] Overall, the experience with PZD and SUZI was that normal fertilization rates were too low. Consequently, only about two-thirds of patients receiving these treatments ever produced embryos (even then, only one or two at a time), such that pregnancy and live birth rates were unacceptably low.[48,52–58]

Intra-cytoplasmic sperm injection (ICSI)

In 1992, our group reported the first pregnancies and births after replacement of embryos generated by a novel procedure of assisted fertilization known as ICSI.[59] In this technique, sperm are injected through the zona pellucida and the oolemma, directly into the oocyte (Fig. 2.11.6c). Prior to this clinical application, ICSI had been used successfully to obtain live offspring in rabbits and cattle.[60] Two other IVF centers had attempted clinical ICSI on a series of 143 oocytes, reporting the transfer of four zygotes in two women and of 11 cleaved embryos in seven others, none of whom became pregnant.[57,61] Our own experience with ICSI has been that the fertilization rate after ICSI is not only significantly better than after SUZI, but that ICSI also leads to the production of more embryos with higher implantation rates.[51,52,62,63] Thus ICSI has been adopted as the technique of choice when assisted fertilization is necessary.

Clinical evaluation of ICSI

General experience with the ICSI procedure is limited because it is such a new clinical technique. Our own experience with ICSI will now be summarized, emphasizing: (a) patient selection, (b) ovarian stimulation and oocyte handling, (c) semen evaluation and preparation, (d) the ICSI procedure itself, (e) oocyte damage and pronuclear status after ICSI, (f) embryo transfer and freezing, and (g) current results of prenatal assessment and a prospective follow-up of the children born after ICSI.

Patient selection

The couples selected for ICSI were all suffering from long-standing infertility. Three categories of couples were treated in 1275 ICSI cycles: First, couples who had undergone at least one, but more frequently two or more standard IVF attempts and failed. After attempting insemination with even high numbers of progressively motile spermatozoa, fertilization had not occurred or had occurred in fewer than 5% of the oocytes. Secondly, couples with such severe male factor that standard IVF treatment was deemed to be futile: semen parameters were hopelessly deficient or the total ejaculate contained fewer than 500 000 progressively motile spermatozoa. Thirdly, couples with obstructive azoospermia due to congenital bilateral absence of the vas deferens (CBAVD) or failed vaso-vasostomy and vasoepididymostomy.

Because the ICSI procedure was clinically unproven, ethics committee review and approval was required to commence this trial. The couples were fully informed about the novelty of the procedure, the uncertainty of its outcome, and the theoretical risk of increased abnormali-

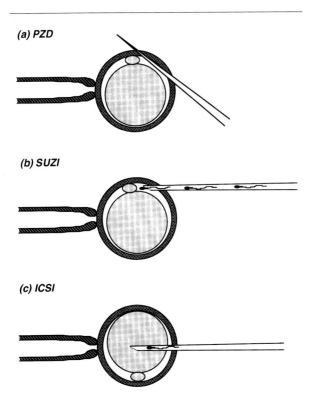

(a) PZD

(b) SUZI

(c) ICSI

Fig. 2.11.6 *Evolution of techniques of assisted fertilization.* **(a)** *Partial zona dissection PZD: the zona pellucida is mechanically breached with a glass micropipette; thereafter the oocyte is inseminated with spermatozoa as for conventional IVF.* **(b)** *Subzonal insemination (SUZI) of a metaphase II oocyte. The oocyte is immobilized with the holding pipette (left) and a variable number (3 to 20) of spermatozoa is injected into the perivitelline space by means of the injection pipette (right).* **(c)** *Intracytoplasmic sperm injection (ICSI) into a metaphase II oocyte. The oocyte is immobilized with the polar body at the 6 o'clock position by means of the holding pipette. A single spermatozoon is aspirated into the injection pipette and injected deep into the cytoplasm of the oocyte after penetrating the zona pellucida and the oolemma (see also Fig. 2.11.4).*

ties arising in any children born to ICSI. After extensive counseling, all patients consented to prenatal diagnosis during any resulting pregnancy and to participate in a prospective follow-up of any child born after ICSI.

Ovarian stimulation and oocyte handling

Controlled ovarian stimulation and oocyte collection were as described above for conventional IVF.[64] A total of 16 109 cumulus enclosed oocytes were retrieved (mean 12.6 oocytes per cycle). The luteal phase was supported from the day after HCG administration by intravaginally administered micronized progesterone.[11,12]

Cumulus cells were removed by incubation for up to one minute in HEPES-buffered Earle's medium containing 60 IU hyaluronidase/ml followed by pipetting in and out of hand-drawn glass pipettes with two different diameters: 250–300 μm followed by 200 μm. The denuded oocytes were then rinsed several times in droplets of HEPES-buffered Earle's and Ménézo's B_2 media and examined microscopically.

Of the 16 109 oocyte complexes collected, 15 387 (95.5%) contained an intact oocyte with an intact zona pellucida and clear cytoplasm. Analysis of the nuclear status of the intact oocytes revealed 85% metaphase-II oocytes that had extruded the first polar body; 11% germinal-vesicle-stage oocytes; and 4% metaphase-I oocytes that had undergone breakdown of the germinal vesicle but not yet extruded the first polar body. The oocytes were then incubated in 25-μl microdrops of B_2 medium covered by lightweight paraffin oil at 37°C in an atmosphere of 5% O_2, 5% CO_2 and 90% N_2. Nuclear maturity was assessed again just prior to the microinjection procedure. ICSI was carried out on all metaphase-II oocytes. ICSI was not carried out in two treatment cycles where no metaphase-II oocytes were observed.

Semen evaluation and preparation

ICSI was carried out using ejaculated sperm in 1194 cycles, deferential sperm in two cycles, freshly collected epididymal sperm in 49 cycles, frozen–thawed epididymal sperm in ten cycles and testicular sperm in 17 cycles. In three treatment cycles, no semen sample was produced. Semen values were considered 'normal'[65,66] if: (a) sperm concentration was at least 20×10^6/ml, (b) progressive sperm motility was at least 40%, and (c) normal sperm morphology was at least 14%.

The characteristics of the 1189 freshly ejaculated semen specimens used for ICSI were as follows: oligo-asthenoteratozoospermia in 50%; two abnormal semen parameters in 29%; one abnormal semen parameter in 15%; and 'normal' semen parameters in the remainder (6%). These last were patients who had unsuccessfully undergone at least two previous IVF cycles in which lack of oocytes was not the cause of failure.

Spermatozoa for ICSI were harvested from ejaculated semen[67] and epididymal fluid[68] by centrifugation on a two-layer Percoll-density gradient, as described above. Epididymal sperm was obtained by micro-epididymal sperm aspiration (MESA): if more sperm were recovered than required for the ICSI procedure, they were stored frozen[69]

for future use. When frozen–thawed epididymal sperm was used for ICSI, it was processed by Percoll density-gradient centrifugation as for ejaculated sperm.

Testicular sperm were used for ICSI if no spermatozoa were found after several MESA attempts or if the epididymis was absent due to previous surgery. Testicular biopsies were shredded in HEPES-buffered Earle's medium and pelleted by centrifugation. Motile spermatozoa were aspirated from a droplet of medium containing the resuspended testicular tissue.

The median number of spermatozoa recovered was 46 000 000 for freshly collected epididymal sperm, 150 000 for frozen–thawed epididymal sperm and 540 000 for testicular sperm. Total and progressive motility rates were 12% and 2% for freshly collected epididymal sperm, whereas very few motile spermatozoa were recovered in frozen–thawed epididymal sperm and testicular sperm.

The motility of all sperm used for ICSI was reduced by adding the sperm suspension to HEPES-buffered Earle's medium containing 10% polyvinylpyrrolidene (PVP).

The ICSI procedure

The preparation of holding and injection pipettes is a critical step in ICSI. Glass capillaries were drawn on a horizontal micro-electrode puller. Holding pipettes were cut and fire-polished on a microforge to produce an outer diameter of 60 μm with an opening of 20 μm. Injection pipettes were prepared on the microforge and ground with a microgrinder to give outer and inner diameters of 7 and 5 μm, respectively, and a bevel angle of 50°. The microforge was used to make a sharp spike on the injection pipette and to bend the edge of the holding and injection pipettes to an angle of about 45°, in order to facilitate the injection procedure in the Petri dish.

Intracytoplasmic sperm injection procedures were carried out on the heated stage (37°C) of an inverted microscope at $\times 400$ magnification. The microscope was equipped with two coarse positioning manipulators and two three-dimensional hydraulic remote-control micromanipulator. The holding and injection pipettes were fitted to a tool holder and connected to a micrometer-type injector. Solution delivery was controlled via a 1 μl resolution vernier micrometer.

A single almost immotile spermatozoon was selected from the droplet containing spermatozoa and was aspirated tail-first into the tip of the injection pipette. The table of the microscope was then moved in order to visualize an oocyte in one of the droplets surrounding the sperm suspension. The oocyte was immobilized by slight negative pressure exerted on the holding pipette. The polar body was held at 12 or 6 o'clock and the micropipette was pushed through the zona pellucida and the oolemma into the ooplasm at 3 o'clock (Fig. 2.11.4a). A single spermatozoon was injected into the ooplasm with about 1–2 pl of medium. The injection pipette was withdrawn gently and the injected oocyte was released from the holding pipette. The aspiration of a single spermatozoon and the injection into the ooplasm was repeated until all metaphase-II oocytes were injected. The injected oocytes were then washed in B_2 medium covered by lightweight paraffin oil.

Oocyte status after ICSI

About 16–18 h after ICSI, the oocytes were examined microscopically for signs of damage that might have been caused by the microinjection procedure (Table 2.11.2). The overall proportion of undamaged oocytes after ICSI on 13 047 metaphase II oocytes was 88.6%. The microinjected oocytes were also checked for fertilization, based on the presence of pronuclei and polar bodies. Normal fertilization occurred in 66.4% of the undamaged oocytes, 58.9% of all the injected oocytes and 47.7% of the total cumulus–oocyte complexes that were recovered. The average number of two-pronuclear oocytes obtained in the 1270 cycles was six per cycle. The normal fertilization rate as expressed as a percentage of the successfully injected oocytes was significantly higher using ejaculated sperm (67.9%) than with epididymal (48.5%) or testicular sperm (49.8%) (Table 2.11.2).

We are continuing to achieve these consistently high fertilization rates in our busy assisted reproduction programme, which carries out three or four ICSI cycles as well as three to four standard IVF procedures per day.

Embryo transfer and freezing

Cleavage of the two pronuclear oocytes was evaluated after a further 24 h of culture in vitro. The cleaving embryos were scored as described above for conventional IVF. Cleaved embryos with less than half of their volume filled with anucleate fragments were eligible for transfer. Up to two, three or, exceptionally, four embryos were loaded with a few microliters of Earle's medium into a Frydman catheter and transferred into the uterine cavity. Embryo replacement was usually performed about 48 h after the microinjection procedure. If excess embryos with <20% anucleate fragments were available, they were cryopreserved on day 2 or day 3 after oocyte retrieval, using the slow-freezing protocol with dimethylsulfoxide.[70,71]

In all, 74% of the two-pronuclear oocytes developed into cleaved embryos with less than 50% of their volume filled with anucleate fragments after a further 24 h of culture in vitro. A total of 5129 embryos (66.8% of the normally fertilized embryos) were transferred or cryopreserved. Significantly more embryos suitable for transfer or freezing developed when ICSI was performed using ejaculated sperm than epididymal sperm or testicular sperm (Table 2.11.3).

Embryo replacement was possible in 1158 (90.8%) of the 1270 treatment cycles, and there was no difference in the numbers of embryos replaced among the four categories of ejaculated semen used (see above). The percentage of transfer cycles resulting in a positive serum HCG was 39.0% for ICSI with ejaculated sperm, 50.9% for ICSI with fresh or frozen–thawed epididymal sperm and 46.2% for ICSI with testicular sperm. The percentage of clinical pregnancies or deliveries per transfer was 30.7% for ICSI with ejaculated sperm, 34.0% for ICSI with epididymal sperm and 38.5% for ICSI with testicular sperm (Table 2.11.3).

Prenatal assessment and pediatric follow-up

At the time of writing (28 January 1995) the number of pregnancies (positive serum HCG) after ICSI-embryos were replaced was 1160, including 64 pregnancies after replacement of frozen–thawed embryos. After chorionic villus sampling or amniocenteseis, 491 fetal karyotypes were obtained. The sex ratio was close to the expected 50/50

Table 2.11.2 Oocyte damage and fertilization rates after ICSI

| | Source of spermatozoa | | |
	Ejaculated	Epididymal	Testicular
No. treatment cycles	1194	59	17
No. mature (M-II) oocytes injected	12 017	759	242
Percentage undamaged oocytes	88.5%	90.0%	89.7%
Pronuclear (PN) status:			
2-PN (normal fertilization)	67.9%[a]	48.5%	49.8%
1-PN (partial fertilization)	4.1%	5.6%	5.5%
3-PN (polyspermy)	4.6%	5.6%	7.4%

[a]Significantly higher fertilization rate than with epididymal or testicular sperm (P=0.0001).

Table 2.11.3 Clinical evaluation of ICSI

| | Source of spermatozoa | | |
	Ejaculated	Epididymal	Testicular
No. fertilized (2-PN) oocytes	7228	331	108
Total embryos transferred or frozen (%)	67.2*[a]	60.7	61.1
Treatment cycles with freezing (%)	43.5**[a]	27.1	29.4
Treatment cycles with transfer (%)	91.3	89.8	76.5
Treatment cycles (per transfer) with positive HCG (%)	39.0	50.9	46.2
Treatment cycles (per transfer) with clinical pregnancy or live birth (%)	30.7	34.0	38.5

[a]Significantly higher rates than with epidiymal or testicular sperm: *P=0.0236; **P=0.0252.

distribution. There were six (1.6%) abnormal karyotypes. So far 669 children have been born. There were 18 major congenital malformations observed in these 669 children, i.e. 2.7% of the children; this percentage is not different from the percentage of abnormalities observed after natural conception or after the standard IVF procedure.

Thus, to-date there has been no indication of an increase in major congenital malformations after replacement of embryos obtained by ICSI.[72] However, it is important to continue with a careful prospective follow-up study of the children born to this new assisted fertilization procedure. This is one of the goals of the 'Task Force on ICSI' that has recently been established by the European Society of Human Reproduction and Embryology (ESHRE).

FUTURE PERSPECTIVES

The efficacy of IVF and related procedures can only be improved by carefully optimizing every step of treat-ment. A component with obvious potential for improvement is the ovarian stimulation protocol. This is likely to be improved with the substitution of 'pure' (recombinant) forms of FSH and LH for existing urinary HMG preparations containing fixed amounts of FSH and LH.[73]

Another area ripe for improvement is the embryo culture medium, which needs to be reformulated to more closely mimic the environment in which embryos develop *in vivo*.

Avoiding the occurrence of multiple pregnancies after IVF remains a major challenge, and the development of non-invasive techniques for objectively assessing embryo quality would allow the selection of fewer, better quality embryos for transfer and/or cryopreservation.

Several aspects of ICSI need to be further refined, including its indications and limitations, the use of testicular spermatozoa, the analysis of fertilization failures and a continuing detailed evaluation of the safety of this novel assisted fertilization technique.[74]

SUMMARY

- IVF/ET is a well-established procedure for the treatment of long-standing infertility due to tubal disease, endometriosis, unexplained infertility or certain types of infertility involving a male factor. IVF can also be applied to couples requiring oocyte donation.
- Conventional IVF involves several related procedures: (a) ovarian stimulation, (b) ultrasound-guided vaginal oocyte retrieval, (c) semen preparation to harvest progressively motile spermatozoa, (d) insemination of the cumulus–oocyte complexes, (e) *in vitro* culture, (f) assessment of fertilization 16–18 h after addition of spermatozoa, (g) assessment of embryo cleavage, (h) replacement to the uterus of two or three morphologically normal embryos, and (i) cryopreservation of excess embryos.
- GIFT and ZIFT are related techniques, suitable in couples with at least one healthy Fallopian tube. In GIFT, up to three oocytes and 100 000 progressively motile spermatozoa can be transferred by laparoscopy into the fimbrial end of the Fallopian tube at the time of oocyte retrieval. In ZIFT, up to three 2-PN oocytes can be transferred into the Fallopian tube on the day after oocyte retrieval.
- IVF, GIFT and ZIFT are all potentially successful procedures in patients with tubal and unexplained infertility. However, fertilization may fail in couples with certain forms of andrological infertility, especially those in which sperm function is severely deficient.
- Techniques of assisted fertilization – partial zona dissection (PZD) and subzonal insemination (SUZI) – have been used with limited success to treat couples with severe andrological infertility who could not be helped by conventional IVF.
- ICSI – the injection of a single spermatozoon into the cytoplasm of a fertilizable metaphase II oocyte – has proved to be more efficient than PZD and ICSI for the alleviation of severe male-factor infertility.
- ICSI with ejaculated sperm can be used to treat couples whose eggs have failed to fertilize after standard IVF, or if there are too few motile spermatozoa in the ejaculate to employ conventional IVF. ICSI with epididymal or testicular spermatozoa can be applied to patients with obstructive azoospermia.
- Crucial technical steps in ICSI are: (a) the preparation of the holding and injection pipettes, (b) removal of the cumulus and corona cells shortly after the oocyte retrieval, and (c) dextrous use of the micromanipulator to pick up and inject a single spermatozoon through the zona pellucida and the oolemma into the cytoplasm of the oocyte without harming it.
- The current experience is that slightly more than 10% of oocytes are damaged by the

microinjection procedure during ICSI. Two-thirds of the oocytes remaining undamaged after ICSI are normally fertilized, of which a further two-thirds cleave into embryos of sufficient morphological quality to be transferred or cryopreserved. The clinical pregnancy rate per transfer is over 30%.

So far, the results of 491 fetal prenatal karyotypes and a prospective follow-up of the first 339 children born to ICSI do not indicate any increase in major congenital malformations. However, the safety of this new clinical procedure needs to be continually reviewed on a much larger scale.

ACKNOWLEDGEMENTS

The authors wish to acknowledge the assistance of the clinical, scientific, nursing and technical staff of the Centres for Reproductive Medicine and Genetics of the Medical Campus of the Dutch-speaking Brussels Free University. Mr Frank Winter of the Language Education Centre reviewed the style of the manuscript and Ms Viviane De Wolf typed the manuscript. The work was supported by grants from the Belgian Fund for Medical Research.

REFERENCES

1. Steptoe PC, Edwards RG, Purdy J. Clinical aspects of pregnancies established with cleaving embryos grown *in vitro*. *Br J Obstet Gynaecol* 1980, **87**: 757–768.
2. Human Fertilisation and Embryology Authority Third Annual Report. HFEA, Paxton House, 30 Artillery Lane, London E1 7LS, UK, 1994.
3. Marrs RP. *Assisted Reproductive Technologies*. Boston: Blackwell Scientific Publications, 1993.
4. Trounson A, Gardner DK. *Handbook of In Vitro Fertilization*. Boca Raton: CRC Press, 1993.
5. Van Steirteghem AC, Pados G, Devroey P, Bonduelle M, Van Assche E, Liebaers I. Oocyte donation for genetic indications. *Reprod Fertil Dev* 1992 **4**: 681–688.
6. Pados G, Camus M, Van Steirteghem A, Bonduelle M, Devroey P. The evolution and outcome of pregnancies from oocyte donation. *Hum Reprod* 1994 **9**: 538–542.
7. Fleming R, Adam AH, Barlow DH, Black WP, MacNaughton MC, Coutts JRT. A new systematic treatment for infertile women with abnormal hormone profiles. *Br J Obstet Gynaecol* 1994 **89**: 80–83.
8. Charbonnel B, Krempf M, Blanchard P, Dano F, Delage C. Induction of ovulation in polycystic ovary syndrome with a combination of a luteinizing hormone-releasing hormone analog and exogenous gonadotropins. *Fertil Steril* 1987 **47**: 920–924.
9. Loumaye E, Vankrieken L, Depreester S, Psalti I, de Cooman S, Thomas K. Hormonal changes induced by short-term administration of a gonadotropin-releasing hormone agonist during ovarian hyperstimulation for *in vitro* fertilization and their consequences for embryo development. *Fertil Steril* 1989 **51**: 105–111.
10. Loumaye E. The control of endogenous secretion of LH by gonadotrophin-releasing hormone agonist during ovarian hyperstimulation for *in-vitro* fertilization and embryo transfer. *Hum Reprod* 1990 **5**: 357–376.
11. Smitz J, Devroey P, Faguer B, Bourgain C, Camus M, Van Steirteghem AC. A prospective randomized comparison of intramuscular or intravaginal progesterone as a luteal phase and early pregnancy supplement. *Hum Reprod* 1992 **7**: 168–175.
12. Smitz J, Bourgain C, Van Waesberghe L, Camus M, Devroey P, Van Steirteghem AC. A prospective randomized study on oestradiol valerate supplementation in addition to intravaginal micronized progesterone in buserelin and HMG induced superovulation. *Hum Reprod* 1993 **8**: 40–45.
13. Kemeter P, Feichtinger W. Pregnancy following *in vitro* fertilization and embryo transfer using pure human serum as culture and transfer medium. *Fertil Steril* 1984 **41**: 936–937.
14. Kruger TF, Stander FSH, Smith K, Van Der Merwe JP, Lombard CJ. The effect of serum supplementation on the cleavage of human embryos. *J In Vitro Fert Embryo Transf* 1987 **4**: 10–12.
15. Shaw JM, Harrison KL, Wilson LM, Breen TM, Shaw G, Cummins JM, Hennessey JF. Results using medium supplemented with either fresh or frozen stored serum in human *in vitro* fertilization. *J In Vitro Fert Embryo Transf* 1987 **4**: 5–9.
16. Leung P, Gronow MJ, Kellow GN, Lopata A, Speirs AL, McBain JC, du Plessis Y, Johnston I. Serum supplement in human *in vitro* fertilization and embryo development. *Fertil Steril* 1984 **41**: 36–39.
17. Ménézo Y, Testart J, Perrone D. Serum is not necessary in human *in vitro* fertilization, early embryo culture and transfer. *Fertil Steril* 1984 **42**: 750–755.
18. Staessen C, Van den Abbeel E, Carlé M, Khan I, Devroey P, Van Steirteghem AC. Comparison between human serum and Albuminar-20 (TM) supplement for *in-vitro* fertilization. *Hum Reprod* 1990 **5**: 336–341.
19. Benadiva CA, Kuczynski-Brown B, Maguire T, Mastroianni L, Flickinger GL. Bovine serum albumin (BSA) can replace patient serum as a protein source in an *in vitro* fertilization (IVF) program. *J In Vitro Fert Embryo Transf* 1989 **6**: 164–167.
20. Drevius LA. The 'sperm rise' test. *J Reprod Fertil* 1972 **24**: 427–432.
21. Mahadevan M, Baker G. Assessment and preparation of semen for *in vitro* fertilization. In Wood C, Trounson A (eds) *Clinical In Vitro Fertilization*. Berlin: Springer-Verlag, 1984: 83.
22. Pertoff H, Laurent TC, Laas T. Density gradients prepared from colloidal silica particles coated by polyvinylpyrrolidone (Percoll). *Anal Biochem* 1978 **88**: 271–277.
23. Arcidiacono A, Walt H, Campana A, Balerna A. The use of Percoll gradients for the preparation of subpopulations of human spermatozoa. *Int J Androl* 1983 **6**: 433–445.
24. Lessley BA, Garner DL. Isolation of motile spermatozoa by density gradient centrifugation in Percoll. *Gamete Res* 1983 **7**: 49–61.
25. Dravland JE, Mortimer D. A simple discontinuous Percoll gradient procedure for washing human spermatozoa. *IRCS Med Sci* 1985 **13**: 16–17.
26. Sapienza F, Verheyen G, Tournaye H, Janssens R, Pletincx I, Derde M-P, Van Steirteghem AC. An auto-controlled study in *in-vitro* fertilization reveals the benefit of Percoll centrifugation to swim-up in the preparation of poor-quality semen. *Hum Reprod* 1993 **8**: 1856–1862.
27. Staessen C, Janssenswillen C, Devroey P, Van Steirteghem AC. Cytogenetic and morphological observations of single

pronucleated human oocytes after *in-vitro* fertilization. *Hum Reprod* 1993 **8**: 221–223.

28. Staessen C, Camus M, Bollen N, Devroey P, Van Steirteghem AC. The relationship between embryo quality and the occurrence of multiple pregnancies. *Fertil Steril* 1992 **57**: 626–630.
29. Staessen C, Camus M, Khan I, Van Waesberghe L, Wisanto A, Devroey P, Van Steirteghem AC. An 18-month survey of infertility treatment by *in vitro* fertilization, gamete and zygote intrafallopian transfer, and replacement of frozen–thawed embryos. *J In Vitro Fert Embryo Transf* 1989 **6**: 22–29.
30. Cummins JM, Breen TM, Harrison KL, Shaw JM, Wilson LM, Hennessey JF. A formula for scoring human embryo growth rates in *in vitro* fertilization: its value in predicting pregnancy and in comparison with visual estimates of embryo quality. *J In Vitro Fert Embryo Transf* 1986 **3**: 284–295.
31. Puissant F, Van Rysselberghe M, Barlow P, Deweze J, Leroy F. Embryo scoring as a prognostic tool in IVF treatment. *Hum Reprod* 1987 **2**: 705–708.
32. Claman P, Armant DR, Seibel MM, Wang TA, Oskowitz SP, Taymor ML. The impact of embryos quality and quantity on implantation and the establishment of viable pregnancies. *J In Vitro Fert Embryo Transf* 1987 **4**: 218–222.
33. Bolton VN, Hawes SM, Taylor CT, Parsons JH. Development of spare human preimplantation embryos *in vitro* and analysis of the correlations among gross morphology, cleavage rates and development to the blastocyst. *J In Vitro Fert Embryo Transf* 1989 **6**: 30–35.
34. Handyside AH, Lesko JG, Tarín JJ, Winston RML, Hughes MR. Birth of a normal girl after *in vitro* fertilization and preimplantation diagnostic testing for cystic fibrosis. *N Engl J Med* 1992 **327**: 905–909.
35. Verlinsky Y *et al.* Preimplantation diagnosis of genetic and chromosomal disorders. *J Assist Reprod Genet* 1994 **11**: 236–243.
36. Staessen C, Janssenswillen C, Van den Abbeel E, Devroey P, Van Steirteghem AC. Avoidance of triplet pregnancies by elective transfer of two good quality embryos. *Hum Reprod* 1993 **8**: 1650–1653.
37. Braeckmans P, Devroey P, Camus M, Khan I, Staessen C, Smitz J, Van Waesberghe L, Wisanto A, Van Steirteghem AC. Gamete intra-Fallopian transfer: evaluation of 100 consecutive attempts. *Hum Reprod* 1987 **2**: 201–205.
38. Devroey P, Braeckmans P, Smitz J, Van Waesberghe L, Wisanto A, Van Steirteghem A, Heytens L, Camu F. Pregnancy after translaparoscopic zygote intrafallopian transfer in a patient with sperm antibodies. *Lancet* 1986 i: 1329.
39. Devroey P, Staessen C, Camus M, De Grauwe E, Wisanto A, Van Steirteghem AC. Zygote intrafallopian transfer as a successful treatment for unexplained infertility. *Fertil Steril* 1989 **52**: 246–249.
40. Palermo G, Devroey P, Camus M, De Grauwe E, Khan I, Staessen C, Wisanto A, Van Steirteghem AC. Zygote intra-Fallopian transfer as an alternative treatment for male infertility. *Hum Reprod* 1989 **4**: 412–415.
41. Devroey P, Camus M, Staessen C, Wisanto A, Bollen N, Henderix P, Van Steirteghem AC. ZIFT: indications and limitations. In Capitanio GL, Asch RH, De Cecco L, Croce S (eds) *GIFT: From Basics to Clinics.* New York: Raven Press, 1990: 333–340.
42. Van Steirteghem A, Van den Abbeel E, Camus M, Devroey P. Cryopreservation of human embryos. *Ballière's Clin Obstet Gynaecol* 1992 **6**: 313–325.
43. Van Steirteghem AC, Van den Abbeel E. Freezing of embryos: early vs late stages. *J Assist Reprod Genet* 1993 **10**: 185–186.
44. SART: Assisted Reproductive Technology in The United States and Canada: 1991 Results from the Society for Assisted Reproductive Technology Generated from the American Fertility Society Registry. *Fertil Steril* 1993 **59**: 956–962.
45. Tournaye H, Devroey P, Camus M, Staessen C, Bollen N, Smitz J, Van Steirteghem AC. Comparison of *in-vitro* fertilization in male and tubal infertility: a 3 year survey. *Hum Reprod* 1992 7: 218–222.
46. Cohen J, Adler A, Alikano M, Ferrara TA, Kissin E, Reing AM, Suzman M, Talansky BE, Rosenwaks Z. Assisted fertilization and abnormal sperm function. *Semin Reprod Endocrinol* 1993 **11**: 83–94.
47. Fishel S, Dowell K, Timson J, Green S, Hall J, Klentzeris L. Micro-assisted fertilization with human gametes. *Hum Reprod* 1993 **8**: 1780–1784.
48. Imoedemhe DAG, Sigue AB. Subzonal multiple sperm injection in the treatment of previous failed human *in vitro* fertilization. *Fertil Steril* 1993 **59**: 172–176.
49. Lippi J, Mortimer D, Jansen RPS. Sub-zonal insemination for extreme male factor infertility. *Hum Reprod* 1993 **8**: 939–944.
50. Palermo G, Joris H, Devroey P, Van Steirteghem AC. Induction of acrosome reaction in human spermatozoa used for subzonal insemination. *Hum Reprod* 1992 7: 248–254.
51. Palermo G, Joris H, Derde MP, Camus M, Devroey P, Van Steirteghem AC. Sperm characteristics and outcome of human assisted fertilization by subzonal insemination and intracytoplasmic sperm injection. *Fertil Steril* 1993 **59**: 826–835.
52. Van Steirteghem AC, Liu J, Nagy Z, Joris H, Tournaye H, Liebaers I, Devroey P. Use of assisted fertilization. *Hum Reprod* 1993 **8**: 1784–1785.
53. Cohen J, Malter H, Wright H, Kort H, Massey J, Mitchell D. Partial zona dissection of human oocytes when failure of zona pellucida penetration is anticipated. *Hum Reprod* 1989 **4**: 435–442.
54. Cohen J, Talansky BE, Malter H, Alikani M, Adler A, Reing A, Berkeley A, Graf M, Davis O, Liu H, Bedford JM, Rosenwaks Z. Microsurgical fertilization and teratozoospermia. *Hum Reprod* 1991 **6**: 118–123.
55. Cohen J, Alikani M, Adler A, Berkely A, Davis O, Ferrara TA, Graf M, Grifo J, Liu H, Malter HE, Reing AM, Suzman M, Talansky BE, Trowbridge J, Rosenwaks Z. Microsurgical fertilization procedures: the absence of stringent criteria for patient selection. *J Assist Reprod Genet* 1992 **9**: 197–206.
56. Fishel S, Timson J, Lisi F, Rinaldi L. Evaluation of 225 patients undergoing subzonal insemination for the procurement of fertilization *in vitro*. *Fertil Steril* 1992 **57**: 840–849.
57. Ng SC, Bongso A, Ratnam SS. Microinjection of human oocytes: a technique for severe oligoasthenoteratozoospermia. *Fertil Steril* 1991 **56**: 1117–1123.
58. Van Steirteghem A, Nagy Z, Liu J, Joris H, Verheyen G, Smitz J, Tournaye H, Liebaers I, Devroey P. Intracytoplasmic sperm injection. *Ballière's Clin Obstet Gynaecol* 1994 **8**: 85–93.
59. Palermo G, Joris H, Devroey P, Van Steirteghem AC. Pregnancies after intracytoplasmic injection of single spermatozoon into an oocyte. *Lancet* 1992 **340**: 17–18.
60. Iritani A. Micromanipulation of gametes for *in vitro* assisted fertilization. *Mol Reprod Dev* 1991 **28**: 199–207.
61. Veeck LL, Oehninger S, Acosta AA, Muasher SJ. Sperm microinjection in a clinical *in vitro* fertilization program. *Proceedings of the 45th Annual Meeting of the American Fertility Society,* San Francisco, 1989.
62. Van Steirteghem AC, Liu J, Joris H, Nagy Z, Janssenswillen C, Tournaye H, Derde MP, Van Assche E, Devroey P. Higher success rate by intracytoplasmic sperm injection than by subzonal insemination. Report of a second series of 300 consecutive treatment cycles. *Hum Reprod* 1993 **8**: 1055–1060.
63. Van Steirteghem AC, Nagy Z, Joris H, Liu J, Staessen C, Smitz J, Wisanto A, Devroey P. High fertilization and implantation rates after intracytoplasmic sperm injection. *Hum Reprod* 1993 **8**: 1061–1066.

64. Smitz J, Devroey P, Camus M, Deschacht J, Khan I, Staessen C, Van Waesberghe L, Wisanto A, Van Steirteghem AC. The luteal phase and early pregnancy after combined GnRH-agonist/HMG treatment for superovulation in IVF or GIFT. *Hum Reprod* 1988 **3**: 585–590.
65. World Health Organization. *WHO Laboratory Manual for the Examination of Human Semen and Sperm Cervical Mucus Interaction.* Cambridge: Cambridge University Press, 1992.
66. Kruger TF, Menkveld R, Stander FSH, Lombard CJ, Van der Merwe JP, van Zyl JA, Smith K. Sperm morphologic features as a prognostic factor in *in vitro* fertilization. *Fertil Steril* 1986 **46**: 1118–1123.
67. Liu J, Nagy Z, Joris H, Tournaye H, Devroey P, Van Steirteghem AC. Intracytoplasmic sperm injection does not require special treatment of the spermatozoa. *Hum Reprod* 1994 **9**: 1127–1130.
68. Silber S, Nagy ZP, Liu J, Godoy H, Devroey P, Van Steirteghem AC. Conventional IVF versus ICSI (intracytoplasmic sperm injection) for patients requiring MESA (microsurgical sperm aspiration). *Hum Reprod* 1994 **9**: 1705–1709.
69. Verheyen G, Pletincx I, Van Steirteghem AC. Effect of freezing method, thawing temperature and post-thaw dilution/washing on motility (CASA) and morphology characteristics of high-quality human sperm. *Hum Reprod* 1993 **8**: 1678–1684.
70. Camus M, Van den Abbeel E, Van Waesberghe L, Wisanto A, Devroey P, Van Steirteghem AC. Human embryo viability after freezing with dimethylsulfoxide as a cryoprotectant. *Fertil Steril* 1989 **51**: 460–465.
71. Van Steirteghem AC, Van der Elst J, Van den Abbeel E, Joris H, Camus M, Devroey P. Cryopreservation of supernumerary multicellular human embryos obtained after intracytoplasmic sperm injection. *Fertil Steril* 1994 **62**: 775–780.
72. Bonduelle M, Desmyttere S, Buysse A, Van Assche E, Schiettecatte J, Devroey P, Van Steirteghem A, Liebaers I. Prospective follow-up study of 55 children born after subzonal insemination and intracytoplasmic sperm injection. *Hum Reprod* 1994 **9**: 1765–1769.
73. Filicori M, Flamignini C (eds). *Ovulation Induction: Basic Science and Clinical Advances.* Amsterdam: Exerpta Medica. International Congress Series 1046, 1994: 395pp.
74. Aitken RJ, Irvine DS. Fertilization without sperm. *Nature* 1996 **379**: 493–494.

2.12

Nutrition, Metabolism and Reproduction in Women

S Franks and S Robinson

INTRODUCTION

It has long been known that nutritional factors can have a profound influence on reproductive function in mammals. In teleological terms, this interrelationship can be regarded as a means of ensuring that reproduction of the species is optimal only when the food supply is adequate to sustain the population. In the field of clinical medicine, the most striking example of the effect of nutrition on reproduction is the effect of weight loss on cyclical ovarian function in women. The amenorrhea which accompanies anorexia nervosa results from a well-characterized, hypothalamic disorder of gonadotropin regulation, although it must be admitted that the precise nature of the metabolic signal that mediates these changes remains unclear.

Anorexia nervosa is an important disease in modern 'developed' societies but obesity and its effects are equally important, and have been recognized for many centuries. The adverse effects of obesity on reproductive function were illustrated with uncanny accuracy in the writings of Hippocrates.[1] In an essay on 'the influence of climate, water supply and situation on health' he describes the Scythians thus: 'The girls get amazingly flabby and podgy. ... People of such constitution cannot be prolific ... fatness and flabbiness are to blame. The womb is unable to receive the semen and they menstruate infrequently and little'. He adds a note on the type of constitution that is associated with normal reproductive performance: 'As good proof of the sort of physical characteristics that are favorable to conception, consider the case of serving wenches. No sooner do they have intercourse with a man than they become pregnant, on account of their sturdy physique and their leanness of flesh'. Modern studies suggest that the mechanism by which obesity affects menstrual function is more complex than is the case for those mediating weight loss-related amenorrhea; peripheral effects of nutritionally related metabolic changes may be more important than those on the hypothalamus. The clinical disorder of polycystic ovary syndrome provides an excel-

lent model for the exploration of these mechanisms. Polycystic ovary syndrome (PCOS) is the most common cause of anovulation and is typically associated with obesity.[2,3] It is now recognized that a disorder of energy expenditure coupled with an abnormality of glucose/insulin homeostasis is a characteristic feature of the syndrome and one which may underpin disordered ovarian function.[4,5] An understanding of the nature of the interrelationship of nutrition, insulin sensitivity and ovarian activity in women with PCOS is important not only for unraveling the complexities of this syndrome but also because of what it may tell us about the physiological role of fuel economy in normal reproductive function.

There are profound metabolic changes during normal pregnancy. As in the non-pregnant state there is a close interrelationship between energy expenditure and insulin sensitivity. The marked reduction in insulin sensitivity and the corresponding fall in postprandial thermogenesis may be of crucial importance in conservation of energy during pregnancy.

This chapter explores the relationship of food intake, insulin action and energy expenditure, firstly, in the context of the maintenance of normal cyclical ovarian function and, secondly, with regard to the adaptive changes of pregnancy.

CURRENT CONCEPTS

Metabolism and ovarian function

Role of nutrition in menarche and ovulation

The onset of menses in the female is clearly related to nutritional status but views of the nature of the causal factors in this relationship continue to provoke considerable controversy. Twenty years ago, Frisch and McArthur[6] put forward the hypothesis that menarche in girls depended on the attainment of a 'critical weight' and this, in turn, led to the idea that ovulation in humans is regulated by body fat. This hypothesis is supported by studies reporting, on the one hand, a correlation between increased gonadotropin secretion and body composition in pubertal girls[7] and, on the other hand, those showing that dieting suppresses menstrual function in adult women.[8,9]

There is, however, a growing body of evidence which suggests that although the role of body fat may be important, it may not be the critical factor determining reproductive capacity.[10] Closer examination of the literature reveals that low body fat in women is not always associated with menstrual disturbance[11,12] and several studies (predominantly in experimental animals) have highlighted the importance of energy intake, *per se*, on reproductive function (reviewed in reference 10). In other words, a certain minimal level of fuel intake appears to be required to initiate and maintain cyclical ovarian function. Body fat composition reflects changes in energy balance and fat tissue itself may, indeed, play a part in the mechanism of reproductive disturbances by affecting, for example, the transport and metabolism of estrogens.[13] Nevertheless, the critical humoral signal(s) which mediate the effect of energy balance on gonadotropin regulation remain unclear. There is some evidence from experimental animals that metabolic fuels may, directly, be capable of modulating the activity of the luteinizing hormone releasing hormone (LHRH) 'pulse generator'.[14] Insulin has been suggested to play a part in regulation of gonadotropins but the available data are somewhat contradictory.[10] It has also been reported that food restriction in lambs results in increased sensitivity of gonadotropins to the negative feedback effect of estradiol but the mechanism underlying this phenomenon is still unknown.[15]

In summary, these observations indicate that energy balance has a critical role in determining the onset of menarche and the maintenance of ovulation (and, therefore, fertility) but much more needs to be learned about the metabolic and hormonal mechanisms which mediate these effects.

Obesity and ovarian function

Restriction of fuel intake may disrupt ovarian function but excess calorie intake may also have adverse effects. Obesity *per se* may be associated with menstrual disturbance in women,[16–18] but the influence of body weight on the ovary is most clearly illustrated in the context of polycystic ovary syndrome. Polycystic ovary syndrome (PCOS) is a disorder of uncertain etiology which, in its most typical form, presents with symptoms of hyperandrogenism (hirsutism, acne, alopecia) and of anovulation (amenorrhea, oligomenorrhea, dysfunctional uterine bleeding, infertility).[2,3] Obesity is also a common feature, occurring in 35–40% of cases in the largest reported series.[3,19,20] The classic biochemical features are hypersecretion of androgens (predominantly of ovarian origin) and of luteinizing hormone. There is, nevertheless, considerable heterogeneity in both clinical and biochemical presentation of women with polycystic ovaries so that the spectrum ranges from anovulation in non-hirsute women (but who are, nevertheless, hyper-

androgenemic) to hirsutism in subjects with regular menses.[3] Importantly, the mode of presentation is influenced by body weight.[20,21] In an analysis of a large series of patients with polycystic ovaries presenting to a gynecological endocrine clinic, it was demonstrated that obese women with polycystic ovaries were more likely to have menstrual disturbance and had a higher prevalence of hirsutism than their lean counterparts.[21] Put simply, the more overweight the subject, the worse were her symptoms.

What, then, is the explanation for the effects of obesity on ovarian function and what is the relevance to reproductive function in women without PCOS? Intriguingly there was no significant difference in gonadotropin or testosterone concentrations between lean and obese women with PCOS.[21] The serum concentration of 'free' testosterone was, however, higher in obese compared with lean subjects and this appeared to reflect lower than normal levels of sex hormone-binding globulin (SHBG), the major binding protein for testosterone in the circulation. Such findings may help to explain the higher frequency of hirsutism in obese compared to lean subjects. There is a striking inverse correlation of SHBG concentrations with body mass index (BMI) in both women with PCOS and normal subjects.[21,22] The humoral factor linking SHBG to BMI is insulin.[22–25] Insulin appears to be the key to understanding the effects of obesity on ovarian function in women with and without PCOS. Similarly, hyperinsulinemia, irrespective of body weight, may be a critical factor in the mechanism of anovulation in women with PCOS.

Insulin and ovarian function

Obesity is well known to be associated with hyperinsulinemia and peripheral insulin resistance but there is now clear evidence that women who present with the classic features of PCOS have higher plasma insulin concentrations and reduced insulin-mediated glucose disposal when compared with weight-matched controls[26–30] (Fig. 2.12.1). Insulin resistance is a feature of lean as well as obese subjects with the syndrome, that is it occurs independently of body weight. This disturbance of insulin action is, of course, magnified in overweight women. Is insulin resistance an obligatory part of PCOS? Recent data suggest that it is characteristic of those women with oligo- or amenorrhea but does not occur in equally hyperandrogenemic women with polycystic ovaries who have regular menses.[5] Put another way, the most obvious biochemical difference between anovulatory and ovulatory women with polycystic ovaries is the presence of hyperinsulinemia and insulin resistance in the former. This association raises the question of whether there is a causal relationship between hyperinsulinemia (or insulin resistance) and anovulation in women with PCOS. Studies showing that amenorrhea induced by pituitary–ovarian suppression in PCOS makes no significant impact on insulin levels or action suggest that it is unlikely that menstrual dysfunction causes insulin resistance.[31,32] There is, however, evidence (albeit indirect) that a significant fall in circulating insulin levels leads to improvement in ovarian cyclicity. Long-term calorie restriction in obese women with PCOS is associated with a

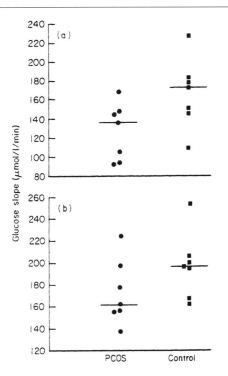

Fig. 2.12.1 *Individual values for insulin sensitivity, as measured by the short insulin tolerance test, in obese (**a**) and lean (**b**) women with PCOS compared with weight-matched controls. (From reference 4 with permission.)*

more regular pattern of menses and, in many cases, fertile cycles.[33,34] The dietary-induced fall in both fasting and glucose-stimulated insulin concentrations can be observed before there is an obvious change in menstrual pattern.[35] The mechanism whereby hyperinsulinemia or insulin resistance affects ovulatory function is not yet known although it is clear that the ovary is indeed a target for insulin action.[36,37] As for the mechanism of the insulin resistance itself, this too remains unclear, although recent evidence points to a defect distal to the insulin receptor.[38,39]

Glucose–insulin homeostasis is intimately related to fuel economy. The thermogenic response to glucose is known to be impaired in insulin resistant states associated with obesity and non-insulin dependent diabetes[40,41] and this has prompted similar studies of energy expenditure in insulin-resistant women with PCOS.

Postprandial thermogenesis and ovarian function

In a study designed to examine the relationship between postprandial thermogenesis and insulin resistance, metabolic rate was measured by continuous indirect calorimetry in two groups of women, those with PCOS and weight-matched controls.[4] Postprandial thermogenesis was calculated by subtracting the calculated energy expenditure after a standard mixed meal from the resting metabolic rate. There was no significant difference in resting energy

expenditure in the two groups but postprandial thermogenesis was significantly reduced in women with PCOS (Fig. 2.12.2). Postprandial thermogenesis correlated negatively with insulin sensitivity in the subjects with PCOS, though not in the controls.

Do these observations have any significance for our understanding of the relationship between energy expenditure and ovarian function, i.e. of a link between metabolism and reproduction? PCOS has a strong genetic basis[42,43] and a high prevalence, thus prompting the speculation that there may be some evolutionary advantage in having PCOS. The reduced energy expenditure after meals may provide a clue to this. In Western societies where food supply is plentiful, reduced insulin sensitivity and postprandial thermogenesis will predispose to weight gain and impaired fertility if food intake is not restricted but at times of food deprivation, this 'fuel economy' may work to the advantage of the population by allowing maintenance of fertility despite shortage of food.

Growth hormone and insulin-like growth factors

Changes in the secretion or action of insulin is by no means the only humoral mechanism by which nutrition can influence reproduction. Growth hormone (GH) and insulin-like growth factors (IGFs) can also be regarded as metabolic hormones which reflect nutritional status and can affect ovarian function.[44] Growth hormone, when administered *in vivo* exerts a gonadotropic action on ovarian folliculogenesis; this effect is accompanied, although not necessarily mediated, by changes in circulating IGF-1.[44-46] Studies *in vitro* have shown that GH has a

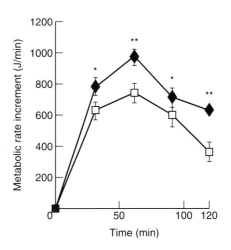

Fig. 2.12.2 *Increment of energy expenditure (EE) after a standard mixed meal (10 kcal/kg lean body mass) in women with PCOS and matched controls. Resting energy expenditure (range 4893–8492 kJ) is standardized to zero so that the values represent the increment in EE after the meal, averaged over 30 min intervals. ♦ Controls; □ PCOS. *P<0.05, **P<0.001. (From reference 4 with permission.)*

direct, stimulatory effect on granulosa cell steroidogenesis,[44,47,48] supporting the concept that it has the potential to act as a 'cogonadotropin' under physiological conditions.[44] Insulin-like growth factor-1 is a potent stimulant of steroid production by human follicular cells and, under certain conditions, interacts synergistically with gonadotropins.[49,50] Recently, it has been shown that, as in the rat follicle, the IGF-binding proteins IGFBP-1 and IGFBP-3 neutralize IGF-activated steroidogenesis by human granulosa cells.[51] Intriguingly, both binding proteins were able to block, partially, the effect of FSH alone. The mechanism of this phenomenon remains unclear but one possibility is that sequestration of endogenous IGFs is involved.

There seems little doubt, therefore, that the GH/IGF system could play a part in human ovarian function, probably by modulation of the action of gonadotropins (Fig. 2.12.3). It is an attractive proposition to consider that this may be of physiological significance, especially during puberty when these effects could provide the means for the necessarily close coordination of somatic growth and reproductive development. There may also be a role for this system in 'fine tuning' of gonadotropin action during the menstrual cycle. Interestingly, recent data suggest that the intraovarian IGF/IGFBP system may subserve the fundamental functions of folliculogenesis and atresia which are not necessarily dependent on cyclical gonadotropin activity.[44,52]

It is tempting to suggest that abnormalities of the GH/IGF-1 axis may play a part in the mechanism of disordered ovarian function, particularly in PCOS but, as yet, there is no clear evidence that this is the case.

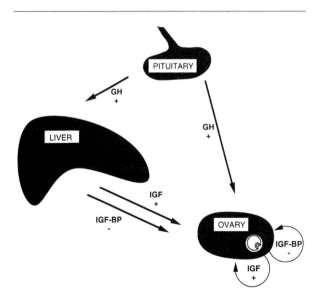

Fig. 2.12.3 *Suggested roles of growth hormone (GH), insulin-like growth factors (IGFs) and IGF-binding proteins (IGF-BPs) in the control of ovarian function. GH acts directly on the liver to stimulate the formation of IGF and IGF-BPs. GH also has the potential to directly stimulate granulosa cell function. Hepatic IGFs circulate in plasma bound to IGF-BPs, which modulate IGF availability at the tissue level. IGFs can act directly on the ovary to augment gonadotropin action. IGFs and IGF-BPs produced within the ovary are also believed to modulate folliculogenesis and steroid hormone biosynthesis.*

Metabolism in pregnancy

The association between pregnancy and derangements of carbohydrate metabolism has been recognized for over 100 years when polyuria and polydypsia presenting in pregnancy were first described. Gestational diabetes is common but resolves after pregnancy, suggesting that pregnancy in some way de-regulates glucose metabolism. Insulin requirements in pregnancy complicated by insulin-dependent diabetes (IDDM) may double or treble in the last trimester, again, implying an effect of pregnancy on insulin action.

The mechanism of these changes in glucose–insulin homeostasis and their precise significance for fetal–maternal nutrition are poorly understood.

Insulin and insulin-resistance in pregnancy

Fasting plasma insulin levels increase through pregnancy, but these changes are not coincident with the well-recognized decrease in fasting plasma glucose concentrations during gestation,[53,54] suggesting that these phenomena are not causally related. Thus, although there are changes in both the response of the pancreatic β cell to glucose and in the sensitivity of peripheral tissues to insulin, these events appear to occur independently.

For a given glucose challenge, the pregnant woman is stimulated to produce more insulin; plasma insulin concentrations may be double the levels in the non-pregnant state.[54,55] Insulin action in normal pregnancy has been studied by the hyperinsulinemic euglycemic clamp technique and resistance to exogenous insulin has been demonstrated in non-diabetic women during the third trimester.[56,57] Endogenous insulin action and β-cell responsiveness have been examined by computation of the results of an intravenous glucose tolerance test.[57] Insulin sensitivity during the third trimester was observed to be one third of that measured in non-pregnant controls. In addition, the first and second phase insulin responses to glucose were three times greater than in non-pregnant women.

Insulin resistance has also been evaluated by assessment of the glucose response to exogenous insulin using the short insulin tolerance test. This repeatable short test correlates well with insulin sensitivity derived from clamp experiments and is a better measure of insulin resistance when the subject is highly insulin-resistant. Using this technique, it can be observed that insulin resistance is already significantly increased by the second trimester of normal pregnancy and increases further in the third trimester.[58] The insulin resistance of pregnancy is the most extreme example of this phenomenon occurring under physiological conditions and is comparable, in degree, with that seen in patients who develop non-insulin dependent diabetes in later life. The insulin resistance in pregnancy involves not only glucose disposal but also extends to the action of insulin in lowering non-esterified fatty acids.[58] What are the implications for fetal–maternal nutrition, of these profound changes in insulin secretion and action during pregnancy?

Intrauterine nutrition

Increased serum triglyceride concentrations in the mother were thought to be an indicator of increased maternal lipid oxidation sparing carbohydrate and protein for fetal use. It has been suggested that the increased ketone body and free fatty acid concentrations in the postabsorptive state represent increased oxidation by the mother of these metabolites and that this more rapid adjustment to fat catabolism allows glucose to be spared for placental transfer.[55,59]

Other workers have interpreted these changes differently. Serum triglyceride concentrations are increased in the second and, still further, in the third trimester of normal pregnancy. Apolipoprotein B (ApoB) levels are similarly increased in the second and third trimesters of pregnancy. This suggests that triglyceride is transported in the form of very-low-density lipoprotein (VLDL) triglyceride. The elevation in serum concentrations of triglyceride and ApoB correlate with the degree of insulin resistance.[58] Based on data obtained from studies in the rat, it was felt that lipid could not cross the placenta in calorically significant quantities. In the guinea pig, however, it has been demonstrated that VLDL triglyceride, presented to the placenta, can be hydrolyzed by placental lipase and that the non-esterified fatty acids, thus produced, can cross the placenta. Furthermore, they can represent a major energy source for the fetus. The insulin resistance of normal pregnancy may therefore be a mechanism of increasing delivery of lipid – which is, after all, a more efficient energy source than glucose – to the fetus.

Energy expenditure in pregnancy

As in the non-pregnant state, energy expenditure in pregnancy can be subdivided into resting energy expenditure (REE), the energy expenditure of exercise and thermogenic activities. Total energy requirements are increased in pregnancy, partly to subserve the extra mass of the fetus, the feto-placental unit and maternal fat stores and partly to provide sufficient caloric intake to support the increased lean body mass. The theoretical energy cost of pregnancy has been estimated at 362 kJ, assuming a 3.4 kg fetus, increased maternal protein of 0.9 kg and an increase in maternal fat stores of 3.8 kg.[60] The question is: is there an adaptive change in REE per unit lean body mass, or do the changes in REE merely represent changes in the lean body mass? All studies report an increase in REE during pregnancy as lean body mass increases, but there are large interpopulation differences varying from 5% in Gambian women to 39% in women from the USA. Resting energy expenditure is related to body weight[61,62] but it is doubtful whether changes in REE during pregnancy can be attributed to weight gain alone.[63] Using the definitive technique of 24 hour calorimetry, it was concluded that there are highly characteristic changes in REE within subjects but large intersubject differences.[64] There was some depression in the metabolic rate up to 24 weeks of gestation; at 36 weeks' gestation, there were increases in REE between +8.6% and +35.4% per unit lean body mass. These changes in REE could not, therefore, be attributed to changes in lean body mass.

Postprandial thermogenesis in pregnancy

Although early studies of postprandial thermogenesis (PPT) showed no obvious effect of gestational age[61] more recent, longitudinal studies have clearly demonstrated a reduction in PPT during pregnancy, being lowest during the third trimester[58,65] (Fig. 2.12.4). In other clinical settings

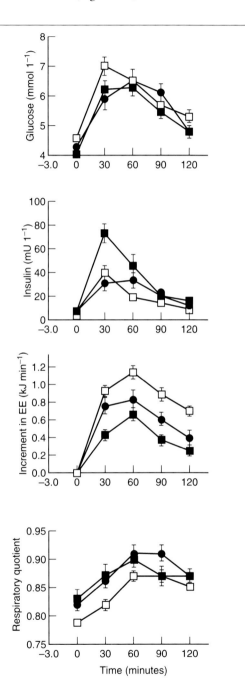

Fig. 2.12.4 *The glucose, insulin and energetic response to a mixed meal (given time 0 min) in normal pregnancy. Values for glucose, energy expenditure (EE) and respiratory quotient are shown as mean +SEM and insulin as median + interquartile range.* □ *Non-pregnant controls;* ● *2nd trimester;* ■ *3rd trimester. Note increasing insulin levels and decreasing postprandial EE with stages of pregnancy. (From reference 58 with permission.)*

(e.g. obesity and PCOS (see above) reduced postprandial thermogenesis is related to insulin resistance. Not surprisingly, therefore, it was found that during normal pregnancy, insulin sensitivity correlated positively with postprandial thermogenesis[58] (Fig. 2.12.5). Using regression analysis, human placental lactogen, prolactin, triglyceride, tri-iodothyronine concentrations, insulin area after the test meal, and body mass index were found to have no significant influence on PPT.

There may be an evolutionary advantage to the insulin insensitivity of pregnancy. Assuming the test meal to represent one-fifth of the daily dietary energy intake, the difference in PPT between controls and the pregnant women would represent an energy saving, over the second and third trimesters, of 38.6 MJ compared to the non-pregnant

state. This represents 13% of the total energy requirement of pregnancy.[63] Since postprandial thermogenesis is closely related to insulin sensitivity, it seems feasible that the decreasing insulin sensitivity during gestation is an important mechanism of conserving energy in pregnancy.

FUTURE PERSPECTIVES

The above observations provide a tantalizing hint of the links between nutrition, metabolism and reproduction. Insulin is clearly an important factor in this complex interrelationship but many questions still remain to be answered. Does insulin mediate the effect of calorie restriction on hypothalamic regulation of gonadotropins? Does insulin action affect postprandial thermogenesis or vice versa? How important is insulin to the normal function of the ovary? What is the mechanism of the putative adverse effect of hyperinsulinemia on the ovary and how does this relate to the cause of anovulation in PCOS? Does the insulin resistance of normal pregnancy indeed have a role in fuel economy during gestation? Given the importance of the topic and the current research activity in these areas, these are questions which are likely to be answered in the near future. A different but equally important perspective, highlighting the possible adverse effects of insulin resistance, has been opened by recent studies of lipid metabolism in PCOS. Anovulatory women with PCOS appear to have a dyslipidemia which is strongly correlated with the degree of insulin resistance and, as in other insulin-resistant states, may indicate an increased long-term risk of cardiovascular disease. We should therefore be able to identify young women at future risk of heart disease by virtue of their presentation during reproductive years with hirsutism and anovulation. The challenge facing us is to establish beyond doubt the connection between the metabolic disturbance associated with PCOS and heart disease and to institute effective methods to reduce the risk of cardiovascular morbidity and mortality.

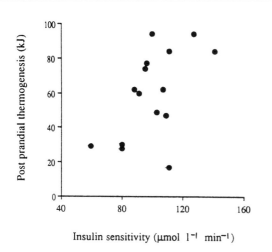

Fig. 2.12.5 *The relationship between insulin sensitivity and postprandial thermogenesis in pregnant women (both 2nd and 3rd trimesters). The correlation coefficient (r) was 0.57 (P<0.05). (From reference 58 with permission.)*

SUMMARY

- Nutrition has a profound effect on reproductive function.
- Calorie restriction, leading to weight loss, results in anovulation. The mechanism involves an effect of nutrients on hypothalamic regulation of gonadotropins but the nature of the metabolic signal which mediates these changes remains unknown.
- Obesity, too, is associated with menstrual disturbance and anovulation. In contrast to weight loss, there is no evidence for a major hypothalamic disturbance in gonadotropin regulation. Hyperinsulinemia and insulin resistance, which

accompany obesity, may be involved in the etiology of anovulation.
- Women with PCOS, the commonest cause of anovulatory infertility, are more hyperinsulinemic and insulin resistant than weight-matched control subjects and have reduced postprandial thermogenesis.
- Calorie restriction in obese women with PCOS results in reduction of hyperinsulinemia and improvement of fertility, again suggesting that insulin may have a role in mediating nutritionally related changes in ovarian function.
- Insulin resistance and reduced postprandial

energy expenditure in PCOS could represent the modern legacy of an adaptive mechanism to enable a subpopulation of women to continue to reproduce at times of food shortage.

- Insulin resistance is a feature of normal pregnancy.
- Insulin affects the transfer of nutrients from mother to fetus but there remains doubt about the nature of the primary fuel source for the fetus. There are data to suggest that fat may be a more important substrate than carbohydrate.

- As in women with PCOS, insulin resistance in pregnancy is linked to reduced postprandial thermogenesis. This could be regarded as a physiological adaptation to maximize energy conservation during pregnancy.
- In some women (presumably those with impaired pancreatic β cell function), the insulin resistance of pregnancy contributes to the development of gestational diabetes.

REFERENCES

1. Hippocrates. Airs, Waters, Places (an essay on the influence of climate, water supply and situation on health). In *Hippocratic Writings; section on Medicine* translated by Chadwick J, Mann WN. London: Penguin Classics 1978 (reprinted 1983), paras 20–21, pp. 164–165.
2. Yen SSC. The polycystic ovary syndrome. *Clin Endocrinol (Oxf)* 1980 **12**: 177–208.
3. Franks S. Polycystic ovary syndrome: a changing perspective. *Clin Endocrinol (Oxf)* 1989 **31**: 87-120.
4. Robinson S, Chan S-P, Spacey S, Anyaoku V, Johnston DG, Franks S. Postprandial thermogenesis is reduced in polycystic ovary syndrome and is associated with increased insulin resistance. *Clin Endocrinol (Oxf)* 1992 **36**: 537–543.
5. Robinson S, Kiddy D, Gelding SV, Willis D, Niththyananthan R, Bush A, Johnston DG, Franks S. The relationship of insulin sensitivity to menstrual pattern in women with hyperandrogenism and polycystic ovaries. *Clin Endocrinol (Oxf)* 1993 **39**: 351–355.
6. Frisch RE, McArthur JW. Menstrual cycles: fatness as a determinant of minimum weight necessary for their maintainance or onset. *Science* 1974 **185**: 949–951.
7. Penny R, Goldstein IP, Frasier SD. Gonadotropin excretion and body composition. *Pediatrics* 1978 **61**: 294–300.
8. Pirke KM, Schweiger U, Lemmel W, Krieg JC, Berger M. The influence of dieting on the menstrual cycle of healthy young women. *J Clin Endocrinol Metab* 1985 **60**: 1174–1179.
9. Loucks AB, Heath EM, Verdun M, Watts JR. Dietary restriction reduces luteinizing hormone (LH) pulses during waking hours and increases LH pulse amplitude during sleep in young menstruating women. *J Clin Endocrinol Metab* 1994 **78**: 910–915.
10. Bronson FH, Manning JM. The energetic regulation of ovulation: a realistic role for body fat (minireview). *Biol Reprod* 1991 **44**: 945–950.
11. Loucks AB, Horvath SM. Athletic amenorrhea: a review. *Med Sci Sports Exerc* 1985 **17**: 56–72.
12. Sinning WE, Little KD. Body composition and menstrual function in athletes. *Sports Med* 1987 **4**: 34–45.
13 Frisch RE. The right weight: body fat, menarche and fertility. *Proc Nutr Soc* 1994 **53**: 113–129.
14. Morin LP. Environment and hamster reproduction: responses to phase specific starvation during the estrus cycle. *Am J Physiol* 1986 **251**: R663–669.
15. Foster DL, Olster DH. Effect of restricted nutrition on puberty in the lamb: pattern of tonic luteinizing hormone (LH) secretion and competence of the LH surge system. *Endocrinology* 1985 **116**: 375–381.
16. Hartz AJ, Barboriak PN, Wong A, Katayama KP, Rimm AA. The association of obesity with infertility and related menstrual abnormalities in women. *Int J Obes* 1979 **3**: 57–73.

17. Kopelman PG, Pilkington TRE, White N, Jeffcoate SL. The effect of weight loss on sex steroid secretion and binding in massively obese women. *Clinical Endocrinol (Oxf)* 1981 **14**: 113–116.
18. Harlass FE, Plymate SR, Farris BL, Belts RP. Weight loss is associated with correction of gonadotropin and sex steroid abnormalities in the obese anovulatory female. *Fertil Steril* 1984 **42**: 649–652.
19. Goldzieher JW, Green JA. The polycystic ovary. 1 Clinical and histological features. *J Clin Endocrinol Metab* 1962 **22**: 325–338.
20. Conway GS, Honour JW, Jacobs HS. Heterogeneity of the polycystic ovary syndrome: clinical, endocrine and ultrasound features in 556 patients. *Clin Endocrinol (Oxf)* 1989 **30**: 459–470.
21. Kiddy DS, Sharp PS, White DM *et al.* Differences in clinical and endocrine features between obese and non-obese subjects with polycystic ovary syndrome: an analysis of 263 consecutive cases. *Clin Endocrinol (Oxf)* 1990 **32**: 213–220.
22. Pugeat M, Crave JC, Elmidani M *et al.* Pathophysiology of sex hormone binding globulin (SHBG): relation to insulin. *J Steroid Biochem Mol Biol* 1991 **40**: 841–849.
23. Sharp PS, Kiddy DS, Reed MJ, Anyaoku V, Johnston DG, Franks S. Correlation of plasma insulin and insulin-like growth factor-I with indices of androgen transport and metabolism in women with polycystic ovary syndrome. *Clin Endocrinol (Oxf)* 1991 **35**: 253–257.
24. Plymate SR, Matej LA, Jones RE, Friedl KE. Inhibition of sex hormone-binding globulin production in human hepatoma (Hep G2) cell line by insulin and prolactin. *J Clin Endocrinol Metab* 1988 **67**: 460–464.
25. Singh A, Hamilton-Fairley D, Koistinen R, Seppala M, James VHT, Franks S, Reed MJ. Effect of insulin-like growth factor type1 and insulin on the secretion of sex hormone-binding globulin and IGF-1 binding protein 1 by human hepatoma cells. *J Endocrinol* 1990 **124 suppl:** R1–R3.
26. Chang RJ, Nakamura RM, Judd HL, Kaplan SA. Insulin resistance in non-obese patients with polycystic ovarian disease. *J Clin Endocrinol Metab* 1983 **57**: 356–359.
27. Jialal I, Naiker P, Reddi K, Moodley J, Joubert SM. Evidence for insulin resistance in nonobese patients with polycystic ovarian disease. *J Clin Endocrinol Metab* 1987 **64**: 1066–1069.
28. Peiris AN, Aiman EJ, Drucker WD, Kissebah AH. The relative contributions of hepatic and peripheral tissues to insulin resistance in hyperandrogenic women. *J Clin Endocrinol Metab* 1989 **68**: 715–720.
29. Dunaif A, Segal KR, Futterweit W, Dobrjansky A. Profound peripheral insulin resistance, independent of obesity, in polycystic ovary syndrome. *Diabetes* 1989 **38**: 1165–1174.
30. Conway GS, Jacobs HS, Holly JMP, Wass JAH. Effects of luteinizing hormone, insulin-like growth factor-1 and insulin-like growth factor binding protein 1 in the polycystic ovary syndrome. *Clin Endocrinol (Oxf)* 1990 **33**: 593–603.

31. Geffner ME, Kaplan SA, Bersch N, Golde DW, Landaw EM, Chang RJ. Persistence of insulin resistance in polycystic ovarian disease after inhibition of ovarian steroid secretion. *Fertil Steril* 1986 **45**: 327–333.

32. Dunaif A, Green G, Futterweit W, Dobrjansky A. Suppression of hyperandrogenism does not improve peripheral or hepatic insulin resistance in the polycystic ovary syndrome. *J Clin Endocrinol Metab* 1990 **70**: 699–704.

33. Pasquali R, Antenucci D, Cassimirri F, Venturoli S, Paradisi R, Fabbri R, Balestra V, Melchionda N, Barbara L. Clinical and hormonal characteristics of obese amenorrheic hyperandrogenemic women before and after weight loss. *J Clin Endocrinol Metab* 1989 **68**: 173–179.

34. Kiddy DS, Hamilton-Fairley D, Bush A, Short F, Anyaoku V, Reed MJ, Franks S. Improvement in endocrine and ovarian function during dietary treatment of obese women with polycystic ovary syndrome. *Clin Endocrinol (Oxf)* 1992 **36**: 105-111.

35. Kiddy DS, Hamiliton-Fairley D, Seppala M, Koistinen R, James VHT, Reed MJ, Franks S. Diet-induced changes in sex hormone-binding globulin and free testosterone in women with normal or polycystic ovaries: correlation with insulin and insulin-like growth factor-I. *Clin Endocrinol (Oxf)* 1989 **31**: 757–763.

36. Garzo VG, Dorrington JH. Aromatase activity in human granulosa cells during follicular development and the modulation by follicle stimulating hormone and insulin. *Am J Obstet Gynecol* 1984 **148**: 657–662.

37. Mason HD, Willis DS, Holly JMP, Franks S. Insulin preincubation enhances insulin-like growth factor-II action on steroidogenesis in human granulosa cells. *J Clin Endocrinol Metab* 1994 **78**: 1265–1267.

38. Dunaif A, Segal KR, Shelley DR, Green G, Dobrjansky A, Licholai T. Evidence for distinctive and intrinsic defects in insulin action in polycystic ovary syndrome. *Diabetes* 1992 **41**: 1257–1266.

39. Ciaraldi TP, El-Roeiy A, Madar Z, Reichart D, Olefsky JM, Yen SSC. Cellular mechanisms of insulin resistance in polycystic ovarian syndrome. *J Clin Endocrinol Metab* 1992 **75**: 577–583.

40. Shetty PS, Jung RT, James WPT, Barrand MA, Callingham BA. Postprandial thermogenesis in obesity. *Clin Sci* 1981 **60**: 519–525.

41. Ravussin E, Bogardus C, Shwartz BS, Robbins DC, Wolfe RR, Horton ES *et al.* Thermic effect of infused glucose and insulin in man: decreased response with increased insulin resistance in obesity and non-insulin-dependent diabetes mellitus. *J Clin Invest* 1983 **72**: 893–902.

42. Simpson JL. Elucidating the genetics of polycystic ovary syndrome. In Dunaif A, Givens JR, Haseltine FP, Merriam GR (eds) *Polycystic Ovary Syndrome.* Oxford: Blackwell Scientific Publications, 1992: 59–77.

43. Carey AH, Chan KL, Short F, White DM, Williamson R, Franks S. Evidence for a single gene effect in polycystic ovaries and male pattern baldness. *Clin Endocrinol (Oxf)* 1993 **38**: 653–658.

44. Katz E, Ricciarelli E, Adashi EY. Review: the potential relevance of growth hormone to female reproductive physiology and pathophysiology. *Fertil Steril* 1993 **59**: 8–34.

45. Homburg R, West C, Torresani T, Jacobs HS. Cotreatment with human growth hormone and gonadotropins for induction of ovulation: a controlled clinical trial. *Fertil Steril* 1990 **53**: 354–360.

46. Burger HG, Kovacs GT, Polson DW, McDonald J, McCloud PI, Harrop M *et al.* Ovarian sensitization to gonadotrophins by human growth hormone. Persistence of the effect beyond the treated cycle. *Clin Endocrinol (Oxf)* 1991 **35**: 119–122.

47. Mason HD, Martikainen H, Beard RW, Anyaoku V, Franks S. Direct gonadotrophic effect of growth hormone on oestradiol production by human granulosa cells. *J Endocrinol* 1990 **126 suppl**: R1–R4.

48. Carlsson B, Bergh C, Bentham J, Olsson J-H, Norman MR, Billig H *et al.* Expression of functional growth hormone receptors in human granolosa cells. *Hum Reprod* 1992 **7**: 1205–1209.

49. Erickson G, Garzo GV, Magoffin D. Insulin-like growth factor-1 regulates aromatase activity in human granulosa and granulosa-luteal cells. *J Clin Endocrinol Metab* 1989 **69**: 716–724.

50. Mason HD, Margara R, Winston RML, Seppala M, Koistinen R, Franks S. Insulin-like growth factor-1 (IGF-1) inhibits production of IGF-binding protein-1 whilst stimulating estradiol secretion in granulosa cells from normal and polycystic ovaries. *J Clin Endocrinol Metab* 1993 **76**: 1275–1279.

51. Mason HD, Willis D, Holly JMP, Cwyfan-Hughes SC, Seppala M, Franks S. Inhibitory effects of insulin-like growth factor-binding proteins on steroidogenesis by human granulosa cells in culture. *Mol Cell Endocrinol* 1992 **89**: R1–R4.

52. Giudice LC. Insulin-like growth factors and ovarian follicular development. *Endocr Rev* 1992 **13**: 641–669.

53. Lind T, Aspigllaga M. Metabolic changes during normal and diabetic pregnancies. In Reece EA, Coustan DR (eds) *Diabetes Mellitus in Pregnancy.* New York: Churchill Livingstone, 1988: 75–102.

54. Kalhan SC, Hertz RH, Rossi KQ, Savin SM. Glucose–alanine relationship in diabetes in human pregnancy. *Metabolism* 1991 **40**: 629–633.

55. Freinkel N. Of pregnancy and progeny. *Diabetes* 1980 **29**: 1023–1035.

56. Ryan EA, O'Sullivan MJ, Skyler JS. Insulin action during pregnancy. Studies with the euglycemic clamp technique. *Diabetes* 1985 **34**: 380–389.

57. Buchanan TA, Metzger BE, Frienkel N, Bergman RN. Insulin sensitivity and β-cell responsiveness to glucose during late pregnancy in lean and moderately obese women with normal glucose tolerance or mild gestational diabetes. *Am J Obstet Gynecol* 1990 **162**: 1008–1014.

58. Robinson S, Viira J, Learner J, Chan S-P, Anyaoku V, Beard RW, Johnston DG. Insulin insensitivity is associated with a decrease in postprandial thermogenesis in normal pregnancy. *Diabet Med* 1992 **10**: 139–145.

59. Metzger BE, Ravinikar V, Vileisis RA, Freinkel N. 'Accelerated starvation' and the skipped breakfast in late normal pregnancy. *Lancet* 1982 **i**: 588–592.

60. Hytten FE. Nutrition. In Hytten FE, Chamberlain G (eds) *Clinical Physiology in Obstetrics.* Oxford: Blackwell Scientific Publications, 1980: 163–192.

61. Nagy LE, King JC. Postprandial energy expenditure and respiratory quotient during early and late pregnancy. *Am J Clin Nutr* 1984 **40**: 1258–1263.

62. Forsum E, Sadurskis A, Wager J. Resting metabolic rate and body composition of healthy Swedish women during pregancy. *Am J Clin Nutr* 1988 **47**: 942–947.

63. van Raaij JMA, Schonk CM, Vermaat-Miedema SH, Peek MEM, Hautvast JGAJ. Body fat mass and basal metabolic rate in Dutch women before, during and after pregnancy: a reappraisal of energy cost of pregnancy. *Am J Clin Nutr* 1989 **49**: 765–772.

64. Prentice AM, Goldberg GR, Davies HL, Murgatroyd PR, Scott W. Energy-sparing adaptations in human pregnancy assessed by whole body calorimetry. *Br J Nutr* 1989 **62**: 5–22.

65. Illingworth PJ, Jung RT, Howie PW, Isles TE. Reduction in postprandial energy expenditure during pregnancy. *Br Med J* 1987 **294**: 1573–1576.

2.13

Menopause

DW Purdie

INTRODUCTION

Menopause is literally the cessation of spontaneous menstrual cycles. It occurs during the climacteric or 'change of life' that spans the transition from the years of fertility to the infertility of older age. The term menopause is often used loosely for the climacteric, of which it is but one constituent event. Although there is no precise temporal definition, the climacteric broadly spans the decade from 45 to 55, beginning when fertility is already low and in steep decline, and ending when the vast majority of women have become menopausal because their ovaries cease to secrete estrogen.[1]

This chapter briefly surveys the causes and consequences of the menopause, emphasizing the effect of estrogen withdrawal on female health and its 'treatment' by hormone replacement therapy (HRT).

CURRENT CONCEPTS

Origin of menopause

Menopause is probably unique to the female of *Homo sapiens*, conferring advantages upon the species through preventing late child-bearing.

Depletion of the oocyte stock

The seeds of the menopause are quite literally sown with the ova in the ovary during utrauterine life. It is the finite number of these ova, the absence of their replacement, and their inevitable numerical exhaustion which locks a female fetus into a ~50 year time-scale, which inevitably results in her climacteric and its attendant menopause.[2,3]

Longevity

The menopause occurs – albeit at variable ages – in all women and no intervention exists that will prevent it. The median age at which ovarian estrogen production ceases to support the menstrual cycle is relatively stable between populations, being estimated at 51 years in Europe[4] and 51.3 years in the USA.[5]

Endocrine correlates of menopause

When fully developed, the menopause is characterized by raised circulating levels of follicle-stimulating hormone (FSH) and luteinizing hormone (LH) and reduced levels of estradiol and inhibin (Fig. 2.13.1).[6-8] FSH is often elevated prior to any change in patterns of menses, apparently due to a relaxation of estrogen restraint upon the pituitary.[9] The rise in LH levels occurs later than that of FSH but is usually apparent after the third month of amenorrhea.

Peripheral aromatization of androgen to estrogen in fatty tissue becomes the principal source of plasma estrogen after the menopause.[10,11] The decline in circulating estrogens at menopause is paralleled by a decline in androgen levels but the postmenopausal ovary continues to secrete appreciable amounts of androgen.[12] Thus, the clinical and metabolic severity of menopause brought on by surgical oophorectomy, in which androgen-producing ovarian stroma is lost as well as the follicles, is greater than that of the natural menopause, consistent with the role of ovarian androgen as a peripheral aromatase substrate.

Menopause and the central nervous system

Hypothalamic thermoregulation

The hot flush is a response to what may best be described as a failure of the CNS thermostat. In the presence of a low or falling plasma estrogen the thermostat, or thermoregulatory center, located in the hypothalamus, undergoes an

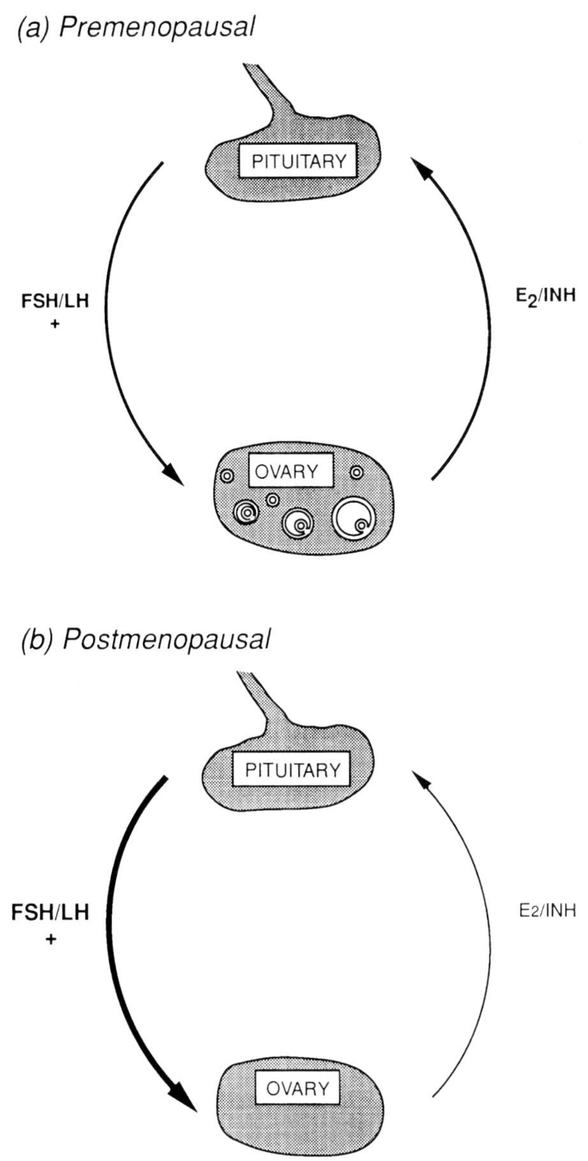

(a) Premenopausal

FSH/LH
+

E₂/INH

(b) Postmenopausal

FSH/LH
+

E2/INH

Fig. 2.13.1 *Ovarian–pituitary axis* **(a)** *before and* **(b)** *after the menopause* (**FSH**, *follicle stimulating hormone;* **LH**, *luteinizing hormone,* **E₂** *estradiol;* **INH**, *inhibin). With depletion of the oocyte stock, follicles no longer develop. Therefore E₂ and inhibin-mediated negative-feedback control of pituitary secretion of FSH and LH is withdrawn and circulating gonadotropin concentrations become chronically elevated.*

Hormones and hot flushes

A primary exposure to estrogen seems to be a necessary prerequisite for flushing as the symptom is not normally observed in prepubertal girls or in patients with ovarian dysgenesis such as Turner's syndrome.[14]

Hot flushes are more common among women of low body weight[15] and may begin prior to the menopause when ovarian estrogen output is still sufficient to maintain a menstrual cycle.[16] Relative falls in estrogen levels rather than reduced estrogen levels as such appear to cause the thermoregulatory center to become unstable.[17,18]

Neuroendocrine mechanisms

Hot flushes and LH pulses can coincide temporally without being causally related.[19,20] Each could result from a hypothalamic neuronal discharge or an event associated with the primary pulsed release of luteinizing hormone-releasing hormone (see Chapter 2.2).

Central neurotransmitters such as endorphins[21] and catecholamines[22] are implicated in the neuroendocrine mechanism through which estrogen deficiency results in vasomotor instability and flushing. Hypothalamic β-endorphin release is stimulated by estrogen and the age-related decline in the number of endorphin-positive cells in the arcuate nucleus of the hypothalamus can be reversed by estrogen.[23] α₂-Adrenergic agonists such as methyldopa reduce the incidence of hot flushes.[24] This effect occurs after a lag-phase that is similar to that following estrogen treatment, consistent with a re-ordering of neurotransmitter synthesis and release in the hypothalamus.

Menopause and the lower genital tract

All gross anatomical tissues of the genital tract, from vulva to ovary, contain estrogen receptors (ER)[25] (see Chapter 2.7). Thus estrogen withdrawal at the menopause has profound effects on the structure and function of these tissues.

Vagina

The vaginal skin is a multilayered, stratified, squamous epithelium that is highly sensitive to estrogen. Climacteric ovarian failure results in a progressive diminution in the layering of the epithelium and a concomitant reduction in the glycogen content of individual cells.[26] The resulting failure of the vaginal skin to support the commensal lactobactillus results in a rise in the pH and an increased likelihood of infection. However, it should be clearly appreciated that the term 'atrophic vaginitis', though hallowed by tradition, is inappropriate for the normal postmenopausal vagina in the absence of inflammation or infection. The term 'vaginal atrophy' should instead be adopted. One result of this vaginal atrophy is that intercourse, in the absence of normal vaginal lubrication provided by the stratified squamous epithelium, may become dry and painful.[27]

Urinary tract

The urinary and lower genital tracts share a common embryological origin and estrogen-sensitive changes in the

acute downset. In other words, the thermostat signals, falsely, that body temperature is too high. This signal entrains a set of adaptive responses designed to rid the body of the centrally perceived excess heat, thereby reducing core temperature to that demanded by the thermostat. The process is akin to that observed in a patient recovering from a pyrexia and in this context it is interesting that a diminution in menopausal flushes has been documented in febrile women.[13]

urethral architecture mirror those in the vagina.[28] The presence of ER in the trigone and proximal urethra is of significance given the increased frequency of urinary problems in perimenopausal women.[29] The effect of estrogen withdrawal seems to be to increase urethral closure pressure.[30]

Menopause and the cardiovascular system

Estrogen has a major beneficial effect on the cardiovascular system, and hormone replacement therapy (HRT) with estrogen reduces the incidence of coronary heart disease in postmenopausal women by ~50%.[31-34] The natural history of cardiovascular disease in the UK shows a markedly higher prevalence in males below the age of 50 years. In older groups, however, the prevalence in females rises such that by the ninth decade the gap is substantially closed (Fig. 2.13.2). One factor which may account for these observations is the climacteric loss of endogenous estrogen.

Cardiovascular effects of estrogen

Studies of cynomolgous monkeys (*Macaca fascicularis*) have shown that coronary atheroma increases after the menopause.[35] Replacement therapy with estradiol alone or in combination with progesterone prevents the increase in atherogenesis caused by oophorectomy.

The action of estrogen is direct upon the coronary arterial wall, primarily due to estrogen-mediated inhibition of uptake and degradation of low-density lipoprotein (LDL) in the coronary vessels. There is epidemiological evidence that estrogen acts in a similar way to prevent cardiovascular disease in women.[36] Estrogen also induces changes in the lipoprotein profile (see below) but it is estimated that only ~30% of the beneficial effect of estrogen is mediated via these changes.[35,36]

The second means by which estrogen may protect

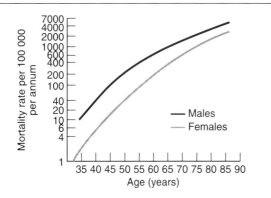

Fig. 2.13.2 *Incidence of cardiovascular disease in men and women: the differential progressively lessens after the menopause – partially due to the loss of the protective effects of estrogen on the cardiovascular system and lipid profile in women. Source: OPCS.*

against cardiovascular disease is at the level of coronary vasospasm. Coronary vasospasm may be induced by a variety of agents such as exercise[37] or cold,[38] operating through endothelium-derived vasoactive agents. Atheromatous coronary arteries are susceptible to paradoxical constriction by acetylcholine – an effect which is preventable by estrogens in the macaque.[39]

Both ER and progesterone receptors (PR) are present in arterial endothelium and smooth muscle,[40,41] consistent with direct actions for both steroids on arterial function. Such actions of estrogen are known to include decreased vascular resistance, increased cardiac output[42] and increased release of endothelium-derived relaxing factor (i.e. nitric oxide).

Animal studies indicate that estrogen withdrawal is likely to cause a modest elevation in blood pressure but there have been no prospective, controlled studies of the effect of natural menopause on blood pressure. HRT stimulates cardiac output but this is balanced by a reduction in peripheral resistance and a modest fall in systolic and diastolic pressure.[42]

Estrogen and plasma lipids

Estrogen withdrawal has effects on lipoprotein biochemistry that are believed to contribute to the increased incidence of cardiovascular disease in postmenopausal women. Total serum cholesterol concentration appears to rise over the climacteric decade such that levels are significantly higher in postmenopausal women.[43,44] The increase in total cholesterol level is paralleled by LDL, which increases with age in women at a substantially greater rate than in men.[45] In contrast, there is little evidence for a significant effect of natural menopause upon high-density lipoprotein cholesterol (HDL) or very low-density lipoprotein cholesterol (VLDL) levels. Bilateral oophorectomy causes changes to lipoprotein profiles in premenopausal women.[46]

Estrogen and the coagulation system

Postmenopausal[47] and oophorectomized women[48] have an increased risk of myocardial infarction and their blood contains increased blood levels of fibrinogen and clotting factors (V, VII and XII)[49-51] as well as plasminogen activator inhibitor (PAI-1) activity.[52] However, postmenopausal increases also occur in antithrombin III (AT III) and protein C concentrations, which would be expected to reduce the occurrence of venous and arterial thromboembolic phenomena.[49]

HRT trials provide an important opportunity to gain more information on the factors that predispose postmenopausal women to coronary artery disease, myocardial infarction and stroke[53,54] (see below).

Menopause and the skeleton

Estrogen withdrawal at the menopause, whether natural or induced, is associated with a series of alterations in bone cell behavior that culminate in bone loss and increased susceptibility to fracture. The principal actions of estrogen on the skeleton are mediated by direct effects on the cells of bone, which will now be considered.

Bone remodeling

The basic sequence of bone turnover – the bone remodeling unit (BRU) – is summarized in Fig. 2.13.3. In each BRU, ~0.5 million cells will be active at any one time. The remodeling cycle begins with the appearance of osteoclasts at a bone surface (Fig. 2.13.3). These marrow-derived cells proceed to excavate a cavity in the underlying bone over a period of 2–3 weeks. This done, the osteoclasts disperse, and after an interval of 2 weeks the excavated cavity becomes lined with osteoblasts – bone forming cells –

which proceed to lay down new bone and mineralize. For the bone to be in balance, the amount of bone formed must be coupled to the amount of bone previously resorbed. This is generally the case in premenopausal women and in healthy men.

The fall in the ambient estradiol level at the menopause results in a decoupling, or imbalance within the BRU, such that the bone removed fails to be matched by the subsequent bone formation. This results in a net loss of bone which, when sufficiently repeated at the same site, leads eventually to a loss of the number, thickness and connectedness of the bone trabeculae. Key sites at which this occurs are legs (femoral), neck, distal radius and spine (Fig. 2.13.4). The trabeculae confer the great engineering strength of trabecular bone, allow it to fulfill its function of

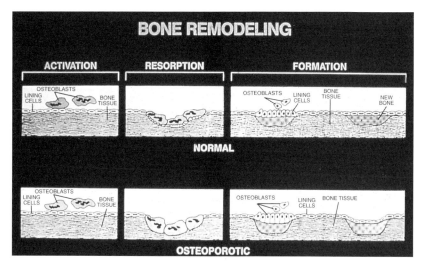

Fig. 2.13.3 *The bone remodeling cycle.* Activation: *remodeling begins with the appearance of osteoclasts at a bone surface.* Resorption: *the osteoclasts excavate a cavity in the underlying bone over a period of 2–3 weeks.* Formation: *The osteoclasts disperse, and after an interval of 2 weeks the excavated cavity becomes lined with osteoblasts – bone forming cells – that proceed to lay down the calcified intercellular substance of bone. Cells (osteocytes) included within bone as it develops are osteoblasts that have ceased to divide and have mineralized. In normal bone* (**upper panel**) *the amount of bone formed is coupled to the amount of bone previously resorbed, whereas in osteoporotic bone* (**lower panel**) *the two processes are uncoupled, and bone progressively deteriorates.*

(a)
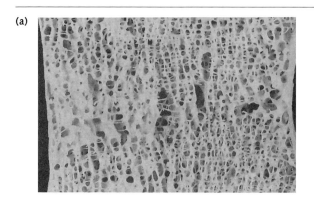

(b)
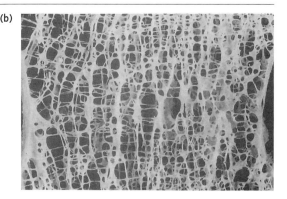

Fig. 2.13.4 *Trabecular architecture of bone.* **(a)** *Normal bone,* **(b)** *osteoporotic bone. Note the overall impression of porosity conveyed by the diminution in trabecular number, thickness and connectedness in osteoporotic bone when compared to the normal pattern.*

shock absorption, and protect it from fracture. Hence the net long-term result of estrogen deficiency is a loss of bone mineral density (BMD) and increased fracturing. When the BMD has fallen to between 1.0 and 2.5 standard deviations below the mean for young normal women in the population, the bone is said to be *osteopenic*, and when the BMD is down to >2.5 standard deviations below the young normal mean, the bone is said to be *osteoporotic*.

Estrogen action on bone cells

Cells of the osteoblast lineage contain ER[55] that are presumably involved in the subcellular mechanism through which estrogen deficiency uncouples bone resorption–formation.

There is experimental evidence that estrogen action on bone cells is mediated by locally produced cytokines and growth factors. In murine hematopoietic marrow precursors, osteoclast development promoted by interleukin-6 (IL-6) was inhibited by estradiol *in vitro*.[56] In the same study, oophorectomy enhanced osteoclast numbers in trabecular bone, which was prevented by giving estradiol or IL-6 antiserum. In human osteoblast-like cell cultures, transferring growth factor-α (TGF-α) and IL-1[57] promoted mitogenesis; however, estradiol was without effect.

Evidence has also been obtained that unconventional, non-nuclear receptors for estrogen mediate estrogen action in bone. Estrogen-stimulated influx of ionized calcium and mobilization of calcium from the endoplasmic reticulum in rat osteoblasts was not inhibited by the estrogen receptor blocker tamoxifen.[58] This might be why treatment of women with tamoxifen does not cause significant bone loss. Thus it may yet prove that tamoxifen and related compounds have a place in the prevention of postmenopausal bone loss.

Calcitropic hormones

The direct effect of estrogen on bone does not account for the full effect of menopause on the skeleton, and there is evidence that calcitropic hormones are also involved.

The three classic calcitropic hormones are parathyroid hormone (PTH), calcitonin and 1,25-dihydroxy vitamin D ($1,25(OH)_2$ D). Slight reductions in circulatory PTH and $1,25(OH)_2$ D levels occur postmenopausally,[59,60] which probably reflect a homeostatic response to the increased release of calcium into the circulation as a consequence of higher bone turnover. Calcitonin has a powerful inhibitory effect on the osteoclasts and has long been thought to be a likely mediator of postmenopausal bone loss. Basal levels of calcitonin are lower in postmenopausal than premenopausal women, and absolute values correlate with ambient estrogen concentrations.[61]

Progesterone levels also fall significantly after the menopause, and it is noteworthy that both progesterone and estrogen have been shown to increase the production of calcitonin by rat thyroid C cells *in vitro*.[62]

Osteoporosis

Clinically, the withdrawal of estrogenic support, whenever and howsoever this occurs, results in a progressive loss of bone tissue. The long duration of human life after menopause means that a woman can expect to lose some 50% of her trabecular bone and some 35% of her cortical bone.[63] The absence of a mid-life male menopause may account in part for the lower incidence of osteoporosis in men at all ages. However, as will now be considered, HRT with estrogen is increasingly seen as a clinical option to restore the balance between bone resorption and bone formation and arrest bone loss, prevent the development of osteoporosis reducing the morbidity from related fractures.

Hormone replacement therapy

The central concept behind HRT is that the replacement of endogenous estrogen with exogenous hormone will allay the immediate, and prevent the longer-term consequences of estrogen deficiency secondary to climacteric ovarian failure.

Estrogen may be delivered locally by direct application to the genital tract or it may be given systemically through a transdermal patch or a subcutaneous implant. However, the most popular route at present remains the oral, with the ingested estrogen traversing the portal circulation and the liver before reaching the systemic circulation and the target organs. Whatever the route of administration the goal is to achieve a physiological plasma level of estrogen >150 pmol/l, i.e. beyond the menopausal range.

As noted above, the principal short-term action of estrogen replacement is to abrogate the vasomotor menopausal symptoms of flushing, sweating and relative insomnia. Locally, in the estrogen-sensitive tissues of the vagina, the effect of HRT is to stimulate replication of squamous epithelial cells and to stimulate epithelial stratification and mucification. To prevent hyperplastic development of the endometrium, it is current practice to induce menstruation, by giving 10–12 days of progestogen in a monthly cycle.[64]

The use of a progestogen results in an inhibition of estrogen-induced endometrial DNA synthesis, thereby retaining the capacity for secretory conversion and hence safe shedding of the endometrium.[65] Withdrawal bleeding is, however, a major reason for non-compliance with HRT in non-hysterectomized women.[66] A major goal of current research into HRT is to identify safe and effective treatment regimens that do not entail a monthly withdrawal bleed. This process has started, and the successful use of continuous combined estrogen preparations has been reported.[67,68] Refinement of this approach should lead to enhanced compliance, assuming that no long-term adverse effects on the breast or cardiovascular system come to light.

FUTURE PERSPECTIVES

HRT and cardiovascular disease There is a need for prospective clinical trials to confirm the safety and benefit of modern combined estrogen–progestogen regimens, particularly in terms of the duration and degree of protection against myocardial infarction and stroke.

HRT and bone metabolism The advent of techniques of precise bone densitometry, such as the new fan-beam, dual-energy, X-ray absorptiometer (DXA), should permit clinical studies to categorize more precisely the protection afforded by HRT against fracture. At the level of basic science, the endocrine and paracrine mechanisms that underpin such protection need to be elucidated.

Which estrogen to use for HRT? The differences in the therapeutic actions of native estradiol and the most popularly used synthetic estrogen, ethinyl estradiol, used in HRT formulations need to be clearly defined. Ethinyl estradiol – the synthetic estrogenic component of most combined oral contraceptive pills – differs in structure and therapeutic action from native estradiol. HRT using natural estradiol would seem to be more physiological and inherently more safe than synthetic estrogen, but research is needed to evaluate this.

What regulates oocyte loss? Finally, almost nothing is known about the factors that control the rate at which oocytes are lost from the ovary to bring about onset of the 'normal' menopause at 45–50 years of age. Even less is known about causes of premature menopause,[69] in which ovarian failure due to depletion of the oocyte stock occurs in ~1% of women younger than 35 or 40 years of age. Possible factors in the etiology of premature ovarian failure are viral infections, ovarian tumor, genetic, chromosomal, autoimmune disorders, galactosemia, cytotoxic drugs or radiation injury. Research to improve understanding of the mechanisms that determine the size of the germ cell stock laid down *in utero* and the rate of its subsequent depletion could have both basic scientific and clinical implications. Whatever the cause of ovarian failure, young women with premature menopause are at considerable risk of osteoporotic problems, and early recognition is important so that preventative HRT can be given.[70]

SUMMARY

- The menopause is universal, and has its origins in the finite number of oocytes located in the ovary during intrauterine life. It occurs in all societies at a median age of around 51 years and a standard deviation of around 18 months.

- The menopause confers advantages upon the species through the prevention of late child bearing and its posterior separation from the effective end of fertility. It is probably unique to the female of *H. sapiens*.

- The menopause causes a set of symptoms prime among which are the vasomotor effects of hot flushing and inappropriate perspiration. These are due to instability of the hypothalamic thermostat, which is estrogen sensitive.

- The withdrawal of estrogen at the climacteric results in substantial changes in the epithelial lining of the lower genital tract, which may result in dyspareunia.

- The menopause may also condition certain changes in the lower urinary tract resulting from reduction in urethral closure pressure.

- The ultimate effect of climacteric ovarian failure is to contribute to the rising trend in ischemic heart disease among women during the sixth decade.

- Estrogens exert substantial effects upon the cardiovascular system through modification of lipid profile and certain hemodynamic parameters including peripheral vascular resistance and cardiac output.

- The skeletal effect of estrogen is mediated through the bone cells, principally osteoblasts and through the calcitropic hormones. Ovarian failure is characterized by an imbalance between bone formation and bone resorption in favor of the latter.

- The ultimate effect of estrogen withdrawal is to increase the prevalence of osteoporosis and its related fractures.

- The menopause should be regarded as a physiological event with pathological consequences which are unique for every individual and which should be investigated and managed on this basis.

REFERENCES

1. Spira A. The decline of fecundity with age. *Maturitas Suppl* 1988 1: 15–22.
2. Styne DM, Grumback MM. Puberty in the male and female: its physiology and disorders. In Yen SSC, Jaffe RB (eds) *Reproductive Endocrinology*. London: WB Saunders, 1986: 313–384.
3. Baker TG. A quantitative and cytological study of germ cells in human ovaries. *Proc R Soc Lond (Biol)* 1963 158: 417–433.
4. Oldenhave A, Jaszmann LJ, Haspels AA, Everaerd WT. Impact of climacteric on well-being. A survey based on 5213 women 39 to 60 years old. *Am J Obstet Gynecol* 1993 168: 772–780.
5. Avis NE, McKinlay SM. A longitudinal analysis of women's attitudes towards the menopause: results from the Massachusetts Women's Health Study. *Maturitas* 1991 13: 65–79.
6. Lee SJ, Lenton EA, Sexton L, Cooke ID. The effect of age on the cyclical patterns of plasma LH, FSH, oestradiol and progesterone in women with regular menstrual cycles. *Hum Reprod* 1988 3: 851–855.
7. McNaughton J, Bangah M, McCloud P, Hee J, Burger HG. Age related changes in follicle stimulating hormone,

luteinizing hormone, estradiol and immunoreactive inhibin in women of reproductive age. *Clin Endocrinol* 1992 **36**: 339–345.

8. Sherman BM, West JH, Korenman SG. The menopausal transition: analysis of LH, FSH, estradiol and progesterone concentrations during menstrual cycles of older women. *J Clin Endocrinol Metab* 1976 **42**: 629–636.

9. Dennerstein L, Smith AKA, Morse C, Burger H, Green A, Hopper J, Ryan M. Menopausal symptoms in Australian women. *Med J Aust* 1993 **159**: 232–236.

10. Franz C, Longcope C. Androgen and estrogen metabolism in male rhesus monkeys. *Endocrinology* 1979 **105**: 869–874.

11. Simpson ER, Merrill JC, Hollub AJ, Graham-Lorence S, Mendelson CR. Regulation of estrogen biosynthesis by human adipose cells. *Endocr Rev* 1989 **10**: 136–148.

12. Longcope C, Hunter R, Franz C. Steroid secretion by the postmenopausal ovary. *Am J Obstet Gynecol* 1980 **138**: 564–570.

13. Barnard RM, Kronenberg F, Downey JA. Effect of fever on menopausal hot flashes. *Maturitas* 1992 **14**: 181–188.

14. Goldfien A, Munroe SE. Ovaries. In Greenspan FS (ed.) *Basic and Clinical Endocrinology*. New Jersey: Hall International, 1991: 442–490.

15. Seidenschnur G, Beck H, Uplegger H, Werner H, Kolmorgen K. Attitude and sex behavior following hysterectomy. *Zentralbl Gynaekol* 1989 **111**: 53–59.

16. Thompson B, Hart SA, Durno D. Menopausal age and symptomatology in a general practice. *J Biosoc Sci* 1973 **5**: 71–82.

17. Voda AM. Climacteric hot flash. *Maturitas* 1981 **3**: 73–90.

18. Aksel S, Schomberg DW, Tyrey L, Hammond CB. Vasomotor symptoms, serum estrogens and gonadotrophin levels in surgical menopause. *Am J Obstet Gynecol* 1976 **126**: 165–169.

19. Kronenberg F, Cote LJ, Linkie DM, Dyrenfurth I, Downey JA. Menopausal hot flashes: thermoregulatory, cardiovascular, and circulating catecholamine and LH changes. *Maturitas* 1984 **6**: 31–43.

20. Shaw RW, Kerr-Wilson RHJ, Fraser HM, McNeilly AS, Howie PW, Sandow J. Effect of an intranasal LHRH agonist on gonadotrophins and hot flushes in post-menopausal women. *Maturitas* 1985 **7**: 161–167.

21. Lightman SL, Jacobs HS, Maguire AK, McGarrick G, Jeffcoate SL. Climacteric flushing: clinical and endocrine response to infusion of naloxone. *Br J Obstet Gynaecol* 1981 **88**: 919–924.

22. Paul SM, Axelford J, Saadvedra JM *et al.* Estrogen-induced efflux of endogenous catecholamines from the hypothalamus *in vitro. Brain Res* 1979 **178**: 499.

23. Tomimatsu N, Hashimoto S, Akasofu K. Effects of oestrogen on hypothalamic-endorphin in ovariectomized and old rats. *Maturitas* 1993 **17**: 5–16.

24. Hammond MG, Hatley L, Talbert LM. A double-blind study to evaluate the effect of methyldopa on menopausal vasomotor flushes. *J Clin Endocrinol Metab* 1984 **58**: 1158.

25. Taylor RW. The mechanism of action of oestrogen in the human female. *J Obstet Gynaecol Br Commonw* 1984 **81**: 856–866.

26. Krouse TB. Menopausal pathology. In Eskin BA (ed.) *The Menopause: Comprehensive Management*. New York: Masson, 1980: 1–46.

27. Leiblum S, Bachmann G, Kemmann E *et al.* Vaginal atrophy with post menopausal women: The importance of sexual activity and hormones. *JAMA* 1983 **249**: 2195.

28. Batra S. Oestrogen and smooth muscle function. *Trends Pharmacol Sci* 1980 **1**: 388–400.

29. Thomas T, Plymat K, Blannin J, Mead J. Prevalence of urinary incontinence. *Br Med J* 1980 **281**: 1243–1245.

30. Beisland HO, Fossberg E, Moer A, Sanders S. Urethral sphincteric insufficiency in postmenopausal females; treatment with phenylpropanolamine and oestriol separately and in combination. *Urol Int* 1984 **39**: 211–216.

31. Findlay I, Cunningham D, Dargie HJ. Coronary heart disease, the menopause, and hormone replacement therapy. *Br Heart J* 1994 **71**: 213–214.

32. Khaw KT. Where are the women in studies of coronary heart disease? *Br Med J* 1993 **306**: 1145–1146.

33. Steingart RM, Packer M, Hamm P *et al.* Sex differences in the management of coronary artery disease. *N Engl J Med* 1991 **325**: 226–230.

34. Petticrew M, McKee M, Jones J. Coronary artery surgery: are women discriminated against? *Br Med J* 1993 **306**: 1164–1166.

35. Adams MR, Kaplan JR, Manuck SB *et al.* Inhibition of coronary artery atherosclerosis by 17-beta estradiol in ovariectomized monkeys: lack of an effect of added progesterone. *Arteriosclerosis* 1990 **10**: 1051–1057.

36. Bush TL, Miller-Bass K. Effect of hormone replacement on cardiovascular disease: an epidemiologic overview. In Christiansen C, Overgaard K (eds) *Osteoporosis*. Proceedings of the Third International Symposium on Osteoporosis, Copenhagen: Osteopress ApS, 1990: 1817–1821.

37. Gage E, Hess OM, Murakami J *et al.* Vasoconstriction of stenotic coronary arteries during dynamic exercise in patients with classical angina pectoris; reversibility by nitroglycerin. *Circulation* 1986 **73**: 865–876.

38. Nabel EG, Ganz P, Gordon JB *et al.* Dilation of normal and constriction of atherosclerotic coronary arteries caused by the cold pressor test. *Circulation* 1988 **77**: 43–52.

39. Williams JK, Adams MR, Klopfenstein HS. Estrogen modulates responses of atherosclerotic coronary arteries. *Circulation* 1990 **81**: 1680–1687.

40. Ingegno MD, Money SR, Thelmo W *et al.* Progesterone receptors in the human heart and great vessels. *Lab Invest* 1988 **59**: 353–356.

41. Lin AL, McGil HC, Shain SA. Hormone receptors of the baboon cardiovascular system. *Circ Res* 1982 **50**: 610–616.

42. Magness RR, Rosenfeld CR. Local and systemic estradiol – 17: effects on uterine and systemic vasodilation. *Am J Physiol* 1989 **256**: (Endocrinol Metabol): E536–542.

43. Colditz GA, Willett WC, Stampfer MJ, Rosner B, Speizer FE, Hennekens CH. Menopause and the risk of coronary heart disease in women. *N Engl J Med* 1987 **316**: 1105–1110.

44. Kannel WB. Metabolic risk factors for coronary artery disease in women: perspective from the Framingham study. *Am Heart J* 1987 **114**: 413–419.

45. Farish E, Fletcher CD, Hart DM, Smith ML. Effects of bilateral oophorectomy on lipoprotein metabolism. *Br J Obstet Gynaecol* 1990 **97**: 78–92.

46. Notelovitz M, Gudat JC, Ware MD, Dougherty MC. Lipids and lipoproteins in women after oophorectomy and the response to oestrogen therapy. *Br J Obstet Gynaecol* 1983 **90**: 171–177.

47. Rosenberg L, Hennekens C, Rosner B, Belanger C, Rothman KJ, Speizer FE. Early menopause and the risk of myocardial infarction. *Am J Obstet Gynecol* 1981 **39**: 47–51.

48. Hamilton PJ, Allardlyce M, Ogston D *et al.* The effect of age upon the coagulation system. *J Clin Pathol* 1974 **27**: 980.

49. Chakrabarti R, Bronzovic M, North WR *et al.* Effects of age on fibrinolytic activity and factors V, VII and VIII. *Proc R Soc Med* 1975 **68**: 267.

50. Lindoff C, Petersson F, Lecander I, Martinsson G, Astedt B. Passage of the menopause is followed by haemostatic changes. *Maturitas* 1993 **17**: 17–22.

51. Wilhelmsen L, Svardsudd K, Korsan-Bengtssen K, Larsson B, Welin L, Tibblin G. Fibrinogen as a risk for stroke and myocardial infarction. *N Engl J Med* 1984 **311**: 501–505.

52. Huber K, Resch I, Stefenelli TH *et al.* Plasminogen activator inhibitor-1 levels in patients with chronic angina pectoris with or without angiographic evidence of coronary sclerosis. *Thromb Haemost* 1990 **63**: 336–339.

53. Bush TL. Extraskeletal effects of estrogen and the prevention of atherosclerosis. *Osteoporosis Int* 1991 **2**: 5–11.

54. Stampfer MJ, Colditz GA. Estrogen replacement therapy and coronary heart disease: a quantitative assessment of the epidemiologic evidence. *Prev Med* 1991 **20**: 47–63.

55. Eriksen EF, Colvard DS, Berg NJ *et al.* Evidence of estrogen receptors in normal human osteoblast-like cells. *Science* 1988 **241**: 84.

56. Jilka RL, Hangoc G, Girasole G *et al.* Increased osteoclast development after estrogen loss: mediation by interleukin-6. *Science* 1992 **257**: 88–91.

57. Rickard DJ, Gowen M, MacDonald BR. Proliferative responses to estradiol, IL-1 alpha and TGF beta by cells expressing alkaline phosphatase in human osteoblast-like cell cultures. *Calcif Tissue Int* 1993 **52**(3): 227–233.

58. Liebeherr M, Grosse B, Kachkache M, Balsan S. Cell signalling and estrogens in female rat osteoblasts: a possible involvement of unconventional nonnuclear receptors. *J Bone Miner Res* 1993 **8**: 1365–1376.

59. Stevenson JC. Vitamin D. in postmenopausal women. In Duusma SA, Sluys Veer Jvd (eds) *Vitamin D.* Wetenschappelijke uitgeverij, Bunge Utrecht, 1983: 43–55.

60. Gallagher JC, Riggs BL, Eisman J, Hamstra A, Arnaud SB, DeLuca HF. Intestinal calcium absorption and serum vitamin D metabolites in normal subjects and osteoporotic patients. *J Clin Invest* 1979 **64**: 729–736.

61. Reginster TY, Deroisy R, Albert A *et al.* Relationship between whole plasma calcitonin levels, calcitonin secretion capacity, and plasma levels of estrone in healthy women and postmenopausal osteoporotics. *J Clin Invest* 1989 **83**: 1073.

62. Greenberg C, Kukreja SC, Bowser EN. Effects of oestradiol and progesterone on calcitonin secretion. *Endocrinology* 1986 **118**: 2594.

63. Riggs BL, Melton LJ. Medical progresss: involutional osteoporosis. *N Engl J Med* 1986 **314**: 1676–1686.

64. Whitehead MI, Fraser D. The effects of estrogens and progestogens on the endometrium: modern approach to treatment. *Obstet Gynecol Clin North Am* 1989 **14**: 299–317.

65. Whitehead MI, Hillard TC, Crook D. The role and use of progestogens. *Obstet Gynecol* 1990 **75**: 59–76S.

66. Ravnikar VA. Compliance with hormone therapy. *Am J Obstet Gynecol* 1987 **156**: 1332–1334.

67. Leather AT, Savvas M, Studd JWW. Endometrial histology and bleeding patterns after 8 years of continuous combined estrogen and progestogen therapy in postmenopausal women. *Obstet Gynecol* 1991 **78**: 1008.

68. Hargrove J, Maxon W, Wentz A, Burnett L. Menopausal hormone replacement therapy with continuous daily oral micronized estradiol and progesterone. *Obstet Gynecol* 1989 **73**: 606–612.

69. Katz E, McClamrock HD, Adashi EY. Ovarian failure including menopause, premature menopause and resistant ovary syndrome and hormonal replacement. *Curr Opin Obstet Gynecol* 1999 **2**: 392–397.

70. Ratcliffe MA, Lanhan SA, Reid DM, Dawson AA. Bone mineral density (BMD) in patients with lymphoma: the effects of chemotherapy, intermittent corticosteroids and premature menopause. *Haematol Oncol* 1992 **10**: 181–187.

Fetal Development and Pregnancy

3.1

The Molecular Basis of Mammalian Embryogenesis

JBL Bard and SE Wedden

INTRODUCTION

The last decade has seen a revolution in our understanding of mammalian embryogenesis, as the techniques and concepts of molecular genetics introduced to study bacteria, but honed on *Drosophila*, have been used to explore mouse – and by extension, human – development. In a relatively short time, we have discovered a set of regulatory molecules that underpin and help explain many aspects of development that had remained opaque after almost a century of research. Such has been the speed of progress, that we are now in a position to pinpoint the molecular lesions responsible for many congenital abnormalities and malignant diseases. By making mouse models with specific molecular lesions, animals with the resulting disease phenotype can be used to develop new forms of therapy, both conventional and genetic.

This molecular revolution stems from our ability to clone and sequence genes (see Chapter 1.1). To clone (i.e. amplify) a DNA sequence such as a gene, the nominated gene is introduced into a host organism (such as the bacterium *Escherichia coli*) using a vector (such as a plasmid). As the bacterium replicates, it generates thousands of copies of the foreign DNA, which can then be separated and used to study the expression and function of the gene during embryogenesis – whether there are related genes in the genome of that or other species, and what happens when that gene is knocked out, overexpressed or mutated. Such studies have, for example, shown that homeobox-containing genes are involved in setting up axial organization, with the homeodomain in the protein binding to specific regions in the genome.[1] Although we still do not know the details of the binding sites or the ways in which homeobox genes control axial development, progress is being made. Indeed, so sophisticated and efficient are these techniques that methods that would have merited a Nobel prize a decade ago, are now standard in undergraduate laboratory programs.

These technological advances have not only opened new fields for medical research, but have also provided deep insights into how evolution has occurred. It transpires that essentially the same regulatory molecules help organize equivalent systems in a very wide range of animals. For example, as we shall see later, very similar homeobox genes are involved in setting up the axial patterns in both mammals and the fruit fly,[1] whereas homologous genes help mediate eye development in these two profoundly different types of organism.[2] As we have to go back 550 million years, to the early Cambrian period,[3] to find a common ancestor for vertebrates and invertebrates, the molecular data are allowing us to integrate evolution and development in a completely revolutionary way.

Such evolutional comparisons have a direct, practical importance in analyzing development. We can now use data obtained from a wide range of organisms to help explain mammalian development with more confidence than ever before. If there are morphological similarities between species with even a weak evolutionary link, similar molecular mechanisms are likely to underpin them. We will use this argument when we come to consider some aspects of mouse early development.

In this short chapter, it is not possible to cover everything that has been discovered about the molecular basis of mammalian development in the last decade. Our intention is merely to describe briefly the tools of molecular genetics and the main types of signaling and other regulatory genes that have been discovered and then to show how they are illuminating some key processes in mammalian development. The chapter ends with a few comments on how technological advances and our knowledge of the molecular basis of development are allowing us to investigate the genetic basis of congenital diseases and explore new ways of treating them.

CURRENT CONCEPTS

Signals, receptors and development

For the mammalian embryologist, the techniques of molecular genetics are illuminating a wide range of phenomena which hitherto had only been discussed in phenomenological terms. Consider, for example, the concept of 'induction', which is traditionally used to cover the events taking place when two distinct tissues interact. A few years ago, such phenomena were analyzed in terms of the need for contact, the physical interactions between the two tissues and the speed and nature of the response phenotype. Today, to take the example of mesoderm induction that will be covered in more detail later, we can sensibly talk of the molecular signals sent by one tissue to another, the receptors to which they bind, the means by which that signal is propagated to the nucleus and the transcription factors which are then activated.[4] Although we still do not know exactly how these factors lead to a change in the phenotype, we can be fairly confident that we will soon.

The same sort of analysis holds for all the other concepts of classical developmental biology. We are starting to understand the molecular basis of 'pattern formation', the process by which cells appreciate their position in, say, the developing neural tube and limb, the nature of 'competence', the ability that subgroups of cells acquire as a result of their developmental history that lets them respond in a particular way to a stimulatory signal, and the basis of 'lineage', the way in which a cell's developmental history dictates its future abilities. Some of these topics will be touched on in the rest of this chapter, but it is important to point out now that the types of molecules involved in these processes seem to belong to a relatively small number of families and classes and that each is used in a range of processes.

The key to understanding these molecular processes is to realize that most developmental phenomena fall into a standard molecular framework (Table 3.1.1). Thus a signal is propagated by one group of cells and recognized by a receptor in another group of cells. The signal is transduced and made available to the nucleus (frequently by a complex biochemical pathway based around protein kinase C and G proteins) (see Chapters 1.4 and 1.5) where it or a secondary signal interacts with a transcription factor that regulates a new set of gene transcription, which then effects the required change in phenotype. Table 3.1.1 lists examples of genes that are involved in signal pathways that will be mentioned later in this chapter.

Table 3.1.1 Regulatory molecules in mammalian development: a small subset of the known genes

Class	Family	Example(s)	Tissues
Signals			
	FGF	FGF-4 (bFGF)	Chick limb growth[5] *Xenopus* mesoderm[4]
	TGF-β	Activin BMP-2,-4,-5,-7 vg-1	Mesoderm induction[4] Osteogenesis[6] Mesoderm induction[4]
	Wnt	*Wnt-1* *Wnt-11*	Midbrain development[7] Mesoderm induction[4]
	Hedgehog	sonic hedgehog	Limb development[8]
	Retinoic acid		Neural axis[9] and limb[10]
Receptor			
cell surface	Receptor tyrosine/ Serine-kinase	EGF receptor	Epidermal differentiation[11]
intracellular	Nuclear	Retinoic acid receptor	Neural axis and limb[12]
Postreceptor	Protein kinase C, G-proteins, etc.	PKC, ras, GRB2	Ubiquitous[1]
	Kinase regulators	14-3-3ε	Mesenchyme differentiation[13]
Transcription factor			
	Homeobox	Hox family goosecoid	Neural axis, limbs organizer, Neurulation[14]
	Pax (paired box)	Pax-2 Pax-3 Pax-6	Nephrogenesis[15] Neural tube closure[16] Eye development[17]
	Pou	Oct-2	Immunoglobin development[18]
		Pit-1	Pituitary development[19]
	Zinc finger	WT-1	Nephrogenesis[20]

The key way in which these signal pathways are being investigated is through examining what happens if the gene is knocked out, either in naturally occurring mutants or in transgenic mice (e.g. where a specific gene is altered by homologous recombination (e.g. 21,22)). It should, however, be said that the effect of knocking out a gene is often much less clear-cut than we might like and this is probably because there is a considerable degree of redundancy in genetic networks. It had, for example, been thought that the adhesion molecule N-CAM* played a key and unique role in ensuring the stability of mesenchyme and neuronal aggregates; quite unexpectedly, mice lacking the *N-CAM* gene turned out to be normal, apart from some minor abnormalities in their olfactory system.[23]

Molecular embryology

Even if the results of molecular studies are not always what we might expect, so detailed are the data emerging from this work that it sometimes highlights weaknesses in our existing information about normal development. As a result, developmental biologists are having to go back to the essential embryology and to re-analyze such examples of normal development as branchial arch formation[24] and somitogenesis.[25] Furthermore, the availability of molecular markers has allowed us to undertake far more sophisticated lineage analyses[1] than had hitherto been possible and it is now possible to study developmental history of a cell type with considerable certainty.

The rest of this chapter will describe some of the recent work that has illuminated our understanding of how the early body plan of the mammalian embryo is laid down.

Early mammalian embryogenesis

Although the morphology of early human and mouse embryos has been carefully described,[1,26] there are a number of molecular and regulatory problems that have to be solved. They focus on the formation and subsequent differentiation of the three germ layers and are attracting considerable attention at the moment. Examples are how primitive ectoderm develops its basal endodermal layer, how some ectoderm migrates through the primitive streak and differentiates into mesoderm which later dorsalizes (i.e. segregates into paraxial, intermediate and lateral mesoderm), how the primitive streak moves posteriorly and how dorsal ectoderm neuralizes. These are key events because, once they have occurred (perhaps day nine in the development of the mouse (E9) and day 21 in the human), the basic structure of the embryo has, if we include early gut formation from the endoderm, been assembled and all the primitive tissues that will later form organs are in place (Fig. 3.1.1).

We now briefly review the current state of understanding in two key areas: how mesoderm is induced and the head–body division achieved, and how the neural tube is partitioned into its various regions.

Gastrulation

The first sign of embryogenesis in the inner cell mass within the blastula that will later form the mammalian embryo is the differentiation of the basal part of the ectoderm into the endoderm. This is followed by gastrulation which is accompanied by the differentiation of a further subgroup of the ectoderm into mesoderm and further endodermal cells. Gastrulation starts with the formation of Henson's node in the future cranial area of the ectoderm and, as this moves caudally creating the primitive streak, presumptive mesoderm and endoderm cells migrate internally (for review, see reference 26). Three events now take place in all vertebrates, although there are, of course, species-specific details in how these events are mediated. First, the mesoderm segregates into different axial, paraxial, intermediate and lateral components by a process called dorsalization: the axial mesoderm differentiates into the notochord, the paraxial component will form the somites (which later give muscle, dermis and vertebrae), the intermediate component will form the urogenital system and the lateral component that forms the heart, limbs and mesothelial tissue. Second, neurulation takes place: this is the process by which a particular domain of early mesoderm (the organizer region in *Xenopus*) induces the dorsal ectoderm to differentiate into the neural plate that will fold to form the neural tube and whose lateral edges will later be the source of neural crest cells. Third, the neural tube segregates into an anterior region that will become the head and a postcranial region that will give the spinal cord (Fig. 3.1.2).

Mesoderm induction

Although our molecular understanding of how mesoderm forms in mammals is still rudimentary, remarkable progress has, over the last five years, been made in elucidating the parallel events in the *Xenopus* embryo which lends itself to easy experimentation. As the evolutionary roots of mammals lie in the amphibia and because the essential topology of the mammalian and *Xenopus* embryos is much the same (although the latter lacks all the extraembryonic paraphernalia of mammals), we can have some confidence that we can use molecular data from the latter to understand the former. This view is strengthened because, as we will see, such molecular data as we have on early mammalian development mesh well with those from amphibia.

Recombination experiments between groups of *Xenopus* cells *in vitro* have now shown that the endoderm induces adjacent ectoderm to form mesoderm through a set of molecular signals, some of which were already present in the unfertilized egg and that later came to be located within the endoderm.[4] Although some of the details still have to be elucidated, the main

*Note on conventions: gene names are in lower case italics, while protein abbreviations are in upper case plain text.

story is now clear. The prime mesoderm-inducing signal seems to be Vg-1, a maternally synthesized protein located in the endoderm, with FGF and activin playing a secondary role, and indeed, if these molecules are added to isolated ectodermal cells, they start to express mesodermal markers.

Neurulation

A small domain of the mesoderm then becomes the 'organizer' region that later induces dorsal ectoderm to become the neural plate. Here, *wnt-11* expression in the endoderm seems to provide the key signal. A further gene, *noggin*,

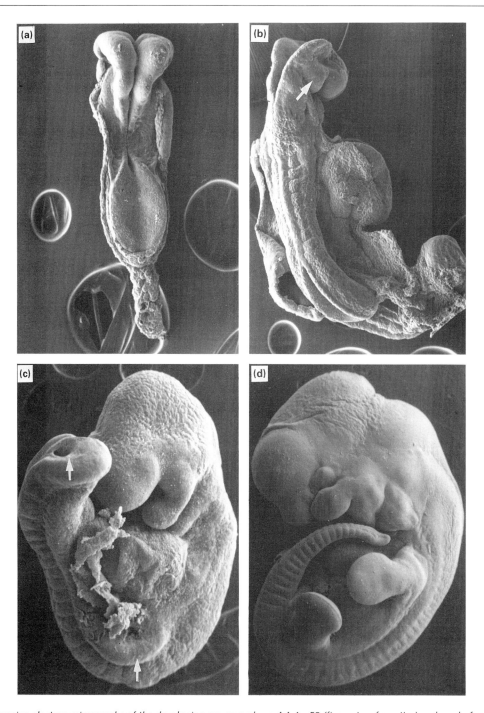

Fig. 3.1.1 *Scanning electron micrographs of the developing mouse embryo.* **(a)** *An E8 (five pairs of somites) embryo before neural tube formation (×68).* **(b)** *An E8.5 (ten pairs of somites) embryo with the neural tube almost closed and the first branchial arch forming (arrow, ×68).* **(c)** *An E9.5 (~20 pairs of somites) embryo with the first sign of a limb ridge (top arrow), an open caudal neuropore (bottom arrow) and a second branchial arch (×57).* **(d)** *An E11.5 embryo with all the major features in place: there are fore- and hind limb buds, the maxillary and mandibular branches of the first branchial arch are extending to become the jaw, and the tail has now grown (×17).*

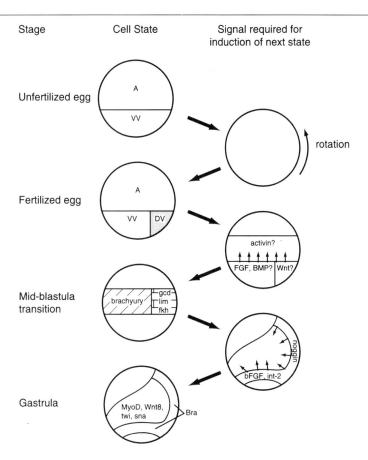

Fig. 3.1.2 *Diagram of the changes that take place in the early development of the* Xenopus *embryo (left) and the underlying molecular events that seem to be responsible. The unfertilized egg has an animal* **(A)** *and a vegetal* **(VV)** *pole and contains Vg-1, Wnt and other signaling molecules. When fertilization takes place, the cortex rotates and, in ways that are still unclear, activates these molecules in the vegetal area and assigns a second region to the 'organizer' or Nieuwkoop center* **(DV)**. *These two regions then induce the ectoderm to form mesoderm at the time of the mid-blastula transition, and a further round of gene expression takes place. A little later, gastrulation starts and the organizer comes to lie under the ectoderm, where it induces neurulation. gcd, goosecoid; fkh, forkhead; sna, snail; twi, twisted; Bra, brachyury. (Redrawn from reference 27.)*

seems to be the signal from the mesoderm that causes ectoderm to neuralize, although loss of activin may also be important here. The noggin protein also appears to be responsible for the dorsalization of the mesoderm, presumably by acting is some concentration-dependent way, although the details have still to be clarified.

Although the signals are the most dramatic part of the story, the cellular response to the signals is equally important and the key events here are the production of a set of domain-specific transcription factors which effect the changes leading to the new phenotype. Perhaps the best known of these is *goosecoid* which is found in the organizer region and, if injected into ectodermal cells, is able to induce a new head.[14]

This experiment and others demonstrate that the initial neural induction process leads to the formation of the anterior part of the head and that a further process, known as caudalization, is required to cause the embryo to elongate and to form the more posterior tissues. Again, the details are not yet clear, but recent work suggests that the upregulation of a gene called *T* plays a key role here. While a homolog of this gene is expressed in *Xenopus* (it is pro-

duced as the embryo elongates but expression ceases when this process ends; for review, see reference 28), most of the work has been done on the mouse because of the availability of the mutants *T* and T^{Wis}.

The T protein is expressed in the nuclei of early mesoderm of the primitive streak and is mutated in the *brachyury* mouse.[28] In the *T/T* mutant mouse, the expression of the gene is abnormal, the mesodermal cells have limited motility and the embryos have no notochord, an abnormal primitive streak and fail to elongate properly. In the T^{Wis}/T^{Wis} mutant, gene expression is normal, but ceases prematurely and at the same time further mesoderm differentiation also ceases.[29] It is thus clear that T is a key factor in regulating mesoderm differentiation and its associated morphogenetic events; unfortunately, here, as in most other cases, we still have little insight into how the gene achieves these effects.

Patterning of the neural axis

The subsequent patterning of the neural tube has turned out to be a sophisticated matter and to involve considerably more than its partition into just cranial and postcranial domains. The cranial region subdivides into a forebrain, midbrain and hindbrain, which recent research has shown to be further broken up into eight transitory rhombomeres (small, distinct domains). Before these hindbrain regions become morphologically distinct, it turns out that each also expresses a unique set of molecular markers, the best known of which are the *Hox* genes (see Fig. 3.1.3; reviewed in reference 30).

The Hox *codes*

Hox genes were first isolated from *Drosophila*, where their mutations are associated with homeotic abnormalities that cause one part of the body to turn into another, and in the mutation *Antennapedia*, for example, limbs form in place of antennae. It is now known that these *Hox* genes are responsible for determining the fate of each segment of the fly.[31] Genetic analysis has shown that they encode transcription factors in which a characteristic region, the 60-amino acid region homeodomain, binds to distinct regions of the genome. In mammals, there are four similar (paralagous) sets of homeobox genes (Fig. 3.1.3) each of which is related to those in *Drosophila*. *In situ* hybridization experiments have shown that both they and their *Drosophila* homologs are expressed in a rostral–caudal direction in the same (3′–5′) order in which they are encoded in the genome. Specific regions of the mammalian neural tube each express a unique subset of these proteins, and this is known as its *Hox* code.[1]

How *Hox* codes are established is currently a matter of debate. The current view is that they are established during gastrulation, with the initial inductive interaction leading to forebrain determination, and posteriorizing factors being responsible for the patterning of the neural tube. One candidate for this role is retinoic acid, and it has been suggested[9] that Henson's node specifies posterior structures by releasing increasing amounts of retinoic acid as it moves posteriorly. To support this view, exogenous retinoic acid has been shown to cause an anteroposterior transformation in the CNS[34] and to alter the *Hox* code in the hindbrain.[35]

The way in which retinoic acid might work also remains unclear, as its pathway of action is extremely complex. However, it is noteworthy that mice in which specific receptors for retinoic acid and its metabolites have been knocked out show an intriguing set of pattern abnormalities.[12] The way in which the *Hox* codes play a patterning role is also unclear, although, again, gene knock-outs show pattern abnormalities (e.g. references 23 and 24). Here, however, it is hard to undertake any detailed analysis because there is considerable redundancy among the four paralagous sets of *Hox* genes and the absence of one, or even more of these genes, can be compensated for by others. Nevertheless, even if the evidence is not as strong as one might like, the clear view of the field is that the *Hox* genes play a key role in cell specification and some of the best evidence here comes from the behavior of cranial neural crest cells.

Neural crest cells and branchial arches

As the neural tube is forming, cells migrate from the dorsal crests of the tube (originally, the lateral edges of the neural plate) and migrate throughout the embryo. In the body, these neural crest cells form the peripheral nervous system, pigment cells, the adrenal medulla and other tissues. In the head, they give rise to the bones, teeth and connective tissues of the face,[36] but most recent attention has been paid to their role in branchial arch development. These arches are in essence a collection of bags (1–6, with 5 being absent) into which cells migrate; their outer surface is skin ectoderm and their inner surface is pharyngeal endoderm. Each contains a mix of head-somite-derived mesenchyme cells and rhombomere-derived neural crest cells and the sole differences between the arches lies in their *Hox* codes which the neural crest cells have carried with them (Fig. 3.1.4).

The specificity associated with the *Hox* genes in the cells of the branchial arches has been demonstrated in gene-knockout experiments. If the *Hox* code specifying neural crest cells in a rhombomere is disrupted genetically, duplicated structures may arise because the cells differentiate according to their new code, irrespective of position or environment (e.g. reference 24). This situation strongly contrasts with the behavior of mesenchymal cells derived from somitomeres (the head equivalent of somites), which also migrate into the arches and eventually differentiate to form muscles. Here, grafting of cells labeled with DiI (a strong fluorescent marker) from one arch to another leads to no abnormal effect and, in contrast to the neural crest cells, the somitomere-derived cells respond to the patterning signals in their new environment.[37]

Later inductive interactions

Patterning in the limb

Of all the systems that are currently under investigation, the one in which the widest range of regulatory systems has been shown to be present is the limb, and it is therefore attracting considerable effort. Although most of this work has been done on the chick (it lends itself to experimentation), recent evidence shows that the same mechanisms operate in the mammalian limb.[38,39] The interactions that have been extensively examined are those that regulate patterning of the structures along the anteroposterior (AP) axis (from thumb to little finger) and the proximodistal axis (from shoulder to finger tips) and these take place within the progress zone of the early limb mesenchyme.[40]

A thickened rim of epithelium at the tip of the developing limb bud, the 'apical ectodermal ridge' (AER), is responsible for maintaining the growth of the underlying domain of progress zone mesenchyme (if the ridge is removed, the limb is truncated). This progress zone, which consists of undifferentiated cells with a high mitotic index, also helps to maintain the capability of the AER through a reciprocal inductive interaction.

Digit specification is under the control of signal(s) emanating from a domain of cells at the posterior margin of the limb known as the 'zone of polarizing activity' (ZPA) or polarizing region.[41] This is shown by a simple experiment: when a ZPA is grafted to the anterior margin, it produces a

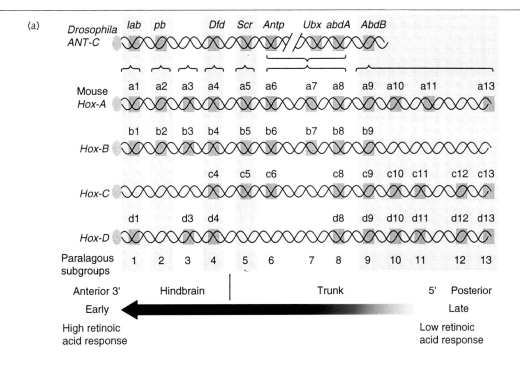

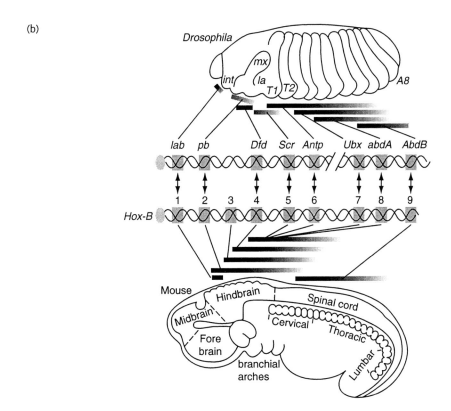

Fig. 3.1.3 **(a)** *Homeotic gene organization on Chromosome 3 of* Drosophila, *together with the four homologous sets of* Hox *genes in the mouse. Paralagous genes with strong similarities are shown in the shaded blocks, representing areas of conservation. In the mouse, the genes are expressed in the 3′–5′ and anterior-to-posterior direction; this pattern seems to be linked to the amounts of retinoic acid present.* **(b)** *The extent of the conservation is shown by the comparison between the expression patterns in* Drosophila *and mouse. (Redrawn from references 1, 32 and 33.)*

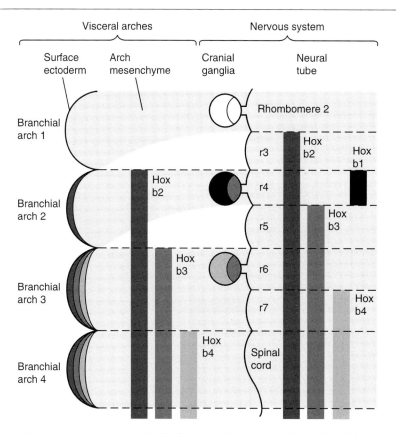

Fig. 3.1.4 Hox *gene expression in the rhombomeres in the hindbrain, and the associated migration of rhombomere-derived neural crest cells into the branchial arches. (Redrawn from references 1 and 33.)*

mirror-image digit pattern duplication in the limb. It is thought that the ZPA produces a diffusible morphogen which forms a concentration gradient along the AP axis, and that mesenchymal cells recognize their position along the AP axis by reference to this morphogen.[42]

These cell-based interactions were established in the 1960s and 1970s, but it is only in the last decade that their molecular basis started to become clear with the discovery that the action of a ZPA graft could be mimicked by all-*trans*-retinoic acid.[43] This observation led to speculation that retinoic acid was the morphogen, but, although retinoic acid is present, and enriched in the anterior half of the limb bud,[10] the story is not as simple as once thought.[12,44]

In the last few years, an extensive search has been made for homeobox and other genes that might be involved in limb patterning (Fig. 3.1.5) and, although the details have yet to be fully worked out, key players so far identified include members of the *Hox d* cluster (previously named *Hox 4* and, before that, *Hox 5*;[45,46]), *Hox b8* (previously named *Hox 2.4*[47]), *Msx 1* and *2* (previously named *Hox 7* and *Hox 8*, respectively[38,48,49]), sonic hedgehog (*Shh*),[8] *Wnt* genes,[49] bone morphogenetic proteins (BMP-2 and BMP-4[50,51]), and FGF-4.[5,52] FGF-4 can direct limb-bud outgrowth and patterning in the absence of the AER[5] and may thus be one of the endogenous ridge signals, but other

genes are important in maintaining the ZPA at the posterior margin. Sonic hedgehog (*Shh*) mRNA localizes with the ZPA and its protein has polarizing activity, so suggesting that SHH protein is the endogenous polarizing signal. Evidence to support this view is that FGF-4 expression in the ridge can be mediated by *Shh*-expressing cells, and that *Shh* expression can be activated by FGF-4 in combination with retinoic acid. Other experiments show that there is also a feedback loop which obviates any further need for retinoic acid once *Shh* expression has been established. This is the first evidence for a molecular basis for feedback between epithelium and mesenchyme.[52]

There is evidence[47] that suggests that *Hox b8* may be involved in the establishment of the ZPA in the forelimb. *Hox b8* is normally only expressed in the posterior half of the mouse forelimb bud, but, when its expression is extended anteriorly (using transgenic technology), mirror-image digit pattern duplications occur. The hindlimb is, however, unaffected, despite the fact that it too expresses *Hox b8* and this observation suggests that the role of *Hox b8* is forelimb specific. Members of the *Hox d* cluster, on the other hand, appear to specify regional differences within all limb buds.[53]

Space limits the analysis that this chapter can provide into other key events taking place as the embryo undergoes organogenesis, but it is worth pointing to two further

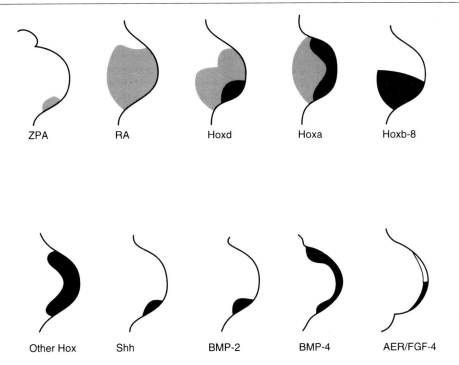

Fig. 3.1.5 *The stage-20 (day 3.5) chick limb bud, showing the expression of key genes involved in outgrowth and digit formation. Note that the ZPA (zone of polarizing activity) is localized at the posterior margin, and that the expression of* sonic hedgehog (Shh) *and bone morphogenetic protein-2 (BMP-2) co-localize with it. Fibroblast growth factor-4 (FGF-4), Msx-2, and BMP-4 are all expressed in the apical ectodermal ridge, whereas Hox genes are expressed as a nested sequence within the mesenchyme. (Redrawn from reference 54.)*

tissues whose development is attracting considerable interest, the notochord and the kidney.

Notochord

For many years, the notochord, the thin, rigid cord of cells subjacent to the neural tube, was thought to be a passive structure responsible for maintaining the straight elongation of the embryo. However, it is now becoming clear from experiments originally done on chick, but more recently on mouse embryos, that signals emanating from the notochord play roles in inducing floor plate and motor neuron development in the neural tube, as well as helping to regulate the differentiation of muscles within the somites, a process mediated by the *MyoD* and *Myf* genes.[55]

The clearest example of the importance of the notochord in mammalian embryogenesis comes from mice embryos lacking both copies of *Hnf-3β*, a gene expressed in the notochord, gut and neural tube.[56] The embryos die on E10–11 with no notochord and showing an absence of floor plate in the ventral neural tube, a grossly malformed gut and poor somitogenesis. The nature of the floor plate-inducing activity has been illuminated by the recent discovery of a member of the *hedgehog* family, *vvh-1*, which is expressed in rat notochord. This signaling gene clearly plays a key role here as, for example, COS cells expressing *vvh-1* induce floor plate and motor neuron activity in neural plate explants.[57] Other experiments have shown that

floor-plate induction requires direct physical contact, whereas motor neuron differentiation is induced by a diffusible factor.[58] As to the signals responsible for making muscles from somitic mesoderm, it seems that these mainly derive from the neural tube, but that the notochord plays a secondary, regulatory role here.[25] The nature of all the signals generated by the notochord has yet to be elucidated, but the speed of progress has been impressive and it should not be too long before the inductive role of this tissue has been elucidated.

Kidney

The last example to be considered here is the development of the metanephros or definitive kidney (Fig. 3.1.6). This forms as a result of a reciprocal inductive interaction between a ureteric bud off the nephric duct and a mesenchymal blastema that appears within the intermediate mesoderm. As a result of this interaction, the bud differentiates into the collecting duct system and the blastema forms epithelialized nephrons in which small aggregates of mesenchyme undergo a mesenchyme-to-epithelial transition to generate polarized tubules. Although something is known of both the cell processes that generate these changes and the genes expressed as they take place,[59,60] little is yet understood of the signals that underpin the inductive interactions.

There has, nevertheless, been one key discovery about

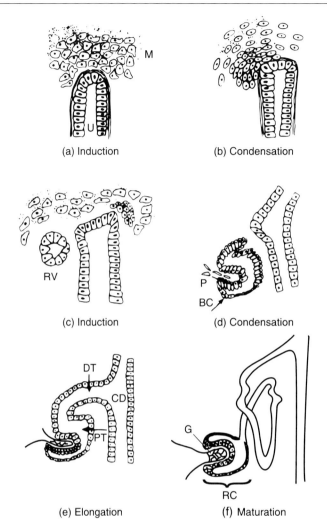

(a) Induction

(b) Condensation

(c) Induction

(d) Condensation

(e) Elongation

(f) Maturation

Fig. 3.1.6 *Kidney morphogenesis. Nephrogenesis is induced* **(a)** *as the ureteric bud* **(U)** *and the metanephric mesenchyme* **(M)** *come into contact. The mesenchyme* **(b)** *condenses into small aggregates that* **(c)** *epithelialize and vesiculate, and then* **(d)** *become S-shaped. The region of the S-shaped body nearest to the ureteric tubule* **(e)** *fuses to the tubule and the tubule elongates to form the proximal* **(PT)** *and distal* **(DT)** *tubules. The cleft distal to the tubule attracts blood vessels* **(f)** *and differentiates into the glomerular region as the nephron matures. As this happens, the uteric tube continues to grow and bifurcate.* **RV,** *renal vesicle;* **P,** *podocyte;* **BC,** *Bowman's capsule;* **RC,** *renal capsule;* **CD,** *collecting duct;* **G,** *glomerulus. (Redrawn from reference 63.)*

the molecular basis of nephrogenesis that is worth mentioning here, as it shows how powerful can be the role of a single regulatory gene in organogenesis. It turns out that the zinc-finger transcription factor *WT1* (for review, see reference 20), which is expressed in the blastema (and later in the developing nephrons), has two effects in early nephrogenesis: it causes the ureteric bud to extend from the nephric duct and then allows the blastema to recognize the inductive signal produced by that bud. This evidence comes from a mouse in which the *WT1* gene has been knocked out,[61] and it is particularly interesting that, in this animal, the blastema forms but the ureteric bud fails to develop and no induction takes place; instead, the blastema undergoes programmed cell death or apoptosis. It is also noteworthy that, when the human form of this gene undergoes mutation, it can either lead to the development of Wilms' tumor, a nephroblastoma in which kidney stem cells undergo uncontrolled proliferation, while failing to differentiate properly, or the Denys–Drash syndrome where, among other anomalies, glomerular differentiation is abnormal.[62]

It is clear that *WT1* is a particularly intriguing transcription factor and the investigation of its molecular role in all stages of nephrogenesis is currently being studied in several laboratories.[20] The kidney is, however, being investigated for two other reasons: its formation involves a wide range of developmental processes and, most unusually, much of kidney development will take place in culture so that the tissue can be studied experimentally with, for a mammalian tissue, relative ease.

FUTURE PERSPECTIVES

This brief survey of some of the regulatory bases of mammalian embryogenesis has demonstrated the strength of genetic technology in providing a molecular explanation for a wide range of developmental phenomena discovered by the techniques of classical embryology – and there is a great deal more to come!

Although a very large number of molecules involved in regulatory pathways remains to be unearthed, their discovery will only be the beginning of the story. The next stage will be finding out how these pathways lead to the changes in cell phenotype that underpin all developmental events, and this will clearly be difficult as we do not, for example, yet understand at the genetic level the action of even a single transcription factor.

Nonetheless, our progress in understanding the molecular underpinnings of the regulatory pathways of development is beginning to have an impact in a far wider area than the fascinating, if limited, domain of mammalian embryogenesis. Our ability to manipulate embryos and control their genetic complement is enabling us to make transgenic mice where almost any gene can be knocked out, mutated or overexpressed so that it is becoming practical to make mouse models of many congenital disorders. The cystic fibrosis mouse is a good example.[22]

The other long-term implication of all this work is that an understanding of the regulatory pathways and the availability of mouse models is going to have profound effects on the way in which drugs are designed and tested. It seems inevitable that the availability of the animal models and new drugs will together revolutionize the practice of medicine. It is an interesting thought that, only a decade ago, mammalian developmental biology was a relatively arcane, academic subject. However, times have changed and it now lies at the heart of modern biomedical research.

SUMMARY

- A flood of molecular data is currently providing new insights into the genetic basis of normal development.
- A set of signaling molecules belonging to a few well-defined families (the FGFs and TGFβs (e.g. activins and BMPs), Wnts, hedgehogs and retinoic acid) seem to be involved in a wide range of tissue interactions.
- Signals sometimes interact directly with transcription factors that control protein synthesis but in other cases they interact with receptor tyrosine kinases at the cell surface that activate a complex kinase-based pathway which, in turn, links to the transcription factors.
- The *Hox* codes defined by the patterns of the four sets of paralagous homeobox genes (examples of transcription factors) provide neural tube and neural crest tissue with position-defining information. The way in which these and other transcription factors work is not well understood.
- The function of some of these genes is being studied in transgenic mice in which one or another factor is functionally blocked, mutated or overexpressed. Progress is limited here, because there is a high degree of genetic redundancy; nevertheless transgenic mice are being made that are good models of human congenital diseases.
- Perhaps the most remarkable feature about all these molecules is that they, or very similar ones, are ubiquitous across the animal kingdom; reciprocal progress is thus being made in the general areas of evolution and development.
- Work on *Xenopus* development is showing how mesoderm is formed and how neurulation is induced.
- Work on chick development is demonstrating how interactions between a detailed set of signals and transcription factors regulate limb development.
- Studies on notochord and kidney development in the mouse are starting to illuminate the mechanisms responsible for forming specific tissues in later development.
- It should not be long before all this information starts to impact on clinical medicine drug design. Here, the use of mouse models of disease will be of central importance.

REFERENCES

1. Gilbert SF. *Developmental Biology*, 4th edn. USA: Sinauer Press, 1994.
2. Quiring R, Waldorff U, Kloter U, Gehring WJ. Homology of the *eyeless* gene of *Drosophila* to the *small-eye* gene in mice and aniridia in humans. *Science* 1994 **265**: 785–789.
3. Whittington HB. *The Burgess Shale*. USA: Yale University Press, 1985.
4. Slack JMW. Inducing factors in *Xenopus* early embryos. *Curr Biol* 1994 4: 116–126.
5. Niswander L, Tickle C, Vogel A, Booth I, Martin GR. FGF-4 replaces the apical ectodermal ridge and directs outgrowth and paterning in the limb. *Cell* 1993 75: 579–587.

6. Lyons KM, Jones CM, Hogan BLM. The DVR gene family in embryonic development. *Trends Genet* 1991 7: 408–412.

7. McMahon AP, Bradley A. The *Wnt-1(int-1)* proto-oncogene is required for the development of a large region of the mouse brain. *Cell* 1990 **62**: 1073–1085.

8. Riddle RD, Johnson RL, Laufer E, Tabin C. *Sonic hedgehog* mediates the polarising activity of the ZPA. *Cell* 1993 **75**: 1401–1416.

9. Hogan BLM, Thaller C, Eichele G. Evidence that Henson's node is a site of retinoic acid synthesis. *Nature* 1992 **359**: 237–241.

10. Thaller C, Eichele G. Identification and spatial distribution of retinoids in the developing chick limb bud. *Nature* 1987 **327**: 625–628.

11. Hunter T. Oncogenes and growth control. *Trends Biochem Sci* 1995 **10**: 275–280.

12. Lownes D, Mark M, Mendelsohn C, Dollé P, Dierich A, Gorry P, Gansmuller A, Chambon P. Function of the retinoic acid receptors (RARs) during development. 1: Craniofacial and skeletal abnormalities in RAR double mutants. *Development* 1994 **120**: 2723–2748.

13. McConnell JE, Armstrong JF, Bard JBL. The mouse 14-3-3ε isoform, a kinase regulator involved in kidney, mesenchyme and neural differentiation. *Dev Biol* 1994 **169**: 218–228.

14. Blumberg B, Wright CVE, De Robertis EM, Cho KWY. Organiser-specific genes in *Xenopus laevis*. *Development* 1991 **103**: 193–209.

15. Rothenpieler UW, Dressler GR. *Pax-2* is required for mesenchyme-to-epithelium conversion during kidney development. *Development* 1993 **119**: 3051–3062.

16. Goulding MD, Chalepakis G, Deutsch U, Erselius J, Gruss P. Pax-3, a novel murine DNA binding protein expressed during early neurogenesis. *EMBO J* 1991 **10**: 1135–1147.

17. Hill RE, Favor J, Hogan BLM, Ton CCT, Saunders GF, Hanson IM *et al.* Mouse small-eye results from mutations in a paired-like homeobox containing gene. *Nature* 1991 **354**: 522–525.

18. Elsholtz HP, Albert VR, Treac MN, Rosenfeld MG. A two-base change in a POU-factor binding site switches pituitary specific to lymphoid specific gene expression. *Genes Dev* 1990 **4**: 43–51.

19. Bodner M, Karin M. A pituitary-specific *trans*-acting factor can stimulate transcription from the growth hormone promoter in extracts of non-expressing cells. *Cell* 1987 **50**: 267–275.

20. Bard JBL, Armstrong JF, Bickmore WA. WT1, a Wilms' tumour gene. *Exp Nephrol* 1993 **1**: 218–223.

21. Capecchi MR. Altering the genome by homologous recombination. *Science* 1989 **244**: 1288–1292.

22. Dorin J, Dickinson P, Alton EFW, Smith SN, Geddes DM, Stevenson BJ *et al.* Cystic fibrosis in the mouse by targeted insertional mutagenesis. *Nature* 1992 **359**: 211–215.

23. Cremer H, Lange R, Christophe A, Plomann M, Vopper G, Roes J *et al.* Inactivation of the *N-CAM* gene in mice results in size reduction of the olfactory bulb and deficits in spatial learning. *Nature* 1994 **367**: 455–459.

24. Rijli FM, Mark M, Lakkaraju S, Dierich A, Dollee P, Chambon P. A homeotic transformation is generated in the rostral branchial region of the head and is generated by disruption of *Hox-a2*, which acts as a selector gene. *Cell* 1993 **75**: 1333–1349.

25. Bober E, Brand-Saberi B, Ebensberger C, Wiltin J, Balling R, Paterson BM, Arnold H-H, Christ B. Initial steps of myogenesis in somites are independent of influence from axial structures. *Development* 1994 **120**: 3073–3078.

26. Kaufman MH. *The Atlas of Mouse Development* (2nd printing). London: Academic Press, 1994.

27. Slack JMW. Embryonic induction. *Mech Dev* 1993 **41**: 91–107.

28. Yamada T. Caudalization by the amphibian organizer: *brachyury*, convergent extension and retinoic acid. *Development* 1994 **120**: 3051–3062.

29. Herrman BG. Expression patterns of the *Brachyury* gene in whole mount T^{Wis}/T^{Wis} mutant embryos. *Development* 1991 113: 913–917.

30. Wilkinson D. Molecular mechanisms of segmental patterning in the verebrate hindbrain and neural crest. *Bioessays* 1993 **15**: 499–505.

31. Lawrence PA. *The Making of a Fly*. Oxford: Blackwell Scientific Publications, 1990.

32. Krumlauf R. Hox genes and axial patterning in the branchial region of the vertebrate head. *Trends Genet* 1993 **9**: 106–112.

33. McGinnis W, Krumlauf R. Homeobox genes and axial patterning. *Cell* 1992 **68**: 283–302.

34. Durston AJ, Timmermans JPM, Hage WJ, Hendricke HFJ, de Vries NJ, Heldeveld M, Nieuwkoop PD. Retinoic acid causes an anteroposterior transformation in the developing nervous system. *Nature* 1989 **340**: 140–144.

35. Marshall H, Nonchev S, Sham MH, Muchamore I, Lumsden A, Krumlauf M. Retinoic acid alters hindbrain *Hox* code and induces transformation of rhombomeres 2/3 into a 4/5 identity. *Nature* 1992 **360**: 737–741.

36. Noden DM. Interactions and fates of avian craniofacial mesenchyme. *Development* 1988 **103** (suppl): 121–140.

37. Trainor PA, Tan S-S, Tam PPL. Cranial paraxial mesoderm: regionalisation of cell fate and impact on craniofacial development in mouse embryos. *Development* 1994 **120**: 2397–2408.

38. Davidson D, Crawley A, Hill RE, Tickle C. Position-dependent expression of two related homeobox genes in the developing vertebrate limbs. *Nature* 1991 **352**: 429–431.

39. Brown JM, Wedden SE, Millburn GH, Robson LG, Hill RE, Davidson DR. Experimental analysis of the control of expression of the homeobox-gene *Msx-1* in the developing limb and face. *Development* 1993 **119**: 41–48.

40. Summerbell D, Lewis DH, Wolpert L. Positional information in chick limb morphogenesis. *Nature* 1973 **244**: 492–496.

41. Saunders JW, Gasseling MT. Ectodermal–mesenchymal interactions in the origin of limb symmetry. In Fleishmajor R, Billingham RE (eds) *Epithelial–Mesenchymal Interactions*. Baltimore: Williams and Wilkins, 1968: 78–97.

42. Tickle C, Summerbell D, Wolpert L. Positional signalling and specification of digits in chick limb morphogenesis. *Nature* 1975 **254**: 199–205.

43. Tickle C, Alberts B, Wolpert L, Lee J. Local application of retinoic acid to limb buds mimics the action of the polarising region. *Nature* 1982 **296**: 654–565.

44. Brockes J. We may not have a morphogen. *Nature* 1991 **350**: 15.

45. Dollé P, Izpisua-Belmonte JC, Falkenstein H, Renucci A, Duboule D. Coordinate expression of the *Hox-5* complex homeobox-containing genes during limb pattern formation. *Nature* 1989 **342**: 767–772.

46. Morgan BA, Izpisua-Belmonte J-C, Duboule D, Tabin CJ. Targeted misexpression of *Hox-4.6* in the avian limb bud causes apparent homeotic transformations. *Nature* 1992 **358**: 236–239.

47. Charité J, de Graaf W, Shen S, Deschamps J. Ectopic expression of *Hoxb-8* causes duplication of the ZPA in the forelimb and homeotic transformation of axial structures. *Cell* 1994 **78**: 589–601.

48. Coelho CD, Krabbenhoft KM, Upholt WB, Fallon JF, Kosher RA. Altered expression of the chicken homeobox-containing genes *Ghox-7* and *Ghox-8* in the limb buds of limbless mutant chick embryos. *Development* 1991 **113**: 1487–1493.

49. Parr BA, Shea M, Vassileva G, McMahon AP. Mouse *Wnt* genes exhibit discrete domains of expression in the early embryonic CNS and limb buds. *Development* 1993 **119**: 247–261.

50. Lyons KM, Pelton RW, Hogan BLM. Organogenesis and pattern formation in the mouse: RNA distribution patterns

suggest a role for *Bone morphogenetic protein-2A* (BMP-2A). *Development* 1990 **109**: 833–844.

51. Jones CM, Lyons KM, Hogan BLM. Involvement of *Bone Morphogenetic Protein-4* (BMP-4) and *Vgr-1* in morphogenesis and neurogenesis in the mouse. *Development* 1991 **111**: 531–542.

52. Niswander L, Jeffrey S, Martin GR, Tickle C. A positive feedback loop coordinates growth and patterning in the vertebrate limb. *Nature* 1994 **371**: 609–610.

53. Izbisua-Belmont J-C, Tickle C, Dollé P, Wolpert L, Duboule D. Expression of the homeobox *Hox-4* genes and the specification of position in chick wing development. *Nature* 1991 **350**: 585–589.

54. Maden M. The limb bud – part two. *Nature* 1994 **371**: 560–561.

55. Lyons GE, Buckingham ME. Developmental regulation of myogenesis in the mouse. *Semin Dev Biol* 1992 **3**: 243–253.

56. Weinstein DC, Altabar AR, Chen WS, Hoodless P, Prezioso UR, Jessel TM, Darnell JE Jr. The winged-helix transcription factor, HNF-3β is required for notochord development in the mouse embryo. *Cell* 1994 **78**: 575–588.

57. Roelink H, Augsburger A, Heemskerk J, Korzh V, Norlin S, Ruiz i. Altaba A *et al.* Floor plate and motor neuron induction by *vvh-1*, a verebrate homolog of *hedgehog* expressed by notochord. *Cell* 1994 **76**: 711–720.

58. Yamada T, Pfaff SL, Edlund T, Jessell TM. Control of cell pattern in the neural tube: motor neuron induction by diffusible factors from notochord and floor plate. *Cell* 1993 **73**: 673–686.

59. Ekblom P. Renal development. In Seldin DW, Giebisch G (eds) *The Kidney: Physiology and Pathophysiology* (2nd edn). New York: Raven Press, 1992: 475–501.

60. Bard J B L, McConnell J E, Davies JA. Towards a genetic basis for kidney development. *Mech Dev* 1994 **48**: 3–11.

61. Kreidberg JA, Sariola H, Loring JM, Maeda M, Pelletier J, Housman D, Jaenisch R. WT-1 is required for early kidney development. *Cell* 1993 **74**: 679–691.

62. Pelletier J, Bruening W, Kashtan CE, Mauer SM, Mauivel JC, Striegel JE *et al.* Germline mutations in the Wilms tumor suppressor gene area associated with abnormal urinogenital development in Denys–Drash syndrome. *Cell* 1991 **7**: 437–447.

63. Mugrauer G, Ekbolm P. Contrasting expression patterns of the *myc* family of proto-oncogenes in the developing and adult mouse kidney. *J Cell Biol* 1991 **112**: 13–25.

3.2

Human Embryogenesis

F Beck

INTRODUCTION

The fertilized ovum is largely dependent on the translation of long-lived mRNA of maternal origin during early cleavage. At the 8-cell stage (>2.5 days postovulatory), the process of compaction is accompanied by the inception of transcription of zygotic DNA. The formation of a morula and blastocyst with concomitant delineation of trophectoderm from the inner cell mass quickly follows. Extra-embryonic tissues are, therefore, specified before the embryo enters the uterus and hatches from the zona pellucida (about 4 and 6 days, respectively). Around day 7 postovulation, the polar trophoblast overlying the inner cell mass becomes attached to the uterine epithelium, usually high up on the posterior uterine wall, and the process of implantation commences. Rapid differentiation of the extra-embryonic membranes follows and abundant raw materials become available for embryonic growth and development following the establishment of placentally mediated histiotrophic and hematotrophic nutrition.

About 7 days after implantation (circa 14 days postovulation), the delineation of the primary germ layers begins with the inception of the primitive streak. This process of gastrulation involves massive cell migration and, together with the succeeding stage of neurulation, results in the laying down of the basic body pattern. It is the single most important event in vertebrate development – one that must be very well controlled with respect to cellular positional information.

Following gastrulation, the central nervous system (CNS) axis is laid down during neurulation; essentially, this marks the beginning of the period known as organogenesis. Morphogenesis of the major body systems is largely completed during this period and the developing embryo is uniquely sensitive to the action of exogenous (potentially teratogenic) agents. For descriptive purposes, organogenesis is essentially completed at 12 weeks with the closure of the secondary palate, but histogenesis and the processes of functional maturation are as yet in their early stages. Histogenesis, particularly of the lung and kidney, is not complete until well into the neonatal period, whereas growth and functional maturation of the nervous system continues into late childhood. Indeed, development, particularly involving the reproductive, musculoskeletal, endocrine and lymphatic systems, is not complete until the end of the adolescent period some 18 to 20 years after birth even though the fetus is theoretically capable of independent existence some 25 weeks after ovulation.

CURRENT CONCEPTS

Some notes on the development of the principal organ systems

Space does not permit comprehensive coverage of developmental anatomy and physiology in a volume of this nature. There follows a series of notes dealing with the timing of the principal events in the embryogenesis of the major organ systems. Comprehensive accounts of human development can be found in references 1–4.

The central nervous system[5-8]

Some 21 days postovulation (a week after the start of gastrulation), the neural groove is well developed and, in the following week, the neural tube forms. By 30 days, the neuropores are closed and fore-, mid- and hindbrain regions are recognizable. The matrix, mantle and marginal layers of the neural tube are histologically distinguishable and the neural crest is beginning to form. Alar (sensory) and basal (motor) regions of the mantle layer are separated by the sulcus limitans (Fig. 3.2.1).

At 5 weeks, the cervical and mesencephalic brain flexures are well marked and the pontine flexure is beginning to appear, cranial and spinal nerves and their ganglia are

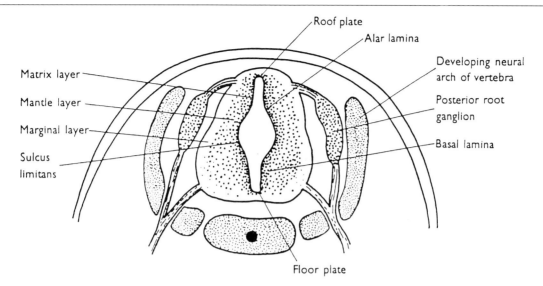

Roof plate

Alar lamina

Matrix layer

Developing neural
arch of vertebra

Mantle layer

Posterior root
ganglion

Marginal layer

Sulcus
limitans

Basal lamina

Floor plate

Fig. 3.2.1 *The developing spinal cord. Neural crest cells form* inter alia *the posterior root ganglia. The three layers of the neural tube are histologically distinguishable from early embryonic stages.*

present and the cerebral vesicles begin to be delineated. The optic vesicle is invaginated by the lens placode (Fig. 3.2.2a).

At 6 weeks, the first macroscopic evidence of cerebellar development is apparent, though this structure is largely intraventricular at this stage (Fig. 3.2.2b). Peripherally, the sympathetic ganglia (derivatives of the neural crest) are formed.

At 7 weeks, the basal ganglia are well formed and a large thalamus is apparent. In the third and fourth month, the brain begins to resemble that of the adult; the cerebral hemispheres cover much of the surface, there is a large cerebellum and the corpus callosum and other commissures are formed (Fig. 3.2.2c). From then on, the cerebral sulci and gyri appear, the insula sinks below the surface covered by the operculae and myelinization commences, though it is not complete until 5 years or so after birth. In recent years, some of the controlling factors responsible for the regional specification of the neural tube and its derivatives have become apparent. Good reviews concerning craniocaudal[9] and dorsoventral[10] differentiation are available.

The external features of the embryo and the musculoskeletal system[11]

The embryonic period extends from conception to about 8 weeks, during which the basic structure of the body is laid down. Crown–rump length can be measured from 4 weeks (4 mm) and the embryo grows at 1 mm per day until it reaches 30 mm. Thereafter, growth is nearer 1.5 mm daily. The early fetal period, between 8 and 28 weeks, is characterized by rapid body growth and histological, as well as functional maturation of its tissues and organs. The second

part of the fetal period is reached when viability commences at 26 to 28 weeks. It is marked by laying down of subcutaneous fat and further maturation, with continuing but relatively minor changes in body form.

The somites are a prominent feature of the early embryo, particularly in the third and fourth weeks after ovulation. They develop from the paraxial mesoderm on either side of the notochord and give rise to the greater part of the axial skeleton and voluntary musculature. The first somite appears at about 20 days and about 30 somites are present by day 30. A total of 42 to 44 somites develop, new ones being added caudally as the cranial ones differentiate into sclerotomes (which give rise to the axial skeleton), dermatomes (from which the dermis of the skin develops) and mytomes (which develop into the voluntary muscles of the adult). Most of the major cell migrations which constitute these processes are completed at about 45 days when the embryo is about 16 mm in crown–rump length (Fig. 3.2.3). The limb buds have appeared at about 26 days and, during the fifth week, they have grown to the extent that the primitive hands and feet are beginning to differentiate from the paddle-shaped extremities. Thereafter, the major landmarks include the primary ossification of the long bones (8 weeks) and the completion of the definitive body wall (12 weeks) which involves the most anterior migration of dermatome to support the surface ectoderm surrounding the umbilicus. Recent experiments have begun to clarify the role of various factors involved in limb morphogenesis.[12] They exemplify the direction of research in modern experimental embryology.

By 3 months, the nails appear and, at 4 months, the first (lanugo) hairs are apparent, whereas, at 7 months, vernix caseosa begins to be secreted by the sebaceous glands of the skin.

The cardiovascular system[13,14]

The heart develops by fusion of a pair of endothelial tubes which fuse and invaginate the primitive pericardial cavity (a subdivision of the intra-embryonic celom). At about 21 days after fertilization, the first heartbeats occur and, at this stage, the heart tube consists of four chambers in series.

These are the sinus venosus (embedded in the septum transversum), atrium, ventricle and bulbus cordis, followed by an outflow channel, the truncus arteriosus, situated in the floor of the foregut (Fig. 3.2.4). By 25 days, the heart forms a characteristic S-shaped loop and the second and succeeding aortic arch arteries begin to develop sequentially. At 32 days, septation into right and left circulations

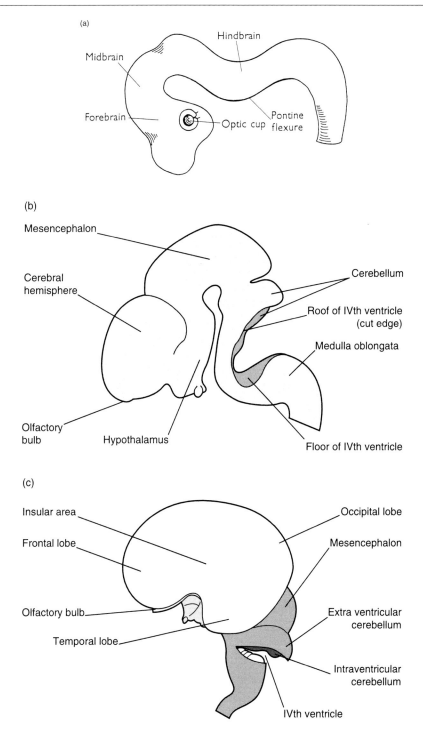

Fig. 3.2.2 (a) *External features of the cranial part of the neural tube at 35 days.* **(b)** *External features of the brain at 42 days.* **(c)** *External features of the brain at 3 months.*

begins with inception of the septum primum, followed, at 37 days, by division of the common atrioventricular canal by fusion of the atrioventricular cushions. At 46 days, the ventricles are separated by fusion of the aorticopulmonary septum and the muscular interventricular septum, together with a contribution from the fused atrioventricular cushions. Septation of the common atrial cavity continues with development of the septum secundum. Communication between the right and left heart is maintained through the foramen ovale until birth and is, in fact, essential for fetal survival. The fetal circulation is illustrated in Fig. 3.2.5. At birth, hemodynamic factors cause the septum primum to be apposed to the septum secundum, thereby separating the atria. This also marks the time at which closure of the

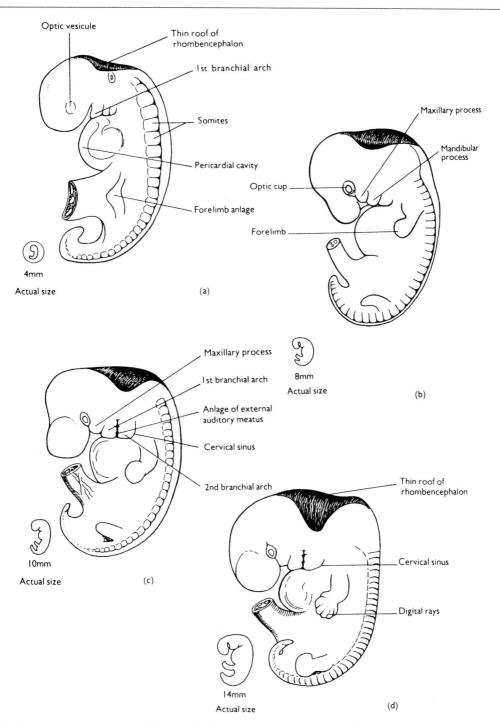

Fig. 3.2.3 *Drawings of human embryos and fetuses at different stages of development. These are not to scale but the approximate actual size of each embryo is shown.* **(a)** *28 days (4 mm),* **(b)** *35 days (8 mm),* **(c)** *37 days (10 mm),* **(d)** *40 days (13.5 mm). (Continued over page)*

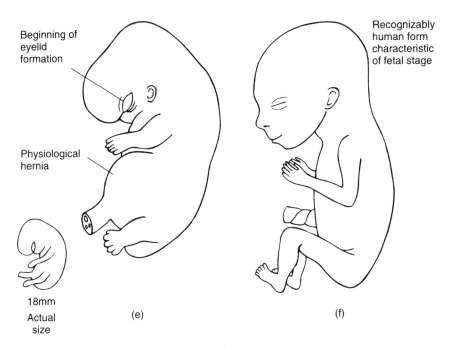

Beginning of
eyelid
formation

Physiological
hernia

Recognizably
human form
characteristic
of fetal stage

18mm
Actual
size

(e)

(f)

Fig. 3.2.3 *Continued.* **(e)** *47 days (18 mm),* **(f)** *110 days (100 mm).*

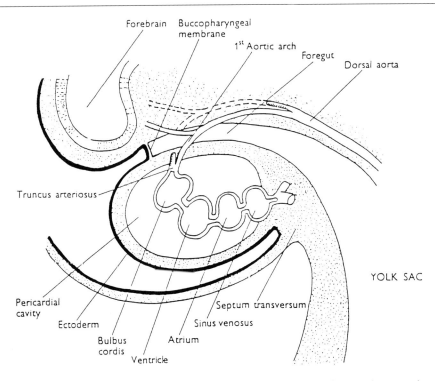

Forebrain   Buccopharyngeal
membrane

1ˢᵗ Aortic arch

Foregut

Dorsal aorta

Truncus arteriosus

YOLK SAC

Pericardial
cavity

Ectoderm

Septum transversum

Sinus venosus

Bulbus
cordis

Atrium

Ventricle

Fig. 3.2.4 *The heart tube becomes subdivided into a number of chambers. From its cranial end a pair of aortic arches pass, one on either side of the foregut, to form the paired dorsal aortae. These fuse more caudally to form a single dorsal aorta.*

ductus arteriosus begins, though some blood may pass through this vessel for some days after birth.

The great vessels develop from the third, fourth and sixth aortic arch arteries which begin to be asymmetrical at 41 days. The right aortic arch begins to disappear at about 52 days, but the adult configuration is not

achieved until the ductus arteriosus closes postnatally.

From 35 days onwards (10 mm crown–rump length), the venous system begins to be asymmetrical and the inferior vena cava develops as a composite vessel on the right side of the body. The brachiocephalic vein serves to shunt blood from the cranial extremity to the right. Final changes

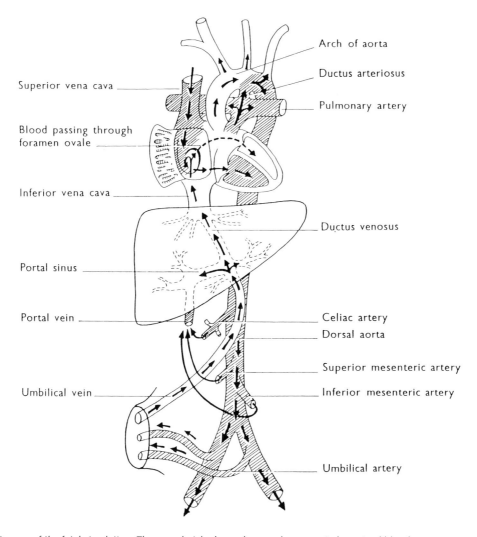

Fig. 3.2.5 *A diagram of the fetal circulation. The cross-hatched vessels carry deoxygenated or mixed blood.*

in the venous system occur after birth with closure of the ductus venosus. Hemodynamic factors are important in determining the structure of the circulatory system and the venous system, in particular, is subject to variation dependent on the nature of these factors.

The branchial region, mouth and face[15,16]

The branchial arch region mesoderm begins to differentiate at around 22 days (seven somites) with the appearance of the mandibular arch swelling. The second (hyoid) arch and groove is apparent at 25 days and the succeeding arches then appear rapidly. By 34 days (6 mm), the second arch is beginning to overlap the more caudal ones and, thus, the cervical sinus becomes established. At about 40 days (13 mm), the caudal lip of the second arch fuses with the pericardial mesoderm, obliterating the cervical sinus and establishing the smooth line of the neck (Fig. 3.2.3).

Table 3.2.1 lists the structures derived from the branchial arch mesoderm and from the endodermal lining of the branchial pouches.

At 5 weeks, the tongue is recognizable. It is formed in the floor of the mouth by fusion of the mesenchyme at the anterior extremity of the third arch with the posterior edge of the first arch, thus burying the second arch. This explains the sensory innervation of the tongue by the mandibular and glossopharyngeal nerves. The tongue musculature invades the mesenchyme from the occipital myotomes (12th cranial nerve). At 5 weeks also, the frontonasal, maxillary and mandibular swellings which go on to form the face have appeared and the nasal sac has formed. At 6 weeks, the primary palate has developed and, by 8 weeks, the upper lip and nostrils have contributed to a recognizably human face. At this stage, too, the palatal processes and the nasal septum begin to fuse and the tongue is fully developed. Palatal fusion is complete at 11 weeks and this marks the end of the organogenetic period of development.

Table 3.2.1 Structures derived from the branchial arch mesoderm and endodermal lining

	Nerve	Dorsal endoderm	Muscle	Ventral endoderm	Skeleton	Artery
1st arch and pouch	• Maxillary and mandibular branches of trigeminal (5th cranial nn) • Chorda tympani (pretrematic branch of facial (7th cranial nn)	Tubotympanic recess and pharyngotympanic tube	• Muscles of mastication • Mylohyoid and anterior belly of digastric • Tensor tympani • Tensor palati	—	• Meckel's cartilage • Sphenomandibular ligament • Malleus • Incus	Largely disappears except for maxillary artery
2nd arch and pouch	Facial nerve (7th cranial nn)	Incorporated into the tubotympanic recess	• Muscles of facial expression • Scalp muscles • Stapedius • Posterior belly of digastric	Palatine tonsil	• Stapes • Styloid process • Stylohyoid ligament • Upper body and lesser cornu of hyoid bone	Largely disappears except for stapedial artery
3rd arch and pouch	Glossopharyngeal (9th cranial nn)	Inferior parathyyroid	Stylopharyngeus	Thymus	Lower body and greater cornu of hyoid bone	Portion of the internal carotid artery
4th arch and pouch	Superior laryngeal branch of vagus[a] (10th cranial nn)	Superior parathyroid	Muscles of larynx and pharynx	—	Contribution to thyroid and cricoid cartilage	• Arch of the aorta • Right subclavian artery
5th arch	← Does not develop in man →					
6th arch	Recurrent laryngeal branch of vagus[a] (10th cranial nn)	—	Muscles of larynx and pharynx	—	Contribution to thyroid and cricoid cartilage	Pulmonary artery and ductus arteriosus

[a]The cranial part of the accessory nerve (11th cranial nn) is developmentally a detached portion of the vagus nerve.

The digestive and respiratory systems[17]

With the development of head and tail folds at 22 days, the foregut and hindgut are delineated (Fig. 3.2.6). Epithelial outgrowths appearing at 25 days at the junction of the foregut and midgut begin to lay down the liver which develops in the substance of the septum transversum, and the pancreas which develops from two buds in the dorsal and ventral gut mesenteries. At about this time, also, the buccopharyngeal membrane ruptures and continuity between the stomatodeum (mouth cavity) and the amniotic cavity is established. At 7 weeks, the stomach forms a fusiform dilatation of the foregut and, a week later, undergoes a 90° clockwise rotation, so that its dorsal surface moves to the left and the duodenal mesentery is obliterated. As a result, the pancreas becomes retroperitoneal.

By 5 weeks, the midgut has acquired a long dorsal mesentery which enables it to develop further in the extraembryonic celom outside the abdominal cavity. Growth of the yolk sac does not keep pace with the gut, so that the former soon becomes an atavistic appendage on the antimesometrial aspect of the midgut loop. At 45 mm (9 weeks), differential growth between the liver and the abdominal wall allows the midgut to return to the intra-embryonic celom where rearrangement of its mesenteric attachments and histo-differentiation result in its forming the intestine between the mid point of the duodenum and a point two-thirds of the way along the transverse colon. The remainder of the large intestine is derived from the hindgut. The terminal portion of the hindgut diverticulum gives rise to the cloaca which becomes partitioned by the urorectal septum into an anterior portion concerned with the urogenital system and a posterior part from which the rectum and the upper part of the anus develop. The cloacal membrane which separates this from the ectodermally lined proctodeum (the lower anal precursor) disappears between 7 and 8 weeks. Fetal gut peristalsis begins at around 10 weeks.

The air passages and lungs develop from a linear groove which appears in the floor of the caudal part of the pharynx and foregut and is known as the laryngo-tracheal groove. It appears at about 22 days and gradually separates from the esophagus so that between 4 and 5 weeks it opens at its cranial extremity around which the larynx develops. At about this time, the lobar bronchi become recognizable at the bilobed caudal end of the diverticulum. At 6 weeks, the segmental bronchi appear and the lung passes successively through so-called glandular (4 months), canalicular (5

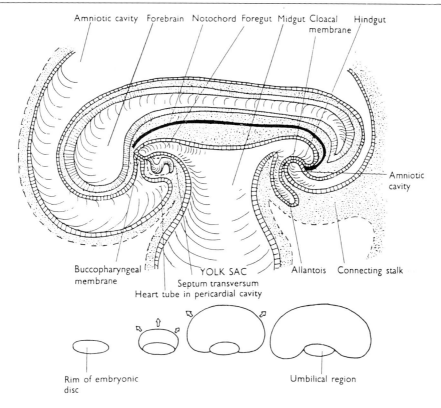

Fig. 3.2.6 *A longitudinal section through the embryonic disc after the formation of the head and tail folds which delineate the foregut and hindgut diverticula.*

months) and alveolar (6–9 months) stages of development. Surfactant becomes biochemically detectable at 7 months with the appearance of type 2 pneumocytes.

The urogenital system[18,19]

The excretory organs arise from the nephrogenic ridge, a portion of the intermediate mesoderm lying between the somites medially and the lateral plate mesoderm. In lower forms and in the embryo, pro- and mesonephric kidneys develop in the cranial part of this structure, but, in adult mammals, this region develops into the ducts associated with the reproductive system (see below) and the metanephric kidneys develop from tissue at its caudal extremity.

The nephrogenic ridge appears at about 24 days and, at the same time, the mesonephric duct draining the transiently functional mesonephric tubes into the cloaca begins to develop. The ureteric bud arises as a diverticulum of the mesonephric duct at about 6 weeks and grows into the metanephric region of the nephrogenic ridge. Here, it organizes the blastema into a functional kidney. This process begins in the eighth week and continues until after birth (Fig. 3.2.7). The mesonephric duct forms the epididymis and vas deferens in the male and atrophies in the female.

The caudal portion of the mesonephric duct distal to the entrance of the ureteric bud is absorbed into the develop-

ing vesico-urethral canal, so that the ureter and (in the male) the vas deferens open independently into the vesico-urethral canal. The latter develops into the bladder and the upper part of the urethra, while inferiorly the remainder of the urethra develops from the definitive urogenital sinus (Fig. 3.2.7). With the perforation of the cloacal membrane at 8 weeks, continuity with the amniotic cavity is established. In the third month, the external genitalia become recognizable as distinctly male or female, the penile urethra is closed inferiorly and the prostate develops around the upper urethra. The gonads develop in the gonadal ridge which is a mass of mesoderm lying along the medial aspect of the intermediate half of the nephrogenic ridge. At about 33 days, primordial germ cells originating in the yolk sac invade the ridges, but it is not possible to distinguish testis from ovary histologically until the ninth week. The genetic basis for sex determination has been clarified recently in remarkable experiments using transgenic mice.[20] In the male, the mesonephric tubes are utilized to carry the sperm from the testis to the mesonephric duct and, therefore, develop into the vasa efferentia. In the female, separate ducts called the paramesonephric (Müllerian) ducts develop alongside the mesonephric ducts during the fifth week. They fuse caudally in the midline and give rise to the uterine tubes, the uterus and the upper portion of the vagina. In the male, the paramesonephric tubes atrophy under the action of Müllerian inhibiting factor secreted by the gonad.

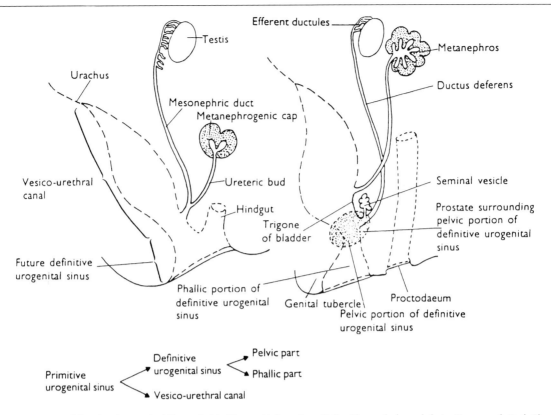

Fig. 3.2.7 *Diagram of the development of the male bladder and internal genitalia. The endodermal derivatives are dotted. The lower end of the mesonephric duct forms the trigone of the bladder and the upper half of the posterior wall of the prostatic urethra. The ureter and mesonephric duct (ductus deferens) now open separately. The 'flow chart' below shows how the primitive urogenital sinus becomes divided.*

FUTURE PERSPECTIVES

With the publication of Keibel and Mall's[1] classic textbook, the basic facts concerning human developmental anatomy were recorded. Since then, close observations have established details of timing, fleshed out the details of histogenesis and (with the help of animal experiments) established the essential details of cell lineage. The classical approach has laid the basis for the modern study of developmental biology which is presently at a most exciting stage. Our increasing understanding of the events governing fertilization and preimplantation development have led to startling practical advances in the field of assisted reproduction. Further, the experimental approach using current techniques of molecular biology and the mouse model have yielded a rich harvest in understanding the principles underlying cell determination and differentiation, morphogenesis and growth. Knowledge in this respect is accelerating rapidly and the first inklings of a practical spin-off are already apparent with the advent of sophisticated prenatal diagnosis and the promise of effective gene therapy. Clearly, the larger possibility of successful cancer therapy is now a realistic hope in the medium-term future.

SUMMARY

Within the framework of current textbooks of embryology, attention has been drawn to the main events which make up human embryogenesis and some attempt has been made to place them in a time frame relative to one another. In a short chapter it is obviously impossible to give an account of human development however abbreviated. The reader is, therefore, referred to standard embryology textbooks (of which there are many) for good accounts of the general processes involved and references to some specialized developmental studies are made. Above all, it is important to be aware that the study of development in the broad context of cell specification and the molecular basis of morphogenesis is now well and truly launched and likely to produce dramatic results in the near future.

REFERENCES

1. Keibel F, Mall FP. *Manual of Human Embryology*, Vols 1 and 2. Philadelphia: Lippincott, 1910, 1912.
2. Moore KL. *The Developing Human*, 4th edn. Philadelphia, London, Toronto: WJ Saunders, 1988.
3. Hamilton WJ, Boyd GD, Mossman H. *Human Embryology*, 4th edn. Baltimore: Williams and Wilkins, 1978.
4. Beck F, Moffat DB, Davies DP. *Human Embryology*, 2nd edn. London: Blackwell, 1985.
5. O'Rahilly R, Gardner E. The timing and sequence of events in the development of the human nervous system during the embryonic period proper. *Z Anat Entw* 1971 **134**: 1–12.
6. O'Rahilly R, Gardner E. The initial development of the human brain. *Acta Anat* 1979 **104**: 123–133.
7. O'Rahilly R, Müller F, Hutchins GM, Moore GW. Computer ranking of the sequence of appearance of 100 features of the brain and related structures in staged human embryos during the first 5 weeks of development. *Am J Anat* 1984 **171**: 243–257.
8. Lemire RJ, Loeser JD, Leech RW, Alvord EC Jr. *Normal and Abnormal Development of the Human Nervous System*. Hagerstown, MD: Harper and Row, 1975.
9. McGinnis W, Krumlauf R. Homeobox genes and axial patterning. *Cell* 1992 **68**: 283–302.
10. Ruiz a Altaba A, Jessel TM. Midline cells and the organisation of the vertebrate neuraxis. *Curr Opin Genet Dev* 1993 **3**: 633–640.
11. O'Rahilly R, Müller F. Stages in early human development. In Feichtinger W, Kermeter P (eds) *Future Aspects in Human In Vitro Fertilisation*, Berlin: Springer, 1987.
12. Smith JC. Hedgehog, the floor plate, and the zone of polarizing activity. *Cell* 1994 **76**: 193–196.
13. O'Rahilly R. The timing and sequence of events in human cardiogenesis. *Acta Anat* 1971 **79**: 70–75.
14. De Haan RL, O'Rahilly R. Embryology of the heart. In Hurst JW, Hogan RB, Schlant RC, Wenger NK (eds) *The Heart*. New York: McGraw Hill, 1978: 6.
15. Sperber GH. *Craniofacial Embryology*. Bristol: John Wright, 1973.
16. Weller GL. Development of the thyroid, parathyroid and thymus glands in man. *Contrib Embryol* 1933 **24**: 93.
17. Grand RJ, Watkins JB, Torti FM. Development of the human gastro-intestinal tract: a review. *Gastroenterology* 1976 **70**: 790.
18. Vaughan ED Jr, Middleton GW. Pertinent genito-urinary embryology, Review for practicing urologists. *Urology* 1975 **6**: 139.
19. Bulmer D. The development of the human vagina. *J Anat* 1957 **91**: 490.
20. Koopman P, Gubbay J, Vivian M, Goodfellow P, Lovell-Badge P. Male development of chromosomally female mice transgenic for SRY. *Nature* 1991 **351**: 117.

3.3

Immunology in Reproduction

PM Johnson and SE Christmas

INTRODUCTION

The primary characteristic of the immune system is an ability to distinguish self from non-self in order to identify and eliminate infectious agents. In the case of the T cell immune system, this is achieved by recognition of foreign antigens in the form of short peptides in association with cell surface molecules of the major histocompatibility complex (human leucocyte antigens, HLA in man). As described earlier (Chapter 1.6), there is extensive variation in these molecules that enables as wide a range as possible of foreign antigenic peptides to be recognized. A consequence is that genetically dissimilar HLA molecules can closely resemble self HLA molecules modified by a foreign antigenic peptide, leading normally to a high frequency of T cells reactive against histoincompatible tissue grafts. The highly polymorphic and outbred nature of most human populations means that, in nearly all pregnancies, there will be a strong antigenic difference between maternal tissues and paternally inherited antigens expressed by the intrauterine fetal tissue 'graft'. It is therefore essential to prevent what might otherwise be expected to be a strong maternal pregnancy-induced immune response from inflicting immunologically mediated damage on the fetoplacental unit. The mechanisms by which this is achieved, as well as immunological involvement in other human reproductive processes that can lead to reproductive immunopathology will now be discussed.

CURRENT CONCEPTS

Antigen expression by trophoblast in extraembryonic membranes

In outbred human populations, almost all pregnancies will involve HLA differences between the mother and the paternally inherited genes of the fetus. Under normal circumstances, the major fetomaternal antigenic difference would be expected to induce a strong allogeneic response but this is avoided in pregnancy by a combination of strategies. Modern investigation has provided real insights into the mechanisms that normally allow the 'transplantation privilege' (unique to the conceptus) of the fetoplacental unit as an intrauterine graft throughout pregnancy. There are two complementary ways of averting immunologically mediated damage to the fetus: primarily, by preventing induction of an anti-fetal response and, secondarily, by invoking mechanisms to block any immune response which does develop.[1,2]

The main point of contact between maternal and fetal tissues occurs at junctions with extraembryonic tissues. Maternal blood bathes the chorionic villi of the placenta and hence has extensive and intimate contact with the apical surface of syncytiotrophoblast (see also Chapter 3.6). Syncytiotrophoblast is a multinucleated unicellular layer overlying the placental chorionic villous structure, including villous cytotrophoblast cells from which syncytiotrophoblast is formed by cell fusion. It is the contact of syncytiotrophoblast with maternal blood that enables the transfer of nutrients (including immunoglobulin (Ig)) and oxygen from maternal to fetal circulation. In early pregnancy, extravillous trophoblast invade through syncytiotrophoblast to create the chorion laeve membrane and rupture uterine spiral arteries in the placental bed to cause their physiological changes that allow the vastly increased blood flow necessary to bathe chorionic villi; these extravillous (or non-villous) cytotrophoblast make extensive contact with maternal decidualized endometrial tissue. It is now clear that specialized features of the fetal trophoblastic cells forming the continuous lining of the placenta and extraembryonic membranes allow the critical protection of this fetal tissue interface from damage by maternal blood-borne or decidual cytotoxic attack.[1-3]

Human trophoblast populations fail to express any classical polymorphic class I or class II human leucocyte antigens (HLA) at all stages of gestation (Table 3.3.1).[1-3] They

Table 3.3.1 Expression of HLA and complement regulatory proteins in the human term placenta

Antigen	Extravillous invasive cytotrophoblast	Syncytiotrophoblast	Villous cytotrophoblast	Hofbauer cells
Class I HLA				
HLA-A, B	−	−	−	+ +
HLA-G	+ +	−	−	−
Class II HLA				
HLA-DR, DQ, DP	−	−	−	+ +
Complement regulatory proteins				
Membrane cofactor				
protein (MCP; CD46)	+ +	+ +	+	(+)
Decay accelerating				
factor (DAF; CD55)	+ +	+ +	+	(+)
Membrane attack				
complex inhibitory				
protein (CD59)	+	+	+	(+)

are therefore resistant to lysis by class I or class II HLA-restricted cytotoxic T cells and to attack by anti-HLA alloantibody. This also provides an explanation as to why fetal syncytiotrophoblastic cellular elements that normally break away into the uterine vein from the implantation site, may lodge in maternal pulmonary sinusoids and persist for some length of time without provoking an overt inflammatory or immune rejection response. In addition, non-trophoblastic placental cells (e.g. Hofbauer cells, placental villous macrophages) will normally express HLA molecules of the fetal tissue type (Table 3.3.1), but these cells are anatomically separated from maternal cells by the HLA-negative trophoblastic barrier.

However, invasive extravillous cytotrophoblast in the placental bed express a non-classical class I HLA molecule which has been identified as HLA-G (Table 3.3.1).[4] This molecule has a similar structure to the classical class I HLA molecules HLA-A, -B and -C and, like these molecules, is non-covalently associated with β_2-microglobulin at the cell surface. The HLA-G heavy chain has a truncated cytoplasmic tail compared with other class I HLA antigens and has a molecular weight of 39 kD rather than 44 kD.[5] HLA-G expression has not been found in adult tissues and hence it may have evolved to fulfill a specialized function of invasive cytotrophoblast that has extensive contact with decidualized endometrium. In view of its high degree of structural homology with other class I HLA molecules, HLA-G is potentially able to bind certain antigenic peptides and present them to CD8+ cytotoxic T cells. Although originally thought to be monomorphic (invariant), it is now appreciated that there is protein polymorphism of HLA-G within the α_1 and particularly the α_2 domain.[6]

Other speculation has focused on a possible immuno-biological role of HLA-G in protecting cytotrophoblast from natural killer (NK) cell-mediated cytolysis, or as an intercellular recognition molecule mediating cell–cell contact. NK cells largely recognize and lyse target cells which are deficient in class I HLA expression;[7] hence selective HLA-G expression (in the absence of HLA-A, -B, -C) may

prevent this, rendering extravillous cytotrophoblast resistant to NK cells. The lack of expression of the classical polymorphic class I HLA antigens would also hinder cytotoxic T lymphocyte(CTL)-mediated lysis, so making this vital fetal tissue interface resistant to both the innate and the adaptive arms of the cell-mediated cytotoxic response.

There are also mechanisms to protect fetal trophoblast against maternal antibody-mediated damage. Three distinct cell surface complement regulatory proteins are selectively expressed at high levels by all trophoblast populations (Table 3.3.1). These are membrane cofactor protein (MCP; CD46), decay-accelerating factor (DAF; CD55) and membrane attack complex inhibitory protein (CD59).[1,3] MCP enhances inactivation of C3b, whereas DAF prevents formation of C3 convertases and accelerates their decay; CD59 disrupts the formation of the cytolytic terminal complement attack complex.[8] The net effect is to frustrate potential complement-mediated damage to trophoblast through either the classical or alternative pathway subsequent to maternal anti-fetal antibody attack or local tissue restructuring and hemostatic alterations, respectively.

Endometrial leucocytes

The mucosal immune system in the Fallopian tube, cervix and vagina involves B and T lymphocytes as well as local IgA production. However, the constitution and relative numbers of leucocytes in the uterine endometrium are unusual (Table 3.3.2).[9] Polymorphonuclear leucocytes and B cells are most uncommon in this tissue, although IgA is present in the endometrial lumen, having passed down from the Fallopian tubes. T cells are a consistent feature, but they become proportionally less of the total when other leucocyte types increase in number in the secretory phase of the menstrual cycle and in early pregnancy. Most of these T cells express the CD8 marker and the vast majority express the common $\alpha\beta$ TCR rather than the rare $\gamma\delta$ form of the TCR.

Table 3.3.2 Immunological cells in human endometrial and decidual tissue

Cell type	Proliferative phase	Secretory phase	First-trimester pregnancy	Term pregnancy
Macrophages	+	+/++	++	++
B cells	−	−	−	−
T cells	+	+	+	+
Endometrial granular leucocytes	+	++	+++	+

Local cellular adaptations in the endometrium, nevertheless, characteristically include the appearance of extensive numbers of leucocytes of the non-adaptive immune system premenstrually and in early pregnancy (Table 3.3.2). These cells can contribute up to 35% of all cells in the endometrium and are either tissue macrophages or, more notably, a novel type of non-B, non-T cell large granulated leucocyte. The macrophage component expresses cell surface markers typical of conventional tissue macrophages. Resident tissue macrophages are also clearly evident in Fallopian tube, cervical and vaginal tissue. However, in pregnancy, decidual macrophages do appear to be highly activated cells and strongly express cellular activation antigens (e.g. class II HLA molecules) as well as spontaneously secreting substantial amounts of the pro-inflammatory cytokine interleukin-1 (IL-1). These activated macrophages are thought to play a vital role in rapid, non-specific host defense to infection at these crucial tissue sites, notably in pregnancy, but can also provide local non-specific immunosuppressive mediators such as prostaglandin E_2.[1]

The most distinctive leucocytic component of first-trimester decidualized endometrium, however, is an unusual granulated leucocyte population of uncertain function.[1,9] These cells are morphologically and phenotypically most similar to peripheral blood large granular lymphocytes (natural killer (NK) cells) in being CD3− and CD56+ (Table 3.3.3) but express much higher levels of the CD56 molecule, an isoform of neural cell adhesion molecule (NCAM), as well as being less responsive to stimulation by IL-2. In addition, they are largely CD16− and, unlike peripheral blood NK cells, exhibit only low

levels of HLA-non-restricted (NK cell-type) killing against tumor cell lines[10] despite containing abundant perforin-containing cytoplasmic granules. They are unlikely therefore to be involved in regulation of trophoblast invasiveness or removal of flawed or otherwise doomed embryos via a lytic mechanism. A more likely role is in cytokine production in response to stimulation by T cell cytokines or following direct interaction with fetal trophoblast. This could involve the production of immunosuppressive factors such as transforming growth factor β_2 (TGF-β_2) or other cytokines with growth regulatory properties for trophoblast. Decidual granulated leucocytes have been shown to express a range of cytokines including interferon(IFN)-γ, tumor necrosis factor (TNF)α, granulocyte, macrophage and granulocyte-macrophage colony stimulating factors (G-, M- and GM-CSFs, respectively) and interleukins (IL)-1, -6, -8 and -10.[11] Syncytiotrophoblast expresses receptors for IFN-γ, TNFα and the CSFs[12] and hence might be susceptible to metabolic modulation by these cytokines produced by maternal cells within decidua.

CD3− granulated leucocytes increase significantly in number in endometrial tissues in early pregnancy, mostly from local proliferation.[9] However, most have disappeared from decidua by term, although it is possible that these cells could have lost their granules and CD56 antigen expression. The appearance of these cells seems to be hormonally regulated in that they occur also in any decidualized tissue in extrauterine ectopic pregnancy. In non-pregnant cycles, considerable numbers are lost by menstruation and hence there is substantial endometrial turnover of these unusual CD3− granulated leucocytes.

Table 3.3.3 Major cell surface antigenic phenotype of endometrial granular leucocytes

Predominant association/specificity of antigen expression	Endometrial granular leucocyte expression
Hematopoietic cell markers	CD45+
Early lymphoid differentiation markers	CD2+, CD7+, CD38+
Mature T cell markers	CD3−, CD4−, CD8−
Mature B cell markers	CD19−, CD20−
Natural killer cell markers	CD11b+, CD16−, CD56+, CD57−
Cell adhesion molecules and integrins	CD11a+, CD18+, CD54+, CD49a+, CD103+/−
Interleukin-2 receptors	CD25−, CD122+
Cell activation markers	Class II HLA−, CD69+

Cellular and antibody transfer between mother and fetus

In addition to syncytiotrophoblastic cellular elements breaking away from the implantation site, there is limited transfer of some fetal lymphocytes into maternal circulation. These latter cells can stimulate the production of maternal pregnancy-induced anti-paternal HLA alloantibody, facilitating their elimination. Such anti-HLA antibodies occur in approximately 15% of all term pregnancies, and up to 60% of multigravidae will have a detectable term lymphocytotoxic anti-HLA antibody with no adverse effects on the fetus. Fetally derived cells in maternal circulation may provide cellular material for prenatal analysis of fetal sex or genetic abnormalities, although such techniques are still in their infancy.[13]

Lymphocyte transfer in the opposite direction, i.e. from mother to fetus, is also possible but more difficult to detect. In this case, potentially alloreactive maternal T cells within the immunologically incompetent fetus could lead to graft-versus-host disease but this has only been found in rare instances of fetal immunodeficiency. Maternal lymphocytes will normally have a single HLA haplotype mismatch with the fetus (i.e. with the paternally inherited haplotype) and, as the alloreactive response is strong, even the immunologically immature fetus or neonate may be able effectively to eliminate maternal cells.

Maternal IgG is selectively transferred across the placenta to the fetus from around week 20 of gestation (Fig. 3.3.1) via $Fc\gamma$ receptors on the surface of syncytiotrophoblast.[14] This provides essential passive immunity to assist postnatal immune protection against infection, prior to antigen-driven expansion of the neonate's own antibody repertoire and total Ig levels. However, potentially harmful maternal IgG anti-fetal HLA antibodies will also be transferred across trophoblast but will then bind efficiently to non-trophoblastic cells bearing fetal HLA within the placental villous tissue core and will not reach the fetal circulation. Any other maternal IgG to fetal antigens expressed in the placenta will be similarly sequestered by binding to

antigen-expressing cells or by binding as soluble immune complexes to high affinity receptors on placental macrophages (Hofbauer cells) and endothelium. Although IgA, IgM and IgD do not cross the placenta (Fig. 3.3.1), they are supplied after birth to the neonate in high concentrations in colostrum.

Red cell incompatibilities

Blood group antigen differences between mother and fetus can lead to the generation of maternal anti-fetal red cell antibodies.[15] Most antibodies in the ABO blood group system are IgM and hence do not cross prenatally into the fetal compartment, although occasional mild neonatal hemolysis may occur in repeated ABO incompatible pregnancies in group O mothers. Severe hemolytic disease can be produced by other blood group incompatibilities, for example the Kell and Duffy antigen systems, although often the density of such minor antigens on fetal red cells is so low as not to produce a cytolytic effect with maternal IgG antibody and only reaches adult levels after birth.

Isoimmunization to rhesus (Rh) D blood group antigens can lead to more common and serious pathological consequences. A proportion of RhD^- mothers of RhD^+ children will become sensitized to RhD and generate an IgG response which, in a subsequent RhD^+ pregnancy with a potential secondary response, can result in hemolytic disease of the newborn following prenatal transfer of the maternal IgG anti-RhD into fetal circulation (Fig. 3.3.2). Primary sensitization may be prevented by the administration of anti-RhD antiserum immediately after the birth of the first RhD^+ child.[16] The presence of this exogenous antibody rapidly clears any fetal red cells that have entered the maternal circulation before these can induce a strong IgG response. ABO blood group incompatibility can be a protective factor for hemolytic disease of the newborn as any pre-existing natural maternal IgM anti-A or anti-B antibodies will rapidly eliminate fetal red cells in a similar manner.

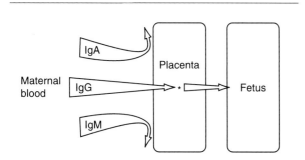

Fig 3.3.1 *Selective transplacental IgG transport at the materno-fetal interface that provides the fetus with passive immunity. *Trapping of any maternal IgG anti-fetal HLA antibodies or any other maternal IgG (auto) antibodies that produce immune complexes with fetal antigen in the placenta.*

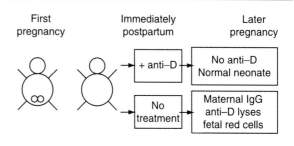

Fig 3.3.2 *Prevention of rhesus hemolytic disease of the newborn. Red blood cells from an RhD^+ fetus can sensitize an RhD^- mother mostly during parturition. This may be prevented by administering anti-RhD antiserum immediately after birth. In a later pregnancy, an untreated mother will mount a damaging secondary response to RhD^+ fetal red cells leading to hemolysis whereas in an anti-D treated mother, a primary response is suppressed and no secondary anti-D response occurs.*

Autoantibodies and autoimmune disease in pregnancy

There are two pertinent factors to consider regarding autoimmune disease in pregnancy: whether there is remission or exacerbation of maternal disease in pregnancy, and whether the fetus is susceptible to disease mediated by maternal IgG autoantibodies transferred across the placenta.[2,17,18] In the case of maternal rheumatoid arthritis, it is well known that most pregnant women undergo significant but transient amelioration of symptoms, although the full mechanism of this effect is unknown. Nevertheless, such observations led to the original identification of glucocorticoids as powerful anti-inflammatory agents. In contrast, in both the organ-specific autoimmune disease diabetes, and the non-organ-specific autoimmune condition systemic lupus erythematosus (SLE), pregnancy often precipitates disease exacerbation. In the former case, this could be indirectly related to hormonal changes during pregnancy and, in the latter, following tissue damage and ensuing autoantigen release during placentation or parturition.

In many autoimmune diseases, potentially pathogenic maternal IgG autoantibodies will be transferred to the fetus via placental uptake.[18-20] Mothers with autoimmune thrombocytopenic purpura have anti-platelet antibodies which may lead to thrombocytopenia in the fetus. Similarly, IgG anti-acetylcholine receptor antibodies may lead to myasthenia gravis in the neonate. Anti-thyroid antibodies that are stimulatory or inhibitory to thyroid function can be transferred to the fetus in autoimmune mothers, leading to transient hyper- or hypothyroidism for the time of retention of prenatally acquired maternal IgG autoantibody in the neonate. Transient symptoms of neonatal SLE are also found in a minority of children whose mothers have SLE. However, children of diabetic mothers actually have a decreased risk of developing diabetes later in life; the reason for this is unknown. In addition to passive transfer of autoimmune disease from mother to fetus, there is also an increased risk of fetal loss or low birth weight associated with autoimmune thrombocytopenia purpura, myasthenia gravis and SLE.

In the latter case, anti-phospholipid antibodies may be the harmful agent. Anti-phospholipid antibodies are directed against negatively charged phospholipids.[18,20,21] These autoantibodies occur in up to 20% of SLE patients and up to 5% of unexplained recurrent spontaneous abortion patients. They are associated with a syndrome that may involve thrombotic episodes, thrombocytopenia and intrauterine fetal loss, sometimes with additional skin or neurological complaints. Their mechanism of action in recurrent fetal loss is probably through induction of a decidual vasculopathy and placental thrombosis. Other less frequently encountered autoantibodies can lead to transient or permanent pathological effects in the fetus or neonate.

Recurrent spontaneous abortion

There has been much recent attention directed towards elucidating any possible immunological basis for women suffering recurrent spontaneous abortion (>3 consecutive first-trimester pregnancy losses; RSA). In over 50% of cases, no predisposing mechanism can be identified and it is unjustified to assume a single cause in all of these cases. The broad hypothesis that hitherto unexplained RSA can be ascribed to failure of active maternal immune adaptation to early pregnancy has provoked extensive debate of controversial concepts.[2,18-20,22]

Initial studies suggested some increased parental HLA tissue-type sharing in RSA although, perhaps inevitably, there have been inconsistencies between studies in patient referral patterns and local patient selection policy: low study numbers, the choice of appropriate control groups, which class I or II HLA loci were involved and the manner of data handling for HLA 'blanks'. Other groups have now reported that increased parental HLA sharing is of uncertain statistical significance and, most importantly, of neither diagnostic nor prognostic value in the assessment of the individual RSA couple.[18,20] A decreased maternal responsiveness to paternal cells in the mixed lymphocyte culture reaction (MLR), which measures the response of viable maternal lymphocytes in response to exposure to inactivated 'foreign' paternal lymphocytes in vitro, for RSA couples compared with controls has also been suggested, although this could result from the marginally increased overall parental HLA sharing.

Furthermore, the production of so-called serum 'blocking factors' which inhibit a variety of in vitro lymphocyte function assays, most notably the MLR, is a common feature of pregnancy.[19] Blocking factors were originally reported to be absent from peripheral blood of RSA women, whether during or after unsuccessful pregnancies. However, doubt remains about these observations since: (a) other pregnancy-related components, notably steroid hormones, may be influential, (b) blocking factors may be the consequence rather than a cause of pregnancy success, (c) there is a shorter exposure time to paternal antigens for RSA women, and (d) the interpretation of results may vary according to the equation used to calculate the MLR inhibitory effect. Thus, early investigations on parental HLA sharing and MLR blocking factors formed much of the original basis for the development of deliberate immunization with paternal or third-party unmatched leucocytes in RSA in order to prime for absent immunoregulatory responses other than by pregnancy itself.

Nevertheless, these considerations led to the formulation of specific immunotherapy protocols in RSA, although the dose, route, timing and frequency of leucocyte immunization has varied significantly between centers, as have patient selection criteria and follow-up rates.[18,20,22] There have been numerous reports of 55–90% subsequent successful pregnancy outcome following immunization, although the majority of these have been uncontrolled open studies. Truly randomized and double-blinded trials can be difficult to perform for leucocyte immunization. An initial randomized trial performed in 1985 showed a significantly better subsequent pregnancy success following immunization with paternal leucocytes compared with administration of control autologous leucocytes. However, more recent reports of randomized control studies have shown little or no statistically significant benefit of paternal leucocyte immunization in RSA and, in these studies, control groups achieved subsequent pregnancy success figures of the order of 65–76%. This variation in live-born delivery rates for control groups in randomized immunotherapy studies has readdressed attention towards the strength of the 'placebo effect' in immunotherapeutic studies in RSA. There may be some clinical risks in administering viable leucocytes to healthy women, such as graft-versus-host disease and sensitization to HLA or other leucocyte antigens, or to platelet or blood group antigens; the latter could compromise a pregnancy following paternal cell immunization. Other transfusion-related risks are potentially increased, notably following third-party immunization, such as cytomegalovirus or human immunodeficiency virus (HIV) transmission.

Immunological infertility

Anti-sperm antibodies occur in some women as well as men and may contribute to infertility by inhibiting spermatogenesis, the motility or other functions of sperm.[18] There is a better correlation of anti-sperm antibodies with clinical infertility in men rather than women. Their presence in the genital secretions of the male or female reproductive tracts is of greater significance than their presence in serum, and IgA appears to be the primary mediator of immunological infertility at these sites.[23] The relevant 'target' antigens on sperm for natural anti-sperm antibodies have not been well characterized although it is clear that spermatozoa do not express class I HLA molecules. The choice of assay is also important and those assays that detect only surface antigens (e.g. tray agglutination test, mixed antiglobulin reaction or immuno-bead binding) perform better in terms of clinical correlation than assays that may also detect cytoplasmic antigens (e.g. ELISA).

Most antibodies to sperm are not donor-specific but, in some instances (no more than 5%), antibodies have been identified with higher titers against autologous or partner's sperm than against unrelated sperm.[23] Excessive exposure to sperm, as in prostitutes, or exposure in inappropriate sites as in homosexual men, increases the risk of developing anti-sperm antibodies.[19] Seminal plasma contains a complex variety of immunosuppressive substances, the function of which may be normally to prevent sensitization to sperm antigens. Serum antibodies against female reproductive tissues or gametes have been described, but are of doubtful relevance to clinical infertility.

Endometriosis

This painful inflammatory condition characterized by the presence of endometrial tissue at ectopic sites, particularly the peritoneal cavity, involves genetic factors although there is no known HLA association.[24] Retrograde menstruation has been implicated in pathogenesis but how this could ever lead to the presence of endometrial tissue away from the peritoneal cavity is unclear. There is some indica-

tion for an autoimmune or 'toxic' cytokine pathogenesis. Severe endometriosis often results in infertility but, in its milder forms, is of little importance in this regard. Peritoneal macrophages are increased in number and state of activation and hence could contribute to infertility associated with endometriosis.[18,24] However, increased macrophage numbers have also been found in subfertile women without endometriosis, and it may be the peritoneal macrophage activation itself which is more important in the endometriosis than in contributing to infertility.

Pre-eclampsia

Pre-eclamptic toxemia (PET) is characterized in the second half of pregnancy by hypertension, edema, proteinuria and activation of the blood coagulation cascade. There are abnormalities of placental development related to inadequacies of cytotrophoblast invasion and disruption of the spiral arteries, leading to deleterious effects on the fetus and, in extreme cases, maternal death. PET can occur in hydatidiform molar pregnancy in the absence of a fetus, and the placenta is of central importance in this condition.[25]

There is a strong genetic component to disease susceptibility and daughters of PET mothers have an increased relative risk of developing the disease. The incidence in first pregnancy is much higher than in subsequent pregnancies and even a prior abortion may confer protection. However, a change of partner in women with at least one previous normal pregnancy also significantly increases the risk of pre-eclampsia in a subsequent pregnancy. This would implicate primi-paternity rather than primi-gravidity and there is current interest in the phenomenon of genetic imprinting where certain paternal genes are preferentially expressed in the placenta. Prior blood transfusions and increased preconceptual exposure to sperm or seminal plasma are also associated with a decreased risk of PET. These lines of evidence could be suggestive of an immunological mechanism and it has been proposed that PET results from an inadequate natural immune adaptation to pregnancy, although these events could be secondary rather than primary to the disease which itself may focus on an endothelial cell dysfunction.[20,25]

Host resistance in pregnancy

There is little evidence for functional systemic immunosuppression during pregnancy and, for most pathogens, there is no increased incidence of infection at sites outside the urogenital tract.[2,19] Some increased susceptibility to certain local infections is well known, but may be more related to exposure and anatomic factors rather than non-specific systemic immunosuppression. Infectious agents can be transmitted from mother to fetus before, during or after birth and, as the fetus or neonate is not fully immunocompetent, it would be more susceptible to an infection acquired in this way. In particular, children of

HIV$^+$ mothers have a 10–40% risk of becoming infected with HIV, largely during parturition or via breast milk rather than via transplacental passage of virus.

FUTURE PERSPECTIVES

With a topic developing as fast as immunology, prophecy can be a dangerous art! In human reproductive immunology, the many interactions of maternal autoimmunity with pregnancy pathology are likely to continue to develop further in areas directly applicable to clinical medicine in line with an ever-better understanding of all aspects of autoimmune diseases. The current focus on recurrent spontaneous abortion may decrease but, together with cytokine involvement, immunological interests in other topics such as endometriosis and clinical infertility may yet expand into more practical clinical involvement. In addition, it has long been suggested that there is a strong interaction between the endocrine and immunological networks and, in this regard, pregnancy would appear to provide the ideal model for its elucidation.

SUMMARY

- In human reproduction, paternal and maternal tissue HLA antigen specificities will usually differ. Under normal circumstances, such histo-incompatibility would be expected to lead to a strong maternal immune rejection response against the fetus which must be avoided during pregnancy.
- A lack of expression of classical HLA molecules (HLA-A, B, DP, DQ, DR) by human sperm and by trophoblast populations at the feto-maternal interface, together with selective expression of HLA-G by extravillous cytotrophoblast, appears to protect these critical tissues against maternal cell-mediated immune attack.
- Extensive trophoblastic expression of complement regulatory proteins protects these cells against damage mediated by local complement activation, including that which might be expected by any maternal antibody against paternal antigens.
- Large numbers of leucocytes occur in the endometrium and decidua, including an extensive unusual non-B, non-T cell population that resembles NK cells. These leucocytes reflect specialized immunological adaptation at this site, particularly in pregnancy. Such cells produce a range of cytokines which may be involved in contributing to local immunosuppression and placental growth regulation.
- Maternal IgG is selectively transferred across the placenta and constitutes the bulk of the protective antibody within fetal circulation in the third trimester of pregnancy and for several months after birth until the neonatal immunoglobulin response is fully developed.
- In mothers with tissue-specific autoimmune disease (e.g. autoimmune thyroiditis), maternal IgG autoantibodies will also be transferred across the placenta, sometimes leading to transient autoimmune pathology in the fetus.
- A rhesus (Rh) D-negative mother bearing an RhD-positive fetus may mount an IgG anti-RhD immune response which could be harmful to a subsequent RhD-positive fetus. RhD sensitization can be prevented by administration of anti-RhD antibody immediately post-partum.
- A proportion of cases of recurrent spontaneous abortion might have an immunological basis, but this is as yet poorly defined, other than a small proportion with maternal anti-phospholipid autoantibodies.
- Antibodies reactive with spermatozoa, present in either the male or female partner, can lead to immunologically mediated clinical infertility.
- In endometriosis and pre-eclamptic toxemia, it is not clear whether immunological involvement is primary or secondary to the clinical condition.

REFERENCES

1. Johnson PM. Reproductive and materno-fetal relations. In Lachmann PJ, Peters DK, Rosen FS, Walport MJ (eds) *Clinical Aspects of Immunology*, 5th edn. Oxford: Blackwell Scientific Publications, 1993: 755–767.
2. Bronson RA, Alexander NJ, Anderson DJ, Branch WD, Kutteh WH (eds). *Reproductive Immunology*. New York: Blackwell Scientific Publications (in press).
3. Hunt JS. Immunobiology of pregnancy. *Curr Opin Immunol* 1992 4: 591–596.
4. Kovats S, Main EK, Librach C, Stubblebine M, Fisher SJ, DeMars R. A class I antigen, HLA-G, expressed in human trophoblasts. *Science* 1990 248: 220–223.
5. Ellis SA, Palmer MS, McMichael A. Human trophoblasts and the choriocarcinoma cell line BeWo express a truncated HLA class I molecule. *J Immunol* 1990 144: 731–735.
6. Van der Ven K, Ober C. HLA-G polymorphisms in African Americans. *J Immunol* 1994 153: 5628–5633.

7. Ljunggren H-G, Karre K. In search of the 'missing self': MHC molecules and natural killer cell recognition. *Immunol Today* 1990 **11**: 237–244.

8. Rooney IA, Ogelesby TJ, Atkinson JP. Complement in human reproduction: activation and control. *Immunol Res* 1993 **12**: 276–294.

9. Bulmer JN. Decidual cellular responses. *Curr Opin Immunol* 1989 **1**: 1141–1147.

10. Deniz G, Christmas SE, Brew R, Johnson PM. Phenotypic and functional cellular differences between human CD3⁻ decidual and peripheral blood leukocytes. *J Immunol* 1994 **152**: 4255–4261.

11. Saito S, Nishikawa K, Morii T *et al.* Cytokine production by CD16⁻ CD56^bright natural killer cells in human early pregnancy decidua. *Int Immunol* 1993 **5**: 559–563.

12. Hampson J, McLaughlin PJ, Johnson PM. Low affinity receptors for TNFα, interferon-γ and GM-CSF are expressed on human placental syncytiotrophoblast. *Immunology* 1993 **79**: 485–490.

13. Adinolfi M. On a non-invasive approach to prenatal diagnosis based on the detection of fetal nucleated cells in maternal blood samples. *Prenat Diagn* 1991 **11**: 799–804.

14. Johnson PM, Brown PJ. Fcγ receptors in the human placenta. *Placenta* 1981 **2**: 355–370.

15. Jones WR, Need JA. Maternal–fetal cell surface antigen incompatibilities. *Bailliere's Clin Immunol Allergy* 1988 **2**: 577–600.

16. Clarke CA. Historical evaluation: rhesus haemolytic disease of the newborn and its prevention. *Br J Haematol* 1982 **52**: 525–536.

17. Scott JS, Bird HA (eds). *Pregnancy Autoimmunity and Connective Tissue Disorders.* Oxford: Oxford University Press, 1990: 346pp.

18. Johnson PM. Reproductive immunopathology. In Lachmann PJ, Peters DK, Rosen FS, Walport MJ (eds) *Clinical Aspects of Immunology*, 5th edn. Oxford: Blackwell Scientific Publications, 1993: 2137–2152.

19. Claman HN. *The Immunology of Pregnancy*, Totowa. NJ: Humana Press, 1993: 219pp.

20. Johnson PM. Immunology of pregnancy. In Chamberlain GVP (ed.) *Turnbull's Obstetrics*, 2nd edn. London: Churchill Livingstone, 1995: 143–159.

21. Mackworth-Young C. Antiphospholipid antibodies: more than just a disease marker. *Immunol Today* 1990 **11**: 60–65.

22. Fraser EJ, Grimes DA, Schulz KF. Immunization as therapy for recurrent spontaneous abortion: a review and meta-analysis. *Obstet Gynecol* 1993 **82**: 854–859.

23. Haas GG. How should sperm antibody tests be used clinically? *Am J Reprod Immunol Microbiol* 1987 **15**: 106–111.

24. Hill JA. Immunological factors in endometriosis and endometriosis-associated reproductive failure. *Infertil Reprod Med Clin North Am* 1992 **3**: 583–596.

25. Roberts JM, Redman CWG. Pre-eclampsia: more than pregnancy-induced hypertension. *Lancet* 1993 **341**: 1447–1451.

3.4

Chromosomes and Reproduction

CM Gosden

INTRODUCTION

Although from the early 1960s it had been appreciated that major chromosomal abnormalities such as trisomies 13, 18 or 21 had severe phenotypic consequences, and that major sex chromosome abnormalities such as 45,X Turner's syndrome or 47,XXY Klinefelter's syndrome had effects on fertility, the importance of cytogenetic abnormalities on other aspects of reproductive medicine, has only emerged more recently. Even apparently minute abnormalities can cause major effects. Aneuploidies such as trisomies or triploidy are often lethal *in utero*, leading to miscarriage, intrauterine death stillbirth or neonatal death. Some of these infants will have major external abnormalities, whereas others may merely seem severely growth retarded. In the most extreme cases of miscarriage with a major chromosomal abnormality, there is only an empty gestational sac with no evidence of an embryo or a cord stump, showing the severe effects some chromosomal abnormalities (such as trisomies for the larger chromosomes such as 2, 3, 4, 5, 6, 7, etc.) may have on development.

In some cases there may be a 'balanced' chromosomal abnormality so that all the genetic material is present, but it is 'rearranged' so that for example for someone who has a reciprocal translocation, the chromosomal material differs slightly from the configuration found in a normal 46,XX or 46,XY individual. As would be expected, these individuals are phenotypically normal, but they may encounter problems when they come to reproduce because of their risks of having progeny with unbalanced forms of the parental rearrangement leading to either miscarriage or handicapped infants. A general introduction which gives details of the different types of cytogenetic abnormalities and how abnormalities arise is given in Chapter 1.7. The spectrum of chromosome abnormalities giving rise to reproductive problems is wide, encompassing a far more extensive and perplexing range of conditions and conse-quences than had been envisaged even 5 years ago. For example, confined placental mosaicism and the way this can influence accuracy in prenatal diagnosis, fetal growth and intrauterine lethality has illustrated the fact that chromosomal abnormalities may not be present in every cell and there may be tissue specific effects. This chapter aims to focus on the ways in which chromosomes may have effects in reproductive medicine and interrelate the clinical aspects of cytogenetics with the underlying scientific mechanisms.

The risk of major cytogenetic abnormalities in the fetus has been the initiative to undertake major screening programs for fetal cytogenetic abnormalities. Initially this started with programs to detect Down's syndrome fetuses in older mothers, but this has now been extended and prenatal karyotyping may be offered to women with abnormal maternal serum biochemical profiles (AFP, HCG and estriol) or to those pregnant women in whom fetal structural markers for chromosome abnormalities are detected on detailed ultrasound scans.

Chromosomal abnormalities can thus affect growth and differentiation, cause early lethality, influence many developmental systems ranging from the brain, heart, kidneys, placenta, germ cells and even though an individual has an apparently balanced karyotype, subtle rearrangements may affect reproduction in a number of different ways. Chromosomal abnormalities are relatively frequent; 1 in 150 newborns has a karyotypic anomaly. Although some of these are lethal or so severely handicapping that affected individuals may not reproduce, in almost all other types of reproductive problems such as infertility, miscarriage and premature menopause, these cytogenetic factors have a major influence. Since the risk of karyotypic anomalies may be high in patients with infertility, recurrent abortion, premature menopause etc, the indications to undertake chromosome and molecular cytogenetic studies on patients, parents, conceptuses, stillbirths or prenatal samples and the range and types of test are increasing dramatically.

CURRENT CONCEPTS

Chromosomes and sex determination including intersexuality

Humans have a chromosomal method of sex determination. Females have a 46,XX chromosomal constitution and males also have 46 chromosomes but with an XY sex chromosome complement. In order to determine whether it is the X or Y chromosome which is crucial in sex determination in man, it is necessary to study dosage effects for sex chromosome abnormalities. Those with a 45,X karyotype are female (with Turner's syndrome); those with a 47,XXX karyotype are female; 47,XXY are male (Klinefelter's syndrome) 48,XXXY are male and even 49,XXXXY are male.

This demonstrates clearly that when a Y chromosome is present, even in the presence of four X chromosomes, the developmental process is along male lines with testes and a penis, even if this is associated with infertility, hypogonadism and hypogenitalism as the number of X chromosomes opposing the Y chromosome increases. When no Y chromosome is present, development is that of a female (this appears to be the default setting for humans). The only exception to this is the case of XX males where Y chromosomal material is actually present but is translocated onto the tip of the short arm of the X chromosome.[1] The situation may also be complicated in other ways. For example, not all the cells in the body have the same chromosomal constitution. If there is mosaicism (with the presence of more than one cell line) then complex interactions of cell lines with and without X and Y chromosomes may occur and some of these may lead to intersexuality and pseudohermaphroditism. There are further influences on sexual and gonadal development such as end organ unresponsiveness to androgen and other hormonal signaling pathways.[2–4]

In testicular feminization syndrome (TFS) the individuals are genetic males with a 46,XY karyotype, but with a female phenotype. Affected males have female external genitalia, female breast development, blind vagina, absent uterus and female adnexa and abdominal or inguinal testes. Patients may present with a presumed inguinal hernia in a female, or primary amenorrhea. The frequency has been estimated to be about 1 in 65 000 males. Familial testicular feminization syndrome may be seen, with two or more affected individuals over several generations due to an X-linked recessive gene. There is a danger in TFS as with some other forms of intersexuality and hermaphroditism, that the gonads may become malignant. It is thus important in abnormal sexual differentiation to detemine gonadal status and location. For example, in cases of blind ending vagina with absent uterus, it is important to distinguish between cases of Rokitanski–Kuster–Hauser syndrome with absence of Müllerian derivatives giving vaginal atresia and rudimentary uterus but with a 46,XX karytoype and normal ovaries, where the risk of malignancy is low, and those of TFS where there is a 46,XY karyotype, blind ending vagina and intra-abdominal testes which have a very high risk of malignancy.[5]

The terms intersex and intersexuality have been used in a wide variety of senses. It has been suggested that the term intersex should be restricted to those patients with ambiguous external genitalia and not used in cases where the genitalia are definitely male or female such as cases of Klinefelter's syndrome or ovarian dysgenesis or cases where the internal organs are gonadal streaks, ovotestes or developed ovaries or testes in an individual with non-corresponding external genitalia. Complex systems of clinical classification have arisen and readers are referred to specialist texts for details. A very simplified version is that true hermaphrodites have both ovarian and testicular tissue present and may have ambiguous external genitalia. If gonads of only one type are present then the terms male and female pseudohermaphrodite are use for testicular and ovarian intersexes, respectively. Thus even if the external genitalia appear to be female or virilized female, if the gonads are testes then the conventional term is male pseudohermaphrodite. Patients with true or pseudohermaphroditism often have iatrogenically induced psychological or emotional problems as a result of medical 'curiosity' about their phenotypic/genotypic/karyotypic correlations and caution about overexamination is crucial. Chromatin positive female pseudohermaphrodites with virilized external genitalia may arise as a result of a genetic abnormality in the fetus such as congenital virilizing adrenal hypoplasia (such as 21 hydroxylase deficiency) or as a result of maternal androgen exposure.

Infertility, the menopause and chromosomes

Infertility

Many chromosomal abnormalities have an effect on fertility, but may affect male and female fertility differently. Sex chromosomal abnormalities such as 45,X and 47,XXY may lead to infertility because of their effects on germ cell production. 47,XYY and 47,XXX individuals are usually fertile, although a proportion will present at subfertility clinics. Females with trisomy 21 are usually fertile, although they have a risk that about 50% of their children will have Down's syndrome. In contrast, males with Down's syndrome are infertile. Translocations and inversions may exert their effects on infertility, by causing recurrent miscarriage or by leading to major handicaps in surviving children. Supernumerary marker chromosomes tend to cause a greater degree of infertility in males than females for the same marker chromosome within the same family.

Karyotype and chromosome pairing is critical for germ cell meiosis and ovulation

The menopause is initiated by a reduction in the number of follicles in the ovary to less than a thousand, rather than chronological age.[6] A number of factors thus influence the age at which the menopause occurs; it has been suggested that mutiple ovulators may have an earlier menopause and it occurs earlier in mothers of twins.[7] Those women who have had repeated ovulation induction to assist conception are thought to be at risk for premature menopause. Women with Turner's syndrome (45,X) are one of the most extreme examples; they do reach the menopause, but this happens before birth. In female fetuses with Turner's syndrome, there are normal numbers of oocytes at fetal gestational ages of 16–20 weeks, but there is only a single X chromosome so this is unable to undergo normal chromosome pairing.[3,8,9] This single unpaired X chromosome thickens and, in trying to find a normal homolog with which to pair, disrupts the early stage of the meiotic division *in utero*. All follicles with unpaired chromosomal regions (i.e. all 45,X containing cells and other cells which have unpaired chromosomal segments, even for autosomes) become atretic, so that if there are no cells with two X chromosomes, all the follicles fail. The ovaries shrink and, because they contain no surviving follicles, become streaks so that the menopause precedes birth.[10]

Females with mosaic Turner's syndrome usually have a less severe phenotype; any follicular cells in the ovary with two X chromosomes survive and aid the formation of normal ovarian structure, in contrast to streak ovaries. This is clearly something particular to human gonadal and follicular development, because the Turner mouse, despite the presence of an unpaired X chromosome in the ovarian follicles, forms normal ovaries and is fertile. Effective chromosome pairing is therefore essential if 'good' oocytes are to be laid down during the intrauterine life of the human female; unpaired segments are responsible for atretic follicles resulting in a reduction of total follicle number and thus premature menopause. Thus in conditions where there is failure of either the autosomes or sex chromosomes to pair satisfactorily, this may result in infertility and possible premature menopause. A number of abnormalities such as chromosomal inversions, some translocations and a number of other anomalies such as aneuploid mosaicism may lead to the carrier having subfertility, early miscarriages or premature menopause (this latter condition appears to be common in 45,X mosaics) depending upon the exact nature of the chromosomal abnormality involved or the proportion of abnormal cells in mosaicism.

Chromosomal abnormalities and their contribution to miscarriage, stillbirth, neonatal death and intrauterine growth retardation (IUGR)

Fetal loss can take place at any stage of gestation, although the majority of losses occur early in the first trimester. The proportion of conceptions with major chromosomal abnormalities is high (in the order of 50%), largely due to errors which have occurred in germ cell formation (in both eggs and sperm), resulting in embryos with major trisomies and triploidy or chromosomal rearrangements. Almost all trisomies for each of the different chromosomes have been found in human miscarriages. Trisomy for the largest human chromosomes from 1 to 12, and a number of other chromosomes such as 14, 15, 16, 17, 19 and 20 appear to cause very early lethality. When the largest chromosomes are involved, the development of the embryo may be limited to that of a blighted ovum or cord stump, or even a completely empty gestational sac, but the growth of the extraembryonic membranes, gestation sac and chorionic villi may be much greater, even to achieving the gestation sac size expected for an embryo of 6–7 weeks gestational age. Each specific chromosomal abnormality may have a characteristic pattern of phenotypic expression (in terms of the size, developmental profile and anomalies of the embryo or fetus). Different malformations or types of pregnancy (such as ectopic pregnancies) may be associated with specific chromosomal abnormalities and there may be different patterns according to gestational age.[11–16] However, overlaid on this basic pattern there are variations according to the different alleles of the genes carried on the chromosomes involved and sometimes with the parent of origin of the abnormal chromosome(s) due to the phenomenon of 'genetic imprinting'.

There is a high rate of attrition *in utero* of chromosomally abnormal conceptuses. This can be deduced from the fact that about 50% of all conceptions are chromosomally abnormal; the majority of these will have been lost by term although about 5% of stillbirths and neonatal deaths have chromosomal abnormalities and about 0.5% of liveborn infants have chromosomal abnormalities. Some chromosomal abnormalities illustrate the paradox of predicting survival for different karyotypic abnormalities.[17] In Turner's syndrome (45,X), about 70% of the conceptuses die *in utero*, some as very early abortions, a further proportion as first trimester losses, and yet more during the second and third trimesters. It appears that a proportion (but not all) of those who survive to term may actually be mosaics having some normal 46,XX or 46,XY cells which dilute the effect of the 45,X Turner cell line.[8,18] Similarly for trisomies 13, 18 and 21 and triploidy; many are lost very early in gestation, a further proportion are lost during the first, second and third trimesters, some are stillborn or die in the neonatal period and yet others survive, in the case of trisomy 21, into adulthood. It has been estimated that 1% of newborns are severely or profoundly retarded, but about half die in the first 7 years. It is, at present, difficult to discern from the karyotype alone what the pattern of survival might be, although it has recently been postulated that, in addition to the fetal karyotype and allelic variation, chromosomal changes in the placenta are critical in fetal growth and development. Knowledge of the karyotype may also help to assess the risks in succeeding pregnancies.[19]

The concept that karyotypic divergence might occur between the fetus and placenta (or even between the different layers of the placenta) and that this might affect the growth and viability of the pregnancy seemed, at first, highly unlikely. However, confined placental mosaicism (a karyotypic abnormality restricted solely to the placenta, while the fetus has a normal karyotype) was first detected in placentae of term pregnancies with severe intrauterine growth retardation. Recognition of the fact that this divergence had both clinical significance and diagnostic relevance came when placental samples from chorionic villus sampling (CVS) were used for early prenatal diagnosis.

The MRC European trial of the safety and accuracy of CVS[20] showed that 1–2% of the CVS samples had confined placental mosaicism so that the placental samples had an abnormal (usually trisomic) karyotype whereas the fetus was normal. Collaborative studies have revealed the types and extent of problems of mosaicism in different prenatal tissues.[21–26]

Some very brilliant and detailed work by Kalousek[27–30] has shown that confined placental mosaicism occurs when the placenta is aneuploid or mosaic or has unequal parental contributions for a particular chromosomal pair, but the fetus is normal. Three types of confined placental mosaicism (CPM) have been recognized using chromosomal, molecular cytogenetics and parental specific gene probes. In type I, the aneuploid cells (usually trisomies) are restricted to the cytotrophoblast. In type II, the aneuploid cells are restricted to the villous stroma and some of these pregnancies result in fetal loss or IUGR. In type III, there is aneuploidy of both villous stroma and cytotrophoblast and when this occurs for certain specific chromosomal abnormalities it is associated with IUGR. A further layer of complexity has been added to these findings. This is that in some placentae where there was IUGR, the placenta originally appeared to have a normal diploid karyotype and did not appear trisomic. However, where special chromosome probes were used which detected differences between those chromosomes derived from mother when compared with those from father it was clear that although there were only two chromosomes from a particular chromosome pair (for example normal disomy for chromosomes 9 or 16), both the chromosomes had actually come from the same parent – a phenomenon described as uniparental disomy (UPD). It is now clear that CPM and UPD play major roles in fetal loss and in growth retardation and that elucidating the role of UPD in early miscarriage of apparently chromosomally normal conceptuses may be important.[26]

Parents who have a stillborn or mentally or physically handicapped child, often seek counseling about the risks of abnormality in future pregnancies. Unfortunately, unless a specific diagnosis is made on the proband such as trisomy, triploidy or chromosomal rearrangement such as deletion or inversion, it is often very difficult to conclude what the recurrence risks are and whether or not prenatal testing could be offered. This is one of the reasons for trying to establish a diagnosis by taking samples and, if necessary collecting and storing samples in a tissue bank in order that definitive testing can be carried out in problem cases when probes or resources become available.[19, 31–35]

Chromosomal abnormalities in prenatal diagnosis including antenatal screening for Down's syndrome

Risk factors and screening in pregnancy

Since the introduction in the early 1970s of fetal karyotyping to detect chromosomal abnormalities in older mothers or those carrying translocations, there has been a rapid expansion of prenatal chromosome studies, and prenatal karyotyping is still numerically the most frequent indication for prenatal diagnosis. There are now many indications for fetal karyotyping, either from amniotic fluid samples, chorionic villi or fetal blood. The most common indications for prenatal chromosome testing are advanced maternal age, a previous child or pregnancy with a major chromosomal disorder, an abnormal maternal serum biochemical screening profile, major structural or growth disorders detected on ultrasound scan, family history of chromosome disorder, or that one of the parents is the carrier of a chromosomal translocation or rearrangement. Maternal anxiety about chromosomal disorders either because of age, family history without a recognizable chromosomal rearrangement, or recurrent miscarriage or because of exposure to irradiation or teratogens may also be an indication for some centers although the exact risks in these cases are difficult to quantify.[36–38]

How to karyotype; which tissues to use?

Prenatal karyotyping can be undertaken on amniotic fluid obtained at amniocentesis, placenta obtained at chorionic villus sampling, or fetal blood at cordocentesis. The safety and accuracy of each of these procedures differs. The indications and risk for each of the methods are complex and depend on patient and obstetrician preference, gestational age, the availability of specialized techniques such as fetal blood sampling, the risks of fetal abnormality and the presence of structural and other anomalies, for example severe oligohydramnios may preclude successful amniocentesis. Patient choice of early first trimester testing (those who want the privacy afforded by early testing and the benefits of a result which make possible early surgical termination of pregnancy should the fetus turn out to be affected, but may be concerned about the problems of safety and accuracy of first trimester testing compared with second trimester amniocentesis), has led to the development of chorionic villus sampling and more recently, early amniocentesis.

Each technique is associated with specific risks of miscarriage and diagnostic problems such as confined placental mosaicism for the CVS samples and culture failure for the early amniocentesis samples. The laboratory aspects of prenatal diagnosis are described in Chapter 3.5. The exact quantitation of these risks of diagnostic accuracy (which encompasses problems such as confined placental mosaicism, false positive and false negative results and maternal cell contamination leading to misdiagnosis) of invasive prenatal testing is complex, as few randomized controlled trials have yet been undertaken.[20] For example, assessment of the background risk of miscarriage, later fetal loss, neonatal and perinatal death and congenital malformations for those who have a risk of chromosomal disorder cannot be undertaken as it would be unethical to randomize patients at risk to a trial arm with no testing at all. Furthermore, the power of any trial increases if all the fetal losses are karyotyped. Tabor et al.[39] carried out a large randomized trial in low risk women which was of help in defining risks in low-risk women; unfortunately, the risks of miscarriage rise with advancing maternal age and with abnormal levels of maternal serum metabolites, so that although it is possible to extrapolate minimum risk figures from the data of Tabor *et al.*, the exact risks for each of the high risk groups require further randomized trials. The problems of testing early in pregnancy may differ from those found in the second trimester and it is thus important to define the exact gestational age ranges involved in randomized studies.[40]

Ultrasound and biochemical markers for aneuploidy

Until recently, most of the indications for karyotyping depended on pre-existing risks for the pregnancy such as advanced maternal age, family history, parental translocation or previous miscarriages. Now the identification of abnormal maternal serum screening parameters[41] and the use of ultrasound markers for fetal chromosomal abnormalities[42] is helping to further refine the risks of karyotypic anomalies in the fetus. This should lead to the avoidance of invasive testing in pregnancy except for those who are actually shown to have high risks, and methods of identification and risk assessment are likely to improve and be refined over the next few years.

Chromosomal abnormalities in prenatal diagnosis

The principal difficulty of prenatal diagnosis of chromosome disorders from amniotic fluid, CVS or fetal blood lies in trying to predict what the phenotypic consequences of specific karyotypic abnormalities might be and, most importantly, trying to assess the probable degree of mental or physical handicap involved. False positive results mean that although the prenatal chromosomal tests indicate a major abnormality, the fetus is karyotypically normal. How could this happen? The reasons for misdiagnosis and incorrect risks of handicap include growing maternal instead of fetal cells, inducing abnormal karyotypes in the cultured cells, karyotyping placental cells with some type of confined placental mosaicism or cells from the placenta of an abnormal twin who died earlier in the pregnancy and mix-up of samples.[43] Terminating a wanted pregnancy because of an abnormality present in the karyotyped cells but not actually in the fetus has serious consequences for the parents, and medicolegally.

False negative results (so that after prenatal testing there is a failure to identify fetuses with major chromosomal abnormalities because the karyotype of the sample appears normal) occur either because of failure to karyotype sufficient cells to recognize that an abnormality is present (especially if this is in mosaic state), or to poor quality chromosomal preparations so that trisomies or small chromosomal deletions or duplications are not identified. Confined placental mosaicism involving trisomic zygote rescue (in certain trisomies the abnormal placenta attempts to compensate by losing the extra chromosome so that placental cells have a normal diploid karyotype whereas the fetus is trisomic),[28,29] is another cause of false positive

results.[44,45] Additional causes include errors in sample identification.

Complexities of predicting the phenotype from the karyotype

Some karyotypes are difficult to interpret and in other cases it is difficult to predict how severe the possible handicap might be. Antenatal diagnosis of sex chromosome abnormalities gives rise to dilemmas for patients and counsellors and causes much controversy. Prediction from biased sources of ascertainment may not be accurate; high risks of mental handicap are often given for Klinfelter's syndrome if these are derived from biased sources, whereas risks from follow-up of sex chromosomal aneuploidies from newborn studies do not give severe predictions of IQ deficits.[46] Even for a karyotype such as that of trisomy 21 (Down's syndrome), there are difficulties in predicting how severe the degree of mental handicap might be or whether or not associated problems such as cardiac abnormalities might lead to early death. Other chromosomal abnormalities can cause much more difficulty. Other karyotypic anomalies such as *de novo* translocations (which are not present in the parents), or other mutant or *de novo* abnormalities, are associated with major problems in trying to predict their phenotypic effects, as the spectrum can vary from normal to severe handicap.[32,46–48]

Chromosomes and their relation to causes of childhood mental and physical handicap

Down's syndrome is the most frequent genetic/cytogenetic cause of mental handicap. Down's syndrome also illustrates the wide-ranging effects of major chromosomal abnormalities in that some individuals with Down's syndrome have major cardiac problems, there is an increased risk of leukemia and many people with Down's syndrome manifest signs of early onset dementia of the Alzheimer type after the age of 30. Most of the other major trisomies are lethal in the pure form, but mosaic individuals in whom there is a mixture of normal and abnormal cells have phenotypes which depend on the proportion of abnormal cells in different tissues and the ameliorating effects of the normal cell lines. For example, for trisomy 8, the degree of mental handicap depends on the proportion of cells with trisomy 8.[49,50] Other partial monosomies and trisomies pinpoint critical chromosomal regions influencing abnormal physical or mental development.[32,51,52] In Turner's syndrome, there is a growing realization that not only survival, but height and ovarian function are crucially dependent on mosaicism of the 45,X line with a normal cell line (which might be either 46,XX or 46,XY). Even a few normal cells present in the ovaries may be sufficient to give some ovarian function, making the search for cytogenetic influences on the phenotype essential in understanding the underlying molecular cytogenetic basis of clinical effects.

As analysis of the chromosomal segments and genes involved in abnormal reproductive phenotypes expands, not only diagnosis but the therapeutic potential can be extended and counseling about the prognosis also has a firmer basis.

FUTURE PERSPECTIVES

New perspectives with chromosome-specific and gene probes: new techniques or new questions?

The realization that there are a number of different mechanisms by which chromosomes may exert their effects is changing the interactions of cytogenetics with obstetrics and reproductive medicine. For example, intrauterine growth retardation may be due to a number of different chromosomal disorders, such as triploidy or trisomy 18, or may be due to true mosaicism, confined placental mosaicism or uniparental disomy. The fact that a greater range of scientific tools such as chromosome and gene specific probes to investigate chromosomal deletions, amplifications and mutations is now available, changes the scientific perspectives for investigation. The clinical tools too have expanded in scope and include ultrasound scanning, color Doppler and other forms of imaging and the ability to sample a range of different tissues enable new initiatives at the clinical/scientific interface.

Interphase karyotyping, in situ hybridization, FISH, PCR and other molecular cytogenetic techniques

One of the most important advances has been in the the ability to 'karyotype' non-dividing interphase cells, using new techniques such as chromosome painting with chromosome-specific probes and fluorescent *in situ* hybridization (FISH). This has enabled studies not previously possible such as studies of gonadal cells, gametes and brain cells not previously amenable to study. It also enables a rapid 'molecular karyotype' to be obtained within a few hours of taking the sample, which will be of value for rapid

karyotyping in prenatal diagnosis. Although at present the accuracy of diagnosis in uncultured cells using some methods and probes may have problems with accuracy in some cases as the probes and knowledge about chromosomes in interphase cells (such as uncultured amniotic fluid samples) increases, the prospects and potential for major future advances are very great.

Mosaicism, confined placental mosaicism and primary prevention of chromosomal abnormalities

Recent use of chromosomal probes to examine the chromosomal complement in gametes and molecular cytogenetic analysis to demonstrate the parental origins of meiotic errors leading to aneuploidy (including the meiotic stage at which errors occur and possible suppression of crossing over during non-disjunction and risks of recurrence). The ability to do such studies on sperm or oocytes may help to elucidate mechanisms of non-disjunction and this in turn may help in advances towards the primary prevention of chromosomal abnormalities rather than the secondary prevention by termination after prenatal diagnosis which is all that can be offered at present.

Preimplantation diagnosis of chromosomal disorders

Studies of early embryos and blastocysts from assisted conception and IVF programs have shown high rates of chromosomal abnormalities and mosaicism. This is in agreement with data from studies of early miscarriages which indicate that for conceptions *in vivo* and *in vitro* there are high rates of chromosomal abnormality. Although the vast majority of chromosomally abnormal conceptuses are lost in early pregnancy, a significant proportion of pregnancies continue. Preimplanation cytogenetic diagnosis using chromosome specific probes would offer options to those parents at high risk of chromosomal disorders for whom prenatal diagnosis and termination would not be an acceptable option.

SUMMARY

- Chromosomal abnormalities are a major cause of mental and physical handicap and may lead to infertility and miscarriage. Even balanced chromosomal rearrangements may cause problems of infertility, miscarriage or stillbirth or handicapped infants. Chromosomal abnormalities are not rare and cause a wide range of effects in reproductive medicine.

- The vast majority of constitutional chromosomal abnormalities arise as errors during meiosis

(non-disjunctional errors) in the formation of eggs or sperm in a parent; about 5% occur as errors during an early cell division in the developing embryo.

- Only 1–2% of parents show chromosomal abnormalities if karyotyped after three or more miscarriages. However, 50% of the products of conception from these miscarriages have chromosomal abnormalities, principally *de novo* abnormalities such as trisomy and triploidy.

There is an increase in the proportion of babies with chromosomal abnormalities with advancing maternal age. As mothers over 35 years have less than 5% of the babies born, despite the increased risks for older mothers, the majority of babies with mutant chromosomal abnormalities are born to younger mothers with no previously identifiable risk factors. There is thus a need to investigate why older mothers have higher risks and to develop new screening methods applicable to all age groups.

Recurrence risks for chromosomal abnormalities after having an affected child depend on the type of chromosomal abnormality and whether the abnormality is mutant (i.e. has occurred *de novo*) or is familial. Risks for chromosomally normal parents who have had a child with a mutant abnormality are approximately 1% (and also depend on the maternal age risks). For parents carrying a translocation these depend on the type of translocation and the chromosomal break points. For example a female carrier of a 14;21 translocation has about a 15% risk of having a child with translocation Down's syndrome.

When screening for chromosomal abnormalities in pregnancy the risks for older mothers increase with advancing age. The risk is not solely for Down's syndrome but includes all chromosome abnormalities such as trisomies 13, 18 and sex chromosome abnormalities such as 47,XXY. Maternal age 35: risk of Down's syndrome, 1 in 280; risk for all chromosome abnormalities, 1 in 80. Maternal age 45: risk of Down's syndrome, 1 in 22; risk for all chromosome abnormalities, 1 in 14.

The risk of chromosome abnormalities when structural anomalies have been detected on ultrasound scan depends on the specific abnormality involved. This is higher when there are multiple defects than for an isolated malformation.

omphalocele	– risk ~ 30% (mainly trisomies and triploidy)
facial cleft	– risk ~ 60% (mainly trisomies)
diaphragmatic hernia	– risk ~ 20%
choroid plexus cysts	– risk ~ 46% with associated defects
	– risk ~ 1–2% when isolated defect

With regard to tissue-specific chromosomal abnormalities, there are certain constraints on tissue for karyotyping. The recognition that certain disorders such as trisomy 18 might lead to false negative results if chorionic villus sampling or placental biopsy is undertaken because of trisomic zygote rescue by the placenta will help to increase diagnostic accuracy by optimizing the tissues used for diagnostic karyotyping.

The identification of confined placental mosaicism and its relationship both to the accuracy of fetal/placental diagnosis and to intrauterine growth retardation and adverse pregnancy outcome is increasing diagnostic accuracy and prognosis in prenatal diagnosis.

For true mosaic abnormalities (excluding confined placental abnormalities) the phenotype depends on the proportion of cells with the abnormality, especially in critical tissues. For example, a 45,X/46,XY mosaic may be male, female or intersex. Even if the proportion of 45, X cells in blood and skin are high, the phenotype will only be Turner-like female or intersex if the proportion of 45,X cells in the ovary exceeds about 60%.

REFERENCES

1. Magenis RE, Casanova M, Fellous M, Olson S, Sheehy R. Further cytologic evidence for Xp-Yp translocation in XX males using *in situ* hybridisation with Y derived probe. *Hum Genet* 1981 75: 228–233.
2. Amrhein JA, Klingensmith GJ, Walsh PC, McKusick VA, Midgeon BJ. Partial androgen sensitivity: the Reifenstein syndrome revisted. *N Engl J Med* 1977 97: 350.
3. Dewhurst J. Fertility in 47, XXX and 45, X patients. *J Med Genet* 1978 15: 132.
4. Brown TR, Lubahn DB, Wison ME, Joseph DR, French FS, Migeon BJ. Deletion of the steroid domain of the human androgen receptor gene in one family with complete androgen insensitivity syndrome: evidence for further genetic heterogeneity in this syndrome. *Proc Natl Acad Sci USA* 1988 85: 8151–8155.
5. Verp MS, Simpson JL. Abnormal sexual differentiation and neoplasia. *Cancer Genet Cytogenet* 1987 25: 191–218.
6. te Velde ER. Disappearing ovarian follicles and reproductive ageing. *Lancet* 1993 341: 1125–1126.
7. Martin NG, Shanley S, Butt K *et al.* Excessive follicular recruitment and growth in mothers of spontaneous dizygotic twins. *Acta Genet Med Gemellol* 1991 40: 291–301.
8. Cockwell A, Mackenzie M, Yoings S, Jacobs P. A cytogenetic study of 45, X fetuses and their parents. *J Med Genet* 1991 28: 151–155.
9. Lindsten J. *The Nature and Origin of X Chromosome Aberration in Turner's Syndrome.* Stockholm: Almquist and Wikseel, 1963.
10. Weiss L. Additional evidence of gradual loss of germ cells in the pathogenesis of streak ovaries in Turner's syndrome. *J Med Genet* 1971 8: 540.
11. Bauld R, Sutherland GR, Bain AD. Chromosome studies in investigation of stillbirths and neonatal deaths. *Arch Dis Child* 1974 49: 782.
12. Bell JE, Gosden CM. Central nervous system abnormalities – contrasting patterns in early and late pregnancy. *Clin Genet* 1978 13: 387–396.
13. Bell JA, Pearn JH, Firman D. Childhood deaths in Down's syndrome. Survival curves and causes of death from a total population study in Queensland Australia 1976–1985. *J Med Genet* 1989 26: 764–768.

14. Elias S, LeBeau M, Simpson JL, Martin AO. Chromosome analysis of ectopic human conceptuses. *Am J Obstet Gynecol* **141**: 698.

15. Kaji T, Ferrier A. Cytogenetics of aborters and abortuses. *Am J Obstet Gynecol* 1977 **131**: 33.

16. Van de Kaa CA, Nelson KAM, Ramaekers FCS, Voojis PG, Hopman AHN. Interphase cytogenetics in paraffin sections of routinely processed hydatidiform moles and hydropic abortions. *J Pathol* 1991 **165**: 281–287.

17. Hook EB, Topol BB, Cross PK. The natural history of cytogenetically abnormal fetuses detected at midtrimester amniocentesis which are not terminated electively: new data and estimates of the excess and relative risk of fetal death associated with 47, +21 and some other abnormal karyotypes. *Am J Hum Genet* 1989 **45**: 855–861.

18. Hassold TJ, Benham F, Leppert M. Cytogenetic and molecular analysis of sex-chromosome monosomy. *Am J Hum Genet* 1988 **42**: 534–551.

19. Boue J, Boue A, Lazar P, Gueguen S. Outcome of pregnancies following a spontaneous abortion with chromosomal anomaly. *Am J Obstet Gynaecol* **116**: 806.

20. MRC Working Party on the Evaluation of Chorion Villus sampling; Meade TW, Ammala P, Aynsley-Green A, Bobrow M, Chalmers I, Coleman D, Elias J, Ferguson-Sith M, Gosden C, Grant A, Hahnemann N, Liu D, MacKenzie I, McPherson K, Milner R, Modell B, O'Toole O, Rodeck C, Stott P, Terzian E, Ward R, Weatherall D. Medical Research Council European Trial of Chorion Villus Sampling. *Lancet* 1991 **337**: 1491–1499.

21. Bui TH, Iselius L, Lindsten J. European collaborative study on prenatal diagnosis: mosaicism, pseudomosaicism and single cell abnormal cells in amniotic fluid cell cultures. *Prenat Diagn* 1984 **4**: 145–162.

22. Ferguson-Smith MA, Yates JRW. Maternal age specific rates for chromosome aberrations and factors influencing them: report of the collaborative European study on 52,965 amniocenteses. *Prenat Diagn* 1984 **4**: 5–44.

23. Hsu LYF, Perlis TE. United States survey on chromosome mosaicism and pseudomosaicism in prenatal diagnosis. *Prenat Diagn* 1984 **4**: 97–130.

24. Vejerslev LO, Mikkelsen M. The European Collaborative Study on mosaicism in chorionic villus sampling: data from 1986–1987. *Prenat Diagn* 1989 **9**: 575–588.

25. Wang BBT, Rubin CH, Williams J. Mosaicism in chorionic villus sampling: an analysis of the incidence and chromosomes involved in 2612 consecutive cases. *Prenat Diagn* 1993 **134**: 179–190.

26. Wolstenholme J, Rooney DE, Davison EV. Confined placental mosaicism, IUGR, and adverse pregnancy outcome: a controlled retrospective UK collaborative study. *Prenat Diagn* 1994 **14**: 345–361.

27. Kalousek DK, Dill FJ. Chromosomal mosaicism confined to the placenta in the human conceptus. *Science* 1983 **221**: 665–667.

28. Kalousek DK, Howard PP, Olson SB, Barrett IJ, Dorfmann A, Black SH, Schulman JD, Wilson RD. Confirmation of CVS mosaicism in term placentae and high frequency of intrauterine growth retardation associated with confined placental mosaicism. *Prenat Diagn* 1991 **11**: 743–750.

29. Kalousek DK, Barrett IJ, Gartner AB. Spontaneous abortion and confined placental mosaicism. *Hum Genet* 1992 **88**: 642–646.

30. Kalousek DK, Langlois S, Barrett IJ, Yam I Wilson DR, Howard-Peebles PN, Johnson MP, Giogiutti E. Uniparental disomy for chromosome 16 in humans. *Am J Hum Genet* 1993 **52**: 8–16.

31. Berr C, Borghi E, Rethore MO, Lejeune J, Alperovitch A. Risk of Down syndrome in relatives of trisomy 21 children. A case control study. *Ann Genet* 1990 **33**: 137–140.

32. Daniel A, Hook EB, Wulf G. Risks of unbalanced progeny at amniocentesis to carriers of chromosome rearrangements: data from United States and Canadian Laboratories. *Am J Med Genet* 1989 **31**: 14–53.

33. Hassold TJ, Jacobs PA. Trisomy in man. *Ann Rev Genet* 1984 **18**: 69–97.

34. Mikkelsen M, Poulsen H, Grinsted J, Lange A. Non-disjunction in trisomy 21: study of chromosomal heteromorphisms in 110 families. *Ann Hum Genet* 1980 **44**: 17–28.

35. Mikkelsen M, Poulsen H, Tommerup N. Genetic risk factors in human trisomy 21. In Hassold TJ, Epstein CJ (eds) *Progress in Clinical and Biological Research. Molecular and Cytogenetic Studies of Non-disjunction*, Vol 311. New York: Alan R Liss 1989: 183–197.

36. Lilford RJ. *Prenatal Diagnosis of Fetal Abnormalities*. London, Boston, Sydney: Butterworths, 1990.

37. Brock DJH, Rodeck CH, Ferguson-Smith MA. *Prenatal Diagnosis and Screening*. Edinburgh, London, New York: Churchill Livingstone, 1992.

38. Neilson JP, Chambers SE. *Obstetric Ultrasound* 1. Oxford: Oxford Medical Publications, Oxford University Press, 1993.

39. Tabor A, Philip J, Madsen M, Bang J, Obel EB, Norgaard-Pedersen B. Randomised controlled trial of genetic amniocentesis in 4606 low-risk women. *Lancet* 1986 i: 1287–1293.

40. Nicolaides K, Brizot M, Patel F, Snijders R. Comparison of chorionic villus sampling and amniocentesis for fetal karyotyping at 10–13 weeks gestation. *Lancet* 1994 **344**: 435–439.

41. Wald NJ, Cuckle HS, Densem JW, Nanchatal K, Royston P, Chard T, Haddow JE, Knight GJ, Palomaki GE, Canick JA. Maternal serum screening for Down's syndrome in early pregnancy. *Br Med J* 1988 **297**: 883–887.

42. Nicolaides KH, Gosden CM, Snijders RJM. Ultrasonographically detectable markers of fetal chromosomal defects. In Neilson JP, Chambers SE (eds) *Obstetric Ultrasound 1*. Oxford, New York, Tokyo: Oxford Medical Publications Oxford University Press, 1993: 41–48.

43. Gosden CM, Nicolaides KH, Rodeck CH. Fetal blood sampling in the investigation of chromosome mosaicism in amniotic fluid cell culture. *Lancet* 1988: 613–617.

44. Gosden CM. Prenatal diagnosis of fetal abnormalities using chorionic villus biopsies. In Drife JO, Donnai D (eds) *Early Prenatal Diagnosis*. London: Springer 1991: 153–167.

45. Gosden CM. Genetic diagnosis, chorionic villus biopsy and placental mosaicism. In Redman CW, Sargent IL, Sankey PM (eds) *The Human Placenta*. London, Edinburgh: Blackwell Scientific, 1992: 113–154.

46. Gosden, CM. Prenatal diagnosis of chromosome anomalies. In Lilford RJ (ed.) *Prenatal Diagnosis of Fetal Abnormalities*. London, Boston, Sydney, Toronto: Butterworths 1990: 104–164.

47. Schinzel A. *Catalogue of Unbalanced Chromosome Aberrations in Man*. New York: Walter de Gruyter, 1984.

48. Warburton D. Outcome of cases of *de novo* structural rearrangements diagnosed at amniocentesis. *Prenat Diagn* 1984 **4**: 69–80.

49. Schinzel A. Trisomy 8 mosaicism syndrome. *Helv Paediatr Acta* 1974 **29**: 531.

50. Warkany J, Passarge E, Smith LB. Congenital malformations in autosomal trisomy syndromes. *Am J Dis Child* 1966 **112**: 502.

51. Bergsma DS. *Birth Defects Atlas and Compendium*, 3rd edn. Baltimore: Williams and Wilkins, 1985.

52. de Grouchy J, Turleau C. *Clinical Atlas of Human Chromosomes*. New York: John Wiley, 1984.

3.5

Laboratory Techniques for Prenatal Diagnosis

LS Martin, Y Ben-Yoseph, SAD Ebrahim and MI Evans

INTRODUCTION

This chapter illustrates the theory and methods required for modern prenatal diagnosis. We will address, in turn, molecular, biochemical and cytogenetic testing.

CURRENT CONCEPTS

Molecular genetics: prenatal diagnosis

Molecular genetics can be defined as the study of human variation (mutation) at the level of the gene: its organization, regulation and expression. It has been estimated that the human genome has 3.0×10^9 base pairs per haploid copy, and contains 50 000–100 000 genes dispersed on 23 chromosomes. Each individual is thought to have 6–10 abnormal genes.

The study of the genetic mechanisms for the expression of inherited information (Chapter 1.1) and their mutant protein products has been facilitated by the investigation of experimental bacterial and animal models. Since the methods used in these experiments (e.g. irradiation or chemical exposure) cannot be used in the human, the study of naturally occurring mutations provides models and insights into the structure–function relationship of the human gene and its environment. These research studies have yielded precise diagnostic tests for many genetic diseases. This section will review the important recombinant molecular genetic diagnostic techniques described in Chapter 1.9 but discussing their use specifically in prenatal diagnosis, together with the diseases that best illustrate them.

History

In 1970 H.O. Smith at the Johns Hopkins University School of Medicine isolated and purified the first restriction endonuclease, Hind II, in *Haemophilus influenzae* for which he, D. Nathans, and W. Arber received the Nobel Prize for Medicine and Physiology in 1978. In 1980, Lawn and Maniatis cloned and sequenced the beta-globin gene, thereby opening the door for DNA mutational analysis.[1] Fortuitously, the beta-globin gene, located on chromosome 11, is only 1600 base pairs (bp) in length; in contrast, the CFTR gene is 250 000 bp in length (of which only 438 bp are of coding sequence). In 1978, the first DNA restriction fragment length polymorphism (RFLP), Hpa 1, was found by W.Y. Kan at the beta-globin locus. This discovery led to the utilization of haplotype analysis in prenatal diagnosis, as markers for gene mapping, for differentiation of mutant alleles, and for the study of the mechanisms of mutation and in forensic and paternity testing.

Southern blot analysis

Localization and identification of specific sequences in the genomic DNA is often performed by the transfer technique described by Southern.[2] Fig. 3.5.1 is a schematic representation of the procedure.

The Southern blot analysis allows one to identify two kinds of mutational differences:

1. Single base pair changes that alter, either obliterate or create, a restriction endonuclease site which results in an altered band size; and/or
2. Insertions or deletions, resulting in the rearrangement of the gene.

Duchenne muscular dystrophy (DMD), a progressive primary disorder of muscle, inherited in an X-linked fashion occurs in one of 3500–4000 males. The dystrophin gene cloned by Kunkel *et al.* in 1987 and one of the largest identified to date (~2.4 million base pairs), is representative of a disease gene which can be examined using the Southern transfer. DMD deletion mutations are detected directly in approximately 60% of affected males. Deletions are clustered into two major regions. Interestingly, Duchenne muscular dystrophy results when deletions alter the

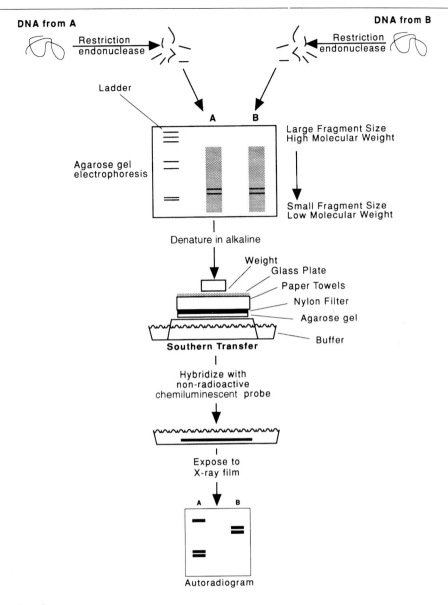

Fig. 3.5.1 *Southern transfer.*

reading frame, whereas Becker muscular dystrophy occurs when the deletions leave the reading frame intact.

Fragile X (Bell) syndrome is the most common inherited form of mental retardation, occurring in approximately one of 1250 males and one of 2500 females. It is inherited in an unusual X-linked fashion, as 30% of carrier females are affected, and 20% of males who carry a fragile X chromosome (Chapter 1.8, p. 86) are phenotypically normal (normal transmitting males). Transmission of the fragile X mutation and phenotypic expression thereafter demands that the X chromosome be inherited through a female. This is known as the 'Sherman Paradox'.

The mutation seen in the fragile X syndrome may be one of two types: small insertions called premutations (~100–600 bp) or large insertions (600–4000 bp) called full mutations. Variation of the length of DNA at the frag-

ile site is found between normal and fragile X individuals and is caused by expansion of a CGG repeat with methylation upstream of the CpG island which appears to correlate with the loss of expression of the FMR-1 mRNA. Methylation of the CpG island alters (obliterates) the restriction site endonuclease activity of Eag 1; thus, the Eag1 and EcoR1 endonuclease restriction digest and Southern transfer is utilized to analyze the methylation pattern and presence or absence of the mutation (Fig. 3.5.2).[3-5]

Linkage

Most variation in DNA is inconsequential with respect to causing disease. The majority of sequences of DNA are not

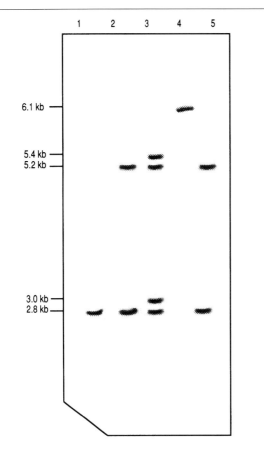

Fig. 3.5.2 *Schematic representation of Southern transfer – EcoR 1 and Eag 1 double digest of genomic DNA; normal male with 2.8 kb fragment (lane 1); normal female with 2.8 and 5.2 kb fragment demonstrating two normal X chromosomes (lane 2); carrier female with premutation alleles with normal fragments, 2.8, 3.0, 5.2 and 5.4 kb (lane 3); affected male with 6.1 kb fragment (lane 4); control female with two normal 2.8 and 5.2 kb fragments (lane 5).*

known to be coding regions; only about 5% of a gene is made up of protein-coding sequence. Within intervening sequences (non-coding regions) one can find a mutation approximately every 200 base pairs. Often, these changes alter or create a restriction endonuclease site, thereby allowing one to discern the change in band size on Southern blot. These variations in sequence are known as DNA polymorphisms. By definition, these alterations should occur in less than 1% of the population. These fragments created by restriction enzymes are termed restriction fragment length polymorphisms (RFLP);. the analysis of the association of RFLPs with disease-producing genes is termed linkage analysis.

The closer the polymorphism is to the disease gene, the less likely is recombination to occur between the two, and hence increase the likelihood that they will be inherited together. This is known as 'tight' linkage. One might imagine that if an alteration were in close proximity to the disease-causing gene, but not necessarily in that gene, one could track the associated fragment (the band on Southern blot) in a given family pedigree. The first such discovered was by Kan and Dozy in 1978 with the Hpa 1 site associated with sickle cell disease. Today, RFLP analysis is used primarily in the diagnosis for diseases in which the gene has yet to be cloned, the mutations are 'private', or DNA sequencing is not practical (Fig. 3.5.3).

Polymerase chain reaction

In 1987, while 'snaking along a moonlit mountain road into northern California's redwood country',[6] Kary B. Mullis conceived of an idea that would revolutionize molecular biology and for which he would ultimately receive the Nobel Prize.[7,8] This discovery is known today as the polymerase chain reaction (PCR). Simply stated, it is a method in which one takes a small aliquot of genomic DNA and

(a)   (b)

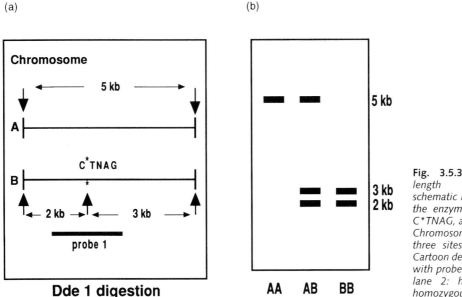

Fig. 3.5.3 (a) *Restriction fragment length polymorphism (RFLP): schematic representation of gene with the enzyme, Dde 1 recognition site, C*TNAG, and resultant fragment sizes. Chromosome A depicts two sites, B three sites as noted by arrows.* **(b)** *Cartoon depicting Southern blot results with probe 1, lane 1: homozygous AA; lane 2: heterozygous AB; lane 3: homozygous BB.*

enzymatically amplifies a specific region of that DNA by, theoretically, 1 billion-fold or, practically, 1 million-fold (Fig. 3.5.4). One can then visualize these fragments of DNA by electrophoresing them through an agarose gel and staining the gel with the fluorescent dye ethidium bromide, which intercalates between the stacked bases of DNA.

The ways in which PCR has been utilized for mutational analysis and diagnostics as it relates to disease genes are multifold.

Recently a number of diseases, e.g. fragile X syndrome, Huntington disease, Kennedy's disease, spinal cerebellar ataxia, dentatorubral-pallidoluysian atrophy (DRPLA) and

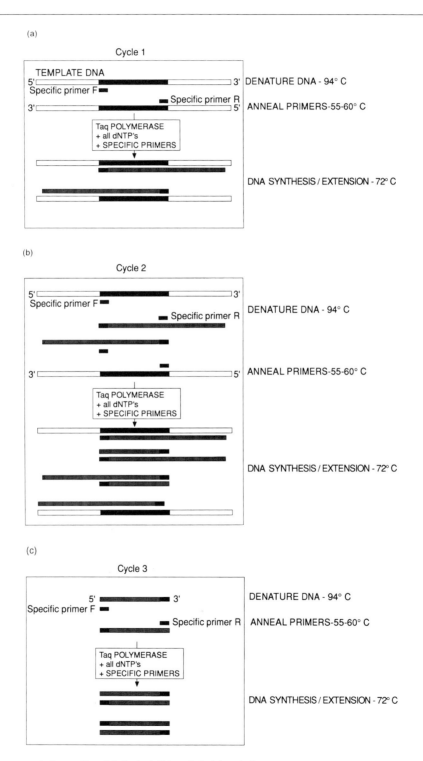

Fig. 3.5.4 *The polymerase chain reaction.* **(a)** *Cycle 1;* **(b)** *cycle 2;* **(c)** *cycle 3.*

myotonic dystrophy, have been found to be the result of an expansion of an unstable region of DNA triplet repeats. Analysis of normal individuals reveals length variation ranging from a low of 6 to a high of 54 repeats in the fragile X gene. As described already, there are two types of mutation: the premutational state in which only a female may pass an allele capable of expanding in an offspring to a full mutation, and the full mutation associated with the fragile X syndrome. The PCR conditions are modified to incorporate radioisotope which allows direct visualization of PCR amplified product after electrophoresis through an acrylamide gel; thus, revealing the size of the repeat, CGG, found in both the normal and premutation state. However, when hundreds of repeats are present as in the full mutation, the region is often too large to be amplified by PCR. This potential problem is resolved using the Southern transfer technique.

Multiplex PCR

Polymerase chain reaction technology allows multiple exons to be amplified simultaneously. This method is known as 'multiplex PCR'. It has the rapidity and sensitivity of the PCR process, and allows us to use small or poor quality samples, i.e. those which might not be sufficient for Southern blot analysis. This technique has been applied to the Duchenne/Becker (DMD/BMD) muscular dystrophy gene, whereby the large, nearly 2400 kb with ~70 exons and 329 deletions, gene may be scanned for deletions in those patients and fetuses at risk for DMD/BMD with detection of over 97% of deletions in DMD and all those with BMD.[9]

Northern blot/reverse transcriptase-PCR (RT-PCR)

Northern blot is the term given to the procedure whereby RNA is separated according to size by electrophoresis through an agarose gel, transferred to a solid support such as a nylon filter, hybridized to radiolabeled or chemiluminescent probe and autoradiography is used to locate the position of the band complementary to the RNA:DNA complex. In some instances, the quantity of RNA is insufficient to be detected in this manner; thus, *reverse transcriptase PCR* methodology permits the identification and isolation of these small quantities of mRNA and thereby the analysis of genes in a more fastidious manner.

Restriction endonuclease allele recognition

Hemoglobinopathies are the qualitative or quantitative disorders of the globin chains: alpha or beta. Sickle cell anemia is the most common disease among these disorders. In the American black population, the frequency of the heterozygous state is 8%, and one in 500 individuals has the disease. The diagnosis can be made readily on examination of a peripheral blood smear. To confirm this diagnosis one must perform a hemoglobin electrophoresis. The beta-globin gene is located on chromosome 11, and the

only responsible mutation is an A to T transition in the second nucleotide of the sixth codon, substituting a valine for glutamic acid; allelic heterogeneity does not exist for this disease. This alteration of DNA obliterates a sequence which the enzyme Dde1 recognizes, CTNAG, which is present in the normal A, CTGAG, and hemoglobin C, CTAAG, allele but not in the S allele, CTGTG, and thus enables one to make the prenatal diagnosis of sickle cell disease or trait by utilizing restriction endonuclease site analysis.

An alternative to relying on naturally occurring phenomena to create or obliterate a restriction endonuclease site is a novel technique called *PCR-mediated site-directed mutagenesis* (PSM), whereby a restriction site is created to facilitate the discrimination of mutations. The general principle is to amplify genomic DNA enzymatically using modified primers containing altered 3′ terminal nucleotide to create these sites. After these primers have been efficiently incorporated into the amplified DNA, the PCR products may than be digested with their respective enzyme. This assay has been applied to the analysis of the β-globin gene to detect the sickle cell mutation,[10] and to the amplification of exon 10 of the CFTR gene for ascertainment of those individuals with the ΔF508 mutation, responsible for ~70% of all cystic fibrosis (CF) chromosomes.[11]

Allele-specific oligonucleotide hybridization (ASO)

Allele-specific oligonucleotide hybridization (ASO) has proven to be a valuable technique which measures the specific binding of short (18–20-mer), radioactively, or non-radioactively, labeled oligonucleotide probes that either match the wild type, normal, DNA sequences exactly or the mutant sequence containing a single base pair substitution under stringent washing conditions. Only the probes that exactly complement the immobilized DNA will remain bound, and thus generate a signal seen on autoradiography. This technique was originally described by Conner *et al.* in 1983 for the detection of sickle cell βs-globin allele[12] without the luxury of PCR amplification of genomic DNA. This technique greatly facilitates the evaluation of genetic disorders in which the gene has to be screened for numerous mutations like thalassemia or cystic fibrosis, or in those where a restriction site is neither created nor obliterated.

Reverse dot blot

The reverse dot blot hybridization procedure which was devised by Saiki in 1989 utilizes membrane-bound oligonucleotides as hybridization targets for amplified genomic DNA.[13] The probe:DNA hybrids may be visualized by non-radioactive chemiluminescent activation or radioactive probes. As one might imagine, it would be more efficient to screen a set of mutations with a sample of amplified genomic DNA rather than screen a patient's DNA sample with a single oligonucleotide as a probe for each of approximately 30 or more allelic mutations. Such a range of potential mutations must be tested to achieve a reasonable level of confidence in a negative test with the unlikelihood of a new mutation.

A prime example for utilization of this methodology would be the diagnosis or screening of the CFTR (cystic fibrosis transmembrane conductance regulator) gene.[14] Cystic fibrosis is a disorder characterized by elevated sweat electrolytes and thick mucous secretions due to abnormal chloride permeability in epithelial tissues. In 1989 a consortium headed by L.C. Tsui cloned and sequenced the cystic fibrosis (CFTR) gene. The incidence of CF varies dramatically among different populations. In the northern European population, one of 2500 individuals will be affected with this autosomal recessively inherited disease (in Northern Ireland one of 1700, in Sweden one of 7700) whereas in Asian and African ethnic groups only one of 110 000 individuals is affected.

The CFTR gene, localized on chromosome 7, comprises approximately 250 000 base pairs of DNA, and is arranged as 27 exons with 26 introns. Exon 11 which encodes the nuclear binding fold (NBF) 1 harbors the more common mutations. One region of exon 11 has at least eleven different sequence alterations clustered in five codons. In contrast, there are several regions in which no mutation has been identified.

To date 30 000 mutant chromosomes have been examined worldwide and 70% carry the delta F508 mutation. However more than 325 different mutations have been defined. Only seven alleles are represented by more than 100 cases; 23 additional mutations by greater than ten cases. Thus, this would be ideally suited to the reverse dot blot method in which multiple alleles need to be examined in order to determine the parental carrier status, and/or fetal genotype.

Sequence analysis

Direct sequencing of the amplified product of a segment of genomic DNA is often the only method for analysis of mutations.[15] This may be due to a previously unrecognized mutation in an affected individual, or in certain diseases for which no allele is predominant: in contrast to the single mutation responsible for sickle cell anemia, or definable but heterogeneous alleles as in the CFTR gene in cystic fibrosis. Manual methods of sequence analysis have been developed and are routinely employed; however, new automated techniques have been exploited to speed the process.

Mutational scanning

Mutational scanning describes a method whereby one scans exons, and intron borders to identify alterations, primarily point mutations, in those genes with a high frequency of sporadic mutation (e.g. X-linked or dominant disorders). Single-stranded conformation polymorphism analysis (SSCP), chemical cleavage of mismatch (CCM) and denaturing gradient gel electrophoresis (DGGE) rep-

resents three modalities of this kind. These applications allow detection of point mutations that alter electrophoretic mobility of radioactively labeled single-stranded DNA in non-denaturing polyacrylamide gels or heteroduplex/homoduplex formation in denaturing gradient gels, respectively.[16-21] These methods have been employed in the prenatal diagnosis of such conditions as hemophilias A and B,[22-23] α-1- antitrypsin deficiency,[24-25] β-thalassemia,[26] and cystic fibrosis.[27] Detection rates vary between 30 and 100% depending upon the method, type of nucleotide change present and gel conditions adopted.

Biochemical genetics

Biochemical tests for diagnosis of genetic disorders are based on:

1. identification of abnormal metabolites; or
2. quantitation of abnormal levels of metabolites; or ultimately
3. identification, quantitation and characterization of the defective or deficient gene product that is responsible for the metabolic block.

Biochemically analyzable gene products include proteins and cofactors such as enzymes, receptors, vitamins, hormones, transporters, activators, stabilizers, structural proteins and inhibitors.[28,29] When the underlying biochemical defect is known and is expressed in readily obtainable fetal tissue (chorionic villi), cells (trophoblasts and amniotic fluid cells) or fluid (amniotic fluid supernatant), the test is based on analysis of the enzyme or other protein primarily involved. In other cases, the test is based on the measurement of secondary biochemical events such as elevation, deficiency or absence of a particular metabolite(s).

Family studies

Definitive diagnosis of an inherited metabolic disorder must be based on clear-cut distinction between the values of affected and unaffected fetuses. In the case of an autosomal recessive disorder, the assay employed should be capable of discriminating affected homozygotes or compound heterozygotes from unaffected heterozygotes or wild-type homozygotes. In the case of an autosomal dominant disorder, the assay should discriminate affected homozygotes or heterozygotes from unaffected wild-type homozygotes. Since variability exists among families due to different mutations and different genomic backgrounds, testing of parents, index cases and unaffected siblings can provide information on the respective values of different genotypes within a particular family. In addition to the benefit in interpretation of the results of the prenatal evaluation, tests may also prove to be reliable means for identification of carriers among members of the extended family.

Pseudo-deficiency

Low levels of enzymic activity in apparently healthy individuals (pseudo-deficiency) make prenatal diagnosis a more difficult task. For example, mutations causing deficiency of arylsulfatase A activity have been identified in unaffected members of families with metachromatic leukodystrophy.[30] Mutations responsible for pseudo-deficiency of hexosaminidase A were identified in individuals with carrier levels of hexosaminidase A.[31]

Prenatal diagnosis cannot be made in such families on tissue or cell extracts but is possible by loading tests that are based on growing intact cells in culture in the presence of the appropriate substrate or its precursor.[32]

Carrier detection

Screening for carriers is usually limited to populations at high risk for a diagnosable disease. Carrier detection for Tay–Sachs disease is routinely offered to all individuals of Ashkenazi Jewish descent, in whom the combined frequency for two common mutations in the α-chain gene of hexosaminidases is 1 in 31. The ultimate benefit of carrier detection programs is the identification of couples at risk prior to having an affected child.[33]

Autosomal dominant conditions

Assays for detection of autosomal dominant diseases such as some of the porphyrias[34] are usually capable of identifying affected homozygotes but sometimes fail to differentiate conclusively affected heterozygotes from unaffected fetuses. Overlap between the normal and heterozygous ranges for enzyme activities are common in most assay systems. This is due in part to variability in assay conditions but mainly to the wide variation found for almost any activity in the normal population. Consequently, the demonstration of decreased enzyme activities compatible with heterozygous forms of autosomal dominant porphyria usually is not considered an indication for termination of pregnancy. Decreased enzyme activities which are consistent with homozygous forms of dominant porphyria might be considered an indication for termination of pregnancy because of their more severe clinical course.

X-linked conditions

X-linked disorders present some specific difficulties in heterozygote detection. Recessive and dominant inheritance refer only to expression of the gene in females and this is often highly variable due to random X inactivation.[35] Depending on the proportions of active mutant and normal X chromosomes in the tissues that are involved in the pathogenesis of the disease, a woman heterozygous for Fabry disease, for example, may be clinically normal or she may have mild or even severe manifestations of the disease.[36] Males, on the other hand, have only one X chromosome and they are either hemizygote affected (with deficient enzyme activity) or hemizygote normal (with activity within the normal range).

Enzyme preparations

Prenatal diagnosis of an enzymic defect may be made by direct assay of fetal tissue or cells when:

1. the particular enzyme is the product of the gene in question; and
2. is expressed in the fetal specimen to be analyzed.

Direct demonstration of abnormality, or deficiency, of the gene (molecular techniques) or the gene product (biochemical techniques) are the preferred diagnostic approaches. Enzyme assays can be performed frequently on tissue and cell extracts but, in some cases, assays must be performed on live cells in culture.[37]

Tissue and cell extracts are prepared by homogenization and sonication, respectively. The duration and intensity of these extracting procedures should be adjusted, depending on the nature of the enzyme to be analyzed. Membranous enzymes, e.g. glucocerebrosidase (Gaucher disease), require effective extraction that is often aided by the use of detergents. Using fresh chorionic villus tissue and freshly harvested trophoblasts and amniotic fluid cells helps to preserve the activity of labile enzymes.[38]

Assay conditions

Assay conditions need to be stringent with respect to optimum pH, incubation time, protein concentration in the enzyme preparations etc., and these should be established for each assay system and for each tissue, cell or fluid type. A typical test consists of duplicates of reaction mixtures containing appropriate dilutions of enzyme preparations from the fetus in question and from at least one normal control. Following incubation, the reactions are terminated and the product is quantitated directly or after its isolation.

Separation and detection methods

Elevated concentrations of amino acids and organic acids in amniotic fluid serve as preliminary indications for several inherited disorders such as amino and organic acidopathies and urea cycle defects. In most cases, however, final diagnosis is made by measuring the actual gene product responsible for the metabolic block. Identification and quantitation of amino acids and organic acids in physiological fluids and in reaction mixtures are performed on amino acid analyzer and gas chromatograph, respectively. Quantities are determined by the ratio between the peak area revealed in the sample and that of the same compound in a calibration mixture of known concentrations. Internal standards are used to correct for any inaccuracies in the amount of sample injected into the instrument. Organic acids need to be extracted and derivatized prior to their separation and quantitation by gas chromatography.

Some natural products of enzymic reactions can be quantitated directly, or following their isolation from the reaction mixtures, based on their physicochemical properties. In other systems substrates are tagged with a colored group, a fluorescent group, or a radioactive group, and thus provide tagged products that can be detected by sensitive colorimetric, fluorometric or radiometric assays, respectively. For example, detection of galactosemia is based on direct measurement of the fluorescence of the reduced natural electron acceptor, NADPH, using a fluorimeter.[39]

Non-enzymic defects

Detection of non-enzymic proteins such as receptors, transporters and activators is more complex than direct enzyme assays in tissue or cell extracts, and usually requires the use of intact cells in culture. Cell cultures have some advantages including the ability to incorporate radioactive precursors, the ability to carry out repeated studies, and the relative ease with which comparative studies can be performed on different patient and control cell lines.

The development of methods for quantitative assessment of the low density lipoprotein (LDL) receptor in cultured cells permitted the prenatal diagnosis of fetuses homozygous for the autosomal dominant disease, familial hypercholesterolemia.[40] Several tests are available for quantitation of the receptor activity, including measurement of the cell surface binding and intracellular uptake of ^{125}I-labeled LDL. In addition, the number of LDL receptors can be determined by immunoblotting or immunoprecipitation of ^{35}S-labeled receptors after supplementing the cell culture with [^{35}S]methionine.

It should be noted, however, that the feasibility of making prenatal diagnosis has been established only for the severe, receptor-negative homozygous familial hypercholesterolemia. It has not yet been established that the diagnosis can be reliably made in those familial hypercholesterolemia homozygotes with the less severe form who have some detectable receptor activity (5–30% of normal). It is unlikely that such homozygotes can be distinguished with sufficient certainty from heterozygotes.

Cystinosis, an autosomal recessive lysosomal storage disease in which cystine accumulation is presumably the result of defective transport across the lysosomal membrane, can be diagnosed prenatally by pulse labeling of cultured cells with [^{35}S]cystine or even by direct measurement of cystine content in chorionic villi.[41]

Cytogenetics

Fetal chromosome analysis may be indicated for advanced maternal age, previous offspring with a chromosomal abnormality, abnormalities of maternal serum biochemical screening, family history of a chromosomal abnormality, detection of abnormalities on ultrasound, exposure to known mutagens or carcinogens, parental anxiety and to confirm the sex of the fetus in X-linked genetic disorders. Cell culture for prenatal cytogenetic studies may be derived from amniotic fluid cells, chorionic villi, and fetal blood obtained by percutaneous umbilical sampling.

Chromosome visualization

In general, cytogenetic analysis involves the examination of dividing cells by blocking cellular division in, or before, metaphase with colchicine, the most commonly used inhibitor of spindle cell formation. Subsequent processing includes treatment with a hypotonic solution at 37°C to swell the cells followed by a series of fixations to preserve the cells and enhance the morphology of the chromosomes.

Staining and banding of the chromosomes is very important to cytogenetic analysis. After appropriate aging and pretreatments, the slides are stained to allow for identification of individual chromosomes and a microscopic analysis is performed. Routine chromosome analysis uses G-banding (trypsin-Giemsa staining) or Q-banding (quinacrine fluorescence staining) or both, which produce differential staining/banding along the chromosomes. Approximately 400–550+ bands resolution level can be obtained by applying these methods. Other staining methods such as C-banding, NOR staining, or T-banding are available for special clinical applications.

Chromosome classification

A brief guide to the 'essentials of chromosomology' is on page 73, Chapter 1.7. Of the 23 homologous pairs (46 chromosomes) found in normal human cells, 22 pairs are the same in both females and males (autosomes). The autosomes are numbered from 1 (the largest) to 22 (the smallest). The twenty-third pair comprise the sex chromosomes, (XX or XY).

Chromosomes are classified according to their lengths, position of the centromere and banding characteristics. Chromosomes have two arms divided by the centromere; the short arm is called p (for petit) and the long arm is called q. When the centromere is located at or near the middle of the chromosome, the chromosome is termed metacentric. When the centromere is located at or near the upper two-thirds of the chromosome, the term submetacentric is applied. If the centromere is located very close to one end of the chromosome, it is known as acrocentric. Each chromosome arm is divided into regions and each region is subdivided into bands. Each homolog has a landmark banding pattern which permits the identification of individual chromosomes.

Chromosomes are cut out from a photographic print or a computer video image and arranged by their matching pairs (karyotype) according to the International System for Human Cytogenetic Nomenclature (Fig. 3.5.5).

Cell culture and karyotypic determination of amniotic fluid

Amniotic fluid containing viable cells arising from the skin, amnion, urogenital, respiratory and alimentary systems can be cultured to give rise to large cell populations for cytogenetic, biochemical, or DNA testing. The optimum gestational age to obtain the amniotic fluid through amniocentesis is 15–18 weeks. A sample of 20 ml of fluid is a reasonable volume for cytogenetic analysis. It is very

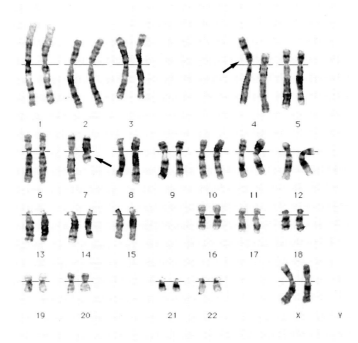

Fig. 3.5.5 *46,XX,t(4;7)(p15;q21). Female karyotype with a translocation between the short arm of chromosome 4 and the long arm of chromosome 7 (arrows).*

important to discard the first 2 ml of amniotic fluid drawn to avoid maternal cell contamination and to split the specimen between two plastic, screw-capped, sterile 15-ml centrifuge tubes, stored at room temperature and sent to the cytogenetic laboratory as soon as possible. The sample must not be frozen or refrigerated. Appropriate clinical and family history, gestational age and indication for study are required to correctly process the specimen.

Amniocentesis samples are subjected to visual inspection, volume measurement, and immediate culture. In the cytogenetics laboratory, the amniotic fluid is centrifuged to separate the amniocytes (pellet) from the fluid. Between 2 and 4 ml of amniotic fluid supernatant is removed and sent for alpha-fetoprotein and/or acetylcholinesterase testing. The pellet is resuspended with Chang/MEM alpha medium (nutrient)[43] and processed for long-term culture using the *in situ* (colony) method[44–45] or the monolayer (flask) method or both. The *in situ* coverslip method is recommended as the preferred technique for culturing amniotic fluid cells for chromosome analysis. The number of culture vessels will depend on the size of the pellet and the gestational age of the sample. Cultures are incubated undisturbed at 37°C with 5% CO_2 for 3–5 days after which they are examined for cellular attachment and cell growth. Harvest for chromosome analysis depends on cell growth and is usually performed after an incubation of 5–10 days. Coverslip cultures (*in situ* method) require no trypsinization (dislodge the cells from surface of the culture

flask) and can be harvested for chromosome analysis as soon as a sufficient number of colonies/cells have grown. Anticondensing agents such as ethidium bromide can be added during the final period of culture. Cells are arrested in mitosis with a spindle inhibitor (colcemid), swollen with hypotonic solution and fixed. The coverslips are placed in a drying hood with 57% humidity and a stream of air to help the spreading of the chromosome. The slides are placed in a drying oven for 2–24 h. The slides can be stained for cytogenetics analysis using the G-banding method or other banding methods. In most cases, the chromosome results are available within 7–10 days.

Cell culture and karyotypic determination of chorionic villus sampling

Chorionic villus sampling (CVS) is a prenatal procedure in which a small amount of tissue from the placenta is collected transvaginally or transabdominally and processed for chromosome, enzymatic, or DNA analysis.[46] Unlike amniotic fluid samples, which require culturing for a few days prior to chromosome harvest, CVS contains spontaneously dividing cells which can be processed for chromosome analysis within 24 h after obtaining the sample (direct preparation). The optimum gestational age to obtain the CVS is 9–12 weeks. A 15–20 mg sample of villi is required for cytogenetic analysis. After removing any blood or blood clots, the villi should be collected in a 15 ml conical centrifuge tube containing 10 ml of transport medium supplemented with heparin and transported to the laboratory at room temperature as soon as possible. The sample must not be frozen or refrigerated.

CVSs are examined microscopically prior to culture to distinguish villi from non-villi material. The villi are carefully cleaned to remove all blood clots and decidua avoiding maternal cell contamination. After the sample is cleaned, the villi are dissociated to obtain a single cell suspension and processed either directly on coverslips (*in situ* method) or in a culture flask for short-term and long-term cultures. Short-term harvests (direct) are attempted when sample volume is sufficient. Cultures are incubated undisturbed at 37°C with 5% CO_2 for 3–5 days after which they are examined for cell growth. Harvests for chromosome analysis are usually obtained after 4–7 days. After treatment with hypotonic solution, followed by a series of fixations, the coverslips are placed in a stream of air to aid the spreading of the chromosome. Chromosome analysis is routinely performed using the G-banding method to ascertain the chromosomal complement of the fetus. In 95% of cases, the chromosome results are available within 8 days. About 1–2% of CVSs show mosaicism and only a very small percentage of these are true fetal mosaicism.[47]

Cell culture and karyotypic determination of fetal blood sample

Percutaneous umbilical blood sample (PUBS) can be used for cytogenetic analysis in special cases when the chromosome results from the amniotic fluid are ambiguous and mosaicism is suspected. The PUBS procedure involves obtaining a small amount (0.5–1 ml) of fetal blood from the umbilical cord to ascertain fetal chromosome complement. The blood should be collected into a sodium heparinized tube at room temperature and sent to the cytogenetic laboratory as soon as possible. The sample must not be frozen.

Fetal blood is cultured for 48–72 h in the presence of a mitogen (phytohemagglutinin), a plant derivative which stimulates the lymphocytes to undergo division. Cells are arrested in mitosis with a spindle inhibitor (colcemid), swollen with hypotonic solution (KCl), fixed and placed on slides. After appropriate slides pretreatments, the slides can be stained by the G-banding method or Q-banding method or both prior to microscopic analysis to ascertain fetal chromosome complement. The chromosome results are available within 48–96 h.

FUTURE PERSPECTIVES

The advanced tools of molecular genetics will continue to improve our understanding of many diseases. A partial list of genetic diseases now amenable to prenatal molecular diagnosis includes: cystic fibrosis, fragile X syndrome, Duchenne/Becker muscular dystrophy, hemophilias A and B, myotonic dystrophy, congenital adrenal hyperplasia, Gaucher disease, Tay–Sachs disease, and the hemoglobinopathies. The sensitivity and specificity of molecular genetic diagnoses are astounding: if the specific mutation has been defined for a disease or an individual family, the result is clear-cut. An understanding of the molecular heterogeneity underlying specific phenotypes allows one to design the most appropriate test for a given situation.

The development of the polymerase chain reaction, increasingly sophisticated electrophoretic methods, positional cloning, recognition of new genetic causes of human disease such as triplet repeats, uniparental disomy, and genetic imprinting all have direct and immediate impact on the practice of reproductive genetics. This new DNA technology has resulted in more definitive diagnosis, utility with extremely small samples, rapid analysis and reporting of results. As increasing numbers of genes are cloned, new techniques, such as solid phase methods and robotics, will allow the routine use of automated, non-radioactive methodologies.

Application of these DNA methods presently allows contemplation of diagnoses based on single cells – fetal cells from maternal blood, or preimplantation genetics. Molecular diagnosis can also replace biochemical diagnosis in informative cases in which the precise mutations are known or when informative linkages have been established in family studies. Molecular diagnosis has the advantage of not requiring that the gene product be expressed in the fetal tissue or cells to be examined, but is impractical, in many instances, to detect all possible mutations directly in the genomic DNA. On the other hand, when available, a single biochemical test can detect the outcome of all the mutations that result in absent, deficient, or defective gene product.

Biochemical diagnostic tests will be expanded to include more non-enzymic entities such as defects in structural proteins, activator proteins, receptors and ion channels. Prenatal biochemical diagnosis will also be established in tissues obtained by procedures other than amniocentesis and chorionic villus sampling. These include fetal blood sampling and the non-invasive isolation of fetal cells from the maternal circulation.

Prenatal detection of chromosomal abnormalities (classical cytogenetics) at the present time relies on analysis of banded metaphases obtained from cell culture of amniotic fluid, chorionic villus and percutaneous umbilical blood sample. Such analysis is reliable for detection of structural and numerical chromosomal abnormalities. The development of exciting new molecular cytogenetic techniques such as chromosomal painting and fluorescent *in situ* hybridization (FISH) permits the expeditious diagnosis of familial translocations, rapid detection of aneuploides, and recognition of microdeletion syndromes such as DiGeorge syndrome. These methods will continue to unlock and identify the lineage of marker chromosomes which can not be identified by classical cytogenetics.

SUMMARY

- Molecular prenatal diagnosis is particular and specific to each disease entity, characterizing the absence or presence of the mutation at the level of the gene.
- DNA diagnosis is possible on scant amounts of tissue (DNA), post-mortem samples, e.g. paraffin-embedded tissue, as well as blood, amniocytes and chorionic villi. Preparation, anticoagulant and sample handling are specific to each laboratory.
- The continued technologic explosion allows for increased sensitivity, specificity, accuracy, rapidity, and diversity of methods in the prenatal diagnosis of genetic disorders.
- Biochemical diagnostic tests are based on quantitation and characterization of the defective or deficient protein which is the product of the mutant allele or quantitation and characterization of metabolites affected by it.
- Prenatal biochemical diagnosis is available when the underlying metabolic defect is known and is expressed in readily obtainable fetal tissue, cells, or fluid.
- Accurate and reliable biochemical diagnosis must clearly distinguish between values of affected and unaffected fetuses, and ideally should be capable of detecting their genotypes.
- Cytogenetic analysis may be performed on almost any fresh tissue, e.g. skin, brain, muscle, renal epithelia, lung, and not only on blood, amniocytes, and chorionic villi.
- Karyotypic analysis is a labor-intensive procedure requiring up to 10 days for results, although with the new molecular cytogenetic techniques on the horizon, turn around times may be dramatically reduced.
- Cytogenetic analysis requires the growth and replication of cells, hence chromosomes; therefore, samples should never be frozen.
- The family history, ethnicity, and intrafamilial relationships are critical for accurate diagnoses.

REFERENCES

1. Lawn RM, Efstratiadis A, O'Connell C, Maniatis T. The nucleotide sequence of the human β-globin gene. *Cell* 1980 **21**: 647–651.
2. Southern EM. Detection of specific sequences among DNA fragments separated by gel electrophoresis. *J Mol Biol* 1975 **98**: 503–517.
3. Oostra BA, Jacky PB, Brown WT, Rousseau F. Guidelines for the diagnosis of fragile X syndrome. *J Med Genet* 1993 **30**: 410–413.
4. Fu PH, Kuhl DP, Pizzuti A, Pieretti M, Sutcliffe JS, Richards S *et al.* Variation of the CGG repeat at the fragile X site results in genetic instability: resolution of the Sherman Paradox. *Cell* 1991 **67**: 1047–1058.
5. Warren ST, Nelson DL. Advances in molecular analysis of fragile X syndrome. (Special Communication). *JAMA* 1994 **271**: 536–542.
6. Mullis KB. The unusual origin of the polymerase chain reaction. *Sci Am*, 1990, April: 56–65.
7. Mullis KB, Faloona FA. Specific synthesis of DNA *in vitro* via a polymerase-catalyzed chain reaction. *Methods Enzymol* 1987 **155**: 335.
8. Saiki RK, Scharf S, Faloona F, Mullis KB, Horn GT, Erlich HA, Arnheim N. Enzymatic amplification of β-globin genomic sequences and restriction site analysis for diagnosis of sickle cell anemia. *Science* 1985 **230**: 1350–1354.
9. Beggs AH, Koenig M, Boyce FM, Kunkel LM. Detection of 98% of DMD/BMD gene deletions by polymerase chain reaction. *Hum Genet* 1990 **86**: 45–48.
10. Hatcher SLS, Trang QT, Robb KM, Teplitz R, Carlson JR. Prenatal diagnosis by enzymatic amplification and restriction endonuclease digestion for detection of haemoglobins A, S and C. *Mol Cell Probes* 1992 **6**: 343–348.
11. Friedman KJ, Highsmith WE Jr, Prior TW, Perry TR, Silverman LM. Cystic fibrosis deletion mutation detected by PCR-mediated site-directed mutagenesis. *Clin Chem* 1990 **36**: 695–696.
12. Conner BJ, Reyes AA, Morin C, Itakura K, Teplitz RL, Wallace RB. Detection of sickle cell βS-globin allele by hybridization with synthetic oligonucleotides. *Proc Natl Acad Sci USA* 1983 **80**: 278–282.
13. Saiki RK, Walsh S, Levenson CH, Erlich HA. Genetic analysis of amplified DNA with immobilized sequence-specific oligonucleotide probes. *Proc Natl Acad Sci USA* 1989 **86**: 6230–6234.
14. Chehab FF, Wall J. Detection of multiple cystic fibrosis mutations by reverse dot blot hybridization: a technology for carrier screening. *Hum Genet* 1992 **89**: 163–168.
15. Maxam AM, Gilbert W. A new method for sequencing DNA. *Proc Natl Acad Sci USA* 1977 **74**: 560.
16. Sekiya T. Detection of mutant sequences by single-strand conformation polymorphism analysis. *Mutat Res* 1993 **288**: 79–83.
17. Cotton RG, Rodrigues NR, Campbell RD. Reactivity of cytosine and thymine in single-base-pair mechanisms with hydroxylamine and osmium tetroxide and its application to the study of mutation. *Proc Natl Acad Sci USA* 1988 **85**: 4397–4401.
18. Smooker PM, Cotton GH. The use of chemical reagents in the detection of DNA mutations. *Mutat Res* 1993 **288**: 65–77.
19. Rossiter BJF, Caskey CT. Molecular scanning methods of mutation detection. (Mini-review). *J Biol Chem* 1990 **265**: 12753–12756.
20. Fan E, Levin DB, Glickman BW, Logan DM. Limitations in the use of SSCP analysis. *Mutat Res* 1993 **288**: 85–92.
21. Myers RM, Lumelsky N, Lerman LS, Maniatis T. Detection of single base substitutions in total genomic DNA. *Nature* 1985 **313**: 459–468.
22. Schwartz M, Cooper DN, Millar DS, Kakkar VV, Scheibel E. Prenatal exclusion of haemophilia A and carrier testing by direct detection of a disease lesion. *Prenat Diagn* 1992 **12**: 861–866.

23. Caprino D, Acquila M, Mori PG. Carrier detection and prenatal diagnosis of hemophilia B with more advanced techniques. *Ann Hematol* 1993 **67**: 289–293.

24. Dubel JR, Fenwick R, Hejtmancik JF. Denaturing gradient gel electrophoresis of the alpha 1-antitrypsin gene: application to prenatal diagnosis. *Am J Med Genet* 1991 **41**: 39–43.

25. Forrest SM, Dry PJ, Cotton RGH. Use of the chemical cleavage of mismatch method for prenatal diagnosis of alpha-1-antitrypsin deficiency. *Prenat Diagn* 1992 **12**: 133–137.

26. Ghanem N, Girodon E, Vidaud M, Martin J, Fanen P, Plassa F, Goossens M. A comprehensive scanning method for rapid detection of beta- globin gene mutations and polymorphisms. *Hum Mutat* 1992 **1**: 229–239.

27. Desgeorges M, Boulot P, Kjellberg P, Lefort G, Rolland M, Demaille J, Claustres M. Prenatal diagnosis for cystic fibrosis using SSCP analysis [letter]. *Prenat Diagn* 1993 **13**: 147–148.

28. Scriver CR, Beaudet AL, Sly WS, Valle D (eds). *The Metabolic Basis of Inherited Disease*, 6th edn, Vols 1 and 2. New York: McGraw-Hill, 1989.

29. McKusick VA. *Mendelian Inheritance in Man*, 10th edn. Baltimore: Johns Hopkins University Press, 1992.

31. Penzien JM, Kappler J, Herschkowitz N, Schuknecht B, Leinekugel P, Propping P *et al*. Compound heterozygosity for metachromatic leukodystrophy and arylsulfatase A pseudodeficiency alleles is not associated with progressive neurological disease. *Am J Hum Genet* 1993 **52**: 557–564.

32. Cao Z, Natowicz MR, Kaback MM, Lim-Steele JST, Prence EM, Brown D, Chabot T, Triggs-Raine BL. A second mutation associated with apparent β-hexosaminidase A pseudodeficiency: identification and frequency estimation. *Am J Hum Genet* 1993 **53**: 1198–1205.

33. Kudeh T, Wenger DA. Diagnosis of metachromatic leukodystrophy, Krabbe disease, and Farber disease after uptake of fatty acid-labeled cerebroside sulfate into cultured skin fibroblasts. *J Clin Invest* 1982 **70**: 89–97.

34. Kaback MM, Lim-Steele J, Dabholkar D, Brown D, Levy N, Zeiger K. Tay–Sachs disease – carrier screening, prenatal diagnosis, and the molecular era. *JAMA* 1993 **270**: 2307–2315.

35. Grandchamp B, Deybach JC, Grelier M, de Verneuil H, Nordmann Y. Studies of porphyrin synthesis in fibroblasts of patients with congenital erythropoietic porphyria and one patient with homozygous coproporphyria. *Biochim Biophys Acta* 1980 **629**: 577–586.

35. Lyon MF. Possible mechanisms of X chromosome inactivation. *Nature* 1971 **232**: 229–232.

36. Broadbent JC, Edwards WD, Gordon H, Hartzler GO, Krawisz JE. Fabry cardiomyopathy in the female confirmed by endomyocardial biopsy. *Mayo Clin Proc* 1981 **56**: 623–628.

37. Ben-Yoseph Y, Mitchell DA. Detection of kinetically abnormal argininosuccinate synthase in neonatal citrullinemia by conversion of citrulline to arginine in intact fibroblasts. *Clin Chim Acta* 1989 **183**: 125–134.

38. Ben-Yoseph Y, Evans MI, Bottoms SF, Pack BA, Mitchell DA, Koppitch FC, Nadler HL. Lysosomal enzyme activities in fresh and frozen chorionic villi and in cultured trophoblasts. *Clin Chim Acta* **161**: 307–313.

39. Copenhaver JH, Bausch LC, Fitzgibbons JF. A fluorometric procedure for estimation of galactose-1-phosphate uridyltransferase activity in red blood cells. *Anal Biochem* 1969 **30**: 327–328.

40. Goldstein JL, Basu SK, Brown MS. Receptor-mediated endocytosis of low density lipoprotein in cultured cells. *Methods Enzymol* 1983 **98**: 241–260.

41. Gahl WA, Dorfmann A, Evans MI, Karson EM, Landsberger EJ, Fabro SE, Schulman JD. Chorionic biopsy in the prenatal diagnosis of nephropathic cystinosis. In Fraccaro M, Simoni G, Brambati G (eds) *First Trimester Fetal Diagnosis*. Berlin: Springer-Verlag, 1985: 260–265.

42. ISCN. In Harnden DG, Klinger HP (eds) *An International System for Human Cytogenetic Nomenclature*. Basel: Karger, 1985.

43. Chang HC, Jones OW. Amniocentesis: cell culture of human amniotic fluid in a hormone supplement. In Sato GH, Pardee AB, Sirbasku DA (eds) *Growth of Cells in Hormonally Defined Media*. Cold Springs Harbor Conferences on Cell Proliferation. 1982: B1187-1192.

44. Hecht F, Peakman DC, Kaiser-McCaw B, Robinson A. Amniocyte clones for prenatal cytogenetics. *Am J Med Genet*, 1981 **10**: 51–54.

45. Spurbeck JL, Carlson RO, Allen JE, Dewald GW. Culturing and robotic harvesting of bone marrow, lymph nodes, peripheral blood, fibroblasts, and solid tumors with the *in situ* techniques. *Cancer Genet Cytogenet* 1988 **32**: 59–66.

46. Evans MI. *Reproductive Risks and Prenatal Diagnosis*. Norwalk: Appleton and Lange, 1992.

47. Mikkelsen M, Ayme S. Chromosomal finding in chorionic villi: a collaborative study. In Vogel F, Sperling K (eds) *Human Genetics*. New York: Springer-Verlag, 1987: 598–606.

3.6

The Placenta

J Kingdom and C Sibley

INTRODUCTION

The placenta has a multiplicity of functions essential to the birth, at term, of a normal baby. It follows that, in pathological pregnancy, a proportion of fetal complications must be due to abnormal placental function. However, despite the common use of the term 'placental insufficiency' it remains almost impossible to directly relate a specific fetal complication with a specific placental abnormality. This reflects the still poor state of knowledge concerning placental function and its relationship with fetal growth and development. Recent epidemiological evidence connecting the size of placenta and fetus at birth with health of the individual 50 or more years later[1] makes it even more urgent that this relationship be understood.

This chapter attempts to summarize the current understanding of placental function; although most topics are covered here the reader interested in placental immunology is referred to references 2 and 3 and Chapter 3.3. Textbook facts about the placenta are relatively few and the continuing fluidity of the field must be borne in mind. An important feature of the placenta is the way in which it changes both morphologically and functionally throughout pregnancy so that a snapshot of one particular moment in gestation, typically of the term placenta, is an inadequate basis for the understanding of adverse outcomes in pregnancy, such as severe pre-eclampsia or intrauterine growth restriction (IUGR), which typically result in delivery before 32 weeks of gestation. For this reason we have been careful to present developmental information where such is available.

One final important general consideration is the very great differences in placentation between species, which makes extrapolation from one mammal to another more dangerous for the placenta than for any other organ.[4] Nevertheless, although this chapter will generally confine itself to the human placenta, some data for mammals other than woman will be presented where we believe it to be applicable.

CURRENT CONCEPTS

Implantation and the first trimester

The blastocyst enters the uterine cavity on day 4 postfertilization when it hatches from the zona pellucida. It can remain free-floating here for up to 48 h or so, but then attaches to the endometrial epithelium to begin the process of implantation. At this stage the blastocyst comprises a shell of cytotrophoblast enclosing the inner cell mass (destined to form the embryo) and the fluid-filled blastocoele. The cytotrophoblast in contact with the uterine epithelium fuses to form a syncytial layer (the syncytiotrophoblast). The uterine epithelium is breached and the developing blastocyst becomes enclosed within the stroma beneath the surface of the uterine epithelium. The syncytiotrophoblast enlarges around the blastocyst and, as it invades the stroma, maternal capillaries are engulfed. Lacunar spaces develop within this syncytiotrophoblast layer and these will coalesce to form the intervillous space. Cytotrophoblast cells grow out radially from the blastocyst to form columns between the lacunae; these structures will form the villi of the placenta. Meantime cytotrophoblast cells invade beyond the leading edge of the syncytiotrophoblast where they have two functions: first to form a trophoblastic shell around the blastocyst and secondly to plug the lumina of maternal vessels which have been invaded. These events will have been accomplished by day 14 postconception and are illustrated in Fig. 3.6.1. This stage is when the next menstrual period would have been expected: but the placenta, together with the surrounding stroma, has already initiated key endocrine events to prevent menstruation.

Continued development of the trophoblastic shell

As the trophoblastic shell is formed it breaches larger vessels within the stroma, but these are plugged by the

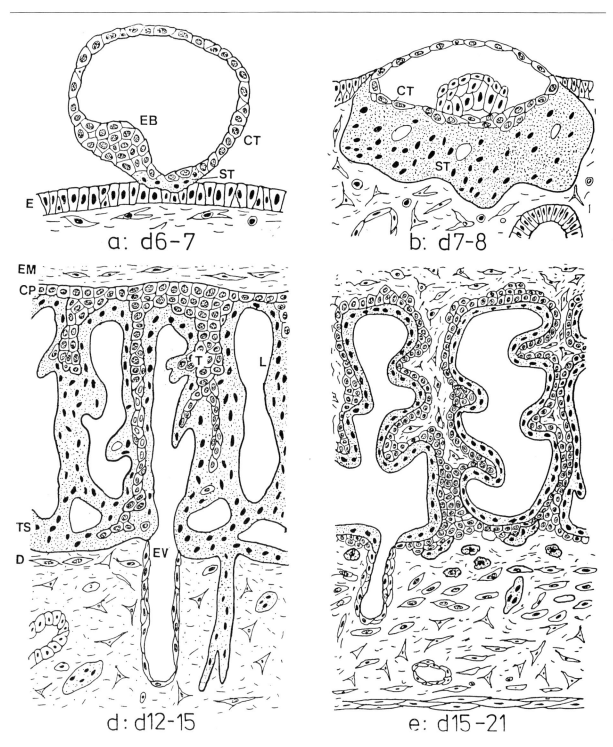

Fig. 3.6.1 *Diagrammatic representation of the typical stages of early placental development.* **(a and b)** *Prelacunar stages;* **(c)** *lacunar stage (on p. 314);* **(d)** *transition from lacunar to primary villous stage;* **(e)** *secondary villous stage;* **(f)** *tertiary villous stage (on p. 314). E, endometrial epithelium; EB, embryoblast; CT, cytotrophoblast; ST, syncytiotrophoblast; EM, extraembryonic mesoderm; CP, chorionic plate; T, trabeculae and primary villi; L, maternal blood lacunae; TS, trophoblastic shell; EV, endometrial vessel; D, decidua; BP, basal plate; PB, placental bed; J, junctional zone. Days in development are postfertilization. (Reproduced with permission from reference 10.) Continued over page.*

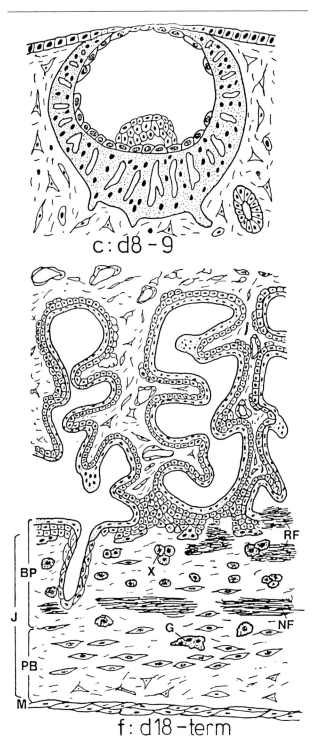

c: d8 - 9

f: d18 - term

Fig. 3.6.1 *continued.*

throughout the period of embryonic development which is completed by 10 weeks of postmenstrual (gestational) age. These histological conclusions are supported by angiographic data[5] and more recently by color flow Doppler ultrasound[6] confirming a lack of intervillous blood flow. An elegant study[7] placing oxygen electrodes in the villous placenta and decidua has demonstrated an oxygen gradient between the two before 10 weeks of gestation; thereafter, the oxygen gradient disappears as maternal spiral arterioles are breached and the intervillous circulation is established.[8]

Embryogenesis therefore takes place in an environment that is relatively hypoxic compared to that of the mother. Failure to plug invaded maternal vessels adequately during early development, with resultant bleeding, may be a mechanism of spontaneous miscarriage.[8] A variant of this process may explain vaginal bleeding at the time of implantation and subsequent episodes of threatened miscarriage; a subchorionic hematoma can occasionally be visualized by ultrasound under these circumstances. Color flow Doppler ultrasound has demonstrated maternal blood flow within the placenta in a proportion of non-viable first trimester pregnancies[6] suggesting a premature rise in oxygen tension within embryonic tissues. Whether this observation could be cause rather than effect in terms of embryo loss is uncertain at present.

Development of the placental villi and the fetoplacental circulation

The central columns of cytotrophoblast cells, covered by syncytiotrophoblast, develop a villous core containing the fetoplacental vessels between days 12 and 21 postfertilization. Central invasion of the villous core by mesenchymal cells derived from the allantoic part of the embryonic disc is followed by the appearance of hemangioblastic cells and the formation of capillaries.[9] By day 28 (6 weeks of gestation) the villi start to be perfused by the fetal circulation. The fetal erythrocytes contain embryonic hemoglobins at this stage, whose properties permit oxygen transfer at low oxygen tension and pH. These villi are the basic structures from which subsequent differentiation and growth take place. For a detailed description of the developing villi the reader is referred to the excellent review by Kaufmann and Burton.[10]

Umbilical artery Doppler

From 7–8 weeks of gestation the umbilical cord can be visualized by color flow Doppler ultrasound. The arterial waveform obtained at this stage is characterized by absent end-diastolic flow velocity (AEDFV);[11] a diastolic component to the umbilical artery waveform appears by 12–14 weeks gestation.[12,13] Thereafter diastolic flow velocity increases progressively towards term.[14] Though several factors (such as cardiac output and blood viscosity) influence the arterial Doppler waveform, the appearance and progressive rise of diastolic flow velocity during normal pregnancy indicates a steady fall in fetoplacental vascular impedance.[15]

extravillous cytotrophoblast cells to prevent hemorrhage from occurring around the implanting blastocyst. The lacunar spaces of the syncytiotrophoblast contain a maternal fluid exudate, rather than blood, and the developing placenta is effectively a barrier between the mother and embryo at this stage. This arrangement persists

Chorionic villus sampling

Abnormalities of chromosome number such as trisomy 21 (Downs syndrome) or of a single gene (such as cystic fibrosis or thalassemia) can be detected in small (typically 20–40 mg) samples of placental villous tissue, obtained using ultrasound guidance after 10 weeks of gestation by one of two routes: transabdominally by needle aspiration, or transcervically using curved biopsy forceps. The latter method is illustrated in Fig. 3.6.2.

The chromosome number is established from rapidly dividing trophoblast cells within 24 hours. The fibroblast cells from the vascular core are grown in explant culture and are stained after about 2 weeks; at this stage G-banding is employed to provide a more accurate assessment of chromosome number and structure (see Chapters 3.4 and 3.5). The latter cells are mesenchymal in origin and therefore reflect the embryo's chromosomal constitution. Occasionally the trophoblast chromosome number is abnormal despite a normal fetal karyotype, a situation referred to as placental mosaicism. This observation is associated with an increased risk of subsequent fetal loss and IUGR.[16] The prenatal diagnosis of single gene disorders is made using DNA extracted from the villi.

The uterine cavity

The developing conceptus is initially embedded within the endometrial stroma, but as it grows in size it begins to bulge centrally into the uterine cavity. The trophoblastic shell which is in contact with the decidua (chorion frondosum) develops into the discoid or mature placenta. That portion of the trophoblastic shell projecting into the uterine cavity (chorion laeve) begins to degenerate and the uterine cavity is finally obliterated by 12 weeks of gestation when the trophoblastic shell comes into contact with the uterine epithelium on the opposite side. The uterine cavity therefore persists during the first trimester and this is of increasing clinical interest since, as has been known for some time, cells of fetal origin can be obtained from within the endocervical canal. Trophoblast cells can be collected by either flushing the cavity or by aspiration and these cells are a potentially 'non-invasive' opportunity for prenatal diagnosis, thus avoiding the 1–2% procedure-related loss from chorionic villous sampling.[17] Techniques such as fluorescent in situ hybridization (FISH) can be used to demonstrate chromosomes 13, 18, 21, X and Y involved in the common aneuploidies[18] and polymerase chain reaction (PCR) amplification of extracted DNA might be capable of detecting single gene disorders such as cystic fibrosis, or fetal blood group in the case of severe red cell allo-immunization[19] (see also Chapters 3.4 and 3.5).

Development of the uteroplacental circulation

Cytotrophoblast cells which migrate from the outer part of the trophoblastic shell into the stroma are known as the

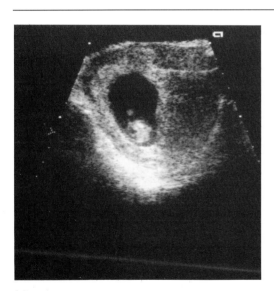

(a)

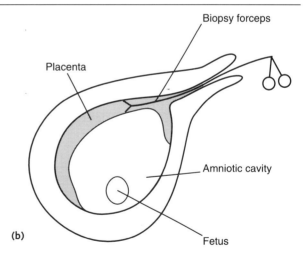

(b)

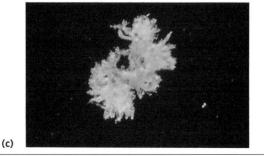

(c)

Fig. 3.6.2 *Transcervical chorionic villus sampling.* **(a and b)** *Transabdominal ultrasound at 10 weeks gestation. The uterus is retroverted and the hyperechoic placenta is anterofundal. The biopsy forceps have entered the placenta and the jaws are open to advance and obtain the sample.* **(c)** *Typical sample of villous placenta. Note the presence of fetal red cells within villous capillaries and the lack of maternal blood contamination since no uteroplacental circulation exists at this gestation (see Plate 4). These samples are excellent for DNA studies. Courtesy of Mr R.H.T. Ward, University College Obstetric Hospital, London.*

extravillous cytotrophoblast. From day 12 postfertilization onwards, these cells begin to invade the capillaries and spiral arterioles of the decidua although this process does not extend into the myometrium until the second trimester. The invasion takes place both intraluminally (initially blocking the vessels, but subsequently replacing the endothelium) and extraluminally (where the arterial medium is replaced).

The second trimester is characterized by invasion of the myometrial portions of the spiral arterioles, converting them into passively dilated channels offering low impedance to blood flow. Maternal cardiac output has increased by over 40% from prepregnant values (Chapter 3.18). The combined effects of these changes are substantial with perhaps a tenfold increase in uteroplacental blood flow to over 500 ml/min. Doppler ultrasound studies of the uterine arteries provide a non-invasive demonstration of these changes. The uterine artery waveform in the prepregnant state and during the first trimester is characterized by low end-diastolic flow velocity and an early dichrotic notch during diastole.[20] However, by 18–20 weeks of gestation the invasion by trophoblast of the uteroplacental arterial vessels results in high diastolic flow velocity and loss of the dichrotic notch (Fig. 3.6.3). This process may fail to occur as discussed on p. 323.

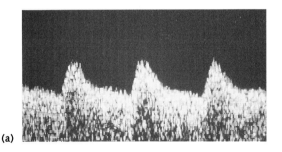

(a)

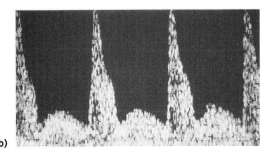

(b)

Fig. 3.6.3 *Doppler ultrasound waveforms from the uterine arteries at 20 weeks' gestation.* **(a)** *Normal waveform demonstrating high end-diastolic velocities and thus low impedance to flow.* **(b)** *Typical abnormal waveform demonstrating an early diastolic notch and low end-diastolic velocities, features associated with high impedance to flow. This observation, particularly if bilateral and persistent at 24 weeks of gestation, is predictive of severe pre-eclampsia and/or IUGR. Courtesy of Dr Susan Bewley, St Thomas's Hospital, London.*

Development of the mature placenta

The uteroplacental circulation is, from an anatomical perspective, largely formed during the first half of gestation. By contrast the fetal villous tree continues to branch and differentiate throughout gestation, a process which probably ensures that the absorptive capacity of the placenta can accommodate the genetically programmed growth potential of the fetus. Placental reserve needs to develop ahead of fetal metabolic requirements in order to avoid hypoxia, lactic acidosis etc. One would therefore expect placental size to increase at least in proportion to that of the fetus, but in fact the opposite is the case – the placental/fetal weight ratio falls as gestation advances.[21] Considerable changes must therefore take place within the placenta to make it an increasingly efficient organ. For hydrophilic solutes this may well involve changes in expression of transport proteins[22] (see also p. 318), but for a gas such as oxygen, transferred by flow-limited simple diffusion, an increased efficiency will predominantly involve ideal maternal and fetal perfusion of the placenta (see p. 318). This concept will now be addressed in detail.

The villous tree

The functional unit within the placenta is the placentome consisting of a fetal villous tree arising from the chorionic plate, perfused centrifugally by a maternal spiral artery. The umbilical arteries ramify across the chorionic plate, penetrating it in about 50 places to start individual villous trees. This basic structure of the fetal placenta is established during the first trimester, with subsequent development being one of growth and differentiation of the individual placentomes. The developmental anatomy of the villous tree is highly complex – a brief description follows and the reader is referred to reference 23 for more detailed information.

The branching pattern within the placentome is illustrated in Fig. 3.6.4. The rami and ramuli chorii represent the muscularized stem villous vessels, often referred to in the clinical literature as primary, secondary and tertiary stem vessels as discussed on p. 323. The development of the villous tree during early gestation takes place by proliferation of the immature intermediate villus forming new generations of muscularized stem villi. Subsequent growth during later gestation is directed towards formation of mature intermediate and terminal villi. Since the latter structures, from morphological appearance, appear to offer little impedance to blood flow[24] the observed increase in fetoplacental blood flow as pregnancy advances (and accompanying change in the umbilical artery Doppler waveform)[15] probably occurs largely as a result of these changes. It is likely that the terminal villi are the major sites of gas and nutrient exchange but this remains to be proved physiologically.

Control of fetoplacental blood flow

In contrast to the adult arrangement, blood leaving the right ventricle of the fetal heart is diverted from the lungs

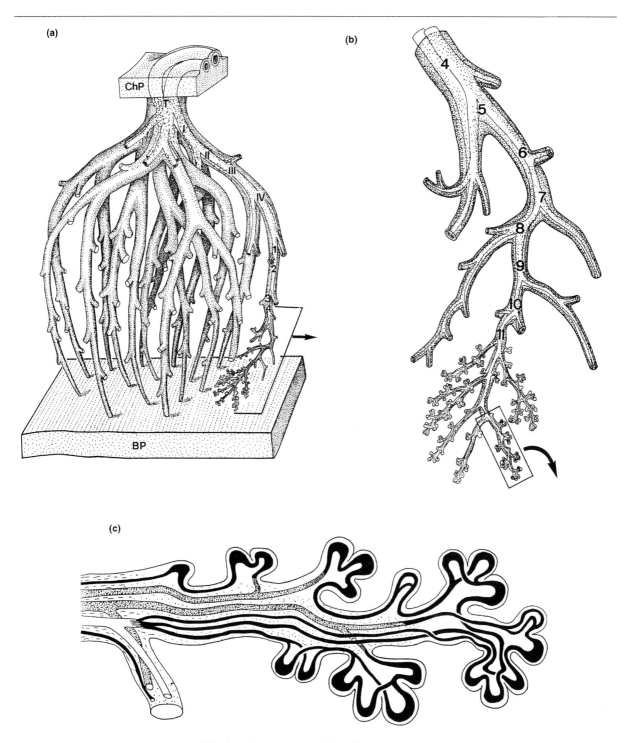

Fig. 3.6.4 *Diagrammatic representation of the branching patterns of the villous tree.* **(a** *and* **b)** *ChP, chorionic plate; BP, basal plate; T, trunchus chorii; I–IV, four generations of rami; 1–11 eleven generations of ramuli. The vessels are shown within the villous tree.* **(c)** *Fetal vessel architecture of an ending stem villus of the last ramulus (line hatched) and a terminal convolute composed of one mature intermediate villus (lightly point shaded) together with its terminal villi (unshaded). Arterioles are point shaded, capillaries are black and venules are unshaded. Note the long capillary loops supplying several terminal villi in series. Terminal villi are abnormally formed and reduced in number in placentae from IUGR pregnancies requiring elective preterm delivery in the fetal interest (see text). (Reproduced with permission from reference 15.)*

to the lower body via the ductus arteriosus. About 40% of aortic blood flow enters the umbilical arteries at term which implies that impedance to blood flow is low compared with the fetal systemic circulation.[25] The fetoplacental circulation is unique since it lacks autonomic innervation[26] and thus the low impedance at term must be conferred either through the anatomical maturation of the villous tree mentioned earlier, or by alterations in the vasomotor control of the smooth muscle cells surrounding the stem villous arterioles.

Vasomotor control

Placental perfusion experiments, pioneered by Panigel[27] have demonstrated that a variety of substances can alter vascular tone within the fetoplacental circulation. Some of these are made locally and may have a paracrine action, whereas others act systemically. The importance of paracrine regulation of vascular tone is increasingly recognized.[28,29] Prostacyclin, the predominant endothelial metabolite of the arachidonic acid pathway, has both anticoagulant and vasodilator properties. However, the physiological role of prostacyclin as a vasodilator within the fetoplacental circulation is questioned since inhibition of synthesis does not raise vascular tone.[30,31] More recently the vascular endothelium has been shown to possess the enzyme nitric oxide synthase (NOS)[32] allowing the local generation of nitric oxide (NO). Evidence of a physiological role for NO in the regulation of vascular tone is more convincing than for prostacyclin.[33] However, it is important to emphasize that the magnitude of NO-mediated relaxation in isolated rings of fetoplacental vessels is much less than in systemic vessels, and some groups have been unable to demonstrate endothelium-dependent relaxation in umbilical cord and chorionic plate vessels.[34,35]

One explanation is that flow-mediated release of NO is more important in the fetoplacental vessels than is receptor-mediated release,[36] the former being demonstrable by placental perfusion.[33] More recent immunohistochemical studies demonstrate the presence of NOS in the umbilical cord and chorionic plate vessels, but with less staining more distally.[37,38] These studies demonstrate strong staining for NOS in the villous syncytiotrophoblast, and thus placental production of NO into the intervillous space (where it may act as an anticoagulant) may be more important than its effects on fetoplacental vascular impedance.

Endothelial cells in addition produce the peptide endothelin (principally endothelin-1) which produces powerful and sustained vasoconstriction.[39,40] The application of ultrastructural immunohistochemical techniques has also demonstrated a large variety of vasoactive substances within endothelial cells of the umbilical cord vessels including substance P, serotonin, ATP, atrial natriuretic peptide and neuropeptide Y[41] but their physiological roles remain unclear. One complicating factor is the heterogeneity of endothelial cells. Another problem is that the necessary *in situ* vasomotor studies, conducted at the level of the small (<90 μm) stem villous arterioles have not as yet been performed. In the authors' opinion the principal functions of these local vasomotor mechanisms, as in the lung, is to

optimize maternal/fetal perfusion overlap – if a villous tree was underperfused on the maternal side, the local effects of hypoxia within the villous tree (reduced NO production, increased endothelin production) would tend to favor vasoconstriction thereby diverting fetoplacental blood to better perfused villous trees. Such a regulatory mechanism would be reversible and therefore serve to keep overall perfusion mismatch to a minimum. Vasomotor control is discussed in more detail by Macara *et al.*[15]

Mechanisms of maternal–fetal exchange across the placenta

Exchange of solutes and water between mother and fetus across the placenta occurs between maternal plasma in the intervillous space and fetal plasma in the capillaries of the villous core (Fig. 3.6.5). Although it is often assumed that most exchange takes place at the level of the terminal villi, because at term these have the shortest distance between capillary and intervillous space and the greatest total surface area,[42] there is no direct evidence that this is true for all solutes. Furthermore, in the first trimester terminal villi have not yet formed[10] (see also above).

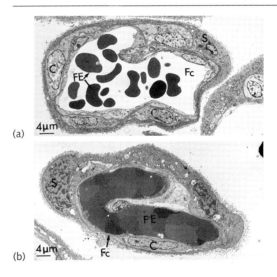

Fig. 3.6.5 (a) *Transmission electron micrographs of a terminal villus from a control.* **(b)** *An IUGR placenta with AEDFV, in other words absent end-diastolic flow velocity in the umbilical artery. There was an increased number of syncytial nuclei in the IUGR villi which were aggregated into syncytial knots. With the fetal capillaries of the IUGR terminal villi there was evidence of antenatal congestion with moulding of the fetal erythrocytes and lysis of the erythrocyte cell membrane.* **S**, *syncytial trophoblast;* **C**, *cytotrophoblast cells,* **FC**, *fetal capillary;* **FE**, *fetal erythrocyte. (From reference 118 with permission.)*

For many biologically important substances the precise mechanism by which they cross the placenta from fetus to mother and vice versa is uncertain, although in several cases individual components of the transfer mechanism have been elucidated. The aim of the following section is to provide an overview of possible mechanisms of transplacental transfer using, as examples, solutes for which the mechanism is fairly well determined. A detailed review of the current knowledge concerning a broad range of substances is provided by Morriss *et al.*[43]

Diffusion

Any solute for which there is a concentration gradient between maternal and fetal plasma at the level of the exchange barrier will show net diffusion across the placenta in the direction dictated by which compartment has the highest concentration. The net rate of diffusion (J_{net}) will be dependent on the properties of the placenta and of the solute in question as described by application of Fick's Law of diffusion:

$$J_{net} = PS\,(C_m - C_f)\ \text{mol s}^{-1}\,\text{g}^{-1}\ \text{placenta} \qquad (3.6.1)$$

where P is the placental permeability, equal to the free diffusion coefficient in water of the solute divided by the diffusion path length between capillary and intervillous space, S is the surface area available for diffusion between the two circulations within 1g of placenta, and C_m and C_f are the mean plasma solute concentrations of the unbound solute in plasma water in maternal and fetal blood, respectively, flowing past the exchange area. Because lipophilic (hydrophobic) solutes are soluble in the plasma membrane there will be effectively considerably more surface area available for diffusion of these than there will be for hydrophilic solutes which cannot partition easily into the plasma membrane. Therefore the rate of diffusion of lipophilic solutes will be much greater than that of hydrophilic solutes. In fact the rate of diffusion of such a lipophilic solute will be so fast that the properties of the placenta itself (S and the diffusional path length part of P in equation (3.6.1)) will be unimportant and the concentration gradient ($C_m - C_f$) will be critical. As, in turn ($C_m - C_f$) is dependent on the rate of maternal and fetal blood flow and the geometrical relationship between these two flows, diffusion of lipophilic solutes is said to be flow limited (Fig. 3.6.6). The geometrical arrangement between the two flows may classically be countercurrent (maternal and fetal blood flowing in opposite directions, the most efficient arrangement), crosscurrent (maternal and fetal blood flows at right angles to each other) or concurrent (maternal and fetal blood flows in the same direction, the least efficient arrangement). The human placental circulation does not fit into one of these standard patterns as blood is squirted fountain-like into the intervillous space and is said to show a multivillous pool flow geometry intermediate in efficiency.[44]

Oxygen is a small, relatively lipophilic molecule and its transfer to the fetus is therefore probably by flow-limited diffusion, as has been shown experimentally in the rabbit and sheep.[43] For gases, C_m and C_f in equation (3.6.1) are replaced by the partial pressures and the driving force for oxygen transfer will therefore be its partial pressure gradient between intervillous space and fetal capillary. Adequate oxygen delivery to the fetus is also aided by the hemoglobin dissociation curve, which is shifted to the left for fetal hemoglobin as compared to adult hemoglobin (see reference 43 for a more detailed discussion). Carbon dioxide transfer is also probably flow limited but is complicated also by the equilibrium

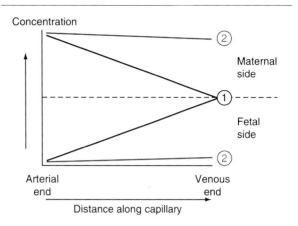

Fig. 3.6.6 *Theoretical plot of the maternal and fetal plasma concentrations of two substances as they pass through the capillary bed on the maternal side (where 'capillary bed' is equivalent to the intervillous space) and fetal side of the placenta from the arterial end to the venous end. Substance 1 is a small hydrophobic molecule such as O_2 which freely diffuses across plasma membranes and so rapidly equilibrates on maternal and fetal sides. Its rate of transfer is only limited by the blood flow supplying or removing it and so is said to be flow limited. Substance 2 is a hydrophilic molecule such as creatinine which cannot easily diffuse across plasma membranes so that its maternal plasma concentration does not approach the fetal plasma concentration. Its rate of transfer is only affected by the surface area of the placenta available for its transfer and the width of the barrier separating maternal and fetal blood and so is said to be diffusion or membrane limited.*

between it and bicarbonate, catalyzed by carbonic anhydrase.[45] Lipophilic drugs will also rapidly cross the placenta, the rate of transfer again only being limited by blood flow rates. For hydrophilic solutes their diffusion coefficient in water (in turn dependent on the size of the molecule), the diffusional path length and S of the placenta will be more important than ($C_m - C_f$) in determining rate of net diffusion and they are said to be 'diffusion limited' or 'membrane limited' (Fig 3.6.6). As these solutes are largely excluded from the intracellular space by the plasma membrane they must diffuse across the placenta through a route continuous with the extracellular space. The anatomical barriers to such exchange, working outwards from the fetal capillary, are: (a) the fetal capillary endothelium, (b) the basement membrane, and (c) the syncytiotrophoblast (Fig. 3.6.5).

The endothelium is typical of the continuous type with intercellular clefts of 4 nm minimum width[46] and functional data[47] suggests that this cellular layer is only an important barrier to proteins of 60 000 mol.wt. and above (e.g. albumin, alphafetoprotein, immunoglobulin G).

Although nothing is known of the permeability properties of the basement membrane of the placenta it may well restrict diffusion of macromolecules.

The syncytiotrophoblast is generally considered to provide the most important barrier because of its syncytial nature and because it is the site of most specific transport mechanisms. However, *in vivo* and *in vitro* measurements of the rate of transfer across the term human placenta of inert hydrophilic solutes have shown that the syncytiotrophoblast does not behave physiologically as a syncytium.[48-53] In these experiments the permeability of the hydrophilic tracers was directly proportional to their coefficients of free diffusion in water. The simplest explanation compatible with this observation is that there is a route(s) of transfer across the syncytiotrophoblast continuous with and containing extracellular fluid through which hydrophilic solutes can diffuse. Thus the syncytiotrophoblast and indeed the entire human placenta is more permeable to hydrophilic solutes than would be suspected on the basis of previously determined morphology; it is feasible that proteins of the size of albumin and alphafetoprotein can diffuse across the placenta in significant amounts.[54]

The identity of the paracellular route in the syncytiotrophoblast is uncertain. It may be provided by areas of syncytial discontinuity which are found in all normal placentae[54] and/or by a system of channels normally too narrow to detect by electron microscopy.[55]

Transport protein mediated exchange

As in other epithelia, the transfer of metabolically important hydrophilic solutes across the syncytiotrophoblast is assisted by insertion into the plasma membrane of specific transport proteins. These will increase the rate of transfer, utilizing the transcellular route, above that expected by paracellular diffusion alone. There are, classically, two types of transport protein:[56] *channels*, which form pores in the plasma membrane allowing diffusion of ions between extracellular and intracellular water, and *carriers* which shuttle solute across the plasma membrane. However, this classification is complicated by recent evidence that some transport proteins may function as both carriers and channels.[57] The two are generally distinguished because, at least physiologically, carriers may be saturated (i.e. every carrier is maximally bound by solute) and show Michaelis–Menten kinetics. Both channels and carriers are selective for specific solutes.

Channels for Cl^- and K^+ have been identified in the microvillous membrane of the human syncytiotrophoblast[58] but their role, if any, in transplacental exchange is not clear. It may be that they only function in the cellular homeostasis of the syncytiotrophoblast itself.

A variety of solute-specific carriers have been identified in both the microvillous and basal plasma membrane of the human syncytiotrophoblast.[43] Vectorial transport in either the maternofetal or fetomaternal direction via these carriers may be accomplished as follows.

By facilitated diffusion

The carrier, in both microvillous and basal plasma membrane, can only shuttle solute in the direction of the prevailing concentration gradient. A good example is glucose, for which there is a transport protein called GLUT-1 in both plasma membranes,[59] one of a family of facilitated glucose transporters.[60] As they are unsaturated at physiological glucose concentrations [61,62] and because maternal plasma glucose concentrations are higher than those in fetal plasma, the transporters will transfer the solute in the maternofetal direction at a rate greater than would be possible by paracellular diffusion alone. Adequate glucose will

thus be supplied both to the placenta, to meet its metabolic requirements, as well as to the fetus.

By pump/leak active transport

Active transport occurs when a solute is transported across the placenta against its electrochemical gradient by direct or indirect input of energy (via ATP). Although, theoretically, energy might be required to transport across both the microvillous plasma membrane and basal membrane of the syncytiotrophoblast, it has generally been found that energy input is at one or other of these sites. In the pump/leak mechanism, solute is pumped across the microvillous membrane so that its concentration in syncytiotrophoblast intracellular water is raised above that in both maternal plasma and fetal plasma. At least some amino acids appear to be transported across the human placenta by such a mechanism. The concentrations of most amino acids are higher in fetal plasma than maternal plasma from at least the second trimester onwards[63] so that, in order to maintain net transport to the fetus for its metabolic and growth needs, energy input to the transporter must occur. There are a number of different amino acid transporters which have been identified on the microvillous plasma membrane, each selective for a different amino acid type, although there is considerable overlap.[43] One such transporter, termed system A, transports amino acids with short polar or linear side chains such as alanine, serine, proline, glycine and methionine. This transporter is sodium-dependent and the inference is that it utilizes the energy in the sodium gradient between the extra- and intracellular water to drive its amino acid substrates into the cell against their concentration gradient. Energy therefore comes indirectly from Na,K-ATPase (Na$^+$ pump) which maintains the sodium gradient. Because the amino acid concentration in the cell is now higher than that in fetal extracellular water, leak down the concentration gradient may take place utilizing other carriers in the basal plasma membrane. However this simple pump/leak model is complicated by the fact that there are also sodium-dependent transporters on the basal plasma membrane which could transport amino acid from fetus into the syncytiotrophoblast. It is thought that net transport in the maternofetal direction is normally maintained by an asymmetry in transporter number: there are more on the microvillous membrane than there are on the basal plasma membrane. Direct evidence for this has been provided for the guinea-pig placenta[64] which is hemomonochorial, very similar to the human.

By leak/pump active transport

Solutes utilizing this mechanism leak into the syncytiotrophoblast across the microvillous plasma membrane down a concentration gradient and energy input occurs at the basal plasma membrane in order to pump them out. Calcium appears to be transported across the human placenta in this way.[65] Thus the concentration of free (ionized) calcium in the syncytiotrophoblast is in the 10^{-7} M range (by analogy to other cells) as compared to that in maternal plasma which is 1–2 mM[66] and the ion diffuses in via a channel or facilitated diffusion type carrier.[67] In order to keep the intracellular concentration of free calcium in the nano-molar range, essential for the normal function of the syncytiotrophoblast, whilst enabling large quantities of the ion to be transported across the cell, it is probably bound by a calcium binding protein which also helps diffusion from the microvillous to the basal plasma membrane. At the basal plasma membrane, calcium is pumped into the extracellular space of the villus core by a high-affinity calcium-dependent ATPase.[68] This pumping is so effective that the ionized calcium concentration in fetal plasma is significantly higher than that in maternal plasma in the human and every other species in which it has been measured.[66]

Solutes such as glucose, at least some amino acids and calcium therefore cross the placenta both by paracellular diffusion and by transcellular transfer utilizing transport proteins. Current evidence suggests that paracellular diffusion is quantitatively the most important mechanism in the human placenta[65,69] whereas in other species with faster growth rates, such as the rat, it is the transcellular component which is most important.[69]

Transfer of macromolecules

As mentioned above the rate of transfer of proteins across the placenta by diffusion may well be finite. However, for some macromolecules there is evidence of additional mechanisms of transfer. Selective transfer of immunoglobulin G seems to occur across the human placenta[70] and confers passive immunity to the fetus. This seems to take place by receptor-mediated endocytosis at the microvillous plasma membrane of the syncytiotrophoblast; Fc receptors in coated pits on this membrane bind IgG which is followed by internalization and formation of coated vesicles.[71–73] Subsequent events are less clear but it seems most likely that binding to receptors in coated vesicles protects IgG from lysosomal digestion (although a large proportion of IgG is still degraded)[74] and that transfer to the fetal side across the basal plasma membrane occurs by exocytosis. Diffusion across the basement membrane and villus core for such a large molecule will be slow and the width of the intercellular spaces between the endothelial cells suggests that only restricted diffusion of IgG could take place by this route; transcytosis across the endothelium might also occur.[73]

Ultrafiltration and water transfer

The net flux of water to the human conceptus must be very large as it forms 80% of the intrauterine contents at term.[75] Although there is a route of water transfer via the amniochorion, 95% of it is transferred via the placenta.[76] There is no doubt that both osmotic and hydrostatic forces are involved in water flux across the human placenta but how net flux is brought about is still uncertain. As the human placenta, and other hemochorial placentae, have a high permeability to hydrophilic solutes it seems likely that the colloid osmotic pressure gradient across the exchange barrier is more important than the total osmotic pressure gradient. Indeed there is evidence that a change of colloid osmotic pressure in the fetal guinea pig can alter its hydra-

tion.[77] However, the osmotic gradient across the exchange barrier *in vivo* is not known. As regards hydrostatic pressures data show that the intervillous space pressure is lower than the umbilical vein pressure[78] suggesting that the gradient across the exchange barrier is such as to drive net water flux in the fetomaternal direction. As this is incompatible with fetal life it is clear that a considerable amount of pertinent information is currently lacking.

A dissolved molecule will be carried with any bulk flow of water across a barrier due to osmotic or hydrostatic pressure gradients, provided that the route taken by the water is permeable to the solute. There is recent evidence that such ultrafiltration does occur in the fetomaternal direction in the rat[79] but the physiological significance of this mechanism of transfer remains to be determined.

Hormone production by the placenta

The human placenta is an endocrine organ of considerable capacity and diversity, producing many hormones which are also produced by other organs. However, the function of most of the hormones produced by the placenta is not known at present. Therefore, this section confines itself to a description of the quantitatively most important placental hormones, which also happen to be those to which some function can be ascribed.

Steroid hormones

All steroid hormones are derived from cholesterol, with its 27 carbon atoms, by a series of reactions which yield 21 carbon progestogens, 19 carbon androgens and finally 18 carbon estrogens. Quantitatively the major steroid products of the human placenta are progesterone and estriol.[80] As can be seen in Fig. 3.6.7 the production of estrogens by the placenta requires precursors from maternal and fetal liver and adrenal, with the fetal steroids being most important; hence the coining of the phrase 'fetoplacental unit'.[81]

The cholesterol used by the human placenta seems to be derived predominantly from low density lipoprotein (LDL) circulating in maternal plasma rather than by *de novo* synthesis from acetate.[80,82] LDL receptors have been identified on the microvillous plasma membrane of the syncytiotrophoblast[83] which would facilitate the uptake of this precursor. Cholesterol is converted into pregnenolone in a reaction catalyzed by cytochrome P-450 cholesterol side chain cleavage enzyme and pregnenolone is readily converted into progesterone because of the abundance in the placenta of 3β-hydroxysteroid dehydrogenase which catalyzes this reaction. In late pregnancy as much as 600 mg of progesterone per day may be produced by the placenta leading to a marked increase in maternal plasma concentrations.[80,82]

Estrogens can only be produced from the C_{19} steroids such as androstenedione and dehydroisoandrosterone, which in turn are synthesized from the C_{21} progesterone and pregnenolone by reactions catalyzed by 17α-hydroxylase and 17,20-desmolase (Fig. 3.6.7). These two enzyme activities are present in one protein, the steroid 17α-

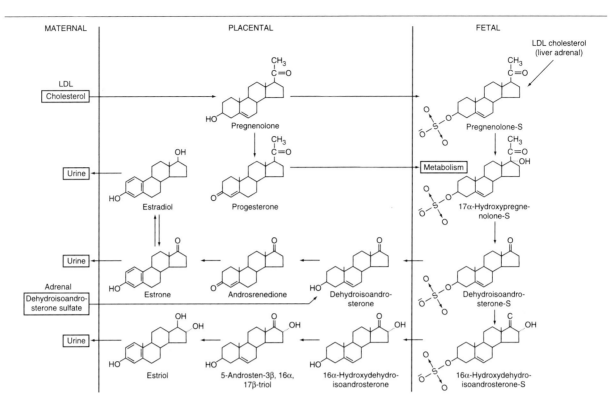

Fig. 3.6.7 *Pathway of synthesis of estrogens in the human fetoplacental unit. (Reproduced with permission from reference 82.)*

hydroxylase. This 17α-hydroxylase is not expressed by the human placenta and therefore its estrogen precursors must be derived from elsewhere. In fact it is now established that estrone and estradiol are produced in the human placenta from dehydroisoandrosterone-sulfate produced equally by the maternal and fetal adrenals; the placenta is rich in sulfatase activity so that non-conjugated dehydroiso-androsterone is readily produced (Fig. 3.6.7). Estriol synthesis requires a 16α-hydroxylation step which is not readily performed by the placenta and again the key reaction is performed elsewhere. This time 16α-hydroxy-dehydroisoandrosterone-sulfate is the key precursor, 90% of which is produced by the fetal adrenal and liver (Fig. 3.6.7). Thus the placental estrogens are produced in cooperative reactions involving uptake of precursors from maternal and fetal plasma.

Most of the progesterone and estrogens so produced are released into maternal plasma where they undoubtedly have major effects on the physiology of the pregnant woman. In fact, as has been recently noted elsewhere,[84] virtually all of the changes in the physiology and metabolism of the pregnant woman have, at some time, been attributed to the high circulating plasma progesterone and estrogen concentrations. Whether this is really the case is less certain.

Polypeptide hormones

Certainly the best studied and probably the most important polypeptide hormones produced by the placenta are human chorionic gonadotrophin (HCG) and human placental lactogen (HPL), the synthesis, secretion and activity of which have been recently reviewed in detail.[85]

HCG

HCG is one of the family of glycoprotein hormones which also includes luteinizing hormone, follicle stimulating hormone and thyroid stimulating hormone. These hormones all consist of two subunits, α and β. The 92 amino acid sequence of the α subunit (molecular weight 14 500) is identical in all four hormones, although the carbohydrate content may differ, whereas the amino acid sequences of the β subunits differ and therefore confer specificity. The β subunit of HCG has 145 amino acids and a molecular weight of about 22 200.[85] The gene for the α subunit is present as a single copy on chromosome 6.[86,87] The β subunit is encoded by a multigene cluster on chromosome 19 composed of six homologous sequences. It seems likely that all these genes are transcribed, although most transcripts in the *in vivo* placenta are from genes 5, 3 and 8.[88]

Intact (dimer) HCG is present in maternal blood within 10 days after the mid-cycle surge of LH, corresponding to the time of implantation of the blastocyst and its first contact with maternal blood. Its concentration then rises dramatically reaching a peak at weeks 10–12 following which it declines to weeks 15–18 from when it remains relatively constant. HCG is also found in amniotic fluid and fetal blood but whereas its concentration in the former compartment is similar to that in maternal blood, at least in the first trimester,[89,90] its concentration in fetal blood is never greater than 3% of its maximum concentration in maternal blood.[90] Free, that is dissociated, α and β subunits are also found in maternal blood. The plasma concentrations of the α subunit increase steadily throughout gestation, reaching a peak at about 36 weeks. However, its concentration at this time is still less than that of intact HCG. Free β subunit concentration in maternal blood follows the pattern of intact HCG, but at a much lower concentration.[91]

Data obtained both *in vivo* and *in vitro* have shown that HCG production is dependent on the stage of differentiation of the trophoblast.[92,93] Thus cytotrophoblast cells produce the HCG α subunit but not the β subunit whereas the more highly differentiated syncytiotrophoblast produces both subunits. Clearly this could partially explain the dramatic rise in dimer HCG production in early pregnancy as syncytiotrophoblast is increasingly formed by fusion of cytotrophoblast cells. However, this also shows that there must be other controlling influences to explain why dimer HCG production then decreases whereas syncytiotrophoblast is still being formed; expression of HCG by term syncytiotrophoblast is certainly lower than that by first trimester syncytiotrophoblast.[94] What these controlling influences are *in vivo* is still not clear although a large number of agents have been shown to affect HCG production by the placenta *in vitro* (see reference 85). This has clinical importance for two reasons: first, maternal serum HCG β subunit concentrations are raised in pregnancies associated with fetal Down's syndrome[95] and secondly, significantly raised (greater than three multiples of the median) maternal serum HCG concentrations are associated with a higher risk of perinatal mortality attributable to pre-eclampsia and intrauterine growth restriction.[96]

The major biological action of HCG is thought to be the maintenance of progesterone production by the corpus luteum until the placenta is able to take over this role. It may have other functions, however, as the peak in HCG production occurs at a time after corpus luteum function has started to decline. One of these might be in promoting male sexual differentiation as plasma HCG correlates well with fetal testosterone production.[97]

HPL

HPL (or HCS) is a non-glycosylated polypeptide of 191 amino acids, molecular weight 22 279. HPL shares about 96% amino acid homology with human growth hormone (HGH) and 67% homology with human prolactin (HPRL). The genes for HGH and HPL form a cluster which spans about 50 kb on chromosome 17. There are actually five genes in the cluster which are, from the 5′ end, HGH-normal(N)/HCS-like (L)/HCS-A/HGH-variant (V)/HCS-B. HGH-N codes for pituitary HGH and is not expressed by the placenta, HGH-V encodes for a variant of HGH expressed by the placenta and HCS-A and HCS-B encode HPL expressed in the placenta; HCS-L is also expressed by the placenta but at the mRNA level only (reviewed in reference 85).

HPL is a product of the differentiated syncytiotrophoblast and HPL mRNA is not found in cytotrophoblast cells.[92] Therefore it is not surprising that the maternal con-

centration of HPL increases during gestation, correlated with placental mass. At term, the production rate of HPL is an incredible 1 g per day; at this time 20% of placental mRNA is HPL mRNA.[80] As with HCG, a large number of agents have been shown to have effects on HPL synthesis and secretion by placental preparations *in vitro*[85] but again it is as yet unclear what the physiological significance of these data might be.

HPL activity has been studied in relation to maternal metabolism, fetal growth, mammary gland function and ovarian function and it does appear to have some effects in all these areas. However, there have been several reports of women having completely normal pregnancies despite the total deletion of the HPL gene. Although there may be possible explanations which still allow for an important role of HPL,[84] the simplest explanation is that HPL does not have an essential role in pregnancy. Left unanswered is the question of why the placenta synthesizes such vast quantities of this hormone?

The placenta and intrauterine growth restriction

Fetal growth is determined by a variety of mechanisms. The 'genetic', or intrinsic growth potential is determined by poorly understood mechanisms related to parental ethnic origin and size.[98] Most low birthweight babies (<2.5 kg) are probably constitutionally small with normal placental function, which has probably obscured our understanding of IUGR itself. A small group of babies are not able to achieve their preprogrammed growth potential. A major chromosomal disorder, congenital viral infection, or other environmental factors (such as smoking, alcohol or substance abuse) may disturb this growth potential;[99] however, the majority of pregnancies complicated by IUGR have none of these associated factors and are thought to be due to 'placental insufficiency'. This section will discuss our current understanding of the placenta and IUGR.

Uteroplacental ischemia

Radioisotope studies during pregnancy indicate that uteroplacental blood flow may be reduced by 60% or more in pregnancies resulting in the birth of small-for-gestation age (SGA) babies.[100] Examination of placental bed biopsies from such pregnancies indicated a failure of trophoblast invasion into the myometrial portions of the spiral arteries.[101] Doppler ultrasound examination of the uterine arteries has demonstrated high-impedance and notched waveforms in pregnancies destined to develop IUGR, similar to the waveform in normal first trimester pregnancy. This non-invasive screening method has been tested at 20–24 weeks of gestation when the changes within the spiral arteries normally would have occurred and the observation of persistent high-impedance waveforms at 24 weeks accompanied by a persistent dichrotic notch was found to be strongly predictive of IUGR[102] and also of other problems thought to have a placental basis such as pre-eclampsia and abruption.

Fetal pathology in IUGR

Ultrasound technology allows the distinction, among small fetuses, between the healthy SGA fetus and one whose growth is restricted (i.e. IUGR).[103] The typical 28–30 week IUGR fetus, whose predicted birthweight is less than the 5th centile, will demonstrate the following features:

1. Substantially reduced fetoplacental perfusion, identified using Doppler ultrasound by the absence of forward end-diastolic flow velocity (AEDFV) in the umbilical artery; and
2. Redistribution of fetal blood flow to the brain at the expense of the lower body. This is associated with reduced urine production and hence a reduction in amniotic fluid volume.

Examination of the fetal environment in such instances has been made possible by the ability to obtain samples of umbilical venous blood under ultrasound guidance. Such studies demonstrate that the preterm IUGR fetus described above may be chronically hypoxic with an elevated plasma erythropoietin,[104] hypercapnic, and, later, acidotic as anaerobic glycolysis occurs.[105] The umbilical cord venous blood concentrations of amino acids are also reduced.[106] These data suggest a widespread defect in placental transport function, accompanied by major adaptive efforts by the fetus to try and maintain cerebral blood flow and oxygenation. These fetuses are at high risk of perinatal death: in a large recent collaborative study, 41% of those with AEDFV died in the perinatal period, rising to 72% if reversed EDFV was observed.[107] Careful monitoring and elective delivery by Caesarean section may reduce this risk of death by as much as half.[108]

Placental pathology in IUGR

The demonstration of strikingly abnormal umbilical artery Doppler waveforms in these preterm IUGR pregnancies prompted several groups to study the stem villous arrangement. A reduction in the numbers of small stem arterioles was observed[109,110] leading to the theory that these vessels had been obliterated by fetal platelets.[111] Fetal sheep studies, in which the umbilical arteries were embolized by microspheres, were able to reproduce the abnormal umbilical artery waveform and so tended to reinforce the obliteration theory.[112] However, the interpretation of vascular tree development from paraffin sections is subject to a number of limitations, in particular that the small arteries, of greatest interest, are difficult to localize.[113] The recent availability of antibodies to localize contractile cells, by the presence of α-smooth muscle action[114] will facilitate more detailed studies of the muscularized vessels. A recent report suggests that there is no selective loss of even the smallest (15 μm diameter) muscularized vessels in IUGR with abnormal umbilical Doppler.[115]

By contrast, more recent stereological studies of placentae from IUGR pregnancies with abnormal umbilical artery Doppler waveforms have indicated a significant reduction in the proportion of placental volume occupied by terminal villi.[116,117] The ultrastructure of these villi is also quite abnormal, demonstrating trophoblast senescence, thickened basal lamina and stromal fibrosis.[118] Vascular casting methods have recently been employed to illustrate the maldevelopment of the terminal villi in severe IUGR demonstrating abnormally coiled and elongated (>200 μM in length) capillaries, with a marked reduction in sinusoidal branching (Kingdom et al., unpublished data). The terminal parts of the placental villous tree, where gaseous diffusion and transport systems probably operate, are clearly very abnormal in IUGR. Thus attention now needs to be focused on the control of villous placental growth and differentiation, in order to characterize the pathology of IUGR in detail.

Placental amino acid transport in IUGR

Measurements on plasma samples obtained from the umbilical vein at cordocentesis have shown that the concentrations of most amino acids are significantly lower in IUGR babies than in normally grown babies.[106,119] Furthermore, experiments in vitro have shown that the activity of the System A amino acid transporter (see p. 318) in the microvillous membrane of placentae of SGA babies is significantly lower than that in the placentae of normally grown babies.[120,121] These data suggest that placental amino acid transport is abnormal when fetal growth is reduced, although it is not yet clear whether this could be causative or whether it is an adaptation. However, it is clear that the activity of the System A transporter in the microvillous membrane of placentae from normal pregnancies increases markedly between first trimester and term[22] and so its lower activity in IUGR pregnancy near to term might, as with the abnormal villous tree, also reflect the failure of normal placental differentiation in this condition.

FUTURE PERSPECTIVES

Compared to most other organs, our understanding of placental biology is still in its infancy. We believe the following are the important questions for future study:

1. What are the key developmental changes in placental biology over the course of gestation? Advances in this field will require the application of in situ techniques to interpret structure and function simultaneously.
2. What are the genetic influences underlying placental development in general and the differentiation of cytotrophoblast cells in particular? Currently nothing is known about placental transcription factors or other genetic elements involved in the induction and attainment of the mature placental phenotype.
3. How are the functions of the placenta controlled in vivo in relation to maternal and/or fetal demands? In some areas, such as maternal–fetal exchange, very little is known from either in vitro or in vivo studies about what controls transport; in other areas, such as placental

hormone synthesis, a great number of agents are known to control production *in vitro*, but it is unclear what the important controlling influences are *in vivo*.

4. Placental pathology needs to be fully characterized both in terms of its relationship with fetal pathology and with Doppler studies. In addition, we need to delineate the way in which the maternal environment acts through the placenta to cause fetal adaptations which may manifest themselves 50 or more years later as, for example, adult hypertension or diabetes mellitus.

SUMMARY

- The properties of the placenta change markedly over gestation.
- There is no maternal blood supply to the placenta until about the 10th week of gestation.
- The umbilical cord can be visualized from 7–8 weeks of gestation by color Doppler.
- During normal pregnancy there is a steady fall in fetoplacental vascular impedance.
- The fetal villous tree continues to branch and differentiate throughout gestation.
- The transfer by diffusion of small lipophilic (hydrophobic) substances will be dependent on placental blood flow: they are flow limited. Diffusional transfer of hydrophilic substances is dependent on the properties of the barrier rather than on blood flow: they are membrane or diffusion limited.

- Hydrophilic substances may also cross the placenta utilizing transport proteins in the plasma membranes or, for very large molecules, endocytosis followed by exocytosis from the syncytiotrophoblast.
- The production of steroid hormones by the placenta is dependent on the supply of precursors from mother and fetus.
- HCG and HPL production is dependent on the stage of placental development and specifically stage of trophoblast differentiation.
- Intrauterine growth restriction may be caused by abnormal villous placental development and differentiation, following inadequate trophoblast invasion of the maternal spiral arteries.

ACKNOWLEDGEMENT

We are very grateful to Mrs Jean French for secretarial assistance.

REFERENCES

1. Barker DJP. *Fetal and Infant Origins of Adult Disease*. London: British Medical Journal, 1992.
2. Redman CWG, Sargent IL, Starkey PM (eds). *The Human Placenta*. Oxford: Blackwell Scientific Publications, 1993.
3. Johnson PJ. Immunology of pregnancy. In Chamberlain GVP (ed.) *Turnbull Obstetrics 2nd edn*. London: Churchill Livingstone, 1995.
4. Leiser R, Kaufmann P. Placental structure: in a comparative aspect. *Exp Clin Endocrinol* 1991 **102**: 122–134.
5. Burchill RC. Arterial blood flow in the human intervillous space. *Am J Obstet Gynecol* 1967 **98**: 303–311.
6. Schaaps JP, Hustin J. *In vivo* aspect of the maternal–trophoblastic border during the first trimester of gestation. *Troph Res* 1988 **3**: 39–48.
7. Rodesh F, Simon P, Donner C, Jauniaux E. Oxygen measurements in endometrial and trophoblastic tissues during early pregnancy. *Obstet Gynecol* 1992 **80**: 283–285.
8. Hustin J, Schaaps JP, Lambotte R. Anatomical studies of the uteroplacental vascularisation in the first trimester of pregnancy. *Troph Res* 1988 **3**: 49–60.
9. Demir R, Kaufmann P, Castellucci M, Erbengi T, Kotowski A. Fetal vasculogenesis and angiogenesis in human placental villi. *Acta Anat* 1989 **136**: 190–203.
10. Kaufmann P, Burton G. Anatomy and genesis of the placenta. In Knobil E, Neil JD (eds) *The Physiology of Reproduction*, Vol. 1, 2nd edn. New York: Raven Press, 1994: 441–484.
11. Fisk NM, MacLachlan N, Ellis C, Tannirandorn Y, Tonge HM, Rodeck CH. Absent end-diastolic flow in first trimester umbilical artery. *Lancet* 1988 ii: 1256–1257.
12. Kurjak A, Zalud I, Salihagic A, Crvenkovic G, Matijevie R. Transvaginal color Doppler in the assessment of abnormal early pregnancy. *J Perinatal Med* 1990 **19**: 155–165.
13. Jauniaux E, Jurkovic D, Campbell S, Hustin J. Doppler ultrasonographic features of the developing placental circulation: correlation with anatomic findings. *Am J Obstet Gynecol* 1992 **166**: 585–587.
14. Hendricks S, Sarasen TK, Wong KY et al. Doppler umbilical artery waveform indices – normal values from fourteen to forty-two weeks. *Am J Obstet Gynecol* 1989 **161**: 761–765.
15. Macara LM, Kingdom JCP, Kaufmann P. Control of the fetoplacental circulation. *Fetal Maternal Med Rev* 1993 **5**: 167–179.
16. Pittalis MC, Dalpra L, Torricelli F et al. The predictive value of cytogenetic diagnosis after CVS based on 4860 cases with both direct and culture methods. *Prenat Diagn* 1994 **14**: 267–278.
17. Kingdom JCP, Sherlok J, Rodeck CH, Adinolfi M. Detection of trophoblast cells in transcervical samples collected by lavage and cytobrush. *Obstet Gynecol* 1995 **86**: 283–288.
18. Adinolfi M, Soothill PW, Rodeck CH. A simple alternative to amniocentesis. *Prenat Diagn* 1994 **14**: 231–233.
19. Adinolfi M, Sherlock J, Kemp T et al. Prenatal detection of fetal RhD DNA sequences in transcervical samples. *Lancet* 1995 **345**: 318–319.
20. Adamson SL, Morrow RJ, Bascom PAJ, Mo LYL, Ritchie

JWK. Effect of placental resistance, arterial diameter, and blood pressure on the uterine arterial velocity waveform: a computer modeling approach. *Ultrasound Med Biol* 1989 **15**: 437–442.

21. Kingdom JCP, Awad H, Fleming JEE, Bowman AW. Obstetrical determinants of relative placental size. *Placenta* 1993 **14**: A36.

22. Mahendran D, Byrne S, Donnai P *et al.* Na$^+$ transport, H$^+$ concentration gradient dissipation and System A amino acid transporter activity in purified microvillous plasma membrane isolated from first trimester human placenta: comparison to the term microvillous membrane. *Am J Obstet Gynecol* 1994 **171**: 1534–1540.

23. Benirschke K, Kaufmann P. *Pathology of the Human Placenta*, 3rd edn. New York: Springer, 1995.

24. Leiser, Kosanke G, Kaufmann P. Human placental vascularization. In Soma H (ed.) *Placenta: Basic Research for Clinical Application*. Basel: Karger, 1991: 32–45.

25. Eik-Nes S, Brubakk AO, Ulstein M. Measurement of human fetal blood flow. *Br Med J* 1980 **i**: 283–284.

26. Reilly FD, Russell PT. Neurohistochemical evidence supporting an absence of adrenergic and cholinergic innervation in the human placenta and umbilical cord. *Anat Rec* 1977 **188**: 277–286.

27. Panigel M. Placental perfusion experiments. *Am J Obstet Gynecol* 1962 **84**: 1664–1683.

28. Vane J, Anggard EE, Botting RM. Regulatory mechanisms of the vascular endothelium. *N Engl J Med* 1990 **323**: 27–36.

29. Myatt L. Control of vascular resistance in the human placenta. *Placenta* 1992 **13**: 329–341.

30. Jacobson RL, Brewer A, Eis A, Siddiqi TA, Myatt L. Transfer of aspirin across the human placental cotyledon. *Am J Obstet Gynecol* 1991 **165**: 939–944.

31. McCarthy AL, Woolfson RG, Evans BJ, Davies DR, Raju SK, Poston L. Functional characteristics of small placental arteries. *Am J Obstet Gynecol* 1994 **170**: 945–951.

32. Anggard E. Nitric oxide: mediator, murderer, and medicine. *Lancet* 1994 **343**: 1190–1206.

33. Myatt L, Brewer A, Brockman DE. The action of nitric oxide in the perfused human fetal–placental circulation. *Am J Obstet Gynecol* 1991 **164**: 687–692.

34. Izumi H, Garfield RE, Makino Y, Shirakawa K, Itoh T. Gestational changes in endothelium-dependent vasorelaxation in human umbilical artery. *Am J Obstet Gynecol* 1994 **170**: 236–245.

35. Templeton AGB, Kingdom JCP, McGrath JC, Whittle MJ. Human umbilical cord and chorionic plate arteries do not demonstrate endothelium-dependent relaxation despite release of nitric oxide – submitted for publication to *Obstetrics & Gynecology*.

36. Learmont JG, Braude PR, Poston L. Flow induced dilation is modulated by nitric oxide in isolated human small fetoplacental arteries. *J Vasc Res* 1994 **31** (Suppl 1): 26.

37. Myatt L, Brockman DE, Eis ALW, Pollock JS. Immunohistochemical localisation of nitric oxide synthase in the human placenta. *Placenta* 1993 **14**: 487–495.

38. Buttery LDK, McCarthy A, Springall DR *et al.* Endothelial nitric oxide synthase in the human placenta: regional distribution and proposed regulatory role at the fetomaternal interface. *Placenta* 1994 **15**: 257–265.

39. Benigni A, Gasparo F, Orisio S *et al.* Human placenta expresses the endothelin gene and the corresponding protein is excreted in the urine in increasing amounts during the course of normal pregnancy. *Am J Obstet Gynecol* 1991 **164**: 844–848.

40. Myatt L, Brewer AS, Brockman DE. The comparative effects of big endothelin-1, endothelin-1, and endothelin-3 in the human fetal-placental circulation. *Am J Obstet Gynecol* 1992 **167**: 1651–1656.

41. Cai WQ, Bodin P, Sexton A, Loesch A, Burnstock G. Localization of neuropeptide Y and atrial natriuretic peptide in the endothelial cells of human umbilical blood vessels. *Cell Tissue Res* 1993 **272**: 175–181.

42. Kaufmann, P. Basic morphology of the fetal and maternal circuits in the human placenta. *Contrib Gynecol Obstet* 1985 **13**: 5–17.

43. Morriss FH, Boyd RDH, Mahendran D. Placental transport. In Knobil E, Neil JD (eds) *The Physiology of Reproduction*, 2nd edn. New York: Raven Press, 1994: 813–862.

44. Schröder H. Structural and functional organisation of the placenta from the physiological point of view. *Bibl Anat* 1982 **22**: 4–12.

45. Mühlhauser J, Crescimanno C, Rajaniemi H *et al.* Immunohistochemistry of carbonic anhydrase in human placenta and fetal membranes. *Histochemistry* 1994 **101**: 91–98.

46. Leach L, Firth JA. Fine structure of the paracellular junctions of terminal villus capillaries in the perfused human placenta. *Cell Tissue Res* 1992 **268**: 447–452.

47. Eaton B, Leach L, Firth JA. Permeability of the fetal villous microvasculature in the isolated perfused term human placenta. *J Physiol* 1993 **463**: 141–156.

48. Willis DM, O'Grady JP, Faber JJ, Thornburg KL. Diffusion permeability of cyanocobalomin in human placenta. *Am J Physiol* 1986 **250**: R459–R464.

49. Thornburg KL, Burry KJ, King-Adams A, Kirk EP, Faber JJ. Permeability of placenta to inulin. *Am J Obstet Gynecol* 1988 **158**: 1165–1169.

50. Bain MD, Copas DK, Landon MJ, Stacey TE. *In vivo* permeability of the human placenta to inulin and mannitol. *J Physiol* 1988 **399**: 313–319.

51. Bain MD, Copas DK, Taylor A, Landon MJ, Stacey TE. Permeability of the human placenta *in vivo* to four nonmetabolized hydrophilic molecules. *J Physiol* 1990 **431**: 505–513.

52. Illsley NP, Hall S, Penfold P, Stacey TE. Diffusional permeability of the human placenta. *Contrib Gynecol Obstet* 1985 **13**: 92–97.

53. Schneider H, Sodha RJ, Progler M, Young MPA. Permeability of the human placenta for hydrophilic substances studied in the isolated dually *in vitro* perfused lobe. *Contrib Gynecol Obstet* 1985 **13**: 98–103.

54. Edwards D, Jones CJP, Sibley CP, Nelson DM. Paracellular permeability pathways in the human placenta. A quantitative and morphological study of maternal fetal transfer of horseradish peroxidase. *Placenta* 1993 **14**: 63–73.

55. Kaufmann P, Schröder H, Leichtweiss HP. Fluid shift across the placenta. II Fetomaternal transfer of horseradish peroxidase in the guinea-pig. *Placenta* 1982 **3**: 339–348.

56. Stein WD. *Channels, Carriers, and Pumps An Introduction to Membrane Transport*. San Diego: Academic Press, 1990.

57. Valverde MA, Diaz M, Sepulveda FV, Gill DR, Hyde SC, Higgins CF. Volume-regulated chloride channels associated with the human multidrug-resistance p-glycoprotein. *Nature* 1992 **355**: 830–833.

58. Greenwood SL, Brown PD, Edwards D, Sibley CP. Patch clamp studies of human placental cytotrophoblast in culture. *Troph Res* 1993 **7**: 53–68.

59. Jansson T, Wennergren M, Illsley N. Glucose transporter protein expression in human placenta throughout gestation and in intrauterine growth retardation. *J Clin Endocrinol Metab* 1993 **77**: 1554–1562.

60. Mueckler M. Facilitative glucose transporters. *Eur J Biochem* 1994 **219**: 713–725.

61. Johnson LW, Smith CH. Monosaccharide transport across microvillous membrane of human placenta. *Am J Physiol* 1980 **238**: C160–C168.

62. Johnson LW, Smith CH. Glucose transport across the basal plasma membrane of human placental syncytiotrophoblast. *Biochim Biophys Acta* 1985 **815**: 44–50.

63. Cetin I, Corbetta C, Sereni LP *et al.* Umbilical amino acid concentrations in normal and growth retarded fetuses sampled *in utero* by cordocentesis. *Am J Obstet Gynecol* 1990 **162**: 253–261.

64. Eaton BM, Yudilevich DL. Uptake and asymmetric efflux of amino acids at maternal and fetal sides of placenta. *Am J Physiol* 1981 **241**: C106–C112.

65. Štulc J, Štulcová B, Šmid M, Šach I. Parallel mechanisms of calcium transfer across the perfused human placental cotyledon. *Am J Obstet Gynecol* 1994 **170**: 162–167.

66. Sibley CP, Boyd RDH. Control of transfer across the mature placenta. In Clarke JR (ed.) *Oxford Reviews of Reproductive Biology* Vol. 10. Oxford: Oxford University Press, 1988: 382–435.

67. Kamath SG, Kelley LK, Friedman AF, Smith CH. Transport and binding in calcium uptake by microvillous membrane of human placenta. *Am J Physiol* 1992 **262**: C789–C794.

68. Kelley LK, Borke JL, Verma AK, Kumar R, Penniston JT, Smith CH. The calcium transporting ATPase and the calcium- or magnesium-dependent nucleotide phosphatase activities of human placental trophoblast basal plasma membrane of separate enzyme activities. *J Biol Chem* 1990 **265**: 5453–5459.

69. Sibley CP. Mechanisms of ion transport by the rat placenta: a model for the human placenta? *Placenta* 1994 **15**: 675–691.

70. Sibley CP, Boyd RDH. Mechanisms of transfer across the human placenta. In Polin RA, Fox WW (eds) *Fetal and Neonatal Physiology*. Philadelphia: W B Saunders, 1992: 62–74.

71. Lin C-T. Immunoelectron microscopic localisation of immunoglobulin G in human placenta. *J Histochem Cytochem* 1980 **28**: 339–346.

72. King BF. Absorption of peroxidase-conjugated immunoglobulin G by human placenta: in vitro study. *Placenta* 1982 **3**: 395–406.

73. Leach L, Eaton BM, Firth JA, Contractor SF. Immunocytochemical and labelled tracer approaches to uptake and intracellular routing of immunoglobulin G (IgG) in the human placenta. *Histochem J* 1991 **23**: 444–449.

74. Contractor SF, Eaton BM, Stannard PJ. Uptake and fate of exogenous immunoglobulin G in the perfused human placenta. *J Reprod Immunol* 1983 **5**: 265–273.

75. Seeds AE. Water metabolism of the fetus. *Am J Obstet Gynecol* 1965 **92**: 727–745.

76. Hutchinson DL, Grey MJ, Plentl AA, Alvarez H, Caldeyro-Barcia R, Lind J. The role of the fetus in the water exchange of the amniotic fluid of normal and hydramniotic patients. *J Clin Invest* 1959 **38**: 971–980.

77. Anderson DF, Faber JJ. Water flux due to colloid osmotic pressures across the haemochorial placenta of the guinea-pig. *J Physiol* 1982 **332**: 521–527.

78. Nicolini U, Fisk NM, Talbert DG *et al*. Intrauterine monometry technique and application to fetal pathology. *Prenat Diagn* 1989 **9**: 243–254.

79. Štulc J, Štulcová B. Asymmetrical transfer of inert hydrophilic solutes across the rat placenta. *Am J Physiol* 1993 **265**: R670–R675.

80. Casey ML, MacDonald PC. Placental endocrinology. In Redman CWG, Sargent IL, Starkey PM (eds) *The Human Placenta*. Oxford: Blackwell Scientific Publications, 1993: 237–272.

81. Diczfalusy E. Endocine functions of the human fetoplacental unit. *Fed Proc* 1964 **23**: 791–798.

82. Solomon S. The primate placenta as an endocrine organ. Steroids. In Knobil E, Neil JD (eds) *The Physiology of Reproduction,* 2nd edn. New York: Raven Press, 1994: 863–873.

83. Alsat E, Mondon F, Rebourcet R *et al*. Identification of specific binding sites for acetylated low-density lipo-protein in microvillous membranes from human placenta. *Mol Cell Endocrinol* 1985 **41**: 229–235.

84. Chard T. Placental hormones and metabolism. In Reece LA, Hobbins JC, Mahoney MJ, Petrie RH (eds) *Medicine of the Fetus and Mother*. Philadelphia: Lippincott, 1992: 88–96.

85. Ogren L, Talamantes F. The placenta as an endocrine organ: polypeptides. In Knobil E, Neil JD (eds) *The Physiology of Reproduction,* 2nd edn. New York: Raven Press, 1994: 875–945.

86. Boothby M, Ruddon RW, Anderson C, McWilliams D, Boime I. A single gonadotropin alpha subunit gene in normal tissue and tumour derived cell lines. *J Biol Chem* 1981 **256**: 5121–5127.

87. Fiddes JC, Goodman HM. The gene encoding the common alpha subunit of the four human glycoprotein hormones. *J Mol Appl Genet* 1981 **1**: 3–18.

88. Bo M, Boime I. Identification of the transcriptionally active genes of the chorionic gonadotropin beta gene cluster *in vivo*. *J Biol Chem* 1992 **267**: 3179–3184.

89. Kletzky OA, Rossman F, Bertoli SI, Platt LD, Mitchell DR. Dynamics of human chorionic gonadotropin, prolactin and growth hormone in serum and amniotic fluid throughout normal human pregnancy. *Am J Obstet Gynecol* 1985 **151**: 878–883.

90. Reyes FI, Boroditsky RS, Winter JSD, Faiman C. Studies on human sexual development II. Fetal and maternal serum gonadotropin and sex steroid concentrations. *J Clin Endocrinol Metab* 1974 **38**: 612–617.

91. Cole LA, Crull TG, Ruddon RW, Hussa RO. Differential occurrence of free beta and free alpha subunits of human chorionic gonadotropin (hCG) in pregnancy sera. *J Clin Endocrinol Metab* 1984 **58**: 1200–1202.

92. Hoshina M, Boothby M, Hussa R, Pattillo R, Camel HM, Boime I. Linkage of human gonadotropin and placental lactogen to trophoblast differentiation and tumorigenesis. *Placenta* 1985 **6**: 163–172.

93. Kliman HJ, Nestler JE, Sermasi E, Sanga JM, Strauss JF. Purification, characterisation and *in vitro* differentiation of cytotrophoblast from human term placenta. *Endocrinology* 1986 **118**: 1567–1582.

94. Hoshina M, Boothby M, Boime I. Cytological localization of chorionic gonadotropin alpha and placental lactogen mRNAs during development of the human placenta. *J Cell Biol* 1982 **93**: 190–198.

95. Spencer K, Coombes J, Mallard SA, Ward MA. Free beta human choriogonadotropin in Down's syndrome screening: a multicentre study of its role compared with other biochemical markers. *Ann Clin Biochem* 1992 **29**: 506–518.

96. Wenstrom KD, Owen J, Boots LR, DuBard MB. Elevated second trimester human chorionic gonadotropin levels in association with poor pregnancy outcome. *Am J Obstet Gynecol* 1994 **171**: 1038–1041.

97. Conley AJ, Mason JI. Endocrine function of the placenta. In Thorburn GD, Harding R (eds) *Textbook of Fetal Physiology*. Oxford: Oxford University Press, 1994: 16–29.

98. Sanderson DA, Wilcox MA, Johnson IR. The individualised birthweight ratio: a new method of identifying intrauterine growth retardation. *Br J Obstet Gynaecol* 1994 **101**: 310–314.

99. Snijders RJM, Sherrod C, Gosden CM, Nicolaides KH. Fetal growth retardation: associated malformations and chromosomal abnormalities. *Am J Obstet Gynecol* 1993 **168**: 547–555.

100. Lunell NO, Sarby B, Lewander R, Nylund L. Comparison of uteroplacental blood flow in normal and intrauterine growth-retarded pregnancy. *Gynecol Obstet Invest* 1979 **10**: 106–118.

101. Khong TY, De Wolf F, Robertson WB, Brosens I. Inadequate maternal vascular response to placentation in pregnancies complicated by pre-eclampsia and by small-for-gestational age infants. *Br J Obstet Gynecol* 1986 **93**: 1049–1059.

102. Bower S, Bewley S, Campbell S. Improved prediction of preeclampsia by two-stage screening of uterine arteries using the early diagnostic notch and color Doppler imaging. *Obstet Gynecol* 1993 **82**: 78–83.

103. Gabbe SG. Intrauterine growth retardation. In Gabbe SG, Niebyl JR, Simpson JL (eds) *Obstetrics: Normal and*

Problem Pregnancies, 2nd edn. New York: Churchill Livingstone: 923–944.

104. Snijders RJM, Abbas A, Melby O, Ireland RM, Nicolaides KH. Fetal plasma erythropoietin concentration in severe growth retardation. *Am J Obstet Gynecol* 1993 **168**: 615–619.

105. Nicolaides KH, Bilardo CM, Soothill PW, Campbell S. Absence of end-diastolic frequencies in the umbilical artery: a sign of fetal hypoxia and acidosis. *Br Med J* 1988 **297**: 1026–1027.

106. Cetin I, Corbetta C, Sereni LP *et al.* Umbilical amino acid concentrations in normal and growth-retarded fetuses sampled *in utero* by cordocentesis. *Am J Obstet Gynecol* 1990 **162**: 253–261.

107. Karsdorp VHM, van Vugt JMG, van Geijn HP *et al.* Clinical significance of absent or reversed end diastolic velocity waveforms in umbilical artery. *Lancet* 1994 **344**: 1664–1668.

108. Pattinson RC, Norman K, Odendall HJ. The role of Doppler velocimetry in the management of high risk pregnancies. *Br J Obstet Gynaecol* 1994 **101**: 114–120.

109. Giles WB, Trudinger BJ, Baird P. Fetal umbilical artery flow velocity waveforms and placental resistance: pathological correlation. *Br J Obstet Gynaecol* 1985 **92**: 31–38.

110. McCowan LM, Mullen BM, Ritchie K. Umbilical artery flow velocity waveforms and the placental vascular bed. *Am J Obstet Gynecol* 1987 **157**: 900–902.

111. Wilcox GR, Trudinger BJ. Fetal platelet consumption: a feature of placental insufficiency. *Obstet Gynecol* 1991 **77**: 616–621.

112. Morrow RJ, Adamson SL, Bull SB, Ritchie JWK. Effect of placental embolization on the umbilical arterial velocity waveform in fetal sheep. *Am J Obstet Gynecol* 1989 **161**: 1055–1060.

113. Jauniaux E, Burton GJ. Correlation of umbilical Doppler features and placental morphometry: the need for uniform methodology. *Ultrasound Obstet Gynaecol* 1993 **3**: 233–235.

114. Skalli O, Ropraz P, Trzeciak A, Benzonana G, Gillessen D, Gabbiani G. A monoclonal antibody against α-smooth muscle actin: a new probe for smooth muscle differentiation. *J Cell Biol* 1986 **103**: 2787–2796.

115. Macara LM, Kingdom JCP, Kohnen G, Bowman AW, Greer IA, Kaufmann P. Elaboration of stem villous vessels in growth-restricted pregnancies with abnormal umbilical artery Doppler waveforms. *Br J Obstet Gynecol* 1995 **102**: 807–812.

116. Hitschold T, Weiss E, Beck T, Hunterfering H, Berle P. Low target birth weight or growth retardation? Umbilical Doppler flow velocity waveforms and histometric analysis of the fetoplacental vascular tree. *Am J Obstet Gynecol* 1993 **168**: 1260–1264.

117. Jackson MR, Walsh AJ, Morrow RJ, Mullen BJ, Lye SJ, Ritchie JWK. Reduced placental villous tree elaboration in small-for-gestational age newborn pregnancies: relationship with umbilical artery Doppler waveforms. *Am J Obstet Gynecol* 1995 **172**: 518–525.

118. Macara LM, Kingdom JCP, Kaufmann P *et al.* Structural analysis of placental terminal villi from growth-restricted pregnancies with abnormal umbilical artery Doppler waveforms. *Placenta* 1996 **17**: 37–48.

119. Bernadini I, Evans M, Nicolaides KH, Economides DL, Gahl WA. The fetal concentrating index as a gestational age independent measure of placental dysfunction in intrauterine growth retardation. *Am J Obstet Gynecol* 1991 **164**: 253–261.

120. Dicke JM, Henderson GI. Placental amino acid uptake in normal and complicated pregnancies. *Am J Med Sci* 1988 **295**: 223–227.

121. Mahendran D, Donnai P, Glazier JD, D'Souza SW, Boyd RDH, Sibley CP. Amino acid (System A) transporter activity in microvillous membrane vesicles from the placentas of appropriate and small for gestational age babies. *Pediatr Res* 1994 **34**: 661–665.

3.7

Control of Fetal Growth

JS Robinson and JA Owens

INTRODUCTION

Growth of the fetus begins when the embryonic period is complete, defined as the end of the eighth week of human pregnancy. Many of the factors regulating fetal growth have their origins or effects earlier than the fetal period, yet are able to influence the trajectory or pattern of fetal growth. It is obvious that genetic effects can be passed through many generations. What has been recognized more recently, is that environmental effects on one generation may have effects on fetal growth persisting for a number of generations. Alternatively, when the environmental insult is present for several generations, a number of generations may be required subsequently to eliminate its effect on growth of the fetus.

Fetal growth rate and development are primarily the result of an interaction between the genetic drive for growth and the nutritional supply that the fetus receives throughout pregnancy. Many disease states, for example pre-eclampsia, alter fetal nutritional state and oxygenation and hence growth. Variations in nutritional supply also modify the internal pattern of fetal growth through a variety of mechanisms, including modulation of organ blood flow, production and action of growth factors, and of the fetal endocrine state. In addition, there is a dynamic interaction throughout pregnancy between the fetus, the placenta and the mother via similar physiological and molecular mechanisms.

This chapter gives an account of the regulation of fetal growth. Emphasis is placed on growth of the human fetus; however, extensive reference is made to experimental studies in large and small animals, since these provide insight of the specific mechanisms regulating human fetal growth. Malformation is only discussed, when it illustrates how specific factor(s) regulate fetal growth. Since the placenta is essential to normal fetal growth, growth and functional development of the placenta and its control of fetal growth are described. The maternal, placental and intrinsic, or fetal, factors influencing or controlling fetal growth are outlined in Tables 3.7.1–3.7.3.

Table 3.7.1 Maternal factors influencing or contributing to the control of fetal growth

Clinical factors controlling fetal growth
  Matrilineal tendency for large or small babies
  Previous history of large or small babies
  Size
    Weight for height
    Prepregnancy weight
    Fat mass
    Weight gain in pregnancy
  Behavioral factors
    Age <16
    Drug use, e.g. smoking
    Socioeconomic status
    Work/exercise
  Environmental agents
    Altitude
    Pollutants
  Medical complications
    Pre-eclampsia
    Complicated hypertension
    Lupus obstetric syndrome
    Anemia
    Diabetes mellitus and glucose intolerance
    Abnormalities of the uterus
    Anorexia nervosa and bulimia
    Malnutrition and undernutrition
    Abnormalities of the uterus
    Cyanotic heart disease
    Severe disease
    Chemotherapy and radiation

Maternal physiological mechanisms regulating fetal growth
  Maternal size
  Prepregnancy nutrition
    Prepregnancy weight and fat mass
  Nutrition in pregnancy
  Nutrient concentrations
  Endocrine e.g. insulin
  Growth factors e.g. insulin-like growth factors
             transforming growth factors β1
  Oxygenation
  Uterine blood flow

Table 3.7.2 Placental factors influencing or contributing to the control of fetal growth

Clinical factors and placental control of fetal growth
  Bleeding in pregnancy
  Placenta praevia
  Focal lesions:
    Infarcts and hematomas
  Chromosomal mosaicism
  Circumvallate placenta
  Placental blood flow

Placentation
  Pre-implantation conditions matching of embryonic and
    uterine development
  Implantation
  Attachment and implantation
  Recruitment of uterine vessels
  Surface area for exchange
  Transport mechanisms

Uterine and umbilical blood flows

Table 3.7.3 Internal fetal factors influencing or contributing to the control of fetal growth

Clinical conditions associated with fetal control of growth
  Multiple pregnancy
  Fetal infections
  Fetal malformation
  Chromosomal anomalies
  Inborn errors of metabolism
  Fetal and amniotic fluids

Fetal factors and control of growth
  Genetic drive to growth:
    Chromosomal anomalies
    Imprinting
    Gene deletion
  Nutrient delivery:
    Glucose, amino acids
    Other nutrients
    Micronutrients
  Oxygen delivery
  Growth factors:
    Insulin-like growth factors
    Maternal rescue: TGFβ1
    Others
  Endocrine factors:
    Insulin
    Thyroid hormones
    Pituitary hormones
  Organ specific regulation:
    Lung, heart, kidney and gut
    Cardiac output and its distribution
  Umbilical blood flow
  Amniotic fluid composition

CURRENT CONCEPTS

Maternal factors regulating fetal growth

Maternal constraint of fetal growth was first demonstrated when large mares were mated with small stallions and vice versa. This effect has now been shown in many species using a variety of techniques including embryo transfer. In these experiments, maternal size is the dominant factor setting the trajectory of fetal growth and hence determines birth weight. However, final adult size reflects its maternal and paternal genetic origins.

Maternal factors account for the majority of parental contribution to the variation of birth weight. The attributable portion of this variation to paternal factors is only ~5% in humans. Other epidemiological studies confirm that maternal size and weight-for-height are important factors for growth of the human fetus. Maternal size is just one component of the constraint of fetal growth in young teenage mothers. It interacts with immaturity, social circumstances, maternal behavior and diseases, particularly pregnancy disorders (Table 3.7.1). For all ages, life events, indicating psychosocial stress, increase the likelihood of low birth weight partly due to preterm birth.

Maternal constraint is also a factor in the size of fetuses of polytoccous species (producing several young at a time). This constraint appears to be mediated, in part, via the insulin-like growth factors (IGFs) because animals selected for high endogenous concentrations of IGF-I, or those given exogenous IGF-I, do not show the reduction of fetal size normally associated with increasing litter size.[1] The role of the IGFs in the fetus is discussed later.

Maternal treatment with IGF-I increases the efficiency of placental function, because fetal weight is increased without change in placental weight.[2] A similar effect is observed when spontaneously hypertensive rats are treated with IGF-I: fetal weight is increased and placental size is reduced.[3] This effect of IGF-I on the fetoplacental weight ratios may require that treatment begins in the first half of pregnancy. Infusion of the mother with IGF-I confined to the second half of pregnancy fails to abolish the effect of litter size and does not reduce growth restriction induced by ligation of one uterine artery.[4,5] Transgenic rats expressing excess growth hormone have increased fecundity, which may relate to the increased size of these animals, in addition to an effect on ovulation, all of which may be partly mediated through a growth hormone (GH)-induced increase in IGF-I production in the mother.[6]

The interaction between maternal nutrition and fetal and placental growth is a complex one. In societies in which mal- or undernutrition is rife, maternal nutritional stores as measured by total body fat or size of a particular fat store correlate with birth weight.[7,8] In wealthier and perhaps all societies, involuntary self starvation in anorexia nervosa and bulimia may prevent pregnancy or lead to poor fetal growth. Maternal starvation throughout pregnancy also inhibits fetal growth, as does undernutrition confined to late pregnancy. These effects of brief or prolonged periods of severe undernutrition were clearly shown by the famines in Holland and Leningrad during the Second World War. More recently, it has been shown that maternal undernutrition in the first half of pregnancy affected the prenatal growth of the grandchildren.[9]

The impact of deficiencies in the maternal diet may be alleviated by changes in energetics in the pregnant compared to the non-pregnant woman. Energy expenditure increases with the duration of pregnancy, but no change is observed when it is expressed per unit of body weight. Postprandial energy expenditure is decreased in the second half of pregnancy, suggesting maternal adaptation, with increased efficiency, when the energy demands of the fetus are high, although the overall daily gain may be small. The energy cost of pregnancy varies between individuals and communities and is remarkably low in Gambian women who have adapted to seasonal famine over many generations.[10] Dietary supplements for these Gambian women led to increased energy expenditure with little or no increase in birth weight. Review of naturally occurring energy sparing strategies, which maintain fetal growth in women, show that those on marginal diets conserve energy by suppressing metabolic rate and by gaining little fat. Further, birth weight is closely related to (maternal weight)$^{0.75}$.[8] Prepregnancy fatness is either closely associated with, or is one of, the components that sets the trajectory of fetal growth. Furthermore, if the latter is correct then the 'satiety factor' that sets body weight (e.g. the *ob* gene product, leptin)[11] may have a role in setting the rate of growth of the fetus. Another interpretation of these data is to suggest that in affluent countries, the energy cost of pregnancy could be met with little or no change in energy intake. Thus the old adage of eating for two may simply lead to 'just getting fat'.

Moderate maternal undernutrition, for 10 to 12 generations in experimental animals, reduces fetal growth and greatly increases the proportion of fetal deaths. Restoration to good nutrition during pregnancy immediately increases the size of the pups, even though the mothers are 40% smaller than controls. However, the outcome of pregnancy remains poor, due to obstructed labor causing fetal death or neurological damage. Three generations of good nutrition are required to restore completely both normal adult size and behavioral outcomes.[12]

Since maternal malnutrition may be the commonest cause of fetal growth restriction, particularly in part of the developing world, many have attempted to improve fetal growth by supplementing the maternal diet for part or all of pregnancy. However, these dietary interventions have generally been disappointing.[13] Indeed a diet too rich in protein reduces, rather than increases, birth weight. Fetal blood sampling by cordocentesis has allowed identification of nutritional and other deficiencies in growth-restricted fetuses. Selected replacements may improve growth of the fetus. For example, it has been suggested that maternal hyperoxia can restore fetal oxygen tension into the normal range and improve fetal outcome.[14] Larger trials of this therapy are required before its efficacy is established. Similar trials will be required for other supplementation to replace identified deficiencies of nutrients. Remarkably, there is still considerable controversy about the requirement for hematinic supplements. In this context, maternal anemia, which is often due to iron deficiency, is associated with alteration in the ratio of fetal weight to placental weight and may have long-term adverse consequences for the subsequent health of the offspring.[15]

Maternal behavioral factors also contribute to maternal constraint of fetal growth (Table 3.7.1). The best known of these is the consequence of smoking cigarettes during pregnancy. The size of this effect is a reduction of birth weight of 13–15 g for each cigarette smoked per day. In Australia, the differences in birth weight across the different socioeconomic groups can largely be attributed to the differences in smoking in the groups.[16] Unfortunately, the incidence of smoking remains high or is even increasing in young teenagers in this society. Education before pregnancy and other factors, such as prohibition of advertising, may have a greater influence than advice during pregnancy on this cause of constraint of fetal growth. However, programs in pregnancy are effective in reducing the impact of smoking. Unfortunately, these programs have least success in the heavier smokers who also tend to be older. These women have a high incidence of low birth weight babies.

Many 'street or social' drugs also adversely affect fetal growth. The recent rise in the incidence of low birth weight in New York has been attributed to the increase in use of heroin and cocaine.[17] Alcohol can also affect fetal growth and there is continuing debate relating to a safe lower limit. High consumption of alcohol, or more than 40–60 g per day, adversely affects fetal growth and increases the risk of the fetal alcohol syndrome. There is even greater controversy over the effects of common substances such as caffeine, which may constrain or, in small amounts in experimental animals, even enhance fetal growth.

Medical complications of pregnancy or obstetric diseases can restrict fetal growth. Although uncomplicated mild to moderate maternal hypertension does not restrict fetal growth, complicated hypertension does, particularly when there is renal disease. In epidemiological studies, preeclampsia remains a major factor restricting fetal growth. The hope that this effect may be reduced by low-dose aspirin was not supported by the recent large randomized trial conducted in 9364 women.[18] Nor does low-dose aspirin improve the growth of pregnancies identified to be at risk by finding abnormal umbilical waveforms[19] although a smaller study had suggested an enormous increase in placental weight.[20] However, low-dose aspirin may have a beneficial role in some subgroups of women. Among these, lupus erythematosus and the obstetric lupus syndrome may benefit most.

Early influences on placental and fetal growth

In vitro manipulation of embryos has highlighted the importance of early influences on the future growth of the fetus and the placenta. Simple media have been either as successful or even more successful than complex ones for embryo culture. Sheep and cattle embryos have been cultured for a few days *in vitro* and then replaced into a recipient for the remainder of pregnancy with some surprising results. The short period of culture *in vitro* has altered both growth rate of the fetus and the length of gestation.[21] In sheep, the largest lamb born after this culture was 11 kg (usual mean 4.5 kg) and the length of gestation increased to a maximum of 160 days (term ~150 ± 2 days). Not too surprisingly, these large lambs have a very high perinatal mortality. The survivors continued to grow rapidly after birth, but few have survived to maturity. These findings are the opposite of those reported for *in vitro* culture of mouse embryos, which leads to reduced birth weight.

Walker *et al.*[21] have considered the factors that contribute to the production of these abnormally large lambs. These include fragmentation of the egg cytoplasm *in vitro*, altered methylation patterns of DNA and abnormal activation of the embryonic genome. A similar enhancement of fetal and placental growth can be achieved in sheep by administration of progesterone to the mother for the first 6 days of pregnancy (Kleeman, Owens, Lok, Seamark and Walker, unpublished observation). Exogenous progesterone has also been used to improve the reproductive performance of well-fed pigs. Gilts on a high feed intake have lower progesterone concentrations. Exogenous progesterone increases embryonic survival in overfed pigs.[22]

It is interesting to speculate that these observations in animals may have parallels in advanced human reproductive technologies. It has been suggested that the timing of the development of the embryo and the endometrium have to be precisely matched to achieve pregnancy.[23] Human IVF pregnancies are associated with increased rates of small-for-gestational age infants. The highest rate of small-for-dates infants occurs with unexplained infertility, as the diagnostic category leading to IVF.[24] This group may have a mismatch of maternal–embryo signaling or development.

Micromanipulation of the genetic constitution of the mouse embryo has shown that normal development of the embryo requires sets of chromosomes from both the mother and father. Parthenogenetic or gynogenetic embryos have poor development of the placenta, although the embryo initially grows normally. Androgenetic embryos show poor embryonic and good placental growth.[25] The human correlate of the androgenetic embryo is the hydatidiform mole which is of paternal origin. Persistence of these tumors, necessitating chemotherapy, is more common when they accompany a normal co-twin.

Attachment, implantation and gene disruption

The process of attachment and invasion of the trophoblast are essential first steps in the formation of the placenta. A brief outline of these processes is given here and the reader is referred to the recent review[26] in which it is noted that implantation proceeds by a series of critical steps. In mice, transient expression of leukemia inhibitory factor (LIF) on day 4 of pregnancy is a requirement for attachment and without this expression or exogenous source of LIF, the embryos remain alive but unattached in the uterine cavity. However, these embryos implant and develop normally when transferred to a uterus that provides the appropriate LIF signal. Similarly, the interleukin-1 receptor is required for implantation and blocking it with the interleukin-1 receptor antagonist causes failure of pregnancy.

The requirement for these two cytokines was discovered in gene knock out experiments using homologous recombination. Other knock out experiments have shown that colony stimulating factor-1 is also required for normal development of pregnancy in the mouse. Similarly, the estrogen receptor is essential and when it is absent, both sexes are infertile. The uterus of the female mouse without an estrogen receptor fails to respond to exogenous estrogen and the ovaries have hemorrhagic cysts.[27] However, fetal expression of the estrogen receptor is not otherwise essential for its growth and development.

Other gene knock out experiments have shown that although a substance may be required for normal development, the mother may provide it throughout pregnancy and lactation, and the deficiency only becomes critical on weaning, as occurs for transforming growth factor β1.[28]

A large number of knock out experiments have been completed, targeting growth factors and their receptors, classical hormones, DNA regulating factors, integrins and newer peptides. For example, an early hemopoietic defect is found in the yolk sac of mouse embryos which are deficient in the transcription factor, GATA-2 and the embryos die of severe anemia between 9.5 and 11.0 days of pregnancy.[29] Many of these factors have specific effects on the developing fetus or its placenta (see reference 26). These knock out experiments have largely been confined to mice since they are facilitated by embryonic stem cell culture, which has, until recently, only been possible for the mouse. If embryonic stem cell cultures are developed for other animals, it will be of interest to test if the same developmental defects occur in other species following gene knock outs. A further complicating factor in the testing of the role of a substance in development is redundancy, which allows similar or closely related substances to subsume the role normally provided by the absent substance.

Growth of the placenta

The human placenta takes the form of a cake, hence its name. The size and development of the placenta is crucial for normal growth of the fetus (Table 3.7.3). The placenta forms after the invasion of the trophoblast into the decidua and the inner layers of the myometrium. Typically, about 100–150 spiral arterioles are recruited to form the maternal vascular supply of the placenta.[30] In the first trimester, the interstitial trophoblast surrounds the spiral arterioles and the endovascular trophoblast invades retrogradely into the lumina and vessels' walls. The intima and media are replaced by trophoblast and fibrinoid to convert these small arterioles into wide-bored flaccid vessels. This process is referred to as the 'physiological changes' and is characteristic of normal pregnancy.[31] At the end of pregnancy, all these vessels show invasion by trophoblast into the decidual portion and 76% show changes in the myometrial segments.[32] The invasion of the trophoblast into these vessels occurs in two waves. In the first trimester, the invasion is limited to the decidua and, late in this period, the plug of trophoblast is withdrawn from the vessel lumen. The latter is probably accompanied by an increase in the blood flow to the intervillous space and a rise in oxygen tension.[33] The timing and nature of these events are consistent with the requirement of the early embryo for low oxygen tension for optimal growth *in vitro*.

The second wave of trophoblast invasion occurs in the second trimester and coincides with the reduction in the vascular resistance measured using Doppler ultrasound. In pregnancies complicated by pre-eclampsia or by idiopathic intrauterine growth restriction, fewer spiral arterioles are recruited. In addition, the physiological changes either do not occur or the invasion is a more superficial one affecting only the decidual proportion of the vessel in such pregnancies.[30,31] In pre-eclampsia, the proportion of vessels invaded by trophoblast is reduced to just 44% in the decidua and to only 18% of the corresponding myometrial segments.[32] Superficial invasion is also associated with spontaneous miscarriage. Late in the third trimester, a third wave of trophoblast invasion may be seen in pre-eclamptic pregnancies. This trophoblast is intraluminal and is rarely seen in normal pregnancies. Presumably, this intravascular plug in a smaller than normal vessel adds to the problem of maternal supply to the placenta and its fetus. Acute atherosis, with reduction in the vessel lumen and loss of the endothelium and thrombosis, further diminishes total placental function.[34]

The microscopic surface area for exchange within the placenta has been determined morphometrically in normal and complicated human pregnancy. Early studies showed that this surface area is about 11 ± 1.3 m^2 in normal pregnancy and is reduced to 6.9 ± 1.6 m^2 in pregnancies with small-for-dates fetuses and to 7.4 ± 2.0 m^2 when hypertension is present (mean $\pm$ SD).[35] However, this reduction in villous surface area is confined to pre-eclamptic pregnancies. The villous surface area of the placenta in women with uncomplicated hypertension may even be significantly increased at term (13.8 ± 1 m^2 vs 11.8 ± 2.0 m^2).[36] Consistent with these patterns of change in functional surface area, reductions in birth weight were confined to the pre-eclamptic group. In addition to the reduction in placental surface area with idiopathic growth retardation, there was a proportionate reduction in parenchymal and non-parenchymal tissues of the placenta.[37] During the period from 22 weeks to term, there is a sevenfold increase in fetal weight and a twofold reduction in surface area relative to fetal weight. At a given gestational age, fetuses with relatively small placentae tend to outgrow their placentae and the fetal weight : placental weight ratio is higher.[38]

The placenta alters its growth and development in response to modest oxygen deficiency. Significant placental adaptation occurs in anemic women and in those living at altitude.[15,39] Lower birth weight occurs at altitude whereas placental weight may be unchanged[39] or increased. The placentae from those living at altitude have larger intervillous spaces and a reduced volume of villi. There is also evidence for a longer-term adaptation or selection of people living at altitude, since Amerindian women had placentae with more trophoblast and more villous stroma than their non-Indian counterparts.[39] Enhancement of oxygen transfer is facilitated by movement of the fetal capillaries to the periphery of the villi[40] and can be defined as increased oxygen diffusive conductance of the villous stroma.[41] Similar adaptations may exist in Tibetans, who have a low incidence of intrauterine growth restriction, consistent with selection for optimization of birth weight at high altitude.[42]

Maternal tobacco smoking also invokes changes in placental structure, but of a different nature, with smaller placentae and thickening of the villous membrane in early pregnancy.[43] In late pregnancy, the capillary volume of the villi is reduced and, at both stages of pregnancy, necrosis of the syncytiotrophoblast is found with maternal smoking.[44] The villi of these placentae also have thickened basement membrane and increased collagen. These structural changes will impact adversely on function and presumably contribute to the reduction in birth weight caused by maternal smoking.

Increased fetal weight occurs in poorly controlled maternal diabetes. The alterations in fetal body proportions reflect sensitivity of various tissues to insulin with increased size of somatic tissues and fat stores. Brain size is not increased. Islet cells of the fetal pancreas may show degranulation suggesting that β-cell function is impaired and this persists postnatally. Maternal diabetes is accompanied by increased placental size and morphometric changes. The surface area of the placenta increased to 17.3 ± 3.6 m^2. This increase is larger than would be expected when the increase in fetal weight of some babies born to diabetic mothers is taken into account.[45] Even when mean weights are similar, the placenta in the diabetic woman has a more voluminous capillary bed, diameter and surface area and shorter diffusion distances.[46] These findings support an earlier suggestion that the placenta may be hypoxic in diabetic mothers and may make adaptations similar to those found in the placenta of women at high altitude.

Ultrasonography has been used to determine placental volume serially in human pregnancy and small placental volumes at mid-gestation were associated with small-for-gestational age babies at term.[47] This abnormal outcome could be predicted with a specificity and sensitivity of about 90%. Furthermore, placental growth retardation always preceded fetal complications or growth retardation by at least three weeks.[48]

There is also an association between placental volume measured by ultrasound at 18 weeks of gestation and placental weight at term. Similarly, there are correlations between estimated fetal weight at this age and birth weight. Placental volume at 18 weeks correlates with maternal height and parity. Interestingly, placental volume is increased in women who are smokers at the time of conception only, but not in those who continued smoking through pregnancy. At 18 weeks' gestation, placental volume also correlates with maternal anemia.[49]

Ultrasonic measurements of placental volume have also shown adaptation by the placenta to maternal exercise and may help to explain the different effects of exercise on birth weight. Placental volumes are significantly greater in women who maintain regular exercise throughout the second trimester. At term, the increased size of the placenta was maintained in those who decreased their exercise, but increasing exercise in the second half of pregnancy reduced both placental size and birth weight.[50]

The high resistance found in the umbilical circulation with Doppler flow velocity waveforms in high risk pregnancies has stimulated examination of the fetal side of the placenta. This increased resistance is associated with poor fetal growth and outcome,[51] although abnormal fetal heart rate patterns immediately before delivery may better predict adverse neurological outcomes.[52–54] The pathological correlation with increased resistance in the umbilical arterial waveforms includes loss of the resistance vessels, the small muscular arteries in tertiary stem villi in the placenta.[55,56] The changes in umbilical arterial waveforms have also been associated with reduced physiological changes in the maternal spiral arterioles.[57] A mathematical model of the umbilical arterial circulation has been developed using the principle of a lumped element electrical circuit, and demonstrates that a large proportion of the resistance vessels need to be obliterated before changes in resistance becomes apparent.[58] It is not too surprising, therefore, that the growth-restricted fetus associated with increased umbilical vascular resistance is often hypoxemic.

These changes have been mimicked in pregnant sheep by repeatedly injecting microspheres into the umbilical arterial circulation to occlude the small resistance vessels. Injecting 9×10^6 15 μm microspheres over 9 days increased placental vascular resistance and an increase in the umbilical artery systolic/diastolic ratio was observed. Umbilical blood flow reduced to 237 ml min⁻¹ compared to 312 ml min⁻¹ in control animals.[59] Embolization of the umbilical circulation can be used to induce fetal growth restriction.[60] Initially, the number of microspheres required to lower oxygen content by 30–35% in the fetus is large, $11.6\pm2.5\times10^6$ on the first day, and then remained on a plateau for several days before declining further to 0.6×10^6 on the 10th day.[61] This suggests that the placental vascular bed opens up or that compensatory growth of the vascular bed occurs during the period that the microspheres are injected. However, the placenta was unable to sustain this (compensatory) process. Alternatively, since the experiment was conducted late in gestation, the onset of a pre-parturient process may have inhibited placental adaptation.

Doppler studies have shown that the umbilical circulation with a high vascular resistance responds to a nitric oxide-donating agent, glyceryl trinitrate.[62] This may be due to inhibition of the vasoconstrictor effects of thromboxane and endothelin.[63] Nitric oxide is reduced in the blood of women with pre-eclampsia and may be partly due to the decrease in the nitric oxide synthetase activity of the placenta. In experimental animals, inhibition of nitric oxide synthesis by administration of amino acids which compete with the endogenous substrate, arginine, cause a syndrome with many features similar to pre-eclampsia including fetal growth restriction.[65] However, caution should be expressed about manipulation of nitric oxide, since it has many actions leading to the comment, 'mediator, murderer and messenger'.[66]

Experimental restriction of placental growth

The methods used to restrict placental growth in experimental animals have been reviewed in more detail elsewhere.[67–70] In sheep, ligation of one uterine horn in early pregnancy effectively halves the number of specific implantation sites or caruncles available for recruitment by the blastocyst. At 120 days (late gestation), both placental and fetal weights were heavier in the ligated group compared to controls. However, at 140 days (just before term), this had reversed and both were lighter in the ligated group. Uterine blood flow was consistently higher in the control group throughout the last 60 days of pregnancy as was the concentration of progesterone in maternal blood.

Reduction of maternal uterine blood flow by either embolization or ligation of the uterine artery can be used to restrict fetal growth.[70,71] In small laboratory animals, ligation of the uterine artery in mid or late gestation restricts fetal growth and alters fetal metabolic state. In the rhesus monkey, which has a bipartite placenta, ligation of the interplacental vessels in mid-gestation causes growth retardation. Similarly, ligation of one umbilical artery in mid-gestation causes fetal growth restriction in sheep. All these methods induce disproportionate growth of the fetus in which there is evidence of chronic hypoxemia. This is also seen in baboons when a uterine artery clamp is applied. These animals also develop a pre-eclamptic syndrome. However, when a uterine artery clamp has been used in sheep to reduce uterine blood flow, fetal growth has been restricted without the induction of concomitant fetal hypoxemia. This suggests that the placenta may produce an inhibitor of fetal growth or that a deficit in a substance, which normally has a small margin of safety for its supply, becomes critical and limits the rate of fetal growth.

Restriction of placental growth can be induced by excising potential placental attachment sites, the endometrial caruncles, from the uterus of non-pregnant ewes. The majority of visible caruncles have to be excised (carunclectomy) to restrict fetal growth significantly. Placental compensation for the reduced number of implantation sites occurs, and includes extension of the implanting conceptus to the extremes of the uterus and increased size of the individual placentomes. Overgrowth of the placentomes, particularly in the body of the uterus, is apparent as early as 77 days of pregnancy. Following restriction, the placentomes assume an everted shape (where fetal tissue appears to overgrow maternal tissue) earlier in gestation. Within the placentomes, there is also an increase in the volume density of the trophoblast and the fetomaternal syncytium following restriction. However, the arithmetic mean thickness of the barrier consisting of the fetomaternal syncytium and the trophoblast, does not change following restricted implantation. The net effect is sufficient to maintain surface area for exchange and fetal growth at 90 days of pregnancy but insufficient at 120 days (term ~150 days)[72] (Chidzanja, unpublished observation). Placental compensation in response to intervention in the first half of pregnancy is common and occurs in many species.

In the placentally restricted sheep, fetal hypoxemia and hypoglycemia become apparent at about 90 days. Fetal hemoglobin concentrations increase but oxygen delivery to the fetus is reduced in proportion to the reduction in placental size. Fetal oxygen consumption per unit weight of fetus is not altered. Placental oxygen and glucose consumption per unit mass of placenta are decreased. However, placental secretion of lactate into the fetal circulation is maintained or increased. The overall result is a progressive decrease in the apparent margin of safety for the supply of oxygen and glucose for the fetus with decreasing placental weight. Not too surprisingly, transient decreases in oxygen delivery due to uterine contractions or increasing consumption with fetal activity induce acute-on-chronic hypoxic episodes characterized by fetal bradycardia and hypertension.[73,74]

The endocrine changes found in these experimentally growth restricted fetuses reflect the reduced supply of essential substrates. The concentrations in fetal blood of the trophic hormones, insulin, thyroid hormones and IGF-I, are reduced and those of catabolic hormones, glucagon, catecholamines and cortisol, are increased. The anabolic and mitogenic actions of the IGFs may also be reduced by changes in the abundance of their binding proteins including increase in IGFBP-1. Although in general, restriction of fetal growth retards development of many key organs and tissues, the high cortisol concentrations and the increased sensitivity of the adrenal to hypoxia in late gestation may induce early maturation of some steroid responsive systems. This may pose a further problem for these fetuses in relation to oxygen supply since there is an early switch from fetal to adult hemoglobin in the growth-restricted fetuses, a change that increases P_{50}. The increased concentrations of myoglobin in the heart with hypoxia[75] may help to protect against this change.

Complex changes are observed in the supply of amino acids. Late in pregnancy the net uptake of most amino acids by the fetus reverses, from one of net fetal accretion and oxidation of amino acids to net fetal loss of amino acids. The pattern of amino acids lost reflects the composition of body protein and includes alanine and the branched-chain amino acids, leucine, isoleucine and valine. The amino acids are taken up by the placenta and although some are metabolized to the branched-chain keto acids, this fraction is reduced. The larger fraction together with amino acids taken up from the maternal uterine circulation are oxidized by the placenta.[69] A consequence of this loss is fetal wasting. Investigations of short-term maternal starvation in this species shows loss of amino acids from the hind limb, probably mostly from skeletal muscle.

Endocrine changes occur in the mother in response to experimental restriction of implantation and include reductions in the concentrations of placental lactogen and progesterone. There is also a reduction in the rate of production of placental lactogen per gram of placenta to 34% of that in control animals. These changes are accompanied by an increase in maternal plasma glucose, but no change in insulin concentrations. Combined with the concomitant fetal hypoglycemia, this increases the transplacental glucose gradient, enhancing glucose transfer. Placental

blood flow per unit mass of placenta is also increased and together with increased extraction of glucose and oxygen, helps to maintain fetal supply of these essential substrates to the fetus. In addition, placental consumption of glucose and oxygen per gram of tissue is reduced. The reduction of supply of nutrients to fetuses, with restriction of placental growth causes the significant correlation between placental weight and fetal weight to emerge at an earlier gestational age than normal. The restriction of substrate supply, and reduced concentrations of those substrates in fetal blood largely account for the endocrine changes that reduce the trophic drive to growth in the fetus.[68]

Supplementation of a limiting substrate in the maternal circulation is one way of attempting to overcome the deficit in supply to the fetus when placental growth is restricted. Maternal hyperoxia increases oxygen tension in the fetus, but does not increase oxygen consumption by the fetus. However, it may have increased the margin of safety between supply and consumption. Glucose infusion into the mother also increases glucose concentration in the growth-retarded fetus; however, the smallest fetuses rapidly become acidotic and die, suggesting that this would be an unwise therapeutic approach!

Human intrauterine fetal growth restriction

In 1987, Peter Soothill et al.[76] published their seminal paper on the metabolic state of the growth-restricted fetus in women. These fetuses were identified by a small abdominal circumference on ultrasound examination. Further studies excluded fetal malformation, infection or chromosomal anomalies. These and later work have led to an exponential growth in our knowledge of oxygenation, metabolism and the endocrine state of the growth-restricted fetus. By and large, these studies, using the technique of cordocentesis, have shown that there is a remarkable similarity between these observations in the growth-restricted human fetus and those in earlier studies of experimental animals, noted above, where fetal blood samples have been obtained from chronically indwelling catheters.[68,76–79] Intrauterine growth restriction is commonly characterized by fetal hypoxemia and hypoglycemia, at least in late gestation. Triglyceride concentrations are higher in the growth-restricted fetus and correlated with the degree of hypoxemia.[80] The growth-restricted human fetus has lowered concentrations of many amino acids in its blood, particularly the branched-chain amino acids, whereas alanine increases. Protein turnover has also been assessed using stable isotopes in normally grown fetuses at the time of Caesarean section.[81] Isoptopically labeled [^{13}C]leucine and phenyl[^{15}N]alanine were used to estimate net uptakes, oxidation and fetal whole body accretion. Fetal whole body protein synthesis is ~13 g kg^{-1} day^{-1}. Importantly, placental supply of these two amino acids exceeds the fetal demand to sustain protein synthesis and oxidation by only a small amount, suggesting that there is only a small margin of safety for these amino acids. Placental transfer to and uptake and utilization of glycine by the small-for-dates fetus is reduced.

The changes in oxygenation and metabolite concentrations are probably responsible for many other changes within the fetus. Soothill *et al.*[76] showed that the number of erythroblasts in the fetal blood relative to white cells was related to the severity of hypoxemia. The endocrine changes in the growth-restricted fetus include lower concentrations of a range of anabolic or growth-promoting hormones including insulin, thyroxine and insulin-like growth factor-I (IGF-I). Stress and catabolic hormones such as β-endorphin, adrenaline, noradrenaline, cortisol and glucagon are elevated. These endocrine changes may account for the slowing of growth and also for the different pattern of growth. These endocrine changes are also likely to influence the timing of maturation of fetal organs.[70]

Internal constraint or enhancement of fetal growth

Multiple pregnancy is associated with reduction in birth weight and the incidence of fetal growth restriction is increased. However, the possibility exists that the growth trajectory for the fetus is lowered early in pregnancy in multiple pregnancy in women, as in polytocous species. Study of birth weight, particularly preterm ones, can not be used to assess this, since many babies born prematurely may be restricted in their growth. Serial ultrasound studies in the first half of pregnancy may resolve this question.

Fetal or placental infection is commonly associated with disturbances of fetal growth. Viral infections including rubella and cytomegalovirus inhibit fetal growth even though there is commonly organomegaly. Varicella can cause limb hypoplasia and hypoplastic digits. Apparent overgrowth of the fetus due to fetal hydrops may occur with fetal parvovirus infection. The current epidemic of the human immunodeficiency virus is not directly associated with fetal growth restriction, but many of the circumstances co-existing with this virus do restrict fetal growth.

Chromosomes, placental and fetal growth

Fetal and placental growth are disrupted in triploid and many trisomic pregnancies (see also Chapter 3.4). More recently, interest has focused on the phenomenon of confined placental mosaicism. The abnormal chromosomal composition may be present in all cellular components of the placenta or limited to just one cell type or layer. This has been found in about 1–2% of human pregnancies and has been highlighted since the introduction of chorion villous biopsy. A high frequency of intrauterine growth restriction has been found at term, when confined placental mosaicism has been confirmed. A more recent estimate of the incidence of this phenomenon is lower and suggests that it contributes about 7% of the cases of early fetal growth restriction.[82] The mosaicism may be confined to the trophoblast, the villous stroma or involve both. Confined placental mosaicism has been reported for chromosomes 2, 3, 7, 8, 9, 13, 14, 15, 16, 18, 22 and X.[83] Intrauterine growth restriction has been found most often

with a confined placental mosaicism with trisomy 16. The extent of the growth restriction relates to the proportion of placental cells with the trisomy. However, the fetuses that survived such pregnancies show catch-up growth and normal development.[84]

Alternatively, the trophoblast may contain normal cells and the fetus, trisomic cells. This has been found in some placentae examined for fetal trisomies 13 and 18 terminated in mid-pregnancy. This can lead to errors in diagnosis (a false negative), when a chorion villus biopsy is normal and the fetus is subsequently found to have a trisomy.[83]

In some of these pregnancies, the embryonic chromosome constitution may be corrected in early pregnancy, a phenomenon known as embryonic chromosome rescue. This can lead to uniparental disomy and imprinting errors in the offspring. Alternatively, recessive genetic disorders have been reported, even though only one parent carries the recessive gene. It is now estimated that there may be as many as 200 imprinted genes and delineation of the effects of uniparental disomy of these are awaited with interest.

The Beckwith–Weidemann syndrome may be due to uniparental disomy, trisomy or relaxation of the normal imprinting process. Excessive body and/or organ growth characterize this syndrome. Later in life, people with this syndrome are prone to tumor formation. The precise mechanisms for the overgrowth are not yet determined. It may be due to overexpression of IGF-II. However, the H19 gene which is thought to function as a tumor suppressor, is oppositely imprinted. It is closely located to the IGF-II gene and both these or part of the intervening 90 kb of DNA may each or separately contribute to the overgrowth. Interestingly, placental abnormalities including overgrowth commonly occur in this syndrome and may be the cause of the high incidence of pre-eclampsia in the mothers of such infants.[85]

Experimental manipulation of fetal growth

The classical approach of ablation of an organ has been used to determine its importance for fetal growth. Removal of the fetal kidney restricts fetal growth and causes oligohydramnios. In the last third of pregnancy of sheep, fetal hypophysectomy does not have a large effect on fetal growth. However, when it is performed in mid-gestation a substantial reduction in growth of some soft tissues and skeleton of the fetus occurs. Part of this deficit in growth is due to hypothyroidism, since the placenta of the sheep is relatively impermeable to thyroid hormones. However, replacement of thyroxine after hypophysectomy only partially restores fetal growth in this species.[86] Similarly fetal thyroidectomy restricts fetal growth and maturation. For example, there is a large delay in osseous maturation. Thyroidectomy also reduces fetal oxygen consumption.[87]

It is well known that insulin and glucose are important factors in determination of fetal size. Macrosomia is common in poorly controlled maternal diabetes mellitus. The role of insulin in fetal growth has also been regarded as central since the rare human fetuses with congenital absence of the pancreas are severely growth restricted.

Further examination of the role of insulin has been possible in fetal sheep. Excision of the fetal pancreas in late gestation reduces body weight by 30% and crown–rump length by 15%.[87] Similar reduction in fetal size occurs when the fetal pancreas has been chemically ablated in several species. The deficit of fetal growth relates to the duration of the hypoinsulinemia. Very recent studies show that deletion of the IRS gene (its product is the link between the insulin receptor and intracellular signaling) reduces fetal growth.[88] Prevention of fetal hypoinsulinemia by an intrafetal infusion of insulin prevents the reduction of fetal size after pancreatectomy. Insulin infusion into pancreatectomized animals also restores oxygen consumption to normal. However, increasing the insulin concentrations to higher concentration than found in normal fetuses does not enhance fetal growth, suggesting that insulin is a facilitator rather than a promoter of growth.[87]

Prolonged glucose infusions, that elevate fetal glucose concentrations, cause variable but higher insulin concentrations. The glucose-infused animals are heavier than normal, principally due to increased deposition of internal and subcutaneous fat.[89] These animals were delivered at term after periods of up to 4 weeks of exogenous glucose; however, in other studies, glucose infusion has led to fetal death.

Insulin-like growth factors

The IGF family, IGF-I and IGF-II, are polypeptide mitogens, that are among the major growth factors controlling mammalian growth before and after birth and during adaptation to changing environments and physiological states.[90] They differ from most other growth factors, in that they are able both to act locally and also in an endocrine fashion. The actions of IGFs are modulated by a family of specific binding proteins (IGFBPs), which generally inhibit, but can also facilitate, their anabolic, mitogenic and differentiative activities on a wide variety of tissues and cell types. Both IGF-I and -II exert many of their actions via the type 1 receptor, whereas IGF-II can also bind to the type 2 receptor, the cation independent mannose-6-phosphate lysosomal enzyme receptor. The IGFs are produced at multiple sites, although the liver has been proposed as the major source of circulating IGF-I postnatally. In pregnancy, circulating IGF-I and -II in the mother increase substantially in early pregnancy and remain high except in rodents where a decline occurs in late pregnancy.

A major role for the insulin-like growth factors-I and -II in the regulation of normal fetal growth is suggested by several observations. Both IGF-I and -II are present in most fetal tissues, as are the two receptors. The type 1 receptor is responsible for most of the anabolic actions of both IGFs. The type 2, the IGF-II, receptor may have an important role in limiting the promotion of fetal growth by competing for IGF-II with the type 1 receptor. Since IGF-II is paternally imprinted and the type 2 receptor maternally imprinted in mice, this has led to the interesting suggestion that there is a conflict between the maternally and paternally derived genomes with the latter enhancing growth

whereas the former cannot allow unregulated growth.[91] Only the IGF-II gene is imprinted in the human, perhaps reflecting the continued greater role for this IGF in the human compared to rodents postnatally.

Targeted disruption of the IGFs in mice has shown that disruption of the IGF-I or IGF-II genes inhibits fetal growth.[92,93] More severe inhibition of fetal growth occurs when disrupted genes for both peptides are present in the fetus. Disruption of the gene for the type 2 receptor results in fetal death at about 9.5 days in the mouse. However, disruption of both IGF-II and the type 2 receptor allows continued development and survival consistent with the proposed role of the type 2 receptor controlling or limiting IGF-II abundance prenatally.[94] Increasing the abundance of IGF-I by intrafetal infusion of IGF-I in sheep increases the growth of many internal organs. The liver, lungs, heart, kidney, spleen, pituitary and adrenal are increased by 16–50% by a ten-day infusion that increases fetal plasma concentrations of IGF-I some threefold.[95] Intrafetal infusion of IGF-I increases placental uptake of amino acids as assessed by α-amino nitrogen. It also changes placental structure reducing the barrier to diffusion by decreasing the thickness of the trophectoderm and reducing the connective tissue core of the villus. The impedance to blood flow measured with Doppler showed a decrease of ~2.5 fold in response to the IGF-I infusion in this species.[96]

Fetal organ growth

Fetal organ growth may be altered by changing mechanical or functional requirements for normal growth. Reducing the effect of fetal breathing movements by abolishing or by reducing negative pressure generated by breathing movements retards lung growth.[97] Draining the lung liquid also reduces lung growth, thus one of the functions of lung liquid in late pregnancy is to hold the fetal lungs at volumes above the functional residual volume, that is observed postnatally. Prenatally, this volume is maintained by functional integrity of breathing movements and the laryngeal sphincter. In the absence of amniotic fluid, fetal swallowing siphons out more lung liquid, reducing lung expansion and lung growth. The result can be severe pulmonary hypoplasia. In contrast, tracheal occlusion preventing lung liquid efflux causes overgrowth of the lung.[97]

Similarly, growth of the gut is dependent on fetal swallowing of fluid that is a mixture of amniotic fluid and lung liquid.[98] Esophageal ligation in the rabbit and esophageal atresia in humans reduces fetal size whereas ligation of the esophagus in the fetal sheep reduces size of the liver and pancreas. It has been estimated that about 10% of protein requirements of the human fetus are obtained by fetal swallowing. Preventing fetal swallowing has its greatest effect on the mucosa, with reduction of the intestinal villi.[98]

The growth of the fetal heart also responds to functional factors, and its growth is partly dependent on afterload. This may account for the increase in size of the heart of the growth-restricted human fetus when afterload due to increased peripheral vasoconstriction and high placental vascular impedance is present. The heart of the infant of the diabetic mother is also large in proportion to body weight, but it may be associated with poor function. Many factors are likely to influence the size of the heart relative to the body and these will include volume loading and in experimental animals, the sodium intake of the mother.

Final comments

In this discussion regulation of growth of the fetus, influential factors have been arbitrarily divided into those derived from external and maternal constraints or promoters of growth and those internal to the fetus. The placenta and the local uterine environment have been considered as separate entities, since they are central to normal fetal growth. However, it needs to be emphasized that there is a dynamic interaction between the external environment and the mother, the uterus and the placenta, the fetus and the placenta, and there are direct links between the fetus and the mother. All these may change growth of the fetus. For example, maternal smoking affects fetal growth and it does this in a multitude of ways. It has been suggested that smoking alters maternal nutritional intake. It certainly affects gas transfer even though this is alleviated by compensatory increases in hemoglobin concentrations in mother and fetus. Vasoconstrictor substances may alter uterine and fetal blood flows and the fetal heart rate rises with maternal smoking. In addition, tobacco smoke contains many substances that inhibit cellular growth including that of the trophoblast and within the placenta the path for diffusion is increased. Thus the inhibition of growth by maternal smoking may occur at many sites, including reduced supply combined with increased energy costs.

FUTURE PERSPECTIVES

The pattern of fetal growth has many long-term implications. Poor neurological outcome is more common in small-for-dates infants born at term. Even higher rates of neurological sequelae occur in preterm infants many of which have poor growth before birth. Recently there has been enormous interest in the association of a variety of indices of fetal growth with common adult diseases suggesting that programming of fetal growth may set the conditions increasing the risk for these diseases. Indeed, the conditions for each stage of development set, or limit, the conditions for all subsequent stages of development.[99] Poor fetal growth is now associated with increased risk for hypertension, coronary artery disease and chronic obstructive airways disease. Both small and large babies are associated with an increased risk for development of adult onset diabetes mellitus. These epidemiological studies initially conducted in England have been confirmed in studies in Australia, India and North America (for review see references 100 and 101).

These epidemiological studies set a major challenge, which is to determine the mechanisms that alter the rate and pattern of fetal growth and how this programs increased risks for the fetus as an adult. There are already a few examples from studies in animals, that the risk for diabetes is increased in animals for up to five generations when diabetes is induced in the first generation. In addition, the prenatal environment can be manipulated experimentally to induce hypertension that persists into adult life. However, it is too early yet to consider intervention studies to alter the rate or pattern of fetal growth with the hope that the risk for an adult disease may be reduced.

SUMMARY

Fetal growth is regulated by extrinsic and intrinsic factors that may constrain or promote growth.

- Common maternal contraints to fetal growth include nutrition, maternal size and weight-for-height, smoking, parity, and pre-eclampsia.
- Maternal diabetes often promotes fetal growth.
- Normal growth and function of the placenta is crucial for fetal growth. The effects of many factors on fetal growth are mediated by the placenta.
- Intrinsic or fetal factors controlling growth include the number of fetuses, genetic and chromosomal disorders, and fetal infections.
- Fetal growth depends on an adequate supply of nutrients. These nutrients modify the fetal endocrine and growth factor environment, which in turn modulates the rate and pattern of fetal growth.
- The insulin-like growth factors are crucial for normal fetal growth. Excess IGFs promote growth and deficits in IGFs result in fetal growth restriction.
- Other growth factors and cytokines are required for normal growth and development of the fetus or its placenta. Critical periods exist during which the presence of some of these factors is essential for continued or normal development.
- The small-for-dates human fetus is often hypoxemic and hypoglycemic. Animal studies show that the margin of safety for supply is reduced when placental size is restricted. Redistribution of nutrients between the fetus and its placenta may help to maintain their supply to the fetus.
- The effects of constraints on the growth or development of the fetus may persist for more than one generation.
- Reduced size and altered phenotype at birth are associated with common adult diseases.

ACKNOWLEDGEMENTS

The authors thank Ms M Brodtmann for help with collation of references and Ms G King for preparation of the manuscript. The authors' research has been generously supported by NHMRC and Ramaciotti Foundation. Dr Owens is an NHMRC Research Fellow.

REFERENCES

1. Morel PCH, Blair HT, Ormsby JE, Breier BH, McCutcheon SN, Gluckman PD. Influence of fetal and maternal genotype for circulating insulin-like growth factor-1 on fetal growth in mice. *J Reprod Fertin* 1994 **101:** 9–14.
2. Gluckman PD, Morel PCH, Ambler BH, Breier HT, McCutcheon SN. Elevating maternal insulin-like growth factor-1 in mice and rats alters the pattern of fetal growth by removing maternal constraint. *J Endocrinol* 1992 **134:** R1–R3.
3. Bassett NS, Currie MJ, Woodall SM, Johnston BM, Batchelor D, Lewis R, Skinner S, Gluckman PD. Maternal IGF-I treatment in spontaneously hypertensive rats reduces placental hypertrophy and enhances fetal growth. *Placenta* 1994 **15:** A4.
4. Gargosky SE, Owens JA, Walton PE, Owens PC, Wallace JC, Ballard FJ. Insulin-like growth factor-1, but not growth hormone, increases maternal weight gain in late pregnancy without affecting fetal or placental growth. *J Endocrinol* 1991 **130:** 395–400.
5. O'Callaghan SP, Katsman AI, Lang RJ, Owens JA, Owens PC, Robinson JS. IGF-I treatment of pregnant rats in late gestation does not prevent fetal growth retardation following unilateral uterine artery ligation. *Placenta* 1994 **15:** A51.
6. Du ZT, Dai YF, Owens PC, Armstrong DT, Seamark RF. Fertility of transgenic female rats expressing pig growth hormone. *Proc Aust Soc Reprod Biol*, Brisbane 1994: 36.
7. Vilar J, Cogswell M, Kestler E, Castillo P, Menendez R, Repke JT. Effect of fat and fat-free mass deposition during pregnancy on birthweight. *Am J Obstet Gynecol* 1992 **167:** 1344–1352.
8. Poppitt SD, Prentice AM, Goldberg GR, Whitehead RG. Energy sparing strategies to protect human fetal growth. *Am J Obstet Gynecol* 1994 **171:** 118–125.
9. Lumey LH. Decreased birthweights in infants after maternal *in utero* exposure to the Dutch famine of 1944–1945. *Paediat Perinatal Epidemiol* 1992 **6:** 240–253.
10. Durnin JVGA. Energy requirements of pregnancy: an integration of the longitudinal data from the five-country study. *Lancet* 1987 **ii,** 1131–1133.
11. Rink TJ. In search of a satiety factor. *Nature* 1994 **372:** 406–407.
12. Stewart RJC, Sheppard H, Preece R, Waterlow JC. The effect of rehabilitation at different stages of development of rats marginally malnourished for ten to twelve generations. *Br J Nutr* 1980 **43:** 403–411.
13. Rush D. Effects of changes in protein and calorie intake during pregnancy on the growth of the human fetus. In Chalmers I, Enkin M, Keirse MJNC (eds) *Effective Care in Pregnancy and Childbirth.* Oxford: Oxford University Press, 1989: 255–280.
14. Battaglia C, Artini PG, Dambrogio G, Galli PA, Segre A, Genazzani AR. Maternal hyperoxygenation in the treatment of intrauterine growth retardation. *Am J Obstet Gynecol* 1992 **167:** 430–435.
15. Godfrey KM, Redman CW, Barker DJ, Osmond C. The effect of maternal anaemia and iron deficiency on the ratio of fetal weight to placental weight. *Br J Obstet Gynaecol* 1991 **98:** 886–891.
16. Lumley J, Correy J, Newnam N, Curran J. Cigarette smoking, alcohol consumption in Tasmania 1981–2. *Aust NZ J Obstet Gynaecol* 1985 **25:** 33–41.
17. Joyce T. The dramatic increase in the rate of low birthweight in New York City: an aggregate time-series analysis. *Am J Public Health* 1990 **80:** 682–684.
18. CLASP. CLASP: a randomised trial of low-dose aspirin for the prevention and treatment of pre-eclampsia among 9364 pregnant women. *Lancet* 1994 **343:** 619–629.
19. Newnham J, Godfrey M, Walters B, Phillips J, Evans S. Low dose aspirin for the treatment of fetal growth restriction: a randomised controlled trial. *Int Meet World Plac Assoc* 1994: W4.8
20. Trudinger BJ, Cook CM, Thompson RS, Giles WB, Connelly A. Low-dose aspirin therapy improves fetal weight in umbilical placental insufficiency. *Am J Obstet Gynecol* 1988 **159:** 681–685.
21. Walker SK, Heard TM, Bee CA, Frensham AB, Warnes DM, Seamark RF. Culture of embryos of farm animals. In Lauria A, Gandolfi, (eds) *Development and Manipulation in Animal Production.* London: Portland Press, 1992: 77–92.
22. Parr RA, Miles MA, Cash MP, Waters JM. Timing of progesterone and embryonic survival in overfed gilts. *Proc Aust Soc Reprod Biol* 1994: 78.
23. Klentzeris LD, Li TC, Dockery P, Cooke ID. Endometrial biopsy as a predictive factor of pregnancy rate in women with unexplained infertility. *Eur J Obst Gynecol Reprod Biol* 1992 **49:** 119–124.
24. Wang JX, Clark AM, Kirby CA, Phillipson G, Petrucco O, Anderson G, Matthews CD. The obstetric outcome of singleton pregnancies following *in vitro* fertilization/gamete intra-Fallopian transfer. *Hum Reprod* 1994 **9:** 141–146.
25. Surani MAH, Barton SC, Norris ML. Experimental reconstruction of mouse eggs and embryos; An analysis of mammalian development. *Biol Reprod* 1987 **36:** 1–16.
26. Cross JC, Werb Z, Fisher S. Implantation and the placenta: key pieces of the development puzzle. *Science* 1994 **266:** 1508–1518.
27. Korach KS. Insights from the study of animals lacking a functional estrogen receptor. *Science* 1994 **266:** 1524–1527.
28. Lettario JJ, Geiser AG, Kulkarni AB, Roche NS, Sporn MB, Roberts AB. Maternal rescue of transforming growth factor-β1 null mice. *Science* 1994 **264:** 1936–1938.
29. Tsai F-Y, Keller G, Kuo FC, Weiss M, Chen J, Rosenblatt M, Alt FW, Orkin SH. An early haemopoietic defect in mice lacking the transcription factor GATA-2. *Nature* 1994 **371:** 221–226.
30. Brosens IA. The utero-placental vessels at term – the distribution and extent of physiological changes. *Troph Res* 1988 **3:** 61–67.
31. Khong TY. The Robertson–Brosens–Dixon Hypothesis – Evidence for the role of haemochorial placentation in pregnancy success – commentary. *Br J Obstet Gynaecol* 1991 **98:** 1195–1199.
32. Meekins JW, Pijnenborg R, Hanssens M, McFadyen IR, van Asshe A. A study of placental bed spiral arteries and trophoblast invasion in normal and severe pre-eclamptic pregnancies. *Br J Obstet Gynaecol* 1994 **101:** 669–674.
33. Rodesch F, Simon P, Donner C, Jauniaux E. Oxygen measurements in endometrial and trophoblastic tissues during early pregnancy. *Obstet Gynaecol* 1992 **80:** 283–285.
34. Khong TY, Mott C. Immunohistologic demonstration of endothelial disruption in acute atherosis in pre-eclampsia. *Eur J Obstet Gynec Reprod Biol* 1993 **51:** 193–197.
35. Aherne W. Effect of insufficiency on the fetus. In Gruenwald P (ed.) *Morphometry. The Placenta and its Maternal Supply Line.* Lancaster: Medical and Technical Publishing Co 1975: 80–97.
36. Boyd PA, Scott A. Quantitative structural studies on

human placentas associated with pre-eclampsia, essential hypertension and intrauterine growth retardation. *Br J Obstet Gynaecol* 1985 **92**: 714–721.

37. Teasdale F. Idiopathic intrauterine growth retardation: Histomorphometry of the human placenta. *Placenta* 1984 **5**: 83–92.

38. Teasdale F. Gestational changes in the functional structure of the human placenta in relation to fetal growth: a morphometric study. *Am J Obstet Gynecol* 1980 **137**: 560–568.

39. Jackson MR, Mayhew TM, Haas JD. Morphometric studies on villi in human term placentae and the effects of altitude, ethnic grouping and sex of newborn. *Placenta* 1987 **8**: 487–495.

40. Jackson MR, Mayhew TM, Haas JD. On the factors which contribute to thinning of the villous membrane in human placentae at high altitude. II. An increase in the degree of peripheralization of fetal capillaries. *Placenta* 1988 **9**: 9–18.

41. Mayhew TM, Jackson MR, Haas JD. Oxygen diffusive conductances of human placentae from term pregnancies at low and high altitudes. *Placenta* 1990 **11**: 493–503.

42. Zamudio S, Droma T, Norkyel KY, Acharya G, Zamudio JA, Niermeyer SN, Moore LG. Protection from intrauterine growth retardation in Tibetans at high altitude. *Am J Phys Anthropol* 1993 **91**: 215–224.

43. Jauniaux E, Burton GJ. The effect of smoking in pregnancy on early placental morphology. *Obstet Gynecol* 1992 **79**: 645–648.

44. Burton GJ, Palmer ME, Dalton KJ. Morphometric differences between the placental vasculature of non-smokers and ex-smokers. *Br J Obst Gynaecol* 1989 **96**: 907–915.

45. Boyd PA, Scott A, Keeling JW. Quantitative structural studies on placentas from pregnancies complicated by diabetes mellitus. *Br J Obstet Gynaecol* 1986 **93**: 31–35.

46. Mayhew TM, Sorensen FB, Klebe JB, Jackson MR. Growth and maturation of villi in placentae from well-controlled diabetic women. *Placenta* 1994 **15**: 57–65.

47. Hoogland HJ, de Haan J, Martin CB. Placental size during early pregnancy and fetal outcome: A preliminary report of a sequential ultrasonographic study. *Am J Obstet Gynecol* 1980 **138**: 441–443.

48. Wolf H, Oosting H, Treffers PE. A longitudinal study of the relationship between placental and fetal growth as measured by ultrasonography. *Am J Obstet Gynecol* 1989 **161**: 1140–1145.

49. Howie DT. Maternal factors, fetal size and placental ratio at 18 weeks: their relationship to final size. In Ward RHT, Smith SK, Donnai D (eds) *Early Fetal Growth and Development*. London: RCOG Press, 1994: 345–355.

50. Clapp JF, Rizk KH. Effect of recreational exercise on mitrimester placental growth. *Am J Obstet Gynecol* 1992 **167**: 1518–1521.

51. Hackett GA, Campbell S, Gamsu H, Cohen-Overbeek T, Pearce JMF. Doppler studies in the growth retarded fetus and prediction of neonatal necrotising enterocolitis, haemorrhage, and neonatal morbidity. *Br Med J* 1987 **294**: 13–16.

52. Todd AL, Trudinger BJ, Cole MJ, Cooney GH. Antenatal tests of fetal welfare and development at age 2 years. *Am J Obstet Gynecol* 1992 **167**: 66–71.

53. Marsal K, Ley D. Intrauterine blood flow and postnatal neurological development in growth-retarded fetuses. *Biol Neonate* 1992 **62**: 258–264.

54. Soothill PW, Ajayi RA, Campbell S, Ross EM, Candy DCA, Snijders RM, Nicolaides KH. Relationship between fetal acidemia at cordocentesis and subsequent neurodevelopment. *Ultrasound Obstet Gynecol* 1992 **2**: 80–83.

55. Giles W, Trudinger BJ, Baird PJ. Fetal umbilical artery flow velocity waveforms and placental resistance: pathological correlation. *Br J Obstet Gynaecol* 1985 **92**: 31–38.

56. McCowan LM, Erskine LA, Ritchie K. Umbilical artery Doppler blood flow studies in the preterm, small for gestational age fetus. *Am J Obstet Gynecol* 1987 **156**: 655–659.

57. McParland P, Pearce JM. Review article: Doppler blood flow in pregnancy. *Placenta* 1988 **9**: 427–450.

58. Thompson RS, Stevens RJ. Mathematical model for interpretation of Doppler velocity waveforms. *Med Biol Eng Comput* 1989 **27**: 269–276.

59. Trudinger BJ, Stevens D, Conelly A, Hales JRS, Alexander G, Bradley L, Fawcett A, Thompson RS. Umbilical artery flow velocity waveforms and placental resistance: The effects of embolization of the umbilical circulation. *Am J Obstet Gynecol* 1987 **157**: 1443–1448.

60. Block BS, Schlafer DH, Wentworth RA, Kreitzer LA, Nathanielsz. Regional blood flow distribution in fetal sheep with intrauterine growth retardation produced by decreased umbilical placental perfusion. *J Dev Physiol* 1990 **13**: 81–85.

61. Gagnon R, Challis JRG, Johnston L, Fraher L. Fetal endocrine responses to chronic placental embolization in the late-gestation ovine fetus. *Am J Obstet Gynecol* 1994 **170**: 929–938.

62. Giles W, O'Callaghan S, Boura A, Walters W. Reduction in human fetal umbilical–placental vascular resistance by glyceryl trinitrate. *Lancet* 1992 **340**: 856.

63. Myatt L, Brewer AS, Langdon G, Brockman DE. Attenuation of the vasoconstrictor effects of thromboxane and endothelin by nitric oxide in the human fetal–placental circulation. *Am J Obstet Gynecol* 1992 **166**: 224–230.

65. Molnar M, Hertelendy F. N-ω-nitro-L-arginine, an inhibitor of nitric oxide synthesis increases blood pressure in rats and reverses the pregnancy induced refractoriness to vasopressor agents. *Am J Obstet Gynecol* 1994 **166**: 1560–1567.

66. Anggard E. Nitric oxide: mediator, murderer and messenger. *Lancet* 1994 **343**: 1199–1206.

67. Owens JA, Robinson JS. The effect of experimental manipulation of placental growth and development. In Cockburn F (ed.) *Fetal and Neonatal Growth*. New York: John Wiley: 1988: 49–77.

68. Owens JA, Owens PC, Robinson JS. Experimental fetal growth retardation. Metabolic and endocrine aspects. In Gluckman P, Johnston B, Nathanielz PW (eds) *The Liggins Symposium – Fetal Physiology and Medicine*. Ithaca, NY: Perinatology Press, 1989: 263–286.

69. Owens JA. Endocrine and substrate control of fetal growth: placental and maternal influences and insulin-like growth factors. *Reprod Fertil Dev* 1991: **3**: 501–517.

70. Owens JA, Owens PC, Robinson JS. Experimental restriction of fetal growth. In: Hanson MA, Spencer JAD, Rodeck CH (eds) *Fetus and Neonate 3 Growth*. Cambridge: Cambridge University Press, 1995: 139–176.

71. Bennett L, Hanson M. Intrauterine compromise. In Ward RHT, Smith SK, Donnai D (eds) *Early Fetal Growth and Development*. London: RCOG Press, 1994: 363–369.

72. Chidzanja ST, Robinson JS, Owens JA. Restricted implantation increases the proportion of fetal villi and trophoblast tissue, and surface density in the ovine placenta. *Proc Aus Soc Reprod Biol* 1992, Abstract 35.

73. Robinson JS, Falconer J, Owens JA. Intrauterine growth retardation: clinical and experimental. *Acta Paediatr Scand Suppl* 1985 **319**: 135–142.

74. Robinson JS, Owens JA, Owens PC. Fetal growth and growth retardation. In Thorburn GD, Harding R (eds) *Textbook of Fetal Physiology*. Oxford: Oxford University Press, 1994: 83–94.

75. Guiang SF, Widness JA, Flanagan KB, Schmidt RL, Radmer WJ, Georgieff MK. The relationship between fetal arterial oxygen saturation and heart and skeletal muscle myoglobin concentrations in the ovine fetus. *J Dev Physiol* 1993 **19**: 99–104.

76. Soothill PW, Nicolaides KH, Campbell S. Prenatal asphyxia, hyperlacticaemia, hypoglycaemia, and erythroblastosis in growth retarded fetuses. *Br Med J* 1987 **294**: 1051–1056.

77. Harding JE, Charlton V. Experimental nutritional supplementation for intrauterine growth retardation. In Harrison MR, Goldbus MS, Filly RA (eds) *The Unborn Patient*. Philadelphia: WB Saunders, 1990: 598–612.

78. Economides DL, Nicolaides KH. Metabolic findings in small-for-gestational-age fetuses. *Contemp Rev Obstet Gynaecol* 1990 **2**: 75–79.
79. Pardi G, Cetin I, Marconi AM, Lanfranchi A, Bozzetti P, Ferrazzi E, Buscaglia M, Battaglia FC. Daignostic vaule of fetal blood sampling in fetuses with growth retardation. *N Eng J Med* 1993 **328**: 692–696.
80. Economides DL, Crook D, Nicolaides KH. Hypertriglyceridemia and hypoxemia in small-for-gestational-age fetuses. *Am J Obstet Gynecol* 1990 **162**: 382–386.
81. Chien PFW, Smith K, Watt PW, Scrimgeour CM, Taylor DJ, Rennie MJ. Protein turnover in the human fetus studied at term using stable isotope tracer amino acids. *Am J Physiol* 1993 **265**: E31–E35.
82. Wolstenholme J, Rooney DE, Davison EV. Confined placental mosaicism, IUGR, and adverse pregnancy outcome: a controlled retrospective UK collaborative survey. *Prenat Diagn* 1994 **14**: 345–361.
83. Kalousek DK. Confined placental mosaicism and intrauterine development. *Placenta* 1994 **15**: 219–230.
84. Fryberg JS, Dimaio MS, Yang-Feng L, Mahoney MJ. Follow-up of pregnancies complicated by placental mosaicism diagnosed by chorionic villous sampling. *Prenat Diagn* 1993 **13**: 481–494.
85. McCowan LME, Becroft DMO. Beckwith–Weidemann syndrome, placental abnormalities, and gestational proteinuric hypertension. *Obstet Gynecol* 1994 **83**: 813–817.
86. Deayton JM, Young IR, Thorburn GD. Early hypophysectomy of sheep fetuses – effects on growth, placental steroidogenesis and prostaglandin production. *J Reprod Fertil* 1993 **97**: 513–520.
87. Fowden AL. Fetal metabolism and energy balance. In Thorburn GD, Harding R (eds) *Textbook of Fetal Physiology*. Oxford: Oxford University Press, 1994: 70–82.
88. Leinhard GF. Life without the IRS. *Nature* 1994 **372**: 128–129.
89. Stevens D, Alexander G, Bell AW. Effect of prolonged glucose infusion into fetal sheep on body growth, fat deposition and gestation. *J Dev Physiol* 1990 **13**: 277–281.
90. Cohick WS, Clemmons DR. The insulin-like growth factors. *Annu Rev Physiol* 1993 **55**: 131–153.
91. Haig D, Graham C. Genomic imprinting and the strange case of the insulin-like growth factor II receptor. *Cell* 1991 **64**: 1045–1046.
92. DeChiara TM, Efstratiadis A, Robertson EJ. A growth-deficiency phenotype in heterozygous mice carrying an insulin-like growth factor II gene disrupted by targeting. *Nature* 1990 **345**: 78–80.
93. Baker J, Liu JP, Robertson EJ, Efstratiadis A. Role of insulin-like growth factors in embryonic and postnatal growth. *Cell* 1993 **75**: 73–82.
94. Wang Z-Q, Fung MR, Barlow DP, Wagner EF. Regulation of embryonic growth and lysomal targeting by the imprinted *lgf2/Mpr* gene. *Nature* 1994 **372**: 464–467.
95. Lok F, Owens JA, Mundy L, Robinson JS, Owens PC. Insulin-like growth factor-l promotes growth in fetal sheep. *Am J Physiol* 1996 (in press).
96. Owens JA, Lok F, Scarpantoni C, O'Callaghan S, Mundy L, Carbone F, Owens PC, Robinson JS. Intravenous infusion of insulin-like growth factor-l into fetal sheep reduces the barrier to diffusion and the impedence of umbilical blood flow. *Placenta* 1994 **15**: A54.
97. Harding R. Development of the respiratory system. In Thorburn GD, Harding R (eds) *Textbook of Fetal Physiology*. Oxford: Oxford University Press, 1994: 140–167.
98. Trahair JF, Harding R. Development of the gastrointestinal tract. In Thorburn GD, Harding R (eds) *Textbook of Fetal Physiology*. Oxford: Oxford University Press, 1994: 219–235.
99. Robinson JS, Seamark RF, Owens JA. Placental function. *Aust NZ J Obstet Gynaecol* 1994 **34**: 240–246.
100. Barker DJP. *Mothers, Babies, and Diseases in Later Life*. London: British Medical Journal, 1994: 180p.
101. Bock R, Whelan J (eds). *The Childhood Environment and Adult Disease*. Ciba Found Symp 156. Chichester: John Wiley, 1991: 243.

3.8

Fetal Cardiovascular Function

L Bennet, DA Giussani and MA Hanson

INTRODUCTION

Once the embryo is more than a few millimeters in size, the transport of gases and nutrients by diffusion from its external surface becomes inadequate for its requirements. Thus, as soon as its most rudimentary elements are present, the circulatory system must function to transport substances around the fetal body. In man, the developing endocardial tube becomes surrounded with myocytes at about 21–22 days (4–8 somites) and begins to contract as soon as it develops. More peripherally, the vitelline arteries and veins supply the yolk sac even before vascularization at the site of implantation is sufficient for exchange to occur there. This is a very rapid time of blood vessel and heart growth. The processes involved are beyond the scope of this chapter, but clearly the turnover of endothelial cells must be extremely high, of the order of a few days, which is greater than occurs postnatally except in parts of the female reproductive tract and in malignant tumors.[1] Early in embryonic life the developing heart can generate a small arterial pressure (about 2.5 mmHg by day 15 in the rat[2]). As it grows, heart rate increases until the time at which adrenergic and cholinergic innervation of the myocardium is complete, after which time heart rate usually declines. This occurs from mid-gestation in the fetal sheep but postnatally in the rat. The developing heart is exquisitely sensitive to the wall stress imposed on it due to its preload and afterload.[3] Thus it is clear that the heart develops morphologically and functionally to meet the demands placed upon it. Disturbances of inflow or outflow tracts produce drastic changes in the morphology and function of the heart.[4]

CURRENT CONCEPTS

Arterial blood pressure and peripheral vascular resistance

The extent to which arterial blood pressure is regulated in the fetus is not known. Needless to say, as fetal body weight increases, so does combined ventricular output and blood volume. There is also a rise in mean arterial blood pressure from the earliest time at which it has been measured – mid-gestation in the sheep.[5] Total peripheral resistance (calculated as mmHg ml^{-1} min^{-1} kg^{-1}) increases from 0.06 at 88 days gestation[6] to 0.09 at 130 days gestation.[7] Over this period, there is a relatively greater increase in arterial blood pressure than in cardiac output. This is due to a relatively greater increase in umbilical than in fetal body vascular resistance (see Table 3.8.1[8]). The fall in umbilical vascular resistance (strictly impedance) in mid-to-late gestation is shown by the change in the shape of the Doppler flow – velocity waveform in normal fetuses[9] such that the end-diastolic component becomes more prominent as gestation proceeds. In the peripheral circulation, the increasing deposition of smooth muscle in the resistance vessel media is offset by the increased vascularity. Whether similar changes in arterial blood pressure occur in the human fetus is not known, as it has not yet been possible to devise a method for measuring arterial blood pressure in the human fetus. It is important to resolve this issue as at present it makes the interpretation of Doppler flow-velocity waveforms difficult. An increase in vascular resistance due to placental pathology may produce an increase in umbilical artery pulsatility index (PI) and also a rise in mean arterial blood pressure. However, it is also true that an increase in mean arterial pressure, due for example to a widespread vasoconstriction in beds other than the umbilical, will produce a fall in umbilical PI as mean frequency increases whereas the systolic–diastolic frequency difference remains relatively constant.

The concept that the placental vascular bed provides a major determinant of peripheral vascular resistance provides a way of interpreting some recent epidemiological findings. It has been found[10] that the incidence of cardiovascular disease is greater in individuals who were born with a relatively large placental–birth weight ratio. The reasons for such an apparent disparity between placental and fetal growth are not clear and we cannot as yet establish cause and effect in the phenomenon. One idea is that

Table 3.8.1 The changes in fetal heart rate, blood pressure, combined ventricular output and vascular resistance with advancing gestational age in the sheep fetus

	Mean gestational age (days)		
	88	98	135[a]
Heart rate (bpm)	224 ± 27	203 ± 16	160 ± 9
Mean arterial blood pressure (mmHg)	31 ± 6	40 ± 3	63 ± 7
Combined ventricular output (ml min^{-1} kg^{-1})	516 ± 95	566 ± 65	497 ± 58
Vascular resistance (mmHg ml min^{-1} kg^{-1})			
Total	0.06 ± 0.02	0.07 ± 0.01	0.09 ± 0.01[b]
Umbilical–placental	0.13 ± 0.05	0.14 ± 0.04	0.18 ± 0.02[b]
Fetal body	0.12 ± 0.03	0.16 ± 0.03	0.15 ± 0.01[b]

Data from references 5, 8[a] and 7[b].

the placenta increases its growth under conditions where fetal growth is compromised due to hypoxemia or nutritional deficiency. Thus, it is interesting that relatively larger placentae have been observed in humans resident at high altitude.[11] Godfrey *et al.*[12] have also reported similar findings in pregnancies associated with maternal anemia during pregnancy. Alternatively, it may be that under these conditions fetal growth is compromised more than placental growth. Whether cause or effect, the relatively larger placental bed may produce a relatively lower peripheral vascular resistance, and it could then be envisaged that fetal blood pressure will be maintained by a more pronounced vasoconstriction in other vascular beds. This increased tone in resistance vessels may lead to changes in the vessel walls as occurs in hypertension postnatally.

After removal of the umbilical circulation at birth, a remodeled vascular tree or a maintained vasoconstriction might lead to a higher basal blood pressure. However, experimental studies have as yet failed to support this idea. Anemia produced either in the sheep or the rat during pregnancy, appears to produce a lower fetal and neonatal blood pressure.[13–15] Furthermore, although reduction of the sites of placentation in the sheep by carunclectomy before pregnancy produces a reduction in fetal growth and some compensatory growth of the remaining placental caruncles, basal fetal arterial blood pressure is lower than in control animals.[16] Finally, repeated exposure of late gestation sheep fetuses (from 110 to 114 days' gestation, term 147 days), to 1 h episodes of acute isocapnic hypoxia on a daily basis for 14 days does not produce any change in development of fetal arterial blood pressure or heart rate.[17] However, it is clear from this study that arterial blood pressure can follow different trajectories in individual fetuses over this period. This appears to be related to fetal weight, including heart and kidney weight, but is not influenced by repeated hypoxemia.[17] It has yet to be examined whether beginning the protocol at a younger age would produce changes in blood pressure or heart rate. Similarly, producing an insult which includes acidosis may induce alterations in blood pressure and heart rate.

There is clearly much more to learn about the processes by which fetal arterial blood pressure is controlled. In particular, we do not know whether remodeling of the peripheral vasculature occurs as for the pulmonary vascula-ture under conditions of persistent pulmonary hypertension.[18]

Heart size and stroke volume

The heart develops in size in relation to the load placed upon it. The factors which determine this are unknown but, as discussed above, disturbances in the pre- or after-load to the heart will produce major disturbances in its growth. Since the heart grows primarily by hyperplasia until after birth in most species,[3,19] the processes must act on myocyte cell division. Postnatally, increases in heart size are by hypertrophy. The processes by which this transition occurs are not known.[3]

Fig. 3.8.1 shows that the stroke volume of the right ventricle is greater than that of the left at any end-diastolic

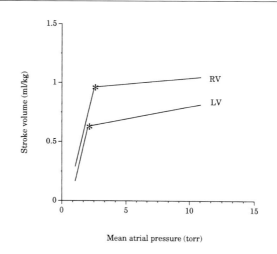

Fig. 3.8.1 *Simultaneous function curves showing right and left ventricular stroke volume of near term fetuses during alterations of mean right atrial pressure produced by rapid hemorrhage and rapid re-infusion. The function curve consists of a steep ascending limb and a plateau limb at elevated atrial pressures. The star on each curve represents the standard deviation of stroke volume and mean atrial pressure at the computer derived breakpoint of the curve (n = 12). (From reference 3 with permission.)*

pressure. Thus the right side of the heart normally contributes more to the combined ventricular output than does the left. Both ventricles operate close to the plateaux of their ventricular function curves so that increases in combined ventricular output are primarily produced via increases in heart rate rather than by heterometric autoregulatory mechanisms. Postnatally, the ventricular function curve of the left ventricle shifts up so that its stroke volume becomes equal to that of the right. This is a necessary prerequisite for the separation of the pulmonary and systemic circulations after closure of the foramen ovale and the ductus arteriosus. The processes by which this upward shift in ventricular function occurs are not known but have been suggested to be due to the removal of mechanical constraints[3] or to endocrine changes at birth.

Heart rate

As in the adult, a plethora of factors act on the fetal heart to maintain its rate above the intrinsic rate of the sino-atrial node. Nervous influences act via the vagus and sympathetic nerves in the late gestation sheep fetus[20] and indirectly via the release of catecholamines from the adrenal medulla.[21] These neural effects, which can form the efferent limb of reflex control of heart rate, appear to play a relatively small role in mid-gestation. In late gestation, hypoxia or asphyxia produces an initial bradycardia followed by a slow increase in heart rate which exceeds its control value over the next few minutes (Fig. 3.8.2). The early bradycardia under these circumstances is chemoreflex in origin as it is abolished by cutting the carotid sinus nerves bilaterally or by

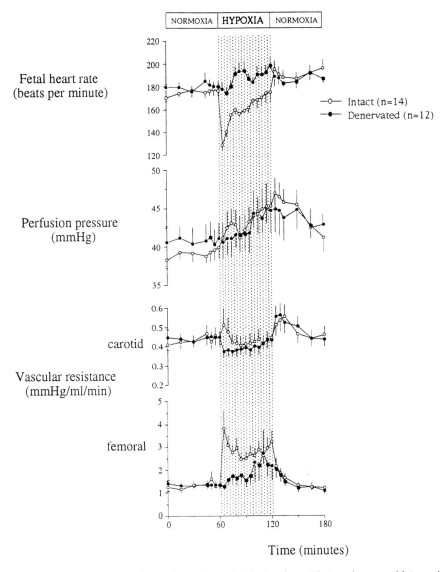

Fig 3.8.2 *Fetal heart rate, perfusion pressure and vascular resistance in intact and carotid-sinus denervated fetuses during acute hypoxemia. Values shown are mean ± S.E.M. (From reference 22.)*

giving atropine.[22] This bradycardia is not baroreflex as it occurs before a rise in arterial pressure has time to develop. Nonetheless, arterial baroreceptors are functional *in utero* and respond to changes in fetal blood pressure. Baroreceptor sensitivity resets to lower levels in late gestation and early neonatal life as blood pressure increases.[23] The delayed increase in fetal heart rate in hypoxemia is due to a β-adrenergic stimulation from the rise in plasma catecholamines.[24] Other humoral agents released in hypoxia or asphyxia may also be involved, but their precise role has yet to be determined. The most well known of these is arginine vasopressin (AVP) which is secreted in large amounts in hypoxia, acidemia, asphyxia or hypertension[25] and has been reported to reduce fetal heart rate.[26]

Hence the so-called 'early decelerations' associated with contractions during normal labour[27] are thought to be via a rapidly acting reflex mediated via vagal efferents. The mechanisms involved in producing 'late decelerations' are not obviously reflex in origin as they are not blocked by atropine.[28] Such decelerations in fetal heart rate are likely to be due to the direct effects of hypoxia on the sino-atrial node or conducting tissue, or possibly to the release of humoral agents which depress the heart. These may be endo-, para- or autocrine.

It is possible to produce prolonged increases in mean fetal heart rate by reflex and non-reflex means, e.g. in pyrexia from fever or from maternal exposure to high environmental temperatures.[29] Hemorrhage also elevates fetal heart rate.[30] However, the presence of an elevated fetal heart rate does not itself imply hypoxemia or acidemia.[31]

Fetal heart rate falls steadily throughout later gestation in the sheep and human fetus due to the rise in stroke volume as the heart grows and possibly secondary to the rise in mean arterial pressure.

Fetal heart rate variation

Interest in fetal heart rate variation has increased enormously over the last 15–20 years and some form of continuous fetal heart rate monitoring is now very common during labor, although its usefulness is debated.[32] A computerized acquisition and analysis system has been developed[33] in order that heart rate variation can be measured. The system reduces inter-observer error and makes judgements more objective. Prolonged loss of fetal heart rate variation and absence of accelerations is commonly held to be a cause for concern either antenatally or intrapartum. However, the possibility that the low variation is simply due to behavioral state has to be taken into account[34] and healthy babies can be born vaginally despite records being taken which did not show accelerations (especially before 34 weeks).

Fetal heart rate variation (FHRV) is reduced in intrauterine growth retardation associated with maternal hypertension or proteinuric pre-eclampsia but reduced variation does not correlate with the presence of acidosis at delivery.[35,36] Smith *et al.*[37] reported that reduced variation was associated with chronic hypoxemia (deduced from lower than normal umbilical artery Pao_2 at delivery). It is also associated with a rise in liquor erythropoietin, hypoglycemia and a rise in plasma alanine. Cordocentesis has also been used to correlate reduced fetal heart rate variation with hypoxemia *in utero*.[38] The degree of the reduction in fetal heart rate variation, and whether both short- and long-term variation are reduced, may indicate the severity of the hypoxemia or the presence of acidemia.[31,33]

However, the physiological processes underlying heart rate variation have not been established. Key studies[39] on the sheep fetus showed that the majority of the variation could be accounted for by fetal body and breathing movements and that variation was greater in the low voltage electrocortical state. Administering neuromuscular blockade to the fetus therefore reduced fetal heart rate variation. However, hypoxia is known to inhibit fetal breathing and body movements, so it would be expected to reduce heart rate variation. But in fact, in the sheep, heart rate variation increases during acute hypoxia[39] and in man variation increases during labor in association with the mild hypoxemia produced by contractions. Therefore, a distinction needs to be drawn between the effect of acute hypoxia, which appears to increase variation in both man and animals, and that of chronic hypoxemia (as in intrauterine growth retardation, rhesus incompatibility) which appears to reduce variation. More work is urgently needed if we are to understand the physiology underlying the difference, which is essential for assessing its clinical significance. For example, we need to know whether the variation normally present is a manifestation of the mechanisms which control fetal heart rate, e.g. baro- and chemoreflexes. Evidence for this in the sheep comes from the work of Itskovitz *et al.*[40] who showed that chemodenervated fetuses had a more variable fetal heart rate than did intact fetuses. Recently, Watanabe *et al.*[41] showed that the increase in FHRV in acute hypoxemia is related to the initial bradycardia which is known to be a carotid chemoreflex.[22] Kozuma *et al.*[42] have further investigated this in intact and carotid sinus denervated fetuses and have shown that the increase in short-term fetal heart rate variation (ST FHRV) during hypoxia is mainly due to a carotid chemoreflex bradycardia. They observed a much smaller increase in ST FHRV and no fall in heart rate in carotid sinus denervated fetuses compared to intact fetuses. The mechanisms determining FHRV during hypoxia in denervated fetuses are currently unknown.

Distribution of combined ventricular output

Table 3.8.1 gives details of the distribution of combined ventricular output in fetal sheep at various stages of gestation. As mentioned above, in late gestation about 44% of the combined ventricular output goes to the placenta. The precise figure for the human fetus at this gestation is not known, although it is likely to be less than the value for the sheep, as the head and neck draw a substantially greater fraction than in the sheep. The figures given for the sheep were determined using the radiolabeled microsphere technique. With this method the microspheres are usually injected intravenously and a reference sample is drawn from an appropriate upper or lower body artery. Flow to small organs, or parts of organs, is hard to determine with this technique as its accuracy depends on the impaction of an adequate number of microspheres. In addition, the method suffers from the disadvantage that flow is only measured at a single point in time. It is possible to use up to six different labels to obtain a sequence of 'snapshots' of blood flow but each will provide a value for a single time point, and the animal must be killed subsequently for measurement of the counts in the tissues. Continuous measurements of blood flow require the implantation of devices for measuring flow. The most widely used were electromagnetic flow meters which suffer from several drawbacks, largely that they must fit tightly around the vessel, and will thus reduce growth, and that they are difficult to calibrate *in vivo* and suffer from baseline drift. More recently, a transit time ultrasound probe (Transonic) has been developed which allows continuous reliable measurements of blood flow from arteries or veins. Transonic have recently introduced a range of microcirculation flow probes which can make blood flow measurements on vessels as small as 250 μm in diameter.

The use of Doppler ultrasonography for measurement of blood flow has been discussed above, and the key point is that it is impossible to extrapolate from measurements of velocity to measurements of flow unless the diameter of the vessel under examination can be measured accurately. As the cross-sectional area of the vessel is proportional to the (radius)^2, any error in the measurement of the radius is magnified substantially. Most recently, laser Doppler instruments have been developed for the estimation of blood flow in various tissues. Basically, these instruments give an estimate of the 'disturbance' of the red cells in a certain volume of blood in the tissue. They are currently only suitable for estimating changes in flow as no absolute calibration is possible. However, the ease with which light can be conducted along optical fibers provides an enormous advantage and the probes can be developed for application to the surface of an organ or to being driven into the organ itself.

Near infrared spectroscopy (NIRS) is also being developed for the study of the fetal circulation and has been used on the fetal scalp during labor.[43] Once again the method is indirect and at present depends on the measurement of total hemoglobin volume (i.e. both saturated and desaturated hemoglobin) as a measurement of blood volume in a tissue. Changes in blood volume can under some circumstances be used to estimate flow. The method has been applied to the fetal sheep brain[44] (Fig. 3.8.3).

Cardiovascular responses to acute isocapnic hypoxemia

Before about 110 days gestation in fetal sheep, isocapnic hypoxemia for an hour produces a rise in heart rate, which continues for an hour, and a small fall in arterial blood pressure.[5,45] Conversely, after about 110 days the initial response to acute hypoxemia is an initial bradycardia, with

a transient increase in arterial blood pressure[22] and an increase in fetal heart rate variability.[46] The magnitude of the heart rate and blood pressure responses depends upon the extent to which the arterial pH and blood gases change. During acute episodes of hypoxemia the combined ventricular output (CVO), the sum of right and left

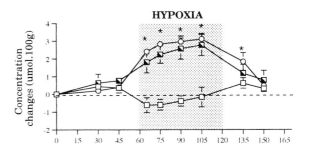

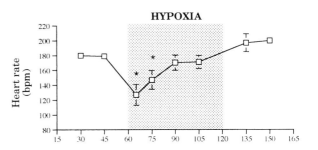

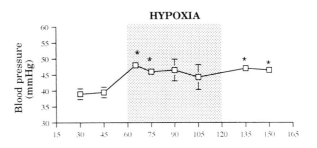

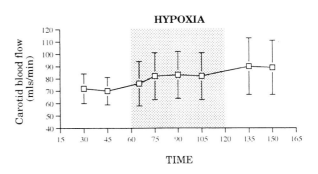

Fig 3.8.3 *This figure shows the effect of 1 h of isocapnic hypoxemia (PaO$_2$ reduced from 20 ± 2.0 to 12 ± 1.5 mmHg) on cerebral oxyhemoglobin (HbO$_2$, □), deoxyhemoglobin (Hb, ○) and thus total hemoglobin (Thb, ◼) and heart rate, blood pressure and carotid blood flow in the late gestation fetal sheep. Values are means ± S.E.M. *P<0.05 hypoxia and recovery versus control. (From reference 44).*

ventricular outputs in the fetus, is redistributed favoring the cerebral, myocardial and adrenal vascular beds at the expense of the gastrointestinal tract, renal, pulmonary, cutaneous and skeletal muscle beds (Fig. 3.8.4). Although blood flow to the umbilical–placental circulation is generally maintained in term fetal sheep during hypoxemia,[47] prior to the last third of gestation acute hypoxemia decreases umbilical–placental blood flow markedly even though mean arterial blood pressure does not change and heart rate increases.[5] This may be clinically important since it suggests an increase in vascular resistance in the placental bed. Although the mechanism mediating this vasoconstrictor action is unknown, hypoxemia may have a direct effect on the placental blood vessels since a decrease in PaO_2 has been shown to decrease blood flow in isolated perfused cotyledons.[48]

A component of the increased peripheral vascular resistance and the increase in arterial blood pressure during hypoxemia is mediated via an increase in plasma vasoconstrictor hormones. Catecholamines are released from the adrenal medulla, due to both increased sympathetic activity and the direct effect of hypoxemia on the gland.[21] In addition, plasma levels of arginine vasopressin (AVP) reach high concentrations during hypoxemia[25,49] (Fig. 3.8.5). Moreover, AVP infusion in normoxemic fetal sheep produces a vasoconstriction in the carcass without significant changes in other organs, and administration of a V_1 antagonist reverses the rise in systemic arterial pressure observed during hypoxemia.[50]

Other humoral systems may also play a role. Plasma renin and angiotensin II (AII) concentrations are high in the fetus compared to the non-pregnant ewe[51] and are thought to produce a tonic vasoconstriction, maintaining umbilical blood flow and gas exchange between the fetal and maternal circulations.[52] Both plasma renin activity[53] and plasma concentrations of AII[54] increase in the sheep fetus in hypoxemia and/or hypercapnia. Furthermore, infusion of AII into the fetal circulation produces a peripheral vasoconstriction.[55]

Studies by Green et al.[56] in intact and carotid sinus denervated fetal sheep (Fig. 3.8.5) showed that the rise in angiotensin II during hypoxemia is not mediated by a carotid chemoreflex. However, AII appears to contribute to the peripheral vasoconstriction more in the denervated than in the intact fetus because the effects on vascular resistance of the angiotensin converting enzyme inhibitor captopril are much greater in the denervated fetus: the effect of AII in intact fetuses is masked by chemoreflex vasoconstrictor mechanisms.

Although plasma concentrations of both adrenocorticotrophic hormone (ACTH) and cortisol are known to be increased during hypoxemic episodes[57,58] (Fig. 3.8.5), whether they have a role in cardiovascular control is little understood. There is some evidence to suggest that increases in plasma cortisol levels may modulate the action of other vasoconstrictor hormones on the peripheral vasculature.[59,60]

Less is known about the actions of other humoral substances, such as neuropeptide Y (NPY), endogenous opioids, prostaglandins and atrial natriuretic factor (ANF) on the fetal cardiovascular responses to hypoxemia. Hypoxemia stimulates β-endorphin release;[61] naloxone potentiates the fall in heart rate during hypoxemia[62] and also modulates the increase in vascular resistance during acute asphyxia.[63] Although ANF has been shown to be increased in hypoxemia, little is known about its possible

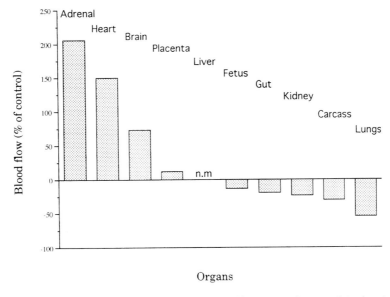

Fig 3.8.4 *Redistribution of organ blood flow (% of control) during maternal hypoxemia (Fio$_2$ = 6%) in chronically prepared fetal sheep near term. Fetal Po$_2$ in the carotid artery was reduced from 21 ± 1 mmHg to 12 ± 1 mmHg with no change in arterial pH. (From reference 6, with permission.)*

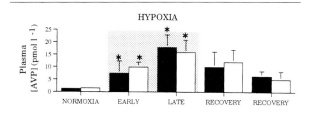

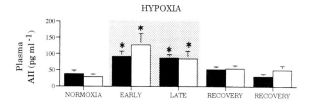

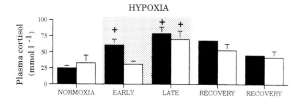

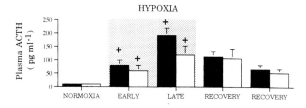

Fig 3.8.5 *This figure shows the effect of one hour of isocapnic hypoxemia (PaO$_2$ reduced from 23 ± 1.5 to 12 ± 1.8 mmHg) on plasma hormone levels in late gestation fetal sheep. Values are means ± S.E.M. for 15 (early) or 45 (late) minutes of hypoxia. *P<0.05 = P <0.01 hypoxia vs control. (From references 49, 56 and 58.)*

effects on the fetal circulation.[64] Green *et al.*[65] have investigated the role of endothelin-1 (ET-1) in peripheral vasoconstriction during acute hypoxia in fetal sheep using an ET$_A$ receptor antagonist. During hypoxia this reduced the femoral vasoconstriction and the carotid vasodilatation suggesting a role for ET-1 in the peripheral vasoconstriction during hypoxemia. There may also be a role for endogenous ET-1 in the tonic regulation of fetal heart rate. This may be via direct action at the SA node, possibly by a nitric oxide-mediated mechanism.[66]

In addition, hypoxemia may act directly on the peripheral circulation via local effects on the synthesis of vasodilators. However, the role played by factors such as adenosine, prostacyclin (PGI$_2$) and nitric oxide (NO) have currently only been discussed for the adult circulation.[67,68] Using the

NO-synthetase inhibitior L-NAME, Green *et al.*[69] have demonstrated a role for endogenous NO in the tonic regulation of FHR and peripheral vascular resistance in both normoxemia and hypoxemia. NO synthesis appears to be responsible for the rise in cerebral blood flow in hypoxemia.

Modulation of cardiovascular responses in sustained/chronic hypoxemia

Although it is now established that the fetus may successfully adapt to a single, acute hypoxemic insult during gestation and/or at birth, little is known about what effects repeated insults of hypoxemia or sustained hypoxemia *in utero* might have on these adaptive mechanisms. This is particularly important since there is increasing clinical evidence to suggest that: (a) prolonged hypoxemia may accompany fetal growth retardation,[70] and (b) antenatal hypoxemia predisposes the fetus to subsequent neurodevelopmental handicap arising from birth asphyxia.[71-73]

Animal studies have used techniques to induce chronic intrauterine hypoxemia such as reduction of uteroplacental blood flow,[74] reduction of placental size,[75,76] induction of maternal anemia,[77] ligation of the umbilical vessels[78] and induction of prolonged maternal hypoxemia.[79,80] With most of these techniques there are difficulties in inducing sustained fetal hypoxemia in a graded, reproducible manner. Other studies have concentrated on reducing uterine blood flow via occlusion of the internal iliac artery.[74, 81-86] Although this technique may allow greater control over the induction of sustained fetal hypoxemia, until recently, it has only been used to induce chronic hypoxemia over a period of 24–48 h. Currently, it is known that if intra-uterine hypoxemia persists for more than 8 h, heart rate,[81] blood pressure[82] and the incidence of body and breathing movements[83] return to normoxemic values even though PaO$_2$ levels remain low. Increases in cerebral, myocardial and adrenal blood flow are maintained. In addition, plasma concentrations of cortisol, prostaglandin E$_2$ and catecholamines are elevated[84,85] and DNA synthesis to the fetal lung, skeletal muscle and thymus[86] is reduced during chronic hypoxemia. A recent report documents the use of this technique for inducing hypoxemia over longer periods of time.[87] Preliminary results suggest that 2 weeks of moderate (about 15 mmHg) sustained hypoxemia enhances the peripheral vasoconstrictory response during a further episode of acute hypoxia. The response is similar to that observed in the llama,[88] a species adapted to the hypoxemia of high altitude.

The physiological processes controlling these behavioral, cardiovascular and endocrine responses to prolonged hypoxemia are currently unknown. In addition, whether 'adaptation' conveys impaired fetal responses to a subsequent superimposed episode of acute hypoxemia, such as may occur in labor, has been little addressed. This is an important area for future research.

FUTURE PERSPECTIVES

Clearly, considerable research now needs to be done to elucidate the mechanisms controlling the fetal cardiovascular system both in the normal and compromised fetus. This research is crucial to the development of future clinical treatment strategies.

In addition to establishing the fundamental physiological processes by which the fetal cardiovascular system develops and is controlled, future research directives will evaluate a number of key aspects of fetal cardiovascular physiology. One example of such future research concerns the mechanisms by which the fetus responds and adapts to alterations to the intrauterine environment. We know that the fetus is capable of adapting to alterations in its oxygen and nutrient supply, but we understand very little about the mechanisms behind this adaptation. Such information is important if we are to be able to assess the consequences of this adaptation for the fetus and newborn and to devise strategies and methods to detect the fetus at risk. For the clinician it is essential to know if the compromised fetus will be able to mount an appropriate cardiovascular response to further episodes of stress such as that seen during labor. It is also important to determine how (or even if) the compromised fetus will be able to cope with potential future treatments such as oxygen and nutrient supplementation and the administration of drugs such as glucocorticoids and thyrotropin releasing hormone (TRH) to enhance lung maturation in expectation of premature delivery.

Ultimately it is clear that the consequences of fetal adaptation to a compromised intrauterine environment do not stop with the fetus and birth. There is now increasing evidence that cardiovascular disease, such as hypertension, in later life may develop as a consequence of adverse events during fetal life. The way in which the fetus responds and adapts may play a key role in the etiology of such disease.

SUMMARY

- The development of the fetal heart is affected by the demands placed upon it. This affects both its structure and its function.
- Fetal blood pressure rises throughout gestation. This is due to both an increase in cardiac output and in vascular resistance.
- In late gestation umbilical vascular resistance becomes a major determinant of total peripheral resistance. This can in part be assessed by umbilical Doppler flow-velocity waveforms, but their precise physiological interpretation is difficult.
- Intrauterine events can have pronounced effects on fetal cardiovascular development: these can have both short-term (e.g. fetal survival, cerebral palsy) and long-term (e.g. adult cardiovascular disease) consequences.
- Fetal and placental growth, both in early and late gestation, profoundly influence fetal cardiovascular development, e.g. in terms of blood pressure and cardiovascular reflexes.
- During fetal life the right ventricle contributes more than the left ventricle to combined ventricular output. At birth, left ventricular output increases due to the change in mechanical conditions, e.g. the inflation of the lungs and neurohumoral influences which increase contractility.

- Fetal heart rate falls during development. The mechanisms controlling this are unknown, as are those determining fetal heart rate variation.
- In late gestation, acute hypoxia induces a chemoreflexly mediated redistribution of combined ventricular output, favoring blood flow to the heart, brain and adrenals at the expense of the fetal kidneys, lungs, gut, skin, muscle etc. These rapidly acting reflexes are reinforced by slower endocrine responses, e.g. the rise in catecholamines, AVP, AII.
- The fetal circulation is also under the control of local modulators of vascular tone. The endothelium plays a major role in the release and they act in a paracrine manner at adjacent vascular smooth muscle. Examples are NO, ET-1, PGI_2 and TXA_2.
- Prolonged fetal hypoxemia, e.g. from placental insufficiency, produces cardiovascular adaptation, whereby heart rate and blood pressure return towards control. However, the cardiovascular reflex, humoral and local control mechanisms (see points above) may be altered. This may impair fetal responses to further episodes of superimposed stress, e.g. acute hypoxemia during labor.

ACKNOWLEDGEMENTS

The authors are grateful to The Wellcome Trust, AFRC and Birthright for research support.

REFERENCES

1. Hudlicka O. What makes blood vessels grow? *J Physiol* 1991 **444**: 1–24.
2. Nakasawa M, Miyagawa S, Ohno T, Miura S, Takao A. Developmental hemodynamic changes in rat embryos at 11 to 15 days of gestation: normal data of blood pressure and the effect of caffeine compared to data from chick embryo. *Pediatr Res* 1988 **23**: 200–205.
3. Thornburg KL, Morton M. Growth and development of the heart. In Hanson MA, Spencer JAD, Rodeck CH (eds) *Fetus and Neonate: Vol. 1: Circulation.* Cambridge: Cambridge University Press, 1993: 137–159.
4. Allan LD. Structural and functional anomalies of the heart. In Hanson MA, Spencer JAD, Rodeck CH (eds) *Fetus and Neonate: Vol. 1: Circulation.* Cambridge: Cambridge University Press, 1993: 365–376.
5. Iwamoto HS, Kaufman T, Keil LC, Rudolph AM. Responses to acute hypoxemia in fetal sheep at 0.6–0.7 gestation. *Am J Physiol* 1989 **256**: H613–H620.
6. Jensen A, Berger R. Regional distribution of cardiac output. In: Hanson MA, Spencer JAD, Rodeck CH (eds) *Fetus and Neonate: Vol. 1: Circulation.* Cambridge: Cambridge University Press, 1993: 23–74.
7. Jensen A, Hanson MA. Circulatory responses to acute asphyxia in intact and chemodenervated fetal sheep near term *Reprod Fertil Dev* 1996 in press.
8. Cohn EH, Sacks EJ, Heymann MA, Rudolph AM. Cardiovascular resposes to hypoxemia and acidemia in fetal lambs. *Am J Obstet Gynecol* 1974 **120**: 817–824.
9. Marsal K. Doppler ultrasonography: techniques. In Hanson MA, Spencer JAD, Rodeck CH (eds) *Fetus and Neonate: Vol. 1: Circulation.* Cambridge: Cambridge University Press, 1993: 296–322.
10. Law C, Barker DJP. Birthweight and blood pressure in childhood and adult life. In Hanson MA, Spencer JAD, Rodeck CH (eds) *The Fetus and Neonate, Vol. I, Circulation.* Cambridge: Cambridge University Press, 1993: 252–265.
11. Kruger A, Arias-Stella J. The placenta of the newborn infant at high altitude. *Am J Obstet Gynecol* 1970 **106**: 586–591.
12. Godfrey KM, Redman CWG, Barker DJP, Osmond C. The effect of maternal anaemia and iron deficiency on the ratio of fetal weight to placental weight. *Br J Obstet Gynaecol* 1991 **98**: 886–891.
13. Davis LE, Hohimer AR. Hemodynamics and organ blood flow in fetal sheep subjected to chronic anaemia. *Am J Physiol* 1991 **261**: R1542–1548.
14. Crowe C, Dandekar P, Bennet L, Hanson MA. The effects of anaemia *in utero* and pre-weaning on heart size and blood pressure in neonatal rats. *20th Meeting of the Society for the Study of Fetal Physiology*, Plymouth, UK, 1993.
15. Crowe C, Dandekar P, Fox M, Dhingra K, Bennet L, Hanson MA. The effects of severe anaemia *in utero* and pre-weaning on heart size, placental to birthweight ratio and blood pressure. *21st Meeting of the Society for the Study of Fetal Physiology*, Cairns, Australia, 1994.
16. Robinson JS, Kingston EJ, Jones CT, Thorburn GD. Studies on experimental growth retardation in sheep. The effects of maternal anaemia. *J Dev Physiol* 1983 **5**: 89–100.
17. Crowe C, Bennet L, Hanson MA. Blood pressure and cardiovascular development in fetal sheep. Relation to hypoxaemia, weight and blood glucose. *Reprod Fertil Dev* 1995 **7**: 553–558.
18. Howarth SG. Persistent fetal circulation: principles of diagnosis and management. In Hanson MA, Spencer JAD, Rodeck CH (eds) *Fetus and Neonate: Volume 1: Circulation.* Cambridge: Cambridge University Press, 1993: 396–424.
19. Oparil S. Pathogenesis of ventricular hypertrophy. *J Am Coll Cardiol* 1985 **5**: 57–65.
20. Hanson MA. The importance of baro- and chemoreflexes in the control of the fetal cardiovascular system. *J Dev Physiol* 1989 **10**: 491–511.
21. Jones CT, Robinson RO. Plasma catecholamines in foetal and adult sheep. *J Physiol* 1975 **248**: 15–33.
22. Giussani DA, Spencer JAD, Moore PJ, Bennet L, Hanson MA. Afferent and efferent components of the cardiovascular reflex responses to acute hypoxia in term fetal sheep. *J Physiol* 1993 **461**: 431–449.
23. Blanco CE, Dawes GS, Hanson MA, McCooke HB. Carotid baroreceptors in fetal and newborn sheep. *Pediatr Res* 1988 **24**: 342–346.
24. Berger R, Jensen A. Fetal circulatory responses to oxygen lack. *J Dev Physiol* 1991 **16**: 181–207.
25. Raffe H, Kane CW, Wood CE. Arginine vasopressin responses to hypoxia and hypercapnia in late-gestation fetal sheep. *Am J Physiol* 1991 **260**: R1077–R1081.
26. Piacquadio KM, Brace RA, Cheung CY. Role of vasopressin in mediation of fetal cardiovascular responses to acute hypoxia. *Am J Obstet Gynecol* 1990 **163**: 1294–1300.
27. Martin CB. Pharmacological aspects of fetal heart rate regulation during hypoxia. In Kunzel W (ed.) *Fetal Heart Rate Monitoring.* Berlin: Springer Verlag, 1985: 170–184.
28. Caldeyro-Barcia R, Mende-Bauer C, Poseiro JJ, Escarna LA, Pose SV, Bieniarz J, Arnt I, Gulin L, Altahabe O. Control of human fetal heart rate during labour. In Cassels DE (ed.) *Heart and Circulation in the Newborn and Infant.* New York: Grune and Stratton, 1966: 7–36.
29. Walker DW. Effects of increased core temperature on breathing movements and electro-cortical activity in fetal sheep. *J Dev Physiol* 1988 **10(6)**: 513–523.
30. Brace RA, Cheung CY. Fetal cardiovascular and endocrine responses to prolonged fetal haemorrhage. *Am J Phys* 1986 **251**: R417–R424.
31. Dawes GS, Rosevear SK, Pello LC, Moulden M, Redman CW. Computerised analysis of episodic changes in fetal heart rate variation in early labour. *Am J Obstet Gynecol* 1991 **165(3)**: 618–624.
32. MacDonald D, Adrian G, Sheridan-Pereira M, Boylan P, Chalmers I. The Dublin randomized controlled trial of intrapartum fetal heart rate monitoring. *Am J Obstet Gynecol* 1985 **152**: 524–539.
33. Dawes GS. Computerized measurement of fetal heart rate variation antenatally and in labour. In *Recent Adv Obstet Gynaecol.* London: Longman, 1991 57–68.
34. Nijhuis JG (ed.) *Fetal Behaviour: Developmental and Perinatal Aspects.* Oxford: Oxford University Press, 1993.
35. Henson GL, Dawes GS, Redman CWG. Antenatal fetal heart-rate variability in relation to fetal acid–base status at caesarean section. *Br J Obstet Gynaecol* 1983 **90**: 516–521.
36. Henson GL, Dawes GS, Redman CWG. Characterization of the reduced heart rate variation in growth-retarded fetuses. *Br J Obstet Gynaecol* 1984 **91**: 751–755.
37. Smith JH, Anand KJS, Cotes PM, Dawes GS, Harkness RA, Howlett TA, Rees LH, Redman CWG. Antenatal fetal heart rate variation in relation to the respiratory and metabolic status of the compromised human fetus. *Br J Obstet Gynaecol* 1988 **95**: 980–989.
38. Visser GHA, Sadovsky G, Nicolaides KH. Antepartum heart rate patterns in small-for-gestational-age third-trimester fetuses: Correlations with blood gas values obtained at cordocentesis. *Am J Obstet Gynecol* 1990 **162**: 698–703.
39. Dalton KJ, Dawes GS, Patrick JE. Diurnal, respiratory and other rhythms of fetal lambs. *Am J Obstet Gynecol* 1977 **127**: 414–424.
40. Itskovitz J, LaGamma EF, Bristow J, Rudolph AM.

Cardiovascular responses to hypoxemia in sino-aortic denervated fetal sheep. *Pediatr Res* 1991 **30**: 381–385.

41. Watanabe T, Bennet L, Green LR, Hanson MA. Change in heart rate variability in acute hypoxaemia in fetal sheep. *The Society for the Study of Fetal Physiology, 20th Annual Meeting*, Plymouth, 1993.

42. Kozuma S, Watanabe T, Bennet L, Green L, Hanson MA. The effect of carotid sinus nerve section on heart rate variability in normoxia and hypoxia in late gestation fetal sheep. *The Society for the Study of Fetal Physiology, 21st Annual Meeting*, Cairns, Australia, 1994.

43. Peebles DM, Edwards AD, Wyatt JS, Bishop AP, Cope M, Delpy T, David T, Reynolds OR. Changes in human fetal cerebral hemoglobin concentration and oxygenation during labor measured by near-infrared spectroscopy. *Am J Obstet Gynecol*, 1992 **166**: 1369–1373.

44. Bennet L, Peebles DM, Edwards AD, Hanson MA. Cerebral haemodynamics changes in unanaesthetized fetal sheep measured by near infra-red spectroscopy (NIRS) in acute hypoxia. *J Physiol* 1994 **479**: 24.

45. Boddy K, Dawes GS, Fisher R, Pinter S, Robinson JS. Foetal respiratory movements, electrocortical and cardiovascular responses to hypoxemia and hypercapnia in sheep. *J Physiol* 1974 **243**: 599–618.

46. Parer JT, Dijkstra HR, Vredebregt PPM, Harris JL, Krueger TR, Reuss ML. Increased fetal heart rate variability with acute hypoxia in chronically instrumented sheep. *Eur J Obstet Gynaecol Reprod Biol* 1980 **10**: 393.

47. Peeters LLH, Sheldon RE, Jones MD, Makowski EL, Meschia G. Blood flow to fetal organs as a function of arterial oxygen content. *Am J Obstet Gynecol* 1979 **135**: 637–646.

48. Howard RB, Hosokawa T, Maguirre MH. Hypoxic induced fetoplacental vasoconstriction in perfused human placental cotyledons. *Am J Obstet Gynecol* 1987 **157**: 1261–1266.

49. Giussani DA, McGarrigle HHG, Spencer JAD, Moore PJ, Bennet L, Hanson MA. Effect of carotid denervation on plasma vasopressin levels during acute hypoxia in the late-gestation sheep fetus. *J Physiol* 1994 **477**: 81–87.

50. Iwamoto HS, Rudolph AM, Keil LC, Heymann MA. Hemodynamic responses of the sheep fetus to vasopressin infusion. *Circ Res* 1979 **44**: 430.

51. Broughton-Pipkin F, Kirkpatrick SML, Lumbers ER, Mott JC. Factors influencing plasma renin and angiotensin II in the conscious pregnant ewe and its foetus. *J Physiol* 1974 **243**: 619–637.

52. Iwamoto HS, Rudolph AM. Effects of endogenous angiotensin II on the fetal circulation. *J Dev Physiol* 1979 **1**: 283–293.

53. Wood CE, Kane C, Raff H. Peripheral chemoreceptor control of fetal renin responses to hypoxia and hypercapnia. *Circ Res* 1990 **67**: 722–732.

54. Martin AA, Kapoor R, Scroop GC. Hormonal factors in the control of heart rate in the normoxaemic and hypoxaemic fetal, neonatal and adult sheep. *J Dev Physiol* 1987 **9**: 465–480.

55. Iwamoto HS, Rudolph AM. Effects of angiotensin II on the blood flow and its distribution in fetal lambs. *Circ Res* 1981 **48**: 183–189.

56. Green LR, McGarrigle HHG, Bennet L, Hanson MA. The effect of acute hypoxaemia on plasma angiotensin II in intact and carotid sinus-denervated fetal sheep. *J Physiol* 1994 **476**: 81P.

57. Jones CT, Boddy K, Robinson JS, Ratcliffe JG. Developmental changes in the response of the adrenal glands of the fetal sheep to endogenous corticotrophin, as indicated by hormone responses to hypoxaemia. *J Endocrinol* 1977 **72**: 279–292.

58. Giussani DA, McGarrigle HHG, Moore PJ, Bennet L, Spencer JAD, Hanson MA. Carotid sinus nerve section and the increase in plasma cortisol during acute hypoxia in fetal sheep. *J Physiol* 1994 **477**(1): 75–80.

59. Tangalakis K, Lumbers ER, Moritz KM, Towstoless MK, Wintour EM. Effect of cortisol on blood pressure and vascular reactivity in the ovine fetus. *Exp Physiol* 1992 **77**: 709–717.

60. Walker BR, Connacher AA, Webb DJ, Edwards CR. Glucocorticoids and blood pressure: a role for the cortisol/cortisone shuttle in the control of vascular tone in man. *Clin Sci* 1992 **83**: 171–178.

61. Stark RI, Wardlaw SL, Daniel SS, Sanocka UM, James LS, van de Wiele RL. Vasopressin secretion induced by hypoxia in sheep: Developmental changes and relationship to β-endorphin release. *Am J Obstet Gynaecol* 1982 **143**: 204–212.

62. LaGamma EF, Itskovitz J, Rudolph AM. Effects of naloxone on fetal circulatory responses to hypoxia. *Am J Obstet Gynaecol* 1982 **143**: 933.

63. Espinoza M, Riquelme R, Germain AM, Tevah J, Parer JT, Llanos AJ. Role of endogenous opioids in the cardiovascular responses to asphyxia in fetal sheep. *Am J Physiol* 1989 **256**: R1063–R1068.

64. Smith FG, Sato T, Varille VA, Robillard JE. Atrial natriuretic factor during fetal and postnatal life; a review. *J Dev Physiol* 1989 **12**(2): 55–62.

65. Green LR, Bennet L, Hanson MA. The role of endothelin-1 in peripheral vasoconstriction during acute hypoxaemia in the late gestation fetal sheep. *Proceedings of the Society for the Study of Fetal Physiology*, Cairns, Australia, 1994.

66. Han X, Shimoni Y, Giles WR. An obligatory role for nitric oxide in autonomic control of mammalian heart rate. *J Physiol* **476**: 309–314.

67. Tenney SM. Hypoxic vasorelaxation. *News in Physiological Sciences* 1990 **5**: 40.

68. Lüscher TF, Dohi Y. Endothelium-derived relaxing factor and endothelin in hypertension. *News in Physiological Sciences* 1992 **7**: 120–123.

69. Green LR, Bennet L, Hanson MA. The role of nitric oxide synthesis in the cardiovascular responses to acute hypoxaemia in the late gestation sheep fetus. *J Physiol* 1996, in press.

70. Nicolaides KH, Economides DL, Soothill PW. Blood gases, pH, and lactate in appropriate- and small-for-gestational-age fetuses. *Am J Obstet Gynecol* 1989 **161**: 996–1001.

71. Dijxhoorn MJ, Visser GHA, Touwen BCL, Huisjes HJ. Apgar score, meconium and acidaemia at birth in small-for-gestational-age infants born at term, and their relation to neurological morbidity. *Br J Obstet Gynaecol* 1987 **94**: 873–879.

72. Hull J, Dodd K. What is birth asphyxia? *Br J Obstet Gynaecol* 1991 **98**: 953–955.

73. Hill A. Current concepts of hypoxic–ischaemic cerebral injury in the newborn. *Ped Neurol* 1991 **7**: 317–325.

74. Clark K, Durnwald M, Austin J. A model for studying chronic reduction in uterine blood flow in pregnant sheep. *Am J Physiol* 1982 **242**: H297–301.

75. Alexander G. Studies on the placenta of the sheep (*Ovis aries* L.): effect of surgical reduction in the number of caruncles. *J Reprod Fertil* 1964 **7**: 307–322.

76. Robinson JS, Kingston EJ, Jones CT, Thorburn GD. The effect of removal of endometrial caruncles on fetal size and metabolism. *J Dev Physiol* 1979 **1**: 379–398.

77. Edelstone DI, Paulone ME, Maljovec JJ, Hagberg M. Effects of maternal anaemia on cardiac output, systemic oxygen consumption and regional blood flow in pregnant sheep. *Am J Obstet Gynecol* 1987 **156**: 740–748.

78. Creasy RK, de Swiet M, Kahanpaa KV, Young WP, Rudolph AM. Pathophysiological changes in the foetal lambs with growth retardation. In Comline RS, Cross KW, Dawes GS, Nathanielsz PW (eds) *Foetal and Neonatal Physiology*. Cambridge: Cambridge University Press, 1973: 398–402.

79. Jacobs R, Robinson JS, Owens JA, Falconer J, Webster MED. The effect of prolonged hypobaric hypoxia on growth in fetal sheep. *J Dev Physiol* 1988 **10**: 97–112.

80. Kitanaka T, Alonso JG, Gilbert RD, Benjamin LS, Clemons GK, Longo LD. Fetal responses to long-term hypoxemia in sheep. *Am J Physiol* 1989 **256**: R1348–R1354.

81. Bocking AD, Harding R, Wickham PJD. Effects of reduced uterine blood flow on accelerations and decelerations in heart rate of fetal sheep. *Am J Obstet Gynecol* 1986 **154**: 329–335.

82. Bocking AD, Gagnon R, White SE, Homan J, Milne KM, Richardson BS. Circulatory responses to prolonged hypoxemia in fetal sheep. *Am J Obstet Gynecol* 1988 **159**: 1418–1424.

83. Bocking AD, White S, Gagnon R, Hansford H. Effect of prolonged hypoxemia on fetal heart rate accelerations and decelerations in sheep. *Am J Obstet Gynecol* 1989 **161**: 722–727.

84. Challis JRG, Fraher L, Oosterhuis J, White SE, Bocking AD. Fetal and maternal endocrine responses to prolonged reductions in uterine blood flow in pregnant sheep. *Am J Obstet Gynaecol* 1989 **160**: 926–932.

85. Hooper SB, Coulter CL, Deayton JM, Harding R, Thorburn GD. Fetal endocrine responses to prolonged hypoxemia in sheep. *Am J Physiol* 1990 **259**: R703–R708.

86. Hooper SB, Bocking AD, White SE, Challis JRG, Han VKM. DNA synthesis is reduced in selected fetal tissues during prolonged hypoxemia. *Am J Physiol* 1991 **261**: R508–R514.

87. Bennet L, Hanson MA. Intra-uterine compromise: physiological consequences. In Donnai D, Smith SK, Ward RHT (eds) *Early Fetal Growth and Development*. London: RCOG Press, 1994: 363–370.

88. Giussani DA, Riquelme RA, Gaete CR, Moraga FA, Sanhueza EM, Hanson MA, Llanos JA. Rapid, intense peripheral vasoconstriction in the llama fetus *in utero* during acute hypoxaemia at 0.6–0.7 of gestation. *J Physiol* 1993 **473**: 64P.

Fetal Lung Development

R Hume

INTRODUCTION

Adequate structural and functional development of the fetal lung *in utero* is essential to allow rapid and successful adaptation of the neonate to extrauterine gas exchange. If fetal lung development is delayed or abnormal, then respiratory insufficiency is likely in the newborn period. For example, respiratory distress syndrome (RDS) is the consequence of failure of fetal lung development and in the UK 6000 preterm infants per annum suffer the severest form of the disease. Ventilatory support is successful for infants at 30 weeks' gestation, where respiratory distress is caused primarily by a deficiency of surfactant. Extreme preterm infants, in addition, have inadequate maturation of the respiratory portion of the lung and from 20 to 30 weeks' gestation, the pattern of survival (0 to 98%) is directly related to that critical stage of lung development when terminal airsacs are being formed.

CURRENT CONCEPTS

Morphology of fetal lung development

Human lung development is dependent on the interaction between an endodermal bud from the developing foregut and the splanchnic mesoderm which it invades. The developmental stages are usually divided into embryonic (3–7 weeks), pseudoglandular (7–16 weeks), canilicular (16–24 weeks) and a terminal sac phase (24 weeks to term).[1]

Embryonic phase

During the embryonic phase, the endodermal outgrowth subdivides at around 4 weeks into two sacs forming the primitive lung buds. The lung buds develop lobar buds corresponding to the mature lung i.e. three on the right, two on the left, and by around 6–7 weeks the lobar buds have further subdivided to form the bronchopulmonary segments.[2]

Pseudoglandular phase

During this phase of development, from 7 to 16 weeks' gestation, the bronchial tree undergoes repeated dichotomous branching resulting in 16–25 generations of presumptive airways (Fig. 3.9.1A). By the end of this phase all the bronchial airways have been formed with the bronchiolar tree ending in terminal bronchii from which three or four orders of respiratory bronchii originate. In turn, the respiratory bronchii end in terminal sacs which are the presumptive alveolar ducts.[1,3]

The branching growth of lung epithelium is regulated by mesenchymal interactions which appear to be specific for different levels of the developing respiratory tree. For example if mesenchyme is removed from around developing lung buds then branching ceases, but if this mesenchyme is grafted onto trachea new outgrowths are induced from the trachea. Conversely mesenchyme from around the trachea will inhibit branching if grafted around developing lung buds. The mesenchymal effects are tissue and organ specific but independent of species.[4]

Canilicular phase

During the late canilicular phase from 20 to 24 weeks' gestation specialization of the respiratory portion of the lung begins with dilatation of the terminal airways and differentiation of the progenitor epithelium to type I (gas exchanging) and type II (surfactant producing) pneumatocytes (Fig. 3.9.1B,C). The progenitor epithelium is in a partially differentiated state, expressing only some of the proteins expected in the fully differentiated cell. The progression of a progenitor cell to a type II pneumatocyte is likely to involve several intermediate cell stages. Many studies have shown that type I and type II pneumatocytes are developmentally related and that type I cells are derived from type

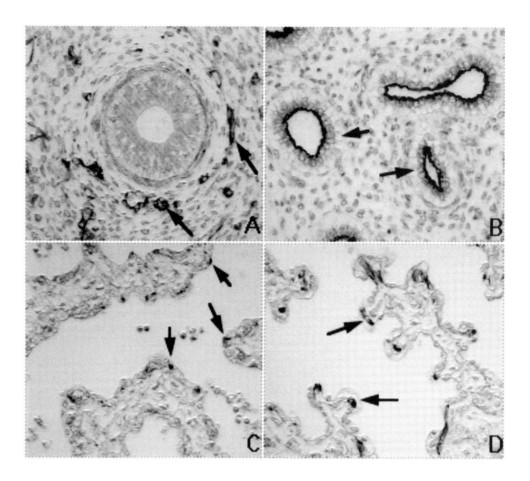

Fig. 3.9.1 *Light photomicrographs of human fetal lung development (×230).* **(A)** *A 9-week gestation lung showing a developing bronchial airway and extensive mesenchymal blood vessel development immunostained with vimentin antibody (arrows).* **(B)** *A 16-week gestation lung showing distal airways lined with partially differentiated columnar cells filled with glycogen (arrows) and apically immunostained with epithelial membrane antigen.* **(C)** *A 23-week gestation lung showing that the distal airways are dilating, that the epithelium is flattening and foci of elastin, stained histochemically, are being deposited (arrows).* **(D)** *A 27-week gestation lung showing the formation of secondary-alveolar crests subdividing the distal airsac at sites of elastin deposition (arrows) (see Plate 2).*

II. The interrelationship and contact between type II cells and an underlying proliferation of mesenchymal capillaries appears to be an important event in the conversion of type II to type I pneumatocytes.[3,5-7]

Terminal sac phase

The development of the respiratory airway continues through the terminal sac phase initially with the formation of dilated saccules separated by primary septae. The next stages in the process of lung maturation are critically dependent on mesenchymal events namely vascularization and elastin deposition.

Elastin as a supporting fibrous network, is present around major airways and lung blood vessels as early as 9–12 weeks' gestation and extends distally along the con-ducting airways to the necks of the dilating saccules. Elastin development around terminal airways is delayed until 23–24 weeks' gestation and the formation of foci of elastin deposition at key points around the dilating saccule is a critical initial event in the subdivision of the saccule and the eventual formation of alveolar spaces (Fig. 3.9.1C).

At around 26–27 weeks' gestation and at those foci of elastin deposition around the dilating saccule, secondary septae containing a capillary loop begin to arise from the primary septae and grow into the lumen of the saccule (Fig. 3.9.1D). Further elongation and thinning of these secondary septae along with the development of a single capillary network, morphologically marks the acquisition of an alveolar structure which can be seen as early as 29 weeks' gestation and is usually present in all lungs by 36 weeks' gestation. At term, alveolar numbers vary widely but human lung has on average 150×10^6 alveoli, around half the adult complement. Alveolar numbers continue to increase through childhood until about eight years of age.[8,9]

Elastin deposition at focal points around the developing saccule appears to be a critical event in the subsequent formation of an alveolar structure but little is known about the regulation of this process. Although epithelial–mesenchymal processes are important in determining the structure of the developing lung, the timing of secondary septal and alveolar formation varies between species, particularly with regard to the differentiation of the respiratory epithelium. For example, mice and rats have simple saccular terminal airways at the time of birth and only develop alveoli postnatally whereas in sheep, alveoli form antenatally before differentiation of the terminal airway epithelium, suggesting that these are independently regulated or species specific processes. Corticosteroids and somatomedins influence elastin formation in blood vessels but have no effect on elastin formation in developing lung. However, recent research suggests that transforming growth factor-beta 1 (TGF-β1) has a role in regulating lung elastin production by increasing levels of soluble elastin mRNA with developing lung more responsive to TGF-β1 than adult.[10,11]

Pulmonary surfactant

Pulmonary surfactant is a lipoprotein complex where glycerophospholipids and several specific proteins interact to reduce surface tension at the air–liquid interface. Surfactant is synthesized by type II pneumatocytes which can be identified as early as 22 weeks' gestation, though amounts of surfactant in amniotic fluid only significantly rise after 30 weeks' gestation.

Surfactant phospholipids

Pulmonary surfactant has a unique composition because it contains a high proportion of dipalmitoylphosphatidylcholine (DPPC), >50% of total surfactant glycerophospholipids and in addition contains large amounts, up to 10%, of phosphatidylglycerol.[12]

The surfactant initially synthesized by fetal lung is rich in DPPC but contains only small amounts of phosphatidylglycerol, although relatively large amounts of another acidic glycerophospholipid, phosphatidylinositol (PI), are present. As gestation proceeds the ratio of phosphatidylglycerol to PI changes, for example in humans from 0.04 at 35 weeks' gestation to 1.75 at term. The role of phosphatidylglycerol in surfactant function has not been clearly defined although the wide variability of content in mammalian surfactant and substitution studies in animals suggest its role is not critical for surfactant function.[13]

The relative proportions of phosphatidylglycerol and phosphatidylinositol synthesized by fetal lung may be under multihormonal control. The evidence for this comes from human fetal lung *in vitro* experiments where glucocorticoids acting in concert with prolactin or insulin stimulate DPPC formation. This hormonal combination also alters the relative rates of synthesis of the two compounds resulting in surfactant rich in phosphatidylglycerol with reduced PI.[14]

Surfactant proteins

Four surfactant-associated proteins, SP-A, SP-B, SP-C and SP-D have been characterized. Their potential importance in the reduction of alveolar surface tension and in endocytosis and reutilization of secreted surfactant by type II cells has stimulated research into the structures of the surfactant proteins and their genes, as well as their developmental and hormonal regulation in fetal lung tissue. The genes encoding SP-A, SP-B and SP-C are expressed in a cell-specific manner and are independently regulated in fetal lung tissue during development.[15,16]

Surfactant protein SP-A

The major surfactant-associated protein, SP-A, is likely to have multiple functions including a role in reduction of alveolar tension but also as a mediator of endocytosis and reutilization of secreted surfactant by binding to high affinity receptors on type II cells. This may in turn act in a negative feedback manner to regulate surfactant synthesis and secretion. In addition, SP-A may, in concert with calcium and the hydrophobic surfactant proteins SP-B and SP-C, assist in the conversion of the physical state of surfactant from the secreted lamellar body into that of tubular myelin.[17–19]

The expression of the SP-A gene is developmentally regulated and in general reflects the appearance and increasing function of type II pneumatocytes with substantial amounts of SP-A only being detected in amniotic fluid after 30 weeks' gestation in parallel with rising levels of DPPC. In amniotic fluid there are no differences in SP-A content based on fetal sex although male infants show reduced lecithin/sphingomyelin (L/S ratios) and DPPC levels compared to females at equivalent gestations. SP-A protein is modified post-translationally by glycosylation and as this process increases with gestational age, it is reflected in an apparent increase in molecular weight of SP-A but the functional consequences of this modification are not clear.[20–22]

SP-A gene expression is exclusively localized to lung and immunohistochemical methods localize the protein to type II cells, non-ciliated bronchiolar cells and alveolar macrophages whereas *in situ* hybridization techniques to detect SP-A mRNA suggest that the main site of production in late gestation is the type II pneumatocyte only. The appearance of SP-A protein but not mRNA in cell types other than type II pneumatocytes is likely to reflect secondary uptake of secreted surfactant although a synthetic role for bronchial cells in earlier gestation has not been excluded.[23,24]

Surfactant proteins SP-B, SP-C and SP-D

The two smaller hydrophobic proteins SP-B, 7–8 kDa, and SP-C, 4–5 kDa, have important functions in reducing surface tension and promoting the conversion of lamellar into tubular myelin. The expression of genes encoding SP-B and

SP-C occurs at an earlier stage of development than SP-A as early as 13 weeks, and thereafter increases with gestation. SP-B mRNA has been detected in type II pneumatocytes and bronchiolar cells. The distribution of gene expression may change with development as SP-C mRNA is found in all epithelial cells prior to the appearance of type II pneumatocytes but the function of this protein in early fetal lung is unknown. Surfactant protein D (SP-D) is a collagenous, surfactant-associated, carbohydrate-binding protein that is synthesized by type II pneumatocytes and non-ciliated bronchiolar cells; in rats, lung and amniotic levels increase prior to birth. Its regulation is currently unknown.[25–28]

Control of lung development

The process of fetal lung development involves the synchronous maturation and interaction of epithelium and mesenchyme in response to hormones and local growth factors. Developmental regulation of the type II pneumatocyte has received most research attention because of the direct link between surfactant deficiency and respiratory distress syndrome. It is becoming clear that surfactant production is regulated by complex interactions between a number of hormones and growth factors and that individual components of surfactant are independently regulated.[15,16]

Hormonal regulation

Glucocorticoids

Since Liggins in 1969 showed that glucocorticoid administration to fetal lambs *in utero* reduced the incidence of respiratory distress, a large number of studies have shown that glucocorticoids accelerate the morphological and biochemical maturation of the lung. In particular, the production of surfactant phospholipid is accelerated by glucocorticoids and this effect is further augmented by agents that increase intracellular cyclic AMP.[15,16,29]

Glucocorticoids act on the lung by binding to cytosolic receptors which are then transported to glucocorticoid responsive elements on the regulatory elements of specific genes where they alter gene transcriptional activity and ultimately increase new protein synthesis. Nucleotide sequences corresponding to glucocorticoid responsive elements have been identified from the gene sequences of SP-A, SP-B and SP-C.[22,25,27]

The effect of glucocorticoids on SP-A levels in lung is species specific and dependent on the stage of lung development. In human fetal lung, glucocorticoids have both stimulatory and inhibitory effects on lung morphological development as well as on surfactant production that are dose and time dependent. In human fetal lung in organ culture, with glucocorticoids at low concentrations (10^{-10}–10^{-9}M), levels of SP-A mRNA and protein are increased whereas at higher concentrations (i.e. 10^{-8}–10^{-7}M), both SP-A mRNA and protein levels are reduced. Paradoxically, glucocorticoids increase SP-A gene transcription, an effect maximal at the higher glucocorti-

coid concentrations, which reduces levels of SP-A mRNA and protein. The dominant effect of glucocorticoids at higher concentrations is therefore to reduce SP-A mRNA stability and the amount of mRNA available for translation to protein. In addition, at early stages in human fetal lung organ culture growth, glucocorticoids are stimulatory with later loss of this positive effect.[16,30,31]

In human fetal lung cultures, glucocorticoids at concentrations that are stimulatory to SP-A mRNA and protein expression increase dilatation of terminal airways and increase the density of type II pneumatocytes whereas at higher concentrations glucocorticoids are not only inhibitory to SP-A protein production but reduce airway volume and the number of type II pneumatocytes.[32]

In contrast to the complex effects on SP-A gene expression, glucocorticoids stimulate increases in the levels of SP-B and SP-C mRNA in a dose dependent manner.[16]

β-Adrenergic receptor agonists

Norepinephrine (noradrenaline) levels increase in fetal plasma with development and catecholamines bind to β-adrenergic receptors on type II pneumatocytes and raise intracellular cyclic AMP levels. The number of β-adrenergic receptors on type II pneumatocytes and their responsiveness to catecholamines increases with gestational age. In addition it has been suggested that the β-adrenergic receptor number can be further increased by administration of corticosteroids although more recent studies in human fetal lung have shown down-regulation of receptors in the presence of corticosteroids.[33–35]

Factors which increase intracellular cyclic AMP levels in fetal lung cells accelerate the morphological maturation of lung and increase the synthesis of surfactant, including the SP-A mRNA and protein components. In contrast to the marked stimulatory effect of cyclic AMP on SP-A, only modest increases are seen in SP-B and SP-C mRNA levels in human lung but without a concomitant rise in the corresponding protein levels. Consensus cyclic AMP-dependent responsive elements have been identified on SP-A, -B and -C genes.[15,16]

Cellular cyclic AMP levels can be increased by a number of routes, for example, through the use of β-adrenergic receptor agonists such as terbutaline or PGE-type prostaglandins or phosphodiesterase inhibitors such as theophylline or adenyl cyclase stimulation by forskolin. In addition, cyclic AMP increases β-adrenergic receptor concentration in human fetal lung and specifically in type II pneumatocytes.[36]

Thyroid hormones

The thyroid hormones triiodothyronine (T3) and thyroxine (T4) enhance fetal lung surfactant phospholipid production, particularly the DPPC component, both *in vivo* and *in vitro* but do not appear to increase surfactant proteins SP-A, SP-B or SP-C.[37,38]

Since neither thyroid hormones nor thyroid-stimulating hormone cross the placenta, thyrotropin releasing hormone (TRH) has been used as a means of elevating fetal T3. TRH increases DPPC in rabbits and lambs and when combined with glucocorticoids, but not alone, increases lung distensibility. In human and animal *in vitro* and *in vivo* studies, glucocorticoids and T3 synergistically increase DPPC synthesis but T3 does not increase the glucocorticoid induction of surfactant proteins synthesis and antagonism exists for other key developmental changes such as the glucocorticoid stimulation of glycogenolysis and fatty acid synthase activity in fetal lung.[39–41]

Prolactin

The balance of evidence from human and animal studies suggests a role for prolactin in lung development. *In vitro* human lung cultures show that prolactin enhances glucocorticoid stimulation of DPPC synthesis and surfactant secretion. In addition prolactin receptors are found in fetal lung. Fetal plasma prolactin levels increase prior to the change in lecithin/sphingomyelin (L/S) ratio and there is a negative correlation of cord plasma prolactin levels and RDS. In lambs the combination of glucocorticoids, T3 and prolactin increases lung distensibility and this may be an important maturation effect.[42–45]

Insulin

Infants of diabetic mothers have an increased incidence of RDS often with normal L/S ratios in amniotic fluid but with reduced or absent PG. Fetal hyperinsulinism has been suggested as inhibitory to fetal lung development. The balance of evidence suggests insulin has no direct effect on PG synthesis but instead is inhibitory to the synthesis of surfactant protein SP-A in human fetal lung. Amniotic fluid levels of SP-A protein are significantly reduced in diabetic pregnancies compared to non-diabetic gestational age-matched controls although in pregnancies where diabetic control is improved amniotic levels are similar to controls.[46,47]

In human fetal lung in organ culture, insulin reduces SP-A synthesis in a dose dependent manner and when combined with glucocorticoid at a concentration of 10^{-7}M has a synergistic effect to further reduce SP-A levels. Phospholipid surfactant synthesis under these conditions is increased and it is suggested that the effect of fetal hyperinsulinemia in diabetic pregnancies is to produce a surfactant with reduced SP-A content. Insulin at higher concentrations inhibits the production of SP-B but has no effect on SP-C.[48]

In addition to hyperinsulinemia, infants of diabetic mothers may have raised levels of α-aminobutyric acid which, in rat lung *in vitro*, inhibits the formation of SP-A but not SP-B.[41]

Androgens, estrogens and fetal sex

Clinical observations suggest that male lung development lags by 1–2 weeks behind females with a corresponding increase in RDS. Androgens delay human lung maturation *in vitro* and the appearance of phospholipid surfactant. Dihydrotestosterone inhibits the dexamethasone-stimulated formation of surfactant phospholipid. A number of mechanisms of action of dihydrotestosterone have been proposed including inhibition of fibroblast pneumocyte factor synthesis (see growth factors) and by delaying the appearance of epithelial EGF receptors during fetal lung development.[49–52]

Estrogens significantly increase phospholipid synthesis when administered to fetal rabbits and also increase surfactant proteins SP-A and SP-B but decrease amounts of SP-C. Estrogen effects are thought to be mediated through the mesenchyme with the transfer of a proposed maturational factor to the fetal epithelium. Estrogen effects on lung maturation in other species and preparations have been inconsistent.[53,54]

Growth factors and lung development

Fibroblast pneumocyte factor

A mesenchymal cell mediator, fibroblast pneumocyte factor (FPF) stimulates surfactant production and SP-A expression in type II pneumatocytes. FPF production is positively regulated by corticosteroids and negatively regulated by TGF-β. In addition dihydrotestosterone interferes with the progression of lung development by delaying the appearance of FPF in developing lung. It is suggested that as part of the proposed reciprocal relationship that exists between epithelial and mesenchymal cells, a factor produced by alveolar cells, possibly IGF-1, stimulates collagen production by fibroblasts.[55–57]

Prostaglandins

Lung primordium is a self-differentiating system in culture and in organ culture from human fetuses as early as 12 weeks' gestation, the epithelium differentiates into type II pneumatocytes containing lamellar bodies of surfactant. In addition, terminal airspaces dilate and the epithelial lining cells flatten to type I pneumatocytes. These morphological changes together with the evidence that surfactant is synthesized confirms that accelerated development has occurred with the morphological appearance of a 26 week' gestation lung. These changes occur in sera-free media in the absences of exogenous hormones or growth factors suggesting the presence of endogenous regulatory factors. Prostaglandins (PGs) are produced in substantial amounts initially by human fetal lung in culture possibly as a result of oxidative and mechanical stresses. Indomethacin inhibits endogenous PG production, the process of accelerated self-development, the spontaneous induction of SP-A gene expression and the increase in levels of SP-A mRNA and protein. Addition of exogenous PGE$_2$ reverses the indomethacin inhibition on morphological development and SP-A expression.[58–61]

Epidermal growth factor

Epidermal growth factor (EGF) both accelerates fetal lung budding and growth. In addition EGF accelerates maturation with the earlier appearance of phospholipid surfactant as well as increases in SP-A mRNA and protein. In contrast, in the presence of anti-EGF antibodies, lung maturation is retarded. Androgens, both *in vivo* and *in vitro*, inhibit lung maturation and it is proposed that part of their mechanism of action is to delay the appearance of EGF receptors in fetal lung.[50,51,62,63]

Transforming growth factor-alpha

Transforming growth factor-alpha (TGF-α), a member of the epidermal growth factor (EGF) family, is a potent mitogen for several cell lines and acts via the EGF receptor. In developing mid-gestation human fetal lung, TGF-α is found in all epithelial cells but particularly in bronchiolar cells suggesting a role in distal airway formation. Consistent with this proposal, ontogenic studies in fetal rat lung have shown that highest levels of TGF-α protein and mRNA are found in canicular lung at a time of distal airway remodeling.[64–66]

Bombesin

Fetal pulmonary neuroendocrine cells contain substantial amounts of mammalian bombesin-like peptides. Bombesin supplementation results in increased growth and maturation of mouse lung both *in vivo* and *in vitro* with increased production of surfactant and SP-A protein, effects antagonized by anti-bombesin receptor antibodies. Bombesin-like peptides are hydrolyzed by a specific neutral endopeptidase expressed in bronchial epithelium and it is suggested that expression of this protease in turn controls the bioavailability of bombesin-like peptides. In studies using monoclonal anti-bombesin antibodies to inhibit bombesin-like peptide action, there is an increase in the number of lung EGF receptors suggesting that there is an interrelationship between these growth factors which have similar effects on developing lung.[67,68]

Transforming growth factor-beta

Transforming growth factor-beta (TGF-β) inhibits the production of SP-A in human fetal lung. The localization of epithelial and mesenchymal TGF-β changes with lung development and parallel alterations in matrix proteins and glycosaminoglycans suggests that TGF-β may have other roles in the control of branching morphogenesis and differentiation.[69–70]

Interferon

Interferon-γ increases SP-A mRNA and protein levels in human fetal lung but has no effect on SP-B , SP-C or phospholipid content. The significance of this effect in the mechanism of physiological control of human fetal lung development is not known.[71]

Oxygen

In human fetal lung in organ culture, the process of self-development is related to ambient oxygen concentrations. For example, at low oxygen concentrations developmental changes in lung morphology are delayed as is SP-A gene expression and the responsiveness of the tissue to cyclic AMP. Oxygen *per se* is thought to play a permissive role to the actions of other lung developmental regulators.[72]

Development of lung antioxidant systems

A proportion of preterm infants requiring mechanical ventilation with oxygen will develop bronchopulmonary dysplasia (BPD), characterized by abnormal epithelial cell proliferation and fibrosis. There are many clinical risk factors which increase the risk of BPD including the duration and concentration of inspired oxygen. Life in oxygen is dependent on effective mechanisms to detoxify active oxygen species and this is achieved by enzymic and non-enzymic methods. Animal studies suggest that failure to detoxify reactive oxygen species is a major determinant of lung damage including effects on peroxidation of membranes and oxidation of DNA.

Antioxidant enzymes

The antioxidant enzymes involved include superoxide dismutase which catalyzes the dismutation of the superoxide radical, and glutathione peroxidase and catalase which detoxify hydrogen peroxide and organic peroxides. In short gestation species such as hamsters, rats, guinea pigs and rabbits as well as sheep, a medium gestation species, fetal lung activities of these antioxidant enzymes increase only late in gestation and almost in parallel with surfactant secretion. These results have led to the proposal that preterm infants at risk of RDS are also vulnerable to increased lung damage through deficiences of lung antioxidant enzyme activities.[73–76]

In fetal animals, glucocorticoids increase the activities of antioxidant enzymes as well as surfactant synthesis. However, when glucocorticoids are combined with TRH in fetal rats, gene transcriptions of lung CuZn SOD(cytosolic), Mn SOD(mitochondial), catalase and glutathione peroxidase are decreased but conversely are unaffected in fetal lambs. The regulation of surfactant and the antioxidant enzyme systems appear to be differentially regulated and species specific.[77–80]

There are fewer studies of the development of lung antioxidant systems in humans. It has been shown that CuZn SOD, Mn SOD and glutathione peroxidase activity measurements and amounts of enzyme are as high in early mid-trimester as adult lung. These results suggest that preterm human infants may be better adapted to life in the relatively oxygen-rich postnatal air environment, when compared to *in utero* oxygen levels, than had previously been thought.[81–82]

This precocious appearance of antioxidant enzymes in human lung, however, does not exclude oxidative damage in the lungs of preterm infants, nor indeed full-term infants, when the dose exposure to oxygen and its reactive species is high enough to saturate available enzymic and non-enzymic routes of detoxification.[82–83]

Lung fluid secretion and absorption in the fetus

Fetal lung secretion

Fetal lung secretion increases linearly with gestational age and substantial rates of production of around 3–5 ml kg^{-1} h^{-1} are reached by term. In a similar manner, lung fluid volume per body weight also increases with development and at term is close to the end-expiratory gas volume of the newborn infant. In addition, given the high compliance of the liquid-filled lung and a positive pressure gradient between the lung lumen and amniotic cavity generated by the secretory mechanism, this is probably sufficient to maintain the lung in an expanded state *in utero*. However, the lung distension pressure generated by the secretory process depends largely on the presence of an outflow resistance with the upper airway, particularly the larynx, acting as a one-way valve allowing ready egress of fluid but offering substantial resistance to the aspiration of amniotic fluid particularly as lung liquid is absorbed in preparation for birth.[84,85]

Fluid volume and lung growth

In diaphragmatic hernia and oligohydramnios syndromes, the developing lung is compressed and this reduction in the space for lung volume expansion results in lung hypoplasia. Lung compression markedly reduces lung cell proliferation and, in parallel, reduces the DNA content per unit dry mass with a reduction in acini formed in early gestation or, if the compression is later, the number of alveoli present. Increasing lung volume expansion, as occurs in laryngeal atresia or experimentally in fetal tracheal ligation, results in lung hyperplasia. The effects of changes in lung volume on fetal lung maturation are less pronounced and may only become obvious if the mitotic activity of the fetal lung has been severely compromised during the canilicular phase.[86-88]

There appears to be no correlation between fetal breathing movements and lung growth. In addition, lung fluid secretion rate is not influenced by fetal breathing movements and the volume changes between periods of apnea and breathing are so small that it is unlikely that fetal breathing influences lung growth through changes in lung fluid secretion or volume.[89]

Mechanism of fetal lung fluid secretion

Lung fluid composition from fetal lambs shows that the ionic composition is not at equilibrium with and differs markedly from that of plasma (Table 3.9.1). Evidence from a number of sources (see reference 84 for a review) suggests that chloride is the most abundant ion present, provides the driving force for lung fluid secretion. In the model for secondary active chloride ion secretion, Cl^- ion transport across the basolateral membrane is driven by an Na^+ gradient and Cl^- enters the cell coupled to Na^+ via a cotransporter that shows Na^+, Cl^- and usually K^+ ion dependence (Fig. 3.9.2a). Once inside the cell, Cl^- exits passively across the apical cell membrane via conductive pathways creating an osmotic gradient for the movement of water into the airway lumen.[90-92]

The alveolar epithelium actively secretes Cl^- and the balance of evidence suggests that this region of the lung is the major source of lung fluid. Alveolar type II cells have apical Cl^- channels and it is likely that these cells are the site of fluid secretion.[93]

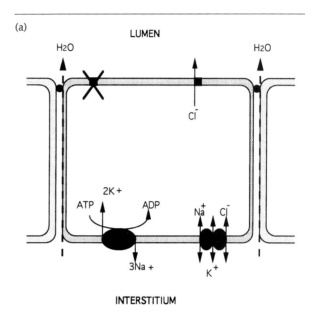

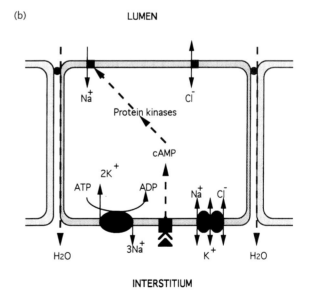

Fig. 3.9.2 *Mechanism of ion transport in the fetal alveolar type II cell. (a) Secretory mode where, under resting conditions, intracellular [Cl^-] is above equilibrium and passes through conductive pathways in the apical membrane. Apical Na^+ permeability is low. (b) Absorptive mode where activation of the cAMP-dependent pathway inserts and/or activates Na^+ channels in the apical membrane. Na^+ permeability is increased and the resultant depolarization of the apical membrane reduces or reverses apical Cl^- flux and fluid flow. (Modified from reference 84.)*

Table 3.9.1 Composition of fetal lung fluid and plasma

	Mean concentration (mmol kg water^{-1})					
	Na$^+$	K$^+$	Ca^{++}	Cl$^-$	HCO$_3^-$	pH
Lung liquid	150	6.3	0.4	157	2.8	6.27
Plasma	150	4.8	3.3	107	24	7.34

Data from fetal sheep 125–147 days' gestation from references 90–92.

Absorption of lung fluid

The transition from intrauterine placental to pulmonary gas exchange postnatally requires a switch from lung secretion to one of absorption of lung liquid and this change in function begins before delivery and continues after birth. In late gestation lung fluid secretion rates decrease, as does lung fluid volume, related to changes in epithelial secretory and absorptive ion transport mechanisms.[94]

Epinephrine (adrenaline) and other β-adrenergic receptor agonists decrease secretion of fetal lung fluid and in late gestation this results in net fluid absorption. Fetal epinephrine levels increase during parturition and are considered to be the predominant factor in initiating and maintaining lung fluid absorption. Delays in activation of this mechanism, as in elective Caesarean section without labor, results in a higher incidence of transient tachypnea of the newborn. In addition, the sensitivity of lung fluid transport to epinephrine increases up to 15-fold in the latter part of gestation and in parallel, the concentration of β-adrenergic receptors increases in the lungs of a variety of species.[95–97]

Fetal arginine vasopressin levels rise in labor and may provide an alternative mechanism for control of lung fluid absorption mediated through cAMP-dependent pathways.[98]

Mechanism of absorption

Cyclic AMP is the likely predominant intracellular signal for epinephrine as well as arginine vasopressin albeit through different receptors and transduction pathways. The role of cAMP is to activate existing or increase the insertion of new Na^+ channels in the apical membrane of lung epithelial cells. In immature lung, the synthesis of new Na^+ channels is the most obvious effect whereas in mature lung activation of existing Na^+ channels predominates.

Increases in apical membrane Na^+ pump activity de-polarizes the membrane and this reduces the electrochemical drive for apical membrane Cl^- secretion. In addition, an increase in the intracellular load of Na^+ stimulates the rate of extrusion of Na^+ by the basal membrane Na^+/K^+ ATPase with Cl^- and water passively following into the interstitial space (Fig. 3.9.2b). The basal membrane Na^+/K^+ ATPase does not change during fetal life although evidence exists for up-regulation around the time of birth. The type II pneumatocyte is the likely site of fluid absorption. Maturation of the absorptive response is synergistically regulated by triiodothyronine and cortisol in part through an increase in the number of β-adrenergic receptors on type II pneumatocytes.[84,99,100]

Modulation of the apical membrane permeability would appear to provide the mechanism for regulation of both lung fluid secretion and absorption.

FUTURE PERSPECTIVES

Glucocorticoids accelerate lung maturation in humans and reduce the incidence of RDS within the constraints of gestational age, and delay and duration of therapeutic effect. Even when antenatal glucocorticoid administration is optimal, some infants still develop RDS. This has stimulated the search for combination therapies including the use of glucocorticoids and TRH which, although it may not increase protection against RDS, may reduce chronic lung disease. At present, the sequential combination of antenatal glucocorticoids followed by postnatal surfactant therapy appears to provide optimal prevention and treatment of RDS. If further, more effective therapeutic stategies are to be developed to accelerate lung development and differentiation *in utero*, particularly before preterm delivery, then this can only be achieved through further understanding of the mechanisms of control of human fetal lung maturation.

SUMMARY

- The process of fetal lung development involves the synchronous maturation and interaction of the epithelium and mesenchyme.
- Lung developmental stages are usually divided into embryonic (3 to 7 weeks), pseudoglandular (7 to 16 weeks), canilicular (16 to 24 weeks) and a terminal sac phase (24 weeks to term).
- The maturational events in the late canilicular and early terminal sac phase between 20 and 30 weeks' gestation, including dilatation of the terminal airsacs, the approximation of capillaries and epithelium and the formation of type I and II pneumatocytes are determinants of gestational age-related survival.
- Surfactant is a lipoprotein complex produced by type II pneumatocytes which reduces airway surface tension and has a unique composition with a high content of dipalmitoylphosphatidylcholine and phosphatidylglycerol and specific proteins SP-A, SP-B, SP-C and SP-D. Individual components are independently regulated.
- The control of fetal lung development is a complex interrelationship between multiple hormones and growth factors.
- Glucocorticoids increase phospholipid surfactant and the synthesis of surfactant proteins SP-A, SP-B and SP-C in human lung as well as accelerating morphological maturation but the effects are dose and time dependent.

- Factors that increase intracellular cyclic AMP levels in fetal lung cells accelerate the morphological maturation of lung and increase the synthesis of surfactant including SP-A mRNA and protein.

- The enzymic mechanisms to detoxify active oxygen species develops in late gestation in animals and, although earlier in humans, this does not exclude oxidative lung damage in preterm or full term infants if the dose exposure to oxygen and its active forms is high.

- Fetal lung fluid secretion involves a mechanism based on secondary active chloride ion secretion and airway fluid distension *in utero* has a role in the control of fetal lung growth.

- The transition from intrauterine placental to pulmonary gas exchange requires a switch from lung secretion to absorption of lung liquid. Epinephrine and, to a lesser extent, vasopressin activate cyclic AMP-dependent pathways that increase sodium ion absorption in the apical membranes of type II pneumatocytes.

REFERENCES

1. Hislop A, Reid L. Development of the acinus in the human lung. *Thorax* 1974 **29**: 90–94.
2. O'Rahilly R. The early prenatal development of the human respiratory system. In Nelson GH (ed.) *Pulmonary Development from Intrauterine to Extrauterine Life. Lung Biology in Health and Disease* Vol 27. New York: Marcel Dekker, 1988: 3–18.
3. Snyder JM, Mendelson CR, Johnston JM. The morphology of lung development in the human fetus. In Nelson GH (ed.) *Pulmonary Development; from Intrauterine to Extrauterine Life. Lung Biology in Health and Disease* Vol 27. New York: Marcel Dekker, 1988: 19–46.
4. Rudnick D. Developmental capabilities of the chick lung in chorioallantoic grafts. *J Exp Zool* 1933 **66**: 125–153.
5. Young SL, Fram EK, Spain CL *et al.* Development of type II pneumocytes in rat lung. *Am J Physiol* 1991 **260**: L113–122.
6. Hansbrough JR, Fine SM, Gordon JI. A transgenic mouse model for studying the lineage relationships and differentiation program of type II pneumocytes at various stages of lung development. *J Biol Chem* 1993 **268**: 9762–9770.
7. Cossar D, Bell J, Lang M *et al.* Development of human fetal lung in organ culture compared with *in utero* ontogeny. *In Vitro Cell Dev Biol* 1993 **29A**: 319–324.
8. Hislop AA, Wigglesworth JS, Desai R. Alveolar development in the human fetus and infant. *Early Hum Dev* 1986 **13**: 1–11.
9. Langsdon C, Kida K, Reed M *et al.* Human lung growth in late gestation and the neonate. *Am Rev Respir Dis* 1984 **129**: 607–613.
10. Foster JA, Curtiss SW. The regulation of lung elastin synthesis. *Am J Physiol* 1990 **3**: L13–L23.
11. McGowan SE. Influences of endogenous and exogenous TGF-beta on elastin in rat lung fibroblasts and aortic smooth muscle cells. *Am J Physiol* 1992 **263**: L257–263.
12. Clements JA, King RJ. Composition of the surface-active material. In Crystal RG (ed.) *The Biochemical Basis of Pulmonary Function.* New York: Marcel Dekker, 1976: 363–387.
13. Oulton M, Martin TR, Faulkner GT *et al.* Developmental study of a lamellar body fraction isolated from human amniotic fluid. *Pediatr Res* 1980 **14**: 722–728.
14. Snyder JM, Longmuir KJ, Johnson JM *et al.* Hormonal regulation of the synthesis of lamellar body phosphatidylglycerol and phosphatidylinositol in fetal lung tissue. *Endocrinology* 1983 **112**: 1012–1018.
15. Gross I. Regulation of fetal lung maturation. *Am J Physiol* 1990 **259**: L337–344.
16. Mendelson CR, Boggaram V. Hormonal control of the surfactant system in fetal lung. *Annu Rev Physiol* 1991 **53**: 415–440.
17. Hawgood S, Benson BJ, Schilling J *et al.* Nucleotide and amino acid sequences of pulmonary surfactant protein SP18 and evidence for cooperation between SP 18 and SP 28–36 in surfactant lipid absorption. *Proc Natl Acad Sci USA* 1987 **84**: 66–70.
18. Ryan RM, Morris RE, Rice WR *et al.* Binding and uptake of pulmonary surfactant protein (SP-A) by pulmonary type II epithelial cells. *J Histochem Cytochem* 1989 **37**: 429–440.
19. Rice WR, Ross GF, Singleton FM *et al.* Surfactant-associated protein inhibits phospholipid secretion from type II cells. *J Appl Physiol* 1987 **63**: 692–698.
20. Torday JS, Nielsen HC, Fencl M *et al.* Sex differences in fetal lung maturation. *Am Rev Respir Dis* 1981 **123**: 205–208.
21. Snyder JM, Kwun JE, O'Brien JA *et al.* The concentration of the 35-kDa surfactant apoprotein in amniotic fluid from normal and diabetic pregnancies. *Pediatr Res* 1988 **24**: 728–734.
22. Mendelson CR, Acarregui MJ, Odom MJ *et al.* Developmental and hormonal regulation of surfactant protein A (SP-A) gene expression in fetal lung. *J Dev Physiol* 1991 **15**: 61–69.
23. Endo H, Oka T. An immunohistochemical study of bronchial cells producing surfactant protein A in the developing human fetal lung. *Early Hum Dev* 1991 **25**: 149–156.
24. Phelps DS, Floros J. Localisation of surfactant protein synthesis in human lung by *in situ* hybridisation. *Am Rev Respir Dis* 1988 939–942.
25. Pilot-Matias TJ, Kister SE, Fox JL *et al.* Structure and organisation of the gene encoding human pulmonary surfactant proteolipid SP-B. *DNA* 1989 **8**: 75–86.
26. Wohlford-Lenane CL, Durham PL, Snyder JM *et al.* Localization of surfactant-associated protein C (SP-C) mRNA in fetal rabbit lung tissue by *in situ* hybridization. *Am J Respir Cell Mol Biol* 1992 **6**: 225–234.
27. Glasser SW, Korfhagen TR, Wert SE *et al.* Genetic element from human surfactant protein SP-C gene confers bronchiolar-alveolar cell specificity in transgenic mice. *Am J Physiol* 1991 **261**: L349–356.
28. Crouch E, Rust K, Marienchek W *et al.* Developmental expression of pulmonary surfactant protein D (SP-D). *Am J Respir Cell Mol Biol* 1991 **5**: 13–18.
29. Liggins GC. Premature delivery of foetal lambs infused with glucocorticoids. *Endocrinology* 1969 **45**: 515–523.
30. Whitsett JA, Pilot T, Clark JC *et al.* Induction of surfactant protein in fetal lung: effects of cAMP and dexamethasone on SAP-35 RNA and synthesis. *J Biol Chem* 1987 **262**: 5256–5261.
31. Liley HG, White RT, Benson B *et al.* Glucocorticoids both stimulate and inhibit production of pulmonary surfactant protein A in fetal human lung. *Proc Natl Acad Sci USA* 1988 **85**: 9096–9100.
32. Odom MJ, Snyder JM, Boggaram V *et al.* Glucocorticoid regulation of the major surfactant-associated protein (SP-A) and its RNA and of morphological development of human fetal lung *in vitro. Endocrinology* 1988 **123**: 1712–1720.
33. Roberts JM, Jacobs MM, Cheng JB *et al.* Fetal pulmonary

beta-adrenergic receptors: characterisation in human and *in vitro* modulation by glucocorticoids. *Pediatr Pulmonol* 1985 **1**: S69–76.

34. Odom MJ, Snyder JM, Mendelson CR. Adenosine 3′,5′-monophosphate analogs and β-adrenergic agonists induce the synthesis of the major apoprotein in human fetal lung *in vitro*. *Endocrinology* 1987 **122**: 1155–1163.

35. Davis DJ, Jacobs MM, Ballard PL *et al.* Beta-adrenergic receptors and cAMP response increase during explant culture of human fetal lung: partial inhibition by dexamethasone. *Pediatr Res* 1990 **28**: 190–195.

36. Duffy DM, Ballard PL, Goldfien A *et al.* Cyclic adenosine 3′,5′-monophosphate increases beta-adrenergic receptor concentration in cultured human fetal lung explants and type II cells. *Endocrinology* 1992 **131**: 841–846.

37. Ballard PL, Hawgood S, Liley HG *et al.* Regulation of pulmonary surfactant apoprotein SP 28–36 gene in fetal human lung. *Proc Natl Acad Sci* 1986 **83**: 9527–9531.

38. Lilly HG, White R, Benson BJ *et al.* Regulation of messenger RNAs for the hydrophobic surfactant proteins in human lung. *J Clin Invest* 1989 **83**: 1191–1197.

39. Whitsett JA, Weaver TE, Clark JC *et al.* Glucocorticoids enhance proteolipid Phe and pVal synthesis and mRNA in fetal lung. *J Biol Chem* 1987 **262**: 15618–15623.

40. Liggins GC, Schellenberg J, Manzai M *et al.* Synergism of cortisol and thyrotropin-releasing hormone on lung maturation in fetal sheep. *J Appl Physiol* 1988 **65**: 1880–1884.

41. Nichols KV, Floros J, Dynia DW *et al.* Regulation of surfactant protein A mRNA by hormones and butyrate in cultured fetal lung. *Am J Physiol* 1990 **259**: L488–L495.

42. Mendelson CR, Johnson JM, MacDonald PC *et al.* Multihormonal regulation of surfactant synthesis by human fetal lung *in vitro*. *J Clin Endocrinol Metab* 1981 **53**: 307–317.

43. Amit T, Barkey RJ, Guy J *et al.* Specific binding sites for prolactin in adult rabbit lung. *Mol Cell Endocrinol* 1987 **49**: 17–24.

44. Gluckman PD, Ballard Pl, Kaplan SL *et al.* Prolactin in umbilical cord blood and the respiratory distress syndrome. *J Pediatr* 1978 **93**: 1011–1014.

45. Schellenberg J, Liggins GC, Manzia M *et al.* Synergistic hormonal effects on lung maturation in fetal sheep. *J Appl Physiol* 1988 **65**: 94–100.

46. Cunningham MD, Desai MS, Thompson SA *et al.* Amniotic fluid phosphatidylglycerol in diabetic pregnancies. *Am J Obstet Gynecol* 1978 **131**: 719–724.

47. Snyder JM, Kwun JE, O'Brien JA *et al.* The concentration of the 35-kDa surfactant apoprotein in amniotic fluid from normal and diabetic pregnancies. *Pediatr Res* 1988 **24**: 278–284.

48. Dekowski SA, Snyder JM. Insulin regulation of messenger ribonucleic acid for the surfactant-associated proteins in human fetal lung *in vitro*. *Endocrinology* 1992 **131**: 669–676.

49. Torday JS. Androgens delay human fetal lung maturation *in vitro*. *Endocrinology* 1990 **126**: 3240–3244.

50. Klein JM, Nielsen HC. Sex-specific differences in rabbit fetal lung maturation in response to epidermal growth factor. *Biochim Biophys Acta* 1992 **1133**: 121–126.

51. Klein JM, Nielsen HC. Androgen regulation of epidermal growth factor receptor binding activity during fetal rabbit lung development. *J Clin Invest* 1993 **91**: 425–431.

52. Nielsen HC, Kellogg CK, Doyle CA. Development of fibroblast-type-II cell communications in fetal rabbit lung organ culture. *Biochim Biophys Acta* 1992 **1175**: 95–99.

53. Connelly IH, Hammond GL, Harding PG *et al.* Levels of surfactant-associated protein messenger ribonucleic acids in rabbit lung during perinatal development and after hormonal treatment. *Endocrinology* 1991 **129**: 2583–2591.

54. Adamson IY, Bakowska J, McMillan E *et al.* Accelerated fetal lung maturation by estrogen is associated with an epithelial–fibroblast interaction. *In Vitro Cell Dev Biol* 1990 **26**: 784–790.

55. Smith BT. Lung maturation in the fetal rat: acceleration by injection of fibroblast pneumocyte factor. *Science* 1979 **204**: 1094–1095.

56. Nielsen HC, Kellogg CK, Doyle CA. Development of fibroblast-type-II cell communications in fetal rabbit lung organ culture. *Biochim Biophys Acta* 1992 **1175**: 95–99.

57. Griffin M, Bhandari R, Hamilton G *et al.* Alveolar type II cell-fibroblast interactions, synthesis and secretion of surfactant and type I collagen. *J Cell Sci* 1993 **105**: 423–432.

58. Hume R, Kelly R, Cossar D *et al.* Self-differentiation of human fetal lung in organ culture: the role of prostaglandins PGE$_2$ and PGF$_{2\alpha}$. *Exp Cell Res* 1991 **194**: 111–117.

59. Accaregui MJ, Snyder JM, Mitchell MD *et al.* Prostaglandins regulate surfactant protein A (SP-A) gene expression in human fetal lung *in vitro*. *Endocrinology* 1990 **127**: 1105–1113.

60. Ballard RL, Gonzales LW, Williams MC *et al.* Differentiation of type II cells during explant culture of human fetal lung is accelerated by endogenous prostanoids and adenosine 3,5-monophosphate. *Endocrinology* 1991 **128**: 2916–2924.

61. Hume R, Bell J, Gourlay M *et al.* Prostaglandin production and metabolism in self-differentiating human fetal lung organ culture. *Exp Lung Res* 1993 **19**: 361–376.

62. St. George JA, Read LC, Cranz DL *et al.* Effect of epidermal growth factor on the fetal development of the tracheobronchial secretory apparatus in rhesus monkey. *Am J Respir Cell Mol Biol* 1991 **2**: 95–101.

63. Yasui S, Nagai A, Oohira A *et al.* Effects of anti-mouse EGF antiserum on prenatal lung development in fetal mice. *Pediatr Pulmonol* 1993 **15**: 251–256.

64. Strandjord TP, Clark JG, Hodson WA *et al.* Expression of transforming growth factor-alpha in mid-gestation human fetal lung. *Am J Respir Cell Mol Biol* 1993 **8**: 266–272.

65. Kubiak J, Mitra MM, Steve AR *et al.* Transforming growth factor-alpha gene expression in late-gestation fetal rat lung. *Pediatr Res* 1992 **31**: 286–290.

66. Brown PI, Lam R, Lakshmanan J *et al.* Transforming growth factor alpha in developing rats. *Am J Physiol* 1990 **259**: E256–260.

67. King KA, Hua J, Torday JS *et al.* CD10/neutral endopeptidase 24.11 regulates fetal lung growth and maturation *in utero* by potentiating endogenous bombesin-like peptides. *J Clin Invest* 1993 **91**: 1969–1973.

68. Sunday MEH, Hua J, Reyes B *et al.* Anti-bombesin monoclonal antibodies modulate fetal mouse lung growth and maturation *in utero* and in organ cultures. *Anat Rec* 1993 **236**: 25–34.

69. Whitsett JA, Weaver TA, Lieberman MA *et al.* Differential effects of epidermal growth factor and transforming growth factor-β on synthesis of Mr = 35,000 surfactant-associated protein in fetal lung. *J Biol Chem* 1987 **262**: 7908–7913.

70. Heine UI, Munoz EF, Flanders KC *et al.* Colocalisation of TGF-beta 1 and collagen I and III, fibronectin and glycosaminoglycans during lung branching morphogenesis. *Development* 1990 **109**: 29–36.

71. Ballard PL, Liley HG, Gonzales MW *et al.* Interferon-gamma and synthesis of surfactant components by cultured human fetal lung. *Am J Respir Cell Mol Biol* 1990 **2**: 137–143.

72. Acarregui MJ, Snyder JM, Mendelson CR. Oxygen modulates the differentiation of human fetal lung *in vitro* and its responsiveness to cAMP. *Am J Physiol* 1993 **264**: L465–474.

73. Frank L, Sosenko IRS. Development of lung antioxidant systems in late gestation: possible implications for the prematurely born infant. *J Pediatr* 1987 **110**: 9–14.

74. Frank L. Prenatal dexamethasone treatment improves survival of newborn rat during prolonged high O$_2$ exposure. *Pediatr Res* 1992 **32**: 215–221.

75. Walther FJ, Wade AB, Warburton D *et al.* Ontogeny of antioxidant enzymes in the fetal lamb lung. *Exp Lung Res* 1991 **17**: 39–45.

76. Minoo P, Segura L, Coalson JJ et al. Alterations in surfactant protein gene expression associated with premature birth and exposure to hyperoxia. Am J Physiol 1991 261: L386–392.

77. Rodriguez MP, Sosenko IR, Antigua MC et al. Prenatal hormone treatment with thyrotropin releasing hormone plus dexamethasone delays antioxidant enzyme maturation but does not inhibit a protective antioxidant enzyme response to hyperoxia in newborn rat lung. Pediatr Res 1991 30: 522–527.

78. Walther FJ, Wabe AB, Warburton D et al. Corticosteroids, thyrotropin-releasing hormone, and antioxidant enzymes in preterm lamb lungs. Pediatr Res 1991 30: 518–521.

79. Chen Y, Whitney P, Frank L. Negative regulation of antioxidant enzyme gene expression in the developing fetal rat lung by prenatal hormonal treatments. Pediatr Res 1993 33: 171–176.

80. Sosenko IR. Antenatal cocaine exposure produces accelerated surfactant maturation without stimulation of antioxidant enzyme development in the late gestation rat. Pediatr Res 1993 33: 327–331.

81. Fryer AA, Hume R, Strange RC. The development of glutathione S-transferase and glutathione peroxidase activities in human lung. Biochim Biophys Acta 1986 833: 448–453.

82. Strange RC, Cotton W, Fryer AA et al. Lipid peroxidation and expression of copper–zinc and manganese superoxide dismutase in lungs of premature infants with hyaline membrane disease and bronchopulmonary dysplasia. J Clin Lab Med 1990 116: 666–673.

83. Ferro TJ, Hocking DC, Johnson A. Tumor necrosis factor-alpha alters pulmonary vasoreactivity via neutrophil-derived oxidants. Am J Physiol 1993 265: L462–471.

84. Olver RE. Fluid secretion and absorption in the fetus. In Effros RM, Chang HK (eds) Fluid and Solute Transport in the Airspaces of the Lungs. Lung Biology in Health and Disease Vol. 70. New York: Marcel Dekker, 1994: 281–302.

85. Fewell JE, Johnson P. Upper airway dynamics during breathing and during apnoea in fetal lambs. J Physiol Lond 1983 339: 495–504.

86. Hislop A, Hey E, Reid L. The lungs in congenital bilateral renal agenesis and dysplasia. Arch Dis Child 1979 54: 32–38.

87. Wigglesworth JS, Desai R. Use of DNA estimation for growth assessment in normal and hypoplastic fetal lungs. Arch Dis Child 1981 56: 601–605.

88. Moessinger AC, Collins MH, Blanc WA et al. Oligohydramnios-induced lung hypoplasia: the influence of timing and duration in gestation. Pediatr Res 1986 20: 951–954.

89. Harding R, Bocking AD, Sigger JN. Upper airway resistances in fetal sheep: the influence of breathing activity. J Appl Physiol 1986 60: 160–165.

90. Adamson TM, Boyd RDH, Platt HS et al. Composition of alveolar liquid in the foetal lamb. J Physiol Lond 1969 204: 159–168.

91. Olver RE, Strang LB. Ion fluxes across the pulmonary epithelium and the secretion of lung liquid in the foetal lamb. J Physiol Lond 1974 315: 395–412.

92. Barker PM, Brown MJ, Ramsden CA et al. The effect of thyroidectomy in the fetal sheep on lung liquid reabsorption induced by adrenaline or cyclic AMP. J Physiol Lond 1988 407: 373–383.

93. McCann JD, Welsh MJ. Regulation of Cl⁻ and K⁺ channels in the airway epithelium. Annu Rev Physiol 1990 52: 115–135.

94. Bland RD, Chapman DL. Absorption of liquid from the lungs at birth. In Effros RM, Chang HK (eds) Fluid and Solute Transport in the Airspaces of the Lungs. Lung Biology in Health and Disease Vol. 70. New York: Marcel Dekker, 1994: 303–322.

95. Walters DV, Olver RE. The role of catecholamines in lung liquid absorption at birth. Pediatr Res 1978 12: 239–242.

96. Brown MJ, Olver RE, Ramsden CA et al. Effects of adrenaline and spontaneous labour on the secretion and absorption of lung liquid in the fetal lamb. J Physiol Lond 1983 344: 137–142.

97. Warburton D, Parton L, Buckley S et al. β-Receptors and surface active material in fetal lamb lung : female advantage. J Appl Physiol 1988 63: 828–833.

98. Perks AM, Cassin S. The effects of arginine vasopressin and epinephrine on fetal lung liquid production in fetal goats. Can J Physiol Pharmacol 1988 77: 491–498.

99. Bland RD, Boyd CAR. Cation transport in lung epithelial cells derived from fetal, newborn, and adult rabbits. J Appl Physiol 1986 61: 507–515.

100. Barker PM, Walters DV, Markiewicz M et al. Synergistic actions of triiodothyronine and hydrocortisone on epinephrine-induced reabsorption of lung liquid in the fetal sheep. Pediatr Res 1990 27: 588–591.

3.10

Parturition

A López Bernal

INTRODUCTION

During pregnancy and labor the uterus has to serve two very different functions. For most of the 40 weeks of pregnancy it is in a relaxed state and gradually increases in size to accommodate the growing fetus. However, at the time of parturition it begins to contract regularly and forcibly, and the cervix progressively effaces and dilates allowing the fetus to descend through the birth canal. Unfortunately, despite the effort of several research groups over more than two decades, the factors controlling uterine relaxation during continuing pregnancy and the transition into uterine contractions at the onset of labor are poorly understood. The clinical relevance of this is of the utmost importance because of the impact of preterm delivery on perinatal mortality and morbidity: the perinatal mortality rate after 36 weeks' gestation is 2 per 1000 births, compared to 26 per 1000 at 32–36 weeks' gestation, and 200 per 1000 at less than 32 weeks.[1] Moreover, although 50% of small preterm babies (weighing between 500 g and 1000 g) now survive, there is a wide range of associated morbidity and the emotional trauma on parents and the burden on intensive care baby units are considerable. The prevention of preterm labor is a major aim of modern obstetrics.

In the early 1970s experimental work in the sheep showed that parturition is initiated by an increase in fetal cortisol secretion which induces 17α-hydroxylase activity in the placenta, resulting in falling progesterone levels and increasing estrogen levels in the maternal circulation.[2,3] Such a strong fetal role in the onset of labor has not been proven in the human, where the placenta lacks an inducible 17α-hydroxylase; there are no steroid changes in the maternal circulation preceding parturition, and the spontaneous onset of labor, although with some loss of precise timing, can occur in anencephaly, without a functional fetal pituitary/adrenal axis.[4] Research into human parturition has gradually moved away from peripheral hormone measurements, to the study of uterine receptors and is now centered on the mechanism of action of hormones

at a cellular level. This chapter reviews recent developments in the physiology and biochemistry of parturition, focusing on changes in the uterine cervix and the control of myometrial contractility, with special emphasis on the role of G proteins and second messengers.

CURRENT CONCEPTS

Functional anatomy

The uterus is formed by bundles of smooth muscle separated by a matrix of connective tissue (collagen and elastin). The collagen fibrils of the matrix facilitate transmission of the contractile forces generated in the individual myometrial cells. The fundus and the corpus uteri have the highest concentration of smooth muscle cells and are responsible for myometrial contractions during labor, whereas the cervix is predominantly fibrous connective tissue with less than 30% muscle cells.[5] There are several smooth muscle layers across the uterus; the innermost layers contain mainly longitudinal fibers and the outermost layers have both longitudinal and circular bundles. The middle layers contain the vascular supply in a mesh of multidirectional muscle fibers. The innervation of the uterus is autonomic. Both adrenergic and cholinergic nerves are present and are more abundant in the cervix than in the fundus. Uterine activity may be modulated physiologically by the autonomic nervous system, but since labor appears to be normal in paraplegic women and in women with bilateral lumbar sympathectomy, neural control must be subordinate to humoral control.

Changes in the connective tissue

Connective tissue changes affect the whole uterus but are more evident in the cervix. Cervical ripening is characterized by softening, effacement and dilatation. The consistency of the cervix becomes softer in preparation for labor and its shape changes from a cylindrical structure 2–3 cm long, to a wide-funneled canal with very thin edges. This softening of the cervical canal is called effacement and in primigravidae is normally completed before the beginning of cervical dilatation, although in multipara effacement and dilatation occur at the same time. These dramatic changes in the cervix result from a combination of structural changes in cervical tissue and the pressure exerted by the membranes or the fetal presenting part.

The softening of the cervix in pregnancy is partly due to increases in vascularity and water content, but mostly to changes in the connective tissue. Cervical connective tissue is made up of collagen fibrils and elastin separated by the ground substance; there are also numerous fibroblasts. The collagen fibril is made up of tropocollagen molecules arranged in a staggered longitudinal way to form the typical striated structure of collagen types I and III. Tropocollagen molecules consist of three polypeptides packed in a triple helix with short, non-helical telopeptides at both ends. About 70% of cervical collagen is type I and the remaining 30% is type III.[5,6] Collagen is resistant to most proteases except collagenase and leucocyte elastase. The ground substance is composed mainly of proteoglycans which are made up of several glycosaminoglycans (GAGs) connected to a protein core. GAGs are acid mucopolysaccharides with a large number of sulfate groups which make the molecule very hydrophilic. Proteoglycans are arranged around the collagen fibrils and modify their physical properties; they may also determine the water content of the tissue. Decorin is the most important proteoglycan in the human cervix; it has a small core protein carrying a single dermatan sulfate or chondroitin sulfate chain; it coats collagen fibrils and is involved in the disorganization of the fibrous network which occurs during cervical dilatation. Dermatan sulfate is probably the most important stabilizer of cervical consistency because of its ability to bind tightly to collagen and fibronectin (a matrix glycoprotein). Another important component of GAGs in human cervical tissue is hyaluronic acid which is not sulfated and does not attach to core proteins. Data obtained from cervical biopsies have shown that near term the collagen concentration decreases by 70% in relation to the concentration in the non-pregnant cervix.[7] At the same time the concentration of GAGs increases about 2.5-fold.[8] At the onset of labor there is a fall in dermatan sulfate and chondroitin sulfate and a steep rise in hyaluronic acid and heparan sulfate.[9] From the onset of labor until full dilatation and the immediate postpartum period, there is a fall in cervical GAG levels resulting mainly from a loss of hyaluronic acid and dermatan sulfate, followed by losses of heparan and dermatan sulfates.[8,9] These changes in the ground substance result in structural disorganization of collagen fibrils which facilitates their enzymatic degradation.

Collagenolysis in the cervix is a complex process balanced by the relative availability of procollagenase (which needs to be cleaved by another protease before it becomes active collagenase), free collagenase, and inhibitory proteins such as α_2-macroglobulin and tissue inhibitor of metalloproteinases (TIMP). The sources of cervical collagenase are the fibroblasts in the connective tissue and infiltrating neutrophils.[10] These two sources produce different types of enzyme with less than 60% amino acid homology. Fibroblast collagenase attacks collagen types I and III and neutrophil collagenase attacks collagen type I. Cervical ripening and dilatation are characterized by increased collagen breakdown as estimated by measurement of extractable hydroxyproline.[7] Biopsies taken from the lower uterine segment at term during Cesarean sections before and after the onset of labor show that active labor is associated with a remarkable 20-fold increase in procollagenase levels, and a loss of 40% of hydroxyproline.[11] By contrast, there is little change in decorin, α_2-macroglobulin and TIMP concentrations. Thus, parturition is associated with an increase in collagenase synthesis and a relative increase in the decorin/hydroxyproline ratio.

Elastin is another important component of uterine connective tissue and during pregnancy its concentration in the human uterus increses eightfold compared to the nonpregnant uterus and then decreases rapidly after parturition.[12] The elastin from the pregnant uterus (corpus and cervix) has a characteristically low content of desmosine (a cross-linker for elastin)[13] and it is thought that their main purpose is to provide elastic recoil coordinated with the contraction–relaxation cycle of the smooth muscle cells. At term there is a significant increase in leucocyte elastase in the cervix which is enhanced by interleukin (IL)-8.[14]

Hormonal control of cervical ripening

The process of cervical ripening is thought to be under hormonal control. Experiments in sheep have shown that despite surgical transection of the cervix, with loss of vascular and mechanical connections with the uterus, cervical softening still occurs in labor.[15] This suggests that the process is independent from uterine contractions but it is strongly synchronized with the onset of labor. In rodents, relaxin of ovarian or decidual origin has an important physiological role in cervical softening, but a similar role is unlikely in higher mammals. Estrogens may be involved and pregnant women with ripe cervices have higher levels of the estrogen precursor dehydroepiandrosterone sulfate (DHAS) than women with unripe cervices;[16] however, the use of estrogens for cervical ripening has been disappointing. Prostaglandins of the E series (PGE) applied locally to the cervix are now used routinely in many centers to ripen unfavorable cervices before the induction of labor.[17] The precise mechanism of action is not known but it is thought that PGE acts by increasing the collagenolytic activity of cervical tissue.[18,19] Cytokines may also be involved; IL-1 increases the levels of collagenase and stromelysin (an endogenous procollagenase activator) while decreasing TIMP levels in human cervical tissue.[20] Paradoxically these effects can be reversed by PGE via cAMP (cyclic adenosine 3',5' monophosphate). The relative increase in hyaluronic acid in the cervix at the initiation of parturition may act as a signal to activate resident macrophages or infiltrating leucocytes to secrete IL-1. IL-1 increases cervical PGE and collagenase production.

Moreover, IL-8, which is produced by human cervical explants, contributes to leucocyte migration and to collagenase and elastase degranulation from neutrophils infiltrating the cervix.[14] Further research is necessary to elucidate the complex biochemical control of cervical collagenolysis and to clarify which changes precede and cause cervical ripening and which are a consequence of the trauma of parturition.

Myometrial contractility

The cytoplasm of uterine smooth muscle cells is largely occupied by the myofilaments actin and myosin, which are not organized as in striated muscle, but occur in long random bundles throughout the muscle cells. Myosin is both a structural protein and an enzyme (Mg^{2+}-ATPase) capable of converting the chemical energy of ATP into the mechanical energy of muscle contraction. Myosin consists of two heavy and four light polypeptide chains; the two heavy chains form a globular head containing the ATPase sites and this is where actin and myosin interaction occurs; the light chains attached to the globular head are the sites of calcium binding and phosphorylation. The actin and myosin filaments slide past each other during contraction and the myosin heads and actin molecules form crossbridges that generate the contractile force of labor.

Role of calcium

Calcium is of fundamental importance in the regulation of actin–myosin interaction but the exact mechanism of this interaction is not completely understood. A well-accepted theory is that smooth muscle contraction is initiated by an increase in intracellular calcium which results in calcium binding to calmodulin (a protein that acts as a calcium sensor and regulates the activities of many intracellular enzymes). The Ca^{2+}-calmodulin complex activates the enzyme myosin light-chain kinase (MLCK) which phosphorylates a light chain (20 kDa) of myosin.[21] Phosphorylated myosin interacts cyclically with actin: this results in activation of myosin ATPase and causes contractions. When calcium is removed, dephosphorylation by myosin phosphatase occurs rapidly and the muscle relaxes (Fig. 3.10.1). In human myometrium there is good correlation between intracellular levels of Ca^{2+} and the extent of myosin light chain phosphorylation, and good temporal relationship between phosphorylation and force development.[21] However, studies in vascular smooth muscle[22,23] have shown that phosphorylation of a single myosin head can stimulate the ATPase activities of other unphosphorylated myosin heads; in other words there is cooperative activation of myosin and as litle as 20% phosphorylation of myosin heads may be sufficient for maximum myosin ATPase activity. It is not known whether positive cooperativity exists in myometrium, but during pregnancy human myometrium becomes more sensitive to the effect of myosin light chain phosphorylation on force development.[24] Smooth muscle contractility can be increased not only by activating MLCK, but also by inhibiting myosin

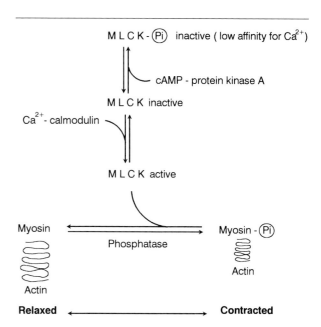

Fig. 3.10.1 *Contractility in myometrial smooth muscle. An increase in intracellular Ca^{2+} leads to the activation of the calcium sensor calmodulin. The Ca^{2+}–calmodulin complex activates the enzyme myosin light chain kinase (MLCK) which phosphorylates myosin. Phosphorylated myosin interacts with actin and produces contractions. The energy for contraction is provided by the hydrolysis of ATP (not shown), catalyzed by the actin–myosin complex. When myosin is dephosphorylated by myosin phosphatase relaxation occurs. Relaxation is also favored by cAMP-dependent protein kinase A, which phosphorylates MLCK thus lowering its affinity for Ca^{2+}–calmodulin and stabilizing its inactive form.*

phosphatase; the latter mechanism has been demonstrated in tracheal smooth muscle using GTP analogs.[25] Thus, some receptors coupled to a G protein (see below) may increase myosin phosphorylation by inhibiting phosphatase activity.

Another role of Ca^{2+} in the regulation of actin and myosin interaction in myometrium involves the proteins caldesmon and calponin;[26] these proteins associate reversibly with actin thin filaments and can modulate Mg^{2+}-ATPase activity.

Agents known to stimulate myometrial contractility, for example prostaglandin $F_{2\alpha}$ and oxytocin, increase both intracellular Ca^{2+} levels and myosin light chain phosphorylation,[21] whereas agents that relax myometrial smooth muscle, for example β-mimetics or prostacyclin, lower intracellular Ca^{2+} by promoting Ca^{2+} uptake by the sarcoplasmic reticulum. Ca^{2+} channel blockers such as nifedipine promote relaxation by preventing Ca^{2+} entry into the cell.

Myometrial cell signaling

Uterine activity can be influenced by many different compounds including hormones (e.g. oxytocin, adrenaline), classical transmitters (acetylcholine, 5-hydroxytryptamine), lipid mediators (prostaglandins, platelet activating factor), ions and even gases (see Table 3.10.1). A common feature in the mechanism of action of these different agonists is that their effects depend on the binding to specific receptors on myometrial cell membranes and the transmission of information to an effector system within the cell (an effector can be an enzyme that generates second messengers, e.g. adenylyl cyclase or phospholipase C, or an ion channel, e.g. certain voltage-sensitive calcium and potassium channels). The link between the receptor and the effector is usually a regulatory GTP-binding protein or 'G protein' (the proteins were discovered for their ability to bind and hydrolyze guanosine triphosphate) which is involved in signal transduction across the plasma membrane. The sequence of events is: hormone → receptor → G protein → effector → second messenger → cellular response. Hence, G proteins play a pivotal role in the flow of information from the outside to the inside of the cell and their function is of major importance in smooth muscle activation and relaxation. G proteins consist of three different subunits (α, β, γ) and are classified into several families according to their α-subunit.[27] Table 3.10.2 summarizes the G proteins present in human myometrium with their effector pathways. An interesting property of G

Table 3.10.1 Second messenger pathways for hormones and other agonists modulating myometrial contractility

	Receptor class	Pathway	Effect
Prostanoids			
PGE_2	EP_1	$InsP_3$/DAG ↑	Contraction
	EP_2	cAMP ↑	Relaxation
	EP_3	$InsP_3$/DAG ↑	Contraction
		cAMP ↓	
$PGF_{2\alpha}$	FP	$InsP_3$/DAG ↑	Contraction
		Phospholipase A_2 ↑	
PGD_2	DP	cAMP ↑	Relaxation
Prostacyclin	IP	cAMP ↑	Relaxation
Thromboxane	TP	$InsP_3$/DAG ↑	Contraction
Peptide hormones			
Oxytocin	OT	$InsP_3$/DAG ↑	Contraction
Vasopressin	V_{1A}	$InsP_3$/DAG ↑	Contraction
Endothelin	ET_A	$InsP_3$/DAG ↑	Contraction
Angiotensin	AT_1	$InsP_3$/DAG ↑	Contraction
		cAMP ↓	
Adrenoceptor agonists			
Epinephrine/norepinephrine	β_2	cAMP ↑	Relaxation
(adrenaline/noradrenaline)		Ca^{2+} channel ↓	
	α_1	$InsP_3$/DAG ↑	Contraction
	α_2	cAMP ↓	Contraction
		Ca^{2+} channel ↓	Relaxation
		K^+ channel ↑	Relaxation
Muscarinic agents			
Acetylcholine	M_1/M_3	$InsP_3$/DAG ↑	Contraction
		cAMP ↓	
Gases			
Nitric oxide	Soluble guanylyl cyclase	cGMP ↑	Relaxation
Other mediators			
Platelet activating factor	PAF	$InsP_3$/DAG ↑	Contraction
Bradykinin	B_2	$InsP_3$/DAG ↑	Contraction
		cAMP ↓	
		Phospholipase A_2 ↑	
5-Hydroxytryptamine	5-HT	$InsP_3$/DAG ↑	Contraction
		cAMP ↓	
Histamine	H_1	$InsP_3$/DAG ↑	Contraction
	H_2	cAMP ↑	Relaxation
Bombesin	BB_2	$InsP_3$/DAG ↑	Contraction

For each receptor the best established pathway is listed first. Less dominant pathways are also given despite some uncertainty as to their presence in human myometrium.

Table 3.10.2 G proteins involved in signal transduction in human myometrium

Family	Subtype	Toxin sensitivity	Effector system
G_s	$\alpha_s{}^a$	CTX (+)	Adenylyl cyclase ↑
			(?) voltage operated Ca^{2+} channel ↑
G_i	α_{i1}, α_{i3}	PTX (−)	Adenylyl cyclase ↓
			(?) Potassium channels ↑
			(?) Ca^{2+} channel ↓
G_q	α_q, α_{11}	—	Phospholipase C ↑
G_z	α_z	—	(?) Phospholipase C
			(?) Phospholipase A_2

[a]Exists as mRNA splice variants. CTX (+): stimulation by cholera toxin; PTX (−): inhibition by pertussis toxin. (?) Denotes uncertainty in human myometrium.

proteins is that some of them are substrates for bacterial exotoxins (the toxins either inhibit or activate the G protein by a reaction that involves ADP-ribosylation) and this property is useful to identify them. The response of the cell to the agonist depends on the number of second messenger molecules generated, and this is a function not only of the number of occupied receptors, but on the degree of coupling between the hormone–receptor complex and the G protein and, above all, on the coupling between the G protein and the effector system. G protein α subunits have enormous versatility and upon activation by an occupied receptor they exchange GDP for GTP, dissociate from the βγ subunits, activate effector molecules, and terminate their own action by hydrolyzing GTP to GDP and reassociating with the βγ subunits to go back to a 'resting' state.[28] Moreover βγ subunits have important roles in their own right, for instance they can stimulate some types of phospholipase C and adenylyl cyclase and they can increase the coupling of some receptors to calcium channels.

Most hormones that influence myometrial contractility use one of two major G protein-mediated pathways: the inositol phospholipid pathway and the cyclic adenosine 3′,5′-monophosphate (cAMP) pathway (Table 3.10.1).

Phosphoinositide hydrolysis

This pathway is used by hormones that stimulate myometrial contractility, for example oxytocin or $PGF_{2\alpha}$ (Table 3.10.1). The hydrolysis of phosphatidylinositol 4,5-bisphosphate (PIP_2, a hormone-sensitive phospholipid present in the cell membrane) by receptor/G protein-activated phospholipase C (PLC) generates two molecules both of which are second messengers: inositol 1,4,5-trisphosphate ($InsP_3$) which mobilizes calcium from the sarcoplasmic reticulum, and 1,2-diacylglycerol (DAG) which activates protein kinase C resulting in the phosphorylation of several target proteins. DAG can be converted into phosphatidic acid and reincorporated into PIP_2, or it can be hydrolyzed by diacyl- and monoacylglycerol lipases. Since DAG contains arachidonic acid in position 2 the latter pathway can generate free arachidonic acid (the precursor for prostaglandins and other eicosanoids). Arachidonate can be more directly generated by calcium/protein kinase activation of phospholipase A_2.

$InsP_3$ binds to receptors in the sarcoplasmic reticulum and promotes calcium release[29] and its action is terminated by rapid stepwise dephosphorylation to inositol which can then be reincorporated into PIP_2. The $InsP_3$ receptor is a calcium channel[30] and several isoforms have been cloned. The receptor in human myometrium is highly specific for the physiological $Ins(1,4,5)P_3$ form, versus the less active $Ins(2,4,5)P_3$ and $Ins(1,3,4)P_3$ isomers and is not occupied by other inositol mono- or polyphosphates.[31] The binding of $InsP_3$ to its receptor is inhibited by Ca^{2+}; moreover, the Ca^{2+} concentration in the sarcoplasmic reticulum can modulate the rate of agonist-stimulated $InsP_3$ synthesis. These regulatory mechanisms may serve to attenuate the response to $InsP_3$ following receptor activation. Ryanodine receptors are structurally and functionally similar to $InsP_3$ receptors[29] and are involved in calcium-induced calcium release, whereby a small influx of calcium through voltage-operated calcium channels triggers a large release of calcium from the sarcoplasmic reticulum; their importance in myometrial function is under investigation.[32]

The nature of the G protein(s) mediating PLC activation in myometrium is not completely elucidated. There are two pathways: one mediated by a pertussis toxin-resistant G protein – most likely a member of the $G_{q/11}$ family[33,34] and another pertussis toxin-sensitive pathway – probably involving a member of the $G_{i/o}$ family.[35,36] As mentioned earlier some types of PLC can be stimulated by βγ-subunits released after $G\alpha_i$ activation (Fig. 3.10.2).

Cyclic nucleotides

A number of myometrial receptors interact with G proteins that stimulate (G_s) or inhibit (G_i) adenylyl cyclase (Table 3.10.1). When intracellular cAMP levels increase, protein kinase A is activated and phosphorylates MLCK. Phosphorylated MLCK lowers its affinity for Ca^{2+}-calmodulin and remains in its inactive form (Fig. 3.10.1). As a consequence the concentration of phosphorylated myosin decreases and the muscle relaxes. In addition, protein kinase A may promote relaxation by lowering intracellular Ca^{2+} by either promoting calcium uptake by the sarcoplasmic reticulum or by inhibiting the formation of $InsP_3$. Hence agonists that increase cAMP levels promote myometrial relaxation and agonists that decrease cAMP

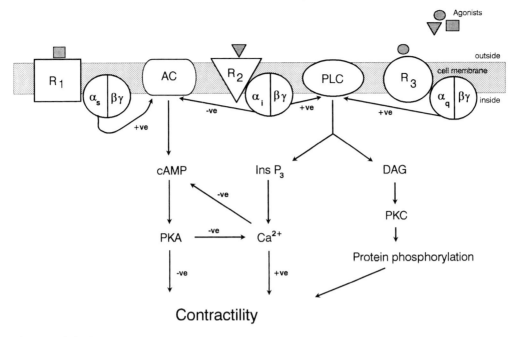

Fig. 3.10.2 *G protein linked receptors and myometrial contractility. Three examples of receptors are shown: R₁ is linked to adenylyl cyclase (AC) stimulation via G_{αs}; R₂ inhibits AC via G_{αi}; R₃ operates through G_{αq}; to stimulate phospholipase C (PLC) resulting in the formation of the two second messengers inositol 1,4,5-trisphosphate (InsP₃) and 1,2-diacylglycerol (DAG). Activation of R₁ promotes myometrial relaxation by increasing cAMP levels. Activation of R₂ has the opposite effect. Activation of R₃ promotes myometrial contractions by increasing intracellular Ca²⁺. In addition, G protein βγ subunits dissociated following activation of R₂ contribute to PLC stimulation. PKA = cAMP dependent protein kinase A. PKC = DAG stimulated protein kinase C. There is evidence for cross-talk between the cAMP and InsP₃ pathways (see text).*

production favor myometrial activation (Table 3.10.1). The action of cAMP is terminated by a phosphodiesterase which in human myometrium is sensitive to Ca^{2+}-calmodulin.[37]

Guanosine 3′,5′-cyclic monophosphate (cGMP) is a very important mediator of smooth muscle relaxation in vascular and bronchopulmonary tissue, but its role in myometrium is controversial.[38,39] Activators of guanylyl cyclase (e.g. nitric oxide donors) diminish the amplitude and frequency of spontaneous contractions in strips of human myometrium,[39,40] and preliminary studies suggest that glyceryl trinitrate may be a useful tocolytic agent in preterm labor[41] but its effectiveness and safety need to be tested in controlled clinical trials. It is thought that cGMP mediates relaxation by decreasing intracellular Ca^{2+} levels and myosin light chain phosphorylation.

myometrial cells contain T- and L-type calcium channels.[44] T-type channels are involved in the transmission of action potentials; they are inhibited by magnesium sulfate, resulting in decreased frequency of contractions. L-type channels participate in calcium transport inside the cell and are blocked by compounds such as nifedipine, resulting in decreased force of contraction. Calcium channel antagonists have been used in the management of preterm labor, but they lack myometrial specificity.

Calcium-activated potassium channels are present in human myometrium.[45,46] Potassium channels contribute to myometrial relaxation by increasing permeability to K^+ and causing membrane hyperpolarization. K^+ channel openers (e.g. L-cromakalim, pinacidil) cause uterine relaxation[47] but their effect is not specific for myometrium as they also relax vascular smooth muscle.

Ion channels in myometrium

Ion channels participate in myometrial activation by bringing extracellular calcium into the cell and by generating electrical signals. Ion channels can be agonist-operated or voltage-operated. In addition, voltage-sensitive channels (e.g. T and L calcium channels) can be regulated by receptor-dependent processes including protein phosphorylation and interaction with G proteins.[42,43] Detailed electrophysiological mechanisms are beyond the scope of this chapter, but it is worth mentioning that human

Gap junctions

Gap junctions play an important role in the regulation of myometrial contractility by facilitating the transmission of electrical stimuli. Measurements of the electrical coupling of human myomerial strips (a measurement of resistance between myometrial cells, presumably reflecting gap junction density) shows that the junctional resistance of nonpregnant myometrium is about 100 Ω cm and decreases to 50 Ω cm in pregnant myometrium at term.[48] These figures compare with approximately 100 Ω cm for stomach,

250 Ω cm for taenia caeci and 400 Ω cm for urinary bladder. The results show that pregnant myometrium is very well coupled compared to other types of smooth muscle. Gap junctions have been demonstrated morphologically in human myometrium where they increase at the time of parturition.[49] Furthermore, the gap junction protein connexin-43 appears to have a high turnover rate in human myometrium in labor.[50] It is interesting to know that gap junctions not only facilitate the transmission of current carrying ions, but also the exchange of second messenger molecules (Ca^{2+}, $InsP_3$) between smooth muscle cells. Thus an increase in gap junction density at the time of parturition would facilitate the spread of excitation and the synchronization of uterine contractions.

Endocrine control of uterine contractility

In some species, notably the sheep, a well-defined sequence of endocrine changes in both fetal and maternal compartments, initiated by increased fetal cortisol secretion, provokes parturition.[2,3] In humans and other primate species there is evidence of gradually increasing fetal adrenal activity towards term (i.e. rising DHAS and cortisol levels in the fetal circulation) but there are no defined endocrine changes in the maternal circulation prior to the onset of labor. This section discusses several endogenous compounds which can modulate uterine activity and are likely to participate in the mechanism of parturition, bearing in mind that none of these compounds has been shown to act as a 'trigger' for the spontaneous onset of labor.

Eicosanoids

Parturition in human and other species is associated with increased intrauterine PG production as demonstrated by the rising levels of PG metabolites in the maternal circulation and urine and in amniotic fluid during progressing labor.[51] The increased PG production is thought to originate in intrauterine tissues (placenta, amnion/chorion/decidua) because following placental separation in the third stage of labor there is an abrupt fall in PG metabolite levels in the maternal circulation.[52,53] Whereas some of this production may be a consequence of the trauma of labor,[54] PGs remain attractive candidates for an important role in parturition because they can be used to ripen the cervix and to induce labor, and PG synthesis inhibitors (e.g. indomethacin) block spontaneous uterine contractions and can be used for the treatment of preterm labor.

PGs are often associated with increased uterine contractility, but these compounds have both stimulatory and inhibitory effects. Binding sites for PGE_2 and $PGF_{2\alpha}$ are present in the uterus.[51] *In vitro* PGE_2 has biphasic effects on human myometrium, being stimulatory at nanomolar concentrations and inhibitory (short contraction followed by prolonged relaxation) at micromolar concentrations.[55,56] PGE_2 increases intracellular Ca^{2+} and activates MLCK,[21] but it also increases cAMP production.[57] This multiplicity of effects can be explained by the presence of three different types of PGE receptors in myometrium:[58] EP_1 receptors are stimulatory and activate PLC; EP_2 receptors are inhibitory and activate adenylyl cyclase; and EP_3 receptors are stimulatory, activating PLC and inhibiting adenylyl cyclase. EP_1, EP_2 and EP_3 receptors have been cloned and possess seven hydrophobic (transmembrane) domains characteristic of the G protein family of receptors.[59] $PGF_{2\alpha}$ is stimulatory and mediates its effect through the FP receptor which activates the phosphoinositide pathway through a pertussis toxin-insensitive G protein, most likely of the $G_{q/11}$ family; the action of $PGF_{2\alpha}$ in the uterus also involves phospholipase A_2 activation.[60] PGD_2 and prostacyclin relax uterine smooth muscle by stimulating adenylyl cyclase through the DP and IP receptors, respectively, linked to G_s. Thromboxane receptors (TP) stimulate contractility probably via $G_{q/11}$ and PLC. Leukotrienes and other arachidonate lipoxygenase products have little influence on myometrial contractility.

Neurohypophyseal hormones

Oxytocin stimulates contraction of uterine smooth muscle, although the physiological significance of this in relation to the spontaneous onset of labor remains uncertain. High affinity oxytocin binding sites are present in human myometrium and increase during pregnancy but not at the onset of labor.[31,61] Messenger RNA levels for the oxytocin receptor in human myometrium are very high towards term indicating increased synthesis of receptor protein. The human oxytocin receptor belongs to the G protein family[62] and its structure is very similar to the V_1 and V_2 vasopressin receptors. The predominant effector pathway for the oxytocin receptor is activation of inositol phospholipid metabolism,[60,63] but the nature of the G proteins involved is not clear, although it is partly pertussis toxin-sensitive in human myometrium.[64] The pertussis toxin-insensitive component is most likely mediated by a G protein of the $G_{q/11}$ class (Fig. 3.10.2). Oxytocin increases intracellular Ca^{2+} in human myometrial cells, mobilizing both intracellular and extracellular sources; intracellular mobilization is mediated by the $InsP_3$ receptor,[64] and extracellular mobilization is probably through an L-type calcium channel.[43] It has been proposed that women who go into preterm labor have higher myometrial sensitivity to oxytocin than women who deliver at term. Whether these changes are due to up-regulation of receptors or to increased G protein coupling, or both is not known, but it is noteworthy that oxytocin antagonists decrease uterine contractility in women in preterm labor.[65] Oxytocin receptors are localized in uterine smooth muscle, myoepithelial cells of the mammary gland and pituitary; this relatively narrow localization of receptors allows the use of oxytocin antagonists in pregnancy with few side-effects.

There are several other peptide hormones that stimulate uterine contractility via the phosphoinositide pathway, e.g. vasopressin, angiotensin, endothelin; however oxytocin remains most closely associated with parturition and it is widely used for the induction and augmentation of labor.

Adrenoceptor agonists

Catecholamines have both stimulatory and inhibitory effects on myometrial contractility; the stimulatory effect is mediated primarily through α_1 receptors and the inhibitory effect through β_2 receptors. Myometrium contains α_1, α_2 and β_2 receptor subtypes all of which operate through G proteins: α_1 adrenoceptors are linked to PLC activation and α_2 receptors are linked to adenylyl cyclase inhibition via G_i.[66,67] Thus α_1 receptors stimulate contractility by increasing $InsP_3$ production and α_2 receptors are also stimulatory because they inhibit cAMP formation. However, α_2 receptors can also provoke relaxation by activating K^+ channels and inhibiting Ca^{2+} channels.[68]

β_2-Adrenoceptors stimulate cAMP formation by coupling to G_s. β-agonists have been used extensively for the management of preterm labor but it is argued[69,70] that their use does not improve perinatal outcome and their main benefit is to allow time for other therapeutic measures (e.g. glucocorticoids to enhance lung maturation) or to transfer the mother to a center with adequate neonatal facilities; their lack of myometrial selectivity can result in serious side-effects. Myometrial tachyphylaxis is a problem with β-agonist tocolysis as these compounds provoke loss of β-receptors in myometrial tissue and increased phosphodiesterase activity leading to lower cAMP levels.[71] In guinea-pig myometrium β-agonists contribute to myometrial relaxation by inhibiting voltage-operated calcium channels and decreasing $InsP_3$ production.[72] This is a cAMP-independent mechanism which seems to involve a pertussis toxin-sensitive G protein.

Cholinergic agents

The muscarinic agents acetylcholine and carbachol stimulate uterine contractility in several species including the human. In the rat, carbachol attenuates cAMP production by stimulating a calcium-dependent phosphodiesterase, but it also stimulates PLC and the formation of $InsP_3$.[73] In the guinea pig, carbachol inhibits the rise in cAMP in response to prostacyclin by a pertussis toxin-sensitive pathway probably involving G_i.[74]

The role of inflammatory mediators

There is an association between inflammation of the fetal membranes (chorioamnionitis) and preterm labor. Chorioamnionitis-associated preterm labor tends to occur very early in gestation (25–30 weeks) and therefore has a very poor neonatal outcome.[1,75] The etiology of chorioamnionitis is most likely, although not conclusively, vaginal bacterial infection. Amnion, chorion, decidua and placenta with histological evidence of inflammation have much higher rates of PGE, $PGF_{2\alpha}$ and leukotriene B_4 production than normal tissues[76,77] and women with intrauterine infection have raised levels of prostanoids and lipoxygenase products in amniotic fluid.[75] It seems plausible that the premature release of PGs within intrauterine tissues in chorioamnionitis triggers the early onset of labor. Other inflammatory mediators that can stimulate uterine contractions include platelet activating factor, bradykinin, histamine and 5-hydroxytryptamine.

Cytokines have recently received a great deal of attention as possible agents in infection-associated preterm labor. IL-1 and TNF (tissue necrosis factor) are produced by human decidua, notably by decidual macrophages, in response to bacterial products.[78,79] They act synergistically to provoke PG release by intrauterine cells, including macrophages themselves.[78,80] Their actions are inhibited by compounds such as TGF-β (transforming growth factor-β) and IL-1ra (interleukin-1 receptor antagonist).[81] In human decidual cells IL-1 potentiates bradykinin-induced $InsP_3$ formation and arachidonate release.[82] In human myometrial cells IL-1 and TNF stimulate arachidonic acid release, probably by direct stimulation of phospholipase A_2;[83] however they also stimulate cAMP production.[84] Other pro-inflammatory cytokines whose levels are increased in the amniotic fluid of women with intrauterine infection include IL-6 and IL-8.[85,86]

FUTURE PERSPECTIVES

Research into human parturition is limited by lack of direct access to experimentation *in vivo*. Nevertheless, there have been considerable advances in our understanding of the cellular mechanisms involved in uterine contractions. G protein-linked receptors undoubtedly have a major role to play in myometrium and it is safe to predict that the expansion in our knowledge of hormonal signaling will continue. It seems likely that parturition is the result of increased sensitivity of the myometrium to stimulation. This could be brought about by several mechanisms such as an up-regulation of stimulatory receptors or a down-regulation of inhibitory ones; by changes in their signal transduction pathways; and by increased electrocoupling between uterine cells. Changes in G protein function in myometrium may acount for uterine quiescence in pregnancy and increased contractility in labor. For example, in pregnancy there is a striking increase in myometrial $G_{\alpha s}$ levels and an increase in PGE_2-stimulated cAMP formation.[87,88] These changes in $G_{\alpha s}$ expression are reversed in spontaneous term or preterm labor. Hence, it is possible that parturition is the result of a switch from a pathway that favors uterine quiescence by increasing $G_{\alpha s}$-mediated cAMP formation, to a pathway that favors contractility through a relative increase in $InsP_3/Ca^{2+}$ availability (Fig. 3.10.3). Further research is required to elucidate the control of G protein expression and its functional coupling in human myometrium, and to identify possible regulatory factors in the maternal or fetal compartments.

Important advances in our knowledge are also likely to derive from the study of contractile proteins and regulatory enzymes in human myometrium. In pregnancy there is hypertrophy of myometrial cells and changes in the regulation of myosin light chain phosphorylation that result in improved force generation in comparison with non-pregnant tissue.[24] In other words, during pregnancy the uterus

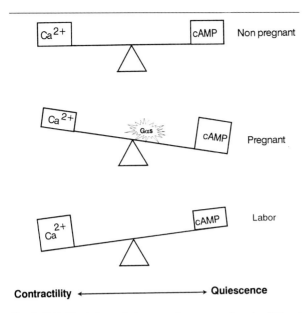

Fig. 3.10.3 *The balance between quiescence and contractility of the uterus. The equilibrium between stimulatory (Ca²⁺) and inhibitory (cAMP) pathways is weighted towards quiescence by increased expression of $G_{\alpha s}$ in pregnancy. The onset of labor could be brought about by the loss of $G_{\alpha s}$ and the relative dominance of pathways that increase intracellular Ca²⁺.*

gets ready for the demands of parturition and our understanding of the biochemical processes underlying these changes is likely to increase in the future. Furthermore, electrophysiological experiments in human myometrial cells have shown that during labor there are changes in the Ca^{2+} dependence and voltage sensitivity of K^+ channels[45] which probably underlie the sequence of synchronized contractions and relaxation characteristic of functional labor. Further investigation of the factors controlling ion channel activity should result in a better understanding of myometrial excitation and relaxation.

In conclusion, there has been a remarkable increase in our understanding of the endocrine and biochemical control of uterine activity, but much remains to be done before the mechanism of human parturition is fully understood. Drugs used to inhibit preterm labor include β-agonists, inhibitors of prostaglandin synthesis, progesterone, magnesium sulfate, calcium antagonists, oxytocin antagonists, nitric oxide donors, etc. Such multipharmacy is a consequence of our ignorance of the regulation of myometrial activity. New developments in our understanding of the cellular mechanisms involved in uterine contractions are likely to result in better therapies for the management of both term and preterm labor.

SUMMARY

- Parturition results from the establishment of intermittent but regular and effective uterine contractions and the softening, effacement and dilatation of the cervix.

- Cervical ripening results from a decrease in collagen cross-links and by changes in the glycosaminoglycans of the ground substance: a decrease in dermatan sulfate and an increase in hyaluronic acid. Collagenase activity in cervical tissue increases in labor.

- Contractions in uterine smooth muscle, are initiated by an increase in intracellular Ca^{2+} which activates MLCK. Activated MLCK phosphorylates myosin light chains, thus increasing myosin ATPase activity and the rate of actomyosin cross-bridge formation which generates the force of labor.

- G proteins play a pivotal role in smooth muscle activation and relaxation by coupling hormone receptors to effector enzymes or ion channels. G_s and G_i stimulate and inhibit adenylyl cyclase, respectively and control cAMP formation. G_q activates phosphoinositide-specific phospholipase C resulting in the formation of two second messengers: $InsP_3$ and diacylgly-

cerol which provoke calcium release and protein kinase C activation, respectively.

- Hormones that influence myometrial activity tend to use either the inositol phospholipid or the cAMP pathways. Agonists that provoke phosphoinositide hydrolysis stimulate myometrial contractiliy by releasing Ca^{2+} from $InsP_3$-sensitive stores in the sarcoplasmic reticulum.

- Agonists that increase cAMP levels (via G_s) promote myometrial relaxation and agonists that decrease cAMP production (via G_i) favor myometrial activation.

- There are complex hormone/second messenger interactions in myometrium: the same agonist (e.g. PGE_2, norepinephrine) can activate both stimulatory and inhibitory receptors; activation of phospholipase C by oxytocin involves both pertussis toxin-resistant ($G_{q/11}$) and pertussis toxin-sensitive (?G_i) pathways; activation of one pathway may attenuate responses through another pathway (cAMP vs $InsP_3/Ca^{2+}$ and vice versa).

- The premature release of inflammatory mediators, e.g. PGs, active peptides, cytokines, within intrauterine tissues triggered by infection can cause preterm labor.

Many hormones are involved in the control of myometrial activity, but the precise role of any of these as triggers for parturition remains undetermined. The increased myometrial contractility characteristic of labor could be brought about by several mechanisms such as an up-regulation of stimulatory receptors or a down-regulation of inhibitory ones; by changes in their signal transduction pathways; or by increased electrocoupling between uterine cells.

ACKNOWLEDGEMENTS

I am grateful to Dr S.M. Sellers for reviewing the manuscript. Work on parturition in the author's laboratory is funded by the MRC and Action Research.

REFERENCES

1. López Bernal A, Watson SP, Phaneuf S, Europe-Finner GN. Biochemistry and physiology of preterm labour and delivery. *Bailliere's Clin Obstet Gynaecol* 1993 7: 523–552.
2. Liggins GC. Initiation of spontaneous labor. *Clin Obstet Gynecol* 1983 26: 47–55.
3. Anderson AB, Flint AP, Turnbull AC. Mechanism of action of glucocorticoids in induction of ovine parturition: effect on placental steroid metabolism. *J Endocrinol* 1975 66: 61–70.
4. Honnebier WJ, Swaab DF. The influence of anencephaly upon intrauterine growth of the fetus and placenta and upon gestation length. *J Obstet Gynaecol Br Commonw* 1973 80: 577–588.
5. Danforth DN. The morphology of the human cervix. *Clin Obstet Gynecol* 1983 26: 7–13.
6. Minamoto T, Arai K, Hirakawa S, Nagai Y. Immunohistochemical studies on collagen types in the uterine cervix in pregnant and nonpregnant states. *Am J Obstet Gynecol* 1987 156: 138–144.
7. Ekman G, Almstrom H, Granstrom L, Malmstrom A, Norman M, Woessner JF. Connective tissue in human cervical ripening. In Leppert PC, Woessner JF (eds) *The Extracellular Matrix of the Uterus, Cervix and Fetal Membranes*. Ithaca, NY: Perinatology Press, 1991: 87–96.
8. Rath W, Osmers R, Szeverenyi M, Stuhlsatz HW, Kuhn W. Changes of glycosaminoglycans in cervical connective tissue during pregnancy and parturition. In Leppert PC, Woessner JF (eds) *The Extracellular Matrix of the Uterus, Cervix and Fetal Membranes*. Ithaca, NY: Perinatology Press, 1991: 105–112.
9. Osmers R, Rath W, Pflanz MA, Kuhn W, Stuhlsatz HW, Szeverenyi M. Glycosaminoglycans in cervical connective tissue during pregnancy and parturition. *Obstet Gynecol* 1993 81: 88–92.
10. Osmers R, Rath W, Adelmann-Grill BC *et al*. Origin of cervical collagenase during parturition. *Am J Obstet Gynecol* 1992 166: 1455–1460.
11. Rechberger T, Woessner JFJ. Collagenase, its inhibitors, and decorin in the lower uterine segment in pregnant women. *Am J Obstet Gynecol* 1993 168: 1598–1603.
12. Gunja Smith Z, Woessner JFJ. Content of the collagen and elastin cross-links pyridinoline and the desmosines in the human uterus in various reproductive states. *Am J Obstet Gynecol* 1985 153: 92–95.
13. Leppert PC, Yu SY. Elastin and collagen in the human uterus and cervix: biochemical and histological correlation. In Leppert PC, Woessner JF (eds) *The Extracellular Matrix of the Uterus, Cervix and Fetal Membranes*. Ithaca, NY: Perinatology Press, 1991: 59–67.
14. Barclay CG, Brennand JE, Kelly RW, Calder AA. Interleukin-8 production by the human cervix. *Am J Obstet Gynecol* 1993 169: 625–632.
15. Ledger WL, Webster M, Harrison LP, Anderson ABM, Turnbull AC. Increase in cervical extensibility during labor induced after isolation of the cervix from the uterus in pregnant ewes. *Am J Obstet Gynecol* 1985 151: 397–402.
16. Zuidema LJ, Khan Dawood F, Dawood MY, Work BAJ. Hormones and cervical ripening: Dehydroepiandrosterone sulfate, estradiol, estriol, and progesterone. *Am J Obstet Gynecol* 1986 155: 1252–1254.
17. MacKenzie IZ, Boland J. Current therapeutic uses of prostaglandins in obstetrics in the United Kingdom. *Contemp Rev Obstet Gynaecol* 1993 5: 9–14.
18. Ekman G, Uldbjerg N, Malmstrom A, Ulmsten U. Increased postpartum collagenolytic activity in cervical connective tissue from women treated with prostaglandin E-2. *Gynecol Obstet Invest* 1983 16: 292–298.
19. Rath W, Osmers R, Adelmann Grill BC, Stuhlsatz HW, Szevereny M, Kuhn W. Biochemical changes in human cervical connective tissue after intracervical application of prostaglandin E$_2$. *Prostaglandins* 1993 45: 375–384.
20. Takahashi S, Ito A, Nagino M, Mori Y, Xie B, Nagase H. Cyclic adenosine 3',5'-monophosphate suppresses interleukin 1-induced synthesis of matrix metalloproteinases but not of tissue inhibitor of metalloproteinases in human uterine cervical fibroblasts. *J Biol Chem* 1991 266: 19894–19899.
21. Mackenzie LW, Word RA, Casey ML, Stull JT. Myosin light chain phosphorylation in human myometrial smooth muscle cells. *Am J Physiol* 1990 258: C92–C98.
22. Vyas TB, Mooers SU, Narayan SR, Witherell JC, Siegman MJ, Butler TM. Cooperative activation of myosin by light chain phosphorylation in permeabilized smooth muscle. *Am J Physiol* 1992 263: C210–C219.
23. Somlyo AV, Goldman YE, Fujimori T, Bond M, Trentham DR, Somlyo AP. Cross-bridge kinetics, cooperativity, and negatively strained cross-bridges in vertebrate smooth muscle. A laser-flash photolysis study. *J Gen Physiol* 1988 91: 165–192.
24. Word RA, Stull JT, Casey ML, Kamm KE. Contractile elements and myosin light chain phosphorylation in myometrial tissue from nonpregnant and pregnant women. *J Clin Invest* 1993 92: 29–37.
25. Kubota Y, Nomura M, Kamm KE, Mumby MC, Stull JT. GTP gamma S-dependent regulation of smooth muscle contractile elements. *Am J Physiol* 1992 262: C405–C410.
26. Marston S. Calcium ion-dependent regulation of uterine smooth muscle thin filaments by caldesmon. *Am J Obstet Gynecol* 1989 160: 252–257.
27. Hepler JR, Gilman AG. G proteins. *Trends Biochem Sci* 1992 17: 383–387.
28. Olate J, Allende JE. Structure and function of G proteins. In Taylor CW (ed.) *Intracellular Messengers*. Oxford: Pergamon Press, 1993: 25–46.
29. Berridge MJ. Inositol trisphosphate and calcium signalling. *Nature* 1993 361: 315–325.
30. Ferris CD, Snyder SH. Inositol 1,4,5-trisphosphate-activated calcium channels. *Annu Rev Physiol* 1992 54: 469–488.
31. Rivera J, López Bernal A, Varney M, Watson SP. Inositol 1,4,5-trisphosphate and oxytocin binding in human myometrium. *Endocrinology* 1990 127: 155–162.
32. Lynn S, Morgan JM, Gillespie JI, Greenwell JR. A novel

ryanodine sensitive calcium release mechanism in cultured human myometrial smooth-muscle cells. *FEBS Lett* 1993 **330:** 227–230.

33. Smrcka AV, Hepler JR, Brown KO, Sternweis PC. Regulation of polyphosphoinositide-specific phospholipase C activity by purified Gq. *Science* 1991 **251:** 804–807.

34. Lee CH, Park D, Wu D, Rhee SG, Simon MI. Members of the Gqα subunit gene family activate phospholipase Cβ isozymes. *J Biol Chem* 1992 **267:** 16044–16047.

35. Camps M, Carozzi A, Schnabel P, Scheer A, Parker PJ, Gierschink P. Isozyme-selective stimulation of phospholipase C-β2 by G protein βτ-subunits. *Nature* 1992 **360:** 684–686.

36. Katz A, Wu D, Simon MI. Subunit βτ of heterotrimeric G protein activate β2 isoform of phospholipase C. *Nature* 1992 **360:** 686–689.

37. Leroy MJ, Cedrin I, Breuiller M, Giovagrandi Y, Ferré F. Correlation between selective inhibition of the cyclic nucleotide phosphodiesterases and the contractile activity in human pregnant myometrium near term. *Biochem Pharmacol* 1989 **38:** 9–15.

38. Diamond J. Beta-adrenoceptors, cyclic AMP, and cyclic GMP in control of uterine motility. In Carsten ME, Miller JD (eds) *Uterine Function. Molecular and Cellular Aspects.* New York: Plenum Press, 1990: 249–275.

39. Word RA, Casey ML, Kamm KE, Stull JT. Effects of cGMP on myosin light chain phosphorylation, and contraction in human myometrium. *Am J Physiol* 1991 **260:** C861–C867.

40. Yallampalli C, Izumi H, Byam Smith M, Garfield RE. An L-arginine–nitric oxide–cyclic guanosine monophosphate system exists in the uterus and inhibits contractility during pregnancy. *Am J Obstet Gynecol* 1994 **170:** 175–185.

41. Lees C, Campbell S, Jauniaux E *et al.* Arrest of preterm labour and prolongation of gestation with glyceryl trinitrate, a nitric oxide donor. *Lancet* 1994 **343:** 1325–1326.

42. Kao CY. Electrophysiological properties of uterine muscle. In Wynn RM, Jollie WP (eds) *The Biology of the Uterus.* New York: Plenum Press, 1989: 403–453.

43. Mironneau J. Ion channels and excitation–contraction coupling in myometrium. In Garfield RE (ed.) *Uterine Contractility.* Norwell, MA: Serono Symposia, USA, 1990: 9–19.

44. Young RC, Smith LH, McLaren MD. T-type and L-type calcium currents in freshly dispersed human uterine smooth muscle cells. *Am J Obstet Gynecol* 1993 **169:** 785–792.

45. Khan RN, Smith SK, Morrison JJ, Ashford ML, Properties of large-conductance K⁺ channels in human myometrium during pregnancy and labour. *Proc R Soc Lond Biol* 1993 **251:** 9–15.

46. Pérez GJ, Toro L, Erulkar SD, Stefani E. Characterization of large-conductance, calcium-activated potassium channels from human myometrium. *Am J Obstet Gynecol* 1993 **168:** 652–660.

47. Piper I, Minshall E, Downing SJ, Hollingsworth M, Sadraei H. Effects of several potassium channel openers and glibenclamide on the uterus of the rat. *Br J Pharmacol* 1990 **101:** 901–907.

48. López Bernal A, Parekh AB, Brading AF. Electrical coupling in human myometrium. *26th British Congress of Obstetrics and Gynaecology* 1992: Abstract.

49. Garfield RE, Blennerhassett MG, Miller SM. Control of myometrial contractility: role and regulation of gap junctions. *Oxf Rev Reprod Biol* 1988 **10:** 436–490.

50. Chow L, Lye SJ. Expression of the gap junction protein connexin-43 is increased in the human myometrium toward term and with the onset of labour. *Am J Obst Gynec* 1994 **170:** 788–795.

51. López Bernal A, Watson SP. Prostaglandins and the control of uterine contractility. Cellular endocrinology. In Drife JO, Calder AA (eds) *Prostaglandins and the Uterus.* London: Springer Verlag, 1992: 213–235.

52. Sellers SM, Hodgson HT, Mitchell MD, Anderson AB, Turnbull AC. Raised prostaglandin levels in the third stage of labor. *Am J Obstet Gynecol* 1982 **144:** 209–212.

53. Noort WA, van Bulck B, Vereecken A, de Zwart FA, Keirse MJ. Changes in plasma levels of PGF₂ alpha and PGI₂ metabolites at and after delivery at term. *Prostaglandins* 1989 **37:** 3–12.

54. MacDonald PC, Casey ML. The accumulation of prostaglandins (PG) in amniotic fluid is an aftereffect of labor and not indicative of a role for PGE₂ or PGF₂ alpha in the initiation of human parturition. *J Clin Endocrinol Metab* 1993 **76:** 1332–1339.

55. Wikland M, Lindblom B, Wilhelmsson L, Wiqvist N. Oxytocin, prostaglandins, and contractility of the human uterus at term pregnancy. *Acta Obstet Gynecol Scand* 1982 **61:** 467–472.

56. Cañete Soler R, López Bernal A. A comparison of leukotriene and prostaglandin binding to human myometrium. *Eicosanoids* 1988 **1:** 79–84.

57. López Bernal A, Buckley S, Rees CMP, Marshall JM. Meclofenamate inhibits prostaglandin E binding and adenylyl cyclase activation in human myometrium. *J Endocrinol* 1991 **129:** 439–445.

58. Senior J, Marshall K, Sangha R, Clayton JK. *In vitro* characterization of prostanoid receptors on human myometrium at term pregnancy. *Br J Pharmacol* 1993 **108:** 501–506.

59. Namba T, Sugimoto T, Negishi M *et al.* Alternative splicing of C-terminal tail of prostaglandin E receptor subtype EP3 determines G-protein specificity. *Nature* 1993 **365:** 166–170.

60. Molnar M, Hertelendy F. Regulation of intracellular free calcium in human myometrial cells by prostaglandin F2 alpha: comparison with oxytocin. *J Clin Endocrinol Metab* 1990 **71:** 1243–1250.

61. Fuchs ARF, Husslein P, Soloff MS. Oxytocin receptors in the human uterus during pregnancy and parturition. *Am J Obstet Gynecol* 1984 **150:** 734–741.

62. Kimura T, Azuma C, Takemura M *et al.* Molecular cloning of a human oxytocin receptor. *Regul Pept* 1993 **45:** 73–77.

63. Schrey MP, Cornford PA, Read AM, Steer PJ. A role for phosphoinositide hydrolysis in human uterine smooth muscle during parturition. *Am J Obstet Gynecol* 1988 **159:** 964–970.

64. Phaneuf S, Europe-Finner GN, Varney M, MacKenzie IZ, Watson SP, López Bernal A. Oxytocin-stimulated phosphoinositide hydrolysis in human myometrial cells: involvement of pertussis toxin-sensitive and -insensitive G-proteins. *J Endocrinol* 1993 **136:** 497–509.

65. Melin P. Oxytocin antagonists in preterm labour and delivery. *Bailliere's Clin Obstet Gynaecol* 1993 **7:** 577–600.

66. Breuiller-Fouche M, Doualla-Bell Kotto Maka F, Geny B, Ferré F. Alpha-1 adrenergic receptor: Binding and phosphoinositide breakdown in human myometrium. *J Pharmacol Exp Ther* 1991 **258:** 82–87.

67. Breuiller M, Rouot B, Litime MH, Leroy MJ, Ferré F. Functional coupling of the alpha 2-adrenergic receptor-adenylate cyclase complex in the pregnant human myometrium. *J Clin Endocrinol Metab* 1990 **70:** 1299–1304.

68. Anwer K, Oberti C, Pérez GJ, Ca²⁺-activated K⁺ channels as modulators of human myometrial contractile activity. *Am J Physiol* 1993 **265:** C976–C985.

69. Keirse MJNC, Grant A, King JF. Preterm labour. In Chalmers I, Enkin M, Keirse MJNC (eds) *Effective Care in Pregnancy and Childbirth.* Oxford: Oxford University Press, 1989: 694–769.

70. The Canadian Preterm Labor Investigators Group. Treatment of preterm labor with the beta-adrenergic agonist ritodrine. *N Engl J Med* 1992 **327:** 308–312.

71. Berg G, Andersson RGG, Ryden G. Beta-adrenergic receptors in human myometrium during pregnancy: Changes in the number of receptors after beta-mimetic treatment. *Am J Obstet Gynecol* 1985 **151:** 392–396.

72. Khac LD, Mokhtari A, Renner M, Harbon S. Activation of beta-adrenergic receptors inhibits Ca^{2+} entry-mediated generation of inositol phosphates in the guinea pig myometrium, a cyclic AMP-independent event. *Mol Pharmacol* 1992 **41**: 509–519.

73. Harbon S, Marc S, Goureau O *et al.* Multiple regulation of the generation of inositol phosphates and cAMP in myometrium. In Garfield RE (ed.) *Uterine Contractility.* Norwell, MA: Serono Symposia, USA, 1990: 123–140.

74. Leiber D, Marc S, Harbon S. Pharmacological evidence for distinct muscarinic receptor subtypes coupled to the inhibition of adenylate cyclase and to the increased generation of inositol phosphates in the guinea pig myometrium. *J Pharmacol Exp Ther* 1990 **252**: 800–809.

75. Gibbs RS, Romero R, Hillier SL, Eschenbach DA, Sweet RL. A review of premature birth and subclinical infection. *Am J Obstet Gynecol* 1992 **166**: 1515–1528.

76. López Bernal A, Hansell DJ, Canete Soler R, Keeling JW, Turnbull AC. Prostaglandins, chorioamnionitis and preterm labour. *Br J Obstet Gynaecol* 1987 **94**: 1156–1158.

77. van der Elst CW, López Bernal A, Sinclair Smith CC. The role of chorioamnionitis and prostaglandins in preterm labor. *Obstet Gynecol* 1991 **77**: 672–676.

78. Mitchell MD, Trautman MS, Dudley DJ. Immuno-endocrinology of preterm labour and delivery. *Baillieres Clin Obstet Gynaecol* 1993 **7**: 553–575.

79. Vince G, Shorter S, Starkey P *et al.* Localization of tumour necrosis factor production in cells at the materno/fetal interface in human pregnancy. *Clin Exp Immunol* 1992 **88**: 174–180.

80. Norwitz ER, López Bernal A, Starkey PM. Tumor necrosis factor-α selectively stimulates prostaglandin $F_{2\alpha}$ production by macrophages in human term decidua. *Am J Obstet Gynecol* 1992 **167**: 815–820.

81. Bry K, Hallman M. Transforming growth factor-beta opposes the stimulatory effects of interleukin-1 and tumor necrosis factor on amnion cell prostaglandin E_2 production: implication for preterm labor. *Am J Obstet Gynecol* 1993 **167**: 222–226.

82. Schrey MP, Holt JR, Cornford PA, Monaghan H, al Ubaidi F. Human decidua is a target tissue for bradykinin and kallikrein: phosphoinositide hydrolysis accompanies arachidonic acid release in uterine decidua cells *in vitro. J Clin Endocrinol Metab* 1992 **74**: 426–435.

83. Molnar M, Romero R, Hertelendy F. Interleukin-1 and tumor necrosis factor stimulate arachidonic acid release and phospholipid metabolism in human myometrial cells. *Am J Obstet Gynecol* 1993 **169**: 825–829.

84. Hertelendy F, Romero R, Molnar M, Todd H, Baldassare JJ. Cytokine-initiated signal transduction in human myometrial cells. *Am J Reprod Immunol* 1993 **30**: 49–57.

85. Romero R, Yoon BH, Kenney JS, Gomez R, Allison AC, Sehgal PB. Amniotic fluid interleukin-6 determinations are of diagnostic and prognostic value in preterm labor. *Am J Reprod Immunol* 1993 **30**: 167–183.

86. Cherouny PH, Pankuch GA, Romero R *et al.* Neutrophil attractant/activating peptide-1/interleukin-8: association with histologic chorioamnionitis, preterm delivery, and bioactive amniotic fluid leukoattractants. *Am J Obstet Gynecol* 1993 **169**: 1299–1303.

87. Europe-Finner GN, Phaneuf S, Watson SP, López Bernal A. Identification and expression of G-proteins in human myometrium: up regulation of Gαs in pregnancy. *Endocrinology* 1993 **132**: 2484–2490.

88. Europe-Finner GN, Phaneuf S, Tolkovsky AM, Watson SP, López Bernal A. Down-regulation of G-alphas and adenylyl cyclase in human myometrium at the onset of labour: a mechanism for parturition. *3rd European Congress of the Society for the Study and Prevention of Infant Deaths* 1993: Abstract.

3.11

Acid–Base Balance in the Fetus

DL Economides

INTRODUCTION

Physiology of acid–base balance

In the fetus acids are produced by normal metabolic processes and various mechanisms ensure that buffering of these acids maintains extracellular pH within a narrow range compatible with life. Two-thirds of an acid or alkali load presented to the fetus will be buffered by intracellular mechanisms. Therefore plasma pH measurements are only estimates of total body acid–base balance. A buffer is a solution that resists the changes in pH produced by adding acid or alkali, and important buffers include bicarbonate in plasma and hemoglobin in erythrocytes. In addition, the placental tissue bicarbonate pool may also play a role in buffering the fetus against changes in maternal pH or blood gas status.

In the adult acid–base balance is achieved by respiratory and renal control of carbon dioxide and bicarbonate concentrations. In the fetus, however, both these processes are carried out by the placenta. Carbon dioxide diffuses across the placenta from the fetal to the maternal vascular compartments while fetal metabolic acids such as lactic and beta-hydroxybutyric acids, diffuse across the intervillous space and are eliminated by the maternal kidneys. Thus, acid–base balance in the fetus depends on normal placental function and adequate perfusion from the uterine and umbilical circulations.

The major energy source of the fetus is oxidation of glucose and fatty acids. In aerobic glycolysis, oxidation of glucose produces carbon dioxide. The erythrocyte enzyme carbonic anhydrase facilitates the hydration of CO_2 to carbonic acid. Most of the free hydrogen ions are formed buffered intracellularly. Bicarbonate re-enters erythrocytes and combines with hydrogen ions to form carbonic acid, which then dissociates to carbon dioxide and water. Carbon dioxide diffuses quickly across the human placenta so that even large quantities produced by the fetus can be rapidly eliminated if maternal respiration, uteroplacental

blood flow, and umbilical blood flow are normal. The $P\text{CO}_2$ gradient between umbilical arterial blood and maternal uteroplacental blood helps the diffusion of carbon dioxide from fetus to mother In pregnancy, maternal $P\text{CO}_2$ is decreased to 34 mmHg from the normal non-pregnant value of 40 mmHg, thus increasing the fetomaternal gradient and facilitating diffusion.

The fetus produces non-carbonic acids by: (a) the incomplete combustion of carbohydrates and fatty acids in the absence of sufficient amounts of oxygen, resulting in production of lactic acid and keto-acids (e.g. beta-hydroxybutyric acid), (b) the utilization of non-sulfur-containing amino acids resulting in uric acid formation. These acids traverse the placenta slowly in comparison with the extremely rapid transit of CO_2. The fetus does have the ability to metabolize accumulated lactate in the presence of sufficient oxygen. However, this is also a slow process and for practical purposes is unlikely to account for a large proportion of lactic acid elimination from the fetal compartment. Fetal renal function is not sufficiently developed to handle excretion of these acids. The maternal kidney excretes non-carbonic acids produced by both maternal and fetal metabolism and in so doing also regenerates bicarbonate.

Factors affecting acid–base balance

Fetal acid–base balance is maintained by the supply of oxygen and removal of carbon dioxide and acid metabolites by the placenta. Thus maternal, placental or fetal factors can affect acid–base homeostasis (Table 3.11.1).

Maternal respiratory acidosis is caused when maternal alveolar ventilation is impaired by either a decrease in minute ventilation or by ventilation–perfusion imbalance. The transplacental carbon dioxide gradient is reduced and the fetus develops respiratory acidosis as a result of decreased carbon dioxide excretion by the maternal lungs. Alternatively, maternal respiratory alkalosis develops when hyperventilation reduces $P\text{CO}_2$ and increases maternal pH.

Table 3.11.1 Factors affecting fetal acid–base balance

Respiratory acidosis
Umbilical perfusion
  cord compression
Placental perfusion
  uterine hyperstimulation, abruptio placentae
Maternal alveolar ventilation
  narcotic overdose
  neuromuscular disorders
  hypokalemia
  magnesium sulfate toxicity
  airways obstruction

Respiratory alkalosis
Maternal hyperventilation
  anxiety
  salicylate poisoning
  sepsis
  pneumonia
  pulmonary emboli

Metabolic acidosis
Umbilical perfusion
  prolonged cord compression
Placental perfusion
  chronic uteroplacental insufficiency
Maternal acidosis
  renal failure
  ketoacidosis, e.g. diabetic, alcoholic, starvation
  lactic acidosis, e.g. drugs
  bicarbonate loss, e.g. diarrhea, renal tubular acidosis

As in respiratory acidosis, restoration of maternal acid–base balance by appropriate treatment results in normalization of fetal blood gases. Increased anion gap metabolic acidosis in the mother can be caused by reduced excretion of inorganic acids as in renal failure, or accumulation of organic acids as in alcoholic, diabetic or starvation ketoacidosis and lactic acidosis. The fetus then develops pure metabolic acidosis provided placental perfusion is normal.

Carbon dioxide removal is dependent on umbilical arterial blood flow to the placenta, diffusion across the placenta, uterine perfusion and elimination from the maternal circulation. Failure of any of these mechanisms can cause carbon dioxide retention and respiratory acidosis. Cord compression, uterine hyperstimulation, and *abruptio placentae* are good examples because they cause a sudden inability of placental respiratory gas exchange secondary to decreased blood flow. If the reduction in blood flow is transient then fetal respiratory acidosis can be reversed within a short time because transport of carbon dioxide and oxygen across the placenta is rapid under normal circumstances. On the other hand if it persists the decrease in PO_2 and anaerobic metabolism leads to an accumulation of lactic acid and a mixed fetal acidosis.

Fetal oxygenation

Although energy may be supplied to the body through anaerobic metabolism, this source is quite limited and ani-mals are therefore dependent on a continuous supply of oxygen for survival. Fetal oxygen supply depends on adequate maternal oxygenation, blood flow to the placenta, transfer across the placenta, fetal oxygenation, and delivery to fetal tissues. Oxygen saturation is a better indicator of fetal oxygenation and oxygen reserves than PO_2 which is a measure of pressure. Because of fetal hemoglobin, the fetal oxygen dissociation curve lies to the left of the maternal and enhances the uptake of oxygen from the maternal blood. The fetal oxygen dissociation curve is also steeper than that of the adult so that fetal blood can unload large quantities of oxygen in a narrow PO_2 range. Furthermore, the oxygen dissociation curve is influenced by changes in pH.

Acute experiments in animal fetuses demonstrated that the fetal PO_2 was much lower than in postnatal life.[1] Several studies in chronically catheterized animals of different species confirmed the observation that the oxygen tension in fetal blood is less than half that in postnatal life.[2] However, even with chronic catheterization studies the emphasis was on fetuses near term and changes with gestational age have not been widely recognized. Nonetheless, early studies in sheep suggested that the fetal PO_2 falls with advancing gestation.[2]

Despite the low fetal PO_2, the high hemoglobin concentration, hemoglobin oxygen affinity and cardiac output allow adequate fetal oxygenation. Indeed, oxygen consumption in fetuses from various species, derived from measurements of umbilical blood flow and arteriovenous blood PO_2 differences, is between 6.0 and 8.5 ml kg^{-1} min^{-1} compared with 3.5 ml kg^{-1} min^{-1} in the adult.[3,4] The high oxygen consumption of the fetus is necessary for the metabolism of a growing organism and in late gestation in the fetal lamb at least 30–40% of oxygen consumption can be attributed to growth needs.[5]

By far the most common cause of fetal acid–base imbalance is a deficient supply of oxygen resulting in acidosis. Maternal causes include hypoxemia or reduced placental perfusion; for example in cyanotic heart disease, hypoventilation, severe anemia, hypotension, placental separation. On the fetal side, anemia or umbilical cord compression with decreased umbilical blood flow can also restrict the availability of oxygen.

CURRENT CONCEPTS

Cordocentesis in the assessment of fetal oxygenation and acid–base balance

Cordocentesis is an ultrasound-guided sampling of the umbilical cord.[6] It is performed as an outpatient technique without maternal fasting or sedation, and it can therefore be used to study the physiology of the relatively undisturbed human fetus. The umbilical cord vessel sampled is identified as artery or vein by the turbulence seen ultrasonically when normal saline is injected through the sampling needle. The usual indications for cordocentesis are prenatal diagnosis of hereditary disorders (e.g. thalassemias, hemophilias), infection (e.g. rubella, toxoplasmosis), chromosomal abnormalities, and the management of red cell alloimmunization. The risk of fetal death after cordocentesis depends on the indication for sampling and the experience of the operator. After excluding pregnancies that were terminated, the fetal loss rates within 2 weeks of sampling were 1, 7, 14 and 25% in groups of structurally normal, structurally abnormal, growth-retarded and hydropic fetuses, respectively.[7] However, no losses were reported in potentially viable fetuses after cordocentesis in 594 cases.[8]

We investigated fetal oxygenation and metabolism in appropriate- (AGA) and small- (SGA) for-gestational age fetuses.[9] The AGA fetuses were shown not to be affected by the condition under investigation, and had appropriate birth weights, whereas in SGA fetuses chromosomal and structural abnormalities were excluded.

In normal fetuses, the blood oxygen tension is much lower than in maternal blood, and this may be caused by incomplete venous equilibration of uterine and umbilical circulations or by high placental oxygen consumption. The umbilical venous and arterial P_{O_2} and pH decrease with gestational age whereas P_{CO_2} increases (Figs 3.11.1–3.11.3 and Table 3.11.2). Despite the decrease in fetal P_{O_2}, the umbilical venous blood oxygen content does not change because the fetal hemoglobin concentration rises with advancing gestation.[18] Simultaneous sampling of human

Table 3.11.2 Mean values of P_{O_2}, P_{CO_2}, pH and lactate in human cord blood from normal pregnancies after vaginal delivery,[10,11] elective Cesarean delivery under spinal,[12] or general anesthetic at term,[13] or after hysterotomy[14,15] and cordocentesis[16,17] in the second trimester

Ref	No	Umbilical vein				Umbilical artery			
		P_{O_2} (mmHg)	P_{CO_2} (mmHg)	pH	Lactate (mmol l⁻¹)	P_{O_2} (mmHg)	P_{CO_2} (mmHg)	pH	Lactate (mmol l⁻¹)
10	25	29	38	7.33		18	45	7.26	
11	52	30	38	7.30	2.1	22	47	7.25	2.5
12	28		41	7.43				7.39	
13	10	35	45	7.32	0.8				
14	23	55	26	7.40		30	38	7.27	
15	19	50	43	7.32		21	55	7.23	
16	48	53	36	7.38	1.2	34	41	7.33	1.2
17	41	37	35	7.40		23	45	7.32	

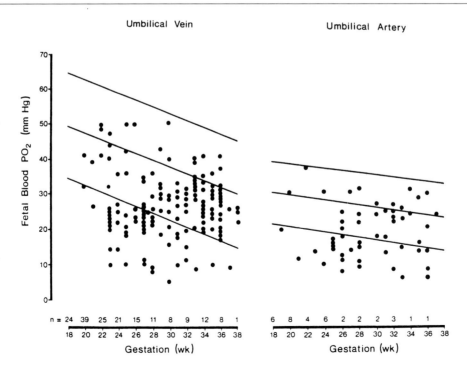

Fig. 3.11.1 *Reference ranges (mean + 2 SD) of umbilical venous and arterial P_{O_2} with gestation constructed from 173 venous and 35 arterial samples obtained from appropriate-for-gestational-age fetuses undergoing prenatal diagnosis. The individual values from 143 venous and 53 arterial samples from small-for-gestational-age fetuses are plotted as closed circles. (From reference 9.)*

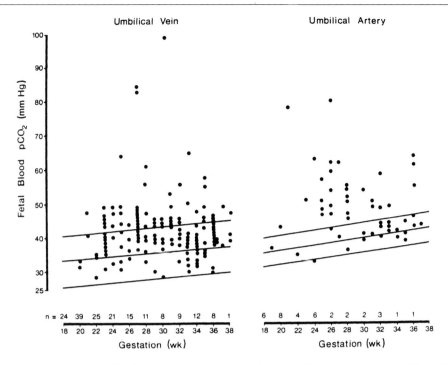

Fig. 3.11.2 *Reference ranges (mean + 2 SD) of umbilical venous and arterial* PCO_2 *with gestation constructed from 173 venous and 35 arterial samples obtained from appropriate-for-gestational-age fetuses undergoing prenatal diagnosis. The individual values from 143 venous and 53 arterial samples from small-for-gestational-age fetusus are plotted as closed circles. (From reference 9.)*

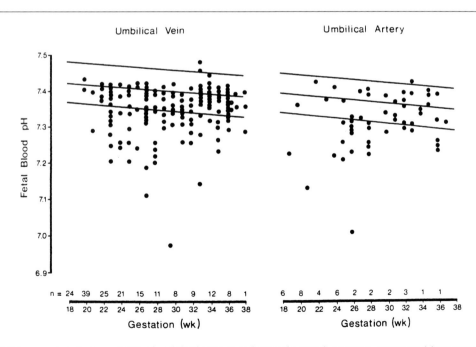

Fig. 3.11.3 *Reference ranges (mean + 2 SD) of umbilical venous and arterial pH with gestation constructed from 173 venous and 35 arterial samples obtained from appropriate-for-gestational-age fetuses undergoing prenatal diagnosis. The individual values from 143 venous and 53 arterial samples from small-for-gestational-age fetusus are plotted as closed circles. (From reference 9.)*

fetal umbilical blood and amniotic fluid in normal pregnancies did not show significant correlations in acid–base values but whether amniotic fluid analysis might be helpful in the assessment of the chronically acidotic fetus remains to be seen.[19]

Blood lactate concentration in cordocentesis samples does not change with gestation[9] and the values are similar to those in samples obtained at elective Cesarean section at term.[20] The umbilical venous blood lactate concentration is higher than the umbilical arterial in unpaired cordocentesis samples, indicating that the normoxemic human fetus is, like the sheep fetus,[21] a net consumer of lactate. Furthermore, the concentration of lactate in umbilical cord blood is higher than in maternal blood and the two are correlated significantly, suggesting that there is a common source of lactate, which is likely to be the placenta. Indeed, the human placenta has been shown to produce lactate that is secreted into both the fetal and maternal circulations.[22]

Some SGA fetuses are hypoxemic, hypercapnic, hyperlacticemic and acidotic,[9] and fetuses of mothers with severe pre-eclampsia are also hypoxemic and acidemic.[23] Both respiratory and metabolic acidosis increase with hypoxemia. In umbilical venous blood mild hypoxemia may be present in the absence of hypercapnia or acidosis (Fig. 3.11.4). In severe uteroplacental insufficiency the rate of clearance of carbon dioxide is exceeded by the rate of production, and hypercapnia and acidosis increase exponentially (Figs 3.11.4 and 3.11.5).[9] The carbon dioxide accumulation is presumably the result of reduced exchange between the uteroplacental and fetal circulations, due to reduced blood flow. Growth-retarded fetuses are hyperlacticemic. Furthermore, there is a significant association between fetal hypoxemia and hyperlacticemia, supporting the concept of reduced oxidative metabolism of lactate being the cause of hyperlacticemia, and under these circumstances the fetus appears to be a net producer of lactate.[9]

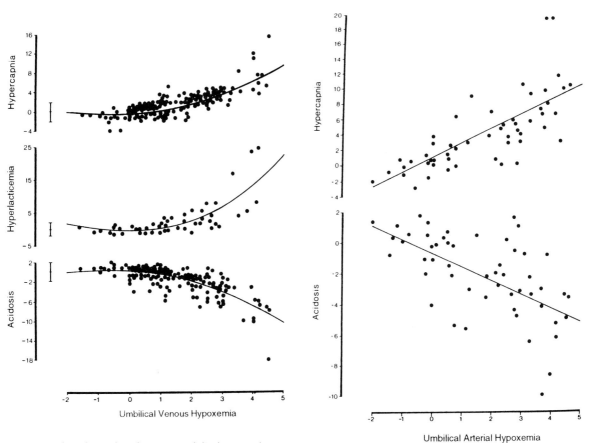

Fig. 3.11.4 *The relationships between umbilical venous hypoxemia and umbilical venous hypercapnia, hyperlacticemia or acidosis (in SDs from the appropriate mean for gestation) in small-for-gestational-age fetuses. Hypercapnia and hyperlacticemia increase and acidosis decreases exponentially with hypoxemia. Both hyperlacticemia and hypercapnia contribute to acidosis. (From reference 9.)*

Fig. 3.11.5 *The relationships between umbilical arterial hypoxemia and hypercapnia or acidosis (in SDs from the appropriate mean for gestation) in small-for-gestational-age fetuses. Hypercapnia and acidosis increase linearly with hypoxemia. (From reference 9.)*

The findings in growth-retarded fetuses demonstrate that asphyxia and hypoglycemia[24] manifested at birth may not be due to the process of birth itself, but rather these may exist antenatally. This may have important clinical and medicolegal implications,[25] as reduced oxygen and glucose supply to fetal brain may cause damage and cerebral dysfunction *in utero*.

Cordocentesis in the assessment of antenatal non-invasive tests of fetal well-being

Cordocentesis has also been used to evaluate non-invasive tests of fetal well-being. When impedance to blood flow in the umbilical artery is increased there is a progressive impairment of placental gas exchange and by the time diastolic flow is lost hypoxemia develops.[26] Indeed, in 59 growth-retarded fetuses with absence of end-diastolic frequencies in the umbilical artery, fetal hypoxemia and acidosis was present in 79% and 46%, respectively.[27] Doppler studies have demonstrated that in fetal hypoxemia there is redistribution of cardiac output that results in a brain-sparing effect at the expense of the peripheral organs. Thus, good correlations were found between the fetal blood gases and the ratio of the common carotid artery to the descending thoracic aorta mean velocity and pulsatility index.[28] This was also true when smaller fetal arteries, identified by color flow mapping, were examined. An increase in the renal artery pulsatility index, and a decrease in the middle cerebral artery pulsatility index with an accompanying increase in mean blood velocity were also related to the degree of fetal hypoxemia and blood oxygen deficit.[29,30] Antepartum fetal heart rate (FHR) patterns in SGA fetuses were found to be abnormal in 79% of those shown to be hypoxemic, acidotic or both, and a repetitive decelerative pattern best identified the hypoxemic fetuses. Fetal PO_2 values in the lower normal range present in many SGA fetuses were associated with a reactive trace.[31] In a small group of highly compromised growth-retarded fetuses the biophysical profile score could predict the degree of fetal acidemia. FHR reactivity and fetal breathing movements are the first whereas fetal gross body movement and tone are the last biophysical activities to be compromised during acidemia.[32]

One of the main challenges of antenatal care is to distinguish between normal small fetuses and growth-retarded fetuses which are at increased risk of intrauterine death or asphyxia. Cordocentesis can certainly distinguish between the two but in the majority of cases non-invasive tests can be used to obtain this information, without the risk of an invasive procedure to the fetus. Cordocentesis has been invaluable in assessing these non-invasive tests and in diagnosing intrauterine asphyxia by obtaining direct information about fetal oxygenation and acid–base balance. However, the acid–base status of growth-retarded fetuses showing absent end-diastolic frequencies was not helpful in predicting perinatal death.[33] An association between chronic fetal acidemia and neurodevelopmental impair-

ment at 12–52 months has recently been demonstrated in a group of 36 children who had prenatal cordocentesis for severe growth retardation.[34]

Acid–base monitoring in labor

The process of labor results in intermittent episodes of fetal hypoxia because during a contraction uterine blood flow is reduced, placental perfusion is transiently compromised and transplacental gaseous exchange is impaired. Between contractions uterine blood flow and oxygen supply is restored to normal. The vast majority of fetuses tolerate labor because they possess good reserve, although with prolonged labor there is progressive reduction in fetal pH, PO_2 and bicarbonate level and increase in PCO_2 and base excess. The fetus may withstand an asphyxial insult without neurological damage because of the fetal cardiovascular adaptation to hypoxemia. Prediction of the significance of an asphyxial insult to the fetus requires a measure of both the duration and degree of asphyxia, as well as an expression of the fetal compensatory response to asphyxia. Monkey fetuses develop central nervous system injury after a period of anoxia of 12 min or relative hypoxia for 2 h.[35] In humans, it appears that the duration of hypoxia is usually in excess of 1 h before the neuropathological damage responsible for motor and cognitive deficits develop.[36] However, neurological injury from hypoxia or trauma accounts for only 8–12% of cases of cerebral palsy.[37] It is important, therefore, to document that the infant is not hypoxic at birth.

Fetal distress is a loose term often applied to abnormal FHR patterns but conventional visual analysis of the FHR pattern as a means of fetal surveillance in labor has been questioned. It was believed that FHR patterns correlated with outcome, as judged by intrapartum fetal death and metabolic acidemia, and so permitted improvements in care. Yet randomized trials of electronic fetal monitoring have not supported this expectation and neither has the prediction of acidemia improved by computerized analysis of the FHR pattern in labor.[38] Fetal scalp sampling was the first method used to assess fetal acid–base balance in labor.[39] A fetal blood sample may be obtained from the scalp or buttocks when indicated. Electronic heart rate monitoring is associated with a high false positive diagnosis of fetal distress, and it has been proposed that use of scalp sampling reduces the risk of Cesarean section.[40]

There are five interdependent variables that may be taken into account when interpreting a fetal blood sample: pH, PCO_2, PO_2, HCO_3, and base excess. In the presence of a low pH, the most important decision is to distinguish between respiratory and metabolic acidosis because this may have a significant impact on patient management. Metabolic acidosis, associated with a scalp pH less than 7.20 and base excess greater than −6.0, requires consideration of delivery, whereas a fetus with respiratory acidosis may benefit from intrauterine resuscitation, and relatively immediate delivery may not be so crucial. Respiratory acidosis can occur with cord compression of uterine hyperstimulation, whereas metabolic acidosis more often represents a chronic condition in the fetus or may result from a long-standing intrapartum hypoxia. Apart from distinguishing between respiratory and metabolic acidosis, it is important to interpret results in the light of clinical circumstances, taking into account stage of labor, color and volume of amniotic fluid, estimated fetal weight, gestational age, parity, and so on. For example, growth-retarded fetuses may not tolerate even the most benign episodes of intrapartum hypoxia without becoming acidotic.

Umbilical cord acid–base measurement

Birth asphyxia remains a poorly defined term, although most obstetric and pediatric practitioners have come to accept a clinical definition that includes both neonatal depression and umbilical cord blood acidemia. A more rigorous definition would also include evidence of neonatal end-organ damage such as early seizures and cardiac or renal dysfunction. It has become increasingly clear that neonatal depression as determined by 1 and 5 minute Apgar scores alone is a poor reflection of birth asphyxia or predictor of long-term neurological deficit.[41-43] Umbilical cord blood pH at delivery provides the most sensitive indication of birth asphyxia and the absence of acidemia excludes this diagnosis.

In interpreting fetal blood gases it is important to distinguish between the umbilical arterial or venous origin of the sample. Umbilical arterial blood represents the fetal condition as this is blood returning from the fetus to the placenta whereas umbilical venous blood represents the state of placental perfusion. Thus, umbilical venous pH and oxygen saturation will be higher and $P\text{CO}_2$ lower than umbilical arterial blood. The definition of an abnormal cord arterial pH has in the past been accepted as <7.20. However, 7.20 falls within the normal range for arterial pH in all the recent large studies. The collective data from almost 19 000 reported deliveries defines the lower limits (2 standard deviations below the mean) for normal arterial cord pH at 7.04–7.10. Although fewer data are available for venous cord blood pH values, the lower limit should be 7.14–7.20 (Table 3.11.3).[44-46]

Although acid–base studies provide an acute assessment of the fetal condition at birth they are not accurate in predicting long-term outcome. Clinically significant acidemia at birth most likely does not occur until arterial pH reaches 7.0,[47] and in over 300 newborns with abnormal arterial pH the only infants with neurological deficit were those with arterial pH values <7.00.[48] In normally grown infants there was no correlation between low umbilical pH values and abnormal neonatal neurological evaluation.[49] A low pH by itself, does not predict abnormal behavior. In follow-up studies of infants for up to six years, acidemia alone at birth did not predict adverse long-term developmental outcome, unless there were other adverse perinatal influences at work.[50,51]

Routine measurement of umbilical cord pH and gases at delivery is becoming increasingly common practice at institutions with large delivery services. Strong consideration should be given to umbilical cord blood gas determinations in all high-risk deliveries and in all infants with unexpected complications in labor. Umbilical cord blood pH at delivery provides the most sensitive reflection of birth asphyxia and the absence of acidemia excludes this diagnosis. Only a cord arterial pH determination is recommended since it reflects fetal or newborn status more accurately than all other measurements.

Newer techniques of assessing acid–base balance in labor

Close correlation between tissue pH and scalp blood pH, and between final tissue pH and umbilical artery pH has been described,[52] but this has been disputed.[53] Tissue pH values are generally lower than arterial pH values by 0.026–0.06 pH units. Tissue pH values below 7.15 are defined as pathological.[54] Technical difficulties, mainly relating to attachment of the electrode to the fetal scalp, have inhibited the widespread acceptance of this method of fetal monitoring in labor. The procedure is invasive and the electrodes available at present are not applicable for routine use.

Continuous O_2 saturation can be measured in the fetus by placing a reflectance pulse oximeter in contact with the

Table 3.11.3 Umbilical cord blood gas and pH values at vaginal delivery

Reference	pH (mean (SD))		Base excess (mEq l⁻¹)		$P\text{O}_2$ (mmHg)		$P\text{CO}_2$ (mmHg)	
	UA	UV	UA	UV	UA	UV	UA	UV
Thorp et al.[44]	7.24 (0.07)	7.32 (0.06)	−4(3)	−3(2)	18(7)	29(7)	56(9)	44(7)
Eskes et al.[45]	7.23 (0.07)	7.32 (0.07)	−13(4)	−6(3)	—	—	—	—
Yeomans et al.[46]	7.28 (0.05)	7.35 (0.05)	—	—	18(6)	29(6)	49(8)	38(6)

Values are mean (SD).
UA, umbilical artery; UV, umbilical vein; $P\text{O}_2$, partial pressure of oxygen; $P\text{CO}_2$, partial pressure of carbon dioxide.

fetal cheek after the membranes are ruptured[55] but there are many limitations on the continuous measurement of fetal P_{O_2} in labor. Fetal oxygen saturation decreases as labor progresses but the signal can be lost during decelerations.[56] Using oxygen saturation measurements during suboptimal FHR patterns may decrease unnecessary interventions.[57] This promising new method of fetal monitoring will increase our understanding of abnormal FHR patterns but needs accurate evaluation before its introduction into clinical practice.

Considering that the electrocardiographic (ECG) changes of myocardial hypoxia are well recognized in adults it is disappointing that similar information cannot be obtained in the fetus. Evaluation of the fetal ECG waveform has been complicated by difficulties in signal acquisition and analysis.[58] However, in the first randomized controlled trial, addition of ECG waveform analysis was associated with significantly fewer operative deliveries for fetal distress but with no significant difference in neonatal outcome.[59] It is clear that considerably more work needs to be done before fetal ECG waveform analysis can be adopted for the purposes of routine fetal monitoring.

FUTURE PERSPECTIVES

Measuring the acid–base status of the fetus remains the only way of determining the presence of asphyxia. However, the techniques used are invasive, especially antenatal fetal blood sampling and it is hoped that non-invasive tests would be able to provide us with useful information of fetal well-being. Doppler blood flow frequencies of the fetal venous circulation (inferior vena cava and ductus venosus) are currently being examined. Further studies are also needed to establish the usefulness of cordocentesis in the management of the growth-retarded fetus and its effect on pregnancy outcome.

Better intrapartum fetal monitoring methods are essential as the current application of electronic fetal monitoring and fetal blood sampling still result in significant false positive and false negative diagnoses of asphyxia. Considering the escalating costs of medical negligence this remains the most urgent priority in modern practice of obstetrics. New pH electrodes appear encouraging with respect to both practicality and reliability but their usefulness needs to be proved in larger and more detailed studies.

SUMMARY

- Acid–base balance in the fetus is dependent on normal placental function, adequate perfusion from the uterine and umbilical circulations and maternal acid–base physiology.
- By far the most common cause of fetal acid–base imbalance is a deficient supply of oxygen resulting in acidosis.
- Some small-for-gestational age fetuses are hypoxemic, hypercapnic, hyperlacticemic and acidotic, as demonstrated in cordocentesis samples; thus, asphyxia manifested at birth may not be due to the process of birth itself, but rather it may exist antenatally.
- Cordocentesis has also been used to assess antenatal non-invasive tests of fetal well-being, e.g. Doppler blow flow studies, biophysical profile, FHR patterns.
- The process of labor results in intermittent episodes of fetal hypoxia because during a contraction uterine blood flow is reduced, placental

perfusion is transiently compromised and transplacental gaseous exchange is impaired.
- Birth asphyxia remains a poorly defined term but clinical definition includes neonatal depression, umbilical cord blood acidemia, and evidence of neonatal end-organ damage such as early seizures and cardiac or renal dysfunction.
- Neurological injury from hypoxia or trauma in labor accounts for only 8–12% of cases of cerebral palsy.
- In interpreting fetal blood gases it is important to distinguish between the umbilical arterial or venous origin of the sample.
- Clinically significant acidemia at birth is unlikely to occur until the arterial pH reaches 7.0.
- Although acid–base studies provide an acute assessment of the fetal condition at birth they are not accurate in predicting long-term developmental outcome.

REFERENCES

1. Huggett A. Fetal blood gas tensions and gas transfusion through the placenta of the goat. *J Physiol* 1927 **62**: 373–384.
2. Battaglia FC, Meschia G. *An Introduction to Fetal Physiology*. London: Academic Press, 1986: 154–167.
3. Comline RS, Silver M. Placental transfer of blood gases. *Br Med Bull* 1975 **31**: 25–30.
4. Keele CA, Neil E, Joels N. *Respiration. Sampson Wright's Applied Physiology*. Oxford: Oxford University Press, 1982: 211–214.
5. Hommes FA, Drost YM, Geraets WXM. The energy requirement for growth. *Pediatr Res* 1975 **9**: 51–55.
6. Nicolaides KH, Soothill PW, Rodeck CH, Campbell S. Ultrasound guided sampling of umbilical cord and placental blood to assess fetal wellbeing. *Lancet* 1986 **i**: 1065–1067.
7. Maxwell DJ, Johnson P, Hurley P, Neales K, Allan L,

Knott P. Fetal blood sampling and pregnancy loss in relation to indication. *Br J Obstet Gynaecol* 1991 **98**: 892–897.

8. Weiner CP, Wenstrom KD, Sipes SL, Williamson RA. Risk factors for cordocentesis and fetal intravascular transfusions. *Am J Obstet Gynecol* 1991 **165**: 1020–1025.

9. Nicolaides KH, Economides DL, Soothill PW. Blood gases and pH and lactate in appropriate and small for gestational age fetuses. *Am J Obstet Gynecol* 1989 161: 996–1001.

10. Rooth G, Sjostedt S, Caligara F. Hydrogen ion concentration, carbon dioxide tension and acid base balance in blood of human umbilical cord and intervillous space of placenta. *Arch Dis Child* 1960 **35**: 278–285.

11. Eguilus A, Bernal L, McPherson K, Parrilla JJ, Abad L. The use of intrapartum fetal blood lactate measurements for the early diagnosis of fetal distress. *Am J Obstet Gynecol* 1983 **147**: 949–954.

12. Crawford JS. Maternal and cord blood at delivery. *Am J Obstet Gynecol* 1965 **93**: 37–43.

13. Cetin I, Marconi AM, Bozzetti P, Sereni LP, Corbetta C, Pardi G *et al*. Umbilical amino-acid concentrations in appropriate and small for gestational age infants: a biochemical difference present *in utero*. *Am J Obstet Gynecol* 1988 **158**: 120–126.

14. Rudolph AM, Heyman MA, Teramo KAW, Barrett CT, Raiha NCR. Studies on the circulation of the previable human fetus. *Pediatr Res* 1971 **5**: 452–465.

15. Morris JA, Hunstead RF, Robinson RG, Haswell GL. Measurement of fetoplacental blood volume in the human previable fetus. *Am J Obstet Gynecol* 1974 **118**: 927–934.

16. Soothill PW, Nicolaides KH, Rodeck CH, Campbell S. Effect of gestational age on fetal and intervillous blood gas and acid–base values in human pregnancy. *Fetal Ther* 1986 **1**: 168–175.

17. Weiner CP. Cordocentesis. *Obstet Gynecol Clin North Am* 1988 **15**: 283–303.

18. Forestier F, Daffos F, Catherine N, Penard M, Andreux JP. Developmental hemopoiesis in normal human fetal blood. *Blood* 1991 77: 2360–2363.

19. Economides DL, Johnson P, MacKenzie IZ. Does amniotic fluid analysis reflect acid base balance in fetal blood? *Am J Obstet Gynecol* 1992 **166**: 970–973.

20. Pardi G, Buscaglia M, Ferrazzi E, Bezzetti P, Marconi AM, Cetin I *et al*. Cord sampling for the evaluation of oxygenation and acid base balance in growth retarded human fetuses. *Am J Obstet Gynecol* 1987 **157**: 1221–1228.

21. Burd LI, Jones MD, Simmons MA. Placental production and fetal utilisation of lactate and pyruvate. *Nature* 1975 **254**: 210–211.

22. Holzman IR, Phillips AF, Battaglia FC. Glucose metabolism, lactate and ammonia production by the human placenta *in vivo*. *Pediatr Res* 1979 **13**: 117–120.

23. Okamura K, Watanabe T, Tanigawara S, Shintaku Y, Endo H, Iwamoto M *et al*. Biochemical evaluation of fetus with hypoxia caused by severe pre-eclampsia using cordocentesis. *J Perinat Med* 1990 **18**: 441–447.

24. Economides DL, Nicolaides KH. Blood glucose and oxygen tension in small for gestational age fetuses. *Am J Obstet Gynecol* 1989 **160**: 385–389.

25. Symonds EM. Antenatal, perinatal or postnatal brain damage? *Br Med J* 1987 **294**: 1046–1047.

26. Weiner CP. The relationship between the umbilical artery systolic/diastolic ratio and umbilical blood gas measurements in specimens obtained by cordocentesis. *Am J Obstet Gynecol* 1990 **162**: 1198–1202.

27. Nicolaides KH, Bilardo CM, Soothill PW, Campbell S. Absence of end-diastolic frequencies in umbilical artery: a sign of fetal hypoxia and acidosis. *Br Med J* 1988 **297**: 1026–1027.

28. Bilardo CM, Nicolaides KH, Campbell S. Doppler measurements of fetal and uteroplacental circulations: Relationship with umbilical venous blood gases measured at cordocentesis. *Am J Obstet Gynecol* 1990 **162**: 115–120.

29. Vyas S, Nicolaides KH, Campbell S. Renal artery flow-

30. Vyas S, Nicolaides KH, Bower S, Campbell S. Middle cerebral artery flow velocity waveforms in fetal hypoxaemia. *Br J Obstet Gynaecol* 1990 **97**: 797–803.

31. Visser GHA, Sadovsky G, Nicolaides KH. Antepartum heart rate patterns in small-for-gestational-age third-trimester fetuses: correlations with blood gas values obtained at cordocentesis. *Am J Obstet Gynecol* 1990 **162**: 698–703.

32. Ribbert LSM, Snijders RJM, Nicolaides KH, Visser GHA. Relationship of fetal biophysical profile and blood gas values at cordocentesis in severely growth-retarded fetuses. *Am J Obstet Gynecol* 1990 **163**: 569–571.

33. Nicolini U, Nicolaidis P, Fisk NM, Vaughan JI, Fusi L, Gleeson R, Rodeck CH. Limited role of fetal blood sampling in prediction of outcome in intrauterine growth retardation. *Lancet* 1990 **336**: 768–772.

34. Soothill PW, Ajayi RA, Campbell S, Ross EM, Candy DCA, Snijders RM, Nicolaides KH. Relationship between fetal acidemia at cordocentesis and subsequent neurodevelopment. *Ultrasound Obstet Gynecol* 1992 **2**: 80–83.

35. Meyers RE. Two patterns of perinatal brain damage and their conditions of occurrence. *Am J Obstet Gynecol* 1972 **112**: 246–253.

36. Low JA, Galbraith RS, Muir DW, Killen HL, Pater EA, Karchmar EJ. Factors associated with motor and cognitive deficits in children following intrapartum fetal hypoxia. *Am J Obstet Gynecol* 1984 **148**: 533–539.

37. Nelson KB. What proportion of cerebral palsy is related to birth asphyxia? *J Pediatr* 1988 **112**: 572–574.

38. Pello LC, Rosevear SK, Dawes GS, Moulden M, Redman CWG. Computerised fetal heart rate analysis in labor. *Obstet Gynecol* 1991 **78**: 602–610.

39. Saling E. Neues Vorgehen zur Untersuchung des Kindes unter Geburt. *Arch Gynak* 1961 **197**: 108–122.

40. Zalar RW, Quilligan EJ. The influence of scalp sampling on the cesarean section for fetal distress. *Am J Obstet Gynecol* 1979 **135**: 239–246.

41. Sykes GS, Johnson P, Ashworth F, Molloy PM, Gu W, Stirrat GM. Do Apgar scores indicate asphyxia? *Lancet* 1982 i: 494–496.

42. Ruth VJ, Raivio KO. Perinatal brain damage predictive value of metabolic acidosis and the Apgar score. *Br Med J* 1988 **297**: 24–27.

43. Marrin M, Paes BA. Birth asphyxia: does the Apgar score have diagnostic value? *Obstet Gynecol* 1988 **72**: 120–123.

44. Thorp JA, Sampson JE, Parisi VM, Creasy RK. Routine umbilical cord blood gas determinations? *Am J Obstet Gynecol* 1989 **161**: 600–605.

45. Eskes TK, Jongsma HW, Houx PC. Percentiles for gas values in human umbilical cord blood. *Eur J Obstet Gynecol Reprod Biol* 1983 **14**: 341–346.

46. Yeomans ER, Hauth JC, Gilstrap LC, Strickland DM. Umbilical cord pH, PCO_2 and bicarbonate following uncomplicated term vaginal deliveries. *Am J Obstet Gynecol* 1985 **151**: 798–800.

47. Gilstrap LC, Leverno KJ, Burris JB, Burris J, Williams ML, Little BB. Diagnoses of birth asphyxia based on fetal pH, Apgar score and newborn cerebral dysfunction. *Am J Obstet Gynecol* 1989 **161**: 825–830.

48. Winkler CL, Haugh JC, Tucker JM, Owen J, Brumfield CG. Neonatal complications at term as related to the degree of umbilical artery acidemia. *Am J Obstet Gynecol* 1991 **164**: 637–641.

49. Dijxhoorn MJ, Visser GHA, Huisjes HJ, Fidler V, Touwen BC. The relation between umbilical pH values and neonatal neurological morbidity in full term appropriate-for-dates infants. *Early Hum Dev* 1985 **11**: 33–42.

50. Touwen BCL, Huisjes HJ, Jurgens-Van Der Zee AD, Bierman-van Eendenburg ME, Smrkorsky M, Olinga AA. Obstetrical condition and neonatal neurological morbidity. An analysis with the help of the optimality concept. *Early Hum Dev* 1980 **4**: 207–228.

51. Touwen BCL, Lok-Meijer TY, Huisjes HJ, Olinga AA. The recovery rate of neurologically deviant newborns. *Early Hum Dev* 1982 7: 131–148.
52. Young BK. Continuous fetal tissue pH monitoring in labour. *J Perinat Med* 1981 **9:** 189.
53. Boos R, Ruttgers H, Muliawan D, Heinrich D, Kubli F. Continuous measurement of tissue pH in the human fetus. *Arch Gynaecol* 1978 **226:** 183.
54. Nickelsen C, Weber T. The current status of intrapartum continuous fetal tissue pH measurements. *J Perinat Med* 1991 **19:** 87–92.
55. Aarnoudse JG, Huisjes HJ, Gordan H, Oeseburg B, Zijlstra WG. Fetal subcutaneous scalp PO_2 and abnormal heart rate during labour. *Am J Obstet Gynecol* 1985 **153:** 565–566.
56. Dildy GA, Clark SL, Loucks CA. Intrapartum fetal pulse oximetry: the effects of normal labor, variable decelerations and maternal oxygen administration on fetal arterial oxygen saturation. *Am J Obstet Gynecol* 1993 **168:** 341.
57. Katz M, Petrick T, Richichi K, Belluomini J. Oxygen saturation (S_aO_2) monitoring in the presence of non-reassuring fetal heart rate (FHR) patterns. *Am J Obstet Gynecol* 1993 **168:** 341.
58. Deans AC, Steer PJ. The use of the fetal electrocardiogram in labour. *Br J Obstet Gynaecol* 1994 **101:** 9–17.
59. Westgate J, Harris M, Curnow JSH, Greene KR. Randomised trial of cardiotocography alone or with ST waveform analysis for intrapartum monitoring. *Lancet* 1992 **340:** 194–198.

3.12

Physiological Adaptation at Birth

RA Silver and RF Soll

INTRODUCTION

At birth, many physiologic changes must take place for the fetus to make the transition from the intrauterine to the extrauterine environment successfully. The most important of these physiologic changes are clearance of fetal lung fluid, initiation of air breathing, conversion from fetal to adult circulation, thermoregulation, and appropriate metabolic changes secondary to loss of placentally derived nutrition.

In asphyxiated infants, these necessary physiologic changes may not occur, resulting in the need for resuscitation in the delivery room and possibly the need for continued intensive care. The ultimate outcome of these infants will be determined by the degree of asphyxia and by the timeliness and appropriateness of neonatal resuscitation. This chapter focuses on the physiology of transition in both the normal newborn and in the asphyxiated infant and reviews the basis and practice of neonatal resuscitation.

CURRENT CONCEPTS

Pulmonary adaptation

For the fetus to begin air breathing successfully, adequate morphologic lung development and development of neuromuscular control of breathing must take place prior to birth. Sufficient alveoli for gas exchange are usually present by 25 weeks' gestation. However, surfactant production is often not sufficient until 35 weeks' gestation.[1] Surfactant deficiency causes decreased alveolar stability and increased fluid leak into the alveoli. It is common to see respiratory distress due to surfactant deficiency in newborns less than 35 weeks' gestation.

The mechanisms of neuromuscular control of breathing are established well before birth. The fetus spends approximately 30% of the time in utero with rapid discordant panting.[2,3] These breathing movements in utero correspond to medullary center output, and are associated with periods of rapid eye movement (REM) sleep.

Near term, the fetus will inhale as much as 600 ml of amniotic fluid per day.[4] The removal of lung fluid is one of the many changes required for successful breathing. At birth, as the infant passes through the birth canal, the thoracic cage is exposed to pressures of 30–160 cm H_2O and as much as 30 ml of amniotic fluid is squeezed out of the airways.[5] Infants born by Cesarean section are not subjected to this squeeze and retain more lung fluid. Retained lung fluid can manifest, clinically, as transient tachypnea of the newborn, which has a higher incidence in infants born by Cesarean section.

Immediately after birth, there is recoil of the thoracic cage which allows for filling with air. An air–liquid interface forms that produces surface retractive forces that would tend to collapse the smaller airways and alveoli if not for the presence of surfactant.[1] Surfactant is produced and secreted in the lung by the type II pneumocyte. Surfactant is made up of phospholipid (primarily dipalmitoyl phosphatidylcholine) and protein (surfactant proteins A, B and C). Surfactant is distributed along the alveoli in a monolayer that reduces alveolar surface retractive forces. The surfactant proteins may be important in the secretion, distribution and re-uptake of surfactant. In addition, surfactant protein B improves the lateral stability of the phospholipid monolayer.[6] The critical amount of surfactant needed to lower alveolar surface tension is 3 mg kg^{-1},[7] although larger surfactant pools are found in term infants.[8]

The initial expansion of the alveoli with air is made easier if there is some fluid retained in the lungs.[9] Inflation of a totally collapsed gas-free lung requires a much greater distending pressure than if the lung is partially filled with fluid[1] (Fig. 3.12.1). Consider the simple analogy of attempting to inflate a totally empty balloon compared to a balloon that is partially distended with water. The inspiratory force generated with the first breath can be as high as 40–80 cm of H_2O pressure. With the first expiration, mobilization and orientation of alveolar surfactant

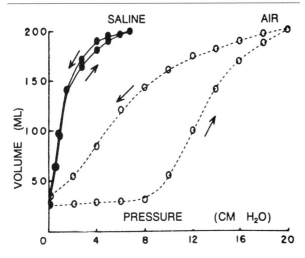

Fig. 3.12.1 *Pressure volume curves demonstrating air (dotted line) versus liquid (solid line) expansion of the lung. (From Redford EP. In Remingan JW (ed.) Tissue Elasticity. Washington, DC: American Physiological Society, 1957.)*

decreases transpulmonary pressure required to maintain lung volume to near 0 cm H_2O,[1] allowing the newborn to maintain a functional residual capacity. Establishment of functional residual capacity significantly decreases the negative inspiratory pressure required for normal inspiration.

The exact reasons why an infant takes its first breaths remain unknown. *In utero*, the fetus usually exhibits breathing movements during periods of REM sleep; at birth and thereafter, the infant has a continuous breathing pattern during sleep and while awake. At birth, the newborn is immediately confronted with multiple new stimuli: cold, light, noise, tactile stimulation, and pain. These factors, in particular the cool environment, play a major role in stimulating the newborn's first breaths. The birth process also results in a fall in arterial pH and arterial P_{O_2}, and a rise in arterial P_{CO_2}. However, these changes do not appear to be primary stimuli for the first breaths.[10]

Continued clearance of lung fluid is enhanced by negative interstitial and intrapleural pressures created by resistance of the chest wall to collapse in opposition to the retractive forces of surface tension. This negative pressure allows for increased pulmonary blood flow which in turn leads to increased capillary hydrostatic pressure. Increased capillary hydrostatic pressure causes fluid to leak into the interstitium.[1] In order to clear this fluid, there is a dramatic increase in lung lymph drainage,[11] during the first 6 hours of life.

In summary, the first breaths allow for the following changes necessary for successful conversion to air breathing:

1. Increased pulmonary blood flow.
2. Increased clearance of fluid from the lungs.
3. Establishment of a functional residual capacity and the characteristic pulmonary function of the newborn infant.[1]

Cardiovascular adaptation

Fetal circulation is strikingly different from adult circulation. During fetal life, the lungs are not used for gas exchange and therefore receive very little of the combined cardiac output. The fetal circulation has a system of shunts that allow the left- and right-sided circulations to act in parallel, as opposed to the separate series circulatory pattern seen in the adult. In the fetus, blood is shunted away from the lungs both at an intracardiac and extracardiac level (Fig. 3.12.2) (see also Chapter 3.2).

Fetal circulation relies on the placenta as the organ for gas exchange. Oxygen rich blood returns from the placenta through the umbilical vein. The umbilical vein joins the portal circulation as the portal vein enters the liver. Much of the umbilical venous return will bypass the hepatic microcirculation by passing through the ductus venosus, which joins the umbilical venous circulation directly to the inferior vena cava. The ductus venosus is one of three shunts present in fetal life that close functionally, shortly after birth.

From the inferior vena cava, mixed venous blood enters the right atrium and joins the systemic venous return from the upper body via the superior vena cava. Due to high pulmonary vascular resistance, right ventricular as well as right atrial pressures are higher than corresponding left-sided pressures. During fetal life, the foramen ovale will allow flow from the right atrium to the left atrium. This shunt may persist in the newborn infant if right-sided pressures remain abnormally high. Since right atrial pressure is higher than left atrial pressure, much of the venous return to the right atrium is shunted across the foramen ovale to the left atrium and then out to the systemic circulation from the left ventricle. Right atrial blood that enters the right ventricle goes out via the main pulmonary artery. In the fetus, the main pulmonary artery and the aorta are connected by the ductus arteriosus. Since the pulmonary vascular resistance remains high, most of this blood is shunted to the aorta through this extracardiac shunt. Between the foramen ovale and the ductus arteriosus, almost all the blood that enters the right side of the heart is shunted to the systemic circulation, so that the pulmonary circulation receives only 4–8% of the fetal cardiac output. Much of the blood flow from the descending aorta that enters the common iliac arteries will enter the umbilical arteries. This blood returns to the placenta to be oxygenated completing the fetal placental circuit.

Due to the mixing of left- and right-sided circulations, the fetal tissues are exposed to arterial blood with a much lower oxygen tension than they are in extrauterine life. The fetus is able to survive in this environment due to high concentrations of fetal hemoglobin. Fetal hemoglobin has a much higher affinity for oxygen than adult hemoglobin. This shifts the oxygen hemoglobin dissociation curve to the left, so that for any given oxygen tension, fetal hemoglobin will have a higher oxygen saturation than adult hemoglobin. The beneficial effects to the fetus are twofold. First, it facilitates oxygen transfer in the placenta from maternal hemoglobin A to fetal hemoglobin F. Second, it increases the oxygen carrying capacity of blood in a low oxygen environment.

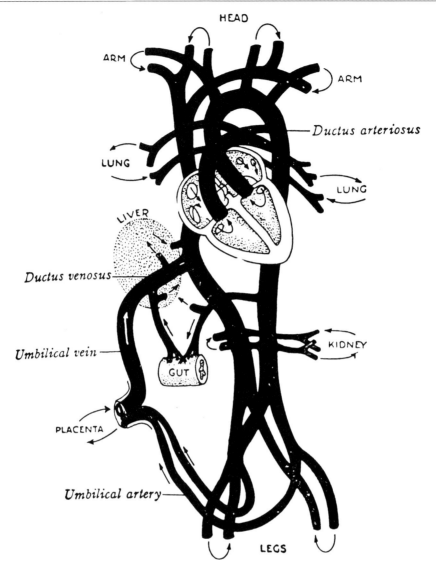

Fig. 3.12.2 *Diagram of fetal circulation. Darker shading indicates more oxygenated blood. (From Rudolph AM.* Congenital Diseases of the Heart. *Chicago, Yearbook Medical Publishers, 1974.)*

When the fetus is born, the organ of gas exchange abruptly changes from the placenta to the lungs. For the fetus successfully to make the transition to air breathing, the circulatory system must also respond to the changes associated with cord clamping and initiation of air breathing. For this to take place, two major changes must occur. First, separation of the left- and right-sided circulations must occur by closure of fetal intra- and extracardiac shunts, and second, an increase in pulmonary blood flow must occur, facilitating gas exchange. In the following section, these two changes will be discussed separately, although they occur simultaneously after birth.

The intra- and extracardiac shunts present during fetal life are no longer necessary in the newborn. The ductus venosus and foramen ovale close simply by the change in the hemodynamic state of the fetus, whereas closure of the ductus arteriosus is mediated by a number of factors. With

clamping of the umbilical cord and initiation of air breathing the following events occur: pulmonary blood flow is established, venous return from the umbilical vein is tremendously diminished, and systemic vascular resistance increases dramatically with the removal of the low resistance placenta. Since umbilical venous flow is greatly diminished, flow through the ductus venosus is also diminished. The ductus venosus will begin to close shortly after birth due to decrease in flow, and in most newborns will be fully closed by the end of the first week of life.[12] With the decrease in venous return to the right atrium and decrease in pulmonary vascular resistance, right atrial pressure falls. Left atrial pressure increases due to increased venous return from the lungs. With left atrial pressure now exceeding right atrial pressure, the flap of the foramen ovale is pushed against the atrial septum, effectively closing this shunt.[12]

The ductus venosus and foramen ovale close simply due

to the altered hemodynamic state of the newborn. Regulation of closure of the ductus arteriosus is much more complex, and the complete mechanism for closure of the duct is not fully understood.[13] There are several factors known to control patency and closure of the ductus arteriosus.

Oxygen is the major stimulus for ductal closure. After birth, there is constriction of ductus arteriosus smooth muscle in response to increased arterial PaO_2. The response to oxygen is not as pronounced in premature babies.[13,14] Although the mechanism is incompletely understood, other mediators have been identified whose presence or absence after birth probably plays a role in ductal closure. Prostaglandin E$_2$ (PGE$_2$), produced in the placenta and in the fetal lung, actively maintains dilation of the ductus arteriosus in the fetus.[15] PGE$_2$ levels fall dramatically at birth, due to removal of the placenta and increase of lung metabolism of PGE$_2$ in response to increased pulmonary blood flow. The absence of PGE$_2$ facilitates the ductal response to oxygen.[12] The ductus arteriosus of premature infants is more sensitive to PGE$_2$, which may help to explain why persistent patency of the ductus arteriosus is more common in preterm infants.[13]

Investigators have proposed a variety of other mechanisms that may effect ductal closure, including mediation by the cytochrome enzyme system, the autonomic nervous system, thromboxane A$_2$, or other vasoactive substances such as bradykinin.[16] Whatever the mechanism, functional closure of the duct will occur in 90% of term newborns by 72 hours of age.[16–18]

Closure of the fetal shunts, with subsequent separation of the pulmonary and systemic circulations is only one of the major circulatory changes that takes place at birth. The other major circulatory change is the increase in pulmonary blood flow. Increased pulmonary blood flow is directly related to pulmonary vascular resistance. At birth,

the fetus makes a change from active pulmonary vasoconstriction to active pulmonary vasodilation.

There are a number of mechanical and chemical factors that maintain pulmonary vasoconstriction in the fetus (Fig. 3.12.3). The fetal and newborn pulmonary arteries have a relatively thick medial smooth muscle layer compared to vessels seen in adults.[14] The medial smooth muscle layer plays a role in creating the increased pulmonary vascular resistance *in utero*. This smooth muscle layer begins to thin at birth and during the next few months after birth.[14] In addition, the fluid-filled fetal lungs tend to compress small pulmonary arteries which increases pulmonary vascular resistance. The relatively low fetal PO$_2$ also has a role in maintaining pulmonary vascular constriction. A number of vasoactive substances are thought to help maintain pulmonary vascular constriction in the fetus. Leukotrienes (LTC$_4$ and LTD$_4$) are pulmonary vasoconstrictors in newborns and adults. Thromboxane A$_2$ and platelet activating factor are also vasoconstrictors. Their role in the maintenance of high pulmonary vascular resistance in the fetus is not completely understood.[14]

Many factors influence the shift to active pulmonary vasodilation which occurs immediately after birth. The decrease in pulmonary vascular resistance seen at birth is due to at least two conditions. First, there is a partial decrease in pulmonary vascular resistance that is produced by physical expansion of the lungs, and second, there is a further decrease in pulmonary vascular resistance produced by an increase in arterial PO$_2$.[19] Both of these components are necessary for successful transition to extrauterine life.[14] Decreased arterial PCO$_2$ and the presence of vasoactive substances also contribute to pulmonary vasodilation, but their mechanisms are not fully known.

Physical expansion of the lungs increases pulmonary blood flow independently of fetal oxygenation. However, lung expansion alone is not sufficient to increase pulmonary blood flow to normal newborn values. The increase in pulmonary blood flow occurs secondary to replacement of lung fluid with air, decreasing the alveolar pressure which tended to collapse the small pulmonary arteries in the fluid-filled lung. The air-filled alveoli produce surface retractive forces which create a negative dilating pressure on small pulmonary arteries. Physical expansion of the lungs leads to the release of vasoactive substances, in particular prostacyclin (PGI$_2$),[20] which also decrease pulmonary vascular resistance.[14]

Ventilation of the lungs with oxygen produces further pulmonary vasodilation.[19] Exposure to increased oxygen in association with physical expansion of the lungs produces full pulmonary vasodilation.[14] Whether oxygen acts directly on the pulmonary vessels is not known. Oxygen stimulates release of bradykinin which acts as a vasodilator. Bradykinin stimulates release of PGI$_2$ and endothelium-derived nitric oxide (EDNO). EDNO is a potent pulmonary vasodilator. In fetal lambs, oxygen-mediated pulmonary vasodilation is blocked by inhibiting EDNO production,[21] supporting the role of EDNO in the maintenance of decreased pulmonary vascular resistance. Acid–base balance also plays a role in oxygen-mediated pulmonary vasodilation. Acidemia by itself will produce an

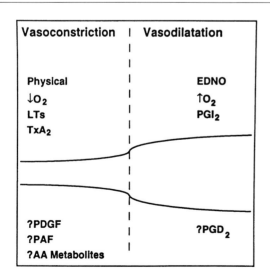

Fig. 3.12.3 *Schematic of factors that control pulmonary blood flow during the fetal and neonatal period. (From reference 14.)*

increase in pulmonary vascular resistance, and acidemia will also potentiate the increase in pulmonary vascular resistance seen in hypoxia.

Thermoregulation

In utero, the fetus is surrounded by a warm environment and certain mechanisms of the thermoregulatory system, such as cold-induced thermogenesis, remain inactive.[22] Heat produced from the fetus by metabolic processes is dissipated through the mother. The majority of heat is dissipated through the placenta, with the remaining heat being lost through the fetal skin, amniotic fluid and abdominal wall.[23] For heat to flow from fetus to mother, the fetus maintains a temperature that is 0.5–1.0° C higher than maternal temperature.[22]

At birth, the infant is immediately exposed to a cool environment. Heat is lost predominantly through the skin. There are four mechanisms by which heat is lost: radiation, convection, conduction, and evaporation. Radiation is heat loss in the form of electromagnetic waves. Factors that determine radiant heat exchange are the surface temperatures of the two objects, areas of orientation of the objects, emissivity (the ratio of radiant energy of a surface to that of a black surface having the same temperature) and reflectivity (the amount of radiant energy reflected by an object).[24]

Convective heat loss is the transference of heat by movement of a liquid or a gas from a warmer to a cooler region. As air over the body is warmed by the body, the warmed air has a tendency to rise and is replaced by cooler air. Determinants of convective heat loss are the temperature difference between the two objects, air movement across the surfaces, and the surface area exposed.[24]

Conductive heat loss is the direct transfer of heat from molecule to molecule between two objects in direct contact with each other. Determinants of conductive heat loss are the surface area in contact between two objects as well as the heat capacity and conductivity of the two objects.[24] Conductive heat loss usually represents a minor source of heat loss in the newborn.

Evaporative heat loss is the heat lost in vaporization of water from the skin or respiratory tract. Evaporative heat loss is determined mostly by the gradient of humidity between objects.[24] At birth, all infants are covered in amniotic fluid. If inadequate attention is paid to drying these newborn infants, evaporative losses can be quite large.

Once adequate attention has been paid to drying the newborn infant, transepidermal loss of water in the term newborn in the indoor environment is quite small due to the stratum corneum of mature skin acting as a barrier to water loss. However, in small premature babies with 'immature' skin lacking a stratum corneum, water loss through the skin can be quite large and may represent not only a major source of heat loss but a source of dehydration as well.

Despite the rapid change in environment at birth, the term newborn infant is able to maintain body temperature at a constant level despite changes in environmental temperature. The mechanism by which newborns maintain body temperature is different from that in the adult (Table 3.12.1). Very premature babies, particularly infants less than 28 weeks' gestation, have little or no ability to maintain their body temperature in varying environmental temperatures. The reasons for the premature infant's inability to maintain body temperature include the previously noted evaporative skin losses, the absence of brown adipose tissue (or brown fat) and the infant's large surface area relative to volume, which greatly increases heat loss from radiation, convection, and conduction.

Brown fat is the major source of energy for heat production in the newborn through the mechanism of non-shivering thermogenesis. In humans, energy is stored in carbohydrates, lipids, and proteins. When these compounds are metabolized, most of the energy is transferred to ATP via the electron transport chain, and the remainder of the energy is dissipated as heat. The energy stored in ATP is then used by the body for biochemical reactions that require energy. The rate of breakdown of these compounds is dependent on the metabolic rate, which is largely determined by the level of thyroid hormone (specifically T_3). In brown fat, lipids are metabolized via the electron transport chain. The mitochondria of brown fat contain a unique protein called thermogenin. Thermogenin uncouples the metabolism of fatty acids in the electron transport chain from production of ATP. Instead, the energy from metabolism of free fatty acids is all dissipated as heat. Brown fat is found in the interscapular and perirenal regions of newborn infants.[24]

In utero, the fetus is unable to produce heat by non-shivering thermogenesis. Since the newborn infant is able to produce heat by non-shivering thermogenesis shortly after cord clamping, it has been hypothesized that the onset of thermogenesis is limited by placental factors.[25,26] After cord clamping, non-shivering thermogenesis becomes

Table 3.12.1 Thermoregulatory thermogenesis in adults, full term and preterm newborn infants

Thermogenesis	Adult	Newborn	
		Fullterm (38–42 wks)	Preterm (28–32 wks)
(1) Voluntary muscle activity	+	−	−
(2) Shivering thermogenesis	+	− or ±	−
(3) Non-shivering thermogenesis	+	+	− or ±

From reference 22.

the main source of heat production in the newborn. Initiation of non-shivering thermogenesis is directly related to the rise in norepinephrine and T_3 seen at birth.[27,28] Regardless of the control of non-shivering thermogenesis, there is a gradual increase in the metabolism of brown fat over the first days of life in term newborns.[25] During the first year of life, shivering thermogenesis replaces non-shivering thermogenesis[22] (Table 3.12.1).

Metabolic adaptation

In utero, the fetus has a steady supply of glucose and nutrients via the placenta. At the time of cord clamping, the supply of nutrients is abruptly cut off. The newborn responds to the abrupt cessation of glucose by mobilizing built up glycogen stores and by gluconeogenesis. In addition to accumulating brown fat stores in the last trimester, the late gestation fetus also diverts much of its glucose to storage as hepatic glycogen.[29–31] The induction of hepatic glycogen synthesis is believed to be dependent on the maturational surge in adrenal corticosteroids.[32,33] Adrenalectomized and hypophysectomized fetal sheep have vastly depleted hepatic glycogen stores.[34] Shortly after the appearance of glycogen synthetic enzymes in the fetus, the enzymes necessary for gluconeogenesis can be demonstrated,[35] although gluconeogenesis has not been shown to take place *in utero*.[32]

The fetus is able to maintain adequate blood glucose levels *in utero* because of constant maternal supply by the placenta. Fetal blood glucose levels are therefore directly dependent on maternal levels. Severe starvation or insulin administration will lower maternal blood glucose levels and have been shown also to lower fetal blood glucose levels.[32]

The stress related to events around birth, namely hypoxia, hypothermia, and hypoglycemia, induce a surge of catecholamines. It is this surge of catechols that induces hepatic phosphorylase and lipase. Hepatic phosphorylase becomes engaged in glycogenolysis. The human fetus has adequate glycogen stores to sustain normal blood glucose levels for the first twelve hours after birth.[1] Lipase activity in adipose tissue metabolizes fat into glycerol and free fatty acids which is made available as a source for gluconeogenesis.[1] Glucose derived from this process will continue to maintain blood sugar levels in the normal range until maternal milk supply is established and the infant is able to receive sufficient glucose enterally.

The premature and small-for-gestational-age infant are at risk for hypoglycemia early in life if they do not receive additional glucose supply. Although their glycogen stores are low, this does not seem to be the major cause for continued hypoglycemia in these infants. These groups of infants have been demonstrated to have high levels of gluconeogenic amino acids despite their hypoglycemia. It has been postulated that they have decreased levels of gluconeogenic enzymes, particularly the rate-limiting enzyme, phosphoenolpyruvate carboxykinase.[36] In some cases these infants may even be hypoglycemic in the delivery room, necessitating immediate intervention.

Abnormal physiology at birth: perinatal asphyxia

Successful transition from the intrauterine to the extrauterine environment may be complicated by a variety of factors, leading to perinatal asphyxia. Perinatal asphyxia is a major concern for obstetricians and pediatricians alike due to its association with poor neonatal outcome including mortality and serious developmental problems. However, our understanding of perinatal asphyxia is clouded by the lack of a clear definition of perinatal asphyxia, resulting in poor identification of infants whose outcome is related to perinatal asphyxia. This section describes the physiology of perinatal asphyxia and reviews current definitions of perinatal asphyxia.

Although the clinical definition of perinatal asphyxia is imprecise, there are clearly defined physiologic changes that occur in the infant undergoing asphyxia around the time of delivery. Asphyxia occurs as a result of failure to provide adequate substrate (mainly glucose) and oxygen required to carry out various metabolic processes. Inadequate glucose and oxygen delivery to fetal tissues results in hypoxia, hypercapnia, and metabolic acidosis. The fetus has a number of mechanisms to compensate for brief periods of asphyxia. When these compensatory mechanisms begin to fail, the infant is at risk for multi-organ system damage and death.

As the fetus begins to experience hypoxia, systemic blood flow will be redistributed such that blood flow is maintained or increased to the brain, heart, and adrenal glands.[37] Furthermore, blood flow to the brain is regulated such that there is increased flow to the brainstem with less flow to the higher centers.[38] To increase flow to these vital organs, blood flow is decreased to the liver, kidneys, gastrointestinal tract, and the extremities. These changes in blood flow are mediated by catecholamines[39] and arginine vasopressin.[40] In response to hypoxia, the fetal heart responds with a vagally mediated bradycardia.

The asphyxiated infant has significantly decreased movement and cessation of respiratory effort. These changes decrease oxygen consumption. Stored glycogen can be released as glucose to increase available substrate. However, under hypoxic conditions, glucose can only be metabolized to pyruvate and lactic acid. Build-up of lactic acid causes the metabolic acidosis seen in asphyxia. Additionally, increasing tissue carbon dioxide will further increase the acidosis. Fortunately, the developing brain has a lower metabolic rate than the adult, which allows the fetus to withstand longer periods of asphyxia before injury will occur.[41]

In severe asphyxia, the cardiovascular adaptive mechanisms fail and shunting of blood to vital organs begins to fall off. There is a drop in cardiac output and in blood pressure. Cerebral autoregulation fails and oxygen delivery to all areas of the brain becomes inadequate. Brain injury is most strongly correlated with fall in blood pressure,[42–44] rather than the degree of acidosis or hypoxia.[41,42,45–47]

Despite our knowledge of the physiologic changes seen in the asphyxiated newborn, the identification and treatment of the asphyxiated newborn is limited. Carter and coworkers describe five principal mechanisms of asphyxia in the human infant during labor, delivery, and the immediate postpartum period. These mechanisms include: (a) interruption of the umbilical circulation (cord accidents or compression); (b) altered placental gas exchange (placental abruption, previa, or insufficiency); (c) inadequate perfusion of the maternal side of the placenta (maternal hypotension, hypertension from any cause, or abnormal uterine contractions); (d) impaired maternal oxygenation (maternal cardiopulmonary disease, or anemia); and (e) failure of the neonate to initiate air breathing and accomplish successful transition.[48]

These investigators emphasize the need to evaluate multiple clinical signs and biochemical indices in order to expediently identify infants at risk of perinatal asphyxia and to make timely interventions to optimize outcome.[48] The following clinical or biochemical signs are the most clinically relevant in defining perinatal asphyxia: acidemia, abnormalities on electronic fetal monitoring (see below), low Apgar scores (for a period >5 minutes), immediate neurologic sequelae, and multiple organ dysfunction. In 1992, The American College of Obstetricians and Gynecologists and The American Academy of Pediatrics Committees on Maternal–Fetal Medicine and Fetus and Newborn defined criteria to help identify the infant who has undergone perinatal asphyxia and may be at risk for long-term neurodevelopmental sequelae.[49] Infants are at increased risk if each of the following criteria are present: (a) profound acidosis (metabolic or a combined metabolic and respiratory acidosis) with pH <7.00; (b) an Apgar score of ≤3 for greater than 5 minutes; (c) clinical neurologic sequelae in the perinatal period including seizures, hypoxic–ischemic encephalopathy, hypotonia, or coma; and (d) evidence of multi-organ system dysfunction.

Portman et al.[50] created a morbidity index scoring system in order to identify infants with perinatal asphyxia. The score is based on three criteria: the 5 minute Apgar score, the initial base deficit, and the fetal heart rate tracing. Scores are assigned based on the parameters detailed in Table 3.12.2. Scores of greater than or equal to 6 points on their morbidity index scoring system were associated with multiple organ system morbidity in infants who may have undergone asphyxia. This scoring system was applied prospectively. The organ systems most commonly involved

include the central nervous system (hypoxic ischemic encephalopathy, cerebral edema, neonatal seizures, and long-term neurodevelopmental delays), the kidneys (oliguria, acute and/or chronic renal failure), the cardiovascular system (tricuspid insufficiency, myocardial necrosis, shock/hypotension), the lungs (pulmonary hypertension, surfactant dysfunction, meconium aspiration), the gastrointestinal system (necrotizing enterocolitis, bowel perforation, hepatic dysfunction), and hematologic complications (thrombocytopenia, DIC).[48]

It is important to emphasize that there is no single physical sign, symptom or laboratory value that will identify perinatal asphyxia in a particular newborn. Neither will a particular single outcome identify perinatal asphyxia retrospectively. Cerebral palsy was at one time thought to be solely attributable to events in the immediate perinatal period. These beliefs have received much criticism in the recent medical literature.[51,52] The crucial issue in the diagnosis of perinatal asphyxia is using the multiple signs and symptoms to identify infants at risk for poor long-term outcome and to make timely and appropriate interventions to optimize outcome.

In summary, perinatal asphyxia changes the pattern of blood flow distribution such that the organs vital to survival, specifically the brain, heart, and adrenal glands, will at first be spared. The organs from which blood is shunted, particularly the kidneys, may show clinical signs of injury even with mild asphyxia. As the asphyxic insult continues, these mechanisms fail and blood pressure and cardiac output can no longer be maintained. The metabolic changes occurring during asphyxia include mixed acidosis as a result of anaerobic glycolysis, and hypoglycemia from rapid utilization of stored glycogen. The normal circulatory changes that occur at birth may not happen secondary to acidosis and hypoxia (see previous section on cardiovascular adaptation at birth). Infants who have undergone asphyxia will be apneic at birth since fetal breathing movements stop with ongoing asphyxia. In order to make the clinical diagnosis of asphyxia in a given infant a number of clinical and laboratory signs must be noted around the time of birth. Attempts to establish the diagnosis retrospectively, based on a particular outcome, have proven to be highly biased and are of little use in our attempts to prevent and treat these infants.

Table 3.12.2 Scoring system for postasphyxia morbidity

	Points			
	0	1	2	3
5-minute Apgar	>6	5–6	3–4	0–2
Base deficit (mEq l⁻¹)	<10	10–14	15–19	≥20
FHR tracing	Normal	Variable decelerations	Severe variables or lates	Prolonged bradycardia

FHR = fetal heart rate.
≥6 points, severe morbidity.
From reference 48.

FUTURE PERSPECTIVES

Future trends pertaining to improving neonatal transition lie mainly in the prevention and treatment of perinatal asphyxia. The major goal of neonatal resuscitation programs is to have proper equipment and properly trained personnel at every delivery in every hospital. Training in the techniques of newborn resuscitation and stabilization must be provided to all health care professionals who will care for newborn infants for this goal to be achieved. Early and appropriate steps in newborn resuscitation and stabilization postresuscitation will optimize recovery from asphyxia. Even in smaller community hospitals without facilities for advanced neonatal care, adequate management can be provided to the infant until transfer of the infant to such a facility can be achieved. Transport services for sick neonates and regionalization of perinatal care are also an integral part of providing optimal care for these infants and their mothers. Nations that provide well-organized systems for perinatal care have lower incidence of perinatal morbidity and mortality.[53]

In developing countries, greater than 90% of deliveries take place where there are not adequate neonatal resuscitation facilities. The World Health Organization and the Commonwealth Association for Mental Handicap and Developmental Disabilities estimates that one million babies die and as many survive with hypoxic encephalopathy each year due to lack of such facilities.[54] Investigators have attempted to modify the recommendations on neonatal resuscitation to better fit these health care situations. Milner et al.[55] devised a face mask resuscitation device that was inexpensive, reusable, and easily used to provide positive pressure ventilation to newborns. Because of these qualities, this device could receive widespread use even by personnel with little experience. Widespread use of such devices might have an impact on the mortality and morbidity of infants born in these circumstances.

Although optimal antepartum and peripartum care reduce the incidence of perinatal asphyxia, there are still many newborns each year who suffer perinatal asphyxia and the long-term adverse neurodevelopmental effects of hypoxic–ischemic encephalopathy. Current therapy mainly consists of fluid restriction for prevention of cerebral edema, correction of metabolic abnormalities to prevent seizures, and aggressive treatment with anticonvulsants for seizures. These therapies are largely aimed at preventing further damage. Newer therapies to treat and reduce the extent of permanent brain injury include the use of oxygen-free radical inhibitors and scavengers, excitatory amino acid antagonists, and calcium channel blockers. A detailed discussion of these is beyond the scope of this chapter. Although none of these therapies are currently accepted for widespread clinical use, there have been some promising results in animal models.[56] Ideally, any of these agents which have been shown to be useful in animal models should be studied in prospective randomized double-blind controlled trials to prove their efficacy in the treatment of perinatal hypoxic–ischemic encephalopathy.

SUMMARY

- Many physiologic changes must occur at birth for successful transition to extrauterine life. The most important physiologic changes at birth are: (a) initiation of air breathing, (b) conversion from fetal to adult circulation, (c) thermoregulation, (d) metabolic adaptation to loss of placentally supplied metabolic substrate.
- Successful conversion to air breathing requires adequate lung development (particularly the presence of pulmonary surfactant) and neuromuscular control of breathing. Both are present by 35 weeks' gestation.
- At birth, successful conversion to air breathing requires the clearance of lung fluid. The fetus has several mechanisms to clear lung fluid during and shortly after birth. In the presence of surfactant, the lungs can fill with air and maintain functional residual capacity.
- For the newborn to receive adequate oxygen from air breathing, the fetal circulation must convert to adult type circulation. This transition requires closure of fetal shunts and dilation of the pulmonary vascular bed. Oxygen is a major stimulant for ductal closure and pulmonary arteriolar dilation.
- Newborn infants have a large surface area relative to volume and therefore lose heat more rapidly than adults. Most heat loss is by conduction and convection. Newborns are able to maintain body temperature by the metabolism of brown fat via non-shivering thermogenesis.
- Normal newborn infants are able to maintain adequate blood sugar levels through the metabolism of hepatic glycogen stored in the last trimester and through increased gluconeogenesis.
- Asphyxiated infants will not make the necessary physiologic changes needed for successful conversion to extrauterine life. Long-term sequelae can develop if periods of hypoxia are prolonged.
- The availability of personnel trained in newborn resuscitation will reduce morbidity and mortality in newborn infants.
- The future of newborn care during transition lies in the areas of preventive health care. Adequate prenatal care and the availability of personnel trained in newborn resuscitation will have the greatest impact in preventing perinatal asphyxia.

REFERENCES

1. Nelson N. Physiology of transition. In Avery GB, Fletcher MA, MacDonald MG (eds) *Neonatology: Pathophysiology and Management of the Newborn*, 4th edn. Philadelphia: JP Lippincott, 1994: 223–249.
2. Patrick J, Natale R, Richardson B. Patterns of human fetal breathing activity at 34–35 wks GA. *Am J Obstet Gynecol* 1978 **132**: 507–513.
3. Boddy K, Mantell CD. Observations of fetal breathing movements transmitted through maternal abdominal wall. *Lancet* 1972 **ii**: 1219–1220.
4. Duenhoelter DV, Pritchard JA. Fetal respiration: quantitative measurements of amniotic fluid inspired near term by human and rhesus fetuses. *Am J Obstet Gynecol* 1976 **125**: 306–309.
5. Saunders RA, Milner AD. Pulmonary pressure/volume relationships during the last phase of delivery and the first postnatal breaths in human subjects. *J Pediatr* 1978 **93**: 667–673.
6. Cochrane CG, Revak SD. Pulmonary SP-B; structure–function relationships. *Science* 1991 **254**: 566–568.
7. Kobayashi T, Shido A, Nitta K. The critical concentration of surfactant in fetal lung liquid at birth. *Resp Physiol* 1990 **80**: 181–192.
8. Notter RH, Shapiro DL. Lung surfactants for replacement therapy: biochemical, biophysical and clinical aspects. *Clin Perinatol* 1987 **14**: 433–479.
9. Faridy EE. Air opening pressure in fetal lungs. *Resp Physiol* 1987 **68**: 293–300.
10. Hagwood S. Respiratory system. In Gluckman PD, Heymann MA (eds) *Perinatal and Pediatric Pathophysiology: A Clinical Perspective*. London: Edward Arnold, 1993: 561–630.
11. Egan EA, Oliver RE, Strang LB. Changes in non-electrolyte permeability of alveoli and the absorption of lung liquid at the start of breathing in the lamb. *J Physiol* 1975 **244**: 161.
12. Friedman AH, Fahey JT. The transition from fetal to neonatal circulation: normal responses and implications for infants with heart disease. *Semin Perinatol* 1993 **17**: 106–121.
13. Valimak I, Airsimaki H, Kozak A. Adaptation of cardio-respiratory control in neonates. *J Perinat Med* 1991 **19(Supp 1)**: 74–79.
14. Heymann MA. Cardiovascular system. In Cluckman PD, Heymann MA (eds) *Perinatal and Pediatric Pathophysiology: A Clinical Perspective*. London: Edward Arnold, 1993: 449–560.
15. Heyman MA. Prostaglandins and leukotrienes in the perinatal period. *Clin Perinatol* 1987 **14**: 857–880.
16. Clyman RI. Ductus arteriosus: current theories of prenatal and postnatal regulation. *Semin Perinatol* 1987 **1**: 64.
17. Gentle R, Stevenson G, Dooley T, Franklin D, Kawabori I, Pearlman A. Pulsed Doppler echocardiographic determination of time of ductal closure in normal newborn infants. *J Pediatr* 1981 **3**: 443.
18. Alenick DS, Holzman I, Ritter SB. The neonatal transitional circulation: a combined non-invasive assessment. *Echocardiography* 1992 **9**: 29.
19. Iwamoto HS, Teitel D, Rudolph AM. Effects of birth related events on blood flow distribution. *Pediatr Res* 1987 **22**: 634–640.
20. Leffler CW, Hessler JR, Green RS. The onset of breathing at birth stimulates pulmonary vascular prostacyclin synthesis. *Pediatr Res* 1987 **18**: 938.
21. Moore P, Velvis H, Fineman JR. EDRF Inhibition attenuates the increase in pulmonary blood flow due to oxygen ventilation in fetal lambs. *J Appl Physiol* 1992 **73**: 2151–2157.
22. Okken A. Postnatal adaptation in thermoregulation. *J Perinat Med* 1991 **19 (Suppl 1)**: 67–73.
23. Gilbert RD, Power CG. Fetal and uteroplacental heat production in sheep. *J Appl Physiol* 1986 **61**: 2018–2022.
24. Gunn TR. Thermoregulation. In Gluckman PD, Heymann MA (eds) *Perinatal and Pediatric Pathophysiology: A Clinical Perspective*. London: Edward Arnold, 1993: 355–372.
25. Symonds ME, Lomax MA. Maternal and environmental influences in thermoregulation in the neonate. *Proc Nutr Soc* 1992 **51**: 165–172.
26. Power GG. Biology of temperature. The mammalian fetus. *J Dev Physiol* 1989 **12**: 295–304.
27. Polk DH. Thyroid hormone effects on neonatal thermogenesis. *Semin Perinatol* 1988 **12**: 151–156.
28. Padbury JF, Martinez AM. Sympathoadrenal system activity at birth: integration of postnatal adaptation. *Semin Perinatol* 1988 **12**: 163–172.
29. Hay, W Jr. Fetal glucose metabolism. *Semin Perinatol* 1979 **3**: 157–176.
30. Shelly HJ. Blood sugars and tissue carbohydrate in foetal and infant lambs and rhesus monkeys. *J Physiol* 1960 **153**: 527–552.
31. Shelly HJ, Bassett JM, Milner RD. Control of carbohydrate metabolism in the fetus and newborn. *Br Med Bull* 1975 **31**: 37–43.
32. Pedbury JF, Ogata ES. Glucose metabolism during the transition to postnatal life. In Polin RA, Fox WW (eds) *Fetal and Neonatal Physiology*. Philadelphia: WB Saunders, 1992: 402–405.
33. Liggins GC. Adrenocortical-related maturational events in the fetus. *Am J Obstet Gynecol* 1976 **126**: 931–941.
34. Barnes RJ, Comline RS, Silver M. Effects of adrenalectomy and hypophysectomy in foetal lambs. *J Physiol (London)* 1976 **254**: 15–16.
35. Sparks JW. Augmentation of the glucose supply in the fetus and newborn. *Semin Perinatol* 1979 **3**: 141–155.
36. Haymond MW, Karl IE, Pagliara AS. Increased gluconeogenic substrate in the small for gestational age infant. *N Engl J Med* 1974 **291**: 322–328.
37. Reid DL, Parer JT, Williams K et al. Effects of severe reduction in maternal placental blood flow on blood flow distribution in the sheep fetus. *J Dev Physiol* 1991 **15**: 183.
38. Jensen A, Hohmann M, Kunzel W. Dynamic changes in organ blood flow and oxygen consumption during acute asphyxia in fetal sheep. *J Dev Physiol* 1987 **9**: 543.
39. Jelinek J, Jensen A. Catecholamine concentrations in plasma and organs of the fetal guinea pig during normoxemia, hypoxemia, and asphyxia. *J Dev Physiol* 1991 **15**: 145.
40. Perez R, Espinoza M, Riquelme R et al. Arginine vasopressin mediates cardiovascular responses to hypoxemia in fetal sheep. *Am J Physiol* 1989 **256**: R1011.
41. Williams CE, Mallard C, Tan W, Gluckman PD. Pathophysiology of perinatal asphyxia. *Clin Perinatol* 1993 **20**: 2.
42. Gunn AJ, Parer JT, Mallard EC et al. Cerebral histological and electrophysiological changes after asphyxia in fetal sheep. *Pediatr Res* 1992 **31**: 486.
43. Mallard EC, Gunn AJ, Williams CE et al. Umbilical cord occlusion causes cerebral damage in the fetal sheep. *Am J Obstet Gynecol* 1992 **167**: 1423.
44. Ting P, Yamaguchi S, Bacher J et al. Hypoxic–ischemic cerebral necrosis in midgestational sheep fetuses: physiopathologic correlations. *Exp Neurol* 1983 **80**: 227.
45. Denis J, Johnson A, Mutch L et al. Acid–base status at birth and neurodevelopmental outcome at four and one half years. *Am J Obstet Gynecol* 1989 **161**: 213.
46. Dijxhoorn M, Visser G, Fidler V et al. Apgar score, meconium and acidaemia at birth in relation to neonatal neurological morbidity. *Br J Obstet Gynaecol* 1986 **93**: 217–222.
47. Marrin M, Paes B. Does the Apgar score have diagnostic value. *Obstet Gynecol* 1988 **72**: 120–123.
48. Carter BS, Haverkamp AD, Merenstein GB. The definition of acute perinatal asphyxia. *Clin Perinatol* 1993 **20**: 287.

49. American Academy of Pediatrics, American College of Obstetricians and Gynecologists Relationship between perinatal factors and neurologic outcome. In Poland RL, Freeman RK (eds) *Guidelines for Perinatal Care* 3rd edn. Elk Grove Village, Illinois: American Academy of Pediatrics, 1992: 221–224.

50. Portman RJ, Carter BS, Gaylord MS *et al.* Predicting neonatal morbidity after perinatal asphyxia: a scoring system. *Am J Obstet Gynecol* 1990 **162**: 174–182.

51. Blair E, Stanly FJ. Intrapartum asphyxia: a rare cause of cerebral palsy. *J Pediatr* 1988 **112**: 515–519.

52. Nelson KB, Leviton A. How much of neonatal encephalopathy is due to birth asphyxia? *Am J Dis Child* 1991 **145**: 1325–1331.

53. Fanaroff AA, Graven SN. Perinatal services and resources. In Fanaroff AA, Martin RJ (eds) *Neonatal–Perinatal Medicine: Diseases of the Fetus and Infant.* St Louis: Mosby-Yearbook 1992: 12–21.

54. Commonwealth Association for Mental Handicap and Developmental Disabilities. Report of the working group for development of a programme on prevention and management of birth asphyxia. *Newsletter* 1988 **8**: 6–8.

55. Milner AD, Upton CJ, Green J, Stokes GM. A device for domiciliary neonatal resuscitation. *Lancet* 1990 **335**: 273–275.

56. Vanucci RC. Current and potentially new management strategies for perinatal hypoxic ischemic encephalopathy. *Pediatrics* 1990 **85**: 961–968.

3.13

Infection During Pregnancy

F Smaill

INTRODUCTION

Both the mother and her unborn child are at risk when infection occurs during pregnancy. The developing fetus is uniquely vulnerable – death, developmental anomalies, congenital infection, preterm delivery, or neonatal sepsis can occur as a consequence of an infection that is trivial for the mother. Likewise, serious maternal disease may result from infection with organisms that are usually associated with mild illness in the non-pregnant woman.

The host–parasite relationship in pregnancy is dynamic. It is important to understand the pathogenicity of the common infecting organisms, their transmission, the basic mechanisms of disease and the role of host defenses. Since a comprehensive review is beyond the scope of this chapter, selected infections will be used to illustrate general principles. HIV infection is discussed in Chapter 3.14.

CURRENT CONCEPTS

Pathogenesis of fetal infection

Most infection that occurs in pregnancy is without consequence for the mother or fetus.[1] The majority of infections in pregnant women involve the upper respiratory tract and gastrointestinal tract and either resolve spontaneously without therapy or are readily treated with antimicrobial agents. Such infection remains localized without affecting the fetus.

For some microorganisms the placenta, rather than serving as a barrier, is the pathway for infection.[2] Although most microorganisms are promptly cleared from the maternal circulation, some will localize within the placenta and spread across the maternal–fetal junction to infect the fetus directly. The factors that permit some microorganisms, and not others, to localize and multiply in the placenta are not well understood.

Damage to the fetus can occur as the result of direct tissue invasion and multiplication of the microorganism or secondary to vascular damage of the placenta. The outcome of infection, whether fetal death and abortion, damage to developing organs, or persistent infection, is partly dependent on the timing of infection relative to placental and fetal development.[3]

Organisms may reach the fetus by ascending from the vagina and endocervix, even before rupture of the fetal membranes. Fetal infection and preterm labor are the likely outcomes. Invasive techniques widely used for *in utero* diagnosis are also potentially associated with fetal infection.[3]

Urinary tract infection

Asymptomatic bacteriuria complicates 5–8% of all pregnancies. The prevalence of asymptomatic bacteriuria in pregnancy is not significantly different from that in non-pregnant women but, without treatment, one third of pregnant women with bacteriuria will develop acute pyelonephritis.[4]

Host: physiological factors

Mechanical factors that obstruct the normal flow of urine are important in the pathogenesis of urinary infection.[5] In pregnancy, urinary obstruction leads to stasis and increases the likelihood that pyelonephritis will complicate asymptomatic bacteriuria.[6]

Mechanical compression from the enlarging uterus is the principal cause of hydroureter and hydronephrosis, but smooth-muscle relaxation induced by progesterone may also play a role.[7] Increased urine output secondary to an increase in glomerular filtration in pregnancy and loss of bladder tone, with incomplete bladder emptying, contribute further to the risk of infection.

Urine acidity and osmolality inhibit the growth of many bacterial organisms, but in pregnancy differences in urine pH and osmolality make the urine more suitable for bacterial growth.[5] Pregnancy-induced glucosuria and aminoaciduria may further facilitate bacterial proliferation.

Organism: virulence factors

Escherichia coli accounts for most urinary infections, with other Gram negative organisms, *Enterococcus faecalis* and group B streptococcus making up the rest.[6] These organisms colonize the vaginal introitus and periurethral area before infection occurs.[5] Uropathogenic bacteria possess specific virulence factors that enhance both colonization and invasion of the urinary tract[8] (Fig. 3.13.1). Certain strains of *E. coli* identified by their surface antigens O, K, or H are more likely to be associated with infection of the urinary tract and cause acute pyelonephritis.[9]

Strains of *E. coli* that cause pyelonephritis adhere better to uroepithelial cells than do strains causing lower tract disease. Bacterial adherence is mediated by surface adhesins known as pili or fimbriae. Most *E. coli* express type I pili which bind to receptors on the surface of cells. Because their attachment to uroepithelial cells is poor, these type I pili are not important virulence factors.[4] However, *E. coli* expressing adhesins referred to as P-fimbriae (because they also bind to the P blood group antigen on erythrocytes) adhere better. A preponderance of *E. coli* expressing P-fimbriae is found in pregnant women with acute pyelonephritis compared to *E. coli* isolated from women with asymptomatic bacteriuria.[10]

Outcome of infection

The association of urinary tract infection with premature delivery and low birth weight demonstrates how maternal infection can adversely affect the development of the fetus, even without direct fetal or placental involvement. Effective treatment of asymptomatic bacteriuria reduces these adverse outcomes.[11]

Very little is known about possible biological mechanisms of preterm labour in women with asymptomatic bacteriuria and how treatment leads to a reduction in preterm delivery.[12] Prevention of pyelonephritis may be part of the explanation. In addition, if asymptomatic bacteriuria is a marker of abnormal cervicovaginal colonization, the observed benefits of treatment may be due to the concurrent eradication, from the lower genital tract, of certain microorganisms associated with prematurity.[13]

Acute pyelonephritis and septic shock

Acute pyelonephritis complicates 1–2% of all pregnancies. With appropriate therapy, most women show rapid clinical improvement, but multisystem organ failure may develop.

The prime mediator of the septic response is endotoxin or lipopolysaccharide (LPS), a component of the outer cell membrane of the Gram-negative bacterium.[14] High levels of circulating endotoxin are associated with organ failure and mortality. The release of endotoxin initiates a cascade

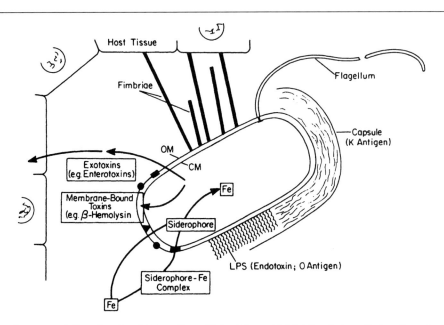

Fig. 3.13.1 *Schematic representation of an E. coli interacting with host tissue, highlighting features that are important in bacterial pathogenicity. Fimbriae (pili) promote adherence to mucosal surfaces; toxins, e.g. β-hemolysins, are cytotoxic and inhibit white cell function; lipopolysaccharide (LPS) mediates host responses to infection; the secretion of iron (Fe)-chelating compounds (siderophores) enhances iron uptake; and the polysaccharide capsule (the K antigen) reduces phagocytosis. OM, outer membrane; CM, cytoplasmic membrane (From reference 8 with permission).*

of inflammatory mediators, including tumor necrosis factor, leading to the physiological alterations seen in the shock syndrome (Fig. 3.13.2).

The spectrum of respiratory insufficiency seen in acute pyelonephritis during pregnancy ranges from transient dyspnea accompanied by pulmonary infiltrates to overt respiratory failure. Transient renal dysfunction and mild hemolysis often occur but are seldom of clinical importance.[4] The possibility of pregnancy-enhanced susceptibility to endotoxin has been suggested but, although demonstrated in animal models, the data are inconclusive in humans.

Listeriosis

The subtle changes in cell-mediated immunity recognized in pregnancy[15] results in decreased resistance to infection with intracellular organisms, such as *Listeria monocytogenes*. Maternal listeriosis is usually characterized by a mild illness that resembles influenza and may not be recognized until preterm labor ensues. When fever and chills predominate, pyelonephritis may be suspected.[16] Listeriosis should also be considered perinatally when a premature infant develops a septicemic illness with respiratory distress, or a full-term infant presents with meningitis.[17]

Listeria monocytogenes is a motile, Gram positive bacillus that is readily isolated in the laboratory. It can, however, be mistaken for a diphtheroid and regarded as a contaminant or confused with group B streptococci, especially if the colonies are β-hemolytic.

Pathogenesis of infection

L. monocytogenes is a facultative, intracellular pathogen that can persist in the cells of the monocyte–macrophage system. Listeriosis is an opportunistic infection in individuals with impaired cell-mediated immunity. A third of listerial infections are perinatal and the remainder are in elderly or immunosuppressed patients.

There are still limited data available on the pathogenesis of listeriosis in pregnancy. The organism appears to have a particular tropism for the gravid endometrium and placenta. Animal studies support the concept that the placenta represents an area of decreased immunocompetence, facilitating transplacental spread.[17] Most cases of listeriosis occur after the fifth month of pregnancy but spontaneous or repeated abortions may occur if infection is earlier. Most fetal infection occurs by transplacental spread following maternal bacteremia.

The gross and microscopic appearance of the placenta in listeriosis are distinctive.[18] Histologically, infection is characterized by the formation of miliary granuloma and focal necrosis or by suppuration in the affected tissues. In cases where perinatal listeriosis is considered, the placenta should always be cultured and examined microscopically. Gram positive rods are usually readily demonstrable within the necrotic centers of villous and decidual microabscesses, as well as within the membranes and umbilical cord.

The fundamental mechanism of the altered T-cell immunity in pregnancy has not been elucidated. Helper T cells, suppressor cells and macrophages are all important in the cell-mediated immune response to *Listeria* and other

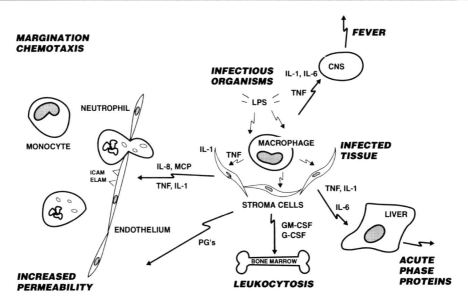

Fig 3.13.2 *Cell and cytokine interaction in the acute phase response to infection. Mediators released from endotoxin (LPS)-stimulated leukocytes interact with multiple tissues and organs to induce the acute phase response. LPS-stimulated mononuclear phagocytes release cytokines IL-1 and TNF and activate the local stromal cells in the infected tissue. The tissue-derived cytokines affect other systemic responses. IL-1, TNF and IL-6 affect the brain and induce fever and mediate the hepatic acute phase response. GM- and G-CSF induce leukocytosis. IL-1 and TNF activate endothelial cells and cause the expression of intracellular adhesion molecules (ICAM) and endothelial leukocyte adhesion molecules (ELAM), and IL-8 and MCP (monocyte chemoattractant protein) cause leukocyte margination and chemotaxis, while prostaglandins (PGs) mediate vascular permeability. CNS, central nervous system.*

intracellular organisms, such as viruses and *Mycobacterium tuberculosis*. Further studies are needed to define the specific immunological changes in pregnancy that increase the susceptibility to such a narrow range of pathogens.

Epidemiology

Listeria are ubiquitous in nature and can be isolated from a variety of sources. Transient gastrointestinal carriage of *Listeria* is common but invasive infection is rare. Pregnancy does not appear to increase the fecal carriage of *L. monocytogenes*. Although most listeriosis is sporadic, clearly defined food-borne outbreaks and clusters of perinatal cases have been reported.[19,20]

Chorioamnionitis and intra-amniotic infection

Preterm birth remains the leading cause of perinatal mortality. Although preterm birth is probably caused by multiple processes, the frequent histological evidence of chorioamnionitis and recovery of microorganisms from amniotic fluid suggest an important role for infection.[21,22] Microbial invasion of the amniotic cavity has been reported in 22% of women in preterm labor with intact membranes who subsequently deliver a preterm infant.[23] The incidence of amniotic fluid infection with preterm rupture of membranes may be as high as 40%.

Normal vaginal microbial flora

Intact fetal membranes provide a physical barrier to the passage of microorganisms. The barrier is not, however, impenetrable. Although infection can occur transplacentally, most intra-amniotic infection occurs by the ascending route when organisms colonizing the lower genital tract cross either intact or ruptured membranes. Some of the organisms present in the genital tract are clearly recognized as pathogens, for example *Neisseria gonorrhoeae*, *Chlamydia trachomatis* and *Trichomonas vaginalis*. More commonly, however, infection involves the indigenous cervicovaginal flora.

The normal vaginal flora consists predominantly of aerobic Gram positive rods and anaerobes, with a predominance of lactobacilli. The function of the normal cervicovaginal flora is complex and the relationship between each microorganism and the host, as well as among microorganisms, is incompletely understood.[24]

The normal flora play an important role in protecting the host from invasion by pathogenic bacteria.[25] The mechanisms by which the normal flora exerts their protective effect include competition for nutrients and space on epithelial attachment sites, the production of compounds toxic to pathogenic organisms, and continued stimulation of the immune system.[26] Although the mechanisms of hormonal control of the vaginal flora remain to be identified, there is no evidence that the protective function of the indigenous flora is altered adversely in pregnancy.[27]

Pathogenesis of preterm labor

There appear to be several mechanisms by which infection can activate preterm labor. Prostaglandins are important in the initiation and progression of labor.[28] Activation of mononuclear cells in response to bacterial infection and secretion of inflammatory mediators (including IL-1α, IL-6, macrophage colony stimulating factor, and tumor necrosis factor) lead to the release of prostaglandins from the decidua, provoking uterine contraction and cervical ripening. Bacterial products, such as lipopolysaccharides and lipoteichoic acid, activate decidual macrophages and, together with cytokines, can be detected in the amniotic fluid of women in preterm labor with intact membranes.

Direct destruction of the fetal membrane by bacterial and inflammatory cell mediators and activation of the prostaglandin pathway with indirect membrane weakening are potential factors in preterm premature rupture of the membranes.[29] Bacteria release proteases that break down the extracellular matrix that gives the membrane its strength. Enzymes released by activated neutrophils, such as collagenase and peroxidase, can further weaken the membrane.

Intrauterine infection is most often subclinical and chorioamnionitis is sometimes only confirmed if the placenta and its membranes are examined histologically (Fig. 3.13.3). The recognition that intrauterine infection precipitating preterm labor can be asymptomatic has led to attempts to improve the early diagnosis of infection. Gram stain and culture of intra-amniotic fluid is relatively insensitive. The measurement of cytokines, particularly IL6, has been shown to predict for microbial invasion in patients both with preterm premature rupture of the membranes[30] and preterm labor with intact membranes.[31]

Outcome of infection

Specific organisms, such as *Chlamydia trachomatis*, *Neisseria gonorrhoeae*, *Trichomonas vaginalis*, *Mycoplasma hominis*, *Ureaplasma urealyticum*, and group B streptococci have been implicated in preterm labor, preterm delivery and preterm rupture of membranes.[32] However, because of

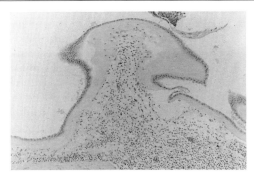

Fig. 3.13.3 *Section of amniotic membrane close to point of rupture with dense neutrophilic exudate; an example of non-specific chorioamnionitis.*

the difficulty in controlling for sociodemographic variables and multiple infections, the association of a specific infection with an adverse pregnancy outcome is sometimes controversial.

There is evidence, however, that certain of these microorganisms can be transmitted to the infant during delivery. Neonatal conjunctivitis is a consequence of maternal infection with *N. gonorrhoea* and *C. trachomatis*. Maternal colonization with group B streptococcus is a risk factor for neonatal group B streptococcal infection and treatment to eradicate maternal infection is associated with decreased neonatal infection.

There is evidence from randomized trials that antibiotic treatment of preterm labor with ruptured membranes improves maternal outcome but not neonatal outcome.[33,34] Studies have, however, failed to show a consistent effect of antibiotic treatment for preterm labor with intact membranes.[35]

Genital mycoplasmas

The genital mycoplasmas, *U. urealyticum* and *M. hominis*, are common inhabitants of the genitourinary tract. Carriage rates of *U. urealyticum* vary from 44% to 81%. Mycoplasmas have no cell wall and are, therefore, fastidious in their growth requirements and resistant to antibiotics that affect the cell wall, e.g. penicillin. The pathogenic potential of *M. hominis* is unclear. There is a significant association between chorioamnionitis and the isolation of *M. hominis*, but most amniotic fluids that are positive for *M. hominis* also contain more virulent bacteria. Endometritis with isolation of *M. hominis* from the bloodstream is recognized as a cause of post-partum fever.[36] *U. urealyticum* does not appear to be consistently associated with placental inflammation. There is an association between infection with *U. urealyticum* and preterm labor and low birth weight, but after adjustment for covariables the association no longer exists.[37] Additionally, erythromycin treatment of maternal infection does not influence neonatal outcomes.[38]

Bacterial vaginosis

Cervicovaginal colonization is a dynamic process. The organisms exist in equilibrium until, by mechanisms that are not clear, the balance is disturbed and disease occurs.

In bacterial vaginosis, a common vaginal infection in women of reproductive age, there is an alteration in the normal flora characterized by replacement of lactobacilli by anaerobes and *Gardnerella vaginalis*.[39] The diagnosis is confirmed if the pH of the vaginal discharge is greater than 4.5 and clue cells (vaginal epithelial cells whose cell border is obscured by bacteria) are seen on wet mount.[40] After correcting for other variables, a relationship between bacterial vaginosis, chorioamnionitis, preterm labour and delivery has been established.[41,42] About half of patients have either no or mild symptoms. If a causal relationship between bacterial vaginosis and prematurity is eventually proven, pregnant women may need to be screened for this infection.[43]

Group B streptococcal infections

Group B streptococci (GBS) constitute part of the normal vaginal flora, colonizing the lower genital tract of up to 30% of women. The rate of vertical transmission from a colonized mother to her infant during labor and delivery is approximately 50%.[44] Reported rates for neonatal disease range from 2 to 3/1000 live births, with considerable geographic variation.[45] The risk of early-onset streptococcal disease is increased in premature and low birth weight babies, and in those pregnancies complicated by prolonged rupture of membranes, prolonged labor, maternal fever or chorioamnionitis. *In utero* infection, through grossly or microscopically compromised membranes, probably explains why half of early-onset infection is clinically apparent at the time of birth.

Late-onset infection, defined as invasive disease occurring after the sixth day of life, occurs more often in a term infant following an uncomplicated pregnancy. The epidemiology and pathogenesis of late-onset disease is much less well-defined than that of early onset infection. Some infection may be nosocomially transmitted. Alternatively, a prior viral upper respiratory tract infection, by altering epithelial cell surfaces, may allow a colonizing strain of GBS to invade the bloodstream.[44]

Pathogenesis

Only a very small percentage of infants exposed to GBS at the time of delivery will develop clinical infection, and the host and bacterial factors that allow for the development of disease have not been fully elucidated. Effective clearance of GBS depends on the presence of type specific antibody, functioning polymorphonuclear leukocytes, and an intact immune system, all of which are deficient to varying degrees in the newborn infant.[46]

The polysaccharide capsule of the organism is an important virulence factor. Phagocytosis of bacteria by macrophages or polymorphs is facilitated by antibody, complement and other serum components, collectively known as opsonins, on the surface of the microorganism.[2] The capsular polysaccharide prevents the effective opsonization of bacteria by preventing the deposition of complement components on the bacterial surface.

Different serotypes of GBS are recognized by the antigenic structure of their polysaccharide capsule. Increased virulence correlates with increased expression of type III capsule.[47] Overall, serotype III strains are associated with about two thirds of invasive group B streptococcal disease, and most infections where there is meningitis. Among neonates with early onset disease, however, there is a more even distribution of the various serotypes and in only a third is infection attributed to serotype III.

When the concentration of antibody to type III polysaccharide antigen is low, there is a higher likelihood that perinatal infection will occur.[48] In the latter half of pregnancy, IgG antibody readily crosses the placenta. About two thirds of pregnant women have been shown to respond to a vaccine made from the type III capsular polysaccharide and protective levels of antibody can be detected in the infants.[49] If attempts to improve the immunogenicity of the vaccine and include other serotypes are successful, widespread implementation of an active immunization program may reduce the mortality and morbidity from group B streptococcal disease.

Current strategies for preventing infection

Because the most obvious determinant of risk for neonatal infection is maternal colonization, eliminating or interrupting maternal carriage of GBS will minimize exposure of the infant.

Attempting to eradicate asymptomatic mucosal infection with GBS antenatally is unsuccessful. The effect of antibiotics is transient and, by the time of delivery, nearly 70% of women are again culture positive.[50] The lower gastrointestinal tract may be the reservoir for GBS. Intrapartum administration of antibiotics to the mother is, however, effective and will block vertical transmission of GBS.[51] The widespread use of antibiotics is not without potential consequences. Apart from allergic reactions and the development of antibiotic-associated colitis, resistant organisms associated with adverse perinatal outcomes can arise.[52]

The publication of guidelines on the management of GBS disease in pregancy[53,54] has only intensified the controversies as to the optimal method of detecting women who are carriers, and to whom chemoprophylaxis should be given. While the risk of neonatal disease is increased in 'at-risk' pregnancies, 70% of early onset group B streptococcal disease occurs in term infants, many of whom have no identifiable risk factors.[55] The intermittent nature of maternal colonization has been emphasized,[56] raising questions about the value of culture early in pregnancy. Unfortunately, the sensitivity of rapid antigen tests to detect maternal colonization during labor continues to be disappointing.[57]

Carefully performed cost-effective analyses[58–60] have not resolved the issue and, until methods to identify 'at risk' pregnancies improve, or an effective vaccine becomes widely available, the controversy will continue.

Viral infections during pregnancy

Several viruses play a major role in perinatal infections. Fetal infection can occur through the placenta, or the infant may be directly exposed at the time of delivery if virus is shed from the mother's genital tract.

Viruses are obligate intracellular parasites that require host cells for replication. Their structure, classification, and biology have been summarized recently by Tyler and Field.[61] Virus particles (virions) contain a core of either DNA or RNA, surrounded by a protein shell of viral capsid proteins. Many viruses, e.g. herpesviruses, also possess a lipid envelope acquired from the host cell, into which are incorporated virally encoded proteins (Fig. 3.13.4).

The first stage of viral infection of target cells begins with attachment of viral proteins to receptors on the cell surface. Following penetration through the plasma membrane of the cell, the viral capsid is removed, making the viral genome accessible to the transcription and translation machinery of the host cell. Double-stranded DNA viruses synthesize viral messenger RNA using host DNA-dependent RNA polymerases. RNA-containing viruses have evolved a number of strategies for the production of

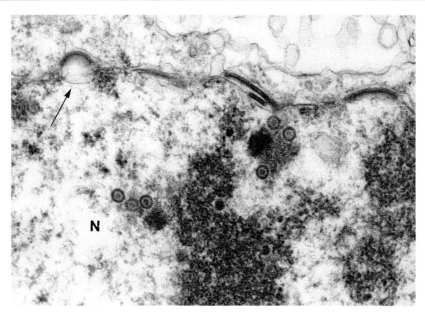

Fig. 3.13.4 *Brain tissue from an infant with herpes simplex encephalitis showing several HSV nucleocapsids within the nucleus (N). A nucleocapsid in the process of budding through the nuclear membrane is seen (arrow). Magnification ×60 000.*

mRNA, that include synthesizing their own transcriptase enzymes and packaging them within the virion. Viral mRNA is translated into virus proteins on cellular ribosomes, assembled with viral genetic material into intact virions and released either when the cell lyses or by budding off from the plasma membrane. While the cell-mediated immune response and cytokines are ordinarily the most important defense mechanisms against viral infections, these factors also contribute to the pathogenesis of viral diseases. When the complex interactions between a virus and host cell are understood better and the process by which viruses cause disease determined at the molecular level, new strategies for preventing and treating viral diseases can be anticipated.

Rubella

Infection with rubella during pregnancy illustrates how a trival maternal infection can have a devastating effect on the fetus.[62] The consequences of maternal rubella infection are directly related to the gestational age of the fetus. Fetal damage is more severe and frequent during the first eight weeks of gestation although why 40% of infants at risk of exposure to the virus during the first trimester remain uninfected is not clear.[63] The factors that influence the effect of gestation on the outcome of infection are unknown. Possibly immature cells are more easily infected and support the growth of virus better.[64] Alternatively, the placenta may become increasingly resistant to infection as it matures, or the development of fetal immunity may help clear the virus.

The release of a mitotic inhibitor from infected cells that inhibits fetal cell growth is the likely explanation for the intrauterine growth retardation and organ malformations that are associated with the congenital rubella syndrome. Infection persists throughout fetal life and sometimes for a year or longer after birth, suggesting a defective immune response to rubella virus.

Maternal immunity to rubella, induced by immunization or natural infection, protects against intrauterine infection although there are rare reports of intrauterine transmission of virus associated with maternal reinfection. Immunity is considered present if the rubella-specific IgG antibody level is >1:8 measured by the hemagglutination inhibition assay.[65] There is, however, no internationally agreed standard level of protective antibody and it remains uncertain whether the minute amounts of antibody detected by some of the new highly sensitive assays are protective. The diagnosis of acute infection in pregnancy is confirmed by the detection of specific IgM antibody, or evidence of a significant antibody rise between acute and convalescent sera.[66] Congenital infection can also be diagnosed by viral culture, with the virus being most readily isolated from nasopharyngeal secretions.[67]

Cytomegalovirus

Cytomegalovirus (CMV) shares with other herpes viruses the properties of latency and reactivation despite the presence of humoral and cell-mediated immunity. Both primary maternal infection and reactivation of latent CMV have been associated with congenital infection, but primary infection is associated with more frequent and more severe neonatal disease.[68]

Intrauterine infection probably occurs after maternal viremia with placental infection and hematogenous dissemination to the fetus. The factors explaining why some infants are severely affected and others remain free of symptoms, and why intrauterine transmisssion occurs in only 30–40% of pregnant women following primary infection, are unknown. Gestational age does not appear to influence the transmission of CMV *in utero*, although symptomatic disease at birth is more often associated with infection early in gestation. Congenital infection that results from reactivation is usually subclinical, suggesting that although antibody may not protect against transmission, tissue damage is minimized. Perinatal infection in a healthy term infant, following exposure to the virus in the maternal genital tract at the time of delivery, is usually asymptomatic and without adverse outcome.

Transmission of CMV occurs through respiratory secretions, infected urine and sexual contact. Seronegative workers in day-care centers[69] or mothers in contact with children excreting CMV are potentially at increased risk of acquiring a primary CMV infection. Overall, however, sexual transmission probably contributes most to the incidence of congenital infection.[70]

While primary CMV infection can be associated with a mononucleosis-like syndrome, most CMV infection is asymptomatic and, unless serial antibody levels are obtained, primary infection goes undiagnosed. Detectable IgM antibody during pregnancy more often reflects reactivation of CMV rather than primary infection and alone cannot be used to make a diagnosis.[71] Prenatal diagnosis of CMV using molecular techniques to detect viral DNA within amniotic fluid has been successful.[72] Without specific therapeutic options, however, routine screening for primary maternal infection or fetal infection during pregnancy is not recommended.[73]

Parvovirus B-19

Human parvovirus B-19 is a single-stranded DNA virus, transmitted through respiratory secretions, and associated with erythema infectiosum or 'fifth disease' in childhood. The virus has a predelicction for erythroid progenitor cells, inhibiting red cell production, which in the fetus can cause severe anemia and congestive cardiac failure, ultimately resulting in hydrops[74] (Fig. 13.3.5). No congenital anomalies or adverse long-term sequelae are known to be associated with fetal infection.[73]

Most women have been exposed to, and are immune to, parvovirus B-19. If infection does occur in pregnancy, fetal loss is uncommon. In women of unknown serologic status, the risk is estimated at 1.5 and 2.5% following school and household exposure respectively.[75] Although diagnostic tests are not routinely available, maternal infection can be confirmed by detecting specific IgM antibody. Where fetal infection is suspected, fetal blood sampling will both quantitate the degree of anemia and confirm infection. The

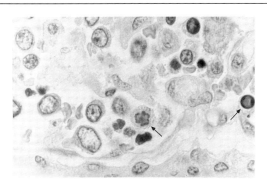

Fig. 3.13.5 *Intranuclear inclusions in immature red cells in chorionic villous capillaries in parvovirus infection. Two 'ground glass' inclusions are arrowed, one of which appears to be disintegrating (left arrow).*

technique of polymerase chain reaction has been successfully used to detect viral DNA in fetal samples.[76]

Varicella zoster

Adults who develop chicken pox have a greater risk of severe disease, particularly pneumonia, when compared to children and in pregnancy the mortality from varicella pneumonia is probably increased.[77,78] Transplacental transmission of varicella can result in the congenital varicella syndrome,[79] with an estimated incidence at about 2% following maternal varicella in the first 20 weeks of pregnancy.[80]

Varicella zoster virus (VZV) is a member of the herpesvirus group. The virus is usually transmitted by the respiratory route and less commonly directly from vesicular fluid. VZV is neurotropic and, after primary infection, becomes latent in the dorsal root ganglia. Zoster or shingles, with lesions that follow the dermatomal distribution of the dorsal root nerve, follows the reactivation of latent infection.

Immunity to VZV is generally lifelong. The passive administration of antibody can protect against primary VZV infection and it is recommended that varicella immune globulin be given to susceptible pregnant women who are exposed to chicken pox.[81]

Herpes simplex

Although fetal infection with herpes simplex virus (HSV) may occur through *in utero* transplacental infection, most neonatal HSV disease is acquired at the time of delivery.[82] Intrapartum transmission of HSV most commonly follows primary maternal genital herpes infection. Most women shedding HSV during labor and most mothers of infants with neonatal herpes, however, do not give a history of symptomatic genital herpes. Unfortunately, the serological assays that are routinely available fail to identify women at risk and none of the currently licensed rapid tests are sensitive enough to be useful for the detection of viral shedding during labor.[83]

HSV is a neurotropic virus that remains latent within neural ganglia. Up to 4% of women with a history of recur-

rent genital herpes infection will shed the virus intermittently during pregnancy, in the absence of clinical lesions. Recurrent HSV infection is, however, rarely associated with neonatal disease, probably because of the protective effect of specific maternal antibody. The management of pregnancies complicated by genital herpes infections has been reviewed recently by Prober *et al.*[83]

Syphilis

The causative agent of syphilis is the spirochete *Treponema pallidum*. Diagnosis of syphilis depends on a positive non-specific antibody test (VDRL or RPR) with a confirmatory specific treponemal test (FTA-Abs or MHA-TP). The specific treponemal antibody tests do not differentiate between active disease and past infection but the non-specific tests are helpful in following the therapeutic response to treatment.

Hematogenous spread of the organism to the fetus may occur at any stage of maternal disease although is more likely during primary or secondary infection than in latent or tertiary infection when, with suppression of infection by a competent immune system, maternal spirochetemia is less.[84] Pregnancy *per se* has little if any effect on the natural course of the disease.

The organism can be transmitted to the fetus at any stage of gestation, including the first trimester, although, because it is generally not until 16 weeks that the fetus can mount an immune response, clinical manifestations are usually not apparent until this time.

The characteristic pathologic changes of syphilis, whether with congenital or acquired infection, are those of a perivascular infiltration of lymphocytes, plasma cells and histiocytes with obliterative endarteritis and extensive fibrosis.[85] The infected placenta is paler, thicker and larger than normal. The spirochete can sometimes be visualized in tissue with a silver stain.

Toxoplasmosis

Toxoplasma gondii is an intracellular protozoan parasite that infects humans and other warm-blooded animals. Differences in the epidemiology of infection in various geographic locales can be explained by differences in exposure to the two main sources of infection, ingestion of the tissue cyst in raw meat or ingestion of the oocyst excreted by cats.[86] Acute maternal infection is usually asymptomatic and parasitemia goes unrecognized. Without an efficient screening programme, establishing a diagnosis of primary infection during pregnancy is difficult. If a sensitive test is available, the presence of IgM antibody usually indicates acute infection, although levels can remain elevated for several months to years following primary infection. Fetal infection can only be confirmed by the recovery of the parasite from fetal blood or amniotic tissue (Fig. 3.13.6). Maternal treatment aims to prevent or reduce congenital infection.[87]

If acute toxoplasmosis is acquired later in the pregnancy, there is a greater possibility that the parasite will infect the

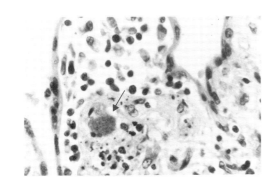

Fig. 3.13.6 *Toxoplasma pseudocyst (arrow) and inflammatory cells in chorionic villous.*

placenta and spread to the fetus than if infection occurs during the first trimester. Neonatal disease can range from obvious systemic involvement to subclinical infection. In the first trimester, although infection is rare, fetal damage is severe. If acute toxoplasmosis occurs in the third trimester, however, infection is usually asymptomatic.

Following primary infection, the organism remains latent in tissues. Whereas reactivation of toxoplasmosis is recognized in severely immunocompromised hosts, e.g. with HIV infection, latent infection in pregnancy is virtually never associated with transmission to the fetus, although exceptions have been reported.[88] A pregnant woman can be reassured that there is no fetal risk if, prior to conception, she has specific IgG antibody.

Malaria

In many developing countries, malaria remains an important health problem. Because of the maternal and fetal consequences of malaria during pregnancy, pregnant women have been identified as a specific target group for malaria control activities by the World Health Organization.

Malaria is a protozoan infection, spread to humans by anopheline mosquitoes.[89] After the bite of the mosquito, sporozoites are injected into the bloodstream. The parasite develops within the hepatocyte to form a schizont which, after a variable period, ruptures to release thousands of merozoites that invade erythrocytes. Within the red cell the ring-form trophozoite matures and, after a period of growth, becomes a schizont when nuclear division occurs. Cyclical fever and chills occur with rupture of the mature schizont and release of inflammatory cytokines. The four species of malaria, of which *Plasmodium falciparum* and *P. vivax* are the most common, can be differentiated by their morphological appearances in a peripheral blood smear.

The immune response to malaria is complex and incompletely understood. In individuals living in areas endemic for malaria, antibodies that block invasion of erythrocytes usually do not appear despite persistent malaria infection.[90] Although clinically immune, these individuals often remain parasitemic which has consequences for the developing fetus. Non-immune individuals are susceptible to

more severe disease. Malaria in a non-immune woman during pregnancy can be complicated by rapid hemolysis, severe anemia, hypoglycemia, high fever and preterm labor. Maternal mortality and fetal losses can be high.[91]

In pregnancy, both the density and prevalence of parasitemia are increased compared with women who are not pregnant.[92] Parasitemia, however, decreases with increasing parity. There is good evidence that maternal parasitemia is associated with low birth weight and adverse infant outcomes and that the degree of placental parasitization correlates with the reduction in birthweight. Anemia and poor nutrition are probably important co-factors. Controlled trials have shown that maternal chemoprophylaxis can improve both maternal outcomes and birth weight.[93]

During normal pregnancy, the immune system is regulated to ensure the fetus is not rejected as a foreign allograft. As a consequence, intraerythrocytic parasites may freely multiply in the placental villous spaces and extraordinarily high levels of parasitemia may be observed.[94] The heavy infiltration of parasites, lymphocytes and macrophages interferes with the circulation of maternal blood through the placenta and likely results in diminished transport of oxygen and nutrients to the fetus. Histologically, the intervillous spaces of infected placentae are packed with lymphoid macrophages which contain phagocytosed pigment in large granules, lymphocytes and immature polymorphonuclear leukocytes.[95] Numerous young and mature schizonts are common.

Despite massive involvement of the placenta, congenital infections are rare. The placenta is a relatively effective barrier and parasites infrequently reach the fetus. Congenital malaria should be suspected in infants born to mothers who have moved from an area endemic for malaria.[96] Congenital malaria is uncommon in infants if maternal immunity is maintained due to frequent exposure. It is probable that passively transferred maternal antibody is important in determining whether parasites that reach the fetal circulation establish infection. The relative importance of transplacental infection or intrapartum transmission during labor as mechanisms by which the infant acquires malaria remain uncertain.

FUTURE PERSPECTIVES

The approach to the management of infections during pregnancy has not changed significantly in the last decade. Advances in care await a better understanding of the dynamic relationships among mother, fetus and infecting organism that are unique to pregnancy.

The role of infection in preterm birth must be clarified and strategies implemented to prevent, diagnose and treat chorioamnionitis effectively. The nature of the subtle immune changes that occur in pregnancy must be defined better. We need to know what factors determine whether fetal infection will occur following maternal infection. We need to improve our ability to diagnose fetal infection early when intervention is possible and, for many infections, we need to develop better therapies.

SUMMARY

- Fetal death, developmental anomalies, congenital infection, preterm delivery or neonatal sepsis can occur as a consequence of maternal infection during pregnancy.
- The outcome of fetal infection is, in part, dependent on the timing of infection relative to placental and fetal development. However, the factors that influence the effect of gestation are not fully understood and, in many instances, the reasons why some infants are infected and others escape infection are unknown.
- The increased risk of pyelonephritis in pregnant women with asymptomatic bacteriuria clearly illustrates the importance of non-specific host defences in the prevention of infection. Physiological changes occurring in the urinary tract during pregnancy prevent the normal flow of urine.
- Some pathogenic microorganisms exhibit specific virulence factors that enhance their ability to colonize and invade (e.g. some strains of *E. coli*) or increase their resistance to phagocytosis (e.g. certain serotypes of group B streptococci).
- The subtle changes in cell-mediated immunity that occur in pregnancy result in an increased risk of infection with intracellular organisms, such as *Listeria*, and more severe viral infections, e.g. varicella.

- Organisms, including those of the normal vaginal flora, may reach the fetus by ascending from the vagina and endocervix, even before rupture of the membranes, to cause infection and preterm labor.
- Infection may activate preterm labor by several possible mechanisms, including activation of mononuclear cells with secretion of inflammatory mediators leading to release of prostaglandins and stimulation of uterine contractions.
- Maternal immunity, whether acquired following natural infection or immunization, is effective in preventing certain fetal infections (e.g. rubella) and, with the passive transfer of maternal antibody across the placenta, may reduce some neonatal infections (e.g. group B streptococcal disease).
- There are some organisms that can persist in the mother in a latent stage, even after the development of an immune response, e.g. syphilis, CMV, and infect the fetus long after the initial maternal infection.
- Many maternal infections associated with fetal infection are asymptomatic, not recognized clinically and difficult to diagnose and treat. Effective management of these infections awaits a better understanding of their pathogenesis.

REFERENCES

1. Klein JO, Remington JS. Current concepts of infections of the fetus and newborn infant. In: Remington JS and Klein JO (eds) *Infectious Diseases of the Fetus and Newborn Infant*, 4th edn, Philadelphia: WB Saunders, 1995: pp 1–19.
2. Mims CA *The Pathogenesis of Infectious Disease*, 3rd edn, London: Academic Press, 1987: 342 pp.
3. MacLean AB. Infection and the antenatal patient. In MacLean AB (ed) *Clinical Infection in Obstetrics and Gynaecology*. Oxford: Blackwell Scientific Publications, 1990: pp 21–38.
4. Cox SM, Cunningham FG. Urinary tract infections. In Charles D (ed) *Obstetric and Perinatal Infections*. St Louis: Mosby – Year Book, 1993: pp 225–234.
5. Sobel JD, Kaye D. Urinary tract infections. In Mandell GL, Bennett JE, Dolin R (eds) *Mandell, Douglas and Bennett's Principles and Practice of Infectious Diseases*, 4th edn. New York: Churchill Livingstone, 1995: pp 662–690.
6. Lucas MJ, Cunningham FG. Urinary infection in pregnancy. *Clin Obstet Gynecol* 1993 **36**: 855–868.
7. Dafnis E, Sabatini S. The effect of pregnancy on renal function: physiology and pathophysiology. *Am J Med Sci* 1992 **303**: 184–205.
8. Eisenstein BI, Jones GW. The spectrum of infectious and pathogenic mechanisms of *Escherichia coli*. *Adv Intern Med* 1988 **33**: 231–252.

9. Mittendorf R, Williams MA, Kass EH. Prevention of preterm delivery and low birth weight associated with asymptomatic bacteriuria. *Clin Infect Dis* 1992 **14**: 927–932.
10. Stenqvist K, Sandberg T, Lidin-Janson G, Ørskov F, Ørskov I, Svanborg-Edén C. Virulence factors of *Escherichia coli* in urinary isolates from pregnant women. *J Infect Dis* 1987 **156**: 870–877.
11. Smaill F. Antibiotic vs no treatment for asymptomatic bacteriuria. In Enkin MW, Keirse MJNC, Renfrew MJ, Neilson JP (eds) Pregnancy and Childbirth module, *Cochrane Database of Systematic Reviews*. Review No. 03170, 22 April 1993. Published through 'Cochrane Updates on Disk', Oxford: Update Software, 1995, Disk issue 2.
12. Romero R, Oyarzun E, Mazor M, Sirtori M, Hobbins JC, Bracken M. Meta-analysis of the relationship between asymptomatic bacteriuria and pre-term delivery/low birth weight. *Obstet Gynecol* 1989 **73**: 576–582.
13. Thomsen AC, Mørup L, Brogaard Hansen K. Antibiotic elimination of group-B streptococci in urine in prevention of preterm labour. *Lancet* 1987 **i**: 591–593.
14. Fein AM, Duvivier R. Sepsis in pregnancy. *Clin Chest Med* 1992 **13**: 709–722.
15. Weinberg ED. Pregnancy-associated depression of cell-mediated immunity. *Rev Infect Dis* 1984 **6**: 814–831.
16. Charles D. Listeriosis. In Charles D (ed) *Obstetric and Perinatal Infections*. St Louis: Mosby – Year Book, 1993: pp 193–209.

17. Bortolussi R, Schlech WF. Listeriosis. In Remington JS and Klein JO (eds) *Infectious Diseases of the Fetus and Newborn Infant*, 4th edn. Philadelphia: WB Saunders, 1995: pp 1055–1073.
18. Topalovski M, Yong SS, Boompasat Y. Listeriosis of the placenta: clinicopathologic study of seven cases. *Am J Obstet Gynecol* 1993 **169**: 616–620.
19. Schlech WF, Lavigne PM, Bortolussi RA *et al.* Epidemic listeriosis – evidence for transmission by food. *N Engl J Med* 1983 **308**: 203–206.
20. Linnan MJ, Mascola L, Lou XD *et al.* Epidemic listeriosis associated with Mexican-style cheese. *N Engl J Med* 1988 **319**: 823–828.
21. Hillier SL, Martius J, Krohn M, Kiviat N, Holmes KK, Eschenbach DA. A case-control study of chorioamnionic infection and histological chorioamnionitis in prematurity. *N Engl J Med* 1988 **319**: 972–978.
22. Romero R, Mazor M. Infection and preterm labour. *Clin Obstet Gynecol* 1988 **31**: 553–584.
23. Romero R, Sirtori M, Oyarzun E, *et al.* Infection and labor. V. Prevalence, microbiology, and clinical significance of intraamniotic infection in women with preterm labor and intact membranes. *Am J Obstet Gynecol* 1989 **161**: 817–824.
24. Larsen B. Microbiology of the female genital tract. In Pastorek JG (ed) *Obstetric and Gynecologic Infectious Disease*. New York: Raven Press, 1994: pp 11–25.
25. Mackowiak PA. The normal microbial flora. *N Engl J Med* 1982 **307**: 83–93.
26. Tramont EC, Hoover DL. General or nonspecific host defense mechanisms. In Mandell GL, Bennett JE, Dolin R (eds). *Mandell, Douglas and Bennett's Principles and Practice of Infectious Diseases*, 4th edn. New York: Churchill Livingstone, 1995: pp 30–35.
27. Larsen B, Galask RP. Vaginal microbial flora: practical and theoretic relevance. *Obstet Gynecol* 1980 **55**: 100S–113S.
28. Mitchell MD, Trautman MS, Dudley DJ. Immunoendocrinology of preterm labour and delivery. *Baillières Clin Obstet Gynaecol* 1993 7: 553–575.
29. Maxwell GL. Preterm premature rupture of membranes. *Obstet Gynecol Surv* 1993 **48**: 576–583.
30. Romero R, Yoon BH, Mazor M *et al.* A comparative study of the diagnostic performance of amniotic fluid glucose, white blood cell count, interleukin-6, and gram stain in the detection of microbial invasion in patients with preterm premature rupture of membranes. *Am J Obstet Gynecol* 1993 **169**: 839–851.
31. Romero R, Yoon BH, Mazor M *et al.* The diagnostic and prognostic value of amniotic fluid white blood cell count, glucose, interleukin-6, and gram stain in patients with preterm labor and intact membranes. *Am J Obstet Gynecol* 1993 **169**: 805–816.
32. Carey JC, Yaffe SJ, Catz C. The vaginal infections and prematurity study: an overview. *Clin Obstet Gynecol* 1993 **36**: 809–820.
33. Owen J, Groome LJ, Hauth JC. Randomized trial of prophylactic antibiotic therapy after preterm amnion rupture. *Am J Obstet Gynecol* 1993 **169**: 976–981.
34. Kirschbaum T. Antibiotics in the treatment of preterm labor. *Am J Obstet Gynecol* 1993 **168**: 1239–1246.
35. Romero R, Sibar B, Caritis S *et al.* Antibiotic treatment of preterm labor with intact membranes: a multicenter, randomized, double-blinded, placebo-controlled trial. *Am J Obstet Gynecol* 1993 **169**: 764–774.
36. Cummings MC, McCormack WM. Genital mycoplasmas. In Charles D (ed) *Obstetric and Perinatal Infections*. St Louis: Mosby – Year Book, 1993: pp 188–192.
37. Carey JC, Blackwelder WC, Nugent RP *et al.* Antepartum cultures for *Ureaplasma urealyticum* are not useful in predicting pregnancy outcome. *Am J Obstet Gynecol* 1991 **164**: 728–733.
38. Eschenbach DA, Nugent RP, Rao AV *et al.* A randomized, placebo-controlled trial of erythromycin for the treatment of *Ureaplasma urealyticum* to prevent premature delivery. *Am J Obstet Gynecol* 1991 **164**: 734–742.
39. Eschenbach DA. Bacterial vaginosis and anaerobes in obstetric-gynecologic infection. *Clin Infect Dis* 1993 **16**: S282–S287.
40. Eschenbach DA, Hillier S, Critchlow C, Stevens C, DeRouen T, Holmes KK. Diagnosis and clinical manifestations of bacterial vaginosis. *Am J Obstet Gynecol* 1988 **158**: 819–828.
41. McGregor JA, French JI, Seo K. Premature rupture of membranes and bacterial vaginosis. *Am J Obstet Gynecol* 1993 **169**: 463–466.
42. Gibbs RS. Chorioamnionitis and bacterial vaginosis. *Am J Obstet Gynecol* 1993 **169**: 460–462.
43. Eschenbach DA. Vaginitis during pregnancy: consequences and treatment. In Charles D (ed) *Obstetric and Perinatal Infections*. St Louis: Mosby – Year Book, 1993: pp 51–59.
44. Baker CJ, Edwards MS. Group B streptococcal infections. In Remington JS and Klein JO (eds) *Infectious Diseases of the Fetus and Newborn Infant*, 4th edn. Philadelphia: WB Saunders, 1995: pp 980–1054.
45. Van Oppen C, Feldman R. Antibiotic prophylaxis of neonatal group B streptococcal infections. *Br Med J* 1993 **306**: 411–412.
46. Lewis DB, Wilson CB. Developmental immunology and role of host defenses in neonatal susceptibility to infection. In Remington JS and Klein JO (eds) *Infectious Diseases of the Fetus and Newborn Infant*, 4th edn Philadelphia: WB Saunders, 1995: pp 20–98.
47. Madoff LC, Kasper DL. Group B streptococcal disease. In Charles D (ed) *Obstetric and Perinatal Infections*. St Louis: Mosby – Year Book, 1993: pp 210–224.
48. Baker CJ, Kasper DL. Correlation of maternal antibody deficiency with susceptibility to neonatal group B streptococcal infection. *N Engl J Med* 1976 **294**: 753–756.
49. Baker CJ, Rench MA, Edwards MS, Carpenter RJ, Hays BM, Kasper DL. Immunization of pregnant women with a polysaccharide vaccine of group B streptococcus. *N Engl J Med* 1988 **319**: 1180–1185.
50. Gardner SE, Yow MD, Leeds LJ, Thompson PK, Mason EO, Clark DJ. Failure of penicillin to eradicate group B streptococcal colonization in the pregnant woman. *Am J Obstet Gynecol* 1979 **135**: 1062–1065.
51. Allen UD, Navas L, King SM. Effectiveness of intrapartum penicillin prophylaxis in preventing early-onset group B streptococcal infection: results of a meta-analysis. *Can Med Assoc J* 1993 **149**: 1659–1665.
52. McDuffie RS, McGregor JA, Gibbs RS. Adverse perinatal outcome and resistant Enterobacteriaceae after antibiotic usage for premature rupture of the membranes and group B streptococcus carriage. *Obstet Gynecol* 1993 **82**: 487–489.
53. American College of Obstetricians and Gynecologists. Group B streptococcal infections in pregnancy. ACOG Technical Bulletin Number 170 – July 1992. *Int J Gynecol Obstet* 1993 **42**: 55–59.
54. Committee on Infectious Diseases and Committee on Fetus and Newborn. Guidelines for prevention of group B streptococcal (GBS) infection by chemoprophylaxis. *Pediatrics* 1992 **90**: 775–778.
55. Schuchat A, Oxtoby M, Cochi S *et al.* Population-based risk factors for neonatal group B streptococcal disease: results of a cohort study in metropolitan Atlanta. *J Infect Dis* 1990 **162**: 672–677.
56. Boyer KM, Gotoff SP. Strategies for chemoprophylaxis of GBS early-onset infections. *Antibiot Chemother* 1985 **35**: 267–280.
57. Green M, Dashefsky B, Wald ER, Laifer S, Harger J, Guthrie R. Comparison of two antigen assays for rapid intrapartum detection of vaginal group B streptococcal colonization. *J Clin Micro* 1983 **31**: 78–82.
58. Strickland DM, Yeomans ER, Hankins GDV. Cost-effectiveness of intrapartum screening and treatment for mater-

nal group B streptococci colonization. *Am J Obstet Gynecol* 1990 **163**: 4–8.

59. Mohle-Boetani JC, Schuchat A, Plikaytis BD, Smith D, Broomes CV. Comparison of prevention strategies for neonatal group B streptococcal infection. A population-based economic analysis. *JAMA* 1993 **270**: 1442–1448.

60. Yancey MK, Duff P. An analysis of the cost-effectiveness of selected protocols for the prevention of neonatal group B streptococcal infection. *Obstet Gynecol* 1994 **83**: 367–371.

61. Tyler KL, Field BN. Introduction to viruses and viral diseases. In Mandell GL, Bennett JE, Dolin R (eds) *Mandell, Douglas and Bennett's Principles and Practice of Infectious Diseases*, 4th edn. New York: Churchill Livingstone, 1995: pp 1314–1325.

62. Freij BJ, South MA, Sever JL. Maternal rubella and the congenital rubella syndrome. *Clin Perinat* 1988 **15**: 247–257.

63. Miller E, Cradock-Watson JE, Pollock TM. Consequences of confirmed maternal rubella at successive stages of pregnancy. *Lancet* 1982 **ii**: 781–784.

64. Cooper LZ, Preblud SR, Alford CA. Rubella. In Remington JS and Klein JO (eds) *Infectious Diseases of the Fetus and Newborn Infant*, 4th edn. Philadelphia: WB Saunders, 1995: pp 268–311.

65. Gabert HA, von Almen W. Rubella. In Pastorek JG (ed) *Obstetric and Gynecologic Infectious Disease*. New York: Raven Press, 1994: pp 353–361.

66. American College of Obstetricians and Gynecologists. Rubella and Pregnancy. ACOG Technical Bulletin Number 171 – August 1992. *Int J Gynecol Obstet* 1993 **42**: 60–66.

67. Dascal A, Libman MD, Mendelson J, Cukor G. Laboratory tests for the diagnosis of viral diseases in pregnancy. *Clin Obstet Gynecol* 1990 **33**: 218–231.

68. Stagno S, Pass RF, Dworsky ME *et al.* Congenital cytomegalovirus infection. The relative importance of primary and recurrent maternal infection. *N Engl J Med* 1982 **306**: 945–949.

69. Adler SP. Cytomegalovirus and child day care. Evidence for an increased infection rate among day-care workers. *N Engl J Med* 1989 **321**: 1290–1296.

70. Fowler KB, Pass RF. Sexually transmitted diseases in mothers of neonates with congenital cytomegalovirus infection. *J Infect Dis* 1991 **164**: 259–264.

71. Cederqvist LL. Cytomegalovirus infection. In Pastorek JG (ed) *Obstetric and Gynecologic Infectious Disease*. New York: Raven Press, 1994: pp 363–369.

72. Donner C, Liesnard C, Content J, Busine A, Aderca J, Rodesch F. Prenatal diagnosis of 52 pregnancies at risk for congenital cytomegalovirus infection. *Obstet Gynecol* 1993 **82**: 481–486.

73. Sison AV, Sever JL. Viral infections. In Charles D (ed) *Obstetric and Perinatal Infections*. St Louis: Mosby – Year Book, 1993: pp 111–148.

74. Morey AL, Keeling JW, Porter HJ, Fleming KA. Clinical and histopathological features of parvovirus B19 infection in the human fetus. *Br J Obstet Gynaecol* 1992 **99**: 566–574.

75. Anderson LJ. Human parvovirus. *J Infect Dis* 1990 **161**: 603–608.

76. Barrett J, Ryan G, Morrow R, Farine D, Kelly E, Mahony J. Human parvovirus B19 during pregnancy. *J Soc Obstet Gynecol Can* 1994 **16**: 1253–1258.

77. Stagno S, Whitley RJ. Herpesvirus infections of pregnancy. Part II: herpes simplex virus and varicella-zoster virus infections. *N Engl J Med* 1985 **313**: 1327–1330.

78. Gershon AA. Chickenpox, measles and mumps. In Remington JS and Klein JO (eds) *Infectious Diseases of the Fetus and Newborn Infant*, 4th edn. Philadelphia: WB Saunders, 1995: pp 565–618.

79. Dickinson J, Gonik B. Teratogenic viral infections. *Clin Obstet Gynecol* 1990 **33**: 242–252.

80. Pastuszak AL, Levy M, Schick B *et al.* Outcome after maternal varicella infection in the first 20 weeks of pregnancy. *N Engl J Med* 1994 **330**: 901–905.

81. Prober CG, Gershon AA, Grose C, McCracken GH, Nelson JD. Consensus: varicella-zoster infections in pregnancy and the perinatal period. *Ped Infect Dis J* 1990 **9**: 865–869.

82. Brown ZA, Vontver LA, Benedetti J *et al.* Effects on infants of a first episode of genital herpes during pregnancy. *N Engl J Med* 1987 **317**: 1246–1251.

83. Prober CG, Corey L, Brown ZA *et al.* The management of pregnancies complicated by genital infection with herpes simplex virus. *Clin Infect Dis.* 1992 **15**: 1031–1038.

84. Charles D. Syphilis. In Charles D (ed) *Obstetric and Perinatal Infections*. St Louis: Mosby – Year Book, 1993: pp 252–269.

85. Ingall D, Sánchez PJ, Musher D. Syphilis. In Remington JS and Klein JO (eds) *Infectious Diseases of the Fetus and Newborn Infant*, 4th edn. Philadelphia: WB Saunders, 1995: pp 529–564.

86. Remington JS, McLeod R, Desmonts G. Toxoplasmosis. In Remington JS and Klein JO (eds) *Infectious Diseases of the Fetus and Newborn Infant*, 4th edn. Philadelphia: WB Saunders, 1995: pp 140–267.

87. Stray-Pedersen B. Treatment of toxoplasmosis in the pregnant mother and newborn child. *Scand J Infect Dis Suppl* 1992 **84**: 23–31.

88. Couvreur J, Thulliez P, Daffos F. Toxoplasmosis. In Charles D (ed) *Obstetric and Perinatal Infections*. St Louis: Mosby – Year Book, 1993: pp 158–180.

89. Strickland GT. Malaria. In Strickland GT (ed) *Hunter's Tropical Medicine*, 7th edn. Philadelphia: WB Saunders, 1991: pp 586–602.

90. Miller LH, Good MF, Milon G. Malaria pathogenesis. *Science* 1994 **264**: 1878–1883.

91. Looareesuwam S, White NJ, Karbwang J *et al.* Quinine and severe falciparum malaria in late pregnancy. *Lancet* 1985 **ii**: 4–8.

92. McGregor IA. Epidemiology, malaria and pregnancy. *Am J Trop Med Hyg* 1984 **33**: 517–525.

93. Mutabingwa TK, Malle LN, de Geus A, Oosting J. Malaria chemosuppression in pregnancy. II. Its effect on maternal haemoglobin levels, placental malaria and birth weight. *Trop Geogr Med* 1993 **45**: 49–55.

94. Ibhanesebhor SE, Okolo AA. Placental malaria and pregnancy outcome. *Int J Gynecol Obstet* 1992 **37**: 247–252.

95. Bulmer JN, Rasheed FN, Morrison L, Francis N, Greenwood BM. Placental malaria. I. Pathological classification. *Histopathology* 1993 **22**: 211–218.

96. Subramanian D, Moise KJ, White AC Jr. Imported malaria in pregnancy: Report of four cases and review of management. *Clin Infect Dis* 1992 **15**: 408–413.

3.14

HIV-1 Infection and AIDS

S Shaunak

INTRODUCTION

The acquired immune deficiency syndrome (AIDS) as defined by the Center for Disease Control (CDC) surveillance criteria, is characterized by the development of opportunistic infections and/or malignancy in patients infected with the human immunodeficiency virus (HIV).[1-3] The main indicator diseases are listed in Table 3.14.1. The laboratory hallmark of HIV infection is a progressive and irreversible decline in the number and function of CD4+ lymphocytes (T-helper subset), with the eventual development of a clinical immunodeficiency state. Death ensues 5–15 years after infection with the virus by which time opportunistic infections and malignancy have supervened to cause additional immunosuppression. Since the description of the original syndrome, HIV-1 and HIV-2 have been identified and successfully cultured, and several strains have been sequenced. Epidemiological studies have defined the modes of transmission. Therapeutic interventions have reduced both morbidity and mortality from HIV and from opportunist infections. Nevertheless the pandemic continues: over half a million people have developed AIDS and millions more carry the virus.[4]

The AIDS pandemic is best viewed as a series of separate epidemics that now overlap in both time and place. There are three broad epidemiological patterns. In regions with pattern 1 (USA, Canada, Western Europe, Australasia, North America and parts of South America) HIV has spread mainly among homosexual and bisexual men and injecting drug users. Those with heterosexually acquired infection form a small proportion of cases. In areas showing pattern 2 epidemiology (Africa and the remainder of South America), most people have acquired HIV heterosexually, and the ratio of infected males to females is approximately one. AIDS has so far had the most profound effects in these regions: for example, 8 million of an estimated 13 million people infected with HIV worldwide reside in sub-Saharan Africa. A third pattern is found in Asia and the Pacific, Eastern Europe, and the Middle East, where HIV was probably introduced rather later than elsewhere. Recent studies however indicate that there is a high incidence of new sero-conversions taking place in these areas. WHO is concerned that the epidemic in Asia may ultimately dwarf all others in scope and in impact.

CURRENT CONCEPTS

The human immunodeficiency viruses

HIV-1 is an RNA virus which belongs to the lentivirus group of the retroviridae family. In common with other members of this group (visna/maedi virus, equine infectious anemia virus, caprine arthritis/encephalitis virus), it is a non-transforming virus which generates a cytopathic or lytic effect on cells *in vitro* and causes a persistent infection following integration of HIV proviral DNA into the host genome. The group now contains the human viruses HIV-1 and HIV-2, the related simian immunodeficiency viruses SIV, and the more distantly related feline leukemia virus (FIV) and bovine leukemia virus (BIV).

Evidence is now emerging which suggests that the *in vivo* biology of HIV-1 and HIV-2 are distinct.[5,6] The lower rate of transmission of HIV-2 during heterosexual transmission may reflect the lower infectivity of HIV-2. This hypothesis is supported by the observation of a longer incubation period and a lower incidence of AIDS caused by HIV-2 than AIDS caused by HIV-1.[7] Data from maternal–infant transmission studies have also shown that this mode of HIV-2 transmission is rare, compared with the 10–30% transmission rate for HIV-1.[8,9]

Structure and protein products

The structure of HIV-1 (Fig. 3.14.1) is representative of the group. Two single-stranded copies of RNA are non-covalently linked to the gag protein p15; p24 is the most abundant core protein and together with p18 they com-

Table 3.14.1 CDC surveillance case definition for AIDS

Diseases diagnosed definitively without confirmation of HIV infection in patients without other causes of immunodeficiency

Candidiasis of the esophagus, trachea, bronchi, or lungs

Cryptococcosis, extrapulmonary

Chronic intestinal cryptosporidiosis > 1 month duration

Cytomegalovirus (CMV) infection of any organ except the liver, spleen, or lymph nodes in patients > 1 month old

Herpes simplex infection, mucocutaneous (> 1 month duration) or of the bronchi, lungs, or esophagus in patients > 1 month duration

Kaposi's sarcoma in patients < 60 years old

Primary CNS lymphoma in patients < 60 years old

Lymphoid interstitial pneumonitis (LIP) and/or pulmonary lymphoid hyperplasia (PLH) in patients < 13 years old

Mycobacterium avium complex or *M. kansaii* disseminated

Pneumocystis carinii pneumonia

Progressive multifocal leukoencephalopathy

Toxoplasmosis of the brain in patients > 1 month old

Invasive cervical carcinoma

Diseases diagnosed definitively with confirmation of HIV infection

Multiple or recurrent pyogenic bacterial infections in patients < 13 years old

Coccidioidomycosis, disseminated or extrapulmonary

Histoplasmosis, disseminated

Chronic intestinal isosporiasis > 1 month duration

Kaposi's sarcoma, any age

Primary CNS lymphoma, any age

Non-Hodgkin's lymphoma – small, non-cleaved lymphoma; Burkitt or non-Burkitt type; or immunoblastic sarcoma

Mycobacterium avium complex or *M. kansaii* disseminated or extrapulmonary *Mycobacterium*, other species or unidentified species, disseminated or extrapulmonary *M. tuberculosis*, any site

Salmonella septicemia, recurrent

Diseases diagnosed presumptively with confirmation of HIV infection

Candidiasis of the esophagus

CMV retinitis

Kaposi's sarcoma

Lipoid interstitial pneumonitis in patients < 13 years old

Disseminated mycobacterial disease (not cultured)

Pneumocystis carinii pneumonia

Toxoplasmosis of the brain in patients >1 month old.

HIV encephalopathy

HIV wasting syndrome

Recurrent pneumonia

Pulmonary tuberculosis

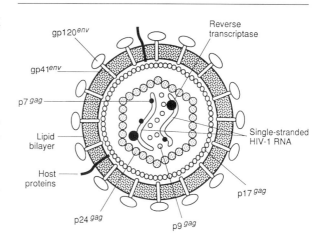

Fig. 3.14.1 *Schematic diagram of the HIV-1 virion. Each of the virion proteins making up the envelope (gp120^{env} and gp41^{env}) and nucleocapsid (p24^{gag}, p17^{gag}, p9^{gag} and p7^{gag}) is identified. In addition, the diploid RNA genome is shown associated with reverse transcriptase, an RNA-dependent DNA polymerase.*

been identified which encode for proteins whose function is to regulate viral replication. Tat (transactivator) proteins accelerate the production of viral proteins (including itself) by as much as 1000 times. The *cis*-acting sequence required for *tat* activity is the transactivation response region (*TAR*) which is located immediately downstream of the cap site residues +1 to +79 and forms part of the 5′ untranslated (U5) region of all the mRNAs encoded by HIV. Interaction of *TAR* and tat facilitates transcriptional elongation, increases mRNA stability and enhances translation.

Nef (negative regulatory factor) was so called because nef proteins were believed to have a negative regulatory effect on viral transcription and replication. However, there are now numerous conflicting reports on whether *nef* has a negative effect, no effect, or a positive effect on viral transcription and replication. Such discrepancies have occurred with researchers using the same virus and the same cell lines. It is likely that any effect of nef on the growth of lentiviruses *in vitro*, is probably small, at least under standard cell culture conditions.

The viral protein rev (regulator of virion protein) serves as a switch which determines whether only non-structural regulatory proteins will be made or whether viral particles can also be made. The role of vif (virion infectivity factor) has not been clearly established, but it seems to have a dramatic effect on virus replication and is thought to play a role in virion infectivity. VpU (viral protein U) allows proper virion assembly, packaging, budding and release of infectious virus. Regulatory proteins therefore affect the production not only of structural gene proteins but also that of regulatory gene proteins including themselves.

Cells arrested in the Go phase (see Chapter 1.3, p. 27) have few if any viral transcripts. Following cellular activation, nuclear factors which activate interleukins and their receptors also lead to the transcription of HIV. Initially, low levels of short viral transcripts are synthesized, with accumulation of tat. On reaching a threshold, tat greatly

prise the major gag structural proteins. RNA-dependent DNA polymerase (reverse transcriptase) encoded by the *pol* gene, is closely associated with the RNA genome. The outer envelope of HIV consists of a lipid and protein membrane which is derived from the host cell membrane and in which a transmembrane glycoprotein (gp41) anchors the extracellular glycosylated protein gp120.

The proviral genome of HIV-1 and HIV-2 is 9–10 kb long (Figs 3.14.2 and 3.14.3). Sequencing data from several different HIV-1 strains have shown that the structural genes *gag* (group antigen) and *pol* (polymerase) are more conserved than *env* (envelope). Several other genes have

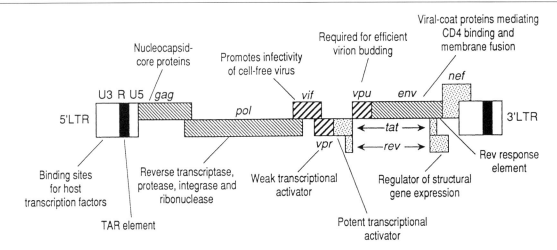

Fig. 3.14.2 *Genomic structure of HIV-1. Each of the nine known genes of HIV-1 are shown, and their recognized primary functions summarized. The 5' and 3' long terminal repeats (LTRs) containing regulatory sequences recognized by various host transcription factors are also depicted, and the positions of the Tat and Rev response elements (TAR (transactivation response) element and Rev RNA response element) are indicated.*

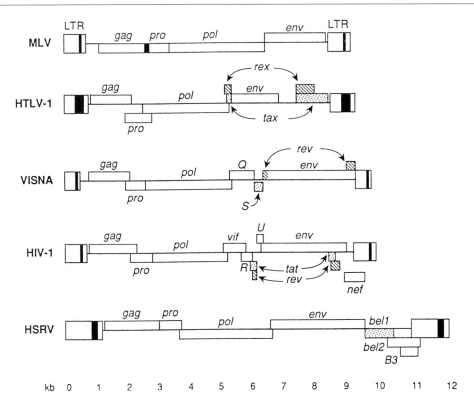

Fig. 3.14.3 *Representative retroviral proviruses. Shown are the genomic organization of MLV, a typical simple retrovirus, and of four representative complex retroviruses. Although all known viral genes are named and drawn approximately to scale, this listing is not exhaustive. Known transcriptional activators are marked by stippling, whereas known post-transcriptional regulators are indicated by hatching. LTRs are indicated by large terminal boxes, with the R region in black. R, Vpr; U, VPU; B3, Bel-3.*

increases the expression of TAR-containing RNA transcripts. Controlled viral replication depends upon a balance being maintained between positive and negative regulatory factors such that when an infected cell dies enough virions are released to infect other cells.

The CD4 receptor for HIV

The CD4 antigen was identified as an essential component of the receptor for infection by HIV following the observation that the development of AIDS was associated with a decline in the CD4+ lymphocyte count. The *in vitro* tropism of HIV for CD4+ lymphocytes was demonstrated using monoclonal antibodies specific for CD4 which blocked HIV infection and syncytium formation, as well as by VSV(HIV) pseudotype plating experiments.[10,11] Transfer of the cDNA for the human CD4 receptor to cells lacking it (HeLa cells) made them susceptible to infection by HIV.[12] In contrast, cDNA inserts of the human CD4 receptor into murine T cells resulted in binding of HIV to the cell surface receptor, but no entry of the virus into cells. These findings suggest that a second cell surface receptor is required for entry of the virus once binding to the CD4 receptor has occurred.

The CD4 antigen acts as the receptor not only for HIV-1, but also for HIV-2 and SIV. It is also present on monocytes and macrophages and is presumed to play a central role in the entry of virus into these cells.[13,14] HIV binds to the CD4 receptor through the gp120 envelope glycoprotein with an affinity constant of 10^{-9} M. The receptor site has been mapped using monoclonal antibodies to a conserved region of gp120 and C3 within amino acid residues 413–456.[15] It is believed that for viral entry to occur gp120 must first bind to CD4. A secondary conformational change in the HIV transmembrane protein gp41 then leads to fusion (in a pH-independent manner) of the virus membrane with that of the host.[16,17]

On brain and bowel cells (which are negative for CD4) galactosyl ceramide is thought to be the receptor for HIV-1.[18,19]

Strain variations

There is increasing evidence to suggest that the biological properties of molecularly cloned viruses vary considerably from clone to clone.[20,21] Active retroviral replication results in changes in the structural genes such that defective virus particles are produced which, although replication incompetent, have been implicated in the pathogenesis of the immunodeficiency syndrome.[22–24] It is now clear that HIV is constantly evolving *in vivo*. Isolates obtained from patients with asymptomatic HIV infection grow slowly, and usually do so only in primary cell cultures. They produce low titres of reverse transcriptase activity and have been termed slow/low viruses. Isolates established from patients with AIDS are capable of continuous viral replication in CD4+ lymphocyte and monocyte cell lines.[24–26] Even isolates obtained sequentially from the same patient show differences in their replicating ability and cytopathic effect,[20,26] and those taken from patients with AIDS having an expanded host cell tropism *in vitro*, faster replication rates and a greater cytopathic effect.[27,28] A large number of related but genotypically distinguishable variants evolve in parallel *in vivo*, with rapid/high variants becoming more common during the course of the infection. The immune mechanisms underlying the emergence of such variants and their relationship to the progression of clinical disease remain to be determined.

Mechanisms of cytopathic effect

A given individual is infected with several different isolates of HIV-1 throughout the course of their disease. Some of these isolates produce high titres of reverse transcriptase and grow rapidly in peripheral blood mononuclear cells (fast/high viruses) whereas others produce low titres of reverse transcriptase activity and grow slowly (slow/low viruses).[25,26] Isolates obtained sequentially from the same patient show differences in their ability to replicate in peripheral blood mononuclear cells and in their cytopathic effect.[20,26] Furthermore, isolates taken from patients with AIDS have an expanded host cell tropism *in vitro*, compared with isolates from patients with asymptomatic HIV infection.[27,28] This difference in the biological properties of viral isolates has been confirmed using molecularly cloned viruses.[20,21]

Although a progressive loss of CD4+ T lymphocytes is central to the immune defect in AIDS, the precise mechanisms underlying the quantitative as well as the functional defects still remain to be defined. Infection *in vitro* of any cell expressing CD4 can lead to one of several possible outcomes.

Syncytia formation

Single cell killing and syncytia formation is through a direct HIV-mediated cytopathic effect.[29,30] Single cell killing may result from the accumulation of unintegrated proviral DNA and/or from defects in post-translational processes which interfere with the processing of heteronuclear cellular RNA and which lead to the arrest of normal cellular processes.[31,32] Syncytium formation involves fusion of the cell membrane of an infected cell with the cell membranes of uninfected CD4+ cells and the formation of multinucleated giant cells. As many as 500 uninfected cells can combine to form a multinucleated giant cell with the subsequent death of both the original infected cell and that of uninfected T cells.

Antibody dependent cellular cytotoxicity

Although the major effect of antibodies against HIV-1 is attributed to their neutralizing properties, some antibodies which are directed against regions of the envelope of HIV-1 may have an additional protective function which is related to their ability to mediate antibody-dependent cellular cytotoxicity. This leads to the death of HIV-infected cells which express viral envelope proteins on their surface.[33]

Autoimmune mechanisms

Non-polymorphic determinants of MHC class II molecules, particularly HLA-DR and HLA-DQ, share some degree of structural homology with the gp120 and gp41 proteins of HIV-1 and antibodies to these HIV-1 proteins can therefore cross-react with MHC class II molecules. Antibodies which react with MHC class II molecules have been found in the serum of patients with HIV-1 infection. These antibodies could therefore prevent the interaction between CD4 and MHC class II molecules on antigen-presenting cells, thereby impairing the cellular interaction which is required for efficient antigen presentation and inhibit the antigen-specific functions which are mediated by helper CD4+ T cells.[34,35]

Anergy

Complexes of gp120–anti-gp120 bind to CD4, and the CD4+ cells then become refractory to further *in vitro* stimulation via their CD3 molecules.[36] Similarly, *in vitro*, peripheral blood mononuclear cells inoculated with HIV-1 do not respond to stimulation with anti-CD3 antibodies.[35] These observations have led to the hypothesis that a negative signal is delivered to CD4+ cells after CD4 has bound to gp120 or to gp120–anti-gp120 complexes.[37] In this regard, anti-gp120 antibodies have been detected on CD4+ T lymphocytes in patients with AIDS.[38]

Superantigens

Several authors have reported that endogenous or exogenous retroviral encoded superantigens stimulate murine CD4+ T cells *in vivo* and that this leads to anergy or deletion of a substantial percentage of CD4+ T cells with specific V_β regions.[39–41] This has led to the hypothesis that a superantigen (either retrovirally encoded or unrelated to HIV-1) may play an important part in the immunopathogenesis of HIV-1 infection.[42] Consistent with this hypothesis have been reports that patients with HIV-1 infection have disturbances of T cell subgroups bearing certain specific V_β regions.[43]

Programed cell death

This is a mechanism whereby the body eliminates autoreactive clones of T cells. Since apoptosis can be induced in mature murine CD4+ T cells after cross-linking CD4 molecules to one another and triggering of the T cell antigen receptor,[44] there has been speculation that cross-linking of the CD4 molecule by gp120 or gp120–anti-gp120 immune complexes prepares the cell for programed cell death which then occurs when an MHC class II molecule complexed to an antigen binds to the T cell antigen receptor.[45] Thus the mere activation of a prepared cell by a specific antigen or superantigen could lead to the death of the cell without direct infection by HIV-1.

Primary HIV-1 infection

Patients with primary HIV infection can present clinically with an abrupt onset of a febrile illness resembling acute mononucleosis. Symptoms can include lymphadenopathy, pharyngitis, rash, myalgia, arthralgia, diarrhea, headache, nausea and vomiting.[46] Shallow ulcers can occur in the mouth, esophagus or in the genital area.[47] Neurological involvement (meningo-encephalitis) also occurs but is uncommon. These symptoms and signs can be associated with a transient leucopenia, atypical lymphocytosis, increased numbers of banded neutrophils and thrombocytopenia.[48] Symptomatic primary HIV-1 infection that comes to medical attention typically occurs 2–6 weeks after exposure to HIV-1 and usually resolves within 1–2 weeks. The symptoms coincide with a high-grade viremia, as indicated by the presence of p24 antigenemia, plasma viremia and a high titre of HIV-1 in peripheral blood mononuclear cells. The HIV strains associated with acute infection are mainly macrophage tropic.[49] Resolution is coincident with the emergence of detectable HIV-specific antibody and an increase in cytotoxic T lymphocytes.[50,51] A host IgM (variable) and IgG response develop within 7–14 days and almost always within 3 months.[52]

The general activation of the immune system during this time is reflected by increases in serum neopterin, a breakdown product secreted from activated macrophages indicating increased cellular activation, β_2-microglobulin, a component of major histocompatibility complex class I indicating increased cellular turnover, and alpha-interferon.[53,54] The activation of the immune response is characterized by the appearance of activated T cells in the circulation.

Responses to antigen and mitogen are impaired during primary HIV-1 infection. Patients have a reduced response to both pokeweed mitogen and to phytohemagglutinin (PHA). Antigen specific responses can remain impaired for up to 6–12 months after the primary infection.[55]

The immunological profile typically shows an initial reduction in total lymphocyte count followed by transient increases in CD8+ lymphocytes and inversion of the CD4:CD8 cell ratio.[51] Although in some subjects the number of CD4+ lymphocytes may recover to the level prior to infection, the overall trend in HIV-infected persons is a progressive decrease in these cells. *In vitro*, autologous CD8+ lymphocytes are capable of suppressing HIV replication in peripheral blood mononuclear cells.[56] Transient increases in the numbers of CD8+ cells and activated CD8+ cells can also be found in acute infections with other viruses such as cytomegalovirus and Epstein–Barr virus and therefore may represent a non-specific immune response against viral infections. However, HIV-1 is the first chronic viral disease associated with prominent cytotoxic T lymphocyte activity.[33]

Although HIV-1 is believed to disseminate widely during the early stages of infection, the immunological response results in a rapid decline in the level of the viraemia within weeks and the acute syndrome subsides. Viral replication is never completely curtailed because it can be detected in lymph nodes during clinically quiescent stages of the disease.[57] The events described above probably occur even in those patients who do not have a clinically recognizable acute seroconversion syndrome.

Following acute infection of T cells by HIV *in vitro*, there is a transient reduction in the expression of HLA DR on the cell surface.[58] Cells which survive the cytopathic effect of the virus have a decreased level of expression of CD4 molecules on their cell surface. Expression of interleukin-2 (IL-2) is also decreased, despite normal expression of the IL-2 receptor gene.[59] This functional defect in the expression of IL-2 may contribute to the antigen-specific defect which requires IL-2 for amplification.

During the early course of asymptomatic HIV infection, the proliferative responses of peripheral blood lymphocytes and purified populations of CD4+ lymphocytes to PHA, tetanus toxoid and/or calcium ionophore do not demonstrate a functional defect in T cell function.[60]

Other as yet undetermined factors are clearly important at this early stage of infection in patients whose acute illness lasts for more than 14 days. The rate of progression to CDC IV within 3 years is eight times higher than that in patients who have mild symptoms. CD4+ lymphocyte counts are similar in these two groups at the time of seroconversion and for a period of 6 months thereafter.[52] It is possible that the severity of symptoms at the time of seroconversion reflect the degree of active viral replication. Similarly, parameters of humoral immunity to HIV at seroconversion affect outcome in terms of disease progression. No immune response to HIV at the time of infection or in the subsequent course of the illness unequivocally clears virus from the host.

Asymptomatic HIV infection

After recovering from their seroconversion illness, most patients have a period of clinical latency during which they are clinically asymptomatic. During this period, which can last for several years, almost all patients have a gradual depletion of their CD4+ T cells. Although it can be difficult to detect virus in the peripheral blood at this time, viral replication continues in lymphoid organs and the spectrum of immunological events which are triggered by the virus are evident within lymph nodes.

Symptomatic HIV infection

The inevitable outcome of the progressive deterioration of the immune system is the development of clinically apparent disease. A re-examination of lymphoid tissue from patients during the early stages of the disease has shown a high burden of HIV-1 in lymphoid tissues, both as extracellular virus trapped in the follicular dendritic cell network of the germinal centers and as intracellular virus.[61,62] HIV replicates, albeit at low levels, during the early, asymptomatic phase of the disease. As the disease progresses, the level of replication of HIV-1 in lymphoid tissue increases.

AIDS

Progression to AIDS is associated with an inversion of both the cytotoxic/suppressor cell ratio and inversion of the CD4/CD8 ratio to less than 1.0. Concomitant infections, especially with cytomegalovirus, cause wide fluctuations in the number of suppressor and cytotoxic T-cells which is reflected in the CD4/CD8 ratio. Consequently the most

consistent indicator of the severity of immune dysfunction is the CD4+ lymphocyte count. The percentage CD4+ lymphocyte count is a more reliable indicator for the longitudinal follow-up of patients than the absolute CD4 count because it is not affected by day-to-day fluctuations in either the total white cell count or the percentage of total lymphocytes.[63] In late-stage AIDS all lymphoid cells including those which are CD8+, are depleted due to both HIV itself as well as to opportunistic infections which may independently cause bone marrow suppression.[64]

In patients with AIDS, the CD4+ lymphocyte is unable to mount a proliferative response to soluble antigens such as tetanus toxoid. This abnormality is seen with both unfractionated cells and with purified CD4+ cells.[65] It is not due to a defect in antigen-presenting cells and implies a selective depletion or a selective functional impairment of a specific subset of T helper/inducer cells. It is also reflected in the defective autologous mixed lymphocyte reaction of peripheral blood mononuclear cells from patients infected with HIV in which CD4+ lymphocytes fail to proliferate.[66] These defects are thought to reflect abnormalities at the level of the cell surface rather than at a subcellular level. gp120 bound to CD4 was thought to interfere with MHC class II function, but this now seems unlikely. Using homolog scanning mutagenesis, it has been found that gp120 binding can be abolished without affecting MHC class II binding and vice versa,[67] indicating that the gp120 and MHC class II binding sites of CD4 are distinct and can be separated.

In assays used to assess the ability of CD4+ cells to help and CD8+ cells to suppress immunoglobulin production by pokeweed mitogen-stimulated B cells in vitro, the CD4+ cells from patients with AIDS demonstrate little or no helper function, in contrast to CD8+ cells from the same patients which exhibit normal suppressor function.[68,69] These results confirm that the overall defect in patients with AIDS remains a failure of helper and inducer cell function rather than increased suppressor cell function.

Lymphoid organs in HIV-1 infection

Lymphoid organs are a major anatomical site in which HIV-1 becomes established and in which it is propagated in both the short and long term. Most studies, of necessity, focus on HIV infection of peripheral blood mononuclear cells, but it is important to remember that the lymphocytes in the peripheral blood at any given time represent only 2% of the total lymphocyte pool.[70] Therefore, in certain pathogenic processes involving lymphoid cells, the peripheral blood may not accurately reflect the status of the disease. Furthermore, specific immune responses are generated predominantly in the lymphoid organs rather than in the peripheral blood.[71] Studies using the standard polymerase chain reaction to detect HIV DNA and reverse transcriptase PCR to detect HIV RNA have found 5–10 times more HIV-infected cells and higher concentrations of both regulatory and structural messenger RNA in the lymphoid organs (lymph nodes, adenoids and tonsils) of patients than in their peripheral blood. This viral burden in lymphoid organs is greater than that in the peripheral blood throughout the period of clinical latency.[72]

In early and intermediate disease, HIV particles, complexed with antibodies and complement, accumulate in lymph nodes, where they are trapped within the network of follicular dendritic cells within germinal centers.[73] Follicular dendritic cells function during the normal immune response to trap antigens in the environment of the germinal center and to allow the presentation of antigen to competent immune cells.[74] This is an efficient means of initiating and propagating an appropriate immune response to antigenic challenge be it microbial or environmental. The progression to clinical HIV-related disease is associated with the degeneration of the network of follicular dendritic cells and the loss of the ability of lymphoid organs to trap HIV particles, thereby contributing to an increase in viremia.

In the late stages of HIV disease, the architecture of the lymph nodes is disrupted and the network of follicular dendritic cells dissolves, removing the mechanisms for trapping virions. HIV is thus free to recirculate, a finding that has been interpreted to be a reflection of a massive increase in the total viral burden in late-stage disease. However, rather than representing a true increase in viral burden, these high levels of viremia in AIDS may reflect, at least in part, the recirculation of HIV particles removed from the constraints of lymph node entrapment.

The increased viral load in lymph nodes has recently been confirmed by culturing mononuclear cells obtained from lymph nodes. The mean titre of virus was 60 times higher in lymph nodes from CDC stage III patients than in blood.[75] Co-cultures of mononuclear cells from lymph nodes also became positive before those from blood.

The gut is another major lymphoid organ in the body and as many as 5–50% of all lymphocytes are contained within it, distributed as Peyer's patches, lamina propria, lymphoid cells and aggregates of intraepithelial lymphocytes. Infection in gut-associated lymphoid tissue is similar to that in peripheral lymph nodes with trapping of virus on follicular dendritic cells which then act as reservoirs of latent and replicating virus.[76] It is likely that reservoirs of HIV exist in other locations within the body and that they also contribute to the total body load of infectious, replicating HIV-1.

Transmission of HIV

HIV-infected lymphocytes and macrophages are present in abundance in normal semen and have been shown to increase in the presence of genital tract inflammation and HIV infection.[77–79] Significant amounts of cell-free virus have also been found in semen,[80] but it still remains to be established whether HIV-1 transmission involves predominantly cell-free virus or cell-associated virus. *In vitro* experiments have shown that cell to cell transmission of HIV-1 is much more efficient and rapid than infection of a cell by cell-free virus. It is possible that Langerhans cells which are present in the vagina and the cervix could be the recipients of HIV-1 during productive infection.[81] However, the

mechanisms underlying transmission of HIV during sexual intercourse and perinatally remain unclear and are currently the subject of considerable research.

FUTURE PERSPECTIVES

Evidence continues to accumulate that the long, clinically latent phase of the disease is not a period of viral inactivity, but an active process in which T-cells are being continuously infected and dying. It is estimated that the rate of CD4+ lymphocyte turnover is 2×10^{10} cells day^{-1}, or about 5% of the total CD4+ lymphocyte population.[81,83] The extraordinarily large number of replication cycles which must therefore occur during the infection of a single individual probably drives both the pathogenic process and the development of genetic variation.

The dynamics of HIV replication *in vivo* are largely unknown, yet they are going to be critical for our understanding of this disease. Researchers are increasingly turning to drugs which inhibit viral replication to study the composite lifespan of both plasma virus and of virus-producing cells. These studies suggest that 30% or more of the total virus population in plasma must be replenished daily. HIV-1 viremia therefore appears to be sustained primarily by a dynamic process which involves continuous rounds of *de novo* infection of CD4+ lymphocytes and a rapid turnover of infected cells.[82,83]

Future studies will continue the use of effective inhibitors of HIV replication with sensitive and accurate quantitative assays of wild-type and mutant genomes in the circulation. Studies of this kind will provide an opportunity to study the dynamics of HIV replication *in vivo* and will also aim to elucidate the relationship between the kinetics of viral replication observed in blood with those in cells at various sites of viral replication. As a result, it should be possible to dissect out the contribution of various populations of infected cells at each stage of the disease.

Our rapidly emerging knowledge about HIV *in vivo* has only served to further complicate attempts at vaccine development. The variability of HIV, especially within the *env* sequence is a major hurdle. However, the observations that certain phenotypes of HIV are selectively transmitted by sexual contact suggest that it may be possible to generate a vaccine which is targeted to specific genotypes and phenotypes of the virus. Considerable effort has also been put into elucidating the immunological basis for protection in SIV and HIV model systems and the findings from these are central to current attempts to develop a vaccine. Detailed studies are also in progress in exposed but uninfected individuals in whom cytotoxic T-cell responses seem to have conferred protection from HIV-1 infection.

The prospect of obtaining results during the course of clinical trials which lead to a real understanding of the process of infection *in vivo* and which also lead to the development of effective therapeutic strategies involving new generations of antiviral drugs is an exciting new prospect for the future.

SUMMARY

- HIV continues to spread with over a million people carrying the virus. Patterns of transmission of the virus vary in different regions of the world.

- HIV-1 and HIV-2 are closely related but their biology *in vivo* appears to be distinct. The rate of transmission of HIV-2 is lower than that of HIV-1 and there is a lower incidence of AIDS with HIV-2.

- The CD4 receptor on T-cells and on macrophages is the major cell surface receptor for HIV-1.

- There are genotypic as well as phenotypic differences between strains of HIV-1. They can be phenotypically distinguished into those viruses which grow slowly and in low titre (non-syncytium inducing) and those which grow fast and in high titre (syncytium inducing).

- Several mechanisms to explain the loss of CD4+ lymphocytes have been postulated for HIV-1. These include syncytia formation, antibody-dependent cellular cytotoxicity, autoimmune mechanisms, anergy, superantigens and programed cell death. The relative contribution of each of these mechanisms *in vivo* remains to be established.

- Primary HIV infection is often asymptomatic but can present with an acute febrile illness resembling acute mononucleosis.

- Although HIV is believed to disseminate widely during the early stages of infection, the immunological response results in a rapid decline in the level of viremia within weeks and the acute syndrome subsides. Viral replication, however, is never curtailed and can be detected in lymph nodes during clinically quiescent stages of the disease.

- Progression from asymptomatic HIV infection to AIDS is associated with the development of either opportunistic infections or malignancy. The diagnosis of AIDS is therefore not dependent on a particular blood test but on the development of one of a predetermined number of clinical disease states.

- The lymphocytes in the peripheral blood represent only 2% of the total lymphocyte pool. Lymphoid organs are therefore the major anatomical site in which HIV-1 becomes established and in which it is propagated in both the short and long term.

- In the latter stages of HIV disease and AIDS, the architecture of the lymph nodes is disrupted and the network of follicular dendritic cells dissolves thereby removing the mechanism within lymph nodes for trapping virions. HIV is then free to recirculate, a finding which has been interpreted to be a reflection of a massive increase in the total viral burden in late-stage disease. However, rather than representing a true increase in viral burden, these high levels of viremia in AIDS may reflect, at least in part, the recirculation of HIV particles removed from the constraints of lymph node entrapment.

REFERENCES

1. Classification system for HTLV III virus infections. *MMWR* 1986 **35**: 334–339.
2. Revision of the CDC surveillance case definition for AIDS. *MMWR* 1987 **36** (Suppl 1): 1–15.
3. CDC surveillance case definition for AIDS. *MMWR* 1992 41 (RR-17).
4. Piot P. World wide epidemiology of HIV infection. In Neu HC, Levy JA, Weiss JA (eds) *Frontiers of Infectious Diseases, Focus on HIV*. New York. Churchill Livingstone, 1993.
5. Chakrabarti L, Guyader M, Alizon M *et al.* Sequence of SIV from macaque and its relationship to other human and simian retroviruses. *Nature* 1987 **328**: 543–547.
6. Franchini G, Gurgo C, Guo HG *et al.* Sequence of SIV and its relationship to HIV. *Nature* 1987 **328**: 539–543.
7. Kanki PJ, Travers KU, Boup S *et al.* Slower heterosexual spread of HIV-2 than HIV-1. *Lancet* 1994 **343**: 943–946.
8. Poulson AG, Kvinesdal BB, Abaaby P *et al.* Lack of evidence of vertical transmission of HIV-2 in a sample of the general population of Bissau. *J Acquir Immune Defic Syndr* 1992 **5**: 25–30.
9. Gayle HD, Gnaore E, Adjorlolo G *et al.* HIV-1 and HIV-2 infection in children in Abidjan, Cote d'Ivoire. *J Acquir Immune Defic Syndr* 1992 **5**: 513–517.
10. Dalgleish AG, Beverley PCL, Clapham PR *et al.* The CD4 antigen is an essential component of the receptor for the AIDS retrovirus. *Nature* 1984 **312**: 763–767.
11. Klatzmann D, Champagne E, Chamaret S *et al.* T-lymphocyte T4 molecule behaves as the receptor for human retrovirus LAV. *Nature* 1984 **312**: 767–768.
12. Maddon PJ, Dalgleish AG, McDougal JS *et al.* The T4 gene encodes the AIDS virus receptor and is expressed in the immune system and the brain. *Cell* 1986 **47**: 333–348.
13. Ho DD, Rota TR, Hirsh MS. Infection of monocyte/macrophages by HTLV III. *J Clin Invest* 1986 **77**: 1712–1715.
14. Crowe S, Mills J, McGrath MS. Quantitative immunocytofluorographic analysis of CD4 antigen expression and HIV infection of human peripheral blood monocyte/macrophages. *AIDS Res Hum Retroviruses* 1987 **3**: 135–138.
15. Lasky LA, Nakamura G, Smith DH *et al.* Delineation of a region of the HIV type I gp 120 glycoprotein critical for interaction with the CD4 receptor. *Cell* 1987 **50**: 975–985.
16. Stein BS, Gowda SD, Lifson JD *et al.* pH-independent HIV entry into CD4+ T cells via virus envelope fusion to the plasma membrane. *Cell* 1987 **49**: 659–668.
17. McClure MO, Marsh M, Weiss RA. HIV-1 virus infection of CD4 bearing cells occurs by a pH independent mechanism. *EMBO J* 1988 **7**: 513–518.
18. Harouse JM, Bhat S, Spitalnik SL *et al.* Inhibition of

19. Yahi N, Baghdiguian S, Moreau H *et al.* Galactosyl ceramide (or a closely related molecule) is the receptor for HIV-1 on human colon epithelial HT 29 cells. *J Virol* 1992 **66**: 4848–4854.

20. Fisher AG, Ensoli B, Looney D *et al.* Biologically diverse molecular variants within a single HIV-1 isolate. *Nature* 1988 **334**: 444–447.

21. Sakai K, Dewhurst S, Ma X *et al.* Differences in cytopathogenicity and host cell range among infectious molecular clones of HIV-1 simultaneously isolated from an individual. *J Virol* 1988 **62**: 4078–4085.

22. Aziz DC, Hanna Z, Jolicoeur P. Severe immunodeficiency disease induced by a defective murine leukaemia virus. *Nature* 1989 **338**: 505–508.

23. Hartley JW, Frederickson TN, Yetter RA *et al.* Retrovirus-induced murine acquired immunodeficiency syndrome; natural history of infection and differing susceptibility of inbred mice strains. *J Virol* 1989 **63**: 1223–1231.

24. Overbaugh J, Donahue PR, Quackenbush SL *et al.* Molecular cloning of a FeLV that induces fatal immunodeficiency disease in cats. *Science* 1988 **239**: 906–910.

25. Asjo B, Morfeldt-Manson L, Albert J *et al.* Replicative capacity of HIV from patients with varying severity of HIV infection. *Lancet* 1986 **ii**: 660–662.

26. Cheng-Mayer C, Seto D, Tateno M, Levy JA. Biologic features of HIV-1 that correlate with virulence in the host. *Science* 1988 **240**: 80–82.

27. Gatner S, Markovits P, Markovitz DM *et al.* The role of mononuclear phagocytes in HTLV III infection. *Science* 1986 **233**: 215–219.

28. Koyanagi Y, Miles S, Mitsuyasu RT *et al.* Dual infection of the central nervous system by AIDS viruses with distinct cellular tropisms. *Science* 1987 **236**: 819–822.

29. Lifson JD, Reyes GR, McGrath MS *et al.* AIDS retrovirus induced cytopathology: giant cell formation and involvement of the CD4 antigen. *Science* 1986 **232**: 1123–1127.

30. Sodroski J, Goh WC, Rosen C, Campbell K, Haseltine WA. Role of the HTLV-3/LAV envelope in syncytium formation and cytopathicity. *Nature* 1986 **322**: 470–474.

31. Levy JA, Kaminsky LS, Morrow WJW *et al.* Infection by the retrovirus associated with AIDS. *Ann Intern Med* 1985 **103**: 694–699.

32. Koya Y, Linstrom E, Fenyo EM *et al.* HIV infection may interfere with hnRNA processing in cells. V International Conference on AIDS. Stockholm June 1988: 2573.

33. Fauci AS. (Moderator) Immunopathogenic mechanisms in HIV-1 infection. *Ann Intern Med.* 1991 **114**: 678–693.

34. Golding H, Robey FA, Gates FT III *et al.* Identification of homologous regions in HIV-1 gp41 and human MHC Class II B1 domain. *J Exp Med* 1988 **167**: 913–923.

35. Golding H, Shearer JM, Hillman K *et al.* Common epitope in HIV-1 gp41 and HLA Class II elicits immunosuppressive autoantibodies capable of contributing to immune dysfunction in HIV-1 infected individuals. *J Clin Invest.* 1989 **83**: 1430–1435.

36. Mittler RS, Holfmann MK. Synergism between HIV-gp 120 and gp120-specific antibody blocking human T cell activation. *Science* 1989 **245**: 1380–1382.

37. Linette GP, Hartzman RJ, Ledbetter JA, June CH. HIV-1 infected T cells show a selective signalling defect after perturbation of the CD3/antigen receptor. *Science.* 1988 **241**: 573–576.

38. Amadori A, de Silvestro G, Zamarchi R *et al.* CD4 epitope masking by gp120 antibody complexes: potential mechanism for CD cell function downregulation in AIDS patients. *J Immunol* 1992 **148**: 2709–2716.

39. Frankel WN. Rudy C, Coffin JM, Huber BT. Linkage of MLS genes to endogenous mammary tumour viruses of inbred mice. *Nature* 1991 **349**: 526–528.

40. Marrack P, Kushnir E, Kappler J. Maternally inherited superantigen coded by a mammary tumour virus. *Nature* 1991 **349**: 524–526.

41. Woodland DL, Happ MP, Gollob AJ, Palmer E. An endogenous retrovirus mediating deletion of T cells? *Nature* 1991 **349**: 529–530.

42. Janeway C. MLS: makes a little sense. *Nature* 1991 **349**: 459–461.

43. Imberti L, Sottini A, Bettinardi A *et al.* Selective depletion in HIV infection of T cells that bear specific T cell receptor V$_B$ sequences. *Science.* 1991 **254**: 860–862.

44. Newell MK, Haughn LJ, Maroun CR, Julius MH. Death of mature T cells by separate ligation of CD4 and the T cell receptor for antigen. *Nature* 1990 **347**: 286–289.

45. Groux A, Torpier G, Monte D *et al.* Activation-induced death by apoptosis in CD4-positive T cells from HIV-1 infected asymptomatic individuals. *J Exp Med.* 1992 **175**: 331–340.

46. Pedersen C, Lindhardt BO, Jensen BL *et al.* Clinical course of primary HIV infection: consequences for subsequent course of infection. *Br Med J* 1989 **299**: 154–156.

47. Gaines H, Sydow M, Pehrson PO *et al.* Clinical picture of primary HIV infection presenting as a glandular fever like illness. *Br Med J* 1988 **297**: 1363–1368.

48. Tindall B, Barker S, Donovan B *et al.* Characterisation of the acute clinical illness associated with HIV infection. *Arch Intern Med* 1988 **148**: 945–949.

49. Zhu T, Mo H, Wang N *et al.* Genotypic and phenotypic characterisation of HIV-1 in patients with primary infection. *Science* 1993 **261**: 1179–1181.

50. Clark SJ, Saag MS, Decker WD *et al.* High titres of cytopathic virus in plasma of patients with symptomatic HIV infections. *N Engl J Med* 1991 **324**: 954–960.

51. Daar ES, Moudgil T, Meyer RD *et al.* Transient high levels of viraemia in patients with primary HIV-1 infection. *N Engl J Med* 1991 **324**: 961–964.

52. Von Sydow M, Gaines H, Sonnerborg A. Antigen detection in primary HIV infection. *Br Med J* 1988 **296**: 238–240.

53. Gaines H, von Sydow MAE, von Stedingk LV *et al.* Immunological changes in primary HIV infection. *AIDS* 1990 **4**: 995–999.

54. Sonnerborg AB, von Stedingk LV, Hansson LO *et al.* Elevated neopterin and β-2 microglobulin levels in blood and cerebrospinal fluid occur early in HIV infection. *AIDS* 1989 **3**: 277–283.

55. Pedersen C, Dickmeiss E, Gaub J *et al.* T cell subset alterations and lymphocyte responsiveness to mitogens and antigen during severe primary infection with HIV: a case series of seven consecutive HIV seroconverters. *AIDS* 1990 **4**: 523–526.

56. Walker CM, Moody DJ, Stites DP *et al.* CD8+ lymphocytes can control HIV infection *in vitro* by suppressing virus replication. *Science* 1986 **234**: 1563–1566.

57. Fauci AS. Multifactorial nature of human immunodeficiency virus disease: implication for therapy. *Science* 1993 **262**: 1011–1018.

58. Mann DL, Lesane F, Blattner WA *et al.* HLA DR is involved in the HIV receptor. III International Conference on AIDS, Washington DC, 1987: 209.

59. Fauci AS. The HIV virus: infectivity and mechanisms of pathogenesis. *Science* 1988 **239**: 617–622.

60. Gurley RJ, Ikeuchi K, Byrn RA *et al.* CD4+ lymphocyte function with early HIV infection. *Proc Natl Acad Sci USA* 1989 **86**: 1993–1997.

61. Pantaleo G, Graziosi C, Demarest JF *et al.* HIV infection is active and progressive in lymphoid tissue during the clinically latent stage of disease. *Nature* 1993 **362**: 355–358.

62. Embretson J, Zupancic M, Ribas JL *et al.* Massive covert infection of helper T lymphocytes and macrophages by HIV during the incubation period of AIDS. *Nature* 1993 **362**: 359–362.

63. Kessler HA, Landay A, Pottage JC Jr *et al.* Absolute number versus percentage of T-helper lymphocytes in HIV infection. *J Infect Dis* 1990 **161**: 356–357.

64. Lane H C, Masur H, Gelmann EP *et al.* Correlation between immunologic function and clinical subpopulations of patients with AIDS. *Am J Med* 1985 **78**: 417–422.

65. Lane HC, Depper JM, Greene WC *et al.* Qualitative analysis of immune function in patients with AIDS : Evidence for a selective defect in soluble antigen recognition. *N Engl J Med* 1985 **313**: 79–84.

66. Gupta S, Safai B. Deficient autologous mixed lymphocyte reaction in Kaposi's Sarcoma associated with a deficiency of Leu 3+ responder T cells. *J Clin Invest* 1983 **71**: 296–300.

67. Lamarre D, Ashkenazi A, Fleury S *et al.* The MHC binding and gp120 binding functions of CD4 are separable. *Science* 1989 **245**: 743–746.

68. Benveniste E, Schroff R, Stevens R H *et al.* Immunoregulatory T cells in men with AIDS. *J Clin Immunol* 1983 **3**: 359–367.

69. Lane HC, Masur H, Edgar LC *et al.* Abnormalities of B cell activation and immunoregulation in patients with AIDS. *N Engl J Med* 1983 **309**: 453–458.

70. Westerman J, Pabst R. Lymphocyte subsets in the blood: a diagnostic window on the lymphoid system? *Immunol Today* 1990 **11**: 406–410.

71. Parrott DM, Wilkinson PC. Lymphocyte locomotion and migration. In de Weck AL (ed.) *Differentiated Lymphocyte Functions. Progress in Allergy*, Vol. 28. Basel: Karger, 1981: 193–284.

72. Wood GS. The immunohistology of lymph nodes in HIV infection: a review. In Rotterdam H, Racz P, Greco MA, Cockerell CJ (eds) *Progress in AIDS Pathology*, Vol. 2. New York: Field and Wood, 1991: 25–32.

73. Speigel H, Herbst H, Niedobitek G *et al.* Follicular dendritic cells are a major reservoir for HIV-1 in lymphoid tissues facilitating infection of CD4+ T helper cells. *Pathology* 1992 **140**: 15–22.

74. Steinman RM. The dendritic cell system and its role in immunogenicity. *Annu Rev Immunol* 1991 **9**: 271–296.

75. Lafeuillade A, Tamalet C, Pellegrino, P *et al.* High viral burden in lymph nodes during early stages of HIV infection. *AIDS* 1993 **11**: 1527–1541.

76. Fox CH, Kotler D, Tierney A, Wilson CS, Fauci AS. Detection of HIV-1 RNA in the lamina propria of patients with AIDS and gastrointestinal disease. *J Infect Dis* 1989 **159**: 467–471.

77. Alexander NJ. Sexual transmission of HIV; virus entry into the male and female genital tract. *Fertil Steril* 1990 **54**: 1218.

78. Anderson DJ. Mechanisms of HIV-1 transmission via semen. *J NIH Res* 1992 **4**: 104–108.

79. Wolff H, Anderson DJ. Male genital tract inflammation associated with increased numbers of potential HIV virus host cells in semen. *Andrologia* 1988 **20**: 297–307.

80. Krieger JN, Coombs RW, Collier AC *et al.* Recovery of HIV-1 from semen; minimal impact of stage of infection and current antiviral chemotherapy. *J Infect Dis* 1991 **163**: 477–482.

81. Hussain LA, Kelly CG, Fellowes R *et al.* Expression and gene transcript of Fc receptors for IGg, HLA class II antigens and Langerhans cells in human cervico-vaginal epithelium. *Clin Exp Immunol* 1992 **90**: 530–538.

82. Wei X, Ghosh SK, Taylor ME, Johnson VA, Emini EA *et al.* Viral dynamics in HIV infection. *Nature* 1995 **373**: 117–122.

83. Ho DD, Neumann AU, Perelson AS, Chen W, Leonard JM, Markowitz M. Rapid turnover of plasma virions and CD4 lymphocytes in HIV-1 infection. *Nature*, 1995: **373**: 123–126.

3.15

Fetal and Placental Pathology

AG Howatson

INTRODUCTION

This chapter outlines general principles of the pathology of the fetus and placenta, highlights areas of specific interest, and seeks to demonstrate the contributions of pathological examination to the delivery of obstetric services.[1,2] Limitations of available space make the content highly selective and topics have been chosen from those emphasized in the pathology component of the syllabus for fetal medicine trainees by the Royal College of Obstetricians and Gynaecologists in the UK.

For the purposes of this discussion, the pathology of the fetus will refer to the postembryonic period (9 weeks' gestation to term). This encompasses pre- or non-viable conceptuses as well as stillbirths (babies born dead after 24 weeks of gestation) and will not include the pathology of the neonatal period.

CURRENT CONCEPTS

Fetal pathology

The postmortem examination of the fetus

Examination of fetal remains, whether resulting from therapeutic abortion (for medical indications), spontaneous abortion or stillbirth, is an important part of the delivery of a competent obstetric service.[3] The information thus obtained contributes to the audit of clinical practice including prenatal diagnostic services, is central to genetic counseling and provides essential information to parents following pregnancy failures. There is no place for the belief that avoidance of autopsy requests and examinations is helpful to grieving parents. The stresses and grief of the acute phase are quickly replaced by questions about the reasons for the loss and the possibility of recurrence in future pregnancies; the information from the autopsy can make counseling more accurate and relevant to individual cases.[4,5]

However, some religious groups, e.g. Orthodox Jews, Christian Scientists, some Orthodox Christians and Muslims, do not approve of autopsy examination. Such opposition is not necessarily absolute and religious leaders and teachers of some of these groups have supported flexibility in permitting examination in specific circumstances, e.g. when required by Civil Law or if it can be demonstrated that there is a clear prospect of benefit to others. In circumstances in which dissection is not acceptable, an external examination conducted by a perinatal pathologist, including measurement, photography and skeletal radiology, can provide useful information. The reader is strongly encouraged to consult the papers by Boglioli and Taft[6] and Geller[7] which review the subject of religious objection. In all circumstances where an autopsy is indicated, and it can be argued that there is seldom a case where it is not, a full explanation of the individual importance and specific value of an examination is more likely to lead to permission being granted for either a full examination or a limited examination of a specific organ system or body region.

When consent is given, the remains should be submitted fresh and as promptly as is practicable in order to facilitate cytogenetic and microbiological investigations if appropriate. The fetus is not a small adult and examination should be performed by a pathologist with relevant training and experience. The provision of adequate clinical information and the highlighting of specific areas of interest to the clinician, prior to the start of the examination, is essential. If these conditions are met then the resulting report will be of enhanced value and, perhaps as important, the report of an absence of positive findings can be valued as a confirmation of the genuine absence of any fetal or placental disorder that might indicate risk of recurrence. The details of the autopsy examination are outwith the scope of this text.

Spontaneous abortion

Spontaneous abortion may be classified as early or late. Early abortion occurs in the embryonic period up to the beginning of the ninth week of development whereas late abortion relates to the loss of the previable fetus and includes the period up to 24 weeks of pregnancy.

It has been calculated that up to 50% of conceptuses will abort spontaneously, with the majority of these losses occurring before the eighth week of development and many indeed before pregnancy is recognized clinically.[8-10] Chromosomal abnormalities probably constitute the largest group in the early spontaneous abortion cases[11,12] whereas in late abortion the etiology is more variable and overlaps with the patterns of disorder to be discussed in the remainder of this chapter.

Patterns of fetal abnormality

A major purpose of the fetal autopsy is to identify abnormal appearances, both generalized and localized, and attribute them to specific conditions, syndromes or sequences, thus permitting clear attribution of cause and providing information as to risk of recurrence.

It is not uncommon for the inexperienced observer to misinterpret changes resulting from maceration as features of dysmorphism.[13] Maceration is a normal process that follows fetal death and is particularly marked if there has been a prolonged period of intrauterine retention of the dead fetus. It is a process of tissue autolysis in the absence of bacterial activity. The result, in the early stages, is skin slippage, laxity of ligaments and generalized tissue oedema. A normal fetus may therefore show marked distortion of skull or facial configuration and generalized subcutaneous fluid excess which may be mistaken for mild hydrops fetalis. These changes increase in severity over a period of a few days. If a dead fetus is retained *in utero* for several weeks, fluid absorption occurs and the fetus becomes reduced in size and the tissues become brown or fawn in color as a result of the breakdown of hemoglobin in the fetal circulation.

Other common pathological disorders which result in a generalized abnormality of a fetus are the edema of hydrops fetalis and intrauterine growth retardation.

Hydrops fetalis results from decreased capillary osmotic pressure, increased capillary hydrostatic pressure or increased capillary fluid leakage.[14] These processes are not mutually exclusive. The degree of fluid accumulation in body cavities and soft tissues is variable and even very gross examples, as detected on ultrasound scanning, can resolve. The causes and associations are very numerous.[15,16]

Intrauterine growth retardation may be classified as symmetrical or asymmetrical.[17,18] The symmetrical form occurs in fetuses with reduced growth potential and the effect is of early onset and is uniform. In the asymmetrical form the cause is generally deficient fetal nutrition as a result of uteroplacental pathology and the onset occurs later in pregnancy. The fetus preferentially 'protects' brain development and the brain is therefore proportionately larger than the other organs in relation to body weight. The more common causes include genetic abnormalities, deficient maternal and fetal nutrition, and infection.

Congenital malformations

Congenital malformations can present as morphological defects of single organs or of regions of the body and are the result of single gene disorders, chromosomal abnormalities, multifactorial disorders involving environmental and genetic factors and teratogenic agents. Individual malformations may occur singly or as part of more complex syndromes and sequences.[19] The following examples serve to highlight the potential complexity of these interrelationships and the need for a careful search for associated defects in individual instances.

Neural tube defects

These are among the commonest patterns of abnormality and are frequently diagnosed antenatally as a result of maternal serum alphafetoprotein level elevation or prenatal ultrasound examination.[20,21] Defects of neural tube closure vary from anencephaly with complete spinal dysraphism (Fig. 3.15.1) to occult defects in the lumbosacral spine.[22] Open neural tube defects (myelocele) are almost invariably associated with the development of hydrocephalus secondary to downward displacement of the cerebellum and

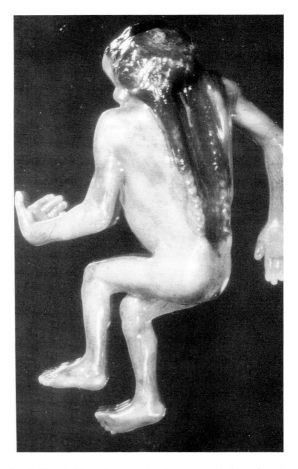

Fig. 3.15.1 *A 16-week fetus showing anencephaly and craniorhachischisis. The brain is a smear of hemorrhagic tissue over the base of the skull, the foramen magnum is absent and most of the length of the neural tube is open.*

brain stem structures through the foramen magnum with resultant obstruction to flow of cerebrospinal fluid through the aqueduct and exit foramina of the fourth ventricle (the Arnold–Chiari malformation).[23] Renal malformations are also common in these cases.[24]

Defects of the skull bones allow protrusion of intracranial contents. In a meningocele only meninges are present whereas an encephalocele will also contain brain tissue. Encephalocele is usually occipital[25] and may indicate a genetic disorder (e.g. Meckel–Gruber syndrome).[26]

Abdominal wall defects

Defects of the anterior abdominal wall present in three forms, namely exomphalos (omphalocele), gastroschisis and body stalk malformation.[27] They must be distinguished from the traumatic abdominal wall disruption not uncommonly seen in macerated fetuses.

Exomphalos results from the failure of the normal physiological reduction of midgut herniation during development and results in a membrane-bound defect involving the base of the umbilical cord (Fig. 3.15.2). The importance of recognizing this abnormality lies in its association with major chromosomal abnormalities (30% of cases) and

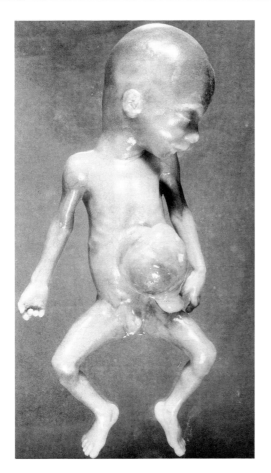

Fig. 3.15.2 *A 20-week fetus showing exomphalos: the abdominal wall defect involves the base of the cord with prolapsed viscera enclosed in a membranous sac.*

other associated major defects (50% of cases). Trisomies 18 and 13 are the most frequent chromosomal abnormalities.[28,29]

Gastroschisis is an abdominal wall defect which is separated from the site of cord attachment to the abdominal wall. Loops of intestine prolapse through the defect and are not enclosed in membranes. Karyotypic abnormalities are not a feature but associated developmental defects, usually of the gastrointestinal tract, are identified in approximately 10% of cases.[30]

Body stalk malformation is part of the spectrum of amnion rupture sequence (see later) and an anterior abdominal wall defect with severe associated spinal and limb deformities are characteristic.

Urinary tract abnormalities

Abnormalities of the urinary tract are frequently identified in prenatal ultrasound examinations. Cystic renal disease can be either sporadic, as in the case of cystic renal dysplasia[31,32] which is part of the spectrum of renal agenesis, or it may be associated with a single gene disorder, as in the case of Meckel–Gruber syndrome or infantile polycystic renal disease. The identification and differentiation of these conditions is vital because of the implications for recurrence (1 in 4 for Meckel–Gruber syndrome and infantile polycystic renal disease).[33] The autosomal recessive conditions highlight the multi-organ involvement of inherited syndromes. In Meckel–Gruber syndrome the characteristic pattern includes encephalocele, polydactyly and polycystic kidneys; congenital hepatic fibrosis is also seen. In infantile polycystic disease, a pattern of congenital hepatic fibrosis is an essential element of the diagnosis and aids separation of this condition from multicystic renal dysplasia and adult polycystic renal disease.[34]

Bladder outlet obstruction as a result of urethral atresia or posterior urethral valves gives rise to urinary tract dilatation and, in particular, enormous dilatation of the bladder. The enlarging bladder causes atrophy of the anterior abdominal wall musculature and this gives rise to the Prune belly syndrome. Survival of a fetus delivered with this syndrome is unusual.[35]

If there is bilateral renal agenesis, aplasia or dysplasia, oligohydramnios will ensue. The result is the characteristic appearance of Potter's facies, talipes equinovarus and associated pulmonary hypoplasia[36] (Fig. 3.15.3).

Osteochondrodysplasia

The correct diagnosis of conditions of skeletal deformity is vitally important.[37] The intrauterine diagnosis by ultrasound of the various conditions resulting in short stature is inaccurate. Clinical photographs are essential in these cases. Postmortem examination, which must include a full radiological skeletal survey, permits the sampling of fetal tissues for genetic studies and aids the identification of the various syndromes and conditions. Bone and epiphyseal growth plate morphology and the associated coexistence of polydactyly and thoracic restriction with pulmonary hypoplasia also help the correct identification of these conditions.

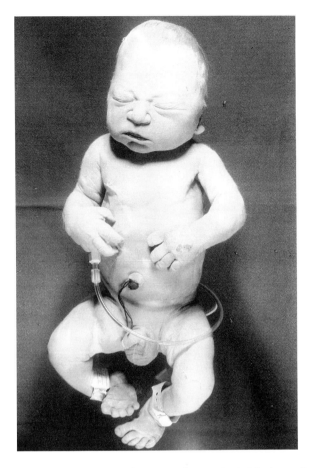

Fig. 3.15.3 *A case of renal agenesis showing typical features of Potter's syndrome: low set ears, flattened nose, small chin, large hands, redundant skin, talipes.*

Amnion rupture sequence

Amnion rupture sequence is a good example of the variability of deformity which can arise when a single disorder occurs at varying times in pregnancy.[38,39] In its more severe form, body stalk malformation with an abnormally short umbilical cord, there is frequently abdominal disruption with reduction limb deformity and spinal deformation. The degree of disorganization of the fetus can be extreme. However, rupture of the amniotic sac can also give rise to patterns of abnormality which are similar to chromosomal defect pathology. This is particularly true of midface clefting which is also frequently seen in Trisomy 13. The correct exclusion of this diagnosis is therefore vital as there is no specific recurrence risk for amnion rupture sequence. Auto-amputation of digits and disruption of the skull vault by amniotic bands, giving rise to encephalocele and anencephalic lesions, is also typical and again should be correctly identified.

Fetal asphyxia and birth injury

The examination of the fetus and placenta in a suspected case of fetal asphyxia or birth injury is greatly aided by the provision of good clinical information regarding the circumstances of the period of labor and delivery.

Various congenital malformations, particularly of the heart and lungs, and intrauterine infections can masquerade as examples of delivery-related asphyxia, a diagnosis which may have medicolegal implications. In cases of fetal asphyxia there may be evidence of umbilical cord obstruction or intrauterine passage of meconium but, more often, no external abnormality is evident. The internal organs are frequently congested and hemorrhages in the thymus, lungs, kidneys and brain are typical. Chronic intrauterine hypoxic stress may be suggested by evidence of thymic involution and adrenal steatosis. Histology may show meconium aspiration or excess amniotic cellular aspirate in the lungs.

Minor birth injuries, bruising, scalp hematoma and skin laceration, are relatively common and are of no clinical consequence. More serious traumatic injuries include nerve palsy and long bone fractures.[40] The pathologist is most likely to see intracranial hemorrhage, with or without skull fractures, as a result of hypoxia with precipitant delivery or instrumentation. Subdural hemorrhage from torn bridging vessels, and tears of the falx and tentorium are the most common of these injuries.

Pathology of the placenta

The placenta should be submitted for examination in all cases of fetal death (whether autopsy is requested or not), in all other pregnancies in which there has been any clinical abnormality, and if a placental abnormality is noted at delivery.

Abnormalities of the umbilical cord

The role of cord abnormalities in fetal loss is frequently controversial. Adequate cord length is necessary for normal fetal passage during vaginal delivery, excessive cord length is associated with increased risk of prolapse through the cervical os or of fetal entanglement with obstruction.[41–43] The cord insertion into the placenta is variable but only the velamentous type (coursing through the membranes prior to insertion into the placental disk) is potentially problematic with a risk of vessel rupture or obstruction and subsequent fetal death.[44–46]

True cord knots occur in up to 2% of pregnancies and most have no clinical sequelae. Obstruction of cord vessels by knots is rare. Cord obstruction secondary to torsion is usually seen at the fetal end and may, rarely, cause fetal death.[47,48]

The presence of a single umbilical artery is seen in up to 1% of births. There is a significantly increased frequency of fetal malformation and chromosomal disorders in such cases.[49–51]

Placental pathology

Abnormalities of the placenta which may compromise fetal well-being can be divided into:

1. disorders of conformation and implantation;
2. focal lesions of placental parenchyma;
3. infections;
4. disorders of hemochorial placentation (excluding gestational trophoblastic disease which is dealt with in Chapter 4.7).

Of these points (3) and (4) constitute the vast majority of significant placental pathologies.

Disorders of conformation and implantation

Variation in placental shape and the presence of accessory lobes have virtually no bearing on the successful outcome of a pregnancy. Size is variable and correlates strongly with fetal size. The placenta has considerable adaptive potential and will increase in size to match increased functional demands.

Extrachorial placentation, i.e. where the surface area of the chorionic plate is less than that of the basal (maternal) surface area, is recognized in two forms, which may coexist in the same placenta. In the circummarginate type, which is of no clinical significance, the transition from chorion to extra-chorionic membrane is a flat ring around the placenta. In the circumvallate type, which is associated with an increased frequency of small for gestational age babies but not with increased fetal loss, the transition is marked by a raised rolled membrane ring.[52]

The site and nature of placental implantation is of more clinical import. In placenta previa, the lower uterine segment implantation increases the risk of antepartum hemorrhage. In placenta accreta, the chorionic villi directly invade the myometrium with no intervening decidua. In these cases there is an increased incidence of incomplete placental separation with postpartum hemorrhage.

Focal lesions of placental parenchyma

Lesions of the parenchyma are common and can be separated into those of clinical significance and those which can be ignored.

Foci of placental calcification (most often seen on the maternal surface), cysts, and small thrombi are of no consequence.[53,54]

Perivillous fibrin deposition, visible as well-demarcated white plaques which appear to replace areas of the placental parenchyma, are seen in over 20% of normal placentae.[54] The deposition of fibrin and the encasement of villi, resulting from turbulent blood flow in the maternal space, excludes them from the process of gaseous exchange but even extensive deposition involving up to 30% of the placental substance does not appear to have any deleterious affect on the fetus. This is an indication of the functional reserve of otherwise normal placentae and contrasts with infarction with loss of placental parenchyma (see below). Some studies have suggested that massive deposition of fibrin involving the villi underlying the maternal surface, so-called maternal floor infarction, is associated with abortion and increased risk of stillbirth.[55,56]

Placental infarcts can be recognized in their fresh state as firm, dark-red foci which become pale, and eventually white, with the passage of time. These lesions are frequently identified in normal placentae but are more common in pregnancies complicated by hypertension or pre-eclampsia and in the placentae of fetuses showing intrauterine growth retardation. If more than 10% of the placental mass has been infarcted, this is indicative of a significant abnormality of uteroplacental blood supply.[54] In these situations the presence of infarcts is a marker of a more deeply seated and basic abnormality of hemochorial placentation (see Chapter 3.6) and the volume of infarction alone is seldom, if ever, sufficient to explain the poor fetal nutrition.

Placental hemorrhage is a result of premature separation of the placenta. Marginal hemorrhages will present as antepartum vaginal bleeding and will be associated with small foci of decidual necrosis. Large retained retroplacental clots with significant placental separation (abruptio placentae) are associated with a high incidence of intrauterine fetal death. These lesions can be recognized macroscopically by a crater or indentation on the maternal surface, which may or may not be filled by blood clot, and histologically by areas of decidual necrosis and disruption with intervillous hemorrhage.[57,58]

Placental hemangiomas or chorangiomas are seen in approximately 1% of all placentae. Most of these lesions are incidental findings, frequently during histological examination of random sections, and are only a few millimeters in diameter. As such, they have no clinical significance. Larger lesions, in excess of 5 cm in diameter, can be associated with fetal compromise as a result of high output cardiac failure secondary to vascular shunting within the hemangioma, or following consumption of platelets or red cells during passage of blood through the lesion. In these instances the fetus may exhibit hydrops or anemia. Hemangiomas are recognized by their dark, congested appearance and are usually well-demarcated from the adjacent parental parenchyma. Histology shows them to have the structure of simple capillary hemangiomas.[54]

Infections

Microorganisms can infect the placenta in three main ways, i.e. by the ascending route from the vagina, by the hematogenous route from the maternal bloodstream, and as a result of invasive investigations, such as amniocentesis, fetoscopy and chorionic villus sampling.

Infection by the ascending route results in development of acute chorioamnionitis with neutrophil polymorphonuclear leucocyte infiltration of the membranes and cord. The presence of membrane infection can lead to premature rupture of membranes and premature labour. Ascending infection is also more likely to occur in situations of premature rupture of membranes and delay in progress of labor. The organisms involved are of the vaginal flora.[59,60]

Hematogenous infection is by organisms present in the maternal bloodstream. These infections give rise to villus inflammation and villitis is recognized in up to 10% of all placentae in various studies.[61–63] Foci of villitis are usually widely scattered. In bacterial infection, such as listeriosis, the inflammatory cells are usually a mixture of lymphocytes and histiocytes. In viral infections the infiltrate is more usually lymphocytic. The presence of focal villitis does not necessarily imply that an organism can be isolated and in most instances of villitis, no microorganism is detectable despite a full series of investigations. The presence of focal villitis, usually of the lymphocytic pattern, is strongly suggestive of viral infection, and may be associated with intrauterine growth retardation.[64]

The increasing use of invasive procedures for therapeutic purposes or genetic studies, exposes the fetal environment to a risk of contamination. Fortunately this is rare but has to be accepted as a risk of these procedures.

Disorders of hemochorial placentation

In recent years our understanding of the pathology of 'placental insufficiency', namely pre-eclampsia, small-for-gestational-age babies, and intrauterine growth retardation has been revolutionized. The pattern of macroscopic and histological abnormalities seen in the placental parenchyma of such cases are now known to be secondary phenomena which result from a primary defect in hemochorial placentation.

The development of an adequate maternal blood flow to the fetus and placenta is dependent on the invasion of muscular maternal spiral arteries by extra-villus or interstitial trophoblast with resultant transformation and replacement of the muscular walls by fibrinoid material which results in the arteries becoming dilated sinusoidal vessels. This process appears to occur in two phases with the decidual phase preceding a similar process in the myometrial segments of these spiral arteries. The whole process is complete by approximately 24 weeks.[65-67]

It is now clear that disturbance of the development of these normal physiological vascular changes is a common feature in a range of clinical obstetric problems which have been regarded as a consequence of inadequate fetal nutrition secondary to 'placental insufficiency'. The defects in hemochorial placentation can occur at any stage in its development and can also be manifest in terms of a deficiency in extent, in which case only a proportion of spiral arteries will undergo physiological changes.[68-70]

The more recent observation of an absence of physiological vascular changes in maternal spiral arterioles identified in products of conception from early pregnancy spontaneous abortion provides further evidence of the central role of this process in determination of successful pregnancy.[71]

The identification of abnormalities of hemochorial placentation is complicated by the variability of this process over the area of placental attachment. Formal placental bed biopsies are clearly not available in normal vaginal deliveries and are very seldom made available during Cesarean section deliveries. It is known that the frequency and intensity of physiological vascular changes decreases towards the periphery of placental attachment. Failure to observe physiological changes at the placental margin may therefore not be significant. However, the presence of unaltered maternal spiral arterioles in the presence of substantial numbers of interstitial trophoblastic cells in a pregnancy with a consistent clinical history can usually be regarded as conclusive evidence of a failure of this basic and vital process.

Pathology of placental insufficiency

In most instances, uteromaternal vessels/maternal spiral arterioles are not included in tissue blocks sampled from placentae of patients with pre-eclampsia or patients who have small-for-gestational-age or intrauterine growth-retarded fetuses. However histological examination frequently reveals a number of abnormalities.[72,73] The normal development of the placental villus architecture and, in particular, the formation of terminal villi may be retarded with the result that the terminal villi are small and show prominent syncytial knots. Other abnormalities include an increase in stromal content in villi, retarded development of villus capillaries and vasculosyncytial membrane formation, a thickening of the trophoblastic basement membranes and an increase in cytotrophoblastic cells in terminal villi. The cytotrophoblast is the generative component of the placenta and proliferation of these cells presumably reflects a response to ischemic injury and a resultant repair mechanism. These features are consistent with a diminished surface area for oxygen and nutritional transport.

In pre-eclampsia, uteromaternal vessels may also show acute atherosis which is characterized by an infiltrate of foamy, lipid-rich, macrophages within the vessel wall with associated fibrinoid necrosis and a variable perivascular lymphocytic infiltrate.[74,75]

FUTURE PERSPECTIVES

The role of the fetal autopsy examination has not diminished in importance with the development of increasingly sophisticated methods of prenatal diagnosis. In fact the reverse is true, as audit of the accuracy of ultrasound and other diagnostic techniques is an important part of obstetric practice. The autopsy provides part of that audit.

As we enter an era of more extensive use of intrauterine therapy, perinatal pathology may expand from its current base in autopsy examination, to include examination of biopsies of fetal tissue taken in life. In addition, new interventions may bring fresh iatrogenic pathology. Obstetricians will require specialist pathology services to assess and understand these processes.

The recent emphasis on the contribution of fetal life and pathology to disease in adult life has opened new areas of research. In many instances the elucidation of the mechanisms will lie in studies of fetal organs and tissues.[76-82]

Other major obstetric problems remain unsolved. The pathogenesis of late intrauterine death remains, for the most part, a mystery and pregnancy failures of this type are perhaps more tragic than most. Investigation of the fetal control of the onset of labour and studies of fetal cell kinetics may well provide useful insights.

In the placenta, the underlying pathogenesis of the failure of development of physiological changes in the walls of the maternal arterioles is a key area for future research. The genetic or environmental basis for a failure of trophoblast to invade or of maternal arterioles to respond to the process of invasion remains to be determined. The possible role of immune interactions between maternal tissues and trophoblast in this process is the source of much conjecture.[83,84] Another major area of interest will be in the regulation of placental angiogenesis and the role of endothelial growth factors. The nature of the vasoactive substances that regulate placental blood flow and fetal vascular tone is the focus of much current research interest. Endothelin[85,86] and atrial naturetic peptide[87,88] are among several molecules that may play an important part in these processes.

SUMMARY

- The fetal autopsy is an important element of the provision of a competent obstetric service.
- The fetal autopsy is central to clinical audit and parental counseling.
- Placental examination is indicated in all cases of fetal autopsy and in all cases of obstetric complications and pregnancy related disorders.
- Provision of adequate clinical information, in advance of the examination, is essential.
- Changes of maceration can be confused with fetal anomaly.
- The presence of fetal anomalies is an indication for karyotypic studies.

- Complex patterns of fetal malformation are not necessarily either of genetic origin or associated with a risk of recurrence.
- Infection remains an important and avoidable cause of pregnancy loss.
- The majority of macroscopic placental lesions, other than infarction and abruption, are of little consequence in terms of fetal well-being.
- Disorders of hemochorial placentation underlie much obstetric pathology from early spontaneous abortion to pregnancy induced hypertension, pre-eclampsia and intrauterine growth retardation.

REFERENCES

1. Keeling JW (ed.) *Fetal and Neonatal Pathology.* London: Springer-Verlag, 1993.
2. Dimmick JE, Kalousek DK (eds) *Developmental Pathology of the Embryo and Fetus.* Phildelphia: JB Lippincott, 1992.
3. Naeye RL. The investigation of perinatal deaths. *N Engl J Med* 1983 **309**: 611–612.
4. Alberman E. Prospects for better perinatal health. *Lancet* 1980 **i**: 189–192.
5. Berger LR. Requesting the autopsy. A pediatric perspective. *Clin Pediatr* 1987 **17**: 445–452.
6. Boglioli LR, Taff ML. Religious objection to autopsy: an ethical dilemma for medical examiners. *Am J Forensic Med Pathol* 1990 **11**: 1–8.
7. Geller SA. Religious attitudes and the autopsy. *Arch Pathol Lab Med* 1984 **108**: 494–498.
8. Wilcox AJ, Weinberg CR, O'Conner JF *et al.* Incidence of early loss of pregnancy. *N Engl J Med* 1988 **319**: 189–194.
9. Yovich JL. Embryo quality and pregnancy rates in in-vitro fertilization. *Lancet* 1985 **i**: 283–284.
10. Opitz JM. Prenatal and perinatal death: the future of developmental pathology. *Paediatr Pathol* 1987 **7**: 363–394.
11. Warburton D, Stein Z, Kline J, Susser M. Chromosomal abnormalities in spontaneous abortion: data from the New York Study. In Porter IH, Hook EB (eds) *Human Embryonic and Fetal Death*, New York: Academic Press, 1980: 261–287.
12. Bouè A, Bouè J, Gropp A. Cytogenetics of pregnancy wastage. *Adv Hum Genet* 1985 **14**: 1–57.
13. Hill LM, Macpherson T, Belfar HL, Kislak S. Role of the perinatal autopsy in evaluating unusual sonographic findings of intrauterine fetal death. *Am J Perinatol* 1986 **6**: 331–333.
14. Giacoia GP. Hydrops fetalis (fetal edema), a survey. *Clin Pediatr* 1980 **19**: 334–339.
15. Machin GA. Hydrops revisited: literature review of 1414 cases published in the 1980's. *Am J Med Genet* 1989 **34**: 366–390.
16. Keeling JW. Hydrops fetalis and other forms of excess fluid collection in the fetus. In Wigglesworth JS, Singer DB (eds) *Textbook of Fetal and Perinatal Pathology.* Oxford: Blackwell Scientific, 1991: 429–454.
17. Evans MI, Lin C-C. Retarded fetal growth. In Lin C-C, Evans MI (eds) *Intrauterine Growth Retardation.* New York: McGraw-Hill, 1984: 55.
18. Pearce JM, Campbell S. Intrauterine growth retardation. *Birth Defects* 1985 **21**: 109.
19. Spranger J, Benirschke K, Hall JG *et al.* Errors of morphogenesis: concepts and terms. Recommendations of an International Working Group. *J Pediatr* 1982 **100**: 160–165.
20. Elwood JM, Elwood JH. *Epidemiology of Anencephaly and Spina Bifida.* Oxford: Oxford University Press, 1980.
21. Laurence KM. The declining incidence of neural tube defects in the UK. *Z Kinderchir* 1989 **41**: 51.
22. Holmes LB, Driscol SG, Atkins L. Etiologic heterogenecity of neural tube defects. *N Engl J Med* 1976 **294**: 365–369.
23. Cameron AH. The Arnold–Chiari and other neuroanatomical malformations associated with spina bifida. *J Pathol Bacteriol* 1957 **73**: 195–211.
24. Cameron AH. Malformations of the neuro-spinal axis urogenital tract and foregut in spina bifida attributable to disturbances of the blastopore. *J Pathol Bacteriol* 1957 **73**: 213–221.
25. Campbell RL, Dayton DH, Sohal GS. Neural tube defects: a review of human and animal studies on the etiology of neural tube defects. *Teratology* 1986 **34**: 171.
26. Fraser FC, Lytwyn A. Spectrum of anomalies in the Meckel syndrome, or: 'maybe there is a malformation syndrome with at least one constant anomaly.' *Am J Med Genet* 1981 **9**: 67–73.
27. Baird PA, McDonald EC. An epidemiologic study of congenital malformations of the anterior abdominal wall in more than half a million consecutive livebirths. *Am J Hum Genet* 1981 **33**: 470–478.

28. Grilbert W, Nicolaides KH. Fetal omphalocoele: associated malformations and chromosomal defects. *Obstet Gynecol* 1987 **70**: 633–635.

29. Torfs C, Curry C, Roeper P. Gastroschisis. *J Pediatr* 1990 **116**: 1–6.

30. Colombani PM, Cunningham MD. Perinatal aspects of omphalocele and gastroschisis. *Am J Dis Child* 1977 **131**: 1386–1388.

31. Risdon RA. Renal dysplasia I. A clinicopathological study of 76 cases. *J Clin Pathol* 1971 **24**: 57–65.

32. Risdon RA. Renal dysplasia II. A necropsy study of 41 cases. *J Clin Pathol* 1971 **24**: 65–71.

33. Risdon RA. Cystic diseases of the kidney and reflux nephropathy. In Anthony PP, MacSween RNM (eds) *Recent Advances in Histopathology*, no 11. Edinburgh: Churchill Livingstone, 1981: 163–184.

34. Bernstein J. Hepatic involvement in hereditary renal syndrome. *Birth Defects* 1987 **23**: 115–130.

35. Wigger HJ, Blanc WA. The prune belly syndrome. *Pathol Annu* 1977 **12**: 17–39.

36. Potter EL. Facial characteristics of infants with bilateral renal agenesis. *Am J Obstet Gynecol* 1946 **51**: 885–888.

37. Gilbert EF, Yang SS, Langer L, Opitz JM, Roskamp JO, Heidelberger KP. Pathologic changes of osteochondrodysplasia in infancy, a review. *Pathol Annu* 1987 **22**: 283–345.

38. Seeds JW, Cefalo RC, Herbert WNP. Amniotic band syndrome. *Am J Obstet Gynecol* 1982 **144**: 243–248.

38. Kalousek DK, Bramforth S. Amnion rupture sequence in previable fetuses. *Am J Med Genet* 1988 **31**: 63–73.

40. Walker CHM. Birth trauma. In Crawford JW (ed.) *Risks of Labour*. Chichester: Wiley 1985: 71–93.

41. Bain C, Elliot BW. Fetal distress in the first stage of labour associated with early fetal heart decelerations and a short umbilical cord. *Aust NZ J Obstet Gynaecol* 1976 **16**: 51–56.

42. Sornes T. Short umbilical cord as a cause of fetal distress. *Acta Obstet Gynecol Scand* 1989 **68**: 609.

43. Spellacy WN, Gravem H, Fisch RO. The umbilical cord complications of true knots, nuchal coils and cords around the body. *Am J Obstet Gynecol* 1966 **94**: 1136.

44. Hovatta O, Lipasti A, Rapola J, Karjalainen O. Causes of stillbirth: a clinicopathologic study of 243 patients. *Br J Obstet Gynaecol* 1983 **90**: 691–696.

45. Kouyoumdjian A. Velamentous insertion of the umbilical cord. *Obstet Gynecol* 1980 **56**: 737–742.

46. Uyanwah-Akpom P, Fox H. The clinical significance of marginal and velamentous insertion of the cord. *Br J Obstet Gynaecol* 1977 **84**: 941–943.

47. Blickstein I, Shoham-Schwartz Z, Lancet M. Predisposing factors in the formation of true knots of the umbilical cord – analysis of morphometric and perinatal data. *Int J Gynaecol Obstet* 1987 **25**: 395–398.

48. Matorras R, Diez J, Pereira JG. True knots in the umbilical cord: clinical findings and fetal consequences. *J Obstet Gynaecol* 1990 **10**: 383–386.

49. Peckham CH, Yerulshamy J. Aplasia of one umbilical artery: incidence by race and certain obstetric factors. *Obstet Gynecol* 1965 **26**: 359–366.

50. Heifetz SA. Single umbilical artery: a statistical analysis of 237 autopsy cases and a review of the literature. *Perspect Pediatr Pathol* 1984 **8**: 345–378.

51. Lilja M. Infants with single umbilical artery studied in a national registry 2. Survival and malformations in infants with single umbilical artery. *Paediatr Perinat Epidemiol* 1991 **5**: 27–36.

52. Fox H, Sen DK. Placenta extrachorialis: a clinico-pathological study. *J Obstet Gynaecol Br Cmwlth* 1972 **79**: 32–35.

53. Tindall VR, Scott JS. Placental calcification: a study of 3025 singleton and multiple pregnancies. *J Obstet Gynaecol Br Cmwlth* 1965 **72**: 356.

54. Fox H. *Pathology of the Placenta*. London: Saunders, 1978.

55. Andres RL, Kuyper W, Resnick R, Piacquadio KM, Benirschke K. The association of maternal floor infarction with adverse perinatal outcome. *Am J Obstet Gynecol* 1990 **163**: 935–938.

56. Clewell WH, Marchester DK. Recurrent maternal floor infarction: a preventable cause of fetal death. *Am J Obstet Gynecol* 1983 **147**: 346–347.

57. Krohn M, Voigt L, McKnight B, Daling JR, Starzyk P, Benedetti TJ. Correlates of placental abruption. *Br J Obstet Gynaecol* 1987 **94**: 333–340.

58. Dommisse J, Tiltman AJ. Placental bed biopsies in placental abruption. *Br J Obstet Gynaecol* 1992 **99**: 651–654.

59. Zaaijma JT, Wilkinson AR, Keeling JW, Mitchell RG, Turnbull AC. Spontaneous premature rupture of the membranes: bacteriology, histology and neonatal outcome. *J Obstet Gynecol* 1982 **2**: 155.

60. Naeye RL. Functionally important disorders of the placenta, umbilical cord and fetal membranes. *Hum Pathol* 1987 **18**: 680–691.

61. Altshuler G, Russell P. The human placental villitides: a review of chronic intrauterine infection. *Curr Top Pathol* 1975 **60**: 63–112.

62. Fox H. Placental involvement in maternal systemic infection. *Perspect Pediatr Pathol* 1981 **6**: 63–81.

63. Knox WF, Fox H. Villitis of unknown aetiology: its incidence in placentae from a British population. *Placenta* 1984 **5**: 394–402.

64. Russell P. Inflammatory lesions of the human placenta. III: the histopathology of villitis of unknown aetiology. *Placenta* 1980 **1**: 227–244.

65. Brosens I, Robertson WB, Dixon HG. The physiological response of the vessels of the placental bed to normal pregnancy. *J Pathol Bacteriol* 1967 **93**: 569–579.

66. Pijnenborg R, Robertson WB, Brosens I, Dixon G. Trophoblast migration and the establishment of haemochorial placentation in man and laboratory animals. *Placenta* 1981 **2**: 71–92.

67. Robertson WB, Khong TY, Brosens I, De Wolf F, Sheppard B, Bonnar J. The placental bed biopsy. A review from three European centers. *Am J Obstet Gynecol* 1986 **155**: 401–412.

68. Brosens I, Robertson WB, Dixon HG. The role of the spiral arteries in the pathogenesis of pre-eclampsia. *Obstet Gynecol Annu* 1972 **1**: 177–191.

69. Adthabe O, Labarrere C, Telenta M. Maternal vascular lesions in placentae of small-for-gestational age infants. *Placenta* 1985 **6**: 265–276.

70. McFadeyn IR, Price AB, Geirrson RT. The relation of birth weight to histological appearances in the vessels of the placental bed. *Br J Obstet Gynaecol* 1986 **93**: 476–481.

71. Khong TY, Liddell HS, Robertson WB. Defective haemochorial placentation as a cause of miscarriage: a preliminary study. *Br J Obstet Gynaecol* 1987 **94**: 649–655.

72. Salafia CM, Vintzileos AM, Silberman L *et al.* Placental pathology of idiopathic intrauterine growth retardation at term. *Am J Perinatol* 1992 **9**: 179–184.

73. Salafia CM, Vogel CA, Bantham KF *et al.* Pre-term delivery: correlations of fetal growth and placental pathology. *Am J Perinatol* 1992 **9**: 190–193.

74. Laberrere CA. Review article: acute atherosis: a histopathological hallmark of immune aggression? *Placenta* 1988 **9**: 95–108.

75. Khong TY. Acute atherosis in pregnancies complicated by hypertension, small-for-gestational age infants and diabetes mellitus. *Arch Pathol Lab Med* 1991 **115**: 722–725.

76. Barker DJP, Osmond C, Goulding J, Kuh D, Wadsworth MEJ. Growth *in utero*, blood pressure in childhood and adult life and mortality from cardiovascular disease. *Br Med J* 1989 **298**: 564–567.

77. Barker DJP, Bull AR, Osmond C, Simmonds SJ. Fetal and placental size and risk of hypertension in adult life. *Br Med J* 1990 **301**: 259–262.

78. Law CM, Barker DJP, Bull AR, Osmond C. Maternal and fetal influences in blood pressure. *Arch Dis Child* 1991 **66:** 1291–1295.
79. Williams S, St George IM, Silva PA. Intrauterine growth retardation and blood pressure at age seven and eighteen. *J Clin Epidemiol* 1992 **345:** 1257–1263.
80. Law CM, de Swiet M, Osmond C *et al.* Initiation of hypertension *in utero* and its amplification throughout life. *Br Med J* 1993 **306:** 24–27.
81. Barker DJP, Martyn CN, Osmond C, Hales CN, Fall CHD. Growth *in utero* and serum cholesterol concentrations in adult life. *Br Med J* 1993 **307:** 1524–1527.
82. Barker DJP. *The Fetal and Infant Origins of Adult Disease.* London: British Medical Journal Books, 1992.
83. Wells M, Bulmer JN. The human placental bed: histology, immunohistochemistry and pathology. *Histopathology* 1988 **13:** 483–498.
84. Bulmer JN. Immune aspects of pathology of the placental bed contributing to pregnancy pathology. *Clin Obstet Gynaecol* 1992 **6:** 461–488.
85. Nakamura T, Kasai K, Konuma S *et al.* Immunoreactive endothelin concentrations in maternal and fetal blood. *Life Sci* 1990 **46:** 1045–1050.
86. Robaut C, Mondon F, Bandet J, Ferre F, Cavero I. Regional distribution and pharmacological characterization of 125-I endothelin-1 binding sites in human fetal placental vessels. *Placenta* 1991 **12:** 55–67.
87. Sen I. Identification and solubilization of atrial naturetic factor receptors in human placenta. *Biochem Biophys Res Commun* 1986 **135:** 480–486.
88. McQueen J, Jardine AG, Kingdom JCP, Templeton A, Whittle MJ, Connell JMC. Interaction of angiotensin II and atrial naturetic peptide in the human fetoplacental unit. *Am J Hypertens* 1990 **3:** 641–644.

Principles of Imaging

WN McDicken

INTRODUCTION

Ultrasonic scanning is by far the most widely applied imaging technique in reproductive medicine. X-ray imaging still finds some application, for example in computerized tomography (CT) pelvimetry, hysterosalpingography and some maternal conditions related to pregnancy, but this is in a very small percentage of cases. Surprisingly little work has been done with magnetic resonance imaging (MRI) in obstetrics. It is thought that this may have value in the study of specific organs such as the fetal lungs and liver, and in growth measurement.[1,2] At present, fetal imaging is achieved with relatively fast scanning techniques which take around 60 s to collect the signals from within the abdomen. More widespread application of MRI may occur when real-time open-field machines become available.[3] The difficulties of patient discomfort and fetal movement are quite severe with present systems. *In vivo* magnetic resonance spectroscopy (MRS) for study of the chemical composition of tissues is just being established for adults. It requires fairly large volumes of tissue (e.g. a cube with sides of 1·5 cm) to provide an adequate signal strength, and it appears to be unsuitable for fetal studies at present.

Because of its importance, the emphasis of this chapter will be on ultrasound.

CURRENT CONCEPTS

Ultrasound

The aspects of diagnostic ultrasound which make it a powerful tool for scientific methods in reproductive medicine are well recognized. Its optimal use requires well-trained staff, quality assurance, and audit schemes.[4]

It is not necessary for the clinical user of medical ultrasound equipment to have a detailed knowledge of the physics and engineering of the technology. However, some knowledge is necessary so that the maximum amount of information can be extracted from the techniques. A basic knowledge is also required so that pitfalls can be avoided and images interpreted accurately.[5-7] All the information which appears in an ultrasonic image has a scientific explanation. As in most fields, a high level of expertise is acquired, step by step, through systematic study. The biggest hazard in this subject is not related to radiation levels but to misdiagnosis.

Transmission and reception of ultrasound by transducers

Ultrasound, like audible sound, is the transmission of mechanical vibrations from a source through a medium such as tissue. The pitch, or frequency, of ultrasound is about 1000 times higher than that which can be heard by the human ear. The source is commonly called a transducer (or a probe) since its active part is a small piezoelectric crystal or plastic element which converts the electrical energy applied to it into mechanical vibrational energy. Even a simple transducer consisting of a single disc-shaped crystal can transmit ultrasound into a narrow region (beam, field) in front of it. This directional capability is unlike our experience with lower frequency audible sound. Modern transducers often have an array of piezoelectric elements which function simultaneously to generate the transmitted ultrasound. The use of an array allows the ultrasound to be transmitted in a narrow zone whose focus can be varied by altering the relative times of excitation of the elements.

The number of oscillations per second which the particles of the medium perform, as the vibration passes, is called the frequency of the ultrasound, for example 500 per second (or 500 Hertz (Hz)) for an audible sound, and 5 000 000 Hz (5 MHz) for ultrasound as used in diagnostic medicine. Sonic vibrations are called 'ultrasound' when their frequency is above the level which the human ear can detect, i.e. above 20 000 Hz (20 kHz). A very important consequence of using ultrasound in the megahertz range (2–30 MHz) is that the wavelengths of the ultrasound in tissue are very short (less than 0.5 mm) compared to the size of the transducer; hence, the spreading out of the transmitted ultrasonic field by the process of diffraction is not a severe problem. Attenuation of the transmitted energy as it passes through tissue determines the frequencies which can be used, e.g. 3 MHz to penetrate 20 cm and 20 MHz for 20 mm; in other words, higher attenuation is experienced at higher frequency. Both pulse-echo and Doppler imaging techniques usually employ short pulses of ultrasound (pulsed wave ultrasound, PW), of a length in tissue 1 mm or less. Some Doppler units use continuous transmission of ultrasound (continuous wave ultrasound, CW).

Echo information from tissues returns to the receiving transducer as a result of a small amount of reflection and scattering of the transmitted ultrasound at large and small tissue boundaries, and even small regions of (weakly reflecting) blood. The magnitude of echoes is determined by the magnitude of the changes in density and rigidity of the tissues at the boundaries. Reception is the converse of transmission and the echo signals are detected from within a narrow reception zone closely resembling the transmission field. Strictly speaking we should use the term 'beam' to describe the combined effect of the narrow transmission field and reception zone to form the region in front of the transducer from which echoes are detected. This narrow beam, typically having a width of 2 or 3 mm at 3 MHz and less at higher frequencies, is normally employed to scan in a plane through body tissues. The narrow beam of small handheld transducers is an exceedingly fortunate feature of ultrasound technology.

Real-time B-mode imaging (pulse-echo imaging)

When an ultrasound beam is directed into tissue, the transducer receives echoes from interfaces, large and small, which lie within the beam. Since the velocity of sound in all soft tissues is close to 1540 m s^{-1}, the time taken for an echo to return to the transducer after transmission can be converted into the depth of the interface which produced the echo. A transducer pointing into complex tissue receives a series of consecutive echoes which can be displayed as a line of bright spots on a display screen. The position of each spot corresponds to the depth of each tissue interface and the degree of brightness (or grayness) to the size of the echo (Fig. 3.16.1). To produce an image the beam is swept through the tissue and for many beam directions, e.g. 200, lines of echoes are displayed in a corresponding direction on the screen. Since the velocity of ultrasound in tissue is extremely high, the echo information for each line is collected virtually instantaneously, e.g. in 0.25 ms, and hence images can be produced rapidly in real-time, e.g. 25 images per second. The real-time feature of ultrasonic imaging has a double bonus in that it enables tissue motion to be viewed directly and also searches

through the abdomen to be carried out with relative ease.

The main requirement of a real-time ultrasonic scanner is that the beam be swept rapidly and repetitively through the plane of scan. One simple way of achieving this is to use a mechanical drive to move a conventional single crystal transducer so that it oscillates, reciprocates or rotates. The narrowness of the beam is normally improved by adding a lens to the front of the crystal to create a focus at a fixed distance from it. A sector-shaped field-of-view is not ideal since a significant part of the fetal anatomy may be close to the transducer and hence only partially imaged.

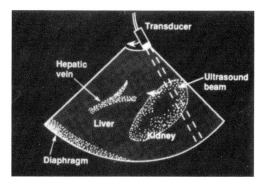

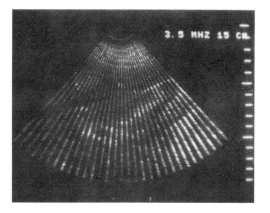

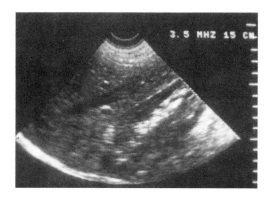

Fig. 3.16.1 *Two-dimensional B-mode image built up from a succession of lines of echo signals. With a large number of lines a complete cross-sectional image is produced.*

Unless it is well-made a transducer with moving parts will be prone to mechanical failure.

A more popular type of transducer for obstetrics is constructed from a number of small piezoelectric elements lying side by side since then it is possible to sweep the beam without moving the transducer. Individual beams are produced by using groups of neighboring elements and the beam is scanned by altering the group used, e.g elements 1 to 32 followed by 2 to 33 and so on. By introducing short time delays between the excitation of the elements the transmitted ultrasound wavefront can be curved, as by a lens, and hence focused. Similarly during reflection, delays introduced to the detected echo signals cause the reception zone to be focused. Indeed during reception an extended focal range can be obtained by altering these delays very rapidly so that the focus always coincides with the depth from which echoes are being received at each instant.[5] Manufacturers put considerable effort into focusing beams since the narrower the beam the sharper the image detail.

Doppler techniques

When ultrasound is reflected from a moving structure or blood cells its frequency is changed due to the Doppler effect.[5,8] For example, 2 MHz ultrasound reflected from blood moving towards the transducer at 30 cm/s would be changed to 2.00078 MHz; for the same speed away from the transducer, the new frequency would be 1.99922 MHz. It can be seen that the Doppler shift in frequency, which is directly proportional to the speed of the target, is only around 1 part in a 1000; however, the electronics of the Doppler instrument, by comparing the transmitted frequency to the received one, can extract a signal at the Doppler shift frequency and also preserve the direction of motion information. A practical situation of a beam interrogating a blood vessel is shown in Fig. 3.16.2. A number of points are worth noting related to the practical use of Doppler.

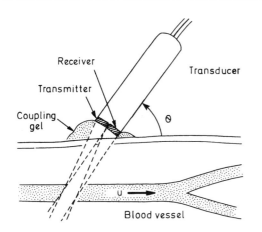

Fig. 3.16.2 *Basic continuous wave (CW) Doppler instrument interrogating a blood vessel lying parallel to the skin surface. If the vessel is not parallel to the skin surface, an imaging mode is required to allow measurement of the beam/vessel angle.*

1. All of the physical factors such as attenuation, refraction, reflection, focusing etc which affect the more familiar pulse-echo B-mode beams also affect Doppler beams.

2. For a beam/vessel angle of $\emptyset$, it is the velocity component, $\mu\cos\emptyset$, along the beam which determines the size of the Doppler shift. At 90°, there is theoretically zero shift since $\cos\emptyset$ is zero and at 0°, the shift is a maximum ($\cos\emptyset=1$). In practise at 90°, a Doppler signal is detected since in a real beam, ultrasound approaches the target from a small range of angles determined by the size of the transducer and the depth of the target.

3. In practice there are rarely blood cells all moving with the same velocity but rather there is a range of velocities in a blood vessel hence a complex Doppler signal is detected containing a range of shift frequencies. Fortunately we have spectrum analysers which can reveal the frequency components in the signal just as the ear analyses audible sound. The frequency components can be converted into absolute velocities if the beam/vessel angle is known and even if this is not possible velocity patterns present at each instant can be deduced.

4. The size of the Doppler shift is dependent on the transmitted ultrasonic frequency i.e. for the same target velocity 5 MHz transmitted ultrasound will produce twice the Doppler shift of 2.5 MHz. This is only a problem if an instrument is changed for one operating at a different ultrasonic frequency.

The simplest Doppler device is the continuous wave (CW) Doppler type which utilizes a double crystal transducer. One crystal transmits and the other receives continuously. Moving structures which fall in the region of overlap of the transmission field and the reception zone give rise to Doppler signals. This region, the sample volume, is quite large and elongated and hence the depth of the moving structure cannot be determined. Despite this limitation CW Doppler devices work well in monitoring of the fetal heart and in the study of patterns of blood velocities in the umbilical cord.

A slightly more complex Doppler device, a pulsed wave (PW) Doppler, emits pulses at regular intervals. These pulses function essentially as samples of a continuous wave and it is possible to process, say 50–100, pulses reflected from a moving target to extract Doppler information. The benefit of the PW principle is that in addition to obtaining velocity information the range of the moving target can be found from the return time of the echoes. Flow at different small sample volumes along the ultrasound beam can be examined by accepting echoes from selected depths, i.e. by moving the small sample volume to sites of interest. Stand-alone PW Doppler units are not used in reproductive medicine but are used in adult cardiac and transcranial studies. Pulsed wave Doppler can be combined with B-mode imaging which allows the Doppler sample volume to be located at any point in the field-of-view of the scanner. This 'duplex' technique was a significant advance which has found application in obstetrics; however, it is now essentially obsolete since it has been replaced by the latest

Doppler technique known as Colour Flow Imaging (CFI).

Doppler information from a number of adjacent sample volumes, say 128, along an ultrasound beam can be obtained by increasing the amount of electronics to handle the additional channels of signal (Fig. 3.16.3). Such multi-gate systems are powerful for the detailed study of hemodynamics where velocity profiles across a vessel are produced in real-time. However, since with PW Doppler, about 50–100 pulses have to be transmitted along each beam direction to provide sufficient samples for the extraction of Doppler shifts the beam cannot be moved quickly enough to collect velocity data for display as an image in real-time. A break-through was made by Kasai[9] who employed faster signal processing to extract the mean velocity in each sample volume using about 10 pulses. Less detailed information on velocities is produced but the mean velocity is obtained about 10 times faster than in PW Doppler processing and hence the beam can be moved reasonably rapidly through the field-of-view. For example, 15 images per second might be produced over a 30° sector scan. The field-of-view and the frame rate are smaller than in pulse-echo B-mode which only requires one pulse per line. Each pixel in the color flow image is usually coded red for flow towards the transducer and blue for flow away. In addition, higher velocity is denoted by making the color brighter.

CFI Doppler makes it much easier to find blood vessels within the body and effectively turns the Doppler technique into a clinical tool for widespread application. As for the duplex mode, a PW sample can be positioned at any point in a color flow image so that a more complete Doppler signal can be obtained and analyzed into its frequency components. This is done by time sharing the beam between the CFI and the PW mode. Indeed, it is possible to present on the display the B-mode echo image, the color image and the output of the spectrum analyzer, the so called 'triplex' mode.

A recently developed type of Doppler image presents the power (energy) of the Doppler signal in each pixel when flow is detected in the corresponding location. In other words, velocity is not displayed but only the magnitude of the Doppler signal detected. This magnitude relates to the amount of blood flow at each location. Interest in this type of image usually relates to the detection of small vessels or to the more complete depiction of regions of flow.

A spectrum analyzer which breaks a Doppler signal down into its frequency components (or velocity components if the beam/vessel angle is known) generates a 'sonogram' or 'spectrogram'. Typically each 5 or 10 ms duration of Doppler signal is analyzed to find the frequency component spectrum present during each short time interval. To generate a sonogram, the first spectrum is displayed with the frequency components as a vertical line of gray shade or color spots and then successive spectra are also placed vertically side by side across the screen so that the horizontal axis represents time. Fig. 3.16.4 shows the sonogram of blood flow in an umbilical artery. It illustrates the importance of keeping the low frequency filter low; otherwise, diastolic flow is artificially cut out. Sonograms are produced in real-time and provide us with highly detailed and quantitative information on blood velocities.

Invasive imaging

As image quality has improved and more clinical information obtained, it has become easier to justify invasive scanning via body orifices and for intraoperative work. The problems of bone, fat, gas and scar tissue are almost completely removed when invasive transducers are employed. In addition, high frequencies are used since the required range of penetration is reduced compared to transabdominal scanning. Typically 5–10 MHz may be used in a transvaginal scanner, and 30 MHz in a catheter scanner for adult intravascular work.[10]

Three-dimensional imaging

Just as a beam can be swept through a plane to create a two-dimensional (2D) image, provided the direction of the

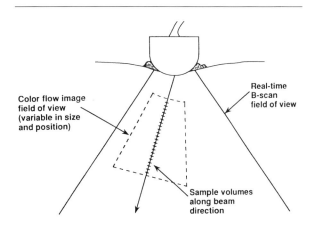

Fig. 3.16.3 *Multiple sample volumes along each beam direction. The beam is swept to produce a color flow image.*

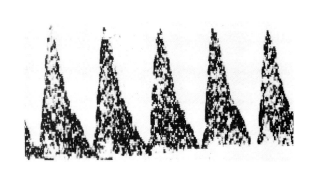

Fig. 3.16.4 *A sonogram from an umbilical artery. The vertical axis is Doppler shift frequency and the horizontal axis is time. The level of the low frequency (wall thump) filter, has been increased manually at successive heart cycles. To show normal flow it is important to display low diastolic flow, i.e. to have the filter set low.*

beam and the return time of the echoes are recorded, a three-dimensional (3D) image can be produced if the direction of the beam and its echo times are recorded as it sweeps through three-dimensional space.[11] While two-dimensional images are readily displayed on a flat TV screen, the display of 3D images is more difficult since the exterior echoes of the scanned volume tend to obscure the interior ones. It is common only to display portions of the collected 3D echo data at any one time. Three-dimensional images are usually generated at present by attaching a motor drive to a 2D scanner so that echo information is collected from a series of parallel scan planes. The 3D transducer scanning system is therefore larger than a typical B-mode array transducer. Three-dimensional systems have also been developed in which a sonic or radio wave transmitter is attached to a normal ultrasound transducer and detecting aerials are located next to the patient. With such systems the beam position and direction can be accurately determined as the transducer is freely moved over the patient.[12,13] Normally, several seconds are required to complete the 3D scan, resulting in a procedure which is not truly real-time. Future developments in transducer technology should make available systems which can scan volumes of interest several times per second. Specialized 3D transducers which can move the beam through 3D space without motion of the whole assembly will be of particular value for invasive imaging since they will help to overcome the loss of flexibility normally associated with internal probes.

One approach to displaying a 3D image is to present a particular view of it on a flat TV screen. It is usually possible to rotate the 3D image to assist interpretation (Fig. 3.16.5). Computer processing can be employed to peel off external echo layers or to smooth echo patterns to create more complete surfaces. However, the full presentation of 3D echo data is difficult. The problem can be eased by displaying a slab of limited thickness of echo data. Perhaps the most useful way of displaying the information is to allow the operator to select any desired slice through the volume. In this mode, slices can be examined which are not accessible to direct scanning due to the presence of bone or the restricted motion of internal transducers. The clinical or scientific value of 3D scanning remains to be ascertained. Accurate volume measurement or depiction of abnormalities are obvious candidates for assessment. Additional planes of scan should also prove valuable since many planes are not accessible to present B-mode techniques.

Color flow Doppler imaging can also be extended to three dimensions. However, as noted above, conventional 2D color flow imaging is already slower than B-mode imaging. A further increase in the data collection time is a consequence of the fact that most arterial flow occurs only during systole. A number of prototype 3D Doppler flow imaging systems have been built and are being assessed in tortuous vascular anatomy and in complex flow patterns within vessels.[14]

Measurement

B-mode and M-mode pulse echo imaging techniques detect echoes from boundaries and are therefore naturally suited to measurement of spatial dimensions. There is an extensive literature on measurement of the developing fetus since it provides direct information on fetal age, growth and abnormalities.[15,16] The accuracy of measurement along the beam direction is typically ~ 0.5 mm for 3 MHz ultrasound and perpendicular to the beam direction ~ 1.0 mm. The accuracy of event timing with real-time B-mode imaging is typically ~ 40 ms for an image

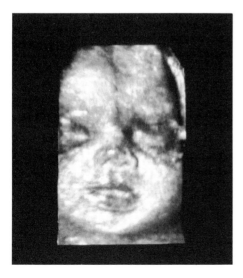
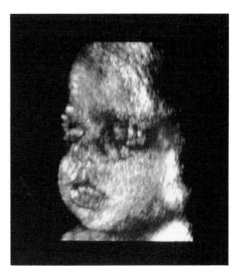

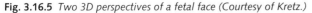

Fig. 3.16.5 *Two 3D perspectives of a fetal face (Courtesy of Kretz.)*

frame rate (sample rate) of 25 s^{-1}. The timing accuracy with M-mode depends on the pulse repetition frequency along the selected beam direction and is typically ~ 2 ms for a PRF of 500 s^{-1}. It could be made smaller by increasing the PRF but 2 ms is more than adequate for most physiological events. Accurate measurement of distance and time obviously allows velocity and acceleration to be calculated. We have seen earlier that an alternative technique for measuring these quantities, particularly blood velocity, exploits the Doppler effect.

Doppler techniques detect the shift in frequency due to the motion of the structure reflecting the ultrasound. As noted, to convert this frequency into velocity, a measure of the angle between the ultrasound beam and the direction of motion needs to be made. The effect of error in this angle measurement on velocity determination depends on the angle being used (Table 3.16.1). The mean velocity measured at a pixel in a color flow image, allowing for beam angle, under ideal conditions can be measured to within about 10%. The peak velocity from a sonogram can be ascertained to within 5%, however 20% is not untypical if sources of error are not minimized. A particular source of error, called 'intrinsic spectral broadening', arises due to the ultrasound in focused beams approaching the moving target at different angles and hence it is not possible to correct for one beam angle in a simple way. It is possible to correct the measurement of peak velocity by determining the smallest angle of approach. As things stand at the moment this large source of error can only be avoided by careful and extensive calibration of the Doppler scanner over its range of operating conditions. Intrinsic spectral broadening is a large source of error in peak velocity measurement when array transducers are strongly focused to produce high resolution images since then a large number of transducer elements (a large aperture) is used as the source of ultrasound. Peak velocities are of prime interest where flow is restricted by a stenosis in a blood vessel or valve orifice.

If it is not required to ascertain velocity absolutely, taking a ratio of velocities, e.g. end-systolic to end-diastolic, can avoid errors due to angle and to intrinsic spectral broadening since they appear in the numerator and denominator and cancel out. The Pulsatility Index and Resistance Index which both relate to the degree of fluctuation in velocity values over the cardiac cycle are commonly used in obstetrics.[17]

Table 3.16.1 Error in velocity at different beam angles for a 3° error in angle measurement

Beam angle	Velocity error (%)
0°	0.1
10°	1.1
20°	2.0
30°	3.1
40°	4.6
50°	6.4
60°	9.2
70°	14.3
80°	29.9

Although ultrasonic techniques are well-suited to measurement, it is essential to have the equipment well-calibrated and to have a strict protocol laid down for performing measurements and checking observer performance.

Needle and catheter guidance

Since needles and catheters are usually made from more rigid and more dense materials than are soft tissues, they normally produce strong echoes which can be observed in an ultrasonic image. The real-time nature of the image allows the tip to be observed as it is guided by the operator through the tissue to the site of interest. For many procedures ultrasonic imaging is the preferred method of guidance.[18] Guidance techniques are commonly employed to sample amniotic fluid, chorion villus and blood from the umbilical cord and conversely to infuse patients. It is also possible to sample fetal tissue. The value of the technique is not only to avoid unsuccessful procedures but also to provide good quality samples for laboratory investigation.

Some care must be exercised in truly identifying the tip of the needle or catheter as distinct from the echo from the rest of their structure. This is particularly true when the 'free-hand' approach is used in which there is no direct physical connection between the needle and the scanning transducer. The operator then needs to develop coordination between the transducer in one hand and the needle in the other. An understanding of where the needle is expected to appear in the image is also required. A more precise, if less flexible, approach is to pass the needle through a guidance channel attached to the transducer ensuring that the needle passes along a defined path in the field-of-view. Guidance channels are intended to attach to transducers without causing undue restrictions; however, since tissue sampling requires manual dexterity they need to be evaluated fully prior to purchase. Added precision can be achieved when a needle is employed which has a small crystal attached to it for detecting when the ultrasound beam is striking the tip.[19,20]

Contrast agents

By far the most successful ultrasonic contrast agents are those based on the very strong scattering of ultrasound by microbubbles, more than a million times stronger than for solid particles of similar size.[21] They have been developed primarily for studies of the heart and the rest of the vascular system (Fig. 3.16.6). At present a few are available commercially and there is a great deal of activity by several companies aimed at producing a range of agents. The very strong scattering of these microbubbles is the result not only of the large difference in acoustic impedance between gas and liquid but also due to the fact that, by coincidence, bubbles of a size which pass through the lung (less than 5 μm) resonate at the low megahertz frequencies used to scan the heart and abdomen.

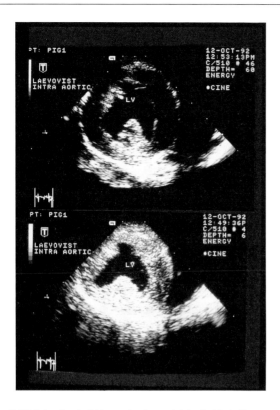

Fig. 3.16.6 *A microbubble contrast agent injected into the coronary of artery of an experimental animal.* **Top,** *low level signals from myocardium.* **Bottom,** *enhanced signal from myocardium due to scatter from the microbubbles.*

Hysterosalpingo-contrast sonography is a technique used in gynecology for determining tubal patency and causes of female sterility. Echo contrast is injected via a transcervical catheter, distending and highlighting the uterine cavity and Fallopian tube lumen. A transvaginal ultrasound probe permits visualization of the passage of contrast through the tubes.[22] The contrast agent used by these investigators consisted of a suspension of soluble galactose microparticles to which air bubbles are bound. The microparticles are suspended in a carrier solution and following injection the galactose microparticles dissolve releasing the bubbles. It remains to be seen if this technique will have an impact on the use of the well-established low-dose X-ray contrast method for delineating the Fallopian tubes.

Contrast agents are essentially a new tool which expands the use of diagnostic ultrasound. No significant toxicity problems have been reported for microbubble agents.[23,24] No reports have been made of their use in the fetus.

Safety

Although at the levels of intensity used in diagnostic machines, ultrasound is not an ionizing radiation like X-rays, it does involve the transmission of energy into the patient.[25] It is therefore important to know the maximum intensity transmitted by each machine/transducer combination and to relate these values to current literature on safety. When we consider that almost the entire population of the Western World is now scanned *in utero* it is obvious that due attention should be paid to radiation safety. The widespread use of ultrasound hinders safety studies since it is difficult to find unexposed control populations.

The intensity of an ultrasonic beam at a point is the rate of flow of energy through unit area placed perpendicularly to the direction of the beam at the point, e.g. 200 mW/cm² at the focus of the beam. The power of a beam is the rate of flow of energy through the whole cross-sectional area of the beam, e.g. 100 mW. The physical parameter most commonly quoted with regard to safety is the intensity averaged over time and measured at the point in the beam where it has its maximum (peak) value, i.e. intensity (spatial peak, temporal average), Ispta. All manufacturers should supply the values of Ispta for the particular machine/transducer combinations which they sell. Both Ispta and power are of interest when consideration is being given to tissue heating. There is also interest in the maximum value of the negative pressure variation in the ultrasound wave as this can generate small bubbles which exhibit cavitation in the transmission medium.[5,25] Cavitation is bubble activity due to resonance or collapse and can damage tissue. It has not been proven to be of significance in tissue for the pressure variations present in diagnostic ultrasound waves. In future it will be easier for operators to have knowledge of exposures when the most appropriate quantities such as intensity and pressure or indices related to heating (thermal index) and cavitation (mechanical index) have been agreed upon and are presented on the display screen.

Several organizations, for example the European Federation of Societies for Ultrasound in Medicine and Biology (EFSUMB) and the American Society of Ultrasound in Medicine, scrutinize the current literature on biological effects and put out statements at regular intervals. In its statement of June 1993 EFSUMB said:

> *Ultrasound imaging for diagnostic purposes in obstetrics has been in extensive clinical use for more than 25 years. Numerous investigations, of various degrees of sophistication, have been undertaken in an endeavour to detect adverse effects. None of these studies have proven that ultrasound at the diagnostic level as used today has led to any deleterious effect to the fetus or mother.[26]*

The statement carries on to say that

> *Routine clinical scanning of every woman during pregnancy using real-time B-mode imaging is not contra-indicated by the evidence currently available from biological investigations and its performance should be left to clinical judgement.*

This is in line with current thinking that the ALARA (as low as reasonably achievable) principle is the best approach to governing the use of radiations in medicine rather than attempting to fix maximum permissible output levels, since the risk should be weighed against the benefit to the patient. No safety threshold levels can be specified from current knowledge but it is generally agreed that Ispta and the negative pressure should be kept below 100 mW cm^{-2} and 4 MPa respectively if possible.

Pulsed Doppler devices in duplex scanners use high pulsing rates with a fixed beam direction to enable them to measure high velocities. EFSUMB considers that since there is a possibility of significant temperature rise in tissues in such an arrangement that

> *routine examinations of the first trimester embryo using pulsed Doppler devices is considered inadvisable at present. It is advisable to minimise exposure time in pulsed Doppler mode during fetal examinations, and particularly when fetal bone structures may lie within the Doppler beam.*

EFSUMB also endorsed the clinical safety statement made by the American Institute of Ultrasound in Medicine.[27] The moving beam of a color flow imager will not produce the significant temperature rise referred to, however care needs to be exercised to ensure that the Doppler duplex mode is not inadvertently used.

The question of the safety of transvaginal scanning has been raised since the embryo or fetus is nearer to the transducer. However, the decreased penetration required allows lower powers to be used, the higher frequency is attenuated faster in intervening tissue and the improved image detail results in reduced scanning time. EFSUMB states that transvaginal B-mode imaging is not contraindicated where clinically indicated or for early pregnancy screening where there are firm clinical grounds. Routine examination of every woman with transvaginal Doppler techniques is not recommended due to the possibility of tissue heating. As for transabdominal scanning, the ALARA principle should be applied for transvaginal scanning.[28]

When invasive techniques are utilized, electrical and mechanical systems should be checked by personnel with expertise in safety of biomedical instrumentation. The hazard from mechanical failure is obvious but it should be borne in mind that very small electrical currents within the body can affect cardiac function or stimulate other muscles. Combinations of scanners and other electronic instruments also require careful checks.

FUTURE PERSPECTIVES

Pulse-echo B-mode imaging to produce two-dimensional images can be regarded as a mature technology and hence the rate of improvement has levelled off in recent years. One area of further improvement will be in the image quality of small portable scanners for use in clinics and the community. On the other hand Doppler technology is relatively immature, the rate of improvement is quite rapid and in addition new techniques are still being introduced. In time, Doppler facilities will be standard features of all scanners. Three-dimensional imaging for both B-mode and Doppler methods are at an early stage of development and can be awkward to use; however no doubt in time the natural evolution of technology will match them better to medical applications. Invasive imaging will benefit from the advance in 3D techniques. The drive for the development of contrast agents comes mainly from cardiology and oncology; if required a new tool could be available for studies in reproductive medicine.

To date ultrasonic techniques have proven remarkably safe. All involved in the design and use of these techniques have a responsibility to keep them safe. If international guidelines are followed, ultrasound should remain a safe and valuable tool.

SUMMARY

- The basic principles of pulse-echo B-mode and Doppler ultrasound techniques were described.
- It was noted that both these types of technology can be incorporated into invasive scanners.
- Three-dimensional imaging is a natural progression in the development of the technology. In time its value will be determined.
- Ultrasonic techniques are well-suited to anatomical and blood flow measurements.
- The real-time interactive nature of the techniques makes them well-suited to needle and catheter guidance.
- Ultrasonic contrast agents are becoming available for medical application.
- Diagnostic ultrasound has no known harmful effects and efforts should be made to ensure that it remains safe in the future.

REFERENCES

1. Powell MC, Worthington BS, Buckley JM, Symonds EM. Magnetic resonance imaging (MRI) in obstetrics. 11. *Br J Obstet Gynaecol* 1988 **95**: 38.
2. Roberts N, Garden AS, Cruz-Orive LM, Whitehouse GH, Edwards RHT. Estimation of fetal volume by magnetic resonance imaging and stereology. *Br J Radiol* 1994 **67**: 1067.
3. Stehling MK, Mansfield P, Ordidge RJ, Coxon R, Chapman B, Blamire A, Gibbs P, Johnson IR, Symonds EM, Worthington BS, Coupland RE. Echo-planar imaging of the human fetus in utero. *Magn Res Med* 1990 **13**: 314.
4. Dudley NJ, Potter R. Quality assurance in obstetric ultrasound. *Br J Radiol* 1993 **66**: 865.
5. McDicken WN. *Diagnostic Ultrasonics: Principles and Use of Instruments*, 3rd edn. Edinburgh: Churchill Livingstone, 1991.
6. Fish P. *Diagnostic Medical Ultrasound*. Chichester: Wiley, 1990.

7. Kremkau FW. *Diagnostic Ultrasound: Principles, Instruments and Exercises*, 4th edn. Philadelphia: Saunders, 1994.

8. Evans DH, McDicken WN, Skidmore R, Woodcock JP. *Doppler Ultrasound: Physics, Instrumentation and Clinical Applications.* Chichester: Wiley, 1989.

9. Kasai C, Namekawa K, Koyano A, Omoto R. Real-time two-dimensional blood flow imaging using an autocorrelation technique. *IEEE Trans Sonics Ultrasonics* 1985 **32**: 458.

10. Bom N, Brommersa PD, Lancee CT. Probes as used in cardiology with emphasis on transesophageal and intravascular applications. In Wells PNT (ed) *Advances in Ultrasound Techniques and Instrumentation*, New York: Churchill Livingstone, 1993.

11. Kirbach D, Whittingham TA. 3D ultrasound – The Kretztechnik Voluson approach. *Eur J Ultrasound* 1994 **1**: 85.

12. Masotti L, Pini R. Three-dimensional ultrasound. In Wells PNT (ed) *Advances in Ultrasound Techniques and Instrumentation*, New York: Churchill Livingstone, 1993.

13. Kelly IMG, Gardener JE, Brett AD, Richards R, Lees WR. Three-dimensional US of the fetus. *Radiology* **192**: 253.

14. Picot PA, Rickey DW, Mitchell R, Rankin RN, Fenster A. Three-dimensional colour Doppler imaging. *Ultrasound Med Biol* 1993 **19**: 95.

15. BMUS. *Clinical Applications of Ultrasonic Fetal Measurement.* London: British Institute of Radiology Publications, 1990.

16. Deter RL, Harrist RB, Birnholz JC, Hadlock FP. *Quantitative Obstetrical Ultrasonography.* New York: Wiley, 1986.

17. Hoskins PR, Haddad NG, Johnstone FD, Chambers SE, McDicken WN. The choice of index for umbilical artery Doppler waveforms. *Ultrasound Med Biol* 1989 **15**: 107.

18. Otto RC, Wellauer J. *Ultrasound-guided Biopsy and Drainage.* Berlin: Springer-Verlag, 1985.

19. Lesny J, Aindow JD. Sonically-sensitive biopsy needles: the Dorchester approach. *Br J Radiol* 1986 **59**: 741.

20. McDicken WN, Anderson T, MacKenzie WE, Dickson H, Scrimgeour JB. Ultrasonic identification of needle tips in amniocentesis. *Lancet* 1984 **ii**: 198.

21. Ophir J, Parker KJ. Contrast agents in diagnostic ultrasound. *Ultrasound Med Biol* 1989 **15**: 319.

22. Schlief R, Diechert U. Hysterosalpingo-contrast sonography of the uterus and fallopian tubes: results of a clinical trial of a new contrast medium in 120 patients. *Radiology* 1991 **178**: 213.

23. Fritzsch Th, Maas B, Muller B, Schobel C, Siegert J, Stevens K. Composition and tolerance of galactose-based echo contrast media. In Katayama HY, Brash RC (eds) *New Dimensions of Contrast Media*, Tokyo: Excerpta Medica, 1991: 156.

24. Feinstein SB, Cheirif J, Ten Cate FJ, Silverman PR, Heidenreich PA, Dick C, Desir RM, Armstrong WF, Quinones MA, Pravin MS. Safety and efficacy of a new transpulmonary ultrasound agent; initial multicenter clinical results. *J Am Coll Cardiol* 1990 **16**: 316.

25. Docker MF, Duck FA. *The safe use of diagnostic ultrasound.* London: British Institute of Radiology Publications, 1991.

26. EFSUMB. Safety statement and reviews of recent literature. *Eur J Ultrasound* 1994 **1**: 95.

27. AIUM. Bioeffects considerations for the safety of diagnostic ultrasound. *J Ultrasound Med* 1988 **7**: no. 9 (suppl).

28. EFSUMB. Transvaginal ultrasonography – safety aspects. *Eur J Ultrasound* 1994 **1**: 355.

Fetal Behavior

JG Nijhuis

INTRODUCTION

'What is fetal behaviour?' asked Levene[1] in his review of the first book on this subject, *Fetal Behaviour: Developmental and Perinatal Aspects.*[2] Behavior may mean 'any or all of a person's total activity' (Dorland's Medical Dictionary) or 'activity that helps an individual interact more efficiently with environmental stimuli' (Churchill's Medical Dictionary). With fetal behavior we mean the total of fetal activities as observed or recorded by the only modality that allows its study, ultrasound equipment. In the first half of pregnancy, fetal activity can be observed with just one ultrasound transducer and simultaneous registration of the fetal heart rate (FHR); cardiotocography (CTG) is not yet possible. In the second half of pregnancy, mostly two ultrasound scanners are needed to observe the fetus, and the FHR should be recorded simultaneously. The combination of observed activity and the simultaneous FHR is a record of 'fetal behavior' (Fig. 3.17.1). In the last weeks of

pregnancy, fetal behavior can almost completely be described in terms of behavioral states, i.e. 'constellations of physiological and behavioral variables (e.g. no eye movements, silent heart rate pattern, and absence of body movements) which are stable over time and recur repeatedly, not only in the same infant, but also in similar forms in all infants' (modified from reference 3). The concept of behavioral states has been used as a descriptive categorization of behavior, and also as an explanatory concept in which states are considered to reflect particular modes of nervous activity which modify the responsiveness of the infant.[4]

Not only in the last trimester, but also in the first and second trimesters fetal behavior can be seen as the output of the fetal central nervous system (CNS). When we discuss 'fetal surveillance' in obstetrical practice, we mean that we want to be informed about the condition of the fetal CNS.

From this background it is important to gain insight in fetal behavior and fetal behavioral states for three main reasons.

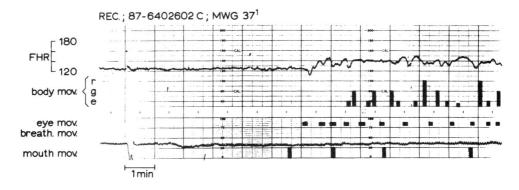

Fig. 3.17.1 *Graphic display of 14 min of a recording of fetal behavior at 37 weeks of gestation. The fetal heart rate (FHR) is recorded in b.p.m. at 3 cm min⁻¹. The presence of body, eye, breathing and mouth movements is indicated with black bars. The first seven minutes have been classified as state 1F, the following seven minutes as state 2F. Mov., movements; r, rotation; g, general movement; e, extremity movement; MWG, menstrual weeks of gestation.*

1. As an obstetrician one should know what 'normal fetal activity' means at a certain gestational age. For example, fetal quiescence during 20–30 min is physiologic in the second and third trimester of pregnancy but indicates pathology in the first trimester;[5] (Table 3.17.1).

2. One should be aware of the association of fetal movements. For example, if body movements are absent, eye movements and also breathing movements are much more likely to be absent than present.[6-9] This may have consequences for biophysical profile testing.

3. As the fetal CNS is still unaccessible, a possible impairment of the CNS can only be measured indirectly by recording fetal behavior. Only if one knows what normal fetal behavior is, is it possible to recognize abnormal fetal behavior.

Because fetal behavior is age-dependent, different aspects of fetal behavior for each trimester of pregnancy will be discussed separately.

Table 3.17.1 Global mean and maximum durations of periods that body movements can be absent when observed with ultrasonography

Gestational age	Mean duration	Maximum duration
8–20 weeks	4 minutes	11 minutes
20–30 weeks	5 minutes	17 minutes
30–36 weeks	10 minutes	35 minutes
36–40 weeks	25 minutes	60 minutes

From reference 5

CURRENT CONCEPTS

The first trimester

The very first 'fetal activity' that can be observed is fetal heart motion which can be observed from 6 weeks of gestation onward (i.e. postmenstrual age). The initial rate of 100 beats per minute (b.p.m.) increases to a mean rate of 167 b.p.m. at nine weeks which will then be followed by a gradual decrease to 156 b.p.m.[10] The next motion to be observed is the 'just discernible movement' at about seven to eight weeks and from this gestational age onward several movements develop rapidly.[11] It were De Vries *et al.*[11] who described the developmental pathway of fetal movements in a longitudinal study of twelve fetuses of healthy nulliparous women (Fig. 3.17.2). They attempted not only to describe a particular movement, but also how these movements were performed in terms of speed and amplitude. Their classification was based on movements that had been noted previously in low-risk preterm and full term infants.[12,13] As already mentioned, 'just discernible movements', lasting 1–2 s, can be seen from 7.5 weeks of gestation. During the following 10 weeks, many more movements appear. Examples are: startles, 8.0–9.5 weeks; general movements, 8.5–9.5 weeks; breathing movements 10.0–11.5 weeks; isolated extremity movements 9.0–10.5 weeks; sucking and swallowing 12.5–14.5 weeks; yawning 11.5–15.5 weeks.[11] Eye movements can be seen from 16 weeks onward.[14]

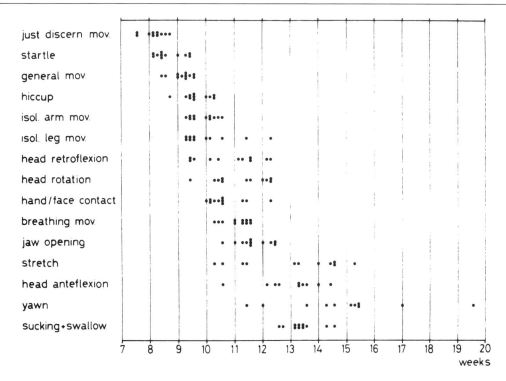

Fig. 3.17.2 *First occurrence of specific fetal movement patterns. Each dot represents an individual. Ages at observations are given in full weeks and days. (Reproduced with permission from reference 11.)*

All fetuses follow a specific sequence in which the different movement patterns are rank-ordered according to the gestational age of their first appearance with a scatter of about 2 weeks. This scatter may be partly due to the observer variability and the fact that only one hour was recorded with one week intervals. De Vries et al.[11] emphasized that most movements patterns vary in amplitude, speed and force. The character of the movements is not jerky, but rather coordinated and graceful. Of course, startles, hiccups, twitches and cloni are, more or less by definition, rather jerky.

In a study which was published in 1985, the same group published observations on quantitative activity of the developing fetus.[15] Their main conclusion was that the fetus shows continual activity over 24 h and that there are no long periods of fetal quiescence. The longest period of quiescence varies from about 12 min at 8 weeks to 5–6 min at 17 weeks.[16]

Fetal motility can be seen as an expression of the quality of the central nervous system. This seems to conflict with the observation by Visser et al. in a study on anencephalic fetuses, that in early life a normal amount of fetal movements can be present. The quality of the observed movements however, differed dramatically when compared with controls.[17] Similarly, in a case with Fanconi anemia, De Vries et al.[18] described qualitatively abnormal fetal motor behavior when the mother reported excessive fetal kicking at 15 weeks of gestation. Postmortem examination after termination at 22 weeks showed a spongy myelinopathy of the CNS. This illustrates again that for the assessment of the integrity of the CNS, quality of movements may be of much greater importance than quantity.

The second trimester

During the second trimester of pregnancy the incidence of body movements gradually decreases and breathing movements increase considerably. The periods of quiescence become longer and eye movements are now clearly visible. The incidence of hiccups, startles and stretches decreases whereas other movement patterns (jaw movements, hand–face contacts, head movements) show no clear developmental changes.[19]

A beginning can be seen of the development of rest–activity cycles, but clear behavioral states are not yet present.[6,7] This can be concluded from studies which show an increased percentage of 'association of state variables'.[6,8,9] This means that if one variable is in the 'off' condition, the other variable is much more likely to be in the 'off' condition than in the 'on' condition (e.g. if eye movements are absent, body movements are much more likely to be absent than present). From a developmental point of view, one could say that in the second trimester development goes on, but no new movements appear for the first time.

The third trimester

In the third trimester, clearly developed behavioral states become present. In 1982 Nijhuis et al.[20] were the first to present the definitions of these fetal behavioral states. The definitions were based on the concept of behavioral states in the neonate, but other criteria had to be used, because of the differences between the fetus and the neonate. For example, regularity of breathing can be used as a state criterion in the neonate. This is not the case in the human fetus, because breathing is not continuously present. Because regularity of breathing is state-dependent, it can be used as a 'state concomitant'.[21] With great similarity to Prechtl's neonatal states 1 through 4,[3] four fetal behavioral states, 1F through 4F, could be defined.[20]

State 1F (similar to state 1 in the neonate): quiescence, which can be regularly interrupted by brief gross body movements, mostly startles. Eye movements are absent. Fetal heart rate pattern (FHRP) 'A' is a stable pattern with a small oscillation bandwidth and no accelerations, except in combination with a startle.

State 2F (similar to state 2 in the neonate): frequent and periodic gross body movements – mainly stretches and retroflexions – and movements of the extremities. Eye movements are present. FHRP B has a wider oscillation bandwidth and frequent accelerations during movements.

State 3F (similar to state 3 in the neonate): gross body movements absent. Eye movements present. FHRP C is stable but with a wider oscillation bandwidth than FHRP A and no accelerations.

State 4F (similar to state 4 in the neonate): vigorous, continual activity including many trunk rotations. Eye movements are present. FHRP D is unstable, with large and long-lasting accelerations, often fused into a sustained tachycardia.

These definitions are summarized in Fig. 3.17.3, which also shows examples of FHRP A through D. Behavioral state 3F ('quiet wakefulness') occurs less than 5% of the recording time. Because of its low incidence, Pillai and James[22] questioned if this state really existed. In the postmature fetus, however, a significant increase of the presence of this state up to 9% has been reported[23] so this may again be an age-related phenomenon.

It is important to emphasize that the existence of states can only be excepted if three requirements are satisfied:

1. a specific combination of variables occurs (e.g. absence of eye movements, absence of body movements and a silent heart rate pattern);
2. which is stable over time (by definition at least 3 min);
3. clear state transitions can be recognized in between, which should be shorter than 3 min.[20]

The concept of behavioral states allows us to get a further insight into the activity of the central nervous system. Examples have been shown in which associations develop later, e.g. in nulliparous women,[24] in growth-

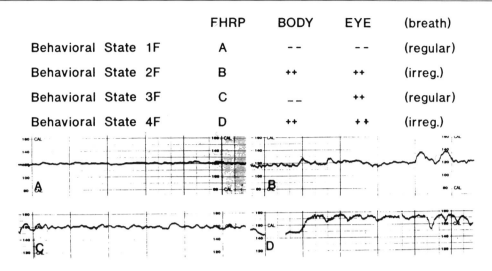

	FHRP	BODY	EYE	(breath)
Behavioral State 1F	A	– –	– –	(regular)
Behavioral State 2F	B	++	++	(irreg.)
Behavioral State 3F	C	_ _	++	(regular)
Behavioral State 4F	D	++	+ +	(irreg.)

Fig. 3.17.3 *Schematic diagram of the definition of behavioral states 1F through 4F and their relation to breathing (if present). In the lower part, an example is given of each of the fetal heart rate patterns A through D, at a recording speed of 3 cm min⁻¹.*

retarded human fetuses,[25,26] and also in type-1-diabetic women.[27]

Some variables cannot be used to define states but are, rather, state-specific. Fetal breathing is such a variable. Because breathing movements are not continuously present, they cannot be used for the definition of states. Yet, their incidence seems to be increased during state 2F as compared to state 1F,[28,29] while in state 1F they seem to be much more regular.[21] Another state-specific movement is 'regular mouthing' and 'sucking'. Regular mouthing consists of short clusters of mouth movements which are fairly superficial. They occur mainly in state 1F when no other movements can be observed. It is perhaps because of the absence of other movements that regular mouthing is known to entrain a small sinusoidal-like fetal heart rate pattern. Stronger mouth movements which seem to be similar to sucking movements after birth are seen during state 3F and cause a much greater sinusoidal-like heart rate pattern.[30,31]

It is now apparent that specific heart-rate patterns can be associated with specific fetal movement patterns. This is important for clinicians, because they use the recording of fetal heart-rate patterns as a technique for fetal surveillance. An example is the sinusoidal heart-rate pattern which is often associated with very sick or anemic fetuses, but a sinusoidal heart-rate pattern can also be seen with fetal sucking movements.[30,31] A differential diagnosis of a sinusoidal CTG should now include fetal anemia, maternal medication, fetal asphyxia, congenital anomalies, but also physiologic fetal sucking behavior.[32]

Fetal stimulation

The fetus can easily be stimulated and tested. Those working in the field of developmental neurology and obstetrics may like to test the fetus for the integrity of its CNS. The observation of a startle response to a vibroacoustic stimulus has not yet been proven to be the final solution.[33] Tas *et al.*[34,35] have shown that the intercostal-to-phrenic-inhibitory reflex can be provoked which leads to arrest of breathing movements in the normal and growth-retarded fetuses. In this study, it appears that the effects in normal and growth-retarded fetuses are similar. It has, however, become clear that stimulation should be done under standardized conditions and one should take the behavioral state into account. As an example, Groome *et al.*[36] who tested 96 normal human fetuses between 37 and 41 weeks using a vibroacoustic stimulus concluded that the response depended on the prestimulus duration of state 1F. Zimmer *et al.*[37] showed not only that the fetus responds to speech stimuli, but also that this response is state-dependent.

FUTURE PERSPECTIVES

The continuity of fetal functions

It has now become clear that the fetus is 'relatively poorly developed' as compared to other primate species before birth. In fact, it may be the case that human pregnancy is actually too short, that fetus' energy demand is such that the mother cannot sustain pregnancy. One of the reasons for this 'expensiveness' is that the fetus has a relatively large brain.[36] Obviously, during evolution the choice could have been to increase the maternal body size or to curtail the duration of pregnancy. The increasing intelligence of the human species made it possible to curtail the duration of pregnancy, because the mothers had the capacity to learn how to look after such an 'immature newborn'.[36,38]

In fact, it is not before six weeks after birth that a real new step in neurodevelopment occurs. Assuming that the mother is capable of nursing the 'immature child', it gives the neonate the possibility to get used to its new environment. During the first weeks after birth much more attention has to be paid to other aspects of life: resetting chemoreceptors because of the increased oxygen saturation, organize continuous breathing without apneas, get used to oral feeding, etc. One could speculate that the fetus devotes more energy to these basic functions in the first weeks. Following that period, there is again time and energy to develop the central nervous system further. Research into this field should continue to compare the fetus and the premature born child. As this research has just started, the field is wide open.

Consequences for clinical practise and research

Once one is prepared to think of a fetus from a behavioral background, it is clear that 'the fetus is but a human being, just as prone as a child or adult to get an accident, a disease or an iatrogenic problem'.[32] Then it is also apparent that birth by itself will not be harmful to the fetus, and that the majority of handicaps result not from parturition but rather the consequence of a condition that was already present before birth or even before conception.[39] As early as 1897 Sigmund Freud stated that 'difficult birth in itself in certain cases is merely a symptom of deeper effects that influenced the development of the fetus'.[40] Therefore, we should focus much more attention to the fetal CNS in clinical thinking and decision-making. Visser *et al.*[41] have developed a scheme in which aspects of fetal behavior are placed in a timescale together with the results of other fetal surveillance tests e.g. CTG, Doppler flow profiles[41] (Fig. 3.17.4). This does not imply that it is necessary to perform a very time-consuming behavioral study in each fetus at risk, but in some specific cases it may prove very useful, for example by demonstrating physical impediments to movement (e.g. arthrogryposis)[42] or cases of 'intrauterine brain death'.[43]

Finally, the study of fetal behavior may also be of use to assess unknown possible effects of medication. For example, maternal betamethasone administration has been advocated for years as a safe drug to stimulate fetal lung maturation. However, it has been shown recently that this medication transiently reduces fetal activity and heart rate variability.[44] Other drugs that have been studied in relation to fetal behavior include anti-epileptic drugs,[45] cocaine[46] and methadone.[47]

In conclusion, the study of fetal behavior has given insights into the output of the fetal CNS. Not only has a beginning been made with the use of recordings of fetal behavior in clinical practise, but also with the first steps toward an intrauterine neurological examination. It is to be expected that the further study of fetal behavior will help achieve better insights still in many aspects of the developing fetal CNS.

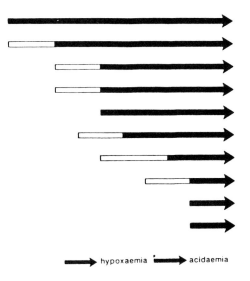

Abnormal umbilical artery waveforms

Abnormal behavioral states development

Qualitative movement changes

Reduced amniotic fluid volume

Heart rate decelerations

Reduced heart rate variation

Reduced general movements

Reduced breathing movements

Absence of movements

Terminal heart rate pattern

hypoxaemia   acidaemia

Fig. 3.17.4 *Suggested rank ordering in which several variables change in growth-retarded human fetuses with progressive deterioration of the fetal condition. (Reproduced with permission from reference 41.)*

SUMMARY

- Fetal movements appear at about seven weeks of pregnancy. All fetuses follow a specific sequence in which the different movement patterns are rank-ordered according to the gestational age.
- All specific movements (breathing, sucking, yawning, eye movements, etc.) develop between 7 and 16 weeks. After this gestational age, periodicity and association of movements changes, but no new movements appear.
- If one wants to judge the fetal condition, quality of movements may be of much greater importance than quantity. Obviously, absence of movements over a prolonged period of time may indeed indicate impending fetal death. The period of time that movements can be absent is age-related and varies from 7 min in the first trimester to 60 min near term.
- In the last weeks of pregnancy fetal behavior can almost completely be described in terms of behavioral states which are similar to sleep states in the neonate.
- From a developmental point of view, birth is not an important issue for the developing fetal CNS. This development can be described as a continuum in which birth by itself does not change the developmental pathway.
- Fetal responsiveness is state-dependent and fetal well-being tests should therefore be standardized for behavioral states.
- A CTG can only be judged properly if one takes fetal behavior and fetal behavioral states into account.
- The fetal CNS is still inaccessible. Fetal behavior is the output of the CNS and the study of fetal behavior comes closest to the study of the activity of the fetal CNS.
- Maternal medication that is supposed to be safe for the fetus may influence fetal behavior and may therefore not be safe for the fetal brain.
- Only if the research of fetal behavior continues will it be possible to develop an intrauterine neurological examination and to get more insight into the development and quality of the fetal 'black box', the fetal central nervous system.

REFERENCES

1. Levene M. Now you see it. . . *Br Med J* 1993 **306**: 344–345.
2. Nijhuis JG. *Fetal Behaviour, Developmental and Perinatal Aspects*. Oxford: Oxford University Press, 1992: 283 pp.
3. Prechtl HFR, Weinmann HM, Akiyama Y. Organization of physiological parameters in normal and neurologically abnormal infants. *Neuropaediatrie* 1969 **1**: 101–129.
4. Prechtl HFR. The behavioural states of the newborn (a review). *Brain Res* 1974 **76**: 185–212.
5. Nijhuis JG. Fetal motility and fetal behaviour. In Van Geijn HP, Copray FJA (eds) *A Critical Appraisal of Fetal Surveillance*. Amsterdam: Elsevier Science BV, 1994: 183–187.
6. Drogtrop AP, Ubels R, Nijhuis JG. The association between fetal body movements, eye movements, and heart rate patterns between 25 and 30 weeks of gestation. *Early Hum Dev* 1990 **23**: 67–73.
7. Visser GHA, Poelman-Weesjes G, Cohen TMN, Bekedam DJ. Fetal behaviour at 30 to 32 weeks of gestation. *Pediatr Res* 1987 **22**: 655–658.
8. Swartjes JM, Van Geijn HP, Mantel R, Van Woerden EE, Schoemaker HC. Coincidence of behavioural state parameters in the human fetus at three gestational ages. *Early Hum Dev* 1990 **23**: 75–83.
9. Nijhuis JG, Pas M van de. Behavioral states and their ontogeny: human studies. *Semin Perinatol* 1992 **16**: 206–210.
10. Heeswijk M van, Nijhuis JG, Hollanders HMG. Fetal heart rate in early pregnancy. *Early Hum Dev* 1990 **22**: 151–156.
11. De Vries JIP, Visser GHA, Prechtl HFR. The emergence of fetal behaviour. I. Qualitative aspects. *Early Hum Dev* 1982 **7**: 301–322.
12. Prechtl HFR. *The Neurological Examination of the Full-term Newborn Infant*, 2nd edn. *Clinics in Developmental Medicine*. London: Heinemann, 1977: 168 pp.
13. Prechtl HFR, Fargel JW. Posture, motility and respiration in low-risk preterm infants. *Dev Med Child Neurol* 1979 **21**: 3–27.
14. Birnholz JC. The development of human fetal eye movement patterns. *Science* 1981 **213**: 679–681.
15. Vries JIP de, Visser GHA, Prechtl HFR. The emergence of fetal behaviour. II. Quantitative Aspects. *Early Hum Dev* 1985 **12**: 99–120.
16. Vries JIP de. Fetal behaviour: the first trimester. In Nijhuis JG (ed.) *Fetal Behaviour, Developmental and Perinatal Aspects*. Oxford: Oxford University Press, 1992: 3–17.
17. Visser GHA, Laurini RN, Vries JIP de, Bekedam DJ, Prechtl HFR. Abnormal motor behaviour in anencephalic fetuses. *Early Hum Dev* 1985 **12**: 173–182.
18. De Vries JIP, Laurini RN, Visser GHA. Abnormal motor behaviour and developmental postmortem findings in a fetus with Fanconi anaemia. *Early Hum Dev* 1994 **36**: 137–142.
19. Visser GHA. The second trimester. In Nijhuis JG (ed.) *Fetal Behaviour, Developmental and Perinatal Aspects*. Oxford: Oxford University Press, 1992: 17–26.
20. Nijhuis JG, Bots RSGM, Martin CB jr, Prechtl HFR. Are there behavioural states in the human fetus? *Early Hum Dev* 1982 **6**: 177–195.
21. Nijhuis JG, Martin CB jr, Gommers S, Bouws P, Bots RSGM, Jongsma HW. The rhythmicity of fetal breathing varies with behavioural state in the human fetus. *Early Hum Dev* 1983 **9**: 1–7.
22. Pillai M, James D. Are the behavioural states of the newborn comparable to those of the fetus? *Early Hum Dev* 1990 **22**: 39–49.
23. Pas M van de, Nijhuis JG, Jongsma HW. Fetal behaviour in uncomplicated pregnancies after term. *Early Hum Dev* 1994 **40**: 29–38.
24. Vliet MAT van, Martin CB jr, Nijhuis JG, Prechtl HFR. Behavioural states in the fetuses of nulliparous women. *Early Hum Dev* 1985 **12**: 21–37.

25. Arduini D, Rizzo G, Caforio L, Romanini C, Mancuso S. Behavioural state transitions in healthy and growth retarded fetuses. *Early Hum Dev* 1989 **19**: 155–165.
26. Vliet MAT van, Martin CB jr, Nijhuis JG, Prechtl HFR. Behavioural states in growth retarded human fetuses. *Early Hum Dev* 1985 **12**: 183–197.
27. Mulder EJH, Visser GHA, Bekedam DJ, Prechtl HFR. Emergence of behavioural states in fetuses of type-1-diabetic women. *Early Hum Dev* 1987 **15**: 231–251.
28. Vliet MAT van, Martin CB jr, Nijhuis JG, Prechtl HFR. The relationship between fetal activity, and behavioural states and fetal breathing movements in normal and growth-retarded fetuses. *Am J Obstet Gynecol* 1985 **153**: 582–588.
29. Mulder EJH, Boersma M, Meeuse M, Van der Wal M, Van de Weerd E, Visser GHA. Patterns of breathing movements in the near-term human fetus: relationship to behavioural states. *Early Hum Dev* 1994 **36**: 127–135.
30. Nijhuis JG, Staisch KJ, Martin CB jr, Prechtl HFR. A sinusoidal-like fetal heart-rate pattern in association with fetal sucking – report of 2 cases. *Eur J Obstet Gynecol Reprod Biol* 1984 **16**: 353–358.
31. Woerden EE van, Geijn HP van, Swartjes JM, Caron FJM, Brons JTJ, Arts NFTh. Fetal heart rhythms during behavioural state 1F. *Eur J Obstet Gynecol Reprod Biol* 1988 **28**: 29–38.
32. Nijhuis JG. Physiological and clinical consequences in relation to the development of fetal behavior and fetal behavioral states. In Lecanuet JP, Krasnegor NA, Fifer WP, Smotherman WP (eds) *Fetal Development: A Psychobiological Perspective*. Hove: Lawrence Erlbaum Associates; 1995: 67–82.
33. Gagnon R. Fetal behaviour in relation to fetal stimulation. In Nijhuis JG (ed.) *Fetal Behaviour, Developmental and Perinatal Aspects*. Oxford: Oxford University Press, 1992: 209–226.
34. Tas BAPJ, Nijhuis JG, Lucas AJ, Folgering HThM. The intercostal-to-phrenic inhibitory reflex in the human fetus near term. *Early Hum Dev* 1990 **22**: 145–149.
35. Tas BAPJ, Nijhuis JG, Nelen W, Willems E. The intercostal-to-phrenic inhibitory reflex in normal and intra-uterine growth-retarded (IUGR) human fetuses from 26–40 weeks of gestation. *Early Hum Dev* 1993 **32**: 177–182.
36. Groome LJ, Bentz LS, Singh KP, Mooney DM. Behavioural state change in normal fetuses following a single vibroacoustic stimulus: effect of duration of quiet sleep prior to stimulation. *Early Hum Dev* 1993 **33**: 21–27.
37. Zimmer EZ, Fifer WP, Kim Y-I, Rey HR, Chao CR, Meyers MM. Response of the premature fetus to stimulation by speech sounds. *Early Hum Dev* 1993 **33**: 207–215.
38. Prechtl HFR. New perspectives in early human development. *Eur J Obstet Gynaecol Reprod Biol* 1986 **21**: 347–355.
39. Nelson KB, Ellenberg JH. Intrapartum events and cerebral palsy. In Kubli FW (ed.) *Prenatal Events and Brain Damage in Surviving Children*. Heidelberg: Springer Verlag, 1988: 139–148.
40. Freud S. Die infantile Cerebrallmung. In Nothnagel H (ed.) *Specielle Pathologie und Therapie*. Vienna: Holder, 1897: 1–327.
41. Visser GHA, Ribbert LSM, Bekedam DJ. Sequential changes in Doppler waveform, fetal heart rate and movement patterns in IUGR fetuses. In Van Geijn HP, Copray FJA (eds) *A Critical Appraisal of Fetal Surveillance*. Amsterdam: Elsevier Science BV, 1994: 193–200.
42. Tas BAPJ, Nijhuis JG. Consequences for fetal monitoring In Nijhuis JG (ed.) *Fetal Behaviour, Developmental and Perinatal Aspects*. Oxford: Oxford University Press, 1992: 258–269.
43. Nijhuis JG, Crevels AJ, Dongen PWJ van. Fetal brain death: the definition of a fetal heart rate pattern and its clinical consequenses. *Obstet Gynecol Surv* 1990 **46**: 229–232.
44. Mulder EJH, Derks JB, Zonneveld MF, Bruinse HW, Visser GHA. Transient reduction in fetal activity and heart rate variation after maternal betamethasone administration. *Early Hum Dev* 1994 **36**: 49–60.
45. Geijn HP van, Swartjes JM van, Woerden EE, Caron FJM, Brons JTJ, Arts NFT. Fetal behavioural states in epileptic pregnancies. *Eur J Obstet Gynecol Reprod Biol* 1986 **21**: 309–314.
46. Hume RF jr, O'Donnell KJ, Stanger CL, Killam AP, Gingras JL. *In utero* cocaine exposure: observations of fetal behavioral state may predict neonatal outcome. *Am J Obstet Gynecol* 1989 **161**: 685–690.
47. Archie CL, Milton IL, Sokol RJ, Norman G. The effects of methadone treatment on the reactivity of the nonstress test. *Obstet Gynecol* 1989 **74**: 254–255.

Maternal Respiratory and Cardiovascular Changes During Pregnancy

SC Robson

RESPIRATORY SYSTEM

INTRODUCTION

Respiratory physiology

The essential function of breathing is to acquire oxygen and eliminate carbon dioxide. Inspiration occurs by active contraction of the diaphragm and intercostal muscles whereas expiration is passive, due to the inherent elastic property of the lung. The strength of the retractive force is related to lung volume. Lung compliance is an expression of the change in lung volume per unit change in transpulmonary (intrapleural) pressure. During breathing bigger changes in intrapleural pressure are observed than would be expected by lung retractive forces alone. This is due to the resistance to airflow offered by the respiratory passages. The greater part of the total airways resistance is situated in the large airways (larynx, trachea and main bronchi).

The total or physiological dead space relates to the volume of gas not participating in gas exchange. This includes the volume of air filling the airways down to the terminal bronchioles (anatomical dead space) plus the volume of gas in alveoli that are underperfused. The remaining alveoli contain alveolar air with the same PCO_2 as arterial blood. Thus, total ventilation can be divided into two hypothetical components; alveolar (effective) ventilation and deadspace (ineffective) ventilation. Deadspace ventilation is normally less than one quarter of the total but the proportion varies with breathing frequency, exercise and other influences.

Four lung volumes are recognized in respiratory physiology:

1. **Tidal volume**; the volume of gas inspired or expired in each respiration;
2. **Inspiratory reserve volume**; the maximum amount of gas that can be inspired beyond the normal tidal inspiration;

3. **Expiratory reserve volume**; the maximum amount of gas that can be expired from the resting end-expiratory position (the position of the chest at the end of quiet expiration when the respiratory muscles are inactive);
4. **Residual volume**; the volume of gas remaining in the lungs, not including the anatomical dead space, at the end of maximal expiration.

Four lung capacities, each of which include two or more of the volumes defined above, are recognized.

1. **Total lung capacity**; the total amount of gas in the lung at the end of maximal inspiration. This includes all four lung volumes.
2. **Vital capacity**; the maximum amount of gas that can be expired after a maximum inspiration. This includes the tidal, inspiratory reserve and expiratory reserve volumes.
3. **Inspiratory capacity**: maximum volume of gas that can be inspired from the resting end-expiratory position. This includes the tidal and inspiratory reserve volumes.
4. **Functional residual capacity**: the amount of gas that remains in the lungs at the resting end-expiratory position and the amount of gas with which the tidal air must mix. This includes the expiratory reserve and residual volumes.

With the exception of residual volume (and the capacities which include it) the remaining lung spaces can be measured by spirometry.

Respiratory changes in pregnancy

Extensive anatomic and functional changes occur in the respiratory system during pregnancy. These are necessary to meet the increased metabolic demands of the mother and fetus. While more recent work has not questioned the general trends reported in early studies,[1] the absolute figures have changed because of technical advances in measuring equipment.[2]

The majority of serial studies of respiratory function during pregnancy have used early postnatal measurements as non-pregnant baseline values. However, for several variables there are clear differences between measurements performed at 6 weeks and at 12 months after delivery.[3] Studies in which 6 week postnatal measurements were taken to represent non-pregnant values may underestimate the size of changes during pregnancy. Ideally women should be recruited prior to conception.[4]

CURRENT CONCEPTS

Anatomical changes

The diaphragm is displaced upwards by 4 cm during pregnancy.[5] This is not secondary to pressure from the gravid uterus because changes are seen well before the third trimester. Radiological studies have shown that the respiratory excursion of the diaphragm is actually increased[5] and therefore there is no evidence that, in the upright position

at least, there is splinting of the diaphragm. There is a compensatory increase in both the transverse and antero-posterior diameters of the thorax so that the circumference of the chest increases by approximately 15 cm. This is associated with flaring of the ribs and an increase in the substernal angle. As a result the internal volume of the thoracic cavity is unchanged.

Lung capacities and volumes

Lung capacities and volumes is non-pregnant and pregnant subjects are shown in Fig. 3.18.1.

Studies of **vital capacity** have shown conflicting results but overall, there is probably a small increase of 100–200 ml in late pregnancy although this is not evident in obese women.[6]

Inspiratory capacity increases progressively during pregnancy from a non-pregnant value of around 2200 to 2500 ml at term.[7] Both residual volume and expiratory reserve volume decrease in pregnancy. This results in a marked reduction in functional residual capacity from 2800 ml in the non-pregnant state to 2300 ml at term.[6–8]

Tidal volume increases by between 150 and 200 ml during pregnancy from a non-pregnant mean of around 500 ml,[9] and 75% of this increase occurs by the end of the first trimester.[10]

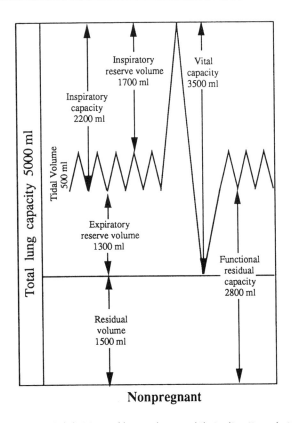

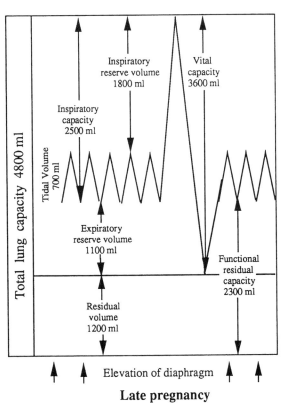

Fig. 3.18.1 *Subdivisions of lung volume and their alterations during pregnancy.*

Respiratory rate, minute ventilation and alveolar ventilation

The **respiratory rate** remains unchanged during pregnancy at 16–18 breaths min[-1].[3] Minute ventilation (the product of respiratory rate and tidal volume) therefore increases in parallel with tidal volume, resulting in an increase above non-pregnant values of around 40%. The major part of this increment is evident as early as 7 weeks of pregnancy.[4] Thus the pregnant woman increases her ventilation by breathing more deeply not by breathing more frequently.

The difference between tidal volume and the volume of the physiological dead space is the alveolar ventilation. Although the physiological dead space increases by about 60 ml in pregnancy,[11] alveolar ventilation is increased dramatically[3] as shown in Fig. 3.18.2.

Pulmonary function

The **forced expiratory volume** in one second (FEV$_1$) remains unchanged during pregnancy in healthy women and in asthmatics.[12] Most studies have suggested that 80–85% of the vital capacity can be forcibly expired in one second in pregnant and non-pregnant subjects.[1] **Peak expiratory flow rate** is also unaffected by pregnancy. Both these indirect measurements depend on airways resistance and lung compliance.

The work done in breathing is divided between the work done in overcoming the total airway resistance of the tracheobronchial tree and the work done in expanding the lungs and chest wall, the compliance. There is a reduction in **airway resistance** during pregnancy possibly due to progesterone-induced relaxation of the bronchial muscles.[13] This reduction may account for the finding that the work of breathing is unchanged in pregnancy, despite the increase in minute ventilation. **Lung compliance** is unaltered during pregnancy.[14]

Pulmonary transfer factor is a measure of the rate at which gas passes from the alveoli to the bloodstream. It is influenced not only by ventilation/perfusion imbalance and the thickness of the alveolar-capillary membrane but also by the pulmonary capillary blood volume and the hemoglobin concentration. Gas transfer is reduced by around 15% and is evident from mid-pregnancy.[15] This fall may be due to the lowered hemoglobin concentration or to an alteration in the mucopolysaccharides of the alveolar wall. The reduction in transfer factor would act against the increase in ventilation to improve the efficiency of gas exchange in pregnancy.[1]

Oxygen consumption and carbon dioxide production

Oxygen consumption increases by between 40 and 50 ml min[-1] during pregnancy,[10,11,16] representing an increase of 15–20%. This increase is necessary to cope with the increased demands of mother and fetus. The major increments in cardiac, respiratory and renal function account for most of the extra oxygen needs in the first two

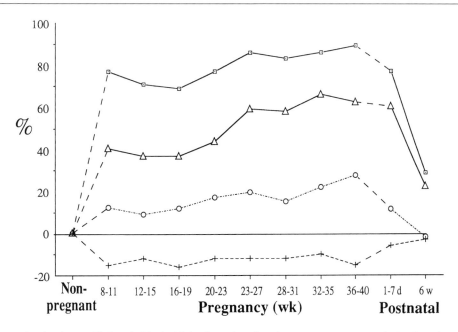

Fig. 3.18.2 *Changes in alveolar ventilation (—□—), tidal volume (–·–○–·–), oxygen consumption (—△—), and PCO_2 (—+—) in 20 women expressed as percentage change from non-pregnant values (determined 12 months after delivery). (Derived from reference 3.)*

trimesters, and almost half of the needs at term; the uterus, placenta, fetus and breasts also have important energy needs.

The output of carbon dioxide by the lungs is dependent not only on its rate of production within the body but also the amount in storage, primarily as bicarbonate. There is a large increase in carbon dioxide production from a non-pregnant median of 160 ml min^{-1} to 265 ml min^{-1} by term.[3]

Blood gases and acid–base balance in pregnancy

P_{CO_2}

The primary alteration in blood gas tension in the pregnant woman is a fall in P_{CO_2}. In people with healthy lungs, alveolar P_{CO_2} (P_{ACO_2}) is virtually equal to arterial P_{CO_2} (P_{aCO_2}). Compared with non-pregnant values, which are generally between 35 and 40 mmHg (4.7–5.3 kPa), values of P_{aCO_2} at the end of pregnancy are between 26 and 34 mmHg (3.5–4.5 kPa).[6,17] Most authors have found a significant decrease in P_{aCO_2} during the first trimester. Women who live at altitude, who normally have a lower P_{CO_2} secondary to hyperventilation, also show a fall in P_{CO_2} during pregnancy.[1] The fetus is more sensitive to CO_2 than the adult and the low maternal P_{CO_2} levels presumably allow an adequate gradient across the placenta for the fetus to dispose of CO_2.

P_{O_2}

The increase in alveolar ventilation may be expected to raise P_{O_2}. Some workers have reported this;[17] others have found little significant change in P_{O_2} during pregnancy. Posture influences P_{O_2} during late pregnancy; changing from the supine to the sitting position increases P_{O_2} by 13 mmHg (1.7 kPa).[18]

Because of the shape of the hemoglobin dissociation curve, any small increment in P_{O_2} will have little effect on hemoglobin saturation. Furthermore, the hemoglobin dissociation curve is shifted to the right in pregnancy.[19]

pH

The decrease in P_{aCO_2} which exists throughout pregnancy results in various compensatory adjustments in an effort to maintain a normal pH. There is a fall in plasma bicarbonate concentration along with other buffer bases. This has the secondary effect of lowering plasma sodium levels and osmolality. However, compensation for the respiratory alkalosis of pregnancy appears to be virtually complete with arterial pH values of 7.40–7.44.

Respiration in labor

Ventilation

Studies in women breathing from an Entonox apparatus suggest that during painful contractions mean tidal volume is 750 ml (range 227–2258 ml) and mean respiratory rate is 34 breaths min^{-1} (range 3–47).[20] Thus, while there is great variability between women, painful labor appears to be associated with significant hyperventilation. When pain is relieved by epidural analgesia the hyperventilation is much reduced.[21] Oxygen consumption also increases during painful contractions but is reduced by epidural analgesia. Pain and the resulting hyperventilation, and not uterine contractions, are the main cause of increased oxygen requirements during painful labor.[22]

Blood gases and acid–base balance

Hyperventilation during painful contractions leads to a further fall in P_{aCO_2}.[21] Values less than 17 mmHg (2.3 kPa) have been recorded in around a third of women.[23] This fall in P_{aCO_2} is not seen in women with continuous epidural analgesia. Associated with hyperventilation, P_{aO_2} also increases during painful contractions.[24] The respiratory alkalosis secondary to hyperventilation during the first stage of labor is accompanied by a progressive rise in lactate and pyruvate concentration.[25] This metabolic acidosis, which may lead to a fall in arterial pH, has been attributed solely to anaerobic metabolism in the uterus and other tissues but effective epidural analgesia appears to greatly reduce or even prevent it.[26] In the second stage of labor there is a significant reduction in pH associated with a further increase in lactate concentration.[25] This appears to be primarily the result of expulsive efforts because the pH changes are much less marked if pushing does not occur.[27]

Mechanism of respiratory changes in pregnancy

The stimulus to the increase in ventilation and the associated decrease in P_{aCO_2} during pregnancy appears to be progesterone which acts through several mechanisms. Progesterone alters the threshold of the respiratory centre to maintain a much lower P_{aCO_2}.[28] This adaptation occurs very early during the first trimester and a similar change is apparent at the end of each normal menstrual cycle. In addition to a lower setting, there is an increased sensitivity of the respiratory center to CO_2 levels.[29] This also appears to be mediated by progesterone[30] although estrogen may also be involved. In addition, progesterone increases the amount of carbonic anhydrase B in red cells;[31] this will facilitate carbon dioxide transfer and decrease P_{aCO_2} independently of any change in ventilation.[1]

CARDIOVASCULAR SYSTEM

INTRODUCTION

Cardiovascular physiology

The circulation is designed to provide tissues with substrate for aerobic respiration and to remove metabolic waste. It is therefore a delivery system which functions by pumping blood through the vascular system. The term hemodynamics refers to the relationship between the motion of blood and the forces acting on this motion. This relationship is described by Poiseuille's Law ($Q=kP\mathrm{d}^4)l$ where Q is volume flow, P is the drop in pressure along a tube of given length (l) and diameter (d) and k is a coefficient related to viscosity). The ratio of mean pressure (P) to mean flow (Q) is thus a measure of the extent to which the system opposes or resists flow; this ratio is called the vascular resistance (R); $R=P/Q$. This equation is valid for laminar flow in straight tubes and therefore represents a gross oversimplification of human hemodynamics. However, it serves to illustrate the essential interrelationships of pressure, flow and resistance and highlights the important point that the key function of the circulatory system, that is to deliver flow, cannot be assessed by measuring blood pressure without knowing cardiac output.

Cardiac output is determined by the product of heart rate and stroke volume. Resting values average 5 l min^{-1} and this can be increased up to threefold during exercise. Cardiac output is influenced by four distinct, although interrelated, mechanisms (Fig 3.18.3):

1. The **preload** (Starling's law of the heart), which is the passive load that establishes the muscle length of the cardiac fibers prior to contraction.
2. The **afterload**, which is the sum of all the loads against which the myocardial fibers must shorten during systole, including the aortic impedance, the arterial resistance, the peripheral vascular resistance, and the end-diastolic volume through the LaPlace relation, as well as the mass of blood in the aorta and great arteries, and the viscosity of blood.
3. The **inotropic** or **contractile state** of the heart, which is reflected in the speed and shortening capacity of the myocardium at a given instantaneous load. At any given end-diastolic volume and afterload, an inotropic stimulus causes a greater shortening, as reflected by a smaller end-systolic size.
4. the **heart rate** or frequency of contraction.

Stroke volume is inversely related to afterload. An increase in myocardial contractility or preload at any given afterload leads to an increase in stroke volume.

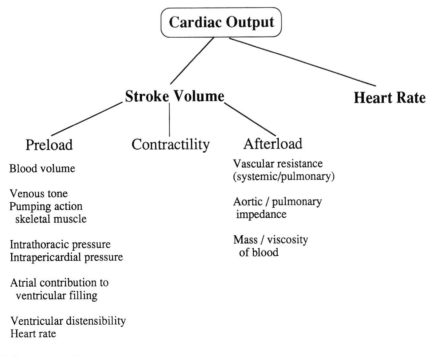

Fig. 3.18.3 *Factors influencing cardiac output.*

Cardiovascular changes during pregnancy

The heart and circulation undergo extensive anatomic and functional changes during pregnancy. Hemodynamic changes include alterations in blood volume, cardiac output, arterial pressure and systemic vascular resistance. The earliest studies of cardiac output employed the indirect Fick method which was very inaccurate. Later, following the development of cardiac catheterization, measurements were performed using the direct Fick and dye-dilution methods. Because of the inherent risks, most studies were cross-sectional in design and were of limited value in view of the wide variations in cardiac output between individuals. More recently, the development of M-mode echocardiography, impedance cardiography and Doppler echocardiography have allowed serial measurements of cardiac output without risk or discomfort to the woman. Of the non-invasive techniques available, combined cross-sectional and Doppler echocardiography appears to be most accurate and reproducible in pregnancy.[32,33] Whereas the impedance technique appears to be the least accurate.[34]

The majority of serial studies of hemodynamics during pregnancy have used postnatal measurements as non-pregnant baseline values. Although some functional adaptations appear to have returned to non-pregnant values by 6 weeks after delivery this does not apply to stroke volume[35] and to structural changes in the heart.[36] Thus, as with studies of respiratory function, some authors who have carried out control measurements during the first 6 weeks of the puerperium may have underestimated the size of changes during pregnancy. Ideally women should be recruited prior to conception. Three detailed longitudinal studies have included preconception hemodynamic measurements.[37-39]

The cardiovascular system is particularly sensitive to posture, activity and anxiety. Measurements must therefore be performed under standard resting conditions. During late pregnancy, inferior caval occlusion by the gravid uterus in the supine position leads to a fall in venous return and hence a reduction in stroke volume and cardiac output.[40] It is therefore necessary to perform all measurements in the lateral position to avoid postural artefacts.

CURRENT CONCEPTS

Cardiac output, heart rate and stroke volume

First trimester

Cardiac output increases early in pregnancy. Atkins et al.[37] were the first to study women prior to conception; cardiac output, measured by impedance cardiography, increased from a non-pregnant mean of 6.5 l min^{-1} to 7.7 l min^{-1} at 12 weeks of pregnancy. The results of the study of Robson et al.[39] in which cardiac output was measured by cross-sectional and Doppler echocardiography at three sites within the heart, are shown in Fig. 3.18.4. The mean non-pregnant cardiac output was 4.9 l min^{-1} and this increased throughout the first trimester reaching a mean of 6.6 l min^{-1} by 12 weeks (an increase of 35%). The increase was statistically significant by 5 weeks after the last menstrual period. The increase in cardiac output appears to result from increases in both heart rate and stroke volume.[38,39] During the menstrual cycle, maximum values of heart rate occur on day 21 and this is followed by a decrease of about 5 beats min^{-1}.[41] This fall is not evident if fertilization occurs and the mean increase in heart rate is 7 beats min^{-1} at 4 weeks and 8 beats min^{-1} at 8 weeks menstrual age.[42] Thus a continued increase in heart rate appears to be the earliest hemodynamic change associated with pregnancy.

Second trimester

Cardiac output increases further during the second trimester. Most studies have shown that maximum values are attained by the end of the second trimester. In the study by Robson et al.[39] cardiac output increased to around 7.1 l min^{-1} at 24 weeks' gestation (Fig. 3.18.4). This represents an increase of 45% over preconception values. The available evidence suggests that stroke volume contributes more than heart rate to the increase in cardiac output during the second trimester.[39,43-45]

Third trimester

There remains controversy about changes in cardiac output during the third trimester. The terminal fall reported by early workers appears to be a postural artefact[40] although Ueland et al.[43] reported a fall in cardiac output, measured by dye dilution in the lateral position, from 7.0 l min^{-1} at 28–32 weeks to 5.7 l min^{-1} at 38–40 weeks. The results of serial M-mode and Doppler echocardiographic studies performed with the subjects in the lateral position are also inconsistent with some showing a further increase in cardiac output[44,46] some showing a decrease[47,48] but most showing no change.[39,40,45]

Most serial studies have suggested that there is a further small increase in heart rate during the third trimester reaching values around 85 beats min^{-1} at term.[39,44-46] Changes in stroke volume are less consistent. Many workers have reported a small decrease of around 5 ml during the third trimester such that stroke volume at term is 80–85 ml.[39,45,47,48] However other workers, using both M-mode and Doppler echocardiography, have reported an increase.[44,46]

Two groups have reported maternal hemodynamic data from normal pregnant women obtained by pulmonary artery catheterization.[49,50] The increases in cardiac output (43%) and heart rate (17%) at 36–38 weeks' gestation were in agreement with non-invasive Doppler data.[39,46,48]

Preload and total blood volume

End-diastolic volume

The term **preload** represents the degree to which the myocardium is stretched before it contracts. The length of

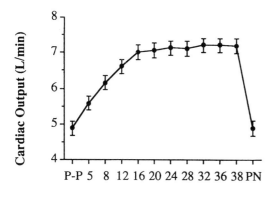

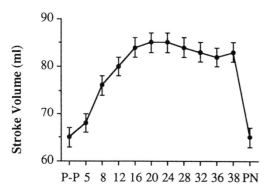

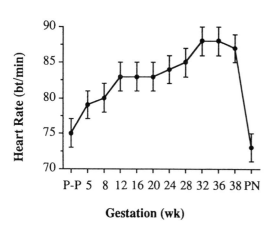

Gestation (wk)

Fig. 3.18.4 *Changes in cardiac output, heart rate and stroke volume during pregnancy measured by cross-sectional and Doppler echocardiography in 13 women studied serially from prior to pregnancy (P-P) to 6 months after delivery (P-N). Values are means ± SE. (Derived from reference 39.)*

the muscle fibers (i.e. the extent of preload) is proportionate to the end-diastolic volume. M-mode and cross-sectional echocardiography studies during pregnancy have shown consistent increases in left and right sided end-diastolic chamber dimensions.[38,39,44,51,52] Left ventricular end-diastolic dimension and left atrial dimension rise during the first and second trimesters and thereafter remain relatively constant.[38,39]

Total blood volume

The **total blood volume** is made up of the plasma volume and the red cell mass. Most studies of plasma volume in pregnancy have used Evans blue dye or radioactive iodinated albumin. The results of two detailed studies performed with subjects in the lateral position are shown in Fig. 3.18.5.[53,54] Both studies confirm that plasma volume increases primarily during the second trimester and that there is no terminal fall as had been suggested by earlier studies performed in the supine position. Plasma volume expansion is slightly greater in multiparous women. The increase in plasma volume is related to fetal size[54] and substantial increases are seen in women with multiple pregnancy; the mean increase in twins being 1940 ml and in triplets 2400 ml.[55]

Red cell mass may be measured directly, using red cells labelled with chromium-51 or phosphorus-32, or indirectly from plasma volume and hematocrit. The extent of the increase in red cell mass during pregnancy is greatly influenced by iron medication (Fig. 3.18.5) Direct studies suggest red cell mass increases by about 250 ml in women not having supplemental iron and by about 400 ml in women taking iron. The mean increase in red cell mass is greater in multiple pregnancy; 684 ml with twins and 902 ml with triplets.[55]

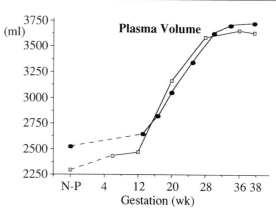

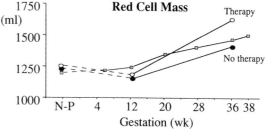

Fig. 3.18.5 *Changes in plasma volume and red cell mass during pregnancy (N-P; non-pregnant). The data on plasma volume were collected in the lateral position. (Reproduced from references 53 ●——● and 54 □——□. Red cell mass data were reproduced from references 54 □——□ and 56 in women given iron and folic acid (○——○) and in women on no therapy (●——●).*

Venous pressure

Although femoral venous pressure has been reported to be elevated in late pregnancy,[57] this reflects obstruction from the gravid uterus and there is no evidence that central venous pressure or pulmonary capillary wedge pressure is increased during pregnancy.[50] Plethysmographic studies in the calf and forearm suggest that venous distensibility and capacitance are increased during pregnancy.[58] These changes are most noticeable during the second trimester and presumably allow the increased blood volume to be accommodated without an increase in venous pressure.

Blood pressure and afterload

Blood pressure

The errors and limitations of blood pressure measurement by sphygmomanometry have been concisely reviewed by de Swiet.[59] Compared with direct intra-arterial measurement, sphygmomanometry gives a reading for systolic pressure which is 3–4 mmHg too low, and a reading for diastolic pressure which is 11 mmHg too high, if K4 (muffling of sounds) is used and 7 mmHg too high if K5 (disappearance of sounds) is used.[59] Comparisons between studies during pregnancy are hindered by variations in subject posture and the time and method of blood pressure measurement. However, the pattern of change appears to be very consistent; there is a small fall in systolic pressure and a marked fall in diastolic pressure, reaching a nadir at around 20 weeks with a progressive increase thereafter[39,60,61] (Fig. 3.18.6). Most studies have shown little difference between blood pressure at term and those in non-pregnant controls. The effect of posture on blood pressure in pregnancy is complex. Several groups have reported that blood pressure is lower in the left lateral position compared to the sitting or supine position.[37,62] However, around 10% of women in late pregnancy have a fall in systolic pressure of greater than 30 mmHg between sitting and lying supine and in some this is associated with the supine hypotensive syndrome.

Vascular resistance

As cardiac output increases and blood pressure falls during the first half of pregnancy vascular resistance must fall dramatically. Robson et al.[39] found that total systemic resistance reached a nadir at 20 weeks' gestation when values were 34% below those calculated prior to conception (Fig. 3.18.6).

Aortic compliance and blood viscosity

Hart et al.[64] demonstrated that the slope of the aortic pressure–area relation was significantly lower in late gestation compared to postpartum. Since the slope is the inverse of compliance, they concluded that the aorta was more compliant during pregnancy. These functional alterations may be related to the marked histological changes seen in the reticulin and elastin fibers of the aortic media during pregnancy.[65]

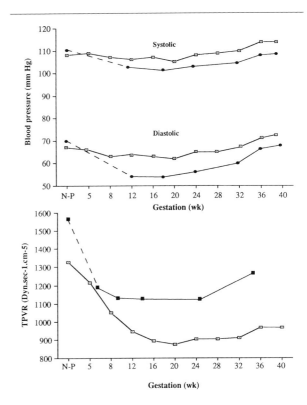

Fig. 3.18.6 *Changes in blood pressure and total peripheral vascular resistance (TPVR) during pregnancy (N-P; non-pregnant). (Reproduced from references 39 □——□, 60 ●——●, and 63 ■——■.*

Hemorheological studies have demonstrated that plasma viscosity is elevated throughout pregnancy, primarily reflecting the increase in fibrinogen levels. Whole blood viscosity falls during the first 24 weeks and then remains stable until the last 6–8 weeks of pregnancy when it increases.[66]

Thus the available evidence suggests that afterload is dramatically decreased during the first half of pregnancy primarily due to the reduction in vascular resistance but with some contribution from the decrease in aortic compliance and blood viscosity. Towards the end of pregnancy vascular resistance, at least on the systemic side of the circulation, and blood viscosity increase, although probably neither returns to non-pregnant levels.

Myocardial contractility

Numerous studies have measured ejection phase indices using M-mode echocardiography during pregnancy. These include fractional shortening, ejection fraction and the mean and peak rates of circumferential fiber shortening (Vcf). These studies suggest that ventricular performance is increased during the first two trimesters and falls towards term.[39,44,45,51,52] However, ejection phase indices, although readily measurable, are dependent not only on contractility but on preload and afterload.

Structural changes in the heart

Ventricular mass can be calculated from M-mode echo-cardiographic measurents of wall thickness. This appears to increase progressively throughout pregnancy reaching values up to 50% above those in the non-pregnant state.[39,44,51] Changes in wall thickness comparable to those seen during pregnancy have been reported in subjects after only 12 weeks of exercise training.[67] It is thought that the increase in cardiac output during training leads to an increase in end-diastolic wall stress, which enlarges the internal diameter and consequently systolic wall stress. The increase in wall thickness serves to normalize systolic wall stress. The same sequence of events may operate during pregnancy.

Valve diameters and areas measured by cross-sectional and M-mode echocardiography increase during pregnancy. This applies for all four cardiac valves[39,64,68] and almost certainly accounts for the increased incidence of regurgitant flow velocities seen during pregnancy.[69,70]

Changes in organ blood flow during pregnancy

Published values for organ blood flow in healthy non-pregnant and pregnant women have varied considerably. A summary of the published literature is given in Table 3.18.1. Peripheral blood flow is increased substantially during pregnancy although this appears to be primarily related to cutaneous vasodilation, there being little or no change in muscle blood flow. Cerebral blood flow is unchanged in pregnancy.[71] No quantitative measurements of mammary or coronary blood flow have been performed during pregnancy. However, it seems likely that both will be increased. Indirect evidence in support of an increase in mammary flow comes from Doppler studies of the mammary branch of the right lateral thoracic artery.[72]

Table 3.18.1 Approximate changes in organ blood flow during pregnancy

Site	Flow (ml min^{-1})	
	Non-pregnant	Pregnant
Kidney	500	900
Uterus	60	500
Skin	500	1000
Skeletal muscle	750	750
Liver	1700	1700
Cerebral	750	750
Breast	Unknown	Unknown
Myocardium	250	Unknown
Other organs	600	Unknown

Hemodynamics changes during labor

Most early studies of **cardiac output** during labor were performed with subjects in the supine position. When measurements are performed in the lateral position in women given pethidine, the increase in cardiac output dur-ing contractions increases throughout the first stage of labor reaching values 34% above baseline by the end of the first stage of labor.[73] Initially, this is due to an increase in stroke volume but later both stroke volume and heart rate increase.[73-76] Basal cardiac output (between contractions) increases by 12% during the first stage of labor due to an increase in stroke volume.[73] Further increases occur during the second stage of labor to produce a cardiac output 49% above prelabour values.[74]

Effective epidural analgesia during labor prevents the increase in heart rate during uterine contractions[73] but has no effect on the increase in stroke volume.[76] This strongly suggests that the increase in heart rate is a sympathetic response to pain. The increase in stroke volume is likely to be secondary to an increase in preload as blood is squeezed into the circulation from the choriodecidual space during uterine contractions. This is supported by the finding that central venous pressure rises by 5 mmHg during contractions.[75]

Both systolic and diastolic pressure increase during uterine contractions.[73,75]

Mechanism of cardiovascular changes in pregnancy

The increase in plasma and extracellular fluid volume, glomerular filtration rate and renal plasma flow has led to the suggestion that pregnancy is a state of volume overload; the so-called 'overfill' hypothesis. This theory proposes that primary hypersecretion of aldosterone leads to sodium and water retention. A more attractive hypothesis proposes that pregnancy is a state of reduced effective blood volume which is accompanied by secondary aldosteronism; the 'underfill' hypothesis. According to this hypothesis arterial vasodilation is the primary circulatory change which leads to underfilling of the circulation. The consequences of this include a decrease in blood pressure, an increase in cardiac output secondary to afterload reduction, stimulation of the renin–angiotensin–aldosterone axis, non-osmotic stimulation of thirst and vasopressin release. This leads to renal sodium and water retention with expansion of the extracellular and plasma volume compartments. Evidence in support of the underfill hypothesis comes from both animal and human studies which have shown that the changes in vascular resistance precede, usually by around 8 weeks, the increase in blood volume.[63,77]

The mechanisms underlying the alterations in vascular resistance are unclear. Estrogens increase cardiac output, primarily by increasing stroke volume and plasma volume, but have an inconsistent effect on blood pressure.[78] Progesterone induces small increases in heart rate but has little effect on blood pressure or cardiac output.[79] Prostacyclin and nitric oxide (endothelium-derived relaxing factor) are two important vasodilators released by the vascular endothelium. There is evidence that the production of both compounds by the endothelium is increased in pregnancy but their relative contribution to peripheral vasodilation remains to be determined.[80,81]

Cardiorespiratory signs and symptoms during pregnancy

Symptoms

The physiological changes in the cardiorespiratory systems are responsible for several symptoms and signs that may simulate disease during pregnancy. Milne *et al.*[82] found the incidence of breathlessness to increase from 15% in the first trimester to about 50% by 20 weeks' gestation and 75% by 28–31 weeks. This does not appear to correlate with any single parameter of respiratory function. Easy fatigability and reduced exercise tolerance are also common in normal pregnancy. Lightheadedness or even syncopal attacks may occur during late pregnancy, presumably as a result of mechanical compression of the enlarged uterus on the inferior vena cava which results in a decrease in venous return and a fall in cardiac output.[83]

Signs

Hyperventilation is a common feature during pregnancy. Compression of the basal parts of the lung by the enlarging uterus may lead to atelectasis and occasional basilar rales. The higher position of the diaphragm displaces the heart and leads to the left ventricular impulse being displaced to the left. A right ventricular impulse can usually be palpated. Cutforth and MacDonald[84] studied cardiac auscultatory findings with phonocardiography during pregnancy.

They found a loud widely split first sound with a tendency for expiratory splitting of the second sound in late pregnancy. A third sound was heard in 84%. Systolic ejection murmurs were found in 92% of pregnant women. These were best heard at the lower left sternal edge and were usually grade 1–3/6. These are thought to represent audible vibrations caused by ejection into the pulmonary artery. A soft early diastolic murmur can also be heard in some women. This may reflect increased flow through the atrioventricular valves.

FUTURE PERSPECTIVES

Although the functional alterations in the cardiovascular and respiratory systems are now reasonably well understood, the mechanisms by which these are brought about warrant more intensive study. This is particularly true of the events which lead to arterial vasodilation. Much attention is currently being directed to nitric oxide (NO). In the non-pregnant state the systemic vascular bed appears to be under constant NO-mediated vasodilator tone and there is preliminary evidence that vascular synthesis of NO is increased during pregnancy. Understanding the mechanism of vasodilation may be of more than physiological interest as in pre-eclampsia the normal cardiovascular adaptations are reversed and there is a marked increase in vascular resistance.

SUMMARY

- Minute ventilation increases by 40% during pregnancy, due to an increase in tidal volume, whereas alveolar ventilation increases by more than 50%. These changes occur early in the first trimester.
- Oxygen consumption increases by 20% during pregnancy to meet the increased demands of the mother and fetus.
- Overbreathing leads to a reduction of $P\text{CO}_2$ by 5–10 mmHg allowing the fetus to offload CO_2. There is a compensatory increase in renal bicarbonate excretion. This leads to a fall in plasma sodium and therefore osmolality.
- The stimulus to the increase in ventilation appears to be progesterone.
- Cardiac output increases by 40–45% during pregnancy due to increases in both stroke volume and heart rate. Maximum values are

attained by mid-pregnancy and thereafter, at least in the lateral position, cardiac output is maintained till term.
- Peripheral arterial vasodilation during the first trimester leads to a fall in blood pressure and a reduction in cardiac afterload.
- Secondary stimulation of the renin–aldosterone axis leads to an increase in blood volume and cardiac preload.
- Myocardial contractility also appears to be increased early in pregnancy.
- The mechanisms responsible for arterial and venous dilation are currently unclear. Nitric oxide and prostacyclin, derived from the vascular endothelium, may be involved.
- The cardiorespiratory changes are among the most dramatic and earliest adaptations seen in pregnancy.

REFERENCES

1. Hytten FE, Leitch I. Respiration. In *The Physiology of Human Pregnancy*, 2nd edn, Oxford: Blackwell Scientific Publications, 1971: 111–131.
2. de Swiet M. The respiratory system. In Hytten FE, Chamberlain G (eds) *Clinical Physiology in Obstetrics* Oxford: Blackwell Scientific Publications, 1991: 83–100.
3. Spatling L, Fallenstein F, Huch A, Huch R, Rooth G. The variability of cardiopulmonary adaptation to pregnancy at rest and during exercise. *Br J Obstet Gynaecol* 1992 **99**: Suppl 8: 1–40.
4. Clapp JF, Seaward BL, Sleamaker RH, Hiser J. Maternal physiologic adaptations to early pregnancy. *Am J Obstet Gynecol* 1988 **159**: 1456–1460.
5. von Mobius W. Atmung und Schwangerschaft. *Munch med Wechr* 1961 **103**: 1389–1396.
6. Eng M, Butler J, Bonica JJ. Respiratory function in pregnant obese women. *Am J Obstet Gynecol* 1975 **123**: 241–245.
7. Gazioglu K, Kaltreider NL, Rosen M, Yu PN. Pulmonary function during pregnancy in normal women and in patients with cardiopulmonary disease. *Thorax* 1970 **25**: 445–450.
8. Knuttgen HG, Emerson K. Physiological response to pregnancy at rest and during exercise. *J Appl Physiol* 1974 **36**: 549–553.
9. Cugell DW, Frank NR, Gaensler EA, Badger TL. Pulmonary function in pregnancy. I. Serial observations in normal women. *Am Rev Tuberculosis* 1953 **67**: 568–597.
10. Lees GR, Broughton Pipkin F, Symonds EM, Patrick JM. A longitudinal study of respiratory changes in normal pregnancy with cross-sectional data on subjects with pregnancy-induced hypertension. *Am J Obstet Gynecol* 1990 **162**: 826–830.
11. Pernoll ML, Metcalfe J, Schlenker TL, Welch JE, Matsumoto JA. Oxygen consumption at rest and during exercise in pregnancy. *Respir Physiol* 1975 **25**: 285–293.
12. Sims CD, Chamberlain GVP, de Swiet M. Lung function tests in bronchial asthma during and after pregnancy. *Br J Obstet Gynaecol* 1976 **83**: 434–437.
13. Gee JBL, Packer BS, Millen JE, Robin ED. Pulmonary mechanics during pregnancy. *J Clin Invest* 1967 **46**: 945–952.
14. Marx GF, Murthy PK, Orkin LR. Static compliance before and after vaginal delivery. *Br J Anaesth* 1970 **42**: 1100–1105.
15. Milne JA, Pack AI, Coutts JRT. Maternal gas exchange and acid base status during normal pregnancy. *Scot Med J* 1977 **22**: 108–114.
16. Alaily AB, Carrol KB. Pulmonary ventilation in pregnancy. *Br J Obstet Gynaecol* 1978 **85**: 518–524.
17. Lucius H, Gahlenbeck H, Kleine HO, Fabel H, Bartels H. Respiratory functions, buffer system and electrolyte concentrations of blood during human pregnancy. *Respir Physiol* 1970 **9**: 311.
18. Ang CK, Tan TH, Walters WAW, Wood C. Postural influences on maternal capillary and carbon dioxide tension. *Br Med J* 1969 **IV**: 20–22.
19. Kamban JR, Handtke RE, Brown WU, Smith BE. Effect of pregnancy on oxygen dissociation. *Anethesiology* 1983 **59**: A359.
20. Crawford JS, Tunstall ME. Notes on respiratory performance during labour. *Br J Anaesth* 1968 **40**: 612–614.
21. Fisher A, Prys-Roberts C. Maternal pulmonary gas exchange. *Anaesthesia* 1968 **23**: 350–356.
22. Hagerdal M, Morgan CW, Summer AE, Gutsche B. Minute ventilation and oxygen consumption during labor and epidural anesthesia. *Anaesthesiology* 1983 **59**: 425–427.
23. Miller FC, Petrie RH, Arce JJ, Paul RH, Hon EH. Hyperventilation during labor. *Am J Obstet Gynecol* 1974 **120**: 489–495.
24. Huch A, Huch R, Lindmark G, Rooth G. Maternal hypoxaemia after pethidine. *J Obstet Gynaecol Br Commonw* 1974 **81**: 608.
25. Marx GF, Greene NM. Maternal lactate, pyruvate and excess lactate production during labor and delivery. *Am J Obstet Gynecol* 1964 **90**: 786–793.
26. Pearson JF, Davies P. The effect of continuous epidural analgesia on maternal acid–base status of maternal arterial blood during the first stage of labour. *J Obstet Gynaecol Br Commonw* 1973 **80**: 218–224.
27. Pearson JF, Davies P. The effect of continuous epidural analgesia on maternal acid–base balance and arterial lactate concentration during the second stage of labour. *J Obstet Gynaecol Br Commonw* 1973 **80**: 225–231.
28. Wilbrand U, Porath C, Matthaes P, Jaster R. Der einfluss der Ovarialsteroide auf die Funktion des Atemzentrums. *Archiv Gynakol* 1952 **191**: 507–509.
29. Prowse CM, Gaensler EA. Respirator and acid base changes during pregnancy. *Anesthesiology* 1965 **26**: 381–392.
30. Lyons HA, Antonio R. The sensitivity of the respiratory centre in pregnancy and after the administration of progesterone. *Trans Assoc Am Phys* 1959 **72**: 173.
31. Schenker JG, Ben-Yoseph Y, Shapira E. Erythrocyte carbonic anhydrase B levels during pregnancy and use of oral contraceptives. *Obstet Gynecol* 1972 **39**: 237–240.
32. Easterling TR, Carlson KL, Schmucker BC, Millard SP. Measurement of cardiac output in pregnancy by Doppler technique. *Am J Perinatol* 1990 **3**: 220–222.
33. Robson SC, Dunlop W, Moore M, Hunter S. Combined Doppler and echocardiographic measurement of cardiac output: theory and application in pregnancy. *Br J Obstet Gynaecol* 1987 **94**: 1014–1027.
34. Secher NJ, Arnsbo P, Heslet Anderson L, Thompson A. Measurement of cardiac stroke volumes in various body positions in pregnancy and during caesarean section: a comparison between thermodilution and impedance cardiography. *Scand J Lab Invest* 1979 **39**: 569–576.
35. Capeless EL, Clapp JF. When do cardiovascular parameters return to their preconception values? *Am J Obstet Gynecol* 1991 **165**: 883–886.
36. Robson SC, Hunter S, Moore M, Dunlop W. Haemodynamic changes during the puerperium: a Doppler and M–mode echocardiographic study. *Br J Obstet Gynaecol* 1987 **94**: 1028–1039.
37. Atkins AJF, Watt JM, Milan P, Davies P, Selwyn Crawford J. A longitudinal study of cardiovascular dynamic changes throughout pregnancy. *Eur J Obstet Gynecol Reprod Biol* 1981 **12**: 215–224.
38. Capeless EL, Clapp JF. Cardiovascular changes in early phase of pregnancy. *Am J Obstet Gynecol* 1989 **161**: 1449–1453.
39. Robson SC, Hunter S, Boys RJ, Dunlop W. Serial study of factors influencing changes in cardiac output during human pregnancy. *Am J Physiol* 1989 **256**: H1060–1065.
40. Lees MM, Scott DB, Kerr MG, Taylor SH. The circulatory effects of recumbent postural change in late pregnancy. *Clin Sci* 1967 **32**: 453–465.
41. Kelleher C, Joyce C, Kelly G, Ferriss JB. Blood pressure alters during the normal menstrual cycle. *Br J Obstet Gynaecol* 1986 **93**: 523–526.
42. Clapp JF. Maternal heart rate in pregnancy. *Am J Obstet Gynecol* 1985 **152**: 859–860.
43. Ueland K, Novy MJ, Peterson EN, Metcalfe J. Maternal cardiovascular dynamics. IV. The influence of gestational age on the maternal cardiovascular response to posture and exercise. *Am J Obstet Gynecol* 1969 **104**: 856–864.
44. Katz R, Karliner JS, Resnik R. Effects of a natural volume overload state (pregnancy) on left ventricular performance in normal human subjects. *Circulation* 1978 **58**: 434–441.
45. Mashini IS, Albbazzaz SJ, Fadel HE *et al.* Serial noninvasive evaluation of cardiovascular hemodynamics during pregnancy. *Am J Obstet Gynecol* 1987 **156**: 1208–1213.
46. Mabie WC, DiSessa TG, Crocker LG, Sibai BM, Arheart

KL. A longitudinal study of cardiac output in normal human pregnancy. *Am J Obstet Gynecol* 1994 **170**: 849–856.

47. Steegers EAP, van Lakwijk HPJM, Benaad T *et al.* Atrial natriuretic peptide (ANP) in normal pregnancy; a longitudinal study. *Clin Exp Hyper Preg* 1990 **B9**: 273–292.

48. Easterling TR, Benedetti TJ, Schmucker BC, Millard SP. Maternal hemodynamics in normal and preeclamptic pregnancies: a longitudinal study. *Obstet Gynecol* 1990 **76**: 1061–1069.

49. Wallenburg HCS. Hemodynamics in hypertensive pregnancy. In Rubin PC (ed.) *Hypertension in Pregnancy* Amsterdam, Elsevier; 1988; 66–101.

50. Clark SL, Cotton DB, Lee W *et al.* Central hemodynamic assessment of normal term pregnancy. *Am J Obstet Gynecol* 1989 **161**: 1439–1442.

51. Laird-Meeter K, Van De Ley G, Bom TH, Wladimiroff JW. Cardiocirculatory adjustments during pregnancy – An echocardiographic study. *Clin Cardiol* 1979 **2**: 328–332.

52. Castillon G, Weissenburger J, Rouffet M, Castillon V, Barrat J. Etude échocardiographique des modifications hémodynamiques de la grossesse. *J Gynecol Obstet Biol Reprod* 1984 **13**: 499–505.

53. Pirani BBK, Campbell DM, Macgillivray I. Plasma volume in normal first pregnancy. *J Obstet Gynaecol Br Commonw* 1973 **80**: 884–887.

54. Lind T. Hematologic system. In *Maternal Physiology* Washington: CREOG, 1985: 7–40.

55. Rovinsky JJ, Jaffin H. Cardiovascular hemodynamics in pregnancy. I. Blood and plasma volumes in multiple pregnancy. *Am J Obstet Gynecol* 1965 **93**: 1–13.

56. Taylor DJ, Lind T. Red cell mass during and after normal pregnancy. *Br J Obstet Gynaecol* 1979 **86**: 364–370.

57. McLennan CE. Antecubital and femoral venous pressure in normal and toxemic pregnancy. *Am J Obstet Gynecol* 1943 **45**: 568–591.

58. Barwin BN, Roddie IC. Venous distensibility during pregnancy determined by graded venous congestion. *Am J Obstet Gynecol* 1976 **125**: 921–923.

59. de Swiet M. The cardiovascular system. In Hytten FE, Chamberlain G (eds) *Clinical Physiology in Obstetrics* Oxford: Blackwell Scientific Publications, 1991: 3–38.

60. MacGillivray I, Rose GA, Rowe B. Blood pressure survey in pregnancy. *Clin Sci* 1969 **37**: 395–407.

61. Schwarz R. Das Verhalten des Kreislaufs in der normalen Schwangersghaft. I. Der arterielle Blutdruck. *Archiv Gynäkol* 1964 **199**: 549–570.

62. Eskes TKAB, Weyer A, Kramer N, Van Elteren P. Arterial blood pressure and posture during pregnancy. A prospective study. *Eur J Obstet Gynec Reprod Biol* 1974 **4**: 87–94.

63. Duvekot JJ, Cheriex EC, Pieters FAA, Menheere PPCA, Peeters LLH. Early pregnancy changes in hemodynamics and volume homeostasis are consecutive adjustments triggered by a primary fall in systemic vascular tone. *Am J Obstet Gynecol* 1993 **169**: 1382–1392.

64. Hart MV, Mortom MJ, Hosenpud JD, Metcalfe J. Aortic function during normal human pregnancy. *Am J Obstet Gynecol* 1986 **154**: 887–891.

65. Manalo-Estrella P, Barker AE. Histopathologic findings in human aortic media associated with pregnancy. *Arch Pathol* 1967 **83**: 336–341.

66. Buchan PC. Maternal and fetal blood viscosity throughout normal pregnancy. *J Obstet Gynaecol* 1984 **4**: 143–150.

67. Lusiani L, Ronsisvalle G, Bonanome A *et al.* Echocardiographic evaluation of the dimensions and systolic properties of the left ventricle in freshman athletes during physical training. *Eur Heart J* 1986 **7**: 196–203.

68. Limacher MC, Ware A, O'Meara ME, Fernandez GC, Young JB. Tricuspid regurgitation during pregnancy: two dimensional and pulsed Doppler echocardiographic observations. *Am J Cardiol* 1985 **55**: 1059–1062.

69. Robson SC, Richley D, Boys RJ, Hunter S. Incidence of Doppler regurgitant flow velocities during normal pregnancy. *Eur Heart J* 1992 **13**: 84–87.

70. Dunlop W. Serial changes in renal haemodynamics during normal pregnancy. *Br J Obstet Gynaecol* 1981 **88**: 1–9.

71. McCall ML. Cerebral blood flow and metabolism in toxemias of pregnancy. *Surg Gynecol Obstet* 1949 **89**: 715–721.

72. Thoresen M, Wesche J. Doppler measurements of changes in human mammary and uterine blood flow during pregnancy and lactation. *Acta Obstet Gynecol Scand* 1988 **67**: 741–745.

73. Robson SC, Dunlop W, Boys RJ, Hunter S. Cardiac output during labour. *Br Med J* 1987 **296**: 1169–1172.

74. Ueland K, Hansen JM. Maternal cardiovascular dynamics. III. Labor and delivery under local and caudal analgesia. *Am J Obstet Gynecol* 1969 **103**: 8–18.

75. Kjeldsen J. Haemodynamic investigations during labour and delivery. *Acta Obstet Gynecol Scand* [Suppl] 1979 **89**: 77–195.

76. Lee W, Rokey R, Cotton DB, Miller JF. Maternal hemodynamic effects of uterine contractions by M-mode and pulsed-Doppler echocardiography. *Am J Obstet Gynecol* 1989 **161**: 974–977.

77. Phippard AF, Horvarth JS, Glynn EM *et al.* Circulatory adaptation to pregnancy – serial studies of haemodynamics, blood volume, renin and aldosterone in the baboon (*Papio hamadryas*). *J Hypertens* 1986 **4**: 773–779.

78. Walters WAW, Lim YL. Cardiovascular dynamics in women receiving oral contraceptive therapy. *Lancet* 1969 **ii**: 879–881.

79. Lumbers ER. Effects on sheep blood pressure of treatment with angiotensin, steroids and salt. *Clin Exp Pharm Physiol* 1990 **17**: 315–319.

80. Lewis PJ. Prostacyclin in pregnancy. *Br Med J* 1980 **ii**: 1581–1582.

81. Conrad KP, Joffe GM, Kruszyna H *et al.* Identification of increased nitric oxide biosynthesis during pregnancy in rats. *FASEB J* 1993 **7**: 566–571.

82. Milne JA, Howie AD, Pack AL. Dyspnoea during normal pregnancy. *Br J Obstet Gynaecol* 1978 **85**: 260.

83. Kerr M. The mechanical effects of the gravid uterus in late pregnancy. *J Obstet Gynaecol Br Commonw* 1965 **72**: 513–529.

84. Cutforth R, MacDonald MB. Heart sounds and murmurs in pregnancy. *Am Heart J* 1966 **71**: 741–747.

Section 4

Reproductive Cancers

4.1

Epidemiology of Reproductive Cancers

J-A Clyma, H Winter, S Wilson and CBJ Woodman

INTRODUCTION

This chapter aims to describe temporal and geographical trends in the incidence, mortality and survival of the three main gynecological malignancies – cancer of the ovary, cervix and uterine body. Information has been drawn from the wide body of data produced at regional and national level by cancer registries and cancer research organizations around the world. In an attempt to improve communication between epidemiologists and clinicians, more reference has been made than is usual to the basic principles which underpin the analysis and interpretation of cancer surveillance data.

The role of cancer registries in assessing the impact of cancer in the general population is an important one, for they hold information on the vast majority of all cancers in defined geographical areas. The totality of this experience cannot be adequately represented by the results of hospital series which, although they may indicate what can be achieved in terms of cancer control, are inevitably subject to biases from case referral and selection.

CURRENT CONCEPTS

Mortality data

One commonly quoted statistic used in monitoring progress towards cancer control, is mortality. However, the interpretation of mortality rates is confounded by three major problems:

1. The certified cause of death is notoriously inaccurate and death certification practises may vary over time and place.
2. Not all patients diagnosed with cancer will die from the cancer. Survival rates vary widely for cancers at different sites; the 5-year survival rate for skin cancer approaches

100% whereas for lung cancer is less than 10%. For most sites of cancer, mortality rates fail to describe adequately the true burden of disease.

3. There is only a limited amount of information on the death certificate. In particular, no information is available concerning the histological type of disease, stage at presentation, type or place of treatment and length of survival – these variables are necessary to describe our progress towards achieving cancer control.

Morbidity data

The incidence of cancer is defined as the number of new primary cancers arising in a defined population during a defined time period. The incidence rate is expressed as the number of new registered cases per 100 000 population per year.

Cancer rates vary greatly with age and the crude (all ages) rate is affected by the age and sex structure of the population. Differences in the age structure of different populations, or between the same population over time, prohibits the use of the crude incidence rate for comparative purposes. In order to compare the pattern of disease in two areas, or over time, it is important to allow for differing population age structures. This is accomplished by age standardization. The age-standardized rate is not as revealing as a thorough examination of age-specific rates but is a useful summary measure. There are two methods of age-standardization in general use – the indirect and direct methods.

Indirect age standardization involves calculating expected numbers of cases by applying a standard set of age-specific rates to the population of interest and comparing them with the numbers actually observed in the population.

Direct standardization results in a theoretical summary rate and is obtained by applying the observed age-specific rates to a reference population. The reference population that is used can be real, e.g. the population of the USA in

1970, or notional, e.g. the World Standard Population or the European Standard Population. The choice of reference population is arbitrary, but, if comparisons are to be made with other published series then the same reference population should be used. The use of different standard populations will provide different values for the standardized rate. Direct age standardization has considerable advantages over the indirect method, the most important of which is that several populations may be compared with each other.

Standardized incidence rates often fail to communicate adequately the absolute risk of an individual developing cancer. Some prefer cumulative risk and although this statistic is itself imperfect, it better indicates the average risk to an individual of developing cancer before a certain age. It is usual to calculate the cumulative risk over the age period 0–74 years as this statistic is based on an approximate formula which becomes more unreliable beyond this age, as the number of deaths from other causes rises with increasing age (Fig. 4.1.1).[1]

This measure has the advantages of removing the arbitrariness of choosing a standard population, is simple to calculate and has a greater intuitive appeal than a standardized incidence rate. However, it should be remembered that the effect of other diseases, such as those occurring in middle age are ignored, and no account is taken of incidence beyond the age of 74 years although one-third of cancer registrations occur in persons aged 75 years or more.

Survival

An alternative method of measuring the effectiveness of cancer care in a population is to examine changes in the survival of individuals diagnosed with cancer. Survival rates may be expressed as the proportion of patients alive at some defined point subsequent to the date of diagnosis of their cancer. The choice of interval is arbitrary, but the 5-year survival rate is conventionally used and is often taken as a measure of cure.

Crude survival estimates the proportion of patients who are still alive at a given point in time after diagnosis. There are, however, two problems with its estimation:

1. Not all cancer patients die from their cancer. Patients who die from other causes should be censored from the analysis at time of death, since the objective is to estimate the mortality from the cancer under consideration.
2. Cases which do not have the required period of follow-up must be excluded from the analysis.

The computation of crude survival rates can be refined by undertaking an actuarial (life-table) analysis. Actuarial methods will allow for differing periods of follow-up. The resultant statistic is often referred to as the Observed Survival Rate.

Survival analysis aims to estimate the force of mortality from the cancer under consideration. Its estimation presents two major difficulties; it is often not possible to decide from routinely collected data whether a patient with cancer has died from the disease or from an unrelated cause, and those deaths from other causes will be more frequent in older people. To overcome these problems, it is now customary when using cancer surveillance data, to estimate a survival rate which allows for deaths from other causes. This is called the Relative Survival Rate. It is calculated as the ratio of the crude survival to that which would be expected from the general mortality experience of the population. The expected survival probabilities for each age and sex category in the general population are obtained

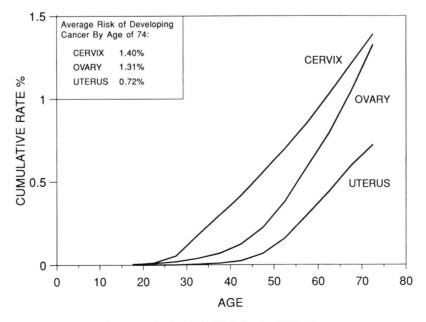

Fig. 4.1.1 *Cumulative incidence rates, North Western Regional Health Authority 1985–89.*

from published Life Tables. The relative survival rate is calculated for each interval of follow-up; this method allows for changes in the age distribution of survivors and the pattern of mortality over time. The five-year survival rate is obtained by multiplying the successive annual probabilities. The difference between observed and relative survival for patients with cancer of the uterine body is shown in Fig. 4.1.2.[1]

Comparisons of 5-year point estimates of survival have been interpreted as suggesting that treatment policies are more effective in certain countries. However, in addition to variation in the access to, or provision of, diagnostic or treatment services, there are other possible explanations for differentials in survival.

Routinely collected surveillance data are subject to two types of error; incomplete ascertainment of cases or deaths and misclassification. The failure of surveillance systems to register all cases of cancer which occur within the defined population may affect estimates of survival. These will be inflated if there is a systematic failure to ascertain deaths, which is more likely in countries that cannot access death certificates. The pathological distinction between what constitutes pre-invasive or invasive cancer may vary over time or between countries, for example, carcinoma in situ of the cervix is a common condition which, if systematically reported as invasive disease will substantially inflate incidence rates for cervical cancer. A further consequence of the systematic designation of pre-malignant conditions as invasive disease would be an apparent improvement in survival.

For many cancers, survival is related to age at diagnosis. This must be taken into account when comparing survival rates. For example, if a district and a region have similar age specific incidence rates for a specified cancer but the district has a substantially younger population, then more cancers in the district will be in younger people. If young age is a favorable prognostic factor then the district will appear to have a better survival rate. It is unfortunately not possible to age stratify international comparisons which are based on published statistics.

Other factors which should be borne in mind when undertaking comparisons of cancer statistics are the efficiency of the local cancer registration process and the date from which survival is measured. The starting point for survival analysis may be either the date of first diagnosis, the date of hospital admission, the date of histological confirmation of disease, or the date of first treatment. Several months can elapse between the primary care practitioner's tentative diagnosis of cancer and the commencement of treatment. The earlier the start date for analysis, the longer the apparent survival.

None of the considerations discussed above invalidate the use of population-based survival rates. They merely illustrate factors that should be taken into account before variations in survival or incidence are used to make assumptions on the effectiveness of health care provision.

Data sources

We have had to exercise a considerable degree of selectivity regarding which data to include in this chapter. Not all countries possess a cancer registration system, few countries have national systems and all of these do not routinely produce survival rates. Those that do include the SEER program in the USA, which covers 13 States, and the Scottish cancer registry. Data from Scotland have recently been published for the period 1968–87 in the form of quinquennial rates.

The most recent survival estimates for England and Wales refer to the survival experience of cancer patients diagnosed during the period 1979–80. We have, therefore, chosen to use estimates of survival derived from local data to enable temporal trends in England to be included. These data, based as they are on large regional populations, should be reasonably representative of the survival of cancer patients in England and Wales as a whole.

Cancer of the uterine corpus

Cancer of the uterine body is estimated to be the eighth most frequently occurring cancer in women worldwide.[2] World standardized age-adjusted incidence rates range from around 2 to 18 per 100 000 women (Fig. 4.1.3).[3] It occurs more frequently in women in developed countries, with the highest incidence rates reported in North America and Northern Europe. Japan appears the only exception, with one of the lowest incidence rates for this tumor worldwide.[3] In the majority of Northern European countries a small rise in incidence has occurred between 1960 and 1985. In North America large increases in incidence occurred between 1965 and 1975, but since 1975 this trend has been reversed (Fig. 4.1.4).[4] It is noteworthy that there was no change in mortality from cancer of the body of the uterus in the US during this period. It is also intriguing that the survival of cases in the US decreased, while a steady improvement in survival had been observed in England and Scotland (Fig. 4.1.5).[1,4,5]

The explanation for these disparate trends may follow

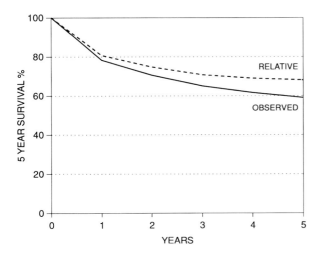

Fig. 4.1.2 *Comparison of observed versus relative survival (uterus), North Western Regional Health Authority, 1985–89.*

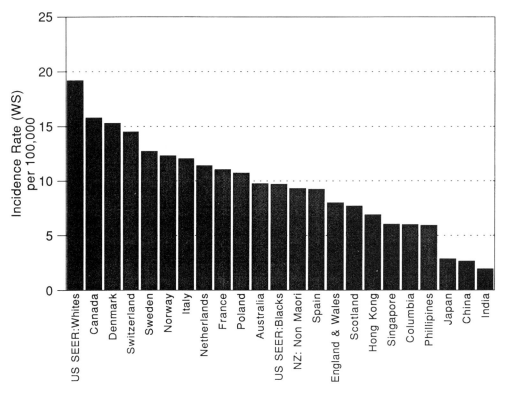

Fig. 4.1.3 *Cancer of the uterus. Geographical trends in incidence, 1983–87.*

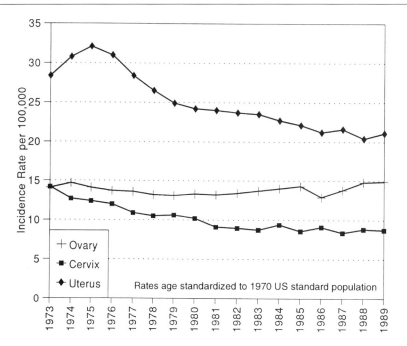

Fig. 4.1.4 *Gynecological cancer in the USA. Temporal trends in incidence 1973–89.*

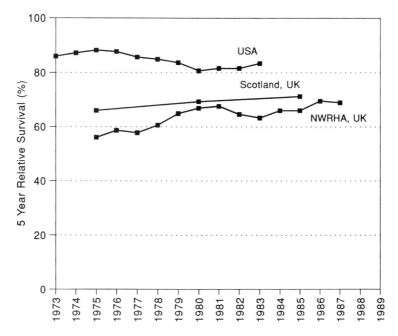

Fig. 4.1.5 *Cancer of the uterus. Temporal trends in survival, 1973–89.*

from transatlantic differences in the prescribing of supplementary or replacement estrogen therapy in the perimenopausal period. An association between the use of hormone replacement therapy (HRT) and the development of endometrial carcinoma has been hypothesized as an explanation of the observed increase in incidence in corpus cancer seen in the US. Initial case control studies supporting this hypothesis were criticized on methodological grounds, in particular the failure to eliminate previous hysterectomy as a potential confounder. Increasingly sophisticated case-control studies, and a few prospective studies, have confirmed a relative risk of approximately 3–4 for ever use of HRT.[6,7] The fall in incidence of corpus cancer which has occurred in the US following the decrease in use of HRT, is regarded as additional evidence of the association. The increased risk of cancer associated with the use of unopposed estrogen therapy is greater for early stage disease, and although this could reflect lead time bias there is evidence to suggest that tumors induced by HRT are better differentiated, less invasive, and therefore associated with a better survival.[8] A reduction in the absolute number of these iatrogenic, good prognosis tumors following a decrease in the use of HRT may explain the apparent worsening of survival in the US in recent years.

Cancer of the ovary

Ovarian cancer is the sixth most common cancer worldwide in women,[2] and the most common cause of death from gynecological cancer in the United Kingdom.[9] World standardized, age-adjusted incidence rates range from 4 to 15 per 100 000, with the highest rates found in the most affluent North European populations (Fig. 4.1.6).[3] Rates

for the period 1955–85 have remained unchanged or have decreased slightly in most European populations, the Americas, Oceania and parts of Asia.[10] There is a suggestion of a recent upward trend in Scotland, some regions of England, and the USA (Figs 4.1.4 and 4.1.7).[4,11] A further period of observation is required in order to determine if this is a true increase in incidence, or simply a reflection of an improvement in diagnosis and accuracy of pathological reporting. Table 4.1.1 shows estimates of relative 5-year survival reported by a number of population-based cancer registries.[4,5,12–17] There is wide international variation in relative survival with a range from 27% to 37%. Fig. 4.1.8 shows that there has been some improvement in relative survival for patients with this disease over the last 20 years, although geographical differences between populations are preserved.[1,4,5]

The aetiology of ovarian cancer is poorly understood, but the theory of 'incessant ovulation' proposed by Fathalla in 1971 as a factor in the genesis of ovarian cancer

Table 4.1.1 Comparative 5-year relative survival rates

Region	Time period	Ovary %	Cervix %	Uterus %
USA (White)	1983–1988	39	68	84
USA (Black)	1983–1988	37	55	54
Finland	1983–1985	37	58	80
S. Australia	1977–1985	35	66	79
Saskatchewan	1980–1986	34	69	82
Denmark	1983–1985	31	64	79
W. Midlands, UK	1981–1985	31	60	72
Yorkshire, UK	1985	30	65	70
Scotland, UK	1983–1987	29	59	71
North West, UK	1985–1989	27	58	70

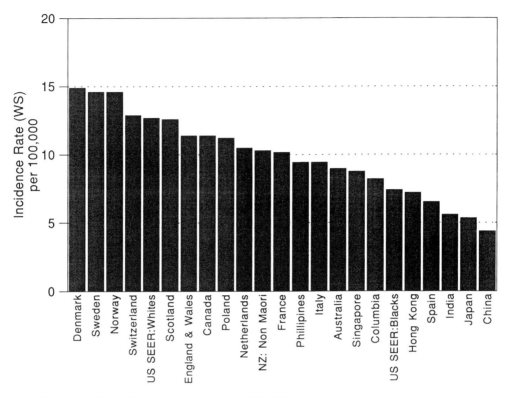

Fig. 4.1.6 *Cancer of the ovary. Geographical trends in incidence, 1983–87.*

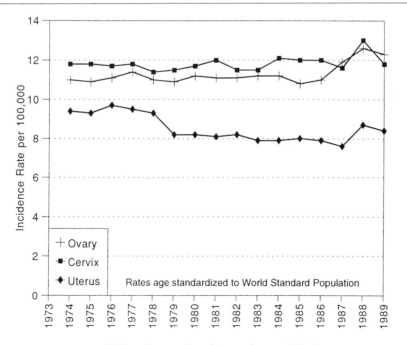

Fig. 4.1.7 *Gynecological cancer in England and Wales. Temporal trends in incidence, 1973–89.*

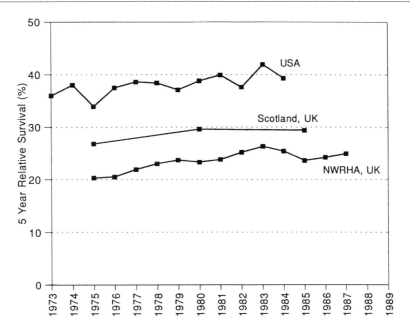

Fig. 4.1.8 *Cancer of the ovary. Temporal trends in survival, 1973–89.*

is compelling.[18] This theory was based on evidence which suggested a possible relationship between the repeated involvement of the ovarian surface epithelium in the process of ovulation and the frequency of development of the common epithelial ovarian neoplasms. In 1979 Casagrande *et al.*[19] calculated a factor called 'protected time' based on all anovulatory periods during a woman's reproductive life. When relative risk was calculated, a statistically significant negative association was found, with risk decreasing with increasing length of protected time. A complementary measure, the ovulatory age (total years of ovulation) was also computed, and this displayed an even stronger association with the risk of developing ovarian cancer, with risk increasing steadily with increasing ovulatory age. Franceschi *et al.*[20] in 1982 also calculated the relative risk associated with total years of ovulation and confirmed this positive association. A further study by La Vecchia *et al.*[21] in 1983 showed that age at menopause was the major determinant of the total number of ovulatory years and that the relative risk of ovarian cancer in relation to age at menopause was as strong as that for ovulatory years. More recent work[22,23] confirms the importance of age at menopause, but also shows that age at menarche does not affect risk. This suggests that the model of exposure time may be more complex than first proposed, and may involve other factors than simply the absolute ovulatory and anovulatory periods during reproductive life.

Although the mechanism of genesis of ovarian carcinoma remains unclear, the strong protective effect endowed by two factors – parity and oral contraceptive use – is universally accepted. Parous women have a lower risk of ovarian cancer than nulliparous women, and risk decreases with each additional pregnancy.[24,25] A strong and significant inverse correlation between average completed family size and mortality ratios for ovarian cancer has been observed across 20 countries and for different generations of women in England and Wales and the USA.[26] This suggests that the observed differences in mortality may be strongly linked to cultural and generational changes in child bearing. Women who have ever used oral contraceptives also have a significant reduction in risk, with risk decreasing as period of use increases.[27] As widespread use of oral contraceptives was not common until the 1960s, it is too early yet to observe a possible cohort effect on incidence and mortality. However, although family size is becoming smaller, the expected increase in risk of ovarian cancer which might be expected to follow from this, may be offset by the protective effect of the increased use of oral contraceptives.

Cancer of the uterine cervix

Cancer of the cervix uteri is the most common cancer in females in developing countries, where 80% of all cervical cancers are diagnosed.[2] In developed countries it is the fifth most common cancer in all women, but the commonest in women under the age of 50 years. World standardized, age-adjusted incidence rates range from 5 to 42 per 100 000 (Fig. 4.1.9).[3]

Trends in the incidence of, and mortality from cervical carcinoma have been extensively examined in Northern Europe.[28,29] In Denmark, Iceland, Finland and Sweden, population-based cervical screening program achieved near complete coverage of their target populations in the mid 1960s and reductions in incidence and mortality were observed soon after this time. Norway, unlike the other Nordic countries, had no organized program in the 1960s and continued to report increased incidence rates into the late 1970s.[30] Similarly, in Aberdeen, where a 5-yearly

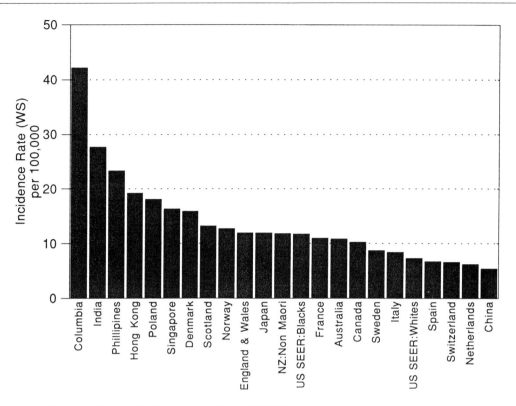

Fig. 4.1.9 *Cancer of the cervix. Geographical trends in incidence, 1973–87.*

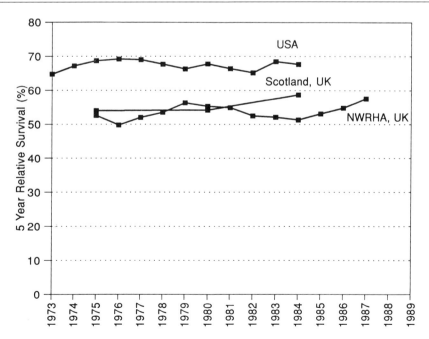

Fig. 4.1.10 *Cancer of the cervix. Temporal trends in survival, 1973–89.*

screening program was introduced in 1960, the incidence rate fell steadily after that time; in 1960 incidence rates in Aberdeen were considerably higher than in the rest of Scotland, but by 1981 the standardized rate was less than 50% of that in Scotland as a whole.[31]

Reductions in mortality which have been attributed to the introduction of screening, have been reported in the Nordic countries, areas of Canada and the USA.[32-35] It is, however, difficult to quantify the contribution that the cervical screening program has made towards reducing the mortality attributable to cervical cancer. Mortality rates have been declining gradually, for many years, in many parts of the world, even in countries with no organized screening program.

In the UK, a reduction in mortality has been observed since the early 1960s, long before organized screening was introduced in 1988. Incidence rates have, however, remained constant over this period. To resolve this apparent paradox, it is necessary to inspect temporal trends in stage-specific survival rates (Fig. 4.1.10). These data are not routinely available on a national basis, but a comprehensive review of cervical cancer in the West Midlands Region of England has identified a well-validated dataset covering a 25-year period which included information on stage of disease.[36] The 5-year survival rates for invasive cancers of the uterine cervix increased from 43% in the period 1957–61 to 55% in 1977–81 (t=5.03, P<0.001). This improvement in survival was attributable to the increased proportion of Stage 1a disease, from 5% in the quinquennia 1962–66 to 22% by 1977–81. When these cases were excluded from the series, the survival rates for the remaining group of patients with clinically invasive disease appeared to remain constant over this 20-year period.

The epidemiological profile of cervical cancer, and its consistent association with early age at first intercourse and number of sexual partners, suggests that this is a sexually transmitted disease and that the infectious agent is almost certainly a virus. A stream of experimental work has now established an impressive set of oncogenic credentials for a role for human papilloma virus (HPV) in the aetiology of cervical neoplasia. Direct evidence for the role of HPV 16 and 18 comes from molecular biological studies which have demonstrated that HPV 16 and 18 can immortalize primary cervical epithelial cells *in vitro*. This effect is mediated by the early E6 and E7 viral genes which are expressed in fresh, HPV-positive cervical carcinoma biopsies and derived cell lines.[37-39] Case control inquiries have revealed that both cervical intraepithelial neoplasia and invasive cervical cancer are strongly associated with the presence of specific HPV DNA sequences in diseased tissue.[40-44] Notwithstanding the strength and consistency of these associations, some reservations remain. The case control studies are of variable quality, with some failing to measure established risk factors of the disease, whereas others have inadequately controlled for these variables in analyses.[43,44] Longitudinal studies currently underway may, more precisely, determine the role of HPV in the etiology of this disease. Other possible determinants of cervical abnormality continue to merit further investigation. An association with cigarette smoking after controling for sexual behavior has been reported by some investigators but not by others.[45] There is experimental and epidemiological evidence which suggests an interaction between HPV and contraceptive use in the genesis of cervical neoplasia,[46] and evidence of an interaction between HPV and sexually transmitted co-factors such as herpes simplex virus type 2[47] in the etiology of this disease. A full discussion of the pathological relationship between HPV and lower genital tract neoplasia can be found in Chapter 4.2.

SUMMARY

- Interpretation of cancer mortality rates is confounded by inaccurate certification, death from a different disease and inadequate information on death certificates about length of survival.
- The incidence of cancer is defined as the number of new primary cancers arising in a defined population during a defined time period. The incidence rate is expressed as the number of new registered cases per 10 000 population per year.
- Direct age standardization, which allows comparison of populations, is obtained by applying observed age-specific rates to a reference popula-tion.
- The relative survival rate from a cancer is calculated as the ratio of the crude survival to that which would be expected from the general mortality experience of the population.

- Cancer of the uterine corpus is the eighth most frequent female cancer. World standardized age-adjusted rates range from 2 to 18 per 100 000 women, with highest rates in developed countries.
- Cancer of the ovary is the sixth most frequent female cancer. World standardized age-adjusted rates range from 4 to 15 per 100 000, with the highest rates in Northern Europe.
- There is a protective effect for ovarian cancer by oral contraception and parity, suggesting that malignant risk increases with the number of ovulating events.
- Worldwide, cervical cancer is the commonest female cancer. World standardized age-adjusted rates range from 5 to 42 per 10 000, the highest rates in developing countries.

Cervical cancer mortality rates have fallen throughout the world, contributed at least in part by cervical screening.

There are strong epidemiological data to support the molecular data associating human papillomavirus with cervical neoplasia.

REFERENCES

1. North Western Regional Cancer Registry, Centre for Cancer Epidemiology, University of Manchester, Christie Hospital, Manchester M20 9QL.
2. Parkin DM, Pisani P, Ferlay J. Estimates of the worldwide incidence of eighteen major cancers in 1985. *Int J Cancer* 1993 **54**: 594–606.
3. Parkin DM, Muir CS, Whelan SL, Gao YT, Ferlay J, Powell J. Cancer incidence in five continents. International Agency for Research on Cancer (WHO) and International Association of Cancer Registries, no. 120, Volume VI, 1992.
4. Miller BA, Ries, LAG, Hankey BF, Kosary CL, Edwards BK (eds) *Cancer Statistics Review: 1973–1989*, National Cancer Institute. NIH Publication No. 92–2789, 1992.
5. Black RJ, Sharp L, Kendrick SW. *Trends in Cancer Survival in Scotland 1968–1990* Information and Statistics Division, Directorate of Information Services, National Health Service in Scotland, 1993.
6. Parazzini F, La Vecchia C, Bocciolone L, Franceschi S. The epidemiology of endometrial cancer. *Gynecol Oncol* 1991 **41**: 1–16.
7. Voight LF, Weiss NS. Epidemiology of endometrial cancer. *Cancer Treat Res* 1989 **49**: 1–21.
8. Schwartzbaum JA, Hulka BS, Fowler WC Jr, Kaufman DG, Hoberman D. The influence of exogenous estrogen use on survival after diagnosis of endometrial cancer. *Am J Epidemiol* 1987 **126**: 851–860.
9. OPCS, Series DH2 no.19, *Mortality Statistics*, 1992.
10. Coleman MP, Esteve J, Damiecki P, Arslan A, Renard H. *Trends in Cancer Incidence and Mortality.* World Health Organisation International Agency for Research on Cancer no. 121, 1993.
11. OPCS, Series MB1 no. 22, *Cancer Statistics Registrations* 1974–1989.
12. Berrino F, Sant M, Verdechia A, Capocaccia R (eds) *Survival of Cancer Patients in Europe: the EUROCARE Study*, ARC Scientific Publications no. 132.
13. *Cancer in Australia 1982.* Australasian Association of Cancer Registries and Australian Institute of Health.
14. Tan LK, Robson DL. *Trends in Cancer Survival in Saskatchewan 1967 to 1986.* Saskatchewan Cancer Registry and Department of Community Health and Epidemiology, University of Saskatchewan, 1991.
15. Woodman C, Wilson S, Prior P, Cummins C, Bowcock M, Redman V, Forrest J. *Cancer in the West Midlands Region 1981–85.* West Midlands Regional Cancer Registry.
16. Joslin C, Rider L, Round C, Smith A, Hilton A, Wilson D. *Yorkshire Cancer Registry Report for the Year 1991 Including Cancer Statistics for 1984–1988.* Yorkshire Regional Cancer Organisation.
17. *Cancer in the North West.* Report by the Centre for Cancer Epidemiology, University of Manchester, 1992.
18. Fathalla MF. Incessant ovulation – a factor in ovarian neoplasia? *Lancet*, 1971 **ii**: 163.
19. Casagrande JT, Louie EW, Pike MC, Roy S, Ross RK, Henderson BE. 'Incessant ovulation' and ovarian cancer. *Lancet*, 1979 **ii**: 170–173.
20. Franceschi S, La Vecchia C, Helmrich S, Mangioni C, Tognoni G. Risk factors for epithelial ovarian cancer in Italy. *Am J Epidemiol* 1982 **115**: 714–719.
21. La Vecchia C, Franceschi S, Gallus G, Decarli A, Liberati A, Tognoni G. Incessant ovulation and ovarian cancer: a critical approach. *Int J Epidemiol* 1983 **12**: 161–164.
22. Booth M, Beral V, Smith P. Risk factors for ovarian cancer: a case-control study. *Br J Cancer* 1989 **60**, 592–598.
23. Franceschi S, La Vecchia C, Booth M *et al.* Pooled analysis of 3 European case-control studies of ovarian cancer: II. Age at menarche and at menopause. *Int J Cancer* 1991 **49**: 57–60.
24. Cramer DW, Hutchison GB, Welch RW, Scully RE, Ryan KJ. Determinants of ovarian cancer risk. I. Reproductive experiences and family history. *J Natl Cancer Inst* 1983 **71**: 711–716.
25. Negri E, Franceschi S, Tzonou A *et al.* Pooled analysis of three European case-control studies: I. Reproductive factors and risk of epithelial ovarian cancer. *Int J Cancer*, 1991 **49**: 50–56.
26. Beral V, Fraser P, Chilvers C. Does pregnancy protect against ovarian cancer? *Lancet* 1978 **ii**: 1083–1086.
27. Franceschi S, Parazzini F, Negri E, Booth M, La Vecchia C, Beral V, Tzonou A, Trichopoulos D. Pooled analysis of 3 European case-control studies of ovarian cancer: III. Oral contraceptive use. *Int J Cancer* 1991 **49**: 61–65.
28. Hakama M. Trends in the incidence of cervical cancer in Nordic countries. In Magnus K (ed.) *Trends in Cancer Incidence, Causes and Practical Implications.* Washington DC, Hemisphere Publishing Corporation, 1982: 279–292.
29. Sigurdsson K. Effect of organised screening on the risk of cervical cancer. Evaluation of screening activity in Iceland 1964–1990. *Int J Cancer* 1993, **54**: 563–570.
30. Bjørge T, Steinar Ø, Thoresen G, Gry B Skare. Incidence, survival and mortality in cervical cancer in Norway, 1956–90. *Eur J Cancer* 1993 **29A**: 2291–2297.
31. MacGregor J, Moss S, Parkin K, Day N. A case-control study of cervical cancer screening in NE Scotland. *Br Med J* 1985 **290**: 1543–1546.
32. Ahluwalia HS, Path MC, Doll R. Mortality from cancer of the cervix uteri in British Columbia and other parts of Canada. *Br J Prev Soc Med* 1968 **22**: 61–164.
33. Läärä E, Day NE, Hakama M. Trends in mortality from cervical cancer in the Nordic countries: association with organised screening programmes. *Lancet* 1987 **i**: 1247–1249.
34. Christopherson WM, Parker JE, Mendez WM, Lundin FE. Cervix cancer death rates and mass cytological screening. *Cancer* 1970 **26**: 808.
35. Cramer DW. The role of cervical cytology in the declining morbidity of cervical cancer. *Cancer* 1974 **34**: 2018–2027.
36. Meanwell CA, Kelly KA, Wilson S, Roginski C, Woodman CBJ, Griffiths R, Blackledge G. Young age as a prognostic factor in cervical cancer: analysis of population based data from 10,022 cases. *Br Med J* 1988 **296**: 386–392.
37. Smotkin D, Wettstein FO. Transcription of human papillomavirus type 16 early genes in a cervical cancer and a cancer-derived cell line and identification of the E7 protein. *Proc Natl Acad Sci USA* 1986 **83**: 4680–4684.
38. Hawley-Nelson P, Vousden KH, Hubbert NL, Lowry DR, Schiller JT. HPV16 E6 and E7 proteins cooperate to immortalise human foreskin keratinocytes. *EMBO J* 1989 **8**: 3905–3910.
39. Munger K, Phelps WC, Bubb V, Howley PM, Schleger R. The E6 and E7 genes of the human papillomavirus type 16 together are necessary and sufficient for transformation of primary human keratinocytes. *J Virol* 1989 **63**: 4417–4421.
40. Meanwell CA, Blackledge G, Cox MF, Maitland NJ HPV16 DNA in normal and malignant cervical epithelium: implications for the aetiology and behaviour of cervical neoplasia. *Lancet* 1987 **i**: 703–707.
41. Morrison EAB, Ho GYF, Vermund SH, Goldberg GL,

Kadish AS, Kelley KF, Burk RD. Human papillomavirus infection and other risk factors for cervical neoplasia: a case-control study. *Int J Cancer* 1991 **49**: 6–13.

42. Muñoz N, Bosch FX, DE Sanjose S, Tafur L, Izarzugaza I, Gili M, Viladiu P, Navarro C, Martos C, Ascunce N, Gonzalez LC, Kaldor JM, Guerrero E, Lörincz A, Santamaria M, De Ruiz PA, Aristizabal N, Shah K. The casual link between human papillomavirus and invasive cervical cancer: a population-based case-control study in Columbia and Spain. *Int J Cancer* 1992 **52**: 743–749.

43. Peng H, Liu S, Mann V, Rohan T, Rawls W. Human papillomavirus types 16 and 33, herpes simplex virus type 2 and other risk factors for cervical cancer in Sichuan province, China. *Int J Cancer* 1991 **47**: 711–716.

44. Schmauz R, Okong P, De Villiers EM, Dennin R, Brade L, Lwanga SK and Owor R. Multiple infections in cases of cervical cancer from a high-incidence area in tropical Africa. *Int J Cancer* 1989 **43**: 805–809.

45. Winkletstein W Jr. Smoking and cervical cancer – Current status: A review. *Am J Epidemiol* 1990 **131**: 945–957.

46. Hildesbeing A, Reeves WC, Brinton LA *et al.* Association of oral contraceptive use and human papillomaviruses in invasive cervical cancer. *Int J Cancer* 1990 **45**: 860–864.

47. Hildesheim A, Mann V, Brinton LA, Szklo M, Reeves WC, Rawls WE. Herpes simplex virus type 2: a possible interaction with human papillomavirus types 16/18 in the development of invasive cervical cancer. *Int J Cancer* 1991 **49**: 335–340.

4.2

Human Papillomavirus and Cervical Neoplasia

DW Visscher and WD Lawrence

INTRODUCTION

Human papilloma virus (HPV) infections have always been an important component of lower female genital tract (LFGT) pathology. One need only consult Papanicolaou's original monograph in order to find artistically rendered drawings of koilocytosis and dyskeratosis, the prototypical cytologic manifestations of cervical HPV infection. Recently acquired knowledge of HPV molecular genetics and pathobiology have furthered our understanding of LFGT neoplasia, especially cervical dysplasia. Perhaps the greatest departure from earlier notions of cervical tumorigenesis and HPV infection is that we now view these processes as being linked. Viral DNA is consistently observed not only in LFGT dysplasias, but also in the primary lesions, metastases and recurrences of carcinomas, implying that viral interactions are fundamentally related to both genesis and maintenance of the malignant state.[1] Current thinking also challenges the classical model of cervical neoplasia progression in which sequential evolution through defined histologic stages occurs over protracted and consistent time intervals. Those stages (mild to moderate to severe dysplasia and carcinoma-in-situ) were not defined in the context of HPV-associated changes, which were considered to be a process separate and independent from dysplasia. Little attention was thus directed toward the epidemiology and natural history of HPV infection.

The technology of molecular genetics is rapidly developing. Its applications and limitations are thus not immediately apparent to the uninitiated. This problem, in conjunction with explosive advancements in cellular pathobiology, have made the HPV field confusing to many anatomical pathologists. There is, however, a common denominator of genetically based techniques employed to study HPV. It is hybridization of viral DNA to synthetic, sequence complementary oligonucleotide probes. Until recently the 'gold standard' was the Southern hybridization procedure, in which sample DNA is purified by extraction in phenol/chloroform and then digested with a restriction

endonuclease. These enzymes cleave DNA at specific points defined by base pair sequence. The restriction fragment products of this reaction are separated on the basis of length by gel electrophoretic mobility to a known HPV positive control, and are then denatured and transferred to a membrane for hybridization with the complimentary DNA probe. Hybridizations are carried out under 'high stringency' conditions, which minimizes non-specific annealing. Signal detection generally employs autoradiography.

Southern hybridization procedures not only detect viral DNA but may be used to distinguish HPV genotypes, since by definition there is less than 50% sequence homology between viral types. A noteworthy limitation of this procedure is sensitivity, especially since the extraction step is associated with loss of DNA. Approximately 1 pg of viral DNA (10^5 genomes) is required to produce a positive signal. In a tissue biopsy sample this correlates with one viral genome per cell. Marginally positive cases produce equivocal hybridization signals. Reproducibility of results using these techniques (both inter- and intralaboratory) constitutes a problem which is infrequently addressed by authors.

Sensitivity issues have been largely resolved by widespread use of the polymerase chain reaction (PCR), in which target DNA from the sample is first amplified 10 000-fold. This is accomplished with use of two hybridization sequences which flank the region of interest. These primers direct repeated transcription cycles of target DNA using an exogenous, thermally controlled, DNA polymerase. Since the reaction product accumulates in excess, electrophoretic separation is unnecessary and detection using a sequence complementary probe is straightforward. A variety of controls, however, are required. These include an internal control reaction employing a second set of primers for a gene which is known to be present (i.e. to confirm success of the amplification reaction) as well as a positive control reaction on a separate sample known to contain the target gene sequence. Finally, an appropriate negative control reaction is critical, since minuscule amounts of contaminant DNA (as little as one copy) may cause a false positive result. Comparison studies with Southern hybridization[2] have confirmed the superior sensitivity of PCR (10^2 genomes); however, the extremely high rates of HPV detection in early PCR reports no doubt reflected failure to prevent contamination.

Other hybridization strategies have been successfully employed, including a commercially available product (Virapap™) which utilizes ^{32}P-labelled RNA 'antisense' probes on digested, denatured specimen DNA applied to nylon filters (so-called 'filter hybridization').[3] Finally, hybridization reactions may be performed *in situ* on intact tissue samples or on cytologic preparations using biotinylated probes.[4] Filter and *in situ* hybridizations are limited by suboptimal sensitivity since amplification is not employed.[5] However, *in situ* hybridizations allow the viral signals to be located within the context of tissue morphology which is a very useful aspect of the technique.[6] Hybridization technology is not necessarily limited to DNA sequences. Availability of sequence complementary mRNA probes make it possible to detect expression of virus-specific genes. This is also adaptable to PCR (i.e. RT-PCR) and *in situ* approaches, however it is limited by specimen handling and processing artefacts, since RNA is susceptible to degradation.

CURRENT CONCEPTS

Molecular biology of HPV infection

The HPV genome is circular, and composed of approximately 8000 base pairs which are functionally divided into the open reading frame (ORF) region and the long control region (LCR). The ORF segment contains seven regulatory gene-encoding sequences, referred to as E (early) genes because they are believed to be expressed early in the virus life cycle. It also contains two L (late) genes which encode for capsid structures. The LCR contains the promoter and enhancer components of ORF gene sequences.

In order to be considered a distinct viral genotype, there must be less than 50% gene sequence homology with other HPV types. Over 60 HPV genotypes have been recognized, twenty of which infect the LFGT. Based on their association with high grade dysplasias or carcinomas, five HPV types are considered 'high risk' or 'oncogenic' (types 16, 18, 31, 33, 35). Two frequently occurring types (6 and 11), in contrast, are considered 'low risk' since they are virtually always associated with exophytic condyloma.

The limited amount of DNA in the HPV genome is insufficient to code for all of the enzymes required for viral replication. Therefore, completion of the viral life cycle entails an intimate molecular-level relationship with host cells. Completion of the HPV life cycle, in fact, is believed to require coordination with the differentiation and proliferation status of the host cell, the various stages of which have divergent gene expression. Specifically, sustaining an HPV infection requires maintenance of a replicative state, but viral assembly and release require a differentiated state.

The complexity of this virus–host relationship has, to date, precluded a full examination of the HPV life cycle *in vitro*.

Using mRNA *in situ* hybridization analyses, Stoler *et al.*[7] have dissected viral gene expression as a function of histology. In condylomas and low-grade cervical dysplasias, all viral ORFs are expressed, however L1 and L2 (i.e. capsid) mRNA is observed only in superficial (i.e. terminally differentiated) cells. This correlates with the morphologic restriction of koilocytosis, a viral cytopathic effect, to the superficial cell layers.

A steady-state infection (i.e. low viral DNA copy number without synthesis of viral particles) is believed to be maintained in the basal cells of the epithelium. In this region of the epithelium viral gene transcription is repressed by the product of E2, one of the early genes. This is mediated via binding interactions with promoter sequences of the remaining viral genome. As infected squamous cells pass through the epithelium and mature, repression of viral gene expression is overcome, possibly by host promoters and transcription factors intrinsic to the differentiated state. Viral gene transcription thus increases as a result of genetic interaction with the host.

The precise nature of host influences on viral gene transcription remain undefined, as do the potential effects of viral promoters on host gene expression. Clearly, the multiplicity of factors (physiologic and pathologic) known to be engaged in epithelial growth and differentiation would suggest that such interactions may be complex. It has been demonstrated that HPV infection is associated with increased expression of progesterone receptors in cervical epithelium.[8] This finding represents a potential mechanism to account for epidemiologic and clinical observations concerning the prevalence and behavior of HPV-associated lesions during pregnancy and oral contraceptive use[9] as well as *in vitro* observations on the influence of progesterone on HPV-induced cell transformation, which suggests that HPV gene expression may be modified by host-derived progestins.[10] The importance of host cell gene expression in HPV-associated lesions may also be appreciated when one considers the differential responses of transformation zone and ectocervix-derived cells to *in vitro* infection. Type 16 infection causes morphologic changes similar to high-grade dysplasia in the former, but only mild dysplastic changes in the latter, analogous to the situation *in vivo*.[11]

Mechanism of HPV carcinogenesis

The role of HPV in carcinogenesis has, of course, been a major subject of recent investigation. Apart from epidemiologic, pathologic and clinical data reviewed elsewhere, this research has focused largely on two other early gene products – E6 and E7. Proteins encoded by E6 and E7 are structurally and functionally analogous to so-called binding proteins elaborated by transforming viruses, such as SV 40. They possess zinc-atom containing motifs which mediate interaction with critical cell cycle regulatory species; p53 in the case of E6 and Rb-1 (retinoblastoma gene product) for E7.[12] Both p53 and Rb-1 gene products act to restrict cell cycle progression and thereby proliferation. As a consequence, cell proliferation becomes uncoupled from physiologic controls (Fig. 4.2.1). Accordingly, proliferative activity is substantially elevated in dysplastic lesions of the cervix, even mild cases.[13]

Apart from the obvious functional implications of inappropriate cell cycling, evidence that E6 and E7 are in some manner related to transformation *in vivo* has been provided by the association between increasing grade of dysplasia with higher levels of expression for these particular genes.[14] Before continuing, we would note that the role of these gene products in (non-dysplastic) condylomatous lesions is undefined. Most investigators agree, however, that the function of these species should not be viewed as limited exclusively to a neoplastic state. Moreover, although E6 and E7 cooperate to immortalize cell lines *in vitro*, they are not sufficient to transform human cells without other genetic lesions. This is analogous to the case *in vivo*, where all available evidence to date suggests HPV is unable to induce malignancy without independent mutations, immunologic deficit or tumor promotion-related factors.

Binding interaction with E6 affects p53 in a variety of ways. In addition to inducing proteolytic degradation of p53, E6 has also been shown to interfere with the transcriptional activation and repressor functions of p53 which require binding to DNA. Convincing evidence of biological relevance for E6 mediated p53 deactivation is the low frequency of p53 mutations in HPV-associated malignancies compared with non-HPV associated LFGT neo-

plasms.[15] This suggests that p53 may be inactivated in one of two ways; by HPV E6 or by mutation.

Functional deactivation of p53 has consequences beyond cell proliferation control. Wild type p53 has been shown to induce apoptosis in cells with DNA damage. Studies *in vitro* suggest that E6 may abrogate this function.[16] If this occurs *in vivo*, it may represent a mechanism for accumulation of genetic defects required for neoplastic progression.

The cellular consequences of E7 activity are also multifunctional. As previously noted, this species preferentially binds, and presumably deactivates, the unphosphorylated (i.e. active) form of Rb-1, thereby releasing at least one constraint to proliferation. E7 also overcomes the inhibition of myc, a growth promoting gene product, by means of a cell growth suppressor – transforming growth factor beta (TGF-β). The myc–TGF–β interaction in normal cells results in G1 growth arrest.[17] Finally, E7 interferes with the DNA-binding capacity of Rb-1.[18] Like Rb-1, the function of E7 is itself dependent on phosphorylation state.[19] This observation implies meaningful interactions between virus encoded proteins and host-derived cell regulatory kinases.

An especially noteworthy aspect of HPV molecular biology is that E6/E7 proteins encoded by 'high risk' types (i.e. those more frequently associated with high grade CIN or carcinoma) function more efficiently than those encoded by 'low risk' types; that is, they have greater binding affinities for p53 and Rb-1, respectively. They also have higher transforming potential in cell line assays.

It will be recalled that this section began by stating that in condyloma, expression of viral genes such as E6/E7 is repressed by viral (and possibly host) transcription factors such as E2. One manner in which E6/E7 expression is thought to be derepressed is via integration of viral DNA into the host genome. This phenomenon is observed in most, if not all, HPV-associated malignancies. Condylomas by contrast always have extrachromosomal (episomal) viral DNA. Viral integration is also associated with non-productive viral infection (i.e. failure to produce and release viral particles) which accounts for lack of koilocytosis or viral capsid expression in high-grade dysplasias and carcinomas.[20] Non-productive infection is believed to reflect disruption or deletion of the E2 encoding sequence during the host–viral recombination event. The resulting proliferative phenotype of the epithelium, caused by E6/E7 derepression, is presumably sufficient to block maturation and differentiation of the squamous epithelium. This in turn inhibits the synthesis of viral particles and results in the growth and differentiation perturbations typical of neoplastic epithelial lesions. The biological importance of E2 disruption is supported by the enhanced transforming ability of cloned HPV DNA which contains disrupted E1/E2 sequences.[17]

It is not known why viral integration occurs, although most authors view it as a mutational event. Possibly, host DNA strand breaks induced by chemical mutagens or other viruses provide sites for recombination between viral and cellular DNA. It is noteworthy that two such mutagenic influences (smoking and Herpes type II infection)

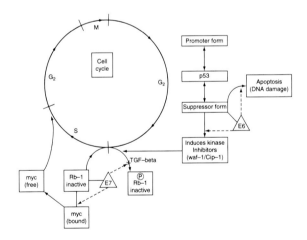

Fig. 4.2.1 *Diagram illustrating the proposed theoretical consequences of HPV gene products E6 and E7 on cell cycle regulation. Near the G₁–S interface, cell cycle progression is opposed by active (unphosphorylated) Rb-1 which also binds the myc oncoprotein. HPV E7 in addition to binding active Rb-1, liberates myc, which then acts as a growth-promoting transcription factor. It also impairs the ability of TGF-beta to stimulate inactivation of Rb-1 via phosphorylation. Phosphorylation of active Rb-1 is also opposed by kinase inhibitors which are induced by p53. E6 binding to the suppressor form of p53 thus not only favors an Rb-1 phosphorylated state but impairs the ability of p53 to induce apoptosis in cells with DNA damage. Note that in this scheme, p53 immunostaining may be accounted for by abnormal accumulation of the promoter form of p53.*

have been epidemiologically correlated with cervical neoplasia. Although the site(s) of integration into the host genome are variable, cytogenetic studies have correlated loci of viral integration with known sites of chromosomal fragility and cancer specific breakpoints.[21] Viral integration also occurs preferentially in the vicinity of oncogene loci, suggesting that this event may promote neoplasia by alteration of host gene expression.[22] It has further been suggested that the host integration sites consist of decondensed (i.e. active) chromatin.[23] Such areas would not only constitute a more 'open' target for recombination, but actively expressed genes in such areas would potentially have a promoting effect on the inserted viral genome.

Many questions about viral integration, in addition to those already cited, remain unsolved. Whether integration predisposes to additional mutational events, for example, is unclear. Mutations may occur in either host or viral DNA.[24] It is also unclear why integration of viral DNA consistently disrupts the E1/E2 region. Finally, it has been established that integrated and episomal DNA may coexist in the same cell.[25] Several studies imply that such 'partial integration' is associated with less aggressive behavior than 'complete integration', possibly due to preservation of E1/E2 function.[26]

What is clear is that integration of viral DNA is a characteristic which is largely, if not exclusively, limited to 'high risk' or 'oncogenic' HPV genotypes. Since the rates of viral integration in high-grade cervical intraepithelial neoplasia approach those of invasive squamous neoplasia, it is evident that other events are required to induce the invasive stage of neoplastic progression.

Pathology of HPV infection

Human papillomavirus infections of the LFGT are generally divided into three categories. Most frequently encountered are the exophytic condylomas and intraepithelial neoplasias (dysplasias and *in situ* carcinomas). About 50% of benign condylomata or intraepithelial neoplasms involve the vulva or cervix alone. Most of the remainder simultaneously involve both areas. Occasionally the LFGT may be afflicted by diffuse, multicentric papillomavirus infection involving cervix, vulva, vagina and perineal/perianal regions.

The second category of HPV-associated LFGT lesion is invasive carcinoma which, as a proportion of all HPV-associated lesions, is rare. Approximately 80–85% of invasive carcinomas are HPV DNA positive.[27] The corresponding frequency in vulvar and perianal malignancies is significantly lower (~ 20–60%), despite the high incidence (70–85%) of HPV DNA in preinvasive lesions from these sites.[28]

Finally, HPV infections may be 'occult', or present without recognizable cytologic or histopathologic manifestations. Various authors have estimated the frequency of such occult cases to be 15–30% (for all HPV types) of the total number of infected patients. It is not yet clear what proportion of such infections represent latent disease, (i.e. stable, non-productive infection without histologic abnormality) early condyloma or intraepithelial neoplasia.

Obviously, the prevalence of 'occult' HPV infection is significantly affected by numerous factors intrinsic to the population which is surveyed. Some have observed, for example, that 'occult' infections are present disproportionately in oral contraceptive users.[29] Whether such an association is causal, or merely a proxy for some other factor correlated with OCP use, is unclear.

Barriers to complete understanding of the natural history of clinical or subclinical HPV infection are formidable. They can be broadly divided into technical and biological issues. First, in addition to suboptimal sensitivity as previously noted, assays for viral DNA may be performed on samples derived by a variety of means; examples include tissue sections, cervical swab, and cervicovaginal lavage. Thus, common problems encountered in many studies are the inability to correlate HPV assay result with the corresponding histology as well as inability to account for, or evaluate, HPV status in multiple, or specific anatomical sites. Concordance rates for viral DNA detection between cervical scrapes and directed biopsy tissue samples is only about 60%.[30] Detection issues extend beyond mere presence or absence of virus since viral copy number per cell may have clinical relevance.

Such technique-related nuances pale insignificance when compared with the issue of biological heterogeneity of HPV-associated disease of the LFGT. In addition to the variety of histologic manifestations, clinical syndromes and list of implicated HPV genotypes, numerous demographic issues complicate analysis of HPV-associated disease. Examples include geographic variation in distribution of HPV types as well as differences within and among study populations in risk factor profiles. Important risk factors for HPV infection and cervical neoplasia include: number of sexual partners, age at first intercourse, cigarette smoking, presence of other sexually transmitted diseases, use of oral contraceptives, and immunosuppression. Moreover, each risk factor may have relevance to different stages of disease progression. Disease co-factors may vary as a function of time, as highlighted by the reported rising incidence of HPV-associated lesions. Finally, the clinical course and outcome of HPV-associated disease may partially be determined by parameters intrinsic to the host genotype, such as histocompatibility antigen profile.[31] For these and many other reasons, consensus has yet to be reached on the clinical relevance of viral DNA detection and typing.

Clinicopathologic studies can be separated into cross-sectional studies, i.e. those performed at one point in time, and longitudinal studies, i.e. those with two or more temporal data points.

Cross-sectional studies of cervical HPV infection

Analyses of this type are designed to address the following issues: (a) the incidence and prevalence of HPV infection, overall as well as for specific genotypes: (b) the correlations between HPV infection and clinical, cytologic or histologic disease manifestations and (c) the epidemiologic factors associated with infection. All cross-sectional analyses are inherently susceptible to biases resulting from study population selection or methodology of HPV detection.

Most publications of this category report the frequency of HPV DNA, usually type specific, in patient groups stratified by Pap smear or cervical biopsy morphology. First, these incidence analyses typically reveal an 80–90% frequency of HPV DNA in high-grade cervical dysplasia, i.e. CIN II or III or high-grade squamous intraepithelial lesion (HGSIL). In contrast, lesions with non-specific histopathologic alterations ('squamous atypia of undetermined significance', or 'changes suspicious, but not diagnostic, for HPV') also harbor HPV, but at significantly lower and more variable frequency (20–40%).[32,33] This is largely a reflection of divergent morphologic criteria utilized for classification of 'low grade' squamous lesions.[34] A sizable number of HPV infections are thereby, almost unavoidably, characterized by cellular changes which overlap with other inflammatory or reactive states. By analogy, colposcopically equivocal lesions also exhibit a 30–50% frequency of HPV DNA detection.[35]

To a certain extent though, presence of HPV DNA in histologically equivocal samples also reflects true (partial or complete) absence of diagnostic cytologic/histologic features in many cases. Although diagnostically specific, koilocytosis and dyskeratosis are evident in Papanicolaou smears from less than 70% of patients with HPV-associated cervical lesions.[36] Nuclear atypia, in fact, is the most sensitive feature for predicting presence of viral DNA.[37] It should be noted that vulvar lesions which are suspicious but lack diagnostic features, also contain HPV DNA in approximately one fourth of cases.[38] Interestingly, 'high risk' HPV types more frequently display 'diagnostic' cytologic features than 'low risk' types.[39]

As noted earlier, clinically and morphologically occult infections are identified with measurable frequency (10–30%) in cross-sectional studies. Some authors have found a higher prevalence of occult disease in younger women.[40] Others report similar incidences of occult infection in premenopausal and postmenopausal women.[41] This discrepancy contrasts with dysplasia and carcinoma, both of which have distinct age distribution patterns. Occult infections also have a relatively high incidence of unusual HPV genotypes[42,43] and, as previously noted, are more frequent in oral contraceptive users and in women with a prior clinical history of dysplasia or HPV infection. They occur with equal frequency in women with and without previous hysterectomy.[29] Taken together, these clinicopathologic associations suggest that at least some occult HPV infections represent a form of carrier state, possibly involving large areas of LFGT mucosa and favored by specific virus or host factors. However, DeVilliers et al.[40] have noted that, in most individuals, viral detection is transient. Accordingly, at least some so-called occult infections may truly represent subclinical disease which is rapidly cleared by the immune system. It must be remembered that in some women with clinically apparent HPV-associated lesions, the virus may also be present in nearby morphologically normal tissues. It has been suggested that this form of latency may account for disease recurrences following local therapy in some patients.[44]

On the basis of viral genotype, exophytic condyloma nearly always contains HPV Type 6/11 DNA. Cervical lesions that are historically and currently included in the low-grade categories of squamous cell dysplasia (mild dysplasia, CIN I, low grade SIL, and so-called 'sqamous atypia of undetermined significance') are more heterogeneous. Approximately one third of such cases that are positive for HPV DNA contain 'oncogenic types' (genotypes 16, 18, 31, 33, 35). Most of the remaining positive cases are either types 6 or 11, although unusual types (42–43, 51–52, 56) account for 15–20% of the total.[45] High-grade cervical lesions (moderate to severe squamous cell dysplasia, CIN II or III, high grade SIL) on the other hand, are infected by 'oncogenic' HPV types in 80–90% of cases. Of the latter, type 16 is by far the most frequent offender, accounting for at least 50–60% of the total in CIN II or III. It must be stated, parenthetically, that significant interseries differences exist in the relative frequency of HPV genotypes. Geographic variation in genotype distribution likely accounts for some differences, but many disparities remain unexplained.

Simultaneous infection by more than one viral genotype is by no means rare, and has been reported in 5–41% of HPV-positive cases. Most available evidence would suggest that synchronous infection with multiple HPV types correlates with clinically multicentric disease (i.e. involve more than two anatomic sites). Beckmann[46] reported a 40% incidence of multitype infection in patients with lesions at two or more LFGT sites. The majority of such cases (63%) demonstrated simultaneous infection by both viral types at more than one anatomic site. Reid et al.[35] have also evaluated simultaneous viral type infection in the context of multicentric (i.e. cervical and vulvar) clinical disease. These authors also found a high frequency of infection by both viruses at both anatomic locations (~60%). Interestingly, multicentric cases infected by only one viral type exhibited concordant degrees of atypia/dysplasia between anatomically separated lesions. Those with multitype infection, in contrast, usually exhibited greater morphologic diversity between anatomically separate lesions; with both infections not necessarily being histologically evident. (One or both infections may be present in histologically normal tissue.) Finally, Lungu et al.[47] reported that synchronous multiple type HPV infection more often occurs in patients with 'low grade' histologic lesions (22%) as opposed to patients with 'high grade' lesions (7%).

It must be noted that non-cervical LFGT HPV-associated lesions are overwhelmingly associated with types 6 and 11. This finding together with the older age distribution of malignancy in such sites as well as other epidemiologic differences from cervical neoplasia would seem to suggest that the biology of cervical and non-cervical LFGT neoplasia may be fundamentally different.

Longitudinal studies of cervical HPV infection

This limited body of literature essentially addresses the clinical relevance of a positive test for HPV DNA in patients who, at the outset of the study, are either clinically normal (i.e. asymptomatic, with a history of negative Pap smears and no history of HPV or CIN) or who present with non-diagnostic morphologic abnormalities. The great advantage of these studies is that they reveal important clues about the natural history of HPV-associated lesions. Such investigations are very difficult and expensive to conduct, however, and may involve smaller cohorts of patients who are more selected than in cross-sectional analyses.

Longitudinal studies also highlight the problem of correlating HPV infection with histologic and cytologic evidence of cervical neoplasia progression. For example, Campion et al.[48] found that the progression rate of untreated mild cervical dysplasias to severe dysplasia was noticeably higher (mean 32%) in series where diagnosis was established with Pap smear only as opposed to biopsy (15% mean progression frequency). Although this may reflect alteration of disease natural history due to tissue sampling, it may also reflect the tendency of undirected Papanicolaou smears to 'undergrade' the disease. Studies which correlate Pap smears with subsequent colposcopically directed biopsy, in fact, suggest 'undergrading' may occur in up to one quarter of cases. The tradeoffs between cytology and histology represent a persistent theme in this literature which, indeed, reflect common problems in clinical practice.

The apparent consensus of the few available longitudinal studies is that presence and type of HPV infection has significant prognostic implications. Koutsky et al.[43] for example, performed both colposcopy and serial HPV DNA testing from cervicovaginal swabs in a set of clinically and pathologically normal women (without history of CIN or HPV infection) presenting for routine annual Pap smears. The incidence of CIN II or III on follow up was 28% in patients with positive HPV tests vs only 3% for patients who remained HPV negative. The importance of this study is that it defines prevalence of HPV in relationship to probable incidence of clinically ominous cervical intraepithelial neoplasias.

Nuovo et al.[49] have analyzed another troublesome subpopulation – patients referred for an abnormal Pap smear but who have a negative colposcopic examination. In this study, a cervical swab sample positive for HPV DNA correlated with the subsequent appearance of dysplasia –55% in HPV+ vs 12% in HPV– (3–12 months follow-up). However, the probability of developing biopsy-proven dysplasia was predicted equally well by a positive Pap smear performed at the time of HPV testing. These data appear to suggest that 'occult' HPV infections may have less potential to 'progress' to dysplasia than those which have manifested overt cellular abnormalities.

The noticeable rapid rate of evolution to dysplasia during the short follow-up interval of this study is compatible with an accelerated time course for progression of some HPV-associated lesions. Additional evidence of this is provided by Koutsky et al.[43] who noted that all CIN II or III lesions developed within 24 months of the initial positive test for HPV. This contrasts with reported transit times of two to three times longer in older literature.[48] What is more noteworthy is that 64% of the high-grade dysplasias in the Koutsky study appeared without evidence of a CIN I stage. However, all of the dysplasias in this series were infected by oncogenic HPV types, so that such data should not be

extended to encompass predictions concerning 'low risk' HPV types.

Finally, Campion et al.[48] have addressed many sampling issues in their prospective study of 100 women who presented with low-grade lesions (CIN I) on Pap smear. No biopsy was performed; however colposcopic examinations were conducted to confirm a cervical lesion. Further, three consecutive Pap smears showing CIN I were required to enter the study, thus minimizing 'undergrading'. The overall prevalence of Type 16 was 35%. However, among the 26 individuals who progressed to CIN III, 22 (85%) were infected with this genotype.

Natural history of HPV infection

The many clinical and morphologic permutations of HPV associated disease as well as the numerous missing pieces of information thus hamper efforts to derive a unified schematic of its natural history. Given what we know to be the relatively high prevalence of infection and the comparatively low incidence of dysplasia, some workers have inferred that most HPV infections are transient. This, presumably, reflects an effective host immune reaction in which the virus is quickly suppressed and eliminated. Such cases may evolve without histologic manifestation or they develop into 'low grade' lesions which spontaneously regress in most instances. This impression is supported in part by data showing that HPV infection is substantially more frequent in younger age groups, even after correction for number of sexual partners.[50] It is also supported by the high 'cure' rate of cryotherapy (~ 90–95%) as well as the observation that 'recurrences' following cryotherapy are generally with a viral genotype different from the initial infection.[51]

In some individuals, though, HPV infections may become persistent. Development of high-grade lesions may then occur on a background of low-grade lesion or possibly de novo. Although this course must be at least partially attributable to infection by 'high risk' viral genotypes, a number of other factors play a significant role. As noted previously, both the incidence of HPV infection and the development of intraepithelial neoplasia or malignancy have been associated with a number of factors.[52] An important role for either local or systemic immunity may be inferred from a variety of evidence, including the higher prevalence and more frequent progression of HPV-associated LFGT lesions in immunosuppressed individuals[53] as well as the association between HPV and postirradiation dysplasia.[54,55] The possible contribution of local tissue immunity is implied by studies which correlate cervical intraepithelial immune cell populations in the cervix to chronic cigarette smoking.[56]

Relationship between HPV type and histology

The question arises; do the various HPV associated lesions display specific histologic features, apart from the grade of

CIN, that might provide clues to the presence of a particular viral genotype? It has been reported for example that macronuclei are significantly more frequent in CIN lesions associated with oncogenic HPV types.[57] This finding is compatible with the observation that 'high risk' HPV types induce aneuploidy in keratinocyte cell lines.[58] Development of DNA aneuploidy may thus represent an important step in cervical neoplasia progression. It is frequently observed in CIN lesions and its presence or degree may correlate with viral integration and risk for clinical disease progression.[59,60] Aneuploidy may also be signalled by the presence of atypical mitotic figures (ATM) since a genome with highly aberrant chromosome count is unable to align metaphase plates appropriately. It has been shown that the frequency of ATM correlates with high-grade dysplasia harboring 'oncogenic' HPV types.[61]

Based on histopathologic differences observed in associated lesions, some investigators have attempted to infer morphologic differences among 'oncogenic' HPV genotypes, particularly 16 and 18, but this remains largely unresolved. Some have proposed that HPV type 18 has a relatively short preinvasive growth phase and thereby results in a 'rapidly progressive' disease.[62] Such an association correlates well with its greater *in vitro* transforming potential and higher rates of integration compared with Type 16.[5] However, Type 18 associated cervical lesions frequently display morphologic features of low-grade CIN.[63,64] Adding to the confusion is the well-established association between HPV 18 and so-called 'bowenoid papulosis', a morphologically high grade but clinically indolent multicentric lesion. Early reports associating type 18 HPV with cervical adenocarcinoma, which may be clinically more aggressive than squamous carcinoma, have not been confirmed by more recent studies, which find types 18 and 16 with equal frequency in glandular neoplasia.[65,66] Type 16 positive endocervical neoplasms, however, often display squamous differentiation, in contrast to type 18 lesions, which exhibit pure glandular histologic features. (It should be noted, by the way, that only 40–60% of endocervical adenocarcinomas are positive for HPV DNA.) Finally, the genotype of associated HPV has not been found to correlate with frequency of nodal metastases in cervical carcinomas.[27]

Conclusions

It is reasonably well established that LFGT infection with 'high risk' HPV types represents a causal factor in the development of epithelial neoplasia at these sites. Recent evidence, moreover, would suggest that perturbations of cell cycle regulation by virus-encoded proteins, as well as genetic consequences of host–viral recombination, are important mechanisms underlying this association. We have repeatedly emphasized, however, the multiplicity of factors which also contribute to this process, either independently or by modulating the virus–host relationship. The reader must bear in mind that progression of LFGT neoplasia may be viewed in the context of many factors, including neovascularization,[67,68] host folate deficiency,[69] DNA hypomethylation,[70] oncogene expression,[71,72] and many others.

The efficacy of HPV DNA detection and typing of clinical specimens, at this date, is unclear. We have seen that, as a screening device, the utility of such testing would be largely negated by the relatively high prevalence of occult infection as well as the low rate for development of clinically serious lesions in 'HPV-positive' individuals. Treatment of such 'high-grade' lesions is guided by clinical manifestations and degree of pathologic dysplasia, the morphologic detection and appearances of which are largely independent of the virus(es) *per se*. Viral detection and typing will therefore most likely be of value in women with lesions of dubious significance. Under such circumstances the presence of a 'high risk' genotype may prompt further diagnostic measures, treatment or closer follow-up. The effectiveness of such algorithms could only be proven by prospective studies which have yet to be performed.

FUTURE PERSPECTIVES

Although perhaps not the only factor in carcinogenesis, HPV nevertheless represents a common demoninator in patients with cervical carcinoma. This suggests that prevention of infection, through vaccination, may represent a useful strategy for lessening the morbidity and mortality of LFGT neoplasia. Until recently, evidence of a humoral response to HPV was evaluated primarily in patients having invasive LFGT malignancies. Antibodies to capsid proteins have been reported, however, in animal models of infection and in some human subjects. Although all evidence would suggest that a cell-mediated response is fundamental to clearing an HPV infection, current investigations are addressing the utility of vaccination approaches to disease prevention.

SUMMARY

- The lower female genital tract may be infected by at least 20 HPV genotypes which are classified on the basis of DNA sequence homology. Based on predominant associations with morphologically defined lesions, 'common' HPV types are grouped as 'high risk' (16, 18, 31, 33, 35 – high-grade dysplasia/carcinoma) or 'low risk' (6, 11 – condyloma/low-grade dysplasia). Less common, so-called 'novel', HPV types (42, 43, 51, 52, 56) collectively account for 15% of HPV infections.

HPV infections of the LFGT are morphologically and clinically occult in 10–30% of cases and simultaneous infection by more than one type occurs frequently (5–40% of cases). In an undefined proportion of cases, pathologic changes in HPV associated lesions overlap with non-viral inflammatory or reactive states.

The natural history of lower female genital tract HPV infection is poorly defined. This reflects differences between HPV genotypes, the multiplicity of co-factors associated with viral transmission, and the complexity of immune and/or genetic factors (individual or population specific) which modulate the course of the infection. Most infections are believed to be transient and are cleared or suppressed by the host.

Longitudinal studies are still at a preliminary stage. However, several have correlated the presence of HPV DNA with morphologic progression of premalignant cervical lesions. These studies have also shown that intervals between infection and development of 'high grade' dysplasia may be shorter than reported in older literature.

HPV detection and genotyping is based on DNA hybridization technologies which are developing and associated with finite sensitivities and specificities as well as limited correlation to pathologic tissue alterations.

The HPV life cycle is inextricably linked to, and coordinated with, epithelial differentiation. There is maturation-specific interaction of viral and host gene expression. A steady-state, non-productive infection occurs in epithelial basal cells. Viral particle assembly with cytopathic effect occurs in superficial, mature cells.

Virus-encoded gene products (E6 and E7) bind to critical molecular species (p53, Rb) which act as physiologic 'checkpoints' on cell cycle progression. This is believed to result in altered cell proliferation. The efficiency of E6 and E7 is greater in the high risk HPV types and their expression is greater in higher grade dysplasias.

HPV-associated malignant transformation correlates with integration of viral DNA into the host genome. It is speculated that this recombination event contributes to malignant phenotype via deranged viral gene expression (by interrupting sequences) as well as by induction of mutation or oncogene activation in host DNA.

Viral integration is a property almost exclusive to high risk genotypes and in high grade intraepithelial lesions. Epidemiologic and experimental data suggest that other factors (immunologic, hormonal, or mutation-related) are necessary for progression of HPV infections to carcinoma.

Between 10 and 15% of cervical carcinomas are HPV-negative. These tumors more frequently display mutations of the p53 gene than HPV-positive cases. This finding, in addition to retention of HPV DNA in metastatic lesions, suggests that viral influences are necessary in order to perpetuate a malignant phenotype.

REFERENCES

1. Burnett AF, Grendys EC, Willett GD, Johnson JC, Barter JF, Barnes WA. Preservation of multiple oncogenic human papillomavirus types in recurrences of early-stage cervical cancers. *Am J Obstet Gynecol* 1994 **170**: 1230–1233.
2. Tham KM, Chow VTK, Singh P, Tock EPC, Ching KC, Lim-Tan SK *et al.* Diagnostic sensitivity of polymerase chain reaction and southern blot hybridization for the detection of human papillomavirus DNA in biopsy specimens from cervical lesions. *Am J Clin Pathol* 1991 **95**: 638–646.
3. Kiviat NB, Koutsky LA, Critchlow CW, Galloway DA, Vernon DA *et al.* Comparison of southern transfer hybridization and dot filter hybridization for detection of cervical human papillomavirus infection with types 6, 11, 16, 18, 31, 33, and 35. *Am J Clin Pathol* 1990 **94**: 561–565.
4. Liang X-M, Wieczorek RL, Koss LG. In situ hybridization with human papillomavirus using biotinylated DNA probes on archival cervical smears. *J Histochem Cytochem* 1991 **39**: 771–775.
5. Burmer GC, Parker JD, Bates J, East K, Kulander BG. Comparative analysis of human papillomavirus detection by polymerase chain reaction and virapap/viratype kits. *Am J Clin Pathol* 1990 **94**: 554–560.
6. Choi YJ. Detection of human papillomavirus DNA on routine Papanicolaou's smears by in situ hybridization with the use of biotinylated probes. *Am J Clin Pathol* 1991 **95**: 475–480.
7. Stoler MH, Mills SE, Gersell DJ, Walker AN. Small cell neuroendocrine carcinoma of the cervix. A human papillomavirus type 18-associated cancer. *Am J Surg Pathol* 1991 **15**: 28–32.
8. Konishi I, Fujii S, Nonogaki H, Nanbu Y, Iwai T, Takahide M. Immunohistochemical analysis of estrogen receptors, progesterone receptors, Ki-67 antigen, and human papillomavirus DNA in normal and neoplastic epithelium of the uterine cervix. *Cancer* 1991 **68**: 1340–1350.
9. Levine AJ, Harper J, Hilborne L, Rosenthal DL, Weismeier E, Haile RW. HPV DNA and the risk of squamous intraepithelial lesions of the uterine cervix in young women. *Am J Clin Pathol* 1993 **100**: 6–11.
10. Nair BS, Radhakrishna P. Review. Oncogenesis of squamous carcinoma of the uterine cervix. *Int J Gynecol Pathol* 1992 **11**: 47–57.
11. Sun Q, Tsutsumi K, Kelleher B, Pater A, Pater MM. Squamous metaplasia of normal and carcinoma in situ of HPV 16-immortalized human endocervical cells. *Cancer Res* 1992 **52**: 4254–4260.
12. Vousden K. Interactions of human papillomavirus trans-

forming proteins with the products of tumor suppressor genes. *FASEB J* 1993 **7**: 872–879.

13. Shurbaji MS, Brooks SK, Thurmond T. Proliferating cell nuclear antigen immunoreactivity in cervical intraepithelial neoplasia and benign cervical epithelium. *Anat Pathol* 1993 **100**: 22–26.

14. Auvinen E, Kujari H, Arstila P, Hukkanen V. Expression of the L2 and E7 gene of the human papillomavirus type 16 in female genital dysplasias. *Am J Pathol* 1992 **141**: 1217–1224.

15. Srivastava S, Tong YA, Devadas K, Zou ZQ, Chen Y, Pirollo KF, Chang EH. The status of the p53 gene in human papilloma virus positive or negative cervical carcinoma cell lines. *Carcinogenesis* 1992 **13**: 1273–1275.

16. Kessis TD, Slebos RJ, Nelson WG, Kastan MB, Plunkett BS, Han SM, Lorincz AT, Hedrick L, Cho KR. Human papillomavirus 16 E6 expression disrupts the p53-mediated cellular response to DNA damage. *Proc Natl Acad Sci USA* 1993 **90**: 3988–3992.

17. Munger K, Scheffner M, Huibregtse JM, Howley PM. Interactions of HPV E6 and E7 oncoproteins with tumour suppressor gene products. *Cancer Surv* 1992 **12**: 197–217.

18. Stirdivant SM, Huber HE, Patrick DR, Defeo-Jones D, McAvoy EM, Garsky VM, Oliff A, Heimbrook DC. Human papillomavirus type 16 E7 protein inhibits DNA binding by the retinoblastoma gene product. *Mol Cell Biol* 1992 **12**: 1905–1914.

19. Firzlaff JM, Luscter B, Eisenman RN. Negative change at the casein human II phosphorylation site is important for transformation but not for Rb protein binding by the E7 protein of HPV type 16. *Proc Natl Acad Sci USA* 1991 **88**: 5187–5191.

20. Ambros RA, Kurman RJ. Current concepts in the relationship of human papillomavirus infection of the pathogenesis and classification of precancerous squamous lesions of the uterine cervix. *Semin Diagn Pathol* 1990 **7**: 158–172.

21. DeBraekeleer M, Sreekantaiah C, Haas O. Herpes simplex virus and human papillomavirus sites correlate with chromosomal breakpoints in human cervical carcinoma. *Cancer Genet Cytogenet* 1992 **59**: 135–137.

22. Popescu NC, DiPaolo JA, Amsbaugh SC. Integration sites of human papillomavirus 18 DNA sequences on HeLa cell chromosomes. *Cytogenet Cell Genet* 1987 **44**: 58–62.

23. Stoler MH, Rhodes CR, Whitbeck A, Wolinsky SM, Chow LT, Broker TR. Human papillomavirus type 16 and 18 gene expression in cervical neoplasias. *Hum Pathol* 1992 **23**: 117–128.

24. Storey A, Greenfield I, Banks L, Pim D, Crook T, Crawford L, Stanley M. Lack of immortalizing activity of a human papillomavirus type 16 variant DNA with a mutation in the E2 gene isolated from normal human cervical keratinocytes. *Oncogene* 1992 **7**: 459–465.

25. Kristiansen E, Jenkins A, Holm R. Coexistence of episomal and integrated HPV16 DNA in squamous cell carcinoma of the cervix. *J Clin Pathol* 1994 **47**: 253–256.

26. Berumen J, Casas L, Segura E, Amezcua JL, Garcia-Carranca A. Genome amplification of HPV types 16 and 18 in cervical carcinomas is related to the retention of E1/E2 genes. *Int J Cancer* 1994 **56**: 640–645.

27. Chen TM, Chen CA, Wu CC, Huang SC, Chang CF, Hsieh CY. The genotypes and prognostic significance of human papillomaviruses in cervical cancer. *Int J Cancer* 1994 **57**: 1881–1884.

28. Rusk D, Sutton GP, Look KY, Roman A. Analysis of invasive squamous cell carcinoma of the vulva and vulvar intraepithelial neoplasia for the presence of human papillomavirus DNA. *Obstet Gynecol* 1991 **77**: 918.

29. Lorincz AT, Schiffman MH, Jaffurs WJ, Marlow J, Quinn AP, Temple GF. Temporal associations of human papillomavirus infection with cervical cytologic abnormalities. *Am J Obstet Gynecol* 1990 **162**: 645–651.

30. Sherlock CH, Anderson GH, Benedet JL, Bowie WR, Coldman AJ *et al*. Human papillomavirus infection of the uterine cervix. Tissue sampling and laboratory methods affect correlations between infection rates and dysplasia. *Am J Clin Pathol* 1992 **97**: 692–698.

31. Gregoire L, Lawrence WD, Kukuruga D, Eisenbrey AB, Lancaster WD. Association between HLA-DQ81 alleles and risk for cervical cancer in African–American women. *Int J Cancer* 1994 **57**: 504–507.

32. Meyer MP, Carbonell RI, Mauser NA, Kanbour AI, Amortegui AJ. Detection of human papillomavirus in cervical swab samples by ViraPap and in cervical biopsy specimens by *in situ* hybridization. *Am J Clin Pathol* 1993 **100**: 12–17.

33. Shroyer KR, Lovelace GS, Abarca ML, Fennell RH, Corkill ME *et al*. Detection of human papillomavirus DNA by *in situ* hybridization and polymerase chain reaction in human papillomavirus equivocal and dysplastic cervical biopsies. *Hum Pathol* 1993 **24**: 1012–1016.

34. Mitchell H. Improving consistency in cervical cytology reporting. *J Natl Cancer Inst* 1993 **85**: 1592–1596.

35. Reid R, Greenberg M, Jenson AB, Husain M, Willett J, Daoud Y, Temple G, Stanhope CR, Sherman AI, Phibbs GD, Lorincz AT. Sexually transmitted papillomaviral infections. I. The anatomic distribution and pathologic grade of neoplastic lesions associated with different viral types. *Am J Obstet Gynecol* 1987 **156**: 212–222.

36. Mayelo V, Garaud P, Renjard L, Dianoux L, Lansac J, Lhuintre Y *et al*. Cell abnormalities associated with human papillomavirus-induced squamous intraepithelial cervical lesions. *Am J Clin Pathol* 1994 **101**: 13–18.

37. Mittal KR, Chan W, Demopoulos RI. Sensitivity and specificity of various morphological features of cervical condylomas. An in situ hybridization study. *Arch Pathol Lab Med* 1990 **114**: 1038–1042.

38. Nuovo GJ. Human papillomavirus DNA in genital tract lesions histologically negative for condylomata. Analysis by in situ, Southern blot hybridization and the polymerase chain reaction. *Am J Surg Pathol* 1990 **14**: 643–651.

39. Nuovo GJ, Walsh LL, Gentile JL, Blanco JS, Koulos J, Heimann A. Correlation of the Papanicolaou smear and human papillomavirus type in women with biopsy-proven cervical squamous intraepithelial lesions. *Am J Clin Pathol* 1991 **96**: 544–548.

40. DeVilliers EM, Schneider A, Miklaw H, Papendick U, Wagner D, Wesch H, Wahrendorf J, Zur Hausen H. Human papillomavirus infections in women with and without abnormal cervical cytology. *Lancet* 1987 **i**: 703–705.

41. Nuovo GJ, Cottral S, Richart RM. Occult human papillomavirus infection of the uterine cervix in postmenopausal women. *Am J Obstet Gynecol* 1989 **160**: 340–344.

42. Cornelissen MTE, Bots T, Briet MA, Jubbink MF, Struyk APHB *et al*. Detection of human papillomavirus types by the polymerase chain reaction and the differentiation between high-risk and low-risk cervical lesions. *Virchows Archiv B Cell Pathol* 1992 **62**: 167–171.

43. Koutsky LA, Holmes KK, Critchlow CW, Stevens CE, Paavonen J *et al*. A cohort study of the risk of cervical intraepithelial neoplasia grade 2 or 3 in relation to papillomavirus infection. *N Engl J Med* 1992 **327**: 1272–1278.

44. Ferenczy A, Mitao M, Nagai N, Silverstein SJ, Crum CP. Latent papillomavirus and recurring genital warts. *N Engl J Med* 1985 **313**: 784–788.

45. Willett GD, Kurman RJ, Reid R, Greenberg M, Jenson AB, Lorincz AT. Correlation of the histologic appearance of intraepithelial neoplasia of the cervix with human papillomavirus types. Emphasis on low grade lesions including so-called flat condyloma. *Int J Gynecol Pathol* 1989 **8**: 18–25.

46. Beckmann AM, Acker R, Christiansen AE, Sherman KJ. Human papillomavirus infection in women with multicentric squamous cell neoplasia. *Am J Obstet Gynecol* 1991 **165**: 1431–1437.

47. Lungu O, Sun XW, Felix J, Richart RM, Silverstein S, Wright TC. Relationship of human papillomavirus type to

grade of cervical intraepithelial neoplasia. *JAMA* 1992 **267** (**18**): 2493–2496.

48. Campion MJ, Cuzick J, McCance DJ, Singer A. Progressive potential of mild cervical atypia: prospective cytological, colposcopic, and virological study. *Lancet* 1986 **i**: 237–240.

49. Nuovo GJ, Moritz J, Walsh LL, MacConnell P, Koulos J. Predictive value of human papillomavirus DNA detection by filter hybridization and polymerase chain reaction in women with negative results of colposcopic examination. *Am J Clin Pathol* 1992 **98**: 489–492.

50. Schiffman MH. Recent progress in defining the epidemiology of human papillomavirus infection and cervical neoplasia. *J Natl Cancer Inst* 1992 **84**: 394–398.

51. Nuovo GJ, Pedemonte BM. Human papillomavirus types and recurrent cervical warts. *JAMA* 1990 **263**: 1223–1226.

52. Dillner J, Lenner P, Lehtinen M, Eklund C, Heino P, Wikluynd F *et al*. A population-based seroepidemiological study of cervical cancer. *Cancer Res* 1994 **54**: 134–141.

53. Williams AB, Darragh TM, Vranizan K, Ochia C, Moss AR, Palefsky JM. Anal and cervical human papillomavirus infection and risk of anal and cervical epithelial abnormalities in human immunodeficiency virus-infected women. *Obstet Gynecol* 1994 **83**: 205–211.

54. Fujimura M, Ostrow RS, Okagaki T. Implication of human papillomavirus in postirradiation dysplasia. *Cancer* 1991 **68**: 2181–2185.

55. Ho GYF, Burk RD, Fleming I, Klein RS. Risk of genital human papillomavirus infection in women with human immunodeficiency virus-induced immunosuppression. *Int J Cancer* 1994 **56**: 788–792.

56. Barton SE, Maddox PH, Jenkins D, Edwards R, Cuzick J, Singer A. Effect of cigarette smoking on cervical epithelial immunity: a mechanism for neoplastic change? *Lancet* 1988 **ii**: 652–654.

57. Kadish AS, Hagan RJ, Ritter DB, Goldberg GL, Romney SL, Kanetsky PA *et al*. Biologic characteristics of specific human papillomavirus types predicted from morphology of cervical lesions. *Hum Pathol* 1992 **23**: 1262–1269.

58. Woodworth CD, Deniju J, DiPaolo JA. Immortalization of human function keratinocytes by various HPV DNAs corresponds to their association with cervical carcinoma. *J Virol* 1989 **63**: 159–164.

59. McCance DJ, Kopan R, Fuchs E, Laimins AL. Human papillomavirus type 16 alters human epithelial cell differentiation *in vitro*. *Proc Natl Acad Sci USA* 1988 **85**: 7167–7173.

60. Hanselaar AGJM, Vooijs GP, Oud PS, Pahlplatz MMM, Beck JLM. DNA ploidy patterns in cervical intraepithelial neoplasia grade III, with and without synchronous invasive squamous cell carcinoma. *Cancer* 1988 **62**: 2537–2545.

61. Claas ECJ, Quint WGV, Pieters WJLM, Burger MPM, Oosterhuis WJW, Lindeman J. Human papillomavirus and the three group metaphase figure as markers of an increased risk for the development of cervical carcinoma. *Am J Pathol* 1992 **140**: 497–502.

62. Arends MJ, Donaldson YK, Duvall E, Wyllie AH, Bird CC. Human papillomavirus type 18 associates with more advanced cervical neoplasia than human papillomavirus type 16. *Hum Pathol* 1993 **24**: 432–437.

63. McLachlin CM, Tate JE, Zitz JC, Sheets EE, Crum CP. Human papillomavirus type 18 and intraepithelial lesions of the cervix. *Am J Pathol* 1994 **144**: 141–147.

64. Genest DR, Stein L, Sheets E, Zitz JC, Crum CP. A binary (Bethesda) system for classifying cervical cancer precursors: criteria, reproducibility, and viral correlates. *Hum Pathol* 1993 **24**: 730–736.

65. Milde-Langosch K, Schreiber C, Becker G, Loning T, Stegner HE. Human papillomavirus detection in cervical adenocarcinoma by polymerase chain reaction. *Hum Pathol* 1993 **24**: 590–594.

66. Duggan MA, Nenoit JL, McGregor SE, Nation JG, Inoue M, Stuart GCE. The human papillomavirus status of 114 endocervical adenocarcinoma cases by dot blot hybridization. *Hum Pathol* 1993 **24**: 121–125.

67. Sillman F, Boyce J, Fruchter R. The significance of atypical vessels and neovascularization in cervical neoplasia. *Am J Obstet Gynecol* 1981 **139**: 154–159.

68. Smith-McCune KK, Weidner. Demonstration and characterization of the angiogenic properties of cervical dysplasia. *Cancer Res* 1994 **54**: 800–804.

69. Butterworth CE, Hatch KD, Macaluso M, Cole P, Sauberlich HE, Soong SJ, Borst M, Baker VV. Folate deficiency and cervical dysplasia. *JAMA* 1992 **267**: 528–533.

70. Kim YI, Giuliano A, Hatch KD, Schneider A, Nour MA, Dallal GE, Selhub J, Mason JB. Global DNA hypomethylation increases progressively in cervical dysplasia and carcinoma. *Cancer* 1994 **74**: 893–899.

71. Riou GF. Proto-oncogenes and prognosis in early carcinoma of the uterine cervix. *Cancer Surv* 1988 **7**: 441–456.

72. Pinion SB, Kennedy JH, Miller RW, MacLean AL. Oncogene expression in cervical intraepithelial neoplasia and invasive cancer of cervix. *Lancet* 1991 **337**: 819–820.

4.3

Hormones and Cancer

NAM De Clercq and JO White

INTRODUCTION

This chapter will focus on the biology of sex-steroid hormones in relation to endometrial and breast cancer. The potential role of endogenous and exogenous sources of estradiol and progesterone will be discussed and will cover recent information on oral contraceptives and hormone replacement therapy. Differences in the biology of endometrial and breast epithelium will be highlighted and discussed in relation to the use of antihormones, in particular the antiestrogen tamoxifen, in the adjuvant and preventive setting. The cellular activity of estradiol and progesterone will be considered by discussion of the structure and function of their respective receptors and the potential interactive pathways that combine to produce tissue specific responses.

CURRENT CONCEPTS

Endogenous hormones

The great majority of cancers of the uterine corpus are adenocarcinomas. The risk factors for this disease include obesity, anovulation, polycystic ovaries, nulliparity, early menarche and late menopause.[1] These risk factors suggest an endocrine component and are consistent with the hypothesis that development of endometrial cancer is related to exposure of the endometrium to mitogenic estrogen stimulation in the absence of natural cyclical progesterone antagonism.[2–4]

Breast cancer is the most common malignancy affecting women, an increased risk of disease being associated with early menarche, late menopause, nulliparity, a late first birth and obesity during the postmenopausal years.[5] The biology of the epithelial cell type from which the majority of breast cancers develop, the terminal duct lobular unit, apparently differs from that of endometrial epithelial cells in response to steroid hormones.[6] Proliferation of this breast epithelium is low in the follicular phase but highest in the mid- to late-secretory phase when the cells are exposed to endocrine stimulation by a combination of estradiol and progesterone of ovarian origin. This contrasts with endometrial epithelium in which proliferation is highest in the follicular phase, which is under estrogen dominance, but diminished in the luteal phase associated with progesterone-induced differentiation. Any possible role for endogenous hormones in the development of breast cancer is therefore considered in the context of a stimulatory, rather than inhibitory, effect of progesterone against a background of estrogenic stimulation. Although such a stimulatory effect of progesterone on breast epithelium may represent a consensus point of view[5,6] there are other data to suggest the antiestrogenic activity of progesterone on human breast cells (reviewed in reference 7). The epidemiological picture for breast cancer is clearly complex and includes a protective effect of early age of first pregnancy, explained by a decrease in the pool of stem cells susceptible to genotoxic insult as a result of development and differentiation of the mammary gland during pregnancy.[8]

Exogenous hormones

The apparent association between endocrine factors and the development of endometrial and breast cancer has led to intensive investigations of any associations between exogenous sex steroids and risk of disease. Oral contraceptives in the reproductive years and hormone replacement therapy, most commonly associated with the perimenopausal and postmenopausal years, are the major sources of exogenous sex steroid hormones. Initial experience with sequential oral contraceptive preparations revealed an increase in the incidence of endometrial cancer[5] that apparently resulted from inadequate progestin antagonism of the estrogen present in the formulation.[9] Sequential oral contraceptives, which contain only an estrogen in the initial phase of the cycle followed by an estrogen plus progestogen, are no longer used in most countries having been replaced by combined oral contraceptives, in which an estrogen and progestogen are taken over a 21-day cycle. Use of combined oral contraceptives reduces the risk of endometrial cancer, the protective effect being related to duration of use and possibly maintained for as long as 15 years after cessation of use.[4] There appears to be no overall increased risk of developing breast cancer in users of combined estrogen plus progestin oral contraceptives although recent studies demonstrate an association between long-term use and breast cancer in younger women. However, such cancers represent a small proportion of all breast cancers.[4]

Hormone replacement therapy (HRT) is used to provide short-term relief of symptoms related to the menopause and longer-term protection from the consequences of estrogen deficiency. The doses of estrogen used in such preparations are sufficient to cause proliferation of the endometrium and in initial studies of estrogen-only replacement therapy a very large relative risk of endometrial cancer became apparent (reviewed in reference 10). The benefit of including a progestin along with estrogen as part of HRT has been clearly established[11,12] and is consistent with the predicted antagonism of the proliferative effects of estrogens on the endometrium.

Long-term estrogen-only HRT is associated with a small increase in the risk of developing breast cancer.[10,13] Much of the data, however, are heterogeneous with an apparent higher risk appearing in European compared with American studies, which may reflect differences in the specific formulations used and the indications for prescribing HRT.[10] Limited data on combination estrogen and progestin HRT suggest that the risk of breast cancer is higher than that of estrogen-only,[14] in support of the mitogenic influence of progestins on breast epithelium. However, this has not been the conclusion of every study.[15]

Antiestrogens and cancer treatment

The antiestrogen tamoxifen (ICI 46,474, Nolvadex), which does not contain a steroid backbone, but has sufficient similarity to estradiol to compete for estrogen receptor-binding, has become the first line endocrine therapy for all stages of breast cancer.[16] Remission rates of approximately 30% have been reported in patients treated for metastatic disease; in these cases tamoxifen is not curative but remission may be maintained for several years.[17,18] An overview analysis of the use of tamoxifen adjuvant to primary surgery for patients with early breast cancer demonstrated a delay in relapse and a reduction in the risk of death by 20–30%.[19] The most prominent response to tamoxifen was observed in postmenopausal women whose tumors had been diagnosed as being estrogen receptor positive, although beneficial effects were also observed in poor prognosis estrogen receptor negative patients. Such effects in receptor poor tumors are not immediately explicable but may be related to the interaction between the surrounding stromal cells and malignant epithelial cells. The control of locally active stimulatory (transform-

ing growth factor alpha, insulin like growth factor-1) and inhibitory (transforming growth factor-beta) growth factors, by estrogen receptor dependent and independent mechanisms, potentially controls proliferative and metastatic potential.[18]

Tamoxifen has been used alone, at various doses, for the treatment of endometrial cancer in recurrent or advanced disease with an overall response rate of approximately 40%.[20] Its use in combination with progestins is based on the ability of tamoxifen to increase the content of progesterone receptors in endometrial cancer.[21,22] Only limited information on the value of such treatment exists and in the best controlled trial there was only a small improvement in survival.[23]

The positive effects of tamoxifen, together with evidence of a reduction in the incidence of contralateral breast cancer,[24] have stimulated the consideration of its use as a chemopreventive agent in patients at high risk of developing breast cancer. The benefits of tamoxifen in the treatment of breast cancer are substantial and proven; however, there is concern about its use in a prophylactic setting based on its potential estrogenic effects in other tissues. Some, but not all, studies have reported an increase in the incidence of endometrial cancer in patients who had received tamoxifen as part of their treatment for breast cancer (reviewed in reference 20). Two more recent studies, one the largest randomized study to date and incorporating a placebo control[25] the other a large case-control study,[26] further support the hypothesis of the potential adverse effects of tamoxifen on the endometrium. The apparent modest increase in risk of developing endometrial cancer will probably have little impact on the risk versus benefit analysis for patients receiving adjuvant treatment for breast cancer but needs consideration in the chemoprevention setting.

Structure and mode of action of steroid receptors

The estrogen (ER) and progesterone receptor (PR) are ligand-inducible transcription factors thus becoming active upon binding of their respective hormones. As members of the steroid and thyroid hormone receptor superfamily they share the same overall modular structure (Fig. 4.3.1). This was revealed by studies using synthetic chimeric receptors in which for example the ligand binding domain of the glucocorticoid receptor (GR) was exchanged for the ligand binding domain of the estrogen receptor turning that GR into an estrogen responsive receptor (reviewed in references 27 and 28). The modular structure is further also partially revealed in the exon/intron structure of their genes, in which there is a very high degree of conservation among different species (human, rodents, chicken).

The most conserved part of all steroid receptors is the DNA binding domain C (Fig. 4.3.1) wherein two zinc fingers, in which the loops are stabilized by the interaction of four cysteine residues with a zinc atom, are responsible for binding of the activated receptor to specific DNA sequences (hormone responsive elements, HREs).[29] These

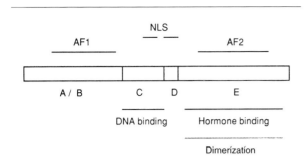

Fig. 4.3.1 *Schematic representation of the modular structure of the steroid hormone receptor. For abbreviations, see text.*

elements were originally defined for the interaction of the glucocorticoid receptor in the mouse mammary tumor virus (MMTV) long terminal repeat (LTR).[30]

Another very well conserved region is the hinge region (region D, Fig. 4.3.1). This region of the receptor contains the main and constitutive nuclear localization signal (NLS).[31] These NLSs are stretches of basic amino acids, mainly arginines and lysines. There is also a second, hormone-dependent NLS, located in the second zinc finger of the DNA binding domain.[31] Recently it has been shown

that the progesterone receptor diffuses into the cytoplasm and is constantly and actively transported back into the nucleus.[32] Preliminary data from the same authors suggest the same happens for estradiol and glucocorticoid receptor.

The less conserved domain E (Fig. 4.3.1) contains the ligand binding pocket, responsible for binding of hormone and antihormones. It also encodes a ligand-dependent transactivation function (AF2)[33] and the region responsible for dimerization of the hormone receptors. The amino-terminal part (domain A/B, Fig. 4.3.1) of all steroid receptors is the least conserved and is mainly involved in gene transactivation through another, ligand-independent, activation function (AF1). It is upon binding of ligand to the receptor and dimerization that conformational changes occur enabling both activation functions to exert their influence on transcription of target genes.

It is generally accepted that steroid receptors occur in cells associated in a multiprotein complex involving several heat shock proteins (hsp) (Fig. 4.3.2), among which the 90 kDa protein (hsp90) is the most extensively studied. As receptors are inactive in the absence of ligand[34] the most plausible role for the hsp90 complex is to prevent unoccupied receptor from activating target genes.[35] There are also

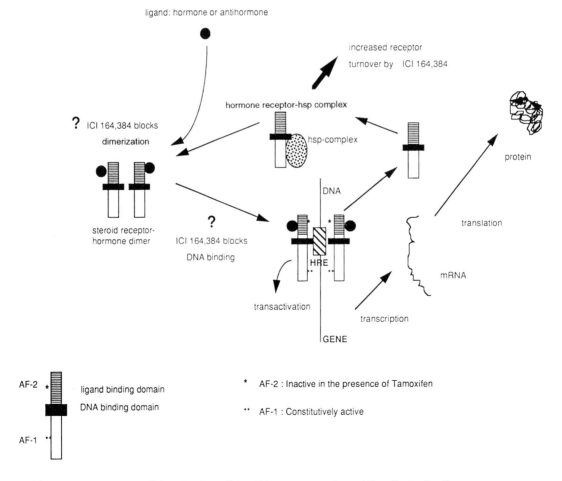

Fig. 4.3.2 *Schematic representation of the activation of steroid hormone receptor and the effects of antihormones.*

recent data suggesting a possible role for hsp90 in nuclear–cytoplasmic shuttling.[36]

Upon binding of the ligand the receptor complex dissociates, the activated receptor dimerizes and this dimer binds to its hormone response element (HRE) (Fig. 4.3.2). These HREs are short nucleotide sequences that contain perfect or imperfect palindromic half sites. Surprisingly, the progesterone receptor was shown to bind to the same responsive element as the glucocorticoid receptor.[37] In fact glucocorticoids, progestins, androgens and mineralocorticoids can all mediate transcription through the response element with the consensus sequence GGTACAnnnTGTTCT. Estrogens on the other hand, act through a similar but different responsive element (ERE: AGGTCAnnnTGACCT). Each of the two receptors in the dimer binds to a half site of the HRE. These HREs are able to render reporter gene constructs responsive to hormone stimulation.[38] Here the HREs are cloned in front of a gene coding for an enzyme (e.g. chloramphenicol acetyl transferase, CAT or luciferase, LUC) which will be switched on as a consequence of the hormone–receptor complex binding to the HRE. The enzyme activity is then a measurement for the hormone responsiveness. However, a full induction can often only be obtained when cooperation of the receptor with other transcription factors, like nuclear factor I (NFI), bound in the vicinity occurs.[39] Many such non-ligand-dependent transcription factors, which bind to very specific response elements, have been characterized to date (reviewed in reference 40).

Action of antiestrogens

Most antihormones act by antagonizing the binding of natural ligand to its cognate receptor. Tamoxifen binds to the ER in the ligand binding domain, prevents estrogen binding to the same receptor and thus interferes with the activation of AF2 which resides within the ligand binding domain. The antagonist activity of tamoxifen has therefore been explained by its inability to induce AF2 activity or by interference with pre-existing AF2 (reviewed in reference 41). Genes that require AF2 activity to be stimulated by hormones are as a consequence not induced in the presence of tamoxifen-liganded ER and hence experience antagonism. The agonistic activity of antiestrogens on the other hand is explained by the fact that tamoxifen-liganded ER still binds to the ERE and can still activate genes that require the activity of AF1, situated in the A/B region of the receptor and therefore ligand independent. Furthermore, higher order protein–protein interactions (i.e. cooperativity) of ER liganded with tamoxifen may differ from those of estradiol-liganded ER and thus contribute to the extent of agonism or antagonism observed in different tissues.[42] For example in endometrial cancer cell lines (Ishikawa cells) agonist activity of tamoxifen, equivalent to that of estradiol, on the induction of cell growth.[43,44] and PR has been reported.[45] A possible explanation for these observations and for the sensitivity of normal endometrial cells[46] may reside in the activity of receptor associated proteins. Such agonist activity of tamoxifen may ultimately contribute to tumor resistance. For example, it is suggested that subpopulations of tumor cells that respond to tamoxifen as an agonist ultimately outgrow the inhibited population of cells such that the overall phenotype of the tumor is altered and is regarded as being tamoxifen resistant.[47]

Tamoxifen-liganded receptor binds to DNA and stimulates transcription of certain responsive genes but not others. However, there are conflicting reports on the mechanism of antiestrogenic action of the new generation of steroidal antiestrogens. These compounds, ICI 164,384 and ICI 182,780, are derivatives of estradiol that carry a 7α-alkylamide side chain, which in the case of ICI 182,780, includes fluorination of the terminal alkyl function to improve drug delivery.[48] Initial reports suggested that ICI 164,384 was able to prevent dimerization and prevent DNA binding of ER (reviewed in reference 41). Recent reports, however, suggest that the binding of ER to an ERE can occur in the absence of ligand and that the role of ligand is to induce protein–protein rather than protein–DNA interactions.[49,50] The nature of such interactions may than depend on the specific conformations adopted by the receptor upon binding of agonist or antagonist. Others have demonstrated that ICI 164,384 increases the turnover of the ER drastically[51] and that this might be due to an impaired receptor dimerization. The antiestrogenic properties of this compound may therefore be related to its ability to decrease ER content. If such differences in the apparent mode of action of two classes of antiestrogen are correct then it might be expected that development of resistance to tamoxifen may not preclude sensitivity to ICI 164,384. Recent evidence clearly illustrates the possibility that different classes of antiestrogens may prove to be efficient second-line treatment of some tamoxifen-resistant tumors. For example, ICI 164,384 retains the ability to inhibit cell proliferation and certain estrogen-responsive genes in a tamoxifen resistant variant of the MCF-7 breast tumor cell line.[52]

Mutation affecting the activity of steroid receptors

Alterations (e.g. point mutations, deletions or insertions) in steroid receptor structure may be, at least in part, responsible for differential responses to antihormones between tissues and the development of resistance. Reports on mutations in hormone receptor genes are numerous for breast cancer but there is limited information on the structure and function of the estrogen receptor in uterine tissues. Although mutations in ER do occur in tamoxifen-resistant tumors they probably do not *per se*, account for the altered phenotype.[53] It remains to be established whether it is the relative amounts of particular receptor variants, that may function in a dominant manner, that contribute to the process of malignant progression and/or acquired resistance to antihormone therapy.

Specific point mutations in distinct domains of the mouse estrogen receptor can confer differential sensitivity to estrogen and tamoxifen.[54] Reese *et al.*[55] demonstrated, using mutation analysis, that the four cysteine residues of the hormone binding domain of the ER are not essential for binding or transactivation activity of estradiol or other reversibly binding estrogen and antiestrogens but these mutations do affect the potency of the covalently attaching antiestrogen tamoxifen aziridine. The functional activity of such variants and their existence in clinical breast cancer material needs to be further investigated. Mutations as a result of exon deletions, leading to truncated receptors are well documented in breast cancer.[56] The existence of an exon 5 deleted variant of ER is associated with the ER negative/PR positive phenotype and may represent a stage in the progression of such cells to autonomy from estrogenic influence.[57]

Progesterone receptor isoforms

The progesterone receptor is unique among the steroid hormone receptors as it exists in the cell as two distinct molecular forms. In humans, hPR-B, 933 amino acids in length (114 kDa) and hPR-A, lacking 164 amino acids from the N-terminus of the receptor (94 kDa), exist.[58,59] The two receptor isoforms are synthesized from nine structurally different mRNAs encompassing two translation start sites.[60] Several authors have identified two promoters in the single copy PR gene. Using transient co-transfection experiments it was demonstrated that both promoters were estrogen inducible.[58] Kraus *et al.*[61] have identified and characterized a weak ERE in the proximal promoter of the rat gene and showed that both promoters of the PR gene are regulated independently. The two forms of the PR have been identified in most species except the rabbit. It is likely that PR-A and PR-B have different physiological functions and that the relative levels of hPR-A and hPR-B in cells is critical for appropriate cellular response to progesterone.[62] In the presence of specific antiprogestins hPR-A acts as a transdominant repressor of hPR-B mediated transcription in promoter- and cell-specific contexts.[63] hPR-A is even capable of influencing glucocorticoid, androgen,[62] and mineralocorticoid receptor[64] mediated gene transcription.

Interaction between signaling pathways

There is increasing evidence of cross-talk between the estrogen receptor pathway and several cell signaling pathways involving protein kinases and growth factors. Aronica and Katzenellenbogen[65] demonstrated that the PR in uterine cells is not only induced by estrogens but also by cAMP and IGF-I. The latter effects of c-AMP and IGF-1 can be suppressed not only by protein kinase inhibitors but also by antiestrogens suggesting mediation by estrogen receptors. Further evidence in support of the involvement of ER is provided by the fact that IGF-I and agents which increase intracellular cAMP (cholera toxin and isobutylmethylxanthine) stimulate ER mediated *trans*-activation and ER phosphorylation.[66] Stimulation of the PK-A signaling pathway (via increasing intracellular

cAMP content) in MCF-7 human breast cancer cells changes the agonist–antagonist activity of tamoxifen and related antiestrogens. Such stimulation enhances estrogen-like agonist activity and reduces the ability of antiestrogens to antagonize the effects of estrogens[67] and may provide a further explanation of the development of tamoxifen resistance in breast cancer. The effects of PK-A activation are promoter specific and are not seen with the pure antiestrogen ICI 164,384. Such apparent discrimination of the PK-A pathway between the activities of different classes of antiestrogens may provide the biological basis for their selective use in the therapy of tamoxifen-resistant breast cancer[52] and an explanation for the pronounced stimulatory effect of tamoxifen in endometrial cancer cell lines.[20]

In conclusion, the cellular responses to steroid hormones requires activation of cognate receptor and regulation of expression of selected target genes. The ability of interactive signaling pathways to modulate the activity of steroid hormone receptors provides a potential mechanism of integrating diverse signals that contribute to cell specific responses. In the context of hormones and cancer, the aberrant activity of second messenger pathways that impinge on steroid hormone receptors may amplify normal physiological responses and hence contribute to transformation events sometimes associated with endogenous and exogenous estrogen and progestogen stimulation.

FUTURE PERSPECTIVES

The products of the protooncogenes *jun* and *fos* have been widely implicated in growth and differentiation. Fos–Jun heterodimers and Jun-Jun homodimers are the principal components of the AP-1 transcription factor family that activate transcription of genes through a defined consensus DNA sequence, termed the AP-1 site or TPA (phorbol ester)-response element (TRE). There is increasing evidence of the modulation of AP-1 activity by estrogens and antiestrogens, involving the estrogen receptor but not requiring the presence of a consensus ERE in the target gene. This may involve the direct interaction of the estrogen receptor with the AP-1 complex or the modulation of an activator/suppressor of AP-1 activity. Thus, in cells exposed to estrogens or antiestrogen the qualitative response may be dependent not only upon interaction of estrogen receptor with its consensus response element but also the status of activators of AP-1. This may, therefore, contribute to the cellular specificity of estrogenic and antiestrogenic activity and provide an explanation for the variable tumor response to antiestrogen therapy, despite the presence of an apparently functional estrogen receptor. Understanding precisely how the estrogen receptor affects AP-1 activity and the range of specificities of existing antiestrogens to modify such interactions is an area which potentially will provide future improvements in therapeutic modalities.

SUMMARY

- Combined oral contraceptives reduce the risk of endometrial cancer.
- There are conflicting data on the link between HRT and cancer.
- The modest increase in risk of developing endometrial cancer as a consequence of tamoxifen administration needs consideration in a chemoprevention setting.
- There is clear evidence for agonistic activity of tamoxifen in endometrial cancer.
- A detailed structural overview of the steroid receptor superfamily is given.
- Possible explanations for the mechanism of tumor resistance to tamoxifen are given.
- New antiestrogens may prove useful alternatives to tamoxifen.
- A possible role in carcinogenesis for mutations in the estrogen receptor is suggested.
- PR isoforms may display different physiological functions.
- Evidence for cross-talk between the estrogen receptor pathway and several cell signaling pathways involving protein kinases and growth factors is discussed.

REFERENCES

1. Kelsey JL, Hildreth NG. *Breast Cancer and Gynaecological Cancer Epidemiology.* Boca Raton: CRC Press, 1983.
2. Ziel HK. Oestrogen's role in endometrial cancer. *Obstet Gynecol* 1982 **60**: 509–515.
3. Key TJ, Pike MC. The dose-effect relationship between unopposed oestrogens and endometrial mitotic rate: its central role in explaining and predicting endometrial cancer risk. *Br J Cancer* 1988 **57**: 205–212.
4. WHO Scientific Group *Oral Contraceptives and Neoplasia.* World Health Organisation Technical Report Series (Geneva): 817; 1992: 1–46.
5. Henderson BE, Ross RK, Pike MC. Hormonal chemoprevention of cancer in women. *Science* 1993 **259**: 633–638.
6. King RJB. Oestrogen and progestin effects in human breast carcinogenesis. *Breast Cancer Res Treat* 1993 **27**: 3–15.
7. Kuttenn F, Malet C, Leygue E, Gompel A, Gol R, Baudot N, Lois-Sylvestre C, Soquet L, Mauvais-Jarvis P. Antioestrogen action of progestogens on human breast cells. In Berg G, Hammar M (eds) *Modern Management of the Menopause.* Lancaster: Parthenon Publishing Group, 1993.
8. Russo J, Tay LK, Russo IH. Differentiation of the mammary gland and susceptibility to carcinogenesis. *Breast Cancer Res Treat* 1982 **2**: 5–73.
9. Gambrell RD Jr. The role of hormones in the aetiology and prevention of endometrial cancer. *Clin Obstet Gynecol* 1986 **13**: 4: 695–724.
10. Hulka BS, Liu ET, Lininger RA. Steroid hormones and risk of breast cancer. *Cancer* 1994 **74**: 1111–1124.
11. Paterson MEL, Wade-Evans T, Sturdee DW, Thom MH, Studd JWW. Endometrial disease after treatment with oestrogens and progestogens in the climacteric. *Br Med J* 1980 **i**: 822–824.
12. Whitehead MI, Hillard TC, Crook D. The role and use of progestogens. *Obstet Gynecol* 1990 **75**: 59S–80S.
13. Steinberg KK, Thacker SB, Smith SJ, Stroup DF, Zack MM, Flanders WD. A meta-analysis of the effect of oestrogen replacement therapy on the risk of breast cancer. *JAMA* 1991 **265** 15: 1985–1990.
14. Bergkvist L, Adami H-O, Persson I, Hoover R, Schairer C. The risk of breast cancer after oestrogen and oestrogen-progestin replacement. *N Engl J Med* 1989 **3321**: 293–297.
15. Gambrell RD, Maier RC, Sanders BI. Decreased incidence of breast cancer in postmenopausal oestrogen-progestogen users. *Obstet Gynecol* 1983 **62**: 435–443.
16. Lerner LJ, Jordan VC. Development of antioestrogens and their use in breast cancer. *Cancer Res* 1990 **50**: 4177–4189.
17. Jones AL, Powles TJ. Chemoprevention of breast cancer. *Rev Endocr Relat Cancer* 1993 **43**: 33–42.
18. Jordan VC. Can all postmenopausal women with a diagnosis of breast cancer benefit from tamoxifen treatment? *Rev Endocr Relat Cancer* 1993 **43**: 23–31.
19. Early Breast Cancer Trialists Collaborative Group. *Lancet* 1992 **339**, 1–15: 71–85.
20. White JO, Owen GI, De Clercq NAM, Soutter WP. Antioestrogens in the treatment of endometrial cancer. *Rev Endocr Relat Cancer* 1993 **44**: 47–57.
21. Mortel R, Levy C, Wolff J-P, Nicolas J-C, Robel P, Baulieu E-E. Female sex steroid receptors in postmenopausal endometrial carcinoma and biochemical response to an antioestrogen. *Cancer Res* 1981 **41**: 1140–1147.
22. Carlson JA, Allegra JC, Day TG and Wittliff JL. Tamoxifen and endometrial carcinoma, alterations in oestrogen and progesterone receptors in untreated patients and combination therapy in advanced neoplasia. *Am J Obstet Gynecol* 1984 **149**: 149–153.
23. Ayoub J, Audet-Lapointe P, Methot Y, Hanley J, Beaulieu R, Chemaly R *et al.* Efficacy of sequential cyclical hormonal therapy in endometrial cancer and its correlation with steroid hormone receptor status. *Gynecol Oncol* 1988 **31**: 327–337.
24. Nayfield SG, Karp JE, Ford LG, Dorr FA, Kramer BS. Potential role of tamoxifen in prevention of breast cancer. *J Natl Cancer Inst* 1991 **83**: 1450–1459.
25. Fisher B, Costantino JP, Redmond CK, Fisher ER, Wickerham DL, Cronin WM. Endometrial Cancer in Tamoxifen-Treated Breast Cancer Patients: Findings from the National Surgical Adjuvant Breast and Bowel Project. *J Natl Cancer Inst* 1994 **86**: 527–537.
26. van Leeuwen FE, Benraadt J, Coebergh JWW, Kiemeney LALM, Gimbrere CHF, Otter R, Schouten LJ, Damhuis RAM, Bontenbal M, Diepenhorst FW, Van den Belt-Dusebout AW, van Tinteren H. Risk of endometrial cancer after tamoxifen treatment of breast cancer. *Lancet* 1994 **343**: 448–452.
27. Gronemeyer H. Transcription activation by estrogen and progesterone receptors. *Annu Rev Genet* 1991 **25**: 89–123.
28. Beato M. Transcriptional control by nuclear receptors. *FASEB J* 1991 **5**: 2044–2051.
29. Berg JM. DNA binding specificity of steroid receptors. *Cell* 1989 **57**: 1065–1068.
30. Scheidereit C, Geisse S, Westphal HM, Beato M. The glucocorticoid binds to defined nucleotide sequences near the promoter of mouse mammary tumour virus. *Nature* 1983 **304**: 749–752.
31. Guiochon-Mantel A, Loosfelt H, Lescop P, Sar S, Atger M, Perrot-Applanat M, Milgrom E. Mechanisms of nuclear localization of the progesterone receptor: evidence for interaction between monomers. *Cell* 1989 **57**: 1147–1154.
32. Guiochon-Mantel A, Delabre K, Lescop P, Perrot-Applanat M, Milgrom E. Cytoplasmic-nuclear trafficking of progesterone receptor. *In vivo* study of the mechanism of action of antiprogestins. *Biochem Pharmacol* 1994 **47**: 21–24.

33. Tora L, White J, Brou C, Tasset D, Webster N, Scheer E, Chambon P. The human estrogen receptor has two independent nonacidic transcriptional activation functions. *Cell* 1989 **59**: 477–487.

34. Danielsen M, Hinck L, Ringold GM. Two amino acids within the knuckle of the first zinc finger specify DNA response element activation by the glucocorticoid receptor. *Cell* 1989 **57**: 1131–1138.

35. Pratt WB, Scherrer LC, Hutchison KA, Dalman FC. A model of glucocorticoid receptor unfolding and stabilization by a heat scock protein complex. *J Steroid Biochem Mol Biol* 1992 **41**: 233–239.

36. Kang KL, Devin J, Cadepond F, Jibard N, Guiochon-Mantel A, Baulieu EE, Catelli MG. *In vivo* functional protein-protein interaction: nuclear targeted hsp90 shifts cytoplasmic steroid receptor mutants into the nucleus. *Proc Natl Acad Sci USA* 1994 **91**: 340–344.

37. von der Ahe D, Janich S, Scheidereit C, Renkawitz R, Schütz G, Beato M. Glucocorticoid and progesterone receptors bind to the same sites in two hormonally regulated promoters. *Nature* 1985 **313**: 706–709.

38. Strähle U, Klock G, Schüte G. A DNA sequence of 15 base pairs is sufficient to mediate both glucocorticoid and progesterone induction of gene expression. *Proc Natl Acad Sci USA* 1987 **84**: 7871–7875.

39. Brüggemeier U, Rogge L, Winnacker E-L, Beato M. Nuclear factor I acts as a transcription factor on the MMTV promoter but competes with steroid hormone receptors for DNA binding. *EMBO J* 1990 **9**: 2233–2239.

40. Faisst S, Meyer S. Compilation of vertebrate-encoded transcription factors. *Nucleic Acids Res* 1992 **20**: 3–26.

41. Gronemeyer H, Benhamou B, Berry M, Bocquel MT, Gofflo D, Garcia T, Lerouge T, Metzger D, Meyer ME, Tora L, Vergezac A, Chambon P. Mechanisms of antihormone action. *J Steroid Biochem Mol Biol* 1992 **41**: 217–221.

42. Klinge CM, Bambara RA, Hilf R. Antioestrogen-liganded oestrogen receptor interaction with oestrogen responsive element DNA *in vitro*. *J Steroid Biochem Mol Biol* 1992 **43**: 249–262.

43. Anzai Y, Holinka CF, Kuramoto H, Gurpide E. Stimulatory effects of 4-hydroxytamoxifen on proliferation of human endometrial adenocarcinoma cells (Ishikawa). *Cancer Res* 1989 **49**: 2362–2365.

44. Croxtall JD, Elder MG, White JO. Hormonal control of proliferation of the Ishikawa endometrial adenocarcinoma cell line. *J Steroid Biochem* 1990 **35**: 665–669.

45. Jamil A, Croxtall JD, White JO. The effect or antioestrogens on cell growth and progesterone receptor concentration in human endometrial cancer cells (Ishikawa). *J Mol Endocrinol* 1991 **6**: 215–221.

46. Cohen I, Rosen DJD, Shapira J, Cordoba M, Gilboa S, Altara MM, Yigael D, Beyth Y. Endometrial changes with tamoxifen: comparison between tamoxifen-treated and nontreated asymptomatic, postmenopausal breast cancer patients. *Gynecol Oncol* 1994 **52**: 185–190.

47. Horwitz KB. How do breast cancers become hormone resistant? *J Steroid Biochem Mol Biol* 1994 **49**: 295–302.

48. Wakeling AE, Dukes M, Bowler J. A potent specific pure anti-estrogen with clinical potential. *Cancer Res* 1991 **51**, 3867–3873.

49. Ylikomi T, Bocquel MT, Berry M, Gronemeyer H, Chambon P. Cooperation of proto-signals for nuclear accumulation of estrogen and progesterone receptors. *EMBO J* 1992 **11**: 3681–3694.

50. Furlow JD, Murdoch FE, Gorski J. High affinity binding of the estrogen receptor to a DNA response element does not require homodimer formation or estrogen. *J Biol Chem* 1993 **268**: 12519–12525.

51. Dauvois S, Daniellan PS, White R, Parker MG. Anitoestrogen ICI 164,384 reduces cellular oestrogen receptor content by increasing its turnover. *Proc Natl Acad Sci USA* 1992 **89**: 4037–4041.

52. Coopman P, Garcia M, Brünner N, Derocq D, Clarke R, Rochefort H. Anti-proliferative and anti-estrogenic effects of ICI 164,384 and ICI 182,780 in 4-OH tamoxifen-resistant human breast cancer cells. *Int J Cancer* 1994 **56**: 295–300.

53. Karnik PS, Kulkarni S, Xiao-Pu L, Budd T, Bukowski RM. Estrogen receptor mutations in tamoxifen-resistant breast cancer. *Cancer Res* 1994 **54**: 349–353.

54. Daniellan PS, White R, Hoare SA, Fawell SE, Parker MG. Identification of residues in the oestrogen receptor that confer differential sensitivity to oestrogen and hydroxytamoxifen. *Mol Endocrinol* 1993 **7**: 232–240.

55. Reese JC, Wooge CH, Katzenellenbogen BS. Identification of two cysteines closely positioned in the ligand-binding pocket of the human estrogen receptor: roles in ligand binding and transcriptional activation. *Mol Endocrinol* 1992 **6**: 2160–2166.

56. McGuire WL, Chamness GC, Fuqua SAW. Abnormal oestrogen receptor in clinical breast cancer. *J Steroid Biochem Mol Biol* 1992 **43**: 243–247.

57. Fuqua SA, Chamness GC, McGuire WL. Estrogen receptor mutations in breast cancer. *J Cell Biochem* 1993 **51**: 135–139.

58. Kastner P, Krust A, Turcotte B, Stropp U, Tora L, Gronemeyer H, Chambon P. Two distinct estrogen-regulated promoters generate transcripts encoding the two functionally different human progesterone receptor forms A and B. *EMBO J* 1990 **9**: 1603–1614.

59. Masrahi M, Venencie P-Y, Saugier-Veber P, Sar S, Dessen P, Milgrom E. Structure of the human progesterone receptor. *Biochim Biophys Acta* 1993 **1216**: 289–292.

60. Wei LL, Gonzalez-Aller C, Wood WM, Miller LA, Horwitz KB. 5′ heterogeneity in human progesterone receptor transcripts predicts a new amino-terminal truncated 'c'-receptor and unique A-receptor messages. *Mol Endocrinol* 1990 **4**: 1833–1844.

61. Kraus WL, Montano MM, Katzenellenbogen BS. Cloning of the rat progesterone gene 5′-region and identification of two functionally distinct promoters. *Mol Endocrinol* 1993 **7**: 1603–1616.

62. Vegeto E, Shahbaz MM, Wen DX, Goldman ME, O'Malley BW, McDonnell DP. Human progesterone receptor A form is a cell- and promoter-specific repressor of human progesterone receptor B function. *Mol Endocrinol* 1993 **7**: 1244–1255.

63. Tung L, Mohamed MK, Hoeffler JP, Takimoto GS, Horwitz KB. Antagonist-occupied human progesterone B-receptors activate transcription without binding to progesterone response elements and are dominantly inhibited by A-receptors. *Mol Endocrinol* 1993 **7**: 1256–1265.

64. McDonnell DP, Shahbdaz MM, Vegeto E, Goldman ME. The human progesterone receptor A-form functions as a transcriptional modulator of mineralocorticoid receptor transcriptional activity. *J Steroid Biochem Mol Biol* 1994 **48**: 425–432.

65. Aronica SM, Katzenellenbogen BS. Progesterone receptor regulation in uterine cells: stimulation by estrogen, cyclic adenosine 3′,5′-monophosphate, and Insulin-Like Growth Factor I and suppression by antioestrogens and protein kinase inhibitors. *Endocrinology* 1991 **128**: 2045–2052.

66. Aronica SM, Katzenellenbogen BS. Stimulation of estrogen receptor mediated transcription and alteration in the phosphorylation state of the rat uterine estrogen receptor by estrogen, cyclic adenosine monophosphate and Insulin-Like Growth Factor-I. *Mol Endocrinol* 1993 **7**: 743–752.

67. Fujimoto N, Katzenellenbogen BS. Alteration in the agonist/antagonist balance of antioestrogens by activation of protein kinase A signalling pathways in breast cancer cells: antioestrogen selectivity and promoter dependence. *Mol Endocrinol* 1994 **8**: 296–304.

Hyperplasias and Epithelial Tumors of the Uterine Corpus and Ovaries

TP Rollason

ENDOMETRIAL HYPERPLASIA AND CARCINOMA

INTRODUCTION

Endometrial hyperplasias and carcinomas are common and present everyday challenges in diagnosis and therapy. Despite longstanding recognition of the important role of hyperplasias generally in the etiology of endometrial carcinoma it is only relatively recently that it has been recognized which specific elements in hyperplasia are of importance in this regard. It is also only in the last 5 years that the different outcome and etiology of various types of endometrial carcinomas has begun to be recognized. The following sections deal specifically with these problems and recent changes in understanding.

CURRENT CONCEPTS

Endometrial hyperplasia

In the past the classification of endometrial hyperplasia has been confused and inconsistent. The classification given in Table 4.4.1 is that accepted by both the WHO and International Society of Gynaecological Pathologists. It will be used in this chapter for that reason but is not the one preferred by the author, whose own preference is for the use of the term 'intra-endometrial neoplasia' rather than 'hyperplasia with atypia'.

Simple hyperplasia (SH) shows a generalized increase in

Table 4.4.1 Classification of endometrial hyperplasias

Simple hyperplasia
Complex hyperplasia
Atypical simple hyperplasia
Atypical complex hyperplasia

glands and stroma (Fig 4.4.1) with preservation of the relative proportions of the two (corresponding to cystic hyperplasia in the older terminologies), but in the WHO terminology areas with mild to moderate degrees of glandular crowding with concomitant reduction in stroma are allowed. Complex hyperplasia (CH) shows a usually focal proliferation of glands at the expense of stroma, producing relative glandular crowding with increased glandular complexity, budding and random glandular orientation. In atypical hyperplasia (ACH), the features of CH are present but with cytological atypia in the glands, i.e. cellular enlargement, loss of polarity, nuclear enlargement and variability, with hyperchromasia and prominent nucleoli (Fig. 4.4.2). The atypia is classically focal. Atypical simple hyperplasia (ASH) shows similar nuclear abnormalities but without the crowding etc. of CH.

The proportion of cases of endometrial carcinoma preceded by hyperplasia is unknown and few epidemiological

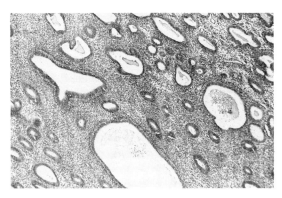

Fig. 4.4.1 *Simple endometrial hyperplasia. The biphasic pattern of cystic and small endometrial glands, with preservation of a gland: stroma ratio similar to proliferative endometrium, is evident. No cellular atypia is seen.*

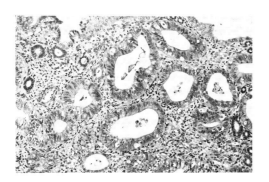

Fig. 4.4.2 *Atypical complex hyperplasia. By comparison with the small, dark, non-atypical glands the marked nuclear pleomorphism and cellular enlargement is clearly evident.*

Table 4.4.2 Classification of endometrial carcinoma

Endometrioid adenocarcinoma
  Typical
  Variants: With squamous differentiation
             Secretory
             Ciliated
Serous papillary adenocarcinoma
Clear cell adenocarcinoma
Mucinous adenocarcinoma
Squamous cell carcinoma
Undifferentiated carcinoma
Mixed carcinoma

studies exist. In the widely quoted study of Kurman *et al.*[1] atypia was clearly shown to be the important feature in prognosis; only 1.6% of cases without atypia progressed to carcinoma whereas 22% of those with atypia did. This work underpins the WHO classification. Only 1% of cases of SH progressed whereas for CH the figure was 3%. Even with atypia it took a mean of 4 years to develop carcinoma. Further recent studies support these findings. The conclusion that has been generally reached is that ACH is a significant precursor of carcinoma, ASH is as yet incompletely defined and SH and CH do not have significant precancerous potential. SH and CH do, however, define a group of patients with significant unopposed estrogenic stimulation.

A problem with the consideration of hyperplasias as precursors of adenocarcinoma is that such conditions appear essentially to be precursors of, and be seen in co-existence with, mainly well-differentiated endometrioid adenocarcinoma, of generally good prognosis. Where a diagnosis of ACH has been made, approximately 12% of patients under 40 years and 28% over 40 will be found on hysterectomy to already have adenocarcinoma. Between 21 and 46% of endometrial carcinomas conversely are associated with synchronous ACH[2,3] (see later). Early assumptions on the likely effectiveness of screening for endometrial hyperplasia have also had to be modified following studies showing a lack of association of aggressive variants of adenocarcinoma with hyperplasia[3] and the fact that, in screening studies, equal proportions of adenocarcinoma and hyperplasia were found, again suggesting that a proportion did not pass through a hyperplasia phase.

Endometrial carcinoma

The most recent WHO/ISGP classification of endometrial carcinoma is given in Table 4.4.2. These individual types have differing prognoses and will be discussed separately.

Endometrioid adenocarcinoma

These make up 80% of endometrial carcinomas.[4] The tumor may occur at virtually any age but is most fre-

quent around or after the menopause. It is the most frequent invasive malignant tumor of the female genital tract in the Western World but is relatively infrequent in Asia and Africa, though the incidence in these countries is rising.[5]

Endometrioid adenocarcinomas are classically composed of tubular, well defined glands with pseudostratified columnar cells, resembling to some extent proliferative endometrial glands (Fig 4.4.3). Mucin is confined to the apical cytoplasm or cell surface. Variant patterns may resemble ovarian Sertoli cell tumors or be lipid-rich. Some take on a villoglandular papillary pattern and ciliated cells may occasionally make up the majority cell type. None of these variants have a clearly different prognosis from the common type.

Squamous differentiation occurs in approximately one quarter of endometrioid adenocarcinomas. In the past these tumours have been termed adenosquamous if the squamous component was cytologically malignant and invasive, and adenocanthoma if it was benign. It was believed that adenosquamous carcinoma had a poorer prognosis than pure adenocarcinoma, and adenoacanthoma a similar or better prognosis.[6] Recently these findings have been questioned and recent work suggests that adenosquamous carcinomas with a poor outcome tend to have a poorly differentiated glandular component whereas 'adenoacanthomas' tend to be associated with a well-differentiated glandular component.[7] These findings still do not explain why the 'benign' squamous components in some

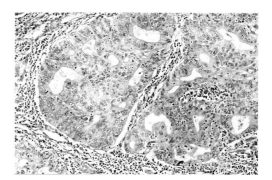

Fig. 4.4.3 *Well differentiated (grade 1) endometrioid adenocarcinoma of the endometrium. The glands are composed of pleomorphic cells with a cribriform pattern evident. The adjacent stroma shows a marked chronic inflammatory cell infiltrate.*

series confer survival advantage. The latest WHO/ISGP classification employs the term adenocarcinoma with squamous differentiation for both variants (with the glandular component graded).

The nature and prognosis of so-called glassy and spindle cell variants of endometrial carcinoma is as yet unclear though they are believed to be variants of 'adenosquamous' carcinoma. Trophoblastic differentiation may be seen rarely in endometrioid adenocarcinomas as in non-genital tract carcinomas and may be extensive enough to suggest choriocarcinoma. HCG secretion may be useful as a serum marker in such tumors. Giant cells, including osteoclast-like cells, are well described but appear to indicate a highly malignant tumor.

Serous papillary adenocarcinoma

This tumor makes up 5–10% of endometrial carcinomas. It tends to occur at an older age than endometrioid carcinomas, the mean being around 70 years, and to have a much less clear association with oestrogen usage. Some cases are associated with previous pelvic irradiation though the interval between irradiation and tumor development may be more than 20 years.[8] These tumors tend to be high stage at presentation; up to 75% are Stage III+IV on surgicopathological staging and between 25 and 57% have nodal metastases.[9]

Histologically these tumors closely resemble ovarian serous carcinomas, showing complex papillae with fibrovascular cores and stratified epithelial cells with pleomorphic nuclei (Fig 4.4.4). Psammoma bodies may be seen. Some are admixed with other patterns of endometrial carcinoma. The adjacent endometrium is usually atrophic. Deep myometrial invasion and vessel invasion is common.

The prognosis of papillary serous adenocarcinoma is much poorer than endometrioid carcinoma, even Grade III. Five-year survival overall is only around 25% and for Stage I tumors is as low as 33% in some series. Even cases with no apparent myometrial invasion may recur.[10]

Clear cell carcinoma

These tumors are closely related to serous carcinomas and admixtures of the two are common. Alone they account for 1–6% of endometrial carcinomas.[9] The tumors occur at an age intermediate between endometrioid and serous carcinomas. As with serous carcinomas, a minority give a history of pelvic irradiation. Almost one third present in Stage II or higher.[11]

Histologically the tumors are typically composed of clear cells producing a tubular, papillary or solid pattern (Fig. 4.4.5). Hobnail cells are a typical feature but oxyphilic cells with abundant cytoplasm are also frequent. Nuclei are typically highly pleomorphic. Frequency of deep myometrial invasion and vessel invasion falls between endometrioid and serous carcinoma.

Prognosis is very similar to serous papillary carcinomas with a 5-year survival around 30–60%.[11] There is also evidence that between 5 and 10 years survival decreases considerably.[11] Stage and the presence or absence of myometrial invasion are the most important prognostic parameters.

Mucinous adenocarcinoma

These are uncommon tumors. As small foci of mucinous differentiation are very common in typical endometrioid carcinomas more than 50–70% of the cells should contain abundant mucin to allow a diagnosis of mucinous adenocarcinoma. Overall prognosis for mucinous adenocarcinoma does not appear to differ from endometrioid adenocarcinoma, stage for stage. Therapy is as for endometrioid adenocarcinoma.

Squamous cell carcinoma

Pure squamous cell carcinoma (SCC) of the endometrium is a rare tumor, with only approximately 40 cases in the literature.[9] Because of the frequency of squamous carcinoma of the cervix most authors require that no co-existent

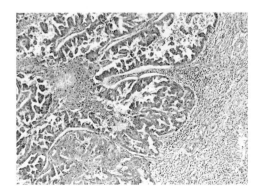

Fig. 4.4.4 *Well differentiated (grade 1) serous adenocarcinoma of the endometrium. The myometrium is infiltrated by broad tongues of tumor composed of serous cells in strikingly papillary arrays.*

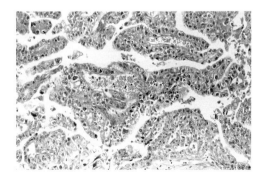

Fig. 4.4.5 *Clear cell carcinoma of the endometrium. The tumor here has a predominantly tubulopapillary pattern. The papillae are covered by cells with clear cytoplasm and pleomorphic nuclei. By nuclear grading, this would be a grade 1 carcinoma.*

cervical carcinoma should be present and no contiguous CIN, no connexion should be present with the cervical squamous epithelium and no co-existent glandular elements should be present (to exclude squamous overgrowth in an adenosquamous carcinoma). If these criteria are applied, endometrial SCCs have a poor prognosis; even in Stage I 40% of patients die of their disease and 50% are Stage III and IV at presentation. The age range is similar to that for endometrioid adenocarcinoma.

Undifferentiated carcinomas

These are relatively uncommon tumors. Some are small cell in type with neuroendocrine markers positive, others are of giant or spindle cell type. Survival figures depend to a large extent on the criteria used to define a tumor as undifferentiated. Overall prognosis is poorer than for endometrioid tumors. Five-year survival for the large cell variant is probably no more than 50%.

Prognostic factors in endometrial carcinoma

Clearly from the previous section it can be seen that tumor type is of major importance in prognosis in endometrial carcinoma. Other classical histological and surgical parameters are examined below. Surgical stage obviously includes some of these and is the most important overall prognostic factor.

Myometrial invasion

In the past, it has been accepted that depth of myometrial invasion is a strong prognostic indicator, with survival rates of 100, 90, 70 and 50% for endometrium only, inner third, mid-third and outer third being typical. Uterine serosal involvement worsens the prognosis further.[4] Variations in the literature relate to the difficulty in distinguishing early myometrial invasion from involvement of adenomyosis or an irregular endomyometrial junction, with occasional studies even showing less than 90% 5-year survival in supposed intra-endometrial tumors.[4]

Recently some doubt has been cast on the independent prognostic value of depth of invasion as this has been shown to be closely associated with grade,[4] vessel invasion[12] and nodal metastasis.[13] Recent studies have also suggested that uninvolved myometrial thickness beneath the serosa may be more important and independent of other variables; 5 mm appears to be the thickness differentiating better and poorer prognostic groups.

Tumor grade

Earlier tumor grading depended on the proportion of non-glandular to glandular areas within the carcinoma. This has been shown to be very useful prognostically,[4] but other studies have shown better correlation with nuclear grade or a combination of nuclear and architectural grade. This has been incorporated into the latest FIGO grading system for endometrioid adenocarcinoma. In older studies most prog-

nostic information related to the poor prognosis of grade 3 compared to grades 1 and 2 and this is unlikely to change. Serous, clear cell and squamous carcinomas are graded only on the nuclear detail and adenosquamous carcinoma only on the glandular component. Mitotic rate may also be useful in prognosis but is less well studied and requires clarification.

Vessel invasion

Several recent studies have shown that vessel invasion is an important prognostic factor.[9] It appears to predict recurrence[14] and outcome and has been suggested to be the most important prognostic feature *within Stage I tumors*. Five-year survivals, for all stages, have differed widely, but are generally between 18 and 66% for cases with invasion and 60–100% for those without. A close correlation exists with other prognostic factors such as grade, myometrial invasion, stage and lymph node status.

Lymph node status and adnexal involvement

The risk of nodal metastasis is highly dependent on histological grade, tumor size, myometrial depth of invasion, vessel status and cervical involvement. Nodal involvement appears to have considerable prognostic importance in studies uncorrected for other variables, with differences in survival in Stage I tumors of 8% and 48% at 5 years. A more recent study, however, has suggested in the absence of other adverse prognostic factors noted above survival was still moderately good in the presence of pelvic node metastases.[13] It would seem that the overwhelming majority of cases with para-aortic node involvement also have other poor prognostic features.[13] Tumors larger than 2 cm diameter appear to have an increased risk of nodal metastases.[15]

Up to 8% of endometrial adenocarcinomas have co-existent ovarian carcinoma. Usually the histological subtype of the two tumors is similar and is endometrioid. Determining which tumor is the primary is then a problem. In most series around 35–55% have been judged independent primaries[16] with an attendant good prognosis; in most of the other cases it was judged that the endometrium was the primary site. The features suggesting metastases to the ovary include small size of the ovarian masses, bilateral ovarian involvement, a multinodular ovarian growth pattern, surface ovarian implants, prominent vessel invasion in the ovary, a high grade endometrial tumor, a non-endometrioid histological subtype, malignant squamous elements, deep myometrial involvement and vessel involvement in the uterus.

Peritoneal cytology

The possible value of positive peritoneal cytology relates essentially to Stage I endometrial adenocarcinoma. Most older studies tend to support its value and recently it has been shown to be useful even in multivariate analysis, with 32% of Stage I tumors with positive cytology developing recurrence, compared to 8.6% of those with negative cytology.[17] By contrast no difference in actuarial survival at 10 years was found by Yazigi *et al.*[18] Lurain[19] concluded that in the absence of disease outside the uterus and/or other poor prognostic variables, cytology probably has no effect on survival. No overall conclusion on the importance of cytology is yet possible.

Other non-histological prognostic factors

Older women and black women tend to have higher stage, higher grade tumors[2] whereas as indicated previously those with a history of previous endometrial unopposed estrogen usage, or with co-existent hyperplasia tend to have well differentiated, endometrioid tumors of low stage.[2] Co-existent hyperplasia appears to be the most important non-tumor prognostic factor, suggesting that two tumor groups may exist – good prognosis, well differentiated, endometrioid tumors in premenopausal women with hyperplasia and poor prognosis in postmenopausal women without hyperplasia.[2]

FUTURE PERSPECTIVES

There are three major areas where understanding of the pathology and molecular biology of endometrial carcinoma is likely to add directly to patient management in the next few years. These are hormone receptor studies, oncogene studies and DNA ploidy and cell turnover analysis. Morphometric analysis may also prove to be of help.

OVARIAN EPITHELIAL TUMORS

INTRODUCTION

It is generally accepted that Müllerian epithelial tumors of the ovary have a common histogenesis, arising from the celomic surface epithelium. Evidence supporting such an origin in fact, however, varies in individual tumor types from convincing to almost non-existent. The development of the Müllerian ducts and derivation from the surface is said to be the reason why ovarian tumors recapitulate Müllerian patterns of differentiation whilst derived from the celomic surface. Such a theory, however useful, cannot explain the development of all 'Müllerian' tumors as, for example, almost all mucinous malignant tumors of the ovary are 'intestinal' in histological type and Brenner and squamous tumors are clearly not Müllerian in differentiation.

Histologically identical tumors to serosal ovarian epithelial tumors have been described elsewhere in the peritoneal cavity and in testicular and paratesticular tissues and it has been suggested that the female genital tract, ovaries and peritoneum should be considered a single organ system. There has also been considerable interest in whether benign proliferations of epithelium such as endosalpingiosis, endometriosis, serosal inclusions and surface epithelial metaplasia may be precursors of carcinomas. This will be further discussed in relation to particular tumors.

Unlike tumors at other sites, it is usual to divide ovarian epithelial tumors into three types: benign, borderline and malignant. The borderline group is most clearly defined for serous and mucinous tumors, but borderline variants have been described for most ovarian epithelial tumour types. What is questionable, however, is the clinical utility of such a diagnosis beyond serous and mucinous tumors as most other 'borderline' tumors appear to have a uniformly good prognosis. For all tumor types an essential defining feature of the borderline variant is the lack of clear stromal invasion.

CURRENT CONCEPTS

Serous ovarian tumors

These tumors are composed of epithelium resembling, to a variable extent, Fallopian tube epithelium. Such serous papillary tumors may be found in most female genital tract sites.[20]

Benign serous cystadenomas characteristically show ciliated cells with surface, but not intracellular, mucin. The cells are well differentiated with little pleomorphism and few, if any, mitoses. These benign tumors fall into three main groups – cystic, surface papillary and adenofibromatous. Most are uni- or pauci-locular. Mean diameter is 10 cm approximately. At the smaller end of the range they become indistinguishable from serosal inclusion cysts.

Borderline serous tumors tend macroscopically to be macrocystic with multiple papillary proliferations often producing masses of friable small nodules projecting into the cyst lumen. Histologically they show epithelial stratification and a complex, fine papillary pattern, often described as lace-like or filigree in form (Fig 4.4.6). Nuclei are larger and more hyperchromatic than in benign tumors but mitoses rarely exceed 4 per 10 HPF.

Frankly invasive adenocarcinomas may be multicystic, particularly when well differentiated, or predominantly solid with necrosis and hemorrhage present. Papillary structures vary from prominent in well-differentiated tumors to non-existent in very poorly differentiated and pleomorphism, mitotic activity, etc. are highly variable (Fig 4.4.7). Grading these tumors is essentially performed either on an architectural basis dependent on the amount of solid tumor (<10% grade 1, 10–50% grade 2, >50% grade 3), on degree of nuclear pleomorphism, or on a combination of both features.

In some patients with serous papillary carcinoma involving the peritoneal surfaces extensively there is minimal ovarian involvement and this is confined to the ovarian serosal surfaces. Such 'serous surface papillary carcinomas'

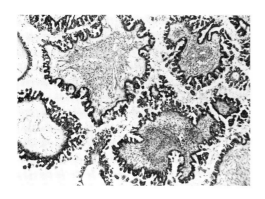

Fig. 4.4.6 *Borderline serous tumor of the ovary. The classical 'filigree' pattern of fine cellular papillae is seen overlying broad, edematous, hypocellular coarse papillae. No invasion of the stroma of the coarse papillae is seen.*

have generally been accepted to have a considerably poorer prognosis than the common serous carcinoma of the ovary with peritoneal spread but recently this conclusion has been questioned and it is unclear whether this tumor, when strictly defined, and with cases closely matched, has a prognosis worse than that for high stage ovarian papillary serous carcinoma.

Extra-ovarian disease

Histological assessment of any extra-ovarian deposits is an integral part of the assessment of serous tumors. These deposits may be benign (endosalpingiosis), borderline (non-invasive), or frankly invasive. It is generally accepted that such deposits, at least when associated with ovarian borderline and benign tumors, most likely arise *de novo*. This is supported by the occasional lack of an ovarian primary and by the fact that those deposits seen in association with borderline and benign tumors cannot by definition be due to metastasis from a non-invasive primary unless the serosa is involved. Recent work on clonality of peritoneal deposits of serous adenocarcinoma has questioned this the-

ory as the evidence to date suggests that the multiple peritoneal deposits are usually monoclonal. This may, however, be explained on the basis of overgrowth of any 'original' tumor foci by a dominant tumor mass as most studies to date have used very advanced and bulky carcinomas. Most would accept that the pattern of the implants relates directly to prognosis, with invasive deposits having a poor prognosis[21] and those with benign or borderline deposits having a favorable outcome.

Mucinous ovarian tumors

Mucinous tumors tend to be the largest ovarian masses. They are commonly up to 25–30 cm in diameter. They make up approximately 20% of ovarian tumors. More than 80% are benign and these are usually unilateral (95%); even borderline and invasive tumors are bilateral in only approximately 10% of cases. The benign tumors tend to occur in the 20–30 year old age group with malignant tumors in the 30–60 age group.

Grossly, benign cystadenomas are often multilocular and are thin walled and mucin filled. Borderline and invasive tumors tend to have solid areas or complex small locules with papillae. Necrosis is common in carcinomas. Classically these tumors, unlike serous, commonly have an admixture of benign, borderline and malignant areas in one tumor and wide sampling is therefore imperative to avoid underdiagnosis. Tumors associated with pseudomyxoma peritonei (see below) are more commonly bilateral.

Mucinous cystadenomas typically have a tall endocervical-type Müllerian mucinous epithelial lining (Fig 4.4.8). Less commonly the lining cells are of intestinal (hind-gut) type with goblet cells prominent and other intestinal type cells, e.g. arygyrophil and Paneth cells, seen. The cells are regular with few mitoses and little pleomorphism. Borderline mucinous tumors are most commonly of intestinal epithelial type and show epithelial atypia, increased mitotic activity, multilayering and papilla formation (Fig 4.4.9). The overall architecture and budding of

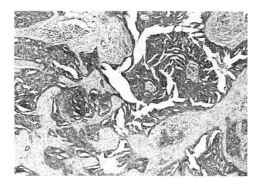

Fig. 4.4.7 *Moderately well differentiated invasive serous carcinoma of the ovary. The tumor retains a partly papillary pattern and the papillae and solid areas are made up of classical serous cells. The sieve-like pattern in the more solid areas is also typical of this tumor type.*

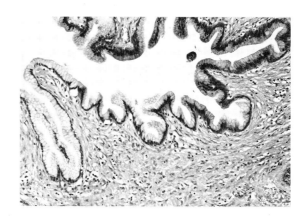

Fig. 4.4.8 *Benign mucinous cystadenoma of the ovary. The cyst lining is composed of mucin-containing cells of Müllerian (endocervical) type without goblet cells. No pleomorphism or fine papilla formation is seen.*

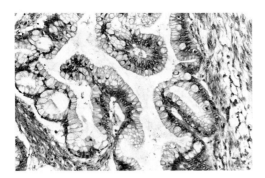

Fig. 4.4.9 *Borderline intestinal-type mucinous tumor of the ovary. The complex infolded epithelium shows moderate nuclear pleomorphism and vacuolated intestinal-type goblet of cells are seen. No stromal destructive invasion is seen. (Reproduced with permission from* Recent Advances in Histopathology, vol. 15 (1992) *Edinburgh: Churchill Livingstone.)*

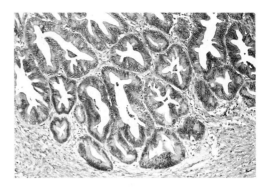

Fig. 4.4.10 *Well differentiated mucinous carcinoma of the ovary. Crowded acini composed of mucin containing cells are seen with considerable nuclear pleomorphism evident. Definite destructive stromal invasion is not evident in this area but was seen elsewhere.*

the epithelium into the stroma makes differentiation from grade I adenocarcinoma very difficult in some cases. The criteria for the differentiation of borderline from malignant tumors are contentious with some using cellular stratification and cribriform areas to indicate carcinoma,[22] others depending on frank invasion. The intestinal type borderline tumor is the ovarian tumor most commonly associated with pseudomyxoma.

Approximately 15% of mucinous borderline tumors are composed of Müllerian type mucinous epithelium or a mixture of Müllerian mucinous, endometrioid and serous types and 30% or more of these tumors have co-existent endometriosis. Histologically such tumors also show the typical 'filigree' papillary pattern of serous tumors and they tend to have a very prominent polymorph infiltrate. Outcome in such tumors appears to be very similar to borderline serous, rather than mucinous, tumors. The tumors are bilateral more frequently than the intestinal type, show discrete peritoneal deposits (with a good long-term outcome) and are not associated with pseudomyxoma peritonei.

Mucinous adenocarcinomas have a complex glandular pattern (Fig 4.4.10) with more marked nuclear pleomorphism, cribriform areas, destructive stromal invasion and a higher mitotic rate, often with abnormal mitoses. It should be noted, however, that some clearly invasive carcinomas may be remarkably well differentiated despite pursuing a frankly malignant course.

A question often posed in epithelial ovarian malignancy is to what extent benign and borderline tumors act as precursors of invasive carcinoma. As previously indicated, it has been suggested that, excepting those arising in association with endometriosis, all ovarian epithelial malignancies arise from small cortical inclusion cysts, either via the formation of benign and borderline tumors or directly. There is, however, little evidence to indicate in what proportion of cases each mechanism operates. Although it is certainly true that some carcinomas appear to arise directly from small atypical inclusions this has not been commonly reported. The overall tumor histology seen in

serous and mucinous tumors suggests that differing processes may occur in each type. Serous and Müllerian mucinous tumors usually are of similar pattern throughout the tumor and admixtures of benign, borderline and malignant tumor, although encountered, are not common. Intestinal type mucinous tumors, by contrast, commonly show benign, borderline and malignant areas in a single ovarian mass. These findings suggest that most serous tumors are 'static' whereas most intestinal-type mucinous tumors are 'evolving', presumably towards malignancy.[23] It is difficult to see how further evidence in humans for tumor evolution will be forthcoming in view of the clinical need for therapy in all multicystic ovarian masses.

Pseudomyxoma peritonei

This condition is due to production of masses of mucin in the peritoneal cavity. Often aggregated or isolated mucinous epithelial cells are seen within the mucin masses. It only appears to occur when there is an associated mucinous lesion of the ovary, appendix or gallbladder. It is most commonly seen in association with an ovarian mucinous tumor of intestinal type, usually borderline but occasionally benign or malignant, and often bilateral (>60% of cases). Appendiceal mucocele is commonly present at the same time and similar epithelial changes may be seen here to those in the ovaries. Pseudomyxoma is almost invariably present at the time of diagnosis of the primary tumor and similar mucinous pools are usually seen in the ovaries (pseudomyxoma ovarii). It is probable that the disease is due to spread of mucin from the primary tumor by breakdown of cyst walls and involvement of the peritoneum but whether mucin alone or mucin and epithelium is needed is unknown.

Endometrioid tumors

These make up 15% of ovarian carcinomas but only 5% of all ovarian tumors. Endometriosis is seen in up to 10% and approximately 30% of carcinomas are accompanied by endometrial tumors of similar type. Benign and borderline endometrioid tumors are very uncommon. All may be cystic or solid and they do not have specific macroscopic features.

All these tumors show tubular glands similar to those of proliferative, hyperplastic or malignant endometrium. The rare benign tumors include endometrial polyp-like lesions arising in endometriotic cysts and endometrioid adenofibromas and cystadenofibromas. There are two main variants of borderline endometrioid tumor. The first is of adenofibromatous pattern but shows nuclear atypia, budding and multilayering of the epithelium. The second (not accepted as a borderline tumor by all workers)[24] resembles ACH of the endometrium but arises in ovarian endometriosis.[23] This second type may also occur in cysts lined by endometrioid epithelium without stroma.[23] As only two cases have had extraovarian tumor[25] it is difficult to define prognostic features etc.

In approximately 25% of cases of endometrioid adenocarcinoma squamous differentiation is seen, either benign or malignant. Other variant patterns may mimic sex-cord stromal tumors, both Sertoli–Leydig and granulosa cell.

Brenner and transitional cell tumors

Brenner tumors account for 2–3% of all ovarian tumors. The great majority are benign with borderline and malignant tumors making up less than 2% of cases. Benign Brenner tumors are usually less than 2 cm diameter and are incidental findings. Less than 10% are bilateral. Up to one quarter appear as nodules in the wall of a mucinous cystadenoma. Histologically they are composed of rounded, well demarcated nests of epithelial cells in an abundant, dense stroma. Often the cell aggregates are solid and closely resemble urothelial transitional epithelium. Central lumina in the cell nests are also frequently seen and are often lined by mucinous epithelium.

Borderline tumors are characteristically cystic with cauliflower-like masses projecting into the cyst lumina (Fig 4.4.11).[26] Malignant tumors may be solid or cystic. The epithelium of borderline tumors is composed of multilayered urothelial transitional-type epithelium closely resembling grade 1 papillary transitional cell carcinoma. No stromal invasion is seen. These borderline tumors appear to have a uniformly good prognosis and further subdivision, although attempted, appears unnecessary.[23] Malignant Brenner tumors are composed of more pleomorphic epithelium of transitional cell type. Squamous differentiation is common and destructive stromal invasion seen.

To diagnose a malignant Brenner tumor histologically, it is generally stated that elements of benign or borderline Brenner must be seen. Those without such components are termed transitional cell carcinoma.[27] Although this may seem to be an arbitrary ruling, it appears to have prognostic importance. Stage for stage, pure transitional cell carcinoma appears to have a considerably poorer prognosis than malignant Brenner tumor after surgery alone, but responds

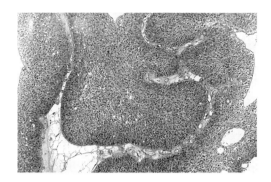

Fig. 4.4.11 *Borderline Brenner tumor of the ovary. The broad, well-defined cords of cells of transitional type are clearly seen. No stromal invasion is evident. The pattern is similar to that seen in well differentiated papillary transitional cell tumors of the urinary tract. (Reproduced with permission from* Recent Advances in Histopathology, *vol. 15 (1992) Edinburgh: Churchill Livingstone.)*

well to chemotherapy.[27] Foci of transitional cell differentiation may be seen in up to 10% of ovarian carcinomas and when this pattern predominates in the primary tumor or metastases it may confer a survival improvement with chemotherapy.

Undifferentiated carcinomas

Approximately 50% of undifferentiated carcinomas are bilateral and the frequency of diagnosis varies widely depending on the diagnostic criteria used. One variant worthy of specific mention is the small cell carcinoma of the ovary. These are highly malignant tumors with a 5-year survival of only 10%. They almost all occur below the age of 40 and two thirds of cases are associated with hypercalcaemia.[28] Their histogenesis remains unclear. A proportion are positive with neuroendocrine markers but they show electron microscopic and other features which appear to differ from small cell anaplastic lung carcinomas. The possibility that two types exist has been suggested, one a neuroendocrine tumor occurring in young patients and the other a non-neuroendocrine tumor in older women. Microscopically they are composed of small, deeply hematoxyphil cells with little cytoplasm. Structures resembling the follicles of granulosa cell tumor may be seen and mucin may be present in occasional cells.

Histological prognostic factors

The detection rate and 5-year survival in epithelial ovarian malignancy has not improved in decades, it has a higher rate of mortality than any other gynecological malignancy and the majority of patients are in an advanced stage at the time of diagnosis, with almost 60% in stages III+IV and with an overall 5-year survival of only 10% for these stages.

The most important prognostic factor in the common ovarian carcinomas is stage of disease using the FIGO system. There has in the past been too ready acceptance of the value of grading, typing etc. as important without critical appraisal of the results of older studies which are often not well controlled for age, therapy, tumor extent etc.[29] Most early studies showed cell type to be important when considered alone, with mucinous and endometrioid tumors having a better prognosis than serous and undifferentiated tumors the worst. Most more recent studies using multivariate analysis find histological type to be less important than other features or even of no importance at all,[29] but tumor type may be very useful in predicting specific response to chemotherapy (e.g. transitional cell carcinomas).

High interobserver variability and lack of uniformity in grading criteria also makes the value of grading difficult to assess. Most studies have found grade to be more important than type but recently, particularly since the use of *cis*-platinum, the position appears less clear. With the exception of Stage I tumors,[30] it is probable that only division into borderline, differentiated and anaplastic groups, in patients without chemotherapy, will be of prognostic use.[29]

The above problems raise the question of what should be included in histological reports on ovarian tumors to attempt to offer more accurate prognosis and more effective comparison of findings in future studies. Clearly accurate diagnosis as benign, borderline or malignant is imperative. Grading and typing of the tumor should be performed and the method employed stated. Ideally typing should be using the latest WHO criteria. No generally accepted grading system is available but the best method in the author's opinion is by a combination of architectural and cellular grading similar to that employed in endometrial carcinomas. The exception is clear cell carcinoma where nuclear grading alone is used. Such grading and typing must also be applied to extraovarian deposits. Tumor macroscopic dimensions must be accurately stated and the presence or absence of ovarian surface tumor and capsular rupture noted, though the significance of this is still unclear.[29] Comment should also be made on the presence or absence of vessel invasion and host lymphoid response though these are at present only useful to allow later comparison of cases.

FUTURE PERSPECTIVES

In many ways expansion of knowledge in epithelial ovarian cancer is occurring along similar pathways to endometrial tumors but the results are, if anything, more contradictory and confusing. A consensus is appearing, however, that both flow cytometry and morphometry are likely to be prognostically important.

SUMMARY

- In endometrial hyperplasia cellular atypia is the major feature of importance leading to an increased risk of development of endometrial adenocarcinoma.
- Endometrial hyperplasias with cellular atypia are in essence part of the spectrum of intra-endometrial neoplasia.
- Tumor type is very important in determining outcome in endometrial carcinoma. Serous and clear cell carcinomas have a poor prognosis.
- Two groups of endometrial carcinomas appear to exist: good prognosis tumors (particularly endometrioid) in association with pre-existing hyperplasia and unopposed estrogen stimulation and poor prognosis occurring predominantly postmenopausally without the above associated factors.
- Tumor stage is the most important prognostic feature in endometrioid endometrial carcinoma but histological parameters including tumor distance from serosa, vessel invasion and tumor grade are also of importance.

- Epithelial ovarian tumors can be divided into three histological groups: benign, borderline and malignant but only in serous and mucinous tumors (and possibly endometrioid) do borderline tumors behave in a manner distinct from benign.
- Extra-ovarian disease in benign and borderline tumors (and in some carcinomas) appears to arise *de novo* and its histological appearances affect prognosis.
- Accurate tumor typing is of considerable importance in some less common ovarian carcinomas, e.g. small cell anaplastic and transitional cell carcinomas, and may have both prognostic and therapeutic implications.
- Stage is again the most important prognostic factor in the common ovarian carcinomas. Grading and to a lesser extent typing are also useful prognostically.
- Flow cytometric and morphometric analyses are likely to be of major prognostic importance in ovarian carcinoma in the future.

REFERENCES

1. Kurman RJ, Kaminski PF, Norris HJ. The behaviour of endometrial hyperplasia. A long term study of 'untreated' hyperplasia in 170 patients. *Cancer* 1985 **56**: 403–412.
2. Beckner ME, Mori T, Silverberg SG. Endometrial carcinoma: non-tumor factors in prognosis. *Int J Gynecol Pathol* 1985 **4**: 131–145.
3. Deligdisch L, Cohen CJ. Histologic correlates and virulence implications of endometrial carcinoma associated with adenomatous hyperplasia. *Cancer* 1985 **56**: 1452–1455.
4. Abeler VM, Kjorstad KE. Endometrial adenocarcinoma in Norway. A study of a total population. *Cancer* 1991 **67**: 3093–3103.
5. Masubuchi K, Nemoto H, Masubuchi S Jr, Fujimoto I, Uchino S. Increasing incidence of endometrial carcinoma in Japan. *Gynecol Oncol* 1975 **3**: 335–346.
6. Silverberg SG, Bolin MG, De Giorgi LS. Adenoacanthoma and mixed adenosquamous carcinoma of the endometrium. A clinicopathologic study. *Cancer* 1972 **30**: 1307–1314.
7. Zaino RJ, Kurman R, Herbold D *et al.* The significance of squamous differentiation in endometrial carcinoma. Data from a Gynecologic Oncology Group study. *Cancer* 1991 **68**: 2293–2302.
8. Parkash V, Carcangiu ML. Uterine papillary serous carcinoma after radiation therapy of carcinoma of the cervix. *Cancer* 1992 **69**: 496–501.
9. Clement PB, Scully RE. Endometrial hyperplasia and carcinoma. In Clement PB, Young RH (eds) *Tumors and Tumorlike Conditions of the Uterine Corpus and Cervix.* New York: Churchill Livingstone, 1993: 181–264.
10. Carcangiu ML, Chambers JT. Uterine papillary serous carcinoma: a study on 108 cases with emphasis on the prognostic significance of associated endometrioid carcinoma, absence of invasion and concomitant ovarian carcinoma. *Gynecol Oncol* 1992 **47**: 298–305.
11. Abeler VM, Kjorstad KE. Clear cell carcinoma of the endometrium: a histopathological and clinical study of 97 cases. *Gynecol Oncol* 1991 **40**: 207–217.
12. Ambros RA, Kurman RJ. Combined assessment of vascular and myometrial invasion as a model to predict prognosis in Stage I endometrioid adenocarcinoma of the uterine corpus. *Cancer* 1992 **69**: 1424–1431.
13. Morrow CP, Bundy RV, Kurman RK *et al.* Relationship between surgicopathological risk factors and outcome in clinical stage I and II carcinoma of the endometrium: a Gynecologic Oncology Group study. *Gynecol Oncol* 1991 **40**: 55–65.
14. Hanson MB, Van Nagell JR Jr, Powell DE *et al.* The prognostic significance of lymph-vascular space invasion in Stage I endometrial cancer. *Cancer* 1985 **55**: 1753–1757.
15. Schink JC, Rademaker AW, Miller DS, Lurain JR. Tumor size in endometrial cancer. *Cancer* 1991 **67**: 2791–2794.
16. Prat J, Matias-Guiu X, Barreto J. Simultaneous carcinoma involving the endometrium and ovary. A clinicopathologic, immunohistochemical, and DNA flow cytometric study of 18 cases. *Cancer* 1991 **68**: 2455–2459.
17. Turner DA, Gershenson DM, Atkinson N *et al.* The prognostic significance of peritoneal cytology for Stage I endometrial cancer. *Obstet Gynecol* 1989 **74**: 775–780.
18. Yazigi R, Piver MS, Blumenson I. Malignant peritoneal cytology in endometrial cancer. *Obstet Gynecol* 1983 **62**: 359–362.
19. Lurain JR. The significance of positive peritoneal cytology in endometrial cancer. *Gynecol Oncol* 1992 **46**: 143–144.
20. Russell P, Bannatyne PM, Solomon HJ, Stoddard LD, Tattersall MHN. Multifocal tumorigenesis in the upper female genital tract – implications for staging and management. *Int J Gynecol Pathol* 1985 **4**: 192–210.
21. Bell DA, Scully RE. Serous borderline tumours of the peritoneum. *Am J Surg Pathol* 1990 **14**: 230–239.
22. Hart WR, Norris HJ. Borderline and malignant mucinous tumours of the ovary. Histogenic criteria and clinical behaviour. *Cancer* 1973 **31**: 1031–1045.
23. Fox H. The concept of borderline malignancy in ovarian tumours: A re-appraisal. *Curr Top Pathol* 1989 **78**: 111–134.
24. Young RH, Clement PB, Scully RE. The ovary. In Sternberg SS, Mills SE (eds) *Surgical Pathology of the Reproductive System and Peritoneum.* New York: Raven Press, 1991: 169–248.
25. Snyder RR, Norris HJ, Tavasolli F. Endometrioid proliferative and low malignant potential tumours of the ovary. *Am J Surg Pathol* 1988 **12**: 661–671.
26. Roth LM, Dallenbach-Hellweg G, Czernobilsky B. Ovarian Brenner tumours. I. Metaplastic, proliferating and of low malignant potential. *Cancer* 1985 **56**: 582–591.
27. Austin RM, Norris HJ. Malignant Brenner tumour and transitional cell carcinoma of the ovary: a comparison. *Int J Gynecol Pathol* 1987 **6**: 29–39.
28. Scully RE. Small cell carcinoma of hypercalcaemic type. *Int J Gynecol Pathol* 1993 **12**: 148–152.
29. Silverberg S. Prognostic significance of pathologic features of ovarian carcinoma. *Curr Top Pathol* 1989 **78**: 85–109.
30. Sevelda P, Vavra N, Schemper M *et al.* Prognostic factors for survival in Stage I epithelial ovarian cancer. *Cancer* 1990 **65**: 2349–2352.

Molecular Genetics of Ovarian Cancer

N Haites, B Milner and L Allan

INTRODUCTION

Ovarian cancer is the leading cause of death from gynecological malignancy in the Western World, and is the most common cancer in women after that of breast, colon and lung.[1] In the United Kingdom, there are just over 5000 cases of ovarian cancer a year. At best, the survival rate is about 80% for patients with tumors that are treated early, but can be under 10% when diagnosis is made after the disease has progressed to the later stages.

The majority of ovarian cancers are serous, endometrioid or mucinous adenocarcinomas. Carcinoma of the ovary arises from the epithelial cells and may originate from the coelomic epithelium. Common epithelial tumors (75% of all ovarian tumors and 95% of the malignant tumors) are derived from the surface epithelium of the ovary. The epithelium is a direct descendant of the celomic epithelium which during embryogenesis contributes to the formation of the Müllerian ducts from which the upper genital organs develop. It is supposed that even in adult life the ovarian epithelium retains its embryonic multipotentiality. This is exemplified by its ability to differentiate along serous, mucinous, endometrioid and mesonephroid lines showing all the differentiation characteristics that are found in epithelial tumors of the ovary. The tumors' histologic heterogeneity is therefore compatible with their common origin.[2]

Many factors are thought to be involved in the epidemiology and etiology of ovarian cancer. Ultimately, however, it is generally accepted that cancer arises as the result of one or an accumulation of genetic changes, occurring either simultaneously or as a chain of events, which divert the cell and its descendants from their particular inherent growth and differentiation program. Clearly, a better understanding of the molecular genetic changes involved in ovarian epithelial tumorigenesis could greatly improve the early diagnosis and prognosis of the disease.

Epithelial ovarian cancer can occur as a sporadic event in women who have no family history but women with ovarian cancer are more likely than expected to have a family history of ovarian neoplasia. Women who do have a family history are at increased risk of suffering from ovarian cancer.

CURRENT CONCEPTS

Genetic epidemiology of ovarian cancer

Familial clustering of cancer has been well documented in the literature, and in fact was first recorded as far back as 100 AD by the Romans who reported the familial aggregation of breast cancer.[3] Two important studies have looked at the occurrence of epithelial ovarian cancer with a large number of other malignancies within families.[4,5] Population based studies suggest that if a woman has one first degree relative affected with ovarian cancer her risk of being similarly affected is increased threefold which corresponds to a 1 in 30 risk of death from ovarian cancer by the age of 70 years.[6,7] If a women has two or more affected close relatives, the lifetime risk may be as high as 30–40%.

Families have been described in which there appears to be autosomal dominant susceptibility to ovarian cancer with a high penetrance of the cancer in predisposed individuals. Epidemiological studies have found evidence for a rare autosomal dominant gene with a high penetrance (80% of female gene carriers develop ovarian cancer by the age of 70 years, 40% by the age of 50 years and 20% by the age of 40 years).[8] This form of ovarian cancer may be site-specific and is characterized by a tendency to early onset with a mean age of diagnosis at 49 years as compared with non-familial cases at 60 years. In addition there is an increased incidence of bilateral ovarian cancer.[9] In such families, cancer indistinguishable from that of the ovary may arise after oophorectomy, leading to the suggestion that the cancer-predisposed tissue may include other derivatives of the celomic epithelium.[10]

The risk for epithelial ovarian cancer was found to be

significantly elevated in patients with first degree relatives with breast cancer (twice the population risk),[11] and similarly the risk for breast cancer was found to be elevated in patients who had first degree relatives with ovarian cancer. No other neoplasm was found to be statistically linked to ovarian cancer in this way.

Inherited predisposition to ovarian cancer

Of the many heritable cancer syndromes which have now been described, there are three distinct types which commonly predispose to ovarian carcinoma. These are:

1. Hereditary site specific ovarian cancer;[12]
2. Familial breast–ovarian cancer;[13]
3. 'Lynch type II', family cancer syndrome or HNPCC (hereditary non-polyposis colon cancer) (as opposed to Lynch syndrome I which presents with site-specific cancer of the colon alone[14]), which is characterized by a familial association of ovarian cancer with colorectal, endometrial and other cancers.

Other genetic disorders are also associated with non-epithelial ovarian cancer. These include:

Gorlin syndrome
Gonadal dysgenesis
Peutz–Jegher syndrome
Ollier disease
Maffucci syndrome

The heterogeneity of hereditary ovarian cancer has been emphasized by a differing age at diagnosis in the three categories mentioned above.[9] The mean age at onset for ovarian cancer in women from families of all three types was found to be significantly lower ($P < 0.05$) than that for the population as a whole (age 59), but of particular interest was the significant difference ($P < 0.05$) between the mean ages of the three cohorts: age 45 in Lynch syndrome II; age 49 in site-specific ovarian cancer; and age 52 in breast/ovarian cancer. This information could be of importance in the development of surveillance and management plans for individual ovarian cancer families.

There has been an increase in the number of reports of familial ovarian cancer in recent years. Before 1970, there were only five cases of familial ovarian cancer in the English language medical literature, beginning with Kimbrough's report of ovarian carcinoma in twins[15] and including the classic report by Liber[16] of a mother and five daughters with ovarian cancer. During the 1970s a further 26 cases were reported, and in a survey done by Piver *et al.*[12] between 1981 and 1983, 94 additional ovarian cancer families were discovered. Previously unreported ovarian cancer families are continually being recorded. A register of families with ovarian cancer in two or more close relatives has been established by the UK Coordinating Committee for Cancer Research.

It seems likely that the apparent increase in incidence of familial clustering of ovarian cancer is due to the increased awareness among clinicians of the significance of hereditary factors in cancer etiology and/or an improvement in data collection, rather than a change in etiological factors. Certainly it has often been noted that, in the past, no family follow-up was carried out on the relatives of ovarian cancer patients.[17] Because ovarian cancer is not nearly as common as, for example, breast and colon cancer, the aggregation of multiple cases of ovarian cancer in successive generations of a family is highly unlikely to be due to chance.[8]

Molecular basis of familial predisposition

When genetic mechanisms which control cellular growth and proliferation are damaged by mutation, cancer can occur. These mutations are usually acquired but can be inherited. Sporadic and inherited counterparts are found for almost all cancers. Genes that are directly involved in cellular growth and differentiation can be divided into two main groups:

1. *Oncogenes* and their normal counterparts *proto-oncogenes* which have a positive effect on growth and proliferation, and
2. *Tumor suppressor genes* which have a negative effect.

A third class of genes involved in *DNA repair* have also been implicated in genetic predisposition to cancer.

Epidemiological studies suggest that malignant transformation is a multistep process resulting from damage to a minimum of four rate limiting steps.[18] Thus for a cancer to develop, a series of mutations needs to accumulate within a cell. Individuals who are predisposed to cancer are born with a mutation in a gene which codes for a product involved in one of these rate limiting steps. Thus the study of cancer predisposition in genetically predisposed families offers the opportunity of identifying some of the genes involved in both cancer predisposition and in the multistep process in sporadic forms.

Genetic linkage studies can be carried out on families with the same apparent disease or predisposition in order to begin to localize the gene which is involved. Such studies indicate that almost all families in which ovarian cancer is associated with young onset breast cancer are due to predisposition at the *BRCA1* locus on chromosome 17q, as are some early onset breast cancer families without ovarian cancer.[19] A typical breast/ovarian cancer pedigree is shown in Fig. 4.5.1. Genetic linkage can be defined as the tendency for alleles that are close together on the same chromosome to be transmitted together from one generation to the next via meiosis. The strength of linkage can then be used to estimate how close two different alleles are and hence begin the process of pinpointing the location of disease causing genes. Where there is strong evidence of linkage, closely linked markers can be used to predict the likelihood of individuals in such families carrying the predisposing gene and hence their risk of expressing it as a cancer.

Genetics of ovarian cancer

The first experimental evidence for the involvement of genetic factors in cancer came from the work of Boveri.[20]

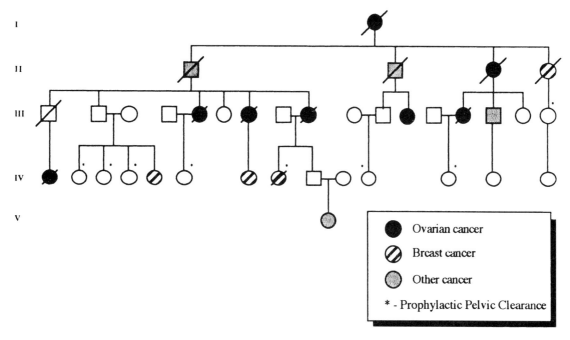

Fig. 4.5.1 *Typical breast/ovarian cancer pedigree.*

He observed that abnormalities in the mitotic cycle of sea urchin eggs frequently produced cells with an altered chromosomal make-up and abnormal growth characteristics. A few years later an inbred strain of mice was developed that was susceptible to leukemia, a trait that was stably transmitted through the germ line.[21] Bearing these studies in mind, and also the hereditary component of cancer susceptibility which was becoming apparent with the discovery of various cases of cancer-prone families, it seemed almost certain that there was some genetic involvement in human cancer.

It has been shown that the appearance of the human cancer phenotype can be associated with many primary causal factors. These include environmental mutagens, certain dietary substances, viral infection (e.g. HPV in cervical cancer[22]), and ionizing radiation.[23] Each of these factors has only an indirect role to play in the etiology of human cancer, the common secondary effect of all of them being the mutational change in an important set of genes which dictate the growth and differentiation pattern of the cell.

Cytogenetics of ovarian cancer

Clonal chromosome abnormalities have been identified in benign tumors of the ovary. Trisomy 12 was the most frequent abnormality detected especially in fibromas and fibrothecomas.[24] The majority of carcinomas have complex karyotypes with massive numerical and structural aberrations and often a near-triploid or hypodiploid modal chromosome number. The most frequent numerical changes were chromosome losses, in particular -X, -17, -22, -13, -14 and -8.[25] Deletions and unbalanced translocations are the most frequent structural aberration. The breakpoints of clonal structural rearrangements clustered to several

bands and segments: 19p13, 19q13, 1p36, 11p13, 3p12–13, 1q23 and 6q21 (the p and q arms of chromosomes are subdivided into segments based on the dark and light banding patterns observed following a standard proteolytic digestion and Giemsa staining procedure, as demonstrated in Fig. 4.5.2).

Cytogenetic analysis of samples obtained from multiple tumor sites, e.g. both ovaries or both ovaries and omental implants, revealed identical baseline karyotypes in all samples obtained from one patient indicating that bilateral ovarian cancer is likely to develop by metastatic spreading.[26] Molecular studies to identify *p53* mutations in bilateral ovarian tumors and their metastases is consistent with ovarian cancers being of uniclonal origin rather than the result of a field change.[27]

Oncogenes and tumor suppressor genes

It is important to understand that both oncogenes and tumor suppressor genes, in their wild-type form, are usually involved in normal cell growth and differentiation processes. The evolutionary conservation of the structure of both types of genes is a measure of their importance.[28] Oncogenes code for vital proteins such as growth factors (*sis*), growth factor receptors (*erbB2*), protein kinases (*abl*), cytoplasmic signal transducers (*ras*), DNA-binding proteins (*myc*), and transcription factors (*jun*).[29] Of the ever-increasing number of candidate tumor suppressor genes, only two (*p53* and *Rb*) have been functionally characterized to any great extent. Both proteins appear to play a central role in cell cycle control and will be further discussed.[30,31]

In general terms, there are two essential differences between oncogenes and tumor suppressor genes. First of

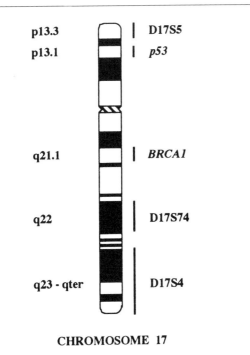

p13.3	D17S5
p13.1	*p53*
q21.1	*BRCA1*
q22	D17S74
q23 - qter	D17S4

CHROMOSOME 17

Fig. 4.5.2 *The five regions of allele loss in ovarian cancer.*

all, at the cellular level, a mutated oncogene acts dominantly in the development of the cancer phenotype, whereas a mutation in a tumor suppressor gene generally acts recessively (having effect only when the normal gene function is homozygously lost). Second, oncogenes tend to acquire 'activating' mutations which affect the cell phenotype directly (e.g. *ras*), whereas tumor suppressor genes are often simply 'inactivated' by mutation such that normal growth control and thus tumor suppression ceases allowing tumorigenesis by an indirect means. These rather simplistic rules of thumb are complicated, though, by the observation that a mutated tumor suppressor gene often adopts the dominant characteristics of a mutated oncogene, the classic example being *p53*.[32]

Oncogene involvement in ovarian cancer

A vast number of oncogenes have now been identified, and there is evidence that one or more of these are involved in most cancer types, including ovarian.[33] Epidermal growth factor receptor (EGFR, the product of the *c-erbB-1* gene) overexpression has been detected, both immunocytochemically and biochemically, at a higher incidence in ovarian metastases than in primary lesions,[34] although no correlation has as yet been made between EGFR status and survival in ovarian cancer. Reports on the prognostic significance of increased expression of the *c-erbB-2* gene product p185 (homologous but not identical to EGFR[35]) in ovarian cancer remain inconclusive. There is evidence to suggest that amplification of the *c-erbB-2* gene is a frequent occurrence in ovarian cancers,[36] and intense p185 immunocytochemical staining has been found to correlate significantly with a lowered survival rate.[37] In opposition to these findings, Imyanitov *et al.*[38] noted a very low incidence

of *c-erbB-2* amplification, and another group found only a very tenuous link between p185 overexpression and ovarian cancer incidence.[39]

The *ras* oncogenes (*H-ras*, *K-ras* and *N-ras*) are probably those most commonly involved in human cancer. The three genes code for structurally and functionally homologous proteins of 21 kDa in size.[40] The protein has been found to be localized to the inner surface of the cell membrane,[41] where it plays a crucial role in the transduction of biochemical signals from membrane to nucleus.[42] In ovarian cancer both the frequency and intensity of p21 immunostaining was found to be increased in malignant as opposed to benign tumors, but no correlation was found between p21 positivity and prognosis.[43] *K-ras* amplification has been reported in ovarian cancer but again was not correlated with extent of disease progression.[44] There is evidence to suggest, from work on colorectal cancer, that *K-ras* mutation is in fact an early event in tumorigenesis,[18] and so its use as a prognostic indicator may be limited.

The involvement of a number of other oncogenes in human ovarian cancer has also been studied. Amplification of the *c-myc* gene, coding for a DNA-binding protein which appears to be involved in the regulation of cell growth,[45] has in general been associated with cancers of a more aggressive nature.[46] Amplified *c-myc* has been detected specifically in invasive ovarian neoplasms but not in benign or borderline tumors,[47] and *c-myc* amplification was found to occur only in tumors of late FIGO stage.[48] Messenger RNA of the *mos* oncogene has been detected by *in situ* hybridization in a proportion of ovarian malignant tumors.[49] The product of *c-mos* is a serine/threonine protein kinase which activates the maturation promoting factor (MPF), an essential cell cycle control element. Finally, there is recent evidence that the gene *AKT2*, which is also a serine/threonine protein kinase, is amplified in ovarian carcinomas and carcinoma cell lines, and it remains to be seen whether this is a characteristic associated with other cancer types.[50]

In summary, it is clear from the studies to date on oncogene expression in ovarian cancer that, as with other solid tumors, despite some clinical correlations for certain oncogenes there is still a considerable amount of heterogeneity within tumor groups. There are no specific consistently detected oncogene markers which can be used as reliable prognostic indicators or that give specific clues as to the etiology of ovarian cancer. However, it is possible that in combination with the more established prognostic indicators, the involvement of the oncogenes discussed above (or of those of as yet unknown status in ovarian cancer) may yet prove useful in providing increasingly accurate prognostic indicators.

Tumor suppressor genes: the retinoblastoma model

Tumor suppressor genes were initially discovered as a result of extensive research on retinoblastoma, a malignant tumor of the retina occurring almost exclusively in children under the age of 5 years. In 1971, Alfred Knudson proposed a model for the etiology of this childhood cancer based on his observations of the disease.[51] He proposed that in sporadically occurring non-hereditary cases, two separate somatic mutations which inactivate a gene must occur, whereas if an already mutated gene for retinoblastoma is transmitted in the germline only one further somatic event is necessary (Fig. 4.5.3). The germline mutation would need to be relatively small in order to produce a viable zygote, and otherwise genetically normal individual. He also found that there was a significantly higher proportion of bilateral tumors in hereditary cases compared to non-hereditary ones. In the absence of a germline mutation constitutional to every cell, it would seem extremely unlikely for a mutation to occur twice, in both eyes, as isolated instances. When a germline mutation is present in every cell in the body, the number of targets for the required single additional mutation is much larger and the chances of two isolated tumors being initiated are far greater. This would also explain why the retinal tumors occurred so early in life. Knudson found that survivors of the bilateral form of the disease were very susceptible to osteosarcoma, a tumor of the bone tissue, and indeed isolated cases of osteosarcoma were later found to have the

same genetic abnormality as that found in retinoblastoma.[52]

Much of the evidence, described above, for the retinoblastoma gene (now called *RB1*) being a tumor suppressor gene is circumstantial. The acid test of tumor suppressor function is to clone the gene and introduce it into tumors lacking a wild-type copy to see if suppression of tumour growth occurs. Tumor suppression by *RB1* has been successfully demonstrated *in vitro* in retinoblastoma, osteosarcoma and bladder cancer cell lines.[53]

The eventual localization and characterization of *RB1* was based on the findings of 'allele loss' or 'loss of heterozygosity (LOH)' analysis.[54] The second 'hit' in a tumor suppressor gene often involves a sizeable DNA deletion or reduction to hemizygosity by some other means with the first 'hit' being a mutation in the other copy of the gene, either constitutive in the case of inherited cancers or a new mutation in sporadic cancers.[51] Therefore, the loss of a DNA marker allele of a known locus in tumor DNA, when compared with normal tissue DNA from the same individual, may be regarded as strongly suggestive of the presence of a tumor suppressor gene at that locus (Fig. 4.5.4). This has become by far the most useful technique as a starting point in the genomic localization and identification of tumor suppressor genes since the discovery of the *RB1* gene.

Mismatch repair genes

Hereditary non-polyposis colorectal cancer is one of the most common genetic diseases of man, affecting as many as one in 200 individuals. Affected individuals develop tumors of the colon, endometrium, ovary and other organs, often before the age of 50 years. A clue to the nature of the genes implicated in this condition came from the discovery, in a subset of sporadic tumors and most colorectal cancers from HNPCC patients, of widespread alterations of short, repeated sequences (microsatellites) distributed throughout the genome.

In approximately 60% of families, the predisposition to cancer is linked to a gene on chromosome 2p called hMSH2. A further 30% of families with this condition are linked to a gene on chromosome 3p called hMLH1. The two genes are part of a DNA repair pathway called 'mismatch repair'. In their normal roles the products of the two genes mentioned above seem able to identify mismatches which occur at point mutations, switching on the enzymes that carry out repair. Results to date are consistent with a model in which a second molecular event is necessary for tumorigenesis. Lymphoblasts from HNPCC patients are repair-deficient at the biochemical level but tumors manifesting microsatellite instability are almost completely devoid of repair activity suggesting that inactivation of both copies of the relevant mismatch repair gene is necessary for tumor formation in HNPCC patients.[55,56]

Once the mutation is identified in a specific gene in a family, this knowledge may be used to predict with great accuracy those in the family who are most at risk.

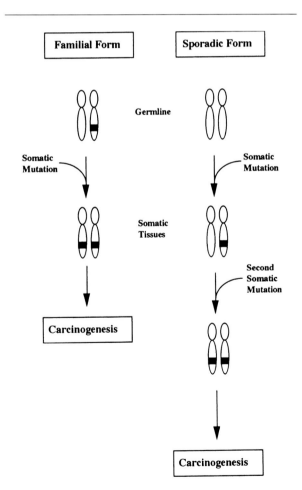

Fig 4.5.3 *The genetic basis of tumorigenesis by tumor suppressor gene loss.* ■ = *mutated tumor suppressor gene.*

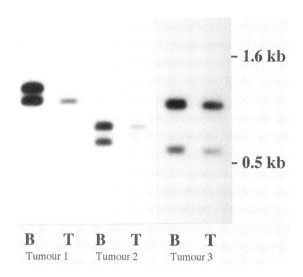

Fig. 4.5.4 *Demonstration of allele loss in tumor DNA using a Southern blot with a chromosome 17 marker probe. In each of cases 1, 2 and 3 a comparison between constitutive and tumor DNA shows that one allele is lost from tumor DNA seen as a reduction in intensity of one of the bands. B = blood; T = tumor.*

Allele loss studies in ovarian cancer

Chromosome 17 in ovarian cancer

Results from molecular analyses on breast cancer now implicate at least five chromosome 17 tumor suppressor loci, two on the p arm of the chromosome and three on the q arm (Fig. 4.5.2).[57] The *p53* tumor suppressor is one of these genes which, having been established as mapping to 17p13.1, is lost in a high proportion of almost all solid cancers including ovarian.[58,59] The second, and as yet completely uncharacterized, tumor suppressor gene lies close to the tip of chromosome 17p at 17p13.3. A higher incidence of LOH has been found in ovarian tumors at this 17p13.3 locus than at the *p53* locus.[58,59] Losses from this new distal region have been confirmed as being independent from the *p53* locus.[57,60] In two other studies in which allele loss on both arms of chromosome 17 was investigated,[61,62] allele loss from a 17q locus was detected, a significant proportion of which had deletions that were restricted to the 17q locus, i.e. in each case, heterozygosity was retained in the tumor DNA for markers on the short arm. The extremely high incidence of loss from this 17q locus, mapping to the region 17q23–q25.3, indicates that a putative tumor-suppressor gene involved in ovarian tumorigenesis is likely to reside there. The two other distinct 17q regions of allele loss have been mapped to 17q22 and 17q21 where the *BRCA1* gene is located.[57,63]

The *BRCA1* gene

In 1990, a locus on the long arm of chromosome 17 was genetically linked to breast cancer predisposition in early-onset families, i.e. those with a mean age at diagnosis below 47 years.[64] The findings of strong linkage to the long arm of chromosome 17 was of great interest since this region had been found to exhibit frequent allele loss in ovarian tumors.[65] Consequently it came as no surprise when it was learnt that the same region on chromosome 17q, identified by Hall *et al.*[64] in breast cancer predisposition, also exhibits strong linkage in almost all breast–ovarian cancer families.[19] An interesting study by Smith *et al.*[66] demonstrated that allele loss from the 17q12–q21 region always involves the non-germline-inherited chromosome in familial breast/ovarian cancers. The gene thought to be responsible for cancer susceptibility in these families has been termed *BRCA1*, and has only recently been isolated and characterized using a variety of sophisticated molecular biological techniques.[67,68] These include loss of heterozygosity and linkage studies as mentioned above, defining the smallest region containing the gene by mapping of cross-overs occurring at meiosis and more recently extensive sequencing of large portions of the genome thought to contain the *BRCA1* gene. The gene codes for a large protein of 1863 amino acids in length, the sequence of which suggests a potential role as a transcription factor. Mutations in the *BRCA1* gene have now been detected in both hereditary cases of breast and ovarian cancer.[69,70]

Preliminary results from the international consortium for the study of families linked to *BRCA1* suggest that:

1. Families may fall into two groups, one in which the disease allele confers a breast cancer risk of 91% and an ovarian cancer risk of 32% by age 70 years, and the other in which the risks are 70% for breast cancer and

84% for ovarian cancer, with the first allele representing 71% of all mutations.

2. There is significant excess of colorectal cancer (approximately 6% by age 70) and possibly prostate cancer (8% by age 70) in 'breast–ovarian' families.[71,72]

3. Mucinous epithelial ovarian cancer does not appear to be a part of the spectrum of cancers caused by this gene.[73]

It is thought that mutations in the *BRCA1* gene account for approximately 45% of familial early-onset breast cancer cases and over 80% of families that have an additional increased incidence of ovarian cancer.[67] A second gene, that has recently been genetically mapped to chromosome 13q, appears to account for a similarly-sized proportion of familial early-onset breast cancer cases to that attributable to the *BRCA1* gene.[74] This gene has been named *BRCA2*.

Only a few extensive families with site-specific ovarian cancer have been described, and it is not clear whether these are genetically distinct.

The *p53* gene

The high level of allele loss from the short arm of chromosome 17 is of great interest as this is the location of the *p53* tumor suppressor gene. The *p53* gene and protein have been researched extensively.[30,75] The wild-type p53 protein is a nuclear phosphoprotein whose expression regulates the cell cycle. It binds DNA specifically as an oligomeric complex that has the ability to transactivate or repress the transcription of other genes (Fig. 4.5.5). Exactly which genes are regulated by p53 has still not entirely been established,

but it is highly likely that they are genes involved in growth inhibition and tumor progression, probably expressed in the G1 and S phases of the cell cycle.

It has recently come to light, however, that the wild-type p53 protein promotes the expression of a newly identified gene, mapping to chromosome 6p21.2 termed *WAF1* (*W*ild-type *p53-A*ctivated *F*ragment *1*), which itself appears to have the characteristics of a tumor suppressor gene with the ability to suppress the growth of human tumor cell lines.[76] The same gene was coincidentally identified by another group who named it *Cip1* (*C*dk-*i*nteracting *p*rotein *1*) as they found that its protein product p21 was a potent inhibitor of cyclin-dependent kinases (Cdks), which themselves are known to inactivate negative regulators of the cell cycle.[77] The chromosome region including 6p21.2 has been previously implicated as a potential tumor suppressor gene site with allele losses from this region in ovarian cancers being a common finding.[78] The involvement of the *p53* gene in ovarian cancer, as is established for most solid cancers, has been confirmed by a number of recent publications. In one of the largest studies on *p53* in ovarian cancer, the gene was found to be mutated in 29 out of 66 malignant carcinomas,[79] and a further eight carcinomas demonstrated abnormally high levels of p53 protein expression apparently not as a direct result of *p53* mutation.[80,81] Of potential significance was the finding that, in contrast to colorectal cancer where *p53* mutation is a late occurrence, in ovarian cancer *p53* mutations are found in both early and late stage tumors thus representing a central molecular event – a finding supported by a similar recent study on early stage ovarian cancers.[82]

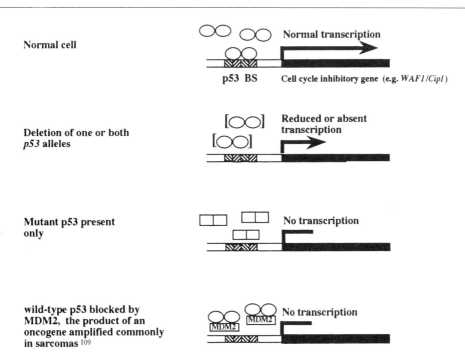

Fig. 4.5.5 *Mechanisms of p53 activation and inactivation. p53 BS = p53 binding site.* ◯ *= wild-type p53;* ▢ *= mutant p53.*

Allele loss from other regions of the genome in ovarian cancer

In recent years allele loss studies have been a popular means of identifying regions that potentially contain tumor suppressor genes in human cancers, so much so that the relevant studies on ovarian cancer have been summarized in Table 4.5.1. This table details the most significant findings of allele loss on many of the chromosome arms (using an arbitrary cut off point of 40% loss), and includes the known or candidate tumor suppressor genes that have been implicated.

Social and ethical implications

The *BRCA1* gene has now been cloned and it is technically possible to identify disease-related mutations within the gene.[67] As a direct result, for many families with the breast/ovarian cancer syndrome, extremely accurate DNA diagnostic tests will become available allowing the identification of those individuals carrying predisposing mutations and hence at high risk of suffering from cancer in their lifetimes. The cloning and characterization of the *BRCA1* gene is exciting as it is certain to improve our understanding of the factors implicated in ovarian and breast cancer predisposition and initiation. In addition, the identification of the product of the normal gene is likely to increase our knowledge of processes involved in maintaining the normal functional status of these tissues and should thus lead to the development of rational and novel forms of therapy in the future.

The cloning of the gene will also raise many clinical, ethical and social questions and until the prevention and management of ovarian and breast cancer improves, may well for some patients cause more problems than it solves. Hence, regardless of the type of predictive test to be offered, all members of families considering such testing must have the opportunity to make their decision free from any form of medical or family coercion, and thus must be fully informed of the possible advantages and disadvantages of their decision. For this to be the case, individuals will need fairly extensive counseling thus allowing a fully informed decision to be made. Where test results indicate that individuals are at a high risk of being predisposed, available management options will need to be carefully discussed with the patient. As management may well involve prophylactic surgery to a well woman, such counseling will need to be multidisciplinary and could appropriately include a gynecological oncologist, breast surgeon and a clinical psychologist.

Future perspectives

With the cloning of the *BRCA1* gene and the characterization of other genes implicated in the progression of ovarian cancer, a more complete picture will emerge of the variety

Table 4.5.1 Allele loss in ovarian cancer

Chromosomal arm with loss	Known or candidate tumor suppressor genes	Reported allele loss in 40% or more tumors (References)
1q	TGFβ2	83
3p	D8	84
4p		83, 85
5q	APC; MCC	83, 86, 87, 88, 89
6p	WAF1/Cip1	82, 83, 84, 85
6q		58, 78, 83, 86
7p		83, 85
8p		86
9p	p16	83, 89
9q		83, 86, 87, 90
11p	WT1; WT2	58, 82, 87, 89, 91, 92, 93, 94
11q	MEN1	95
13q	RB1; BRUSH1	83, 86, 96, 97, 98, 99
14q	TGFβ3	83, 86, 87
15q		83, 87
16q		83
17p	p53	58, 59, 83, 85, 86, 87, 89, 98, 100, 101
17q	BRCA1; nme1; nme2; PHB; NF1; THRA1; RARA	58, 59, 65, 83, 86, 87, 89, 98, 100, 102, 103, 104, 105, 106, 107, 108
18q	DCC	83, 86
19p		83, 87
22q	NF2	83, 86
Xp		87, 97, 98
Xq		83

of proteins whose dysfunction can contribute to transformation of the ovarian epithelium. In a parallel fashion it is to be hoped that alternate forms of therapy: gene therapy, immunotherapy or the use of antisense probes, will be introduced either as separate entities or in conjunction with current chemotherapeutic regimes.

SUMMARY

- Ovarian cancer is a genetic disease.
- In 5–10% of cases it may occur as a part of an inherited predisposition to breast/ovarian cancer, to site specific ovarian cancer or as a part of Lynch syndrome II (HNPCC) with colorectal, endometrial and other cancers in the family.
- The majority of breast/ovarian cancer families are due to a mutation in the *BRCA1* gene on chromosome 17q21.
- In Lynch syndrome II the defective genes have been shown to be mismatch repair genes.
- In some families it is now possible to use linked markers or mutation detection in Lynch syndrome II to predict those in the family at highest risk.

- The risk of epithelial ovarian cancer is increased in any woman who has a close affected relative but especially if the relative is less than 55 years of age.
- Both oncogenes and other tumor suppressor genes appear to be implicated in progression of ovarian cancer.
- *p53* mutations are implicated in around 44% of epithelial ovarian cancers.
- There appear to be four or five genes on chromosome 17 (including *BRCA1* and *p53*) involved in ovarian cancer from LOH studies.
- It is likely that a knowledge of the molecular events involved in ovarian cancer will lead to improved prognostic indicators and to alternative forms of therapy.

REFERENCES

1. Ruddon RW. Cancer biology, 2nd edn. Oxford: Oxford University Press, 1987.
2. Lauchlan SC. The secondary Mullerian system. *Obstet Gynecol Surv* 1972 **27**: 133–146.
3. Lynch HT, Albano WA, Lynch JF, Lynch PM, Campbell A. Surveillance and management of patients at high genetic risk for ovarian carcinoma. *Obstet Gynecol* 1982 **59**: 589–596.
4. Schildkraut JM, Thompson WD. Relationship of epithelial ovarian cancer to other malignancies within families. *Genet Epidemiol* 1988 **5**: 355–367.
5. Schildkraut JM, Risch N, Thompson WD. Evaluating genetic association among ovarian, breast, and endometrial cancer: evidence for a breast/ovarian cancer relationship. *Am J Hum Genet* 1989 **45**: 521–529.
6. Ponder B. Report of a Meeting of Physicians and Scientists, Institute of Cancer Research and the Royal Marsden Hospital, London. In Non-surgical aspects of ovarian cancer. *Lancet* 1994 **343**: 335–340.
7. Greggi CA, Ponder BAJ, Mancuso S. Establishment of a European Register for familial ovarian cancer. *Eur J Cancer* 1991 **27**: 113–115.
8. Easton D, Peto J. The contribution of inherited predisposition to cancer incidence. *Cancer Surv* 1990 **9**: 395–416.
9. Lynch HT, Watson P, Bewtra C *et al.* Hereditary ovarian cancer. Heterozygosity in age at diagnosis. *Cancer* 1991 **67**: 1460–1466.
10. Lynch HT, Bewtra C, Lynch JF. Familial peritoneal ovarian carcinomatosis: a new clinical entity? *Med Hypothesis* 1986 **21**: 171–177.
11. Muderspach LI. In Cameron RB (ed.) *Practical Oncology* Englewood Cliffs, NJ: Prentice-Hall International, 1994.
12. Piver MS, Mettlin CJ, Tsukada Y *et al.* Familial ovarian cancer registry. *Obstet Gynecol* 1984 **64**: 195-199.
13. Fraumeni Jr AF, Grundy GW, Creagan ET, Everson RB. Six families prone to ovarian cancer. *Cancer* 1975 **36**: 364–369.
14. Lynch HT, Lynch PM. Tumor variation in the cancer family syndrome: ovarian cancer. *Am J Surg* 1979 **138**: 439–442.
15. Kimbrough Jr RA Coincident carcinoma of the ovary in twins. *Am J Obstet Gynecol* 1929 **18**: 148–149.
16. Liber AF Ovarian cancer in mother and five daughters. *Arch Pathol Lab Med* 1950 **49**: 280–290.
17. Nevo S Familial ovarian carcinoma: a problem in genetic counselling. *Clin Genet* 1978 **14**: 219–222.
18. Vogelstein B, Fearon ER, Hamilton SR *et al.* Genetic alterations during colorectal-tumor development. *N Engl J Med* 1988 **319**: 525–532.
19. Easton DF, Bishop DT, Ford D, Crockford GP. Genetic linkage analysis in familial breast and ovarian cancer – results from 214 families. *Am J Hum Genet* 1993 **52**: 678–701.
20. Boveri T. *The Origin of Malignant Tumors.* Baltimore: Williams & Wilkins, 1929.
21. Furth J, Seibold HR, Rathbone RR. Experimental studies on lymphomatosis of mice. *Am J Cancer* 1933 **19**: 521–604.
22. Sebbelov AM, Kjorstad KE, Abeler VM, Norrild B. The prevalence of human papilloma virus type 16 and 18 DNA in cervical cancer in different age groups: a study on the incidental cases of cervical cancer in Norway in 1983. *Gynecol Oncol* 1991 **41**: 141–148.
23. Finch S, Moriyama I. The delayed effects of radiation exposure among atomic bomb survivors, Hiroshima and Nagasaki, 1945–1979. *Radiat Effects Res Found TR* 1980 **11**: 16–78.
24. Pejovic T, Heim S, Mandahl N *et al.* Trisomy 12 is a consistent chromosomal aberration in benign ovarian tumors. *Genes Chromosomes Cancer* 1990 **2**: 48–52.
25. Pejovic T, Heim S, Mandahl N *et al.* Chromosome aberrations in 35 primary ovarian carcinomas. *Genes Chromosomes Cancer* 1992 **4**: 58–68.
26. Pejovic T, Heim S, Mandahl M *et al.* Bilateral ovarian carcinoma: cytogenetic evidence of unicentric origin. *Int J Cancer* 1991 **47**: 358–361.
27. Mok C-H, Tsao S-W, Knapp RC, Fishbaugh PM, Lau CC.

Unifocal origin of advanced human epithelial ovarian cancers. *Cancer Res* 1992 **52**: 5119–5122.

28. Chiao PJ, Bischoff FZ, Strong LC, Tainsky MA. The current state of oncogenes and cancer: experimental approaches for analysing oncogenetic events in human cancer. *Cancer Metast Rev* 1990 **9**: 63–80.

29. Bishop JM. Cellular oncogenes and retroviruses. *Annu Rev Biochem* 1983 **52**: 301–354.

30. Levine AJ. The *p53* tumour suppressor gene and product. *Cancer Surv* 1992 **12**: 59–79.

31. Weinberg RA. The retinoblastoma gene and gene product. *Cancer Surv* 1992 **12**: 43–57.

32. Lane DP, Benchimol S. *p53*: oncogene or anti-oncogene? *Gene Dev* 1990 **4**: 1–8.

33. Field JK, Spandidos DA. The role of *ras* and *myc* oncogenes in human solid tumours and their relevance in diagnosis and prognosis (review). *Anticancer Res* 1990 **10**: 1–22.

34. Henzen-Logmans SC, Berns EMJJ, Klijn JGM *et al.* Epidermal growth factor receptor in ovarian tumours: correlation of immunocytochemistry with ligand binding assay. *Br J Cancer* 1992 **66**: 1015–1021.

35. Yamamoto T, Ikawa S, Akiyama T *et al.* Similarity of protein encoded by the human *c-erb-B-2* gene to epidermal growth factor gene. *Nature* 1986 **319**: 230–234.

36. Hung M-C, Zhang X, Yan D-H *et al.* Aberrant expression of the *c-erbB-2/neu* proto-oncogene in ovarian cancer. *Cancer Lett* 1992 **61**: 95–103.

37. Berchuck A, Kamel A, Whitaker R *et al.* Overexpression of *HER-2/neu* is associated with poor survival in advanced epithelial ovarian cancer. *Cancer Res* 1990 **50**: 4087–4091.

38. Imyanitov EN, Chernitsa OI, Serova OM, Knyazev PG. Rare occurrence of amplification of *HER-2* (*erbB-2/neu*) oncogene in ovarian cancer patients. *Eur J Cancer* 1992 **28A**: 1300.

39. Kacinski BM, Mayer AG, King BL, Carter D, Chambers SK. NEU protein overexpression in benign, borderline, and malignant ovarian neoplasms. *Gynecol Oncol* 1992 **44**: 245–253.

40. Sigal IS, Marshall MS, Schaber MD *et al.* Structure/function studies of the ras protein. *Cold Spring Harbor Symp Quant Biol* 1988 **LIII**: 863–869.

41. Willingham MC, Pastan I, Shih TY, Scolnick EM. Localization of the *src* gene product of the Harvey strain of MSV to the plasma membrane of transformed cells by electron microscope immunocytochemistry. *Cell* 1980 **19**: 1005–1014.

42. Marshall CJ, Lloyd AC, Morris JDH *et al.* Signal transduction by p21ras. *Int J Cancer* 1989 **44**: 29–31.

43. Yaginuma Y, Yamashita K, Kuzumaki N, Fujita M, Shimizo T. *ras* oncogene product p21 expression and prognosis of human ovarian tumors. *Gynecol Oncol* 1992 **46**: 45–50.

44. van't Veer LJ, Hermens R, van den Berg-Bakker LAM *et al.* *ras* oncogene activation in human ovarian carcinoma. *Oncogene* 1988 **2**: 157–165.

45. Cole MD The *myc* oncogene: its role in transformation and differentiation. *Annu Rev Genet* 1987 **20**: 361–384.

46. Yokota J, Tsunetsugu-Yokota Y, Battifora H, Lefevre C, Cline MJ. Alterations of the *myc*, *myb*, and *ras-Ha* protooncogenes in cancers are frequent and show clinical correlation. *Science* 1986 **231**: 261–265.

47. Sasano H, Garrett CT, Wilkinson DS *et al.* Protooncogene amplification and tumor ploidy in human ovarian neoplasms. *Hum Pathol* 1990 **21**: 382–391.

48. Baker VV, Borst MP, Dixon D *et al.* *c-myc* amplification in ovarian cancer. *Gynecol Oncol* 1990 **38**: 340–342.

49. Xerri L, Charpin C, Hassoun J, Birnbaum D, Delapeyriere O. *Mos* oncogene expression in human ovarian cancer. *Anticancer Res* 1991 **11**: 1629–1634.

50. Cheng JQ, Godwin AK, Bellacosa A *et al.* *AKT2*, a putative oncogene encoding a member of a subfamily of protein-serine/threonine kinases, is amplified in human ovarian carcinomas. *Proc Natl Acad Sci USA* 1992 **89**: 9267–9271.

51. Knudson AG. Mutation and cancer: statistical study of retinoblastoma. *Proc Natl Acad Sci USA* 1971 **68**: 820–823.

52. Toguchida J, Ishizaki K, Sasaki MS *et al.* Chromosome reorganization for the expression of recessive mutation of the retinoblastoma susceptibility gene in the development of osteosarcoma. *Cancer Res* 1988 **48**: 3939–3943.

53. Banerjee A, Xu H-J, Hu S-X *et al.* Changes in growth and tumorigenicity following reconstitution of retinoblastoma gene function in various human cancer cell types by microcell transfer of chromosome 13. *Cancer Res* 1992 **52**: 6297–6304.

54. Dryja TP, Cavenee WK, White R *et al.* Homozygosity of chromosome 13 in retinoblastoma. *N Engl J Med* 1984 **310**: 550–553.

55. Leach FS, Nocholaides NC, Papadopoulos N *et al.* Mutations of a *mutS* homolog in hereditary non-polyposis colon cancer. *Cell* 1993 **75**: 1215–1225.

56. Papadopoulos N, Nicolaides NC, Wei YF *et al.* Mutation of a *mutL* homolog in hereditary colon cancer. *Science* 1993 **63**: 1625–1629.

57. Kirchweger R, Zeillinger R, Schneeberger C, Speiser P, Louason G, Theillet C. Patterns of allele losses suggest the existence of five distinct regions of LOH on chromosome 17 in breast cancer. *Int J Cancer* 1994 **56**: 193–199.

58. Lee JH, Kavanagh JJ, Wildrick DM, Wharton JT, Blick M. Frequent loss of heterozygosity on chromosomes 6q, 11 and 17 in human ovarian carcinomas. *Cancer Res* 1990 **50**: 2724–2728.

59. Eccles DM, Russell SEH, Haites NE *et al.* Early loss of heterozygosity on 17q in ovarian cancer. *Oncogene* 1992 **7**: 2069–2072.

60. Coles C, Thompson AP, Elder PA *et al.* Evidence indicating at least two genes on chromosome 17p in breast carcinogenesis. *Lancet* 1990 **336**: 761–763.

61. Eccles DM, Cranston G, Steel CM, Nakamura Y, Leonard RCF. Allele losses on chromosome 17 in human epithelial ovarian cancer. *Oncogene* 1990 **5**: 1599–1601.

62. Russell SEH, Hickey GI, Lowry WS, White P, Atkinson RJ. Allele loss from chromosome 17 in ovarian cancer. *Oncogene* 1990 **5**: 1581–1583.

63. Jacobs IJ, Smith SA, Wiseman RW *et al.* A deletion unit on chromosome 17q in epithelial ovarian tumors distal to the familial breast/ovarian cancer locus. *Cancer Res* 1993 **53**: 1218–1221.

64. Hall JM, Lee MK, Newman B *et al.* Linkage of early-onset familial breast cancer to chromosome 17q21. *Science* 1990 **250**: 1684–1689.

65. Saito H, Inazawa J, Saito S *et al.* Detailed deletion mapping of chromosome 17q in ovarian and breast cancers: 2-cM region on 17q21.3 often and commonly deleted in tumors. *Cancer Res* 1993 **53**: 3382–3385.

66. Smith SA, Easton DF, Evans DGR, Ponder BAJ. Allele losses in the region 17q12-21 in familial breast and ovarian cancer involve the wild-type chromosome. *Nature Genet* 1992 **2**: 128–131.

67. Miki Y, Swensen J, Shattuck-Eidens D *et al.* A strong candidate for the breast and ovarian cancer susceptibility gene *BRCA1*. *Science* 1994 **266**: 66–71.

68. Gelehrter TD, Collins FS. *Principles of Medical Genetics* Baltimore: Williams & Wilkins, 1990: pp 208–217.

69. Futreal PA, Liu Q, Shattuck-Eidens D *et al.* *BRCA1* mutations in primary breast and ovarian carcinomas. *Science* 1994 **266**: 120–122.

70. Merajver SD, Pham TM, Caduff RF et al. Somatic mutations in the *BRCA1* gene in sporadic ovarian tumours. *Nature Genet* 1995 **9**: 439-443.

71. Ford D, Easton DF, Bishop DT, Narod SA, Goldgar DE and the Breast Cancer Linkage Consortium. Risks of cancer in *BRCA1* mutation carriers. *Lancet* 1994 **343**: 692–695.

72. Easton DF, Ford D, Bishop DT and the Breast Cancer Linkage Consortium. Breast and ovarian cancer incidence in *BRCA1* mutation carriers. *Am J Hum Genet* 1995 **56**: 265–271.

73. Narod S, Tonin P, Lynch H, Watson P, Feunteun J, Lenoir G. Histology of *BRCA1*-associated ovarian tumours. *Lancet* 1994 **343**: 236.

74. Wooster R, Neuhausen SL, Mangion J *et al.* Localization of a breast cancer susceptibility gene, *BRCA2*, to chromosome 13q12-13. *Science* 1994 **265**: 2088–2090.

75. Vogelstein B & Kinzler KW *p53* function and dysfunction. *Cell* 1992 **70**: 523–526.

76. El-Deiry WS, Tokino T. Velculescu VE *et al. WAF1*, a potential mediator of tumour suppression. *Cell* 1993 **75**: 817–825.

77. Harper JW, Adami GR, Wei N, Keyomarsi K, Elledge SJ. The p21 Cdk-interacting protein Cip1 is a potent inhibitor of G1 cyclin-dependent kinases. *Cell* 1993 **75**: 805–816.

78. Foulkes WD, Ragoussis J, Stamp GWH, Trowsdale J. Frequent loss of heterozygosity on chromosome 6 in human ovarian carcinoma. *Br J Cancer* 1993 **67**: 551–559.

79. Milner BJ, Allan LA, Eccles DM *et al. p53* mutation is a common genetic event in ovarian carcinoma. *Cancer Res* 1993 **53**: 2128–2132.

80. Eccles DM, Brett L, Lessells A *et al.* Overexpression of the p53 protein and allele loss at 17p13 in ovarian carcinoma. *Br J Cancer* 1992 **65**: 40–44.

81. Milner BJ. Unpublished results.

82. Kohler MF, Kerns BJ, Humphrey PA, Marks JR, Bast RC, Berchuck A. Mutations and overexpression of *p53* in early stage epithelial ovarian cancer. *Obstet Gynecol* 1993 **81**: 643–650.

83. Dodson MK, Hartmann LC, Cliby WA *et al.* Comparison of loss of heterozygosity patterns in invasive low-grade and high-grade epithelial ovarian carcinomas. *Cancer Res* 1993 **53**: 4456–4460.

84. Zheng J, Robinson WR, Ehlen T, Yu MC, Dubeau L. Distinction of low grade from high grade human ovarian carcinomas on the basis of losses of heterozygosity on chromosomes 3, 6 and 11 and *HER-2/neu* gene amplification. *Cancer Res* 1991 **51**: 4045–4051.

85. Sato T, Saito H, Morita R, Koi S, Lee JH, Nakamura Y. Allelotype of human ovarian cancer. *Cancer Res* 1991 **51**: 5118–5122.

86. Cliby W, Ritland S, Hartman L *et al.* Human epithelial ovarian cancer allelotype. *Cancer Res* 1993 **53**: 2393-2398.

87. Osborne RJ, Leech V. Polymerase chain reaction allelotyping of human ovarian cancer. *Br J Cancer* 1994 **69**: 429–438.

88. Allan GJ, Cottrell S, Trowsdale J, Foulkes WD. Loss of heterozygosity on chromosome 5 in sporadic ovarian carcinoma is a late event and is not associated with mutations in *APC* at 5q21-22. *Human Mutation* 1994 **3**: 283–291.

89. Weitzel JN, Patel J, Smith DM, Goodman A, Safaii H, Ball HG. Molecular genetic changes associated with ovarian cancer. *Gynecologic Oncology* 1994 **55**: 245–252.

90. Schultz DC, Vanderveer L, Buetow KH. Characterization of chromosome 9 in human ovarian neoplasia identifies frequent genetic imbalance on 9q and rare alterations involving 9p, including *CDKN2*. *Cancer Research* 1995 **55**: 2150–2157.

91. Lee JH, Kavanagh JJ, Wharton JT, Wildrick DM, Blick M. Allele loss at the *c-Ha-ras1* locus in human ovarian cancer. *Cancer Res* 1989 **49**: 1220–1222.

92. Eccles DM, Gruber L, Stewart L, Steel CM, Leonard RCF. Allele loss on chromosome 11p is associated with poor survival in ovarian cancer. *Dis Markers* 1992 **10**: 95–99.

93. Vandamme B, Lissens W, Amfo K *et al.* Deletion of chromosome 11p13–11p15.5 sequences in invasive human ovarian cancer is a subclonal progression factor. *Cancer Res* 1992 **52**: 6646–6652.

94. Viel A, Giannini F, Tumiotto L, Sopracordevole F, Visentin MC, Boiocchi M. Chromosomal localisation of two putative 11p oncosuppressor genes involved in human ovarian tumours. *Br J Cancer* 1992 **66**: 1030–1036.

95. Foulkes WD, Campbell IG, Stamp GWH, Trowsdale J. Loss of heterozygosity and amplification on chromosome 11q in human ovarian cancer. *Br J Cancer* 1993 **67**: 268–273.

96. Gallion HH, Powell DE, Morrow JK *et al.* Molecular genetic changes in human epithelial ovarian malignancies. *Gynecol Oncol* 1992 **47**: 137–142.

97. Yang-Feng TL, Li S, Han H, Schwartz PE. Frequent loss of heterozygosity on chromosomes Xp and 13q in human ovarian cancer. *Int J Cancer* 1992 **52**: 575–580.

98. Yang-Feng TL, Han H, Chen KC *et al.* Allelic loss in ovarian cancer. *Int J Cancer* 1993 **54**: 546–551.

99. Liu Y, Heyman M, Wang Y *et al.* Molecular analysis of the retinoblastoma gene in primary ovarian cancer cells. *International Journal of Cancer* 1994 **58**: 663–667.

100. Phillips N, Ziegler M, Saha B, Xynos F. Allelic loss on chromosome 17 in human ovarian cancer. *Int J Cancer* 1993 **54**: 85–91.

101. McManus DT, Yap EPH, Maxwell P, Russell SEH, Toner PG, McGee JOD. *p53* expression, mutation, and allelic deletion in ovarian cancer. *Journal of Pathology* 1994 **174**: 159–168.

102. Foulkes WD, Black DM, Stamp GW, Solomon E, Trowsdale J. Very frequent loss of heterozygosity throughout chromosome 17 in sporadic ovarian carcinoma. *Int J Cancer* 1993 **54**: 220–225.

103. Godwin AK, Vanderveer L, Schultz DC *et al.* A common region of deletion on chromosome 17q in both sporadic and familial epithelial ovarian tumors distal to *BRCA1*. *American Journal of Human Genetics* 1994 **55**: 666–677.

104. Leary JA, Kerr J, Chenevix-Trench G *et al.* Increased expression of the *NME1* gene is associated with metastasis in epithelial ovarian cancer. *International Journal of Cancer* 1995 **64**: 189–195.

105. Cornelis RS, Neuhausen SL, Johansson O *et al.* High allele loss rates at 17q12-q21 in breast and ovarian tumors from *BRCA1*-linked families. *Genes Chromosomes and Cancer* 1995 **13**: 203–210.

106. Viel A, DallAgnese L, Canzonieri V *et al.* Suppressive role of the metastasis-related *nm23-H1* gene in human ovarian carcinomas: Association of high messenger RNA expression with lack of lymph node metastasis. *Cancer Research* 1995 **55**: 2645–2650.

107. Merajver SD, Frank TS, Xu J *et al.* Germline *BRCA1* mutations and loss of the wild-type allele in tumors from families with early onset breast and ovarian cancer. *Clinical Cancer Research* 1995 **1**: 539–544.

108. Schildkraut JM, Collins NK, Dent GA *et al.* Loss of heterozygosity on chromosome 17q11-21 in cancers of women who have both breast and ovarian cancer. *American Journal of Obstetrics and Gynecology* 1995 **172**: 908–913.

109. Oliner JD, Kinzler KW, Meltzer PS, George DL, Vogelstein B. Amplification of a gene encoding a p53-associated protein in human sarcomas. *Nature* 1992 **358**: 80–83.

4.6

Growth Factors and Oncogenes

JMS Bartlett

INTRODUCTION

Within any normal tissue cellular populations are in a constant state of flux. As cells senesce and die they are replaced by a complex process of cellular proliferation and differentiation. These processes are under the control of many diverse factors affecting proliferation, differentiation and cellular function. Imbalances in this process often manifest as disease. In particular imbalances in cellular proliferation and cell death can result in tumor formation. Either an increase in cellular proliferation or a decrease in the rate of cell death may lead to tumor formation by disturbing the normal physiological balance between these two events. The scope of this chapter is to review the role of growth factors and oncogenes in this process in relation to gynecological malignancies.

Growth factors are small polypeptides which are, as their name implies, implicated in the regulation of cellular proliferation. However, their functions often extend far beyond simple induction of cell division. Oncogenes are genes which have been implicated in the formation of tumors, these often include growth factors, their receptors or proteins involved in cellular signaling.[1,2] This overlap can lead to confusion as some growth factors and their receptors were either first identified as oncogenes or have oncogenic homologs. In addition the identification of tumor suppressor genes (often called anti-oncogenes[3,4]) has further complicated this picture; the role of such anti-oncogenes is, however, outwith the scope of this chapter.

The majority of tumors arising in humans are now thought to result from inactivation or activation of normal cellular genes which regulate cellular proliferation. These can function in two ways: genes which show activation in cancers generally act as inducers of cellular proliferation via diverse mechanisms, activation of such oncogenes requires only one dominant mutation, the second copy of a gene may remain unaltered in many situations. Genes which are inactivated in cancer often encode for proteins which normally act by inhibiting proliferation, inactivation of these

tumor suppresser genes (or anti-oncogenes) may require both alleles to be inactivated to elicit tumorigenesis.[4]

CURRENT CONCEPTS

Growth factors and their receptors

Polypeptide growth factors mediate their actions by binding to cell surface proteins (receptors), which are thereby activated and 'transduce' the signal within the cell cytoplasm, to the cell nucleus. This appears to be such a central step in control of cell function that many of these 'signal transducers' are implicated as oncogenes. The central role of not just growth factors and their receptors but also these 'second messengers' in tumor biology forms the main theme of this review. An overview of the normal functions of these factors is given to provide a background crucial to the understanding of the consequences of oncogenic activation of these cell regulatory proteins. Growth factor-induced changes in cellular status are multistage processes. Induction of growth factor synthesis, delivery to the target cell and the response of the cell itself all play a role in growth factor action. In many transformed tissues, particularly hormonally responsive tumors (breast, ovarian and endometrial cancers), steroid or other hormones may regulate tumor growth factor production. Growth factors, once synthesized, interact at many levels with their target tissues (Fig. 4.6.1). In endocrine regulation the factor is produced within one organ such that targets cells in other organs having passed through the circulatory system (Fig. 4.6.1a). Paracrine regulation involves regulation of one cell type within an organ by factors produced by an adjacent cell population (Fig. 4.6.1b). Autocrine regulation occurs when a factor produced by a cell population regulates the same population of cells (Fig. 4.6.1c). Growth factors may act by one or all of these routes to affect cellular function. More recent evidence suggests that in some cases externalization and release of growth factors may not be required

(a) Endocrine

Tissue A

(b) Paracrine

Cell A

(c) Autocrine

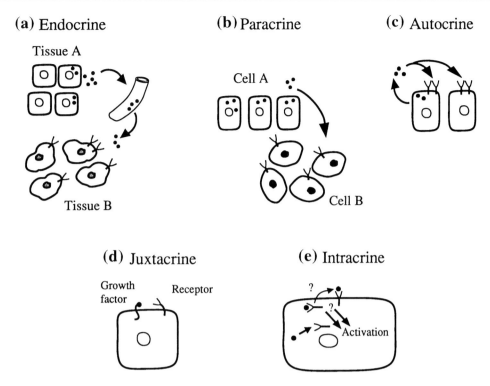

Tissue B

Cell B

(d) Juxtacrine

Growth factor   Receptor

(e) Intracrine

?

?

Activation

Fig. 4.6.1 *Cellular communication. Diagrammatic representation of the diverse mechanisms of intracellular communications occurring between cells.*

for signaling to take place. Interactions between growth factors and receptors either while both are anchored in the cell membrane (juxtacrine regulation) or indeed while both are still within the cell cytoplasm (intracrine regulation) have been postulated to explain some of the interactions seen between growth factors with transmembrane domains (juxtacrine, Fig. 4.6.1d) or those lacking sequences required for cellular release (intracrine, Fig. 4.6.1e). Such proposed mechanisms are extremely difficult to distinguish experimentally from autocrine regulation, and often such distinctions may be more mechanistic than functional. Often a feature of transformed cells is the acquisition of autocrine growth control, mediated by tumor cells producing their own growth factors, which releases them from control by normal physiological regulators of proliferation.

As intimated above, growth factors are pluripotent peptides with many diverse functions. Growth factors may have both positive and negative effects on cell proliferation, differentiation and function (Fig. 4.6.2). Cells may respond to growth factor stimulation by increased proliferation (Fig. 4.6.2a), modified function (Fig. 4.6.2b) or by entering a programed series of events leading to cell death (Fig. 4.6.2c). All three processes described here are under control of one or more growth factor pathways. The balance between different pathways is most clearly illustrated by the current understanding of regulation of cell apoptosis. This involves the integration of both positive and negative growth factor-mediated signals to direct cells towards either proliferation or cell death.[5] Which of these pathways is utilized by a particular cell may depend on the panel of

growth stimulatory events to which it is exposed, its own status with regard to the cell cycle and the duration and 'strength' of the signal received. It can be seen that growth factors have enormous potential for regulation of both normal and transformed cell behavior. As can be seen below the multiplicity of growth factor signals and intracellular mediators of such signalling makes this an extremely complex picture to investigate and elucidate.

Similarities in structure or function of many of the growth factors and their receptors have led to a classification of the majority of receptors into families and subclasses. Currently three major divisions of growth factor receptors have been identified, based on the primary mechanisms by which they mediate their effects. Growth factor receptors are, almost exclusively, expressed on the outer surface of cells, growth factors bind at this point and the signal is mediated by either the intracellular domain or proteins associated with the receptor within the cell. This process is the start of 'signal transduction'.[6–9] Signal transduction mechanisms involve many diverse biochemical changes, but the initial event is usually clearly identifiable for any particular receptor family. It is this event which is used to classify receptors into subclasses. For many receptors the initial signaling event which occurs following ligand binding is the activation of a 'kinase'. Kinases induce phosphorylation (i.e. the addition of a phosphate group) of specific sites in target proteins. This phosphorylation causes marked changes in the conformation and activity of such targets often initiating a cascade of events leading to modification of cellular proteins and activation of nuclear

(a) Proliferation

(b) Differentiation

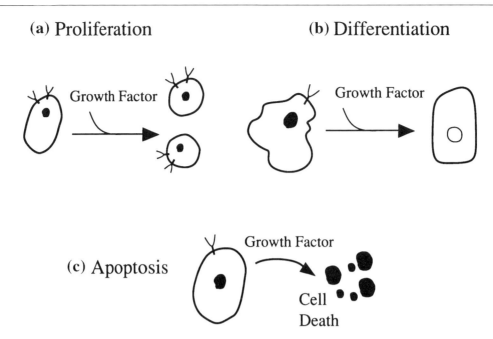

(c) Apoptosis

Fig. 4.6.2 *Growth factor-mediated events. Growth factors mediate multiple functions relating to cellular proliferation, differentiation and apoptosis.*

transcription factors which initiate the synthesis of novel proteins.

Tyrosine kinase receptors

As their name implies these receptors initiate signaling by phosphorylation of tyrosine residues, usually within the receptor itself. These phosphorylated tyrosines are then crucial to the transduction of the receptor signal.[8,10]

Serine–threonine kinase receptors

As with tyrosine kinase receptors the initial signaling event mediated by this class of receptors involves phosphorylation of amino acid residues within the receptor; in this case however, serine and threonine residues are targeted.[9]

G-protein-linked receptors (or seven-transmembrane receptors)

G-protein-linked receptors mediate their action via association with a family of adenyl cyclase and kinase regulating proteins. Activation of the receptor leads to inactivation of these regulatory proteins and subsequent activation of intracellular signal pathways.[6]

Within each receptor family are many subdivisions into subclasses of receptors each often with the potential to interact with multiple ligands. Of these differing types of receptors the tyrosine kinase and G-protein linked receptors have been most widely studied. The serine threonine kinase receptors are a relatively recently identified class of receptors about which relatively little is known. Allied to each family of receptors and often providing means by

which different receptors may communicate within the cell are a plethora of intracellular signaling pathways which themselves involve non-receptor tyrosine and serine/threonine kinase activities.

Tyrosine kinase receptors

Over 50 receptor tyrosine kinases grouped into 14 or more subfamilies have been identified to date. The level of information available ranges from knowledge of the protein and cDNA sequence only to a detailed understanding of the intracellular signaling mechanisms and receptor–ligand interaction and function. Extensive data are, however, only available for a relatively small number of these receptors which provide a model for the understanding of how this class of receptors exert their functions.

The great diversity of tyrosine kinase receptor associated growth factors has intensified interest in the mechanisms by which their receptors mediate their actions. As research into these mechanisms has progressed the central involvement of many known oncogenes in the process of cellular signaling has become apparent. Much of the data described below is applicable to signaling mechanisms mediated via many tyrosine kinase receptors although the specific example described relates to EGF receptor.

Activation of receptor tyrosine kinase and receptor phosphorylation

The type I receptor tyrosine kinases share a similar response to binding of ligand (Fig. 4.6.3) involving activation of the receptor kinase domain and phosphorylation of

(a) Receptor Dimerization

(b) Autophosphorylation

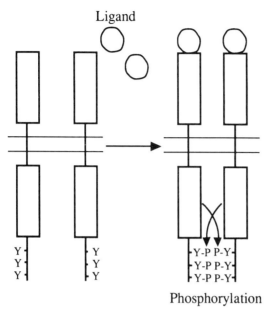

Ligand

Phosphorylation

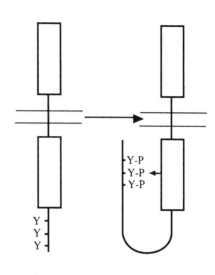

Fig. 4.6.3 *Tyrosine kinase growth factor receptors: the role of autophosphorylation.* **(a)** *Many of the tyrosine kinase growth factor receptors mediate their action by ligand binding and receptor dimerization. Dimerization of receptor and the conformational changes induced by ligand binding result in the activation of receptor tyrosine kinase domains. Following such activation, tyrosine residues (Y) on each receptor are modified by the opposing kinase domain by addition of phosphate (P). This phosphorylation initiates the subsequent signaling events shown in Fig. 4.6.4 (see text for details).* **(b)** *Autophosphorylation of cell surface or cytoplasmic tyrosine kinases may result in partial inactivation of the kinase domain. Alternatively c-src appears to exist in an autophosphorylated (inactive) state from which it is released by receptor-mediated or oncogenic activation.*

specific receptor tyrosine residues. To date the most widely studied mechanism for such phosphorylation invariably implicated two receptors with kinase domains cross phosphorylating each other.

First, following ligand binding, receptor pairing or dimerization is promoted by conformational changes in receptor structure (Fig. 4.6.3a). Following this dimerization the tyrosine kinase signaling activity of each receptor is activated and each receptor phosphorylates a number of tyrosine residues on its partner, a process known as cross-phosphorylation (Fig. 4.6.3a). Dimerization of receptors is accomplished by a variety of means. EGF receptors (and other type I receptors) show increased affinity for similar receptors following ligand binding and this promotes dimerization and activation. However, type II receptors (insulin etc.) exist as linked dimeric units, whereas type III receptors (PDGFs) are dimerized by a linked ligand.

Despite the preponderance of evidence suggesting that receptor dimerization is essential for activation in many classes of receptor tyrosine kinases, evidence from Src related tyrosine kinases suggests that partial autophosphorylation may inhibit activity of other members of the tyrosine kinase family. Such autophosphorylation seems to be particularly important in the Src-related protein tyrosine kinases, in this instance free Src may exist in an inactive autophosphorylated form (Fig. 4.6.3b) from which it is released by receptor-mediated or oncogenic activation.[8,11]

Oncogenic activation of receptors may involve changes to extracellular or intracellular domains which result in permanent activation of the receptor, or increased expression of the normal protein may lead to oncogenic transformation.[10]

Signal transduction

A complex series of events has been identified involving multiple signaling pathways by which growth factors modify cellular activity following ligand binding at the cell surface. A generalized system by which the majority of these receptors act is described using the EGF receptor as an example, since such a system is useful for the understanding of many of the events which result in tissue transformation. Although the mechanisms by which different receptor-linked tyrosine kinases mediate these effects differ[12-14] the central signaling mechanisms appear to be consistent between different receptors of this type.

The purpose of a multistage intracellular signaling mechanism appears twofold. First, as the signal from the cell surface is transferred towards the cell nucleus the signal strength is amplified at specific points in the pathway enabling a seemingly slight effect at the cell surface to produce fundamental changes is cellular behavior. Secondly, each signal transduction pathway has multiple checkpoints at which interaction with other cell surface receptors and intracellular systems allow either amplification of appropriate signals or modification or cancellation of inappropriate signals. In this way interactions between multiple growth factors produce a complex sequence of events to control cellular proliferation.

In the case of tyrosine kinase receptors, the initial signaling event is phosphorylation of the receptor itself on multiple tyrosine residues. This causes activation of several distinct signaling mechanisms, which together modify cellular behavior. The most clearly understood mechanisms by which tyrosine kinase receptors modify protein behavior are:

1. Translocation
2. Conformational change
3. Phosphorylation

These mechanisms initiate a series of protein modifications resulting in activation of cellular signals leading ultimately to modification of cellular function and also activation of specific nuclear transcription factors resulting in *de novo* protein synthesis. Examples for each of the above are given.

Translocation mediated activation of the MAP kinase phosphorylation cascade

Following receptor phosphorylation it has been clear for some time that the cytosolic serine/threonine kinases known as MAP kinases (mitogen activated protein kinases)

are activated. The mechanism by which these proteins are activated has recently been elucidated and involves several complex steps (Fig. 4.6.4a).

First, a complex of two cytosolic proteins Grb-2 and SOS is bound via the Grb-2 SH2 domain to the phosphorylated receptor (SH2 domains have a high affinity for phosphorylated tyrosine residues). This translocation of the SOS protein to the cell membrane results in the exchange of GDP for GTP bound to membrane-associated p21 RAS leading to activation of a protein kinase cascade which in turn leads to activation of nuclear transcription factors including myc, fos and jun.[10,11–15,16]

Alternative mechanisms for activation of the MAP kinase pathway by different receptors include the use of further intermediary proteins in PDGF receptor mediated signaling which lacks a Grb-2 binding site[16] and the use of an alternate intermediary IRS-1 in IGF-mediated signaling.[11–13] Thus a great diversity in receptor-mediated activation of the MAP pathway can be envisaged.

Other signal transduction pathways may also be activated by translocation of the initiating intracellular proteins. Following binding of interferon to its receptor the JAK kinase is translocated to the membrane and activated. Translocation of intracellular signal proteins therefore represents a common event in many of the tyrosine kinase-mediated signal pathways.

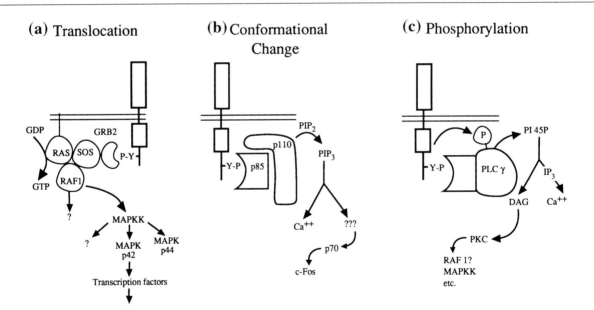

(a) Translocation (b) Conformational Change (c) Phosphorylation

Fig. 4.6.4 *Tyrosine kinase-mediated intracellular signaling mechanisms. **(a)** Following receptor-ligand binding and phosphorylation (Fig. 4.6.3) the intermediary receptor binding Grb-2/SOS complex binds to phosphorylated tyrosines (P-Y). This interaction facilitates the association of p21 RAS (RAS) with the receptor and activation of RAS by exchange of guanosine diphosphate (GDP) for guanosine triphosphate (GTP). RAS then activates the protein kinase RAF-1 which in turn activates proteins including MAP kinase kinase (MAPKK). MAPKK then activates isoforms of MAP kinase (MAPK) which leads to nuclear translocation and activation of transcription factors. (See text for details.) **(b)** The p85 subunit (p85) of phosphatidylinositol 3′ kinase has an affinity site for phosphorylated tyrosines. Binding of the p85:p110 heterodimeric protein results in phosphorylation of phosphatidylinositol (PIP) to phosphatidylinositol 3′ phosphate (PIP₃). This molecule acts as a soluble intracellular message resulting in mobilization of calcium and (possibly) activation of p70^{56K} (p70) and the c-Fos transcription factor. **(c)** Binding of phospholipase C (PLC) to phosphorylated tyrosines on receptor tyrosine kinases results in the phosphorylation (P) of this enzyme by the tyrosine kinase domain of the receptor. This results in enzyme activation and the cleavage of the membrane phospholipid phosphatidylinositol diphosphate (PI45P) to form diacyl glycerol (DAG) and inositol triphosphate (IP₃). Diacyl glycerol formation results in the activation of protein kinase C (PKC) and subsequent activation of RAF1 and the MAP kinase kinase pathway shown in panel A. IP₃ causes the mobilization of intracellular calcium (see text for details).*

Conformational activation of phosphatidylinositol 3' kinase

The exact role of phosphatidylinositol 3' kinase (PI3-K) in intracellular signaling is unclear. The main function of the enzyme is phosphorylation of the second messenger phosphatidylinositol phosphate (PIP). PI3-K exists as a heterodimeric protein with two subunits of 85 (p85) and 110 kDa (p110). On phosphorylation of receptor tyrosine residues the p85 subunit binds to these sites and a conformational activation of the p110 subunit occurs leading to increased PIP phosphorylation (Fig. 4.6.4b). The significant events downstream of PIP in modifying cell function remain unclear: two possible pathways have been identified. Firstly, PIP acts by liberating intracellular calcium, a known modifier of many functional cellular proteins, there is, however, little evidence for involvement of this activity in modulating cellular proliferation. Secondly, there is potential for induction of the c-fos transcription factor and other mitogenic signals via p70[S6K]; however, the steps by which PI3-K might activate p70[S6K] remain unknown.

Phosphorylation mediated phospholipase C activation

Phospholipase C is recruited following EGF binding[17] and acts via cleavage of phosphatidylinositol diphosphate, a membrane phospholipid, to produce inositol triphosphate (ITP) and diacylglycerol (DAG), both of which have potent signaling activities.

ITP is involved via a specific intracellular receptor-mediated interaction in mobilization of intracellular calcium whereas DAG activates some members of the protein kinase C (PKC) family of proteins (Fig. 4.6.4b). Although the role of calcium mobilization in activation of mitogenic pathways remains unclear, PKC activation has among its consequences activation of the MAP kinase phosphorylation cascade described above possibly via direct phosphorylation of RAF-1.[18] This in addition to other potential PKC-mediated events may be the route by which PKC impacts on cellular proliferation.

The diversity of effects mediated by different members of this family of intracellular protein kinases provides yet another level of diversification of receptor mediated signals.

The signaling pathways described above illustrate the diversity of function of receptor tyrosine kinases and the wide range of intracellular responses which they mediate. It is likely to be some years before a clear understanding of individual signaling pathways and their effects is attained.

The diversity and redundancy built into these systems may explain the diversity of function between receptor families all of which utilize similar signaling pathways. In addition the potential for oncogenic activation of the cell signaling pathway is highlighted by the central role of oncogenes such as *SOS*, *RAS*, *RAF*, *myc* and the nuclear transcription factors jun and fos involved in this process.

Serine–threonine receptor kinases

Of all the receptor kinases described to date those which apparently signal via serine–threonine kinases are the least understood at this time. The TGFβ receptor superfamily which includes receptors for the related peptides, activin, inhibin and Müllerian inhibitory substance, has only recently been identified. Over the past 2–3 years significant progress in the understanding of ligand–receptor interactions has been made and it is now clear that different receptors for TGFβ interact to transduce signals within the cell.[19–23] The type II receptors appear to supply ligand specificity whereas it is suggested that type I receptors initiate intracellular signaling.[19–23] There is some evidence to implicate guanine nucleotides in the intracellular signal transduction pathways involved in TGFβ signaling, however, to date no clear understanding of such pathways has emerged.[9] The involvement of proteins downstream of the cell surface receptor in the regulation of proteins central to the control of the cell cycle have recently been documented, and this represents an important step towards increasing our understanding of how TGFβ receptors influence cell function.

G-protein linked receptors

This superfamily of membrane receptors now includes in excess of 40 subfamilies among which are included receptors for the neurotransmitters, vasoregulators, glycoprotein hormones and LHRH. Intracellular signaling via these receptors is mediated not by the receptor but by associated G-protein complexes which functionally regulate the primary effectors of these receptors – the adenyl-cyclases. The primary signaling event in G-protein-linked receptor signal transduction depends on the GTPase activity of G-proteins.[6,7]

In the unstimulated state G-proteins exist as heterotrimeric complexes composed of alpha, beta and gamma subunits loosely associated with the cell membrane but not associated with receptors. The GTPase containing alpha subunit exists in this complex with GDP bound to a specific guanine nucleotide binding site. On ligand binding to the cell surface receptors the G-proteins complex with the receptor complex and the GDP dissociates from the alpha subunit. This provides a site on the G-protein complex which allows binding of GTP to the guanine nucleotide binding site. The current consensus then supports dissociation of the GTP bound alpha subunit from a dimeric beta-gamma subunit. These units are associated with activation of a variety of signal transduction pathways downstream from the receptor. The role of G-protein heterodimeric beta-gamma subunit in downstream signaling remains controversial. The main function of this subunit appears to be to stabilize the G-alpha-GDP complex and to promote binding of the heterotrimeric G-protein to the activated receptor.[6]

Deactivation of G-proteins occurs via the intrinsic GTPase activity associated with the G-alpha subunits; this enzyme activity cleaves GTP to GDP which remains bound to the G-alpha subunit. This facilitates the reformation of the G-protein heterotrimeric alpha–beta–gamma complex which is functionally inactive. The rate of this enzymatic cleavage of GTP regulates the signal transduction effects mediated by ligand binding, depending on the particular G-alpha subunit present this rate of cleavage may vary up to 100-fold. This variation in the rate of G-protein deactivation is central to the diversity of signaling functions mediated by the G-protein-linked receptor superfamily.[6]

In addition to the diversity of receptors within this family multiple forms of the components of the G-protein complexes and different isoforms of adenyl-cyclase mediate the diversity of cellular responses to this receptor family. The primary form of diversity of function in signaling relates again to the multiple isoforms of the G-protein alpha subunits. These proteins are loosely grouped according to structure into four subfamilies G_{ai}, G_{as}, G_{aq}, and G_{a12}. Although the functional diversity of these proteins and their effects on signal transduction are outwith the scope of this review the effects of the G_i and G_s families of proteins serve to highlight the complexity of this system. Whereas many of the functions of these proteins are similar, they have differing effects on the main signal transduction pathway mediated by G-proteins, via adenyl-cyclases, G_i proteins inhibit whereas G_s proteins stimulate this important cellular activity. This variation in response markedly alters the pattern of responses which can be mediated via ligand binding to receptors.[6]

Intracellular signal transduction systems mediated via this receptor family share some similarities with those described downstream of the receptor tyrosine kinases, and there is potential for both negative and positive cooperation between these receptor families. Binding of ligand to its receptor can activate a series of intracellular messengers including phospholipase C, and protein kinases A and C. Which specific enzyme isoform activated and thereby cellular response, is determined by the components of the G-protein complex associated with the receptor.[6]

On binding of ligand to receptor the heterotrimeric G-protein complex dissociates releasing GDP and binding GTP, the G-alpha subunit then binds to adenyl cyclase or PLC in an isoform-specific interaction. Activation of PLC leads to production signals similar to those seen with tyrosine kinases, ITP, DAG leading to protein kinase C activation and calcium release (Fig. 4.6.5). Binding of G proteins to adenyl cyclase may lead to either enzyme activation or inhibition dependent on subunit type. In the case of enzyme activation the second messenger cyclic adenosine monophosphate (cAMP) is produced and binds to cAMP binding proteins associated with PKA (Fig. 4.6.5). This results in release of active PKA which mediates a number of further events including destabilization of some mRNAs, initiation of DNA transcription via the cAMP response element and phosphorylation and inhibition of the G-protein receptor in a negative feedback loop (Fig. 4.6.5). More recently cAMP mediated activation of

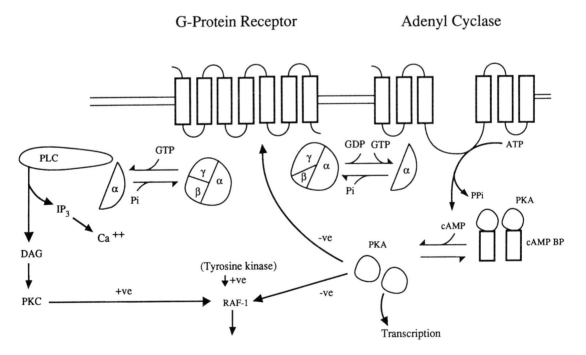

Fig. 4.6.5 *G-protein receptor mediated signaling. Binding of ligand to G-protein receptors results in the dissociation of the hetero-trimeric G-protein complex involving the exchange of GDP and GTP by the alpha subunit of this complex. This alpha subunit then mediates the activation of either adenyl cyclase or phospholipase C (or both). Reassociation of the alpha, beta and gamma subunits of the G-protein complex is mediated by cleavage of bound GTP to GDP by the alpha subunit. PLC activation results in mobilization of intracellular calcium and activation of protein kinase C (Fig. 4.6.4c), leading to activation of RAF-1 among other events. Activation of adenyl cyclase results in the cleavage of adenosine triphosphate (ATP) to a cyclic adenosine monophosphate (cAMP) with the release of a diphosphate (PPi). cAMP acts as a second messenger binding to the regulatory subunits (cAMP BP) of the protein kinase A (PKA) complex, causing dissociation and activation of PKA. PKA then initiates a series of events leading to activation of nuclear transcription factors. Interestingly PKA may also negatively regulate RAF-1 activity leading to a decrease in tyrosine kinase mediated signaling. PKA also inhibits further activation of G-protein receptors (negative feedback) by phosphorylation of the receptor (see text for details).*

PKA has been implicated in the negative control of signaling via tyrosine kinase receptors via inhibition of raf-1 kinase activity.[6]

This summary of signal transduction by G-protein receptors precludes detailed discussion of the immense diversity of signaling mediated by these receptors predominantly through the complex interactions of multiple forms of G-protein complexes and effector enzyme isoforms. For such discussions, the reader is directed to a wealth of literature on this topic.[6]

Growth factors and oncogenes in gynecological cancers

Growth factors and their signaling mechanisms are of central importance in the control of cellular function in normal tissues.[8-11,15,16] The sensitive nature of such controls is demonstrated by the oncogenic potential of many of these normally expressed proteins which when modified or inappropriately expressed give rise to tumorigenic changes in cellular behavior. A clearer understanding of the role of so-called 'oncogenes' in normal cellular function and of the central role played by growth factors in such processes will provide a crucial background for those seeking to understand the role of growth factors, their receptors and oncogenes in the disease processes associated with cancers. Many of the associations between growth factor receptor and oncogene overexpression and disease progression and outcome may well become more readily understandable in the light of the progress made in the understanding of growth factor function described above.

Erb B receptor tyrosine kinases and cancer

The mammalian type I tyrosine kinase receptors include the epidermal growth factor receptor (EGFr, C-erbB-1) and three proteins with similar function C-erbB-2, B-3 and B-4 with considerable sequence homology between family members and with the viral oncogene *v-erb*. Each receptor has been shown to interact with soluble polypeptide growth factors and for some members of the family, such as the epidermal growth factor receptor, a number of different ligands have been identified including epidermal growth factor (EGF), heparin binding epidermal growth factor, transforming growth factor alpha, cripto and amphiregulin, all of which share a common structure.[24] Although EGF receptor and its homologs are classical growth factor receptors with important functions in normal physiology, when transfected into or overexpressed in normal cells they have oncogenic properties.[25] Perhaps most widely studied in breast cancer (data on over 5000 patients for EGF receptor are available[26]) the role of EGF receptor and c-erbB-2 in gynecological malignancies has also been extensively investigated.[27,28] Although data on c-erbB-3 and c-erbB-4 are sparse at present it is already clear that members of this growth factor family have a major role to play in many diverse tumor types both as prognostic markers and as potential therapeutic targets.[27,29,30] The

strong links between expression of members of this growth factor and disease outcome argues for their role as mediators of disease progression.

Studies on *in vitro* models of ovarian, cervical and endometrial cancer have confirmed the importance of EGF receptor-mediated autocrine regulation of cell proliferation in these systems, co-expression of ligand and receptors and ligand-mediated proliferation have been confirmed using cell lines and primary human material.[31-34] Evidence is emerging that cooperation between receptors within this family may be mediated by heterodimerization of different receptors. Co-expression of ligands for the EGF receptor with the receptor itself have been confirmed in many studies relating to ovarian cancer.[35,36] These studies have established the importance of autocrine regulation of cancer growth by members of the type I receptor tyrosine kinase family.

Expression of EGF receptor and c-erbB-2 in gynecological malignancies has also been extensively studied and related to disease outcome. Evidence from early studies with small numbers of patients was conflicting, however with increasing numbers of patients available, a clear relationship between growth factor receptor expression and poor disease outcome has emerged. Although in common with other solid neoplasms amplification of the c-erbB-2 receptor has been implicated in a proportion of ovarian cancers, there remains some controversy as to the extent to which this event is seen in ovarian tumors. c-erbB-2 amplification rates approaching 25–40% have been seen in some studies, but another large series of tumors showed rates as low as 3%. This discrepancy may reflect methodological and possibly patient-derived heterogeneity. Expression of EGF receptor occurs in 30–90% with c-erbB-2 overexpression observed in around 30% of ovarian tumors.[31,35,37,38] Gene amplification and protein overexpression for c-erbB-2 have been related to poor prognosis in ovarian carcinoma and cervical adenocarcinoma.[31,35,37-39] Rates of receptor expression in endometrial cancer vary widely between reports,[40] with only a single report revealing a link between EGF receptor expression and a decrease in disease-free survival. EGF receptor and c-erbB-2 expression appear to be correlated with more aggressive forms of cervical carcinoma and with mortality,[39,41] although studies on earlier forms of disease suggest that the rate of expression in carcinoma is much lower than that seen in dysplasia.[42] Generally data on prognosis related to type I tyrosine kinase receptor expression for endometrial or cervical carcinoma remains preliminary and requires extensive study. The picture is becoming much clearer with respect to ovarian cancer where both EGF receptor and c-erb-B-2 expression have been linked to decreased survival in a number of large patient studies.[36,43]

Although much work remains to be carried out in some areas, there is a clear consensus, especially with respect to ovarian tumors, that type I tyrosine kinase receptors have an important role in mediating tumor growth in gynecological malignancies. Following these data, efforts are being made to exploit expression of such growth factors in diagnostic and therapeutic management. Evidence is growing that c-erbB-2 detected in serum may reflect tumor growth factor status in a proportion of patients providing a potential tool for rapidly detecting patients with expression of this growth factor. More significantly evidence is emerging that c-erbB-2 may represent a useful clinical target. Experimental evidence has shown that treatment with antibodies to c-erbB-2 results in inhibition of tumor growth; addition of cytotoxic agents in conjunction with such treatments can significantly enhance tumor kill mediated by the toxins.[44] Such approaches are now being successfully tested in clinical situations.[29] The potential of growth factor receptors as therapeutic targets is now widely accepted and investigations are underway to determine the best means of exploiting this potential. When such approaches bear fruit the type I receptor tyrosine kinases are likely to be among the first to be tested and as such patients with malignancies which are known to express such receptors will be the earliest to benefit.

Type II IGF receptor tyrosine kinases and cancer

The type II receptor tyrosine kinases include both the insulin (IR) and type I insulin-like growth factor receptors (IGFIR). The IGF-II receptor is a discrete entity. There is close homology between insulin and IGFIR receptors both structurally, and functionally some cross-reactivity between the receptors is evidenced by binding of other members of the growth factor family (insulin, insulin-like growth factor-I and -II) with lower affinity to both the insulin and IGF type I receptor. Activity of these growth factors is markedly modified by a series of growth factor binding proteins (IGF-BPs).

Growth factors acting on these, receptors, particularly IGF-I, have been shown to stimulate cellular proliferation in ovarian and endometrial tumour cells *in vitro*.[45] Expression of IGFIR, IGF-BPs and IGF-I itself have been identified in endometrial and ovarian carcinomas.[46–49] No clear link to disease outcome has yet been established for these variables, probably due to the low numbers of patients studied to date. However, laboratory studies would suggest that there is evidence for a central role of IGFs in both ovarian and endometrial cancers, but further investigations are required before a clear understanding of the importance of this family of growth factors and receptors is forthcoming.

Type III receptor tyrosine kinases: platelet-derived growth factor and colony-stimulating growth factor receptors

Type III receptor tyrosine kinases include platelet-derived growth factor receptors, the colony-stimulating factor type I receptor (CSFr) and also the *c-kit* oncogene. Classically regarded as being members of the hemopoetic growth factor system, evidence is growing to relate CSFr and other cytokines (such as the interleukins, tumor necrosis factor) directly to tumor cell regulation.[50] Recent evidence on the relationship between M-CSF receptors and IL-2 and IL-5 receptors may classify this group as a distinct receptor subfamily.

Almost nothing is known of the role PDGF plays in gynecological cancers. In view of the central role this family of growth factor plays in many other tumor types, this area may require attention in future.[51] Concomitant expression of PDGF and PDGFr has been linked to disease progression in a study of 45 ovarian cancers where approximately 30% of tumors showed a gain of PDGF expression in conjunction with PDGF receptor.

Macrophage-colony stimulating factor (M-CSF) and its receptor (*c-fms* oncogene) have been identified in ovarian and endometrial tumors.[52] In some cases circulating M-CSF has proven useful in the monitoring of ovarian cancer as a tumor marker.[53,54] Production of M-CSF receptor has been established in cell lines from both ovarian and endometrial cancers.[28] The related cytokine granulocyte–macrophage colony stimulating factor has been shown to stimulate growth of ovarian tumor cells *in vitro*.[53]

Type IV receptor tyrosine kinases: fibroblast growth factor receptors

The major component of the type IV receptor tyrosine kinase receptor family is the diverse group of fibroblast growth factors (FGFs) and their receptors. Four members of this growth factor receptor family have been identified to date, all displaying affinity for members of the FGF family. Activation of these receptors also involves receptor dimerization and transphosphorylation, probably via the mediation of non-FGF molecules. Evidence shows that proteoglycans on the cell surface, and specifically their heparin and heparin sulfate carbohydrate chains are essential to FGF activity. It appears that such molecules cause dimerization of FGFs to promote receptor dimerization and activation. As with PDGFs heterodimerization of receptors appears to be facilitated by heterologous pairing of the seven known FGF peptides each with differing patterns of affinity for the five identified FGF receptors. As with other growth factors there are strong oncogenic links with a number of the receptors being initially identified as oncogenes (flg, bek, cek 1,2,3) and three of their ligands (int-2, hst-1 and FGF5) also initially identified as oncogenes.

Little is known of the biology of FGF receptor in gynecological malignancies or of its role in tumor proliferation or function. Interest in this family of growth factors stems from the finding that amplification of Int-2 or FGF receptor 3 is a relatively frequent event in breast cancer.[26] There is increasing evidence that amplification of this receptor family, and particularly of int-2/FGFR3 is also a common event in ovarian cancer. Amplification of FGFR3 has been identified in approximately 20% of ovarian cancers. Gene amplification is low level (less than five copies) and appears to be significantly related to disease stage but not to any other variable.[55]

Tumour necrosis factor (TNF) and interleukin (IL) in metastatic spread of ovarian cancer

TNFalpha has been implicated as an autocrine regulator of ovarian carcinoma growth.[56] A series of studies involving tumor models of ovarian cancer have suggested a role for both IL-1 and TNFα in promoting tumor metastatic spread in ovarian cancer.[56,57] Expression of IL-1, IL-6 and TNFalpha mRNA has been demonstrated in small numbers of ovarian cancer cell lines and in some primary tumors. IL-2 receptor, which is released into serum in a soluble form, has been shown to be a marker of tumor growth in patients with ovarian, cervical and endometrial cancer.[58] Both IL-4 and IL-6 have been shown to be autocrine regulators of tumor cell proliferation. IL-4 decreased growth in ovarian cancer cell lines while enhancing MHC class II expression whereas IL-6 potentiates growth in cervical cancer cells. Future studies may well implicate a wider range of cytokines in the regulation of tumor behavior. However it is already clear that interleukins and TNF may play a role not only in modulating *in vivo* response to tumors mediated through the immune system but also as tumor growth regulators in their own right.[58]

Transforming growth factor beta

Transforming growth factor beta (TGFβ) and its receptors have been shown to be involved in the autocrine inhibition of ovarian and endometrial carcinoma cell proliferation *in vitro*[59-61] although not all cell lines were responsive. Expression of TGFβ and its receptors in ovarian tumors has been documented in a series of over 100 ovarian tumors (Bartlett, unpublished observations) showing that the majority (>85%) of ovarian tumors express TGFβ receptors with one or more isoforms of TGFβ being present in over 50% of tumors. Although there are few data available at present, it would appear that TGFβ may also play a role in the regulation of tumor growth by acting directly on tumor cells. ·

Oncogenes related to receptor signaling

Amplified expression of a number of transcription factors and oncogenes have been described in both endometrial and ovarian tumor cell lines and primary tumors. Transcription factors such as fos and jun together with regulatory factors such as myc and myb have been shown to be overexpressed in cell lines and primary tumors.[28,38,62] All of these oncogenes have been implicated in the signal transduction pathway initiated by EGF receptors (see above). The importance of events, such as myc overexpression leading to apoptosis and modification of transcription factors such as jun and fos to tumor progression have been widely discussed. It is of interest that modification of other oncogenes are now seen to impact on these important events also.[4,5]

The best example of this fact involves the *p21 ras* oncogene which appears central to many signaling pathways involving receptor tyrosine kinases. Ras transformation of cells is closely linked with receptor tyrosine kinase signaling.[63,64] Mutations in both *Ha-ras* and *K-ras* have been identified in ovarian and endometrial tumors[65] with overexpression of *p21 ras* being observed also in cervical carcinomas.[66] *K-ras* mutations have been associated with severity of disease in ovarian cancer, with higher frequencies of *K-ras* mutations seen in mucinous as opposed to serous carcinomas,[67] and in endometrial cancer where *K-ras* mutations may confer a worse prognosis.[68] The frequent association of oncogenic proteins with central events in cellular signaling underlines the importance of these mechanisms to the control of normal cellular function and the damaging effects of changes in these signaling pathways.

Conclusion

Aberrant expression or function of growth factors, their receptors or proteins involved in signal transduction are clearly events of central importance in a wide range of cancers. As our understanding of growth factor function grows so does the potential number of oncogenic events we can envisage. Although some areas relating to these events are relatively well understood there remain large areas about which we know virtually nothing. Despite this lack of knowledge it is already clear that even within single tumor types a multiplicity of aberrant signals may exist mediated by overexpression of growth factors or their receptors, dysfunction of receptor kinases and signaling pathways.

FUTURE PERSPECTIVES

The challenge ahead is clearly twofold, first, to initiate a systematic and comprehensive evaluation of tumor growth control, and secondly to exploit these controls as therapeutic targets and to provide new treatments for those with cancer. We are now in a position to relate the expression of particular oncogenes to their normal cellular function and to understand, at least in part, how their aberrant expression may lead to loss of normal control of cellular proliferation and function. Such opportunities will increase as our knowledge of the mechanisms by which such growth factors act continues to grow.

The second challenge which we are increasingly equipped to meet is that of exploiting the knowledge gained to develop novel therapies specifically directed against oncogenic events. An understanding of the way in which transformation is mediated facilitates rational investigation of mechanisms by which transformed cells can be targeted. Considerable progress has already been made in the investigation of a number of mechanisms directed at specific growth factor receptors. Such approaches have included antibody mediated blockade of the extracellular signal, intracellular inhibition of cell signaling and molecular intervention aimed at preventing growth factor expression.

Research into potential gene therapy is well established and the cellular mechanisms discussed in this chapter represent potential targets.[69-73]

SUMMARY

- Growth factors and their receptor signaling pathways regulate a complex system of cellular functions in both normal and transformed tissues.
- Oncogenic events frequently represent aberrations in growth factor receptors or receptor signaling pathways.
- A clear understanding of the physiological role of oncogenes and their cellular homologs in these processes is emerging in the current literature.
- Multiple oncogenic events are involved in proliferation and progression of most tumor types.
- Despite an increasing understanding of these mechanisms much remains to be done to clarify the relative importance of individual growth factors/ oncogenes in tumor biology.
- The current understanding of oncogene and growth factor biology has identified a number of novel therapeutic approaches which may bear fruit in the near future.

REFERENCES

1. Goustin AS, Leof EB, Shipley GD, Moses HL. Growth factors and cancer. *Cancer Res* 1986 **46**: 1015–1029.
2. Pawson T, Hunter T. Oncogenes and cell proliferation. Editorial overview: Signal transduction and growth control in normal and cancer cells. *Curr Opin Genet Dev* 1994 **4**: 1–4.
3. Carbone DP, Minna JD. Antioncogenes and human cancer. *Annu Rev Med* 1993 **44**: 431–464.
4. Hinds PW, Weinberg RA. Tumor suppressor genes. *Curr Opin Genet Dev* 1994 **4**: 135–141.
5. Harrington EA, Fanidi A, Evan GI. Oncogenes and cell death. *Curr Opin Genet Dev* 1994 **4**: 120–129.
6. Watson S, Arkinstall S. *The G-protein Linked Receptor Factsbook*. London: Academic Press, 1993.
7. Birnbaumer L, Birnbaumer M. Signal transduction by G proteins: 1994 edition *J Recept Signal Transduct Res* 1995 **15**: 213–252.
8. Cantley LC, Auger KR, Carpenter C *et al*. Oncogenes and signal transduction. *Cell* 1991 **64**: 281–302.
9. Roberts AB, Flanders KC, Heine UI *et al*. Transforming growth factor-beta: multifunctional regulator of differentiation and development. *Philos Trans R Soc Lond Biol* 1990 **327**: 145–154.
10. Kazlaukas A. Receptor tyrosine kinases and their targets. *Curr Opin Genet Dev* 1994 **4**: 5–14.
11. Rodrigues GA, Park M. Oncogenic activation of tyrosine kinases. *Curr Opin Genet Dev* 1994 **4**: 15–24.
12. SanchezMargalet V, Zoratti R, Sung CK. Insulin-like growth factor-1 stimulation of cells induces formation of complexes containing phosphatidylinositol-3-kinase, guanosine triphosphatase-activating protein (GAP), and p62 GAP-associated protein. *Endocrinology* 1995 **136**: 316–321.
13. Werner H, LeRoith D. Insulin-like growth factor I receptor: structure, signal transduction, and function. *Diabet Rev* 1995 **3**: 28–37.
14. Erpel T, Courtneidge SA. Src family protein tyrosine kinases and cellular signal transduction pathways. *Curr Opin Cell Biol* 1995 **7**: 176–182.
15. McCormick F. Activators and effectors of ras p21 protein. *Curr Opin Genet Dev* 1994 **4**: 71–76.
16. McCormick F. How receptors turn ras on. *Nature* 1993 **363**: 15–16.
17. Diakonova M, Payrastre B, Van Velzen AG, Hage WJ, Van Bergen en Henegouwen PMP, Boonstra J *et al*. Epidermal growth factor induces rapid and transient association of phospholipase C-gamma 1 with EGF-receptor and filamentous actin at membrane ruffles of A431 cells. *J Cell Sci* 1995 **108**: 2499–2509.
18. Kolch W, Heidecker G, Kochs G, Hummel R *et al*. Protein kinase Calpha activates RAF-1 by direct phosphorylation. *Nature* 1993 **364**: 249–252.
19. Chen F, Weinberg RA. Biochemical evidence for the autophosphorylation and transphosphorylation of transforming growth factor beta receptor kinases. *Proc Natl Acad Sci USA* 1995 **92**: 1565–1569.
20. Chen RH, Moses HL, Maruoka EM, Derynck R, Kawabata M. Phosphorylation-dependent interaction of the cytoplasmic domains of the type I and type II transforming growth factor-beta receptors. *J Biol Chem* 1995 **270**: 12235–12241.
21. Franzen P, Heldin CH, Miyazono K. The GS domain of the transforming growth factor-beta type I receptor is important in signal transduction. *Biochem Biophys Res Commun* 1995 **207**: 682–689.
22. Halstead J, Kemp K, Ignotz RA. Evidence for involvement of phosphatidylcholine-phospholipase C and protein kinase C in transforming growth factor-beta signaling. *J Biol Chem* 1995 **270**: 13600–13603.
23. Lin HY, Moustakas A, Knaus, P, Wells RG, Henis YI, Lodish HF. The soluble exoplasmic domain of the type II transforming growth factor (TGF)-beta receptor. A heterogeneously glycosylated protein with high affinity and selectivity for TGF-beta ligands. *J Biol Chem* 1995 **270**: 2747–2754.
24. Bacus SS, Huberman E, Chin D *et al*. A ligand for the erbb-2 oncogene product (gp30) induces differentiation of human breast-cancer cells. *Cell Growth Diff* 1992 **3**: 401–411.
25. Di Fiore PP, Kraus MH. Mechanisms involving an expanding erbB/EGF receptor family of tyrosine kinases in human neoplasia. *Cancer Treat Res* 1992 **61**: 139–160.
26. Klijn JGM, Berns PMJJ, Schmitz PIM, Foekens JA. The clinical significance of epidermal growth-factor receptor (egf-r) in human breast cancer – a review on 5232 patients. *Endocr Rev* 1992 **13**: 3–17.
27. Miyazawa K. Role of epidermal growth factor in obstetrics and gynecology. *Obstet Gynecol* 1992 **79**: 1032–1040.
28. Gurpide E. Endometrial cancer: biochemical and clinical correlates. *J Natl Cancer Inst* 1991 **83**: 405–416.
29. Wiener JR, Berchuck A, Bast RJ. Biology and therapy with biologic agents in gynecologic cancer. *Curr Opin Oncol* 1992 **4**: 946–954.
30. Simpson BJB, Phillips HA, Lessells AM, Langdon SP, Miller WR. C-erbB growth-factor-receptor proteins in ovarian tumours. *Int J Cancer* 1995 **64**: 202–206.
31. Bast RCJ, Boyer CM, Jacobs I *et al*. Cell growth regulation in epithelial ovarian cancer. *Cancer* 1993 **71**: 1597–1601.
32. Stromberg K, Collins TJ, Gordon AW, Jackson CL, Johnson GR. Transforming growth factor-alpha acts as an autocrine growth-factor in ovarian-carcinoma cell-lines. *Cancer Res* 1992 **52**: 341–347.
33. Crew AJ, Langdon SP, Miller EP, Miller WR. Mitogenic effects of epidermal growth-factor and transforming growth factor-alpha on egf-receptor positive human ovarian carcinoma cell-lines. *Eur J Cancer* 1992 **28**: 337–341.
34. Morishige KI, Kurachi H, Amemiya K *et al*. Evidence for the involvement of transforming growth factor-alpha and epidermal growth-factor receptor autocrine growth-mecha-

nism in primary human ovarian cancers *in vitro. Cancer Res* 1991 **51**: 5322–5328.

35. Bauknecht T, Angel P, Kohler M *et al.* Gene structure and expression analysis of the epidermal growth factor receptor, transforming growth factor-alpha, myc, jun, and metallothionein in human ovarian carcinomas. Classification of malignant phenotypes. *Cancer* 1993 **71**: 419–429.

36. Leake RE, Owens O. The prognostic value of steroid receptors, growth factors and growth factor receptors in ovarian cancer. In Sharp F, Mason WP, Leake RE (eds) *Ovarian Cancer Biological and Therapeutic Challenges,* Vol. 1. London: Chapman and Hall Medical, 1990: 69–75.

37. Owens OJ, Leake RE. Growth factor content in normal and benign ovarian tumours. *Eur J Obstet Gynecol Reprod Biol* 1992 **47**: 223–228.

38. Berchuck A, Kohler MF, Boente MP, Rodriguez GC, Whitaker RS, Bast RJ. Growth regulation and transformation of ovarian epithelium. *Cancer* 1993 **71**: 545–551.

39. Kihana T, Tsuda H, Teshima S *et al.* Prognostic significance of the overexpression of c-erbB-2 protein in adenocarcinoma of the uterine cervix. *Cancer* 1994 **73**: 148–153.

40. Wang D, Konishi I, Koshiyama M *et al.* Expression of c-erbB 2 protein and epidermal growth receptor in endometrial carcinomas. Correlation with clinicopathologic and sex steroid receptor status. *Cancer* 1993 **72**: 2628–2637.

41. Hale RJ, Buckley CH, Gullick WJ, Fox H, Williams J, Wilcox FL. Prognostic value of epidermal growth factor receptor expression in cervical carcinoma. *J Clin Pathol* 1993 **46**: 149–153.

42. Chapman WB, Lorincz AT, Willett GD, Wright VC, Kurman RJ. Epidermal growth factor receptor expression and the presence of human papillomavirus in cervical squamous intraepithelial lesions. *Int J Gynecol Pathol* 1992 **11**: 221–226.

43. Meden H, Marx D, Rath W, Kuhn W, Hinney B, Schauer A. (Overexpression of c-erbB-2 oncogene in primary ovarian cancers: incidence and prognostic significance in 243 patients). *Geburtshilfe Frauenheilkd* 1992 **52**: 667–673.

44. Hancock MC, Langton BC, Chan T *et al.* A monoclonal-antibody against the c-erbb-2 protein enhances the cytotoxicity of *cis*-diamminedichloroplatinum against human breast and ovarian tumor-cell lines. *Cancer Res* 1991 **51**: 4575–4580.

45. Yee D, Morales FR, Hamilton TC, Vonhoff DD. Expression of insulin-like growth factor-i, its binding-proteins, and its receptor in ovarian cancer. *Cancer Res* 1991 **51**: 5107–5112.

46. Nagamani M, Stuart CA, Dunhardt PA, Doherty MG. Specific binding sites for insulin and insulin-like growth factor I in human endometrial cancer. *Am J Obstet Gynecol* 1991 **165**: 1865–1871.

47. Berns EM, Klijn JG, Henzen LSC, Rodenburg CJ, van dBME, Foekens JA. Receptors for hormones and growth factors and (onco)-gene amplification in human ovarian cancer. *Int J Cancer* 1992 **52**: 218–224.

48. Beck EP, Russo P, Gliozzo B, Jaeger W, Papa V, Wildt L *et al.* Identification of insulin and insulin-like growth factor I (IGF I) receptors in ovarian cancer tissue. *Gynecol Oncol* 1994 **53**: 196–201.

49. Van Dam PA, Vergote IB, Lowe DG, Watson JV, Van Damme P, Van der Auwera JC *et al.* Expression of c-erbB-2, c-myc, and c-ras oncoproteins, insulin-like growth factor receptor I, and epidermal growth factor receptor in ovarian carcinoma. *J Clin Pathol* 1994 **47**: 914–919.

50. Kacinski BM. CSF-1 and its receptor in ovarian, endometrial and breast cancer. *Ann Med* 1995 **27**: 79–85.

51. Henriksen R, Funa K, Wilander E, Backstrom T, Ridderheim M, Oberg K. Expression and prognostic significance of platelet-derived growth factor and its receptors in epithelial ovarian neoplasms. *Cancer Res* 1993 **53**: 4550–4554.

52. Baiocchi G, Kavanagh JJ, Talpaz M, Wharton JT, Gutterman JU, Kurzrock R. Expression of the macrophage colony-stimulating factor and its receptor in gynecologic malignancies. *Cancer* 1991 **67**: 990–996.

53. Xu FJ, Ramakrishnan S, Daly L *et al.* Increased serum levels of macrophage colony-stimulating factor in ovarian cancer. *Am J Obstet Gynecol* 1991 **165**: 1356–1362.

54. Elg SA, Yu Y, Carson LF *et al.* Serum levels of macrophage colony-stimulating factor in patients with ovarian cancer undergoing second-look laparotomy. *Am J Obstet Gynecol* 1992 **166**: 134–137.

55. Rosen A, Sevelda P, Klein M *et al.* First experience with FGF-3 (INT-2) amplification in women with epithelial ovarian cancer. *Br J Cancer* 1993 **67**: 1122–1125.

56. Wu S, Boyer CM, Whitaker RS *et al.* Tumor necrosis factor alpha as an autocrine and paracrine growth factor for ovarian cancer: monokine induction of tumor cell proliferation and tumor necrosis factor alpha expression. *Cancer Res* 1993 **53**: 1939–1944.

57. Balkwill FR. Tumour necrosis factor. *Br Med Bull* 1989 **454**: 389–400.

58. Owens OJ, Taggart C, Wilson R, Walker JJ, McKillop JH, Kennedy JH. Interleukin-2 receptor and ovarian cancer. *Br J Cancer* 1993 **68**: 364–367.

59. Havrilesky LJ, Hurteau JA, Whitaker RS, Elbendary A, Wu S, Rodriguez GC *et al.* Regulation of apoptosis in normal and malignant ovarian epithelial cells by transforming growth factor beta. *Cancer Res* 1995 **55**: 944–948.

60. Bartlett JMS, Rabiasz GJ, Scott WN, Langdon SP, Smyth JF, Miller WR. Transforming growth-factor-beta messenger-RNA expression and growth-control of human ovarian-carcinoma cells. *Br J Cancer* 1992 **65**: 655–660.

61. Sakata M, Kurachi H, Ikegami H *et al.* Autocrine growth mechanism by transforming growth factor (TGF)-beta 1 and TGF-beta 1-receptor regulation by epidermal growth factor in a human endometrial cancer cell line IK-90. *Int J Cancer* 1993 **54**: 862–867.

62. Levine AJ, Broach JR. Oncogenes and cell proliferation. *Curr Opin Genet Dev* 1995 **5**: 1–4.

63. Chiao PJ, Kannan P, Yim SO *et al.* Susceptibility to *ras* oncogene transformation is coregulated with signal transduction through growth factor receptors. *Oncogene* 1991 **6**: 713–720.

64. Chien C, Chen F. Estrogen and growth-factors regulation of c-myc and c-fos expression in human ovarian-cancer. *Am J Hum Genet* 1991 **49**: 425.

65. Teneriello MG, Ebina M, Linnoila RI *et al. p53* and *Ki-ras* gene mutations in epithelial ovarian neoplasms. *Cancer Res* 1993 **53**: 3103–3108.

66. Hayashi Y, Hachisuga T, Iwasaka T *et al.* Expression of *ras* oncogene product and EGF receptor in cervical squamous cell carcinomas and its relationship to lymph node involvement. *Gynecol Oncol* 1991 **40**: 147–151.

67. Ichikawa Y, Nishida M, Suzuki H *et al.* Mutation of *K-ras* protooncogene is associated with histological subtypes in human mucinous ovarian tumors. *Cancer Res* 1994 **54**: 33–35.

68. Mizuuchi H, Nasim S, Kudo R, Silverberg SG, Greenhouse S, Garrett CT. Clinical implications of *K-ras* mutations in malignant epithelial tumors of the endometrium. *Cancer Res* 1992 **52**: 2777–2781.

69. Workman P, D'Incalci M, Berdel WE *et al.* New approaches in cancer pharmacology: drug design and development. *Eur J Cancer* 1992 **28A**: 1190–1200.

70. Calabretta B, Skorski T, Szczylik C, Zon G. Prospect for gene-directed therapy with antisense oligodeoxynucleotides. *Cancer Treat Rev* 1993 **19**: 169–179.

71. Neckers L, Whitesell L. Antisense technology: biological utility and practical considerations. *Am J Physiol* 1993 **265**: L1–L12.

72. Hung MC, Matin A, Zhang Y, Xing X, Sorgi F, Huang L *et al.* HER-2/neu-targeting gene therapy – a review. *Gene* 1995 **159**: 65–71.

73. Helm CW, Shrestha K, Thomas S, Shingleton HM, Miller DM. A unique c-myc-targeted triplex-forming oligonucleotide inhibits the growth of ovarian and cervical carcinomas *in vitro. Gynecol Oncol* 1993 **49**: 339–343.

4.7

Pathology of Gestational Trophoblastic Disease

H Fox

INTRODUCTION

The term 'gestational trophoblastic disease' could, in theory, be applied to any abnormality of the trophoblast but is, by convention, restricted to a small number of conditions, the classification of which is given in Table 4.7.1. This classification is based principally on morphology but, perhaps somewhat illogically, includes one non-morphological component, namely 'persistent trophoblastic disease'; this term is applied to a biochemical abnormality, i.e. an elevated level of human chorionic gonadotrophin (HCG) following a molar pregnancy, and this diagnosis not only lacks any specific morphological connotation but becomes invalid if a morphological diagnosis is achieved.

The term 'gestational trophoblastic neoplasia' is sometimes used as an alternative to gestational trophoblastic disease and indeed many seem to feel, often at a subliminal level, that these various conditions represent a neoplastic spectrum, with moles at the benign end of this spectrum, choriocarcinoma at the malignant extreme and invasive hydatidiform mole being equivalent to a neoplasm of borderline malignancy. This is a totally misleading approach for there is nothing to suggest that a hydatidiform mole, of any type, is a form of neoplasia; it is, without question, a specific form of abortion. A choriocarcinoma is usually considered to be neoplastic but, as will be discussed later, even this may be no more than an unusual type of abortus in some cases and the only undoubtedly neoplastic entity

Table 4.7.1 Classification of gestational trophoblastic disease

Hydatidiform mole
  Complete
  Partial
Invasive hydatidiform mole
Persistent trophoblastic disease
Choriocarcinoma
Placental site trophoblastic tumor

within this group of conditions is the placental site trophoblastic tumor.

CURRENT CONCEPTS

Hydatidiform moles

During the last few decades molar disease has been divided into complete and partial hydatidiform moles, the distinction between these two entities being based on their differing morphological and cytogenetic features.[1-3] The later application to moles of such techniques as flow cytometry and DNA fingerprinting, although largely confirming the existence of two differing types of molar pregnancy, has, however, tended to blur somewhat the sharpness of the distinction between the two forms.

Epidemiology

There is a striking geographic variation in the incidence of molar disease[4,5] with it generally being thought that the incidence of hydatidiform moles is much higher in Asia, Latin America and Africa than in Europe and North America. The degree of this difference is, however, difficult to estimate because of the serious flaws that have characterized all but the most recent of epidemiological studies of molar pregnancies. Nevertheless it is now clear that molar gestations occur four times more frequently in Japan[6] and in the United Arab Emirates[7] than in the United Kingdom.[8] The reasons for this geographic variation remain, however, obscure. Molar disease tends to occur most frequently at the extremes of a woman's reproductive life and therefore populations in which pregnancy occurs at an early age and in which child-bearing continues until late in life would be expected to have a higher incidence of molar disease than those in which pregnancies usually occur within a more restricted age range. This could explain some of the observed regional differences but certainly not all and attempts to define an ethnic, nutritional or socioeconomic basis for this variability have not met with success.[5]

Morphology

A complete mole is characterized by diffuse vesicular change which involves, to a greater or lesser degree, the entire villous population, thus producing the classical 'bunch of grapes' appearance. The mass of villous tissue is markedly increased, to the extent that an *in situ* mole can fill or even distend the uterus (Fig. 4.7.1), with neither a remnant of a normal placental shape discernible nor a fetus nor gestational sac present. Histological examination confirms that all the villi are swollen and edematous, some very markedly so but others only minimally (Fig. 4.7.2); central cistern formation is common. It is usually maintained that trophoblastic hyperplasia is a characteristic feature of a complete mole but, in reality, the degree of trophoblastic proliferation in such lesions is often no greater, and sometimes less, than that seen in the normal first trimester placenta. It is the pattern, rather than the degree, of trophoblastic proliferation which is abnormal in a complete mole; whereas in a normal pregnancy trophoblast proliferates along one side or at one pole of a villus in a complete mole the villous trophoblastic proliferation is

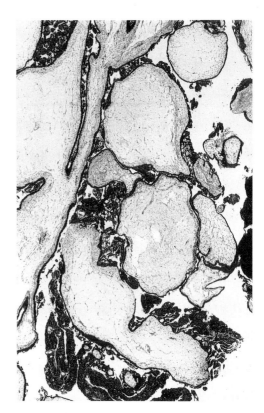

Fig. 4.7.2 *Complete hydatidiform mole. The villi are distended and there is atypical trophoblastic proliferation. From* Textbook of Gynecologic Oncology *by GRP Blackledge, JA Jordan and HM Shingleton.*

either circumferential or multifocal. A moderate degree of nuclear atypia is commonly present in molar trophoblast though this is often no more marked than that seen in the trophoblast of placentae from normal first trimester pregnancies. Because of the use of ultrasound, anembryonic gestations and hence molar pregnancies, are now being diagnosed at an earlier stage of gestation than in the past: in these early lesions the classical gross appearances of a complete mole may not be apparent and in such cases the abnormal pattern of trophoblastic proliferation becomes the key factor in the recognition of a molar pregnancy.

A partial mole differs in numerous respects from a complete mole: it is commonly associated with a fetus, retains a placental shape and does not have an increased villous mass. Only a proportion of the villi show gross vesicular change, these being scattered within normal placental tissue. Histologically (Fig. 4.7.3) the presence of both edematous swollen villi and villi of normal size, albeit often with an unusually fibrotic or cellular stroma, is confirmed. The vesicular villi commonly have a very irregular, scalloped outline, this resulting in the 'Norwegian fjord' appearance: cutting of some of these deep indentations in cross-section results in the presence of so-called 'trophoblastic inclusions' within the villous stroma. There is abnormal trophoblastic proliferation, which, as with com-

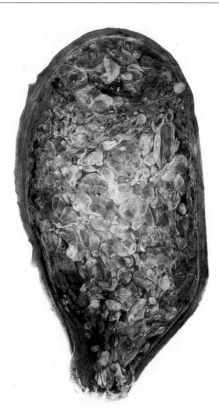

Fig. 4.7.1 *A complete hydatidiform mole which is distending the uterus. There is diffuse villous vesicular change. From* Textbook of Gynecologic Oncology *by GRP Blackledge, JA Jordan and HM Shingleton.*

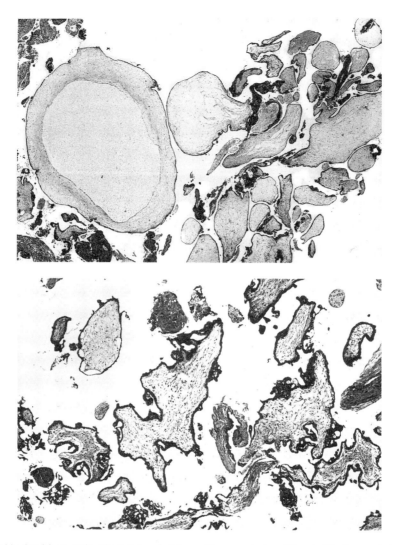

Fig. 4.7.3 Upper: *partial hydatidiform mole. There is an admixture of large vesicular villi and villi of normal size.* **Lower:** *partial hyda-tidiform mole. The villi are of markedly irregular outline: there is an atypical pattern of trophoblastic proliferation. From* Textbook of Gynecologic Oncology *by GPR Blackledge, JA Jordan and HM Shingleton.*

plete moles, is usually either circumferential or multifocal; the degree of trophoblastic proliferation is usually not only less than that seen in complete moles but is less than that encountered in normal first trimester placentae. The villous trophoblast frequently has a somewhat vacuolated, or 'lacy', appearance. It is often maintained that partial moles are characterized by 'syncytiotrophoblastic hyperplasia' but it is, of course, quite impossible for the villous syncytiotrophoblast to be hyperplastic for this is a postmitotic, terminally differentiated tissue which is incapable of DNA synthesis and cell division. It should be noted that the use of the word 'partial' to describe a mole does not mean that one portion of the placenta is normal and another portion molar. This latter situation is encountered if a complete mole is part of a dizygotic twin pregnancy and associated with a normal twin;[9] in such pregnancies one placenta is molar and the other non-molar. In a true partial mole there is an intermingling of molar and non-

molar villi with the molar villi distributed throughout the entire placenta.

Cytogenetics

It has been recognized for some time that complete moles are androgenetic, i.e. all their nuclear DNA is paternally derived;[10] furthermore, approximately 95% of complete moles have a 46XX chromosomal constitution the remainder having a 46XY karotype.[2] Banding studies have shown that the vast majority of 46XX complete moles are derived from a single sperm (monospermic or homozygous moles) whereas all 46XY moles and a small minority of 46XX moles are derived from two sperms (dispermic or heterozygous moles). A hypothetical model has been proposed to explain these findings, namely that homozygous moles are due to fertilization of a 'dead' ovum (i.e. one containing no viable genomic material) by a single haploid sperm which then undergoes endoreduplication of its genetic material without cell division[11] and that heterozygous moles result from entry into a 'dead' ovum of two haploid sperms which then fuse and replicate.[12] It has to be stressed that this concept is purely theoretical and that the true nature of a 'dead' ovum has never been determined and, indeed, such an ovum has never been identified.

Partial moles contain both paternal and maternal genomic material, and the vast majority are chromosomally triploid, usually 69XXY but sometimes 69XXX or 69XYY.[13] It is of course known that not all triploid gestations are associated with molar change in the placenta and it is now clear that if the extra chromosomal load is of paternal origin a partial mole will result whereas if the extra chromosomal content is contributed from the mother a non-molar placenta will develop.[14] It is thought that paternally derived triploidy is usually the result of two haploid sperms fertilizing a haploid ovum but that a few cases may be due to fertilization of a haploid ovum by a diploid 46XX sperm.

This relatively simple subdivision into androgenetic diploid complete moles and biparentally derived triploid partial moles is not, however, the whole story. Cytogenetic studies have yielded a few instances of triploid and tetraploid complete moles and of diploid and tetraploid partial moles.[15–18] Further, flow cytometric studies, although in general confirming that most complete moles are diploid and most partial moles triploid, have nevertheless rather consistently revealed small subpopulations of diploid partial moles and triploid complete moles.[19–22] To complicate the matter still further there have been very occasional instances of androgenetic partial moles and biparentally derived complete moles[17] entities for which there is, at the moment, no very plausible explanation.

It should be noted that these anomalies have been detected in moles for which a rigorous morphological diagnosis had been made. Triploid complete moles may well be due to three haploid sperms entering a 'dead' ovum but many of the reported diploid partial moles have, in reality, been examples of a complete mole with an accompanying concomitant non-molar twin pregnancy; nevertheless, a distinct entity of diploid partial mole does exist which, it has been suggested, merits consideration as a separate third type of molar pregnancy,[23] such cases possibly being a result of uniparental disomy. The fact that not all molar gestations fit neatly into a rigid classification raises the question as to how the different varieties of mole should be defined; should the diagnosis rest on the morphological findings or upon the cytogenetic data or, alternatively, is there any point to be served in trying to differentiate these two forms of molar disease and should a pregnancy simply be considered as molar or non-molar?

The cytogenetic findings in molar pregnancy suggest strongly that paternal genes play a dominant role in placental development and growth and that maternal genes largely exert their influence on fetal development: this differential function of paternal and maternal genes has been confirmed by experimental animal studies[24,25] and is an excellent example of the phenomenon of genomic imprinting.

Postmolar disease

In the United Kingdom about 8% of patients who have had a complete mole will develop persistent trophoblastic disease:[8,26] the figure in the United States is rather higher because of the use of different diagnostic criteria. The actual cause of persistent trophoblastic disease is generally unknown. There may have been incomplete removal of the mole but it is equally possible that many of these cases are invasive hydatidiform moles with residual invasive molar tissue within the myometrium or its vasculature; it is also possible that some are early cases of choriocarcinoma. It is thought that the risk of development of a clinically overt choriocarcinoma following a complete mole is in the region of 5%.

The incidence of persistent trophoblastic disease following a partial mole has been much disputed but there is now no doubt that it occurs, though the magnitude of the risk is very much lower than is that for complete moles.[27–30] The eventual risk of choriocarcinoma in patients with partial moles is also unknown: choriocarcinomas have been reported following partial moles[27,31,32] but this, in itself, does not necessarily mean that this condition increases the risk of a choriocarcinoma for this can follow a normal pregnancy.

Prognostic factors

As it is widely agreed that all women who have had a molar pregnancy should enter a follow-up surveillance program there is no practical point in attempting to define those cases at most risk of developing postmolar disease. Nevertheless, from a purely theoretical viewpoint it is of interest to consider if a high-risk group can be defined. It was at one time considered that the risk of eventual postmolar disease was directly related to the degree of trophoblastic proliferation in the mole[33] but this has proved not to be the case[34,35] and 'grading' of moles in terms of their degree of trophoblastic proliferation has now been abandoned. Attempts to forecast those cases at greatest risk for postmolar disease by the use of cell proliferation markers and flow cytometry[36–38] have failed but it has been maintained that heterozygous (dispermic) moles have a much higher risk of subsequent postmolar complications than do homozygous (monospermic) moles.[39] Doubts have, however, been cast upon this claim by the failure to find any association between the presence of a Y chromosome, detected by the polymerase chain reaction, in a mole and an excess incidence of postmolar disease.[40]

Invasive hydatidiform mole

An invasive hydatidiform mole is one which penetrates into the myometrium or invades the uterine vasculature. A deeply invasive mole usually becomes clinically evident several weeks after apparently complete evacuation of a mole from the uterus, the patient usually presenting with hemorrhage. If a hysterectomy is performed at this stage the appearances range from at one extreme, only a small hemorrhagic focus in the myometrium to, at the other end of the spectrum, a large deeply cavitating hemorrhagic lesion of the uterine wall (Fig. 4.7.4) which mimics a choriocarcinoma. Rarely, a mole does penetrate the full thickness of the myometrium, leading either to uterine perforation or to extension of the mole into adjacent structures, such as the broad ligament. The histological distinction from a choriocarcinoma is dependent on the finding of molar villi within the uterine wall, these more commonly being seen in the myometrial vascular channels than between the myometrial fibers. The molar villi show a very variable degree of trophoblastic proliferation and sometimes this is far from being a conspicuous feature.

Invasive moles have, in the past, caused death from uterine bleeding or perforation but their mortality rate is now virtually zero because of the success achieved in their treatment by a limited course of chemotherapy. In fact the

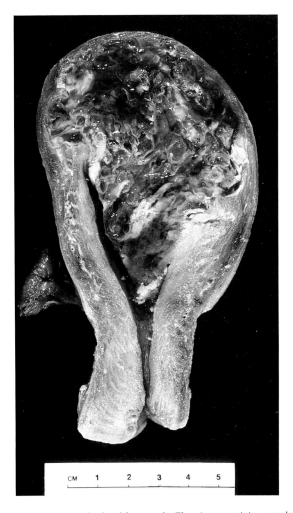

Fig. 4.7.4 *Invasive hydatidiform mole. The uterus contains a mole which is invading deeply into the myometrium. (Courtesy of Professor D. O'B. Hourihane, Dublin.) From* Textbook of Gynecologic Oncology *by GRP Blackledge, JA Jordan and HM Shingleton.*

diagnosis of an invasive mole, which can only be made with certainty on a hysterectomy specimen, is now almost obsolete because nearly all invasive moles are subsumed into the category of persistent trophoblastic disease.

It has to be stressed that the invasive capacity of some moles is not an indication that they are neoplastic. Normal trophoblast has the ability to invade both the myometrium and the uterine vessels[41,42] whereas villi from a normal placenta can invade deeply into, or even through, the uterine wall to give rise to a placenta increta or a placenta percreta,[43] both of which are the exact non-molar equivalents of an invasive mole.[44]

Molar tissue can be transported via the bloodstream to extrauterine sites, particularly to the vagina and lungs. The transported molar trophoblast can then grow in these sites to form nodules that are either clinically or radiologically detectable. The development of 'metastatic' lesions implies that molar trophoblast has entered the uterine vessels and hence their presence is taken as *de facto* evidence of the presence of an invasive mole; the 'metastatic' nodules are not, however, usually associated with evidence of molar invasion of the myometrial tissues.

The 'metastatic' nodules usually appear several weeks after evacuation of a mole from the uterus but may occur concurrently with a mole or can be the presenting symptom of such a lesion. Vaginal lesions form hemorrhagic submucous nodules, the true nature of which only becomes apparent when microscopy reveals the presence of villous structures,[45] a finding which rules out a diagnosis of choriocarcinoma. Pulmonary lesions can cause hemoptysis but are usually an asymptomatic radiological finding, and histological examination of these lesions will also reveal their content of villi.[46,47] These extrauterine lesions may resolve spontaneously but are commonly treated with limited chemotherapy which achieves excellent results.

The fact that molar trophoblast is transported to extrauterine sites is not an indication of neoplastic behavior. Trophoblast enters the maternal bloodstream in every normal pregnancy[48] and is transported to sites such as the lung.[49] This transported trophoblast only gives rise to detectable lesions if it is molar in nature.

Choriocarcinoma

Approximately 50% of choriocarcinomas follow a molar pregnancy, 30% occur after an abortion and 20% follow an apparently normal gestation. The time interval between the antecedent pregnancy and the clinical presentation of a choriocarcinoma is very variable, ranging from a few weeks or months to 15 years.

The variation in the incidence of choriocarcinoma is at least as great as that for molar disease with those geographic areas having a high incidence of hydatidiform moles also having a high incidence of choriocarcinoma. However, whether the excess of choriocarcinoma in these regions is simply a reflection of the high incidence of moles or whether it indicates that the same factors which predispose to a molar gestation also predispose to choriocarcinoma is a moot point.

Morphology

Within the uterus a choriocarcinoma forms single or multiple hemorrhagic nodules which are often accompanied by local metastases to the cervix and vagina. The neoplastic masses consist of a central area of hemorrhagic necrosis and, usually though not invariably, a peripheral rim of viable tumor tissue. The central, sometimes complete, necrosis of the neoplastic tissue is a reflection of the fact that a choriocarcinoma has no intrinsic blood supply, relying for its oxygenation on its ability to invade the uterine blood vessels: it is therefore only the growing edge of the tumor which is adequately oxygenated, the remainder undergoing ischemic necrosis.

Histologically, a choriocarcinoma has a biphasic structure that recapitulates, often to a striking degree, that of the trophoblast of the normal implanting blastocyst, central sheets or cores of cytotrophoblast being 'capped' by a peripheral rim of syncytiotrophoblast (Fig. 4.7.5). The trophoblastic cells in a choriocarcinoma commonly show no greater degree of atypia and mitotic activity than is seen in an implanting blastocyst. Villi are never present in an extraplacental choriocarcinoma and, indeed, the presence of villous structures negates a diagnosis of choriocarcinoma.

Because of the need to obtain an oxygen supply a choriocarcinoma is avariciously invasive of vascular chan-

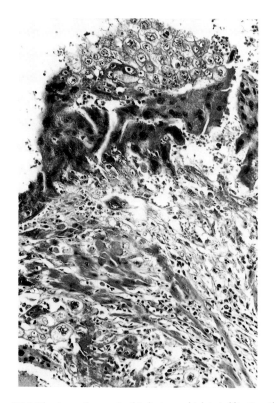

Fig. 4.7.5 *Choriocarcinoma. In this lesion, which is infiltrating the myometrium, the biphasic differentiation into cytotrophoblast and syncytiotrophoblast is clearly apparent. From* Textbook of Gynecologic Oncology *by GRP Blackledge, JA Jordan and HM Shingleton.*

nels in the myometrium, vessels which, it should be noted, are also invaded by trophoblast during the process of normal implantation. The tumor cells tend to form solid plugs within the myometrial vasculature and, although there is often extravascular extension, the malignant trophoblast tends to infiltrate between the muscle fibers with very little tissue destruction. The propensity for vascular invasion is the basis for the predominantly hematogenous dissemination of a choriocarcinoma to sites such as the lungs, brain, liver, kidney and gastrointestinal tract: large tumor emboli may impact within the pulmonary arteries. Lymph node deposits of a choriocarcinoma are usually tertiary metastases from a large extrauterine lesion.

Origin

There are many puzzling aspects of choriocarcinoma such as their status as an allograft (which they must be because of their content of paternal antigens), their increased frequency in women of blood groups A with group O spouses and in group O women with group A spouses[50–52] and their rather strange, almost bizarre, epidemiological risk factors, which include dieting, a family history of dizygotic twins, more than one marriage and infrequent sexual intercourse:[53] by far the most perplexing problem they pose is, however, their origin. As already remarked choriocarcinomas may follow either a normal or a molar pregnancy, more commonly the latter, and there is a considerable gap in our knowledge as to the relationship between the previous pregnancy and the subsequent choriocarcinoma. Is the neoplasm actually derived from the trophoblast of the prior pregnancy and, if so, what has been happening to this trophoblast during the intervening months or years? The application of genetic techniques, such as the study of cytogenetic polymorphism,[54] DNA restriction fragment-length polymorphism assays[55–57] or the study of tandem repeat regions amplified by the polymerase chain reaction[58] has shown that some, but by no means all, choriocarcinomas are androgenetic. It has been presumed that these androgenetic tumors were derived from a previous molar gestation despite the fact that in two such cases there had been a full-term normal delivery intervening between the molar pregnancy and the development of the choriocarcinoma.[57,58] In one of these cases the time interval between the mole and the choriocarcinoma was 10 years[57] and it is difficult to understand how tissue from the mole remained in the uterus for that length of time, and throughout a later normal pregnancy, to then subsequently undergo a neoplastic resurgence. This typifies the questions posed by this enigmatic lesion.

Some points are, however, becoming clearer. It is seeming increasingly probable that many, possibly most or even all, choriocarcinomas that follow an apparently normal pregnancy are, in reality, metastases from an undetected small intraplacental choriocarcinoma. Only a small number of intraplacental choriocarcinomas have been described[59–66] and in nearly all the choriocarcinoma was very small and easily overlooked unless the placenta was meticulously examined. In most cases the placenta had been subjected to such examination because metastases had developed in the mother during pregnancy and in only two cases had the tumor been detected in the absence of such complications.[59,63] One case[64] is of particular interest in so far as a patient developed an apparently primary choriocarcinoma soon after a normal pregnancy: re-examination of the placenta at that time revealed a tiny intraplacental choriocarcinoma. Intraplacental choriocarcinomas are histologically identical to extraplacental choriocarcinomas but are often separated from the normal villous population by villi with a surrounding mantle of choriocarcinoma-like trophoblast which has replaced the normal trophoblast. This therefore confirms the long held opinion, based largely on the ability of choriocarcinomas to secrete HCG, that a choriocarcinoma is a lesion of villous trophoblast despite the invariable absence of villi from extraplacental tumors.

If choriocarcinomas following a normal pregnancy are in reality metastases from an intraplacental choriocarcinoma, are those which follow a molar gestation similarly derived from an intramolar choriocarcinoma? This is certainly a possibility, for one such lesion has been described,[67] though it was not associated with subsequent disease. The prolonged time interval, in many cases, between a molar pregnancy and the development of an overt choriocarcinoma does, however, suggest that by no means all postmolar choriocarcinomas are derived from intramolar lesions and it is certainly conceivable that some such choriocarcinomas are new pregnancies, the choriocarcinoma *ab initio* that has long been considered as a possibility.[68] There seems no good reason why a pregnancy, androgenetic or otherwise, should not evolve directly into a choriocarcinoma and there is an excellent precedent for the belief that a pregnancy can appear to be neoplastic, namely the now generally agreed concept that a teratoma is a parthogenetic pregnancy.[69] This raises the question, however, as to whether such pregnancies should be considered as truly neoplastic or simply as aberrant gestations. It is true that they invade vessels and spread to distant sites but so does normal trophoblast. They resemble acutely the trophoblast of the normal implanting blastocyst and their response to methotrexate, although quite different from that of virtually every other neoplasm, is not unlike that of a normal, but ectopic, early gestation. This is, of course, pure speculation but nevertheless the possibility that some choriocarcinomas are simply abnormal pregnancies should not be dismissed too lightly.

Placental site trophoblastic tumor

This is an uncommon tumor that is derived from the extravillous trophoblast of the placental bed (sometimes referred to as 'intermediate trophoblast'). In the vast majority of cases the neoplasm develops after a normal pregnancy, only 5% occurring after a molar gestation.[70] Patients present at anything from a few weeks to 18 months after the antecedent pregnancy with a complaint of irregular vaginal bleeding or, perhaps more commonly, amenorrhea: a small proportion of patients develop a nephrotic syndrome which appears to be due to chronic

intravascular coagulation initiated by factors released from the tumor.[70] The uterus is commonly enlarged but a pregnancy test is positive in only one-third of patients, this reflecting the fact that the principal secretory product of extravillous trophoblast is human placental lactogen (HPL) rather than HCG.

The tumors tend to form tan, white or yellow masses within the myometrium and often protrude into the endometrial cavity, sometimes forming a polypoidal mass. Histologically, the tumor replicates, in an anarchic form, the appearances seen in the normal placental bed. The tumor is formed principally of mononuclear cytotrophoblastic cells with an irregular and inconsistent admixture of multinucleated cells, the latter resembling the multinucleated cells of the placental bed rather than true syncytiotrophoblast. The tumor cells infiltrate between, and dissect, the myometrial fibers as cords and sheets with a striking absence of necrosis and hemorrhage (Fig. 4.7.6). Invasion of vessels by tumor cells is common but the massive intravascular growth that characterizes a choriocarcinoma is not seen and some vessels within the tumor are surrounded, but not invaded, by neoplastic cells. Noninfiltrated vessels often show fibrinoid necrosis of their wall, whereas a pseudodecidual change, and sometimes an Arias–Stella reaction, may be apparent in the adjacent endometrium.

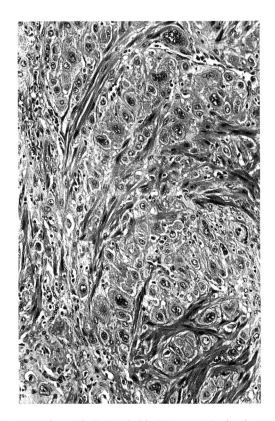

Fig. 4.7.6 *Placental site trophoblastic tumor. Cords of cytotrophoblastic cells infiltrate between the smooth muscle fibers of the myometrium. From* Textbook of Gynecologic Oncology *by GRP Blackledge, JA Jordan and HM Shingleton.*

About 15–20% of placental site trophoblastic tumors behave in a malignant fashion[71] and either recur locally or spread to such distant sites as the liver, lung and central nervous system. Assessment of the degree of malignancy of any individual neoplasm is, however, difficult for although those which have run a malignant course have usually had a high mitotic count this is not an invariable rule[72] and a low mitotic count should not necessarily engender a sense of security.

It is noteworthy that the placental site trophoblastic tumor responds very poorly to the cytotoxic drug therapy which is so successful in choriocarcinoma;[71] indeed the response to any form of chemotherapy is unsatisfactory and surgery is the basis of treatment.

Flow cytometry of placental site trophoblastic tumor has been performed only rarely but most of the tumors appear to be diploid;[73] there has been one triploid neoplasm which, very surprisingly, followed a normal term pregnancy.

KEY POINTS FOR CLINICAL PRACTICE

- Hydatidiform moles, of all types, are a form of abortion.
- Partial hydatidiform moles can be complicated by persistent trophoblastic disease and by choriocarcinoma: patients with such moles should be followed up.
- Normal trophoblasts are invasive and metastatic: invasive moles share these qualities which are not an indication of malignancy or neoplasia.
- Choriocarcinoma can be derived from a hydatidiform mole despite an intervening normal pregnancy.
- Choriocarcinoma following a normal pregnancy may be a metastasis from an unnoticed intraplacental choriocarcinoma.
- Some choriocarcinomas may be new pregnancies.
- About 15–20% of placental site trophoblastic tumors behave in a malignant fashion.
- Features suggesting that a placental site trophoblastic tumor may behave in an aggressive fashion are, a high mitotic count, deep myometrial invasion and many cells with clear cytoplasm. Tumors, however, may be malignant in the absence of any of these features.

FUTURE PERSPECTIVES

Future approaches to gestational trophoblastic disease are quite clearly defined. There is a need for epidemiological surveys which study carefully selected populations and are based on rigorous histological diagnoses in order to elucidate the true geographic variability of molar disease and to seek an explanation for such variance. Further genetic studies of moles and choriocarcinoma are required in order to define more clearly the relationship between the two forms of molar disease and between molar disease and choriocarcinoma. A definitive answer must be sought to the question of whether dispermic moles are particularly likely to be complicated by postmolar disease and there should be a more vigorous search for intraplacental and intramolar choriocarcinomas. The concept of trophoblastic 'hyperplasia' in moles needs to be reconsidered and thought should be given to the view that some choriocarcinomas are simply abnormal pregnancies.

REFERENCES

1. Vassilakos P, Riotton G, Kajii T. Hydatidiform mole: two entities: a morphologic and cytogenetic study with some clinical considerations. *Am J Obstet Gynecol* 1977 **127**: 167–170.
2. Szulman AE, Surti U. The syndromes of hydatidiform mole. I. cytogenetic and morphologic correlations. *Am J Obstet Gynecol* 1978 **131**: 665–671.
3. Szulman AE, Surti U. The syndromes of hydatidiform mole. II. Morphologic evolution of the complete and partial mole. *Am J Obstet Gynecol* 1978 **132**: 20–27.
4. Grimes DA. Epidemiology of gestational trophoblastic disease. *Am J Obstet Gynecol* 1984 **150**: 309–318.
5. Bracken MB. Incidence and aetiology of hydatidiform mole: an epidemiological review. *Br J Obstet Gynaecol* 1987 **94**: 1123–1135.
6. Ishizuka N. Studies of trophoblastic neoplasia. *Gann* 1976 **18**: 203–216.
7. Graham IH, Fajardo AM, Richards RL. Epidemiological study of complete and partial hydatidiform moles in Abu Dhabi: influence of maternal age and ethnic group. *J Clin Pathol* 1990 **43**: 661–664.
8. Womack C, Elston CW. Hydatidiform mole in Nottingham: a 12 year retrospective epidemiological and morphological study. *Placenta* 1985 **6**: 95–105.
9. Miller D, Jackson R, Ehein T, McMuurtrie E. Complete hydatidiform mole coexistent with a twin live fetus: clinical course of four cases with complete cytogenetic analysis. *Gynecol Oncol* 1993 **50**: 119–123.
10. Kajii T, Ohama K. Androgenetic origin of hydatidiform mole. *Nature* 1977 **268**: 633–634.
11. Jacobs PA, Wilson CM, Sprenkle JA, Rosenhein NB, Migson BR. Mechanisms of origin of complete hydatidiform mole. *Nature* 1980 **286**: 714–716.
12. Surti U, Szulman AE, O'Brien S. Dispermic origin and clinical outcome of three complete hydatidiform moles with 46XY karotype. *Am J Obstet Gynecol* 1982 **144**: 84–87.
13. Lawler SD, Fisher RA, Pickhall VJ, Povey S, Evans MW. Genetic studies on hydatidiform moles. I. The origin of partial moles. *Cancer Genet Cytogenet* 1982 **5**: 309–320.
14. Jacobs PA, Szulman AE, Funkmouska J, Maatsura JS, Wilson CC. Human triploidy: relationship between paternal origin of the additional haploid complement and development of partial hydatidiform mole. *Ann Hum Genet* 1982 **46**: 223–231.
15. Teng NNH, Ballon SC. Partial hydatidiform mole with diploid karotype: report of three cases. *Am J Obstet Gynecol* 1984 **150**: 961–964.
16. Surti U, Szulman AE, Wagner K, Leppert M, O'Brien SJ. Tetraploid partial hydatidiform moles: two cases with a triple paternal contribution and a 92 XXXY karotype. *Hum Genet* 1986 **72**: 15–21.
17. Vejerslev LO, Fisher RA, Surti U, Walke N. Hydatidiform mole: cytogenetically unusual cases and their implications for the present classification. *Am J Obstet Gynecol* 1987 **157**: 180–184.
18. Lage JM, Weinberg JS, Yavner DL *et al.* Tetraploid partial hydatidiform moles: histopathology, cytogenetics, and flow cytometry. *Hum Pathol* 1989 **20**: 419–425.

19. Hemming JD, Quirke P, Womack C, Wells M, Elston CW. Diagnosis of molar pregnancy and persistent trophoblastic disease by flow cytometry. *J Clin Pathol* 1987 **40**: 615–620.

20. Lage JM, Mark SD, Roberts DJ *et al.* A flow cytometric study of 137 fresh hydropic placentas: correlation between types of hydatidiform moles and nuclear DNA ploidy. *Obstet Gynecol* 1992 **79**: 403–410.

21. Koenig C, Demopoulos RI, Vamvakas EC, Mittal KR, Feiner HD, Espiritu B. Flow cytometric DNA ploidy and quantitative histopathology in partial moles. *Int J Gynecol Pathol* 1993 **12**: 235–240.

22. Lage JM, Popek EJ. The role of DNA flow cytometry in evaluation of partial and complete hydatidiform moles and hydropic abortions. *Semin Diagn Pathol* 1993 **10**: 267–274.

23. Verjeslev LO, Sunde L, Hansen BF, Larsen JK, Christensen IJ, Larsen J. Hydatidiform mole and fetus with normal karotype: support of a separate entity. *Obstet Gynecol* 1991 **77**: 868–874.

24. Barton SC, Surani MAH, Norris ML. Role of paternal and maternal genomes in mouse development. *Nature* 1984 **311**: 374–376.

25. Kaufman MH, Lee KKH, Speirs S. Influence of diandric and digynic triploid genotypes on early mouse embryogenesis. *Development* 1989 **105**: 137–145.

26. Bagshawe KD, Dent J, Webb J. Hydatidiform mole in England and Wales 1973–83. *Lancet* 1986 **ii**: 673–677.

27. Bagshawe KD, Lawler SD, Paradinas F, Dent J, Brown P, Boxer GM. Gestational trophoblastic tumours following initial diagnosis of partial hydatidiform mole. *Lancet* 1990 **335**: 1074–1076.

28. Rice LW, Berkowitz RS, Lage JM, Goldstein DP, Bernstein MR. Persistent gestational trophoblastic tumor after partial hydatidiform mole. *Gynecol Oncol* 1990 **36**: 358–362.

29. Lage JM, Berkowitz RS, Rice LW, Goldstein DP, Bernstein MR, Weinberg DS. Flow cytometric analysis of DNA content in partial hydatidiform moles with persistent gestational trophoblastic tumor. *Obstet Gynecol* 1991 **77**: 111–115.

30. Goto S, Yamada A, Ishizuka T, Tomoda Y. Development of postmolar trophoblastic disease after partial molar pregnancy. *Gynecol Oncol* 1993 **48**: 165–170.

31. Looi LM, Sivanesaratnam A. Malignant evolution with fatal outcome in a patient with partial hydatidiform mole. *Aust NZ J Obstet Gynaecol* 1981 **21**: 51–52.

32. Gardner HAR, Lage JL. Choriocarcinoma following a partial mole: a case report. *Hum Pathol* 1992 **23**: 468–471.

33. Hertig AT, Sheldon WH. Hydatidiform mole: a pathologicoclinical correlation of 200 cases. *Am J Obstet Gynecol* 1947 **53**: 1–36.

34. Elston CW, Bagshawe KD. The value of histological grading in the management of hydatidiform mole. *J Obstet Gynaecol Br Cmmwlth* 1972 **79**: 717–724.

35. Genest DG, Laborde O, Berkowitz RS *et al.* A clinical-pathologic study of 153 cases of complete hydatidiform mole (1980–1990): histologic grade lacks prognostic significance. *Obstet Gynecol* 1991 **77**: 111–115.

36. Hemming JD, Quirke P, Womack C, Wells M, Elston CW, Pennington GW. Flow cytometry in persistent trophoblastic disease. *Placenta* 1988 **9**: 615–621.

37. Fukunaga M, Ushigome S, Fukunaga M, Sugishita M. Application of flow cytometry in diagnosis of hydatidiform moles. *Mod Pathol* 1993 **6**: 353–359.

38. Cheung AN, Ngan HY, Chen WZ, Loke SL, Collins RJ. The significance of proliferating cell nuclear antigen in human trophoblastic disease: an immunohistochemical study. *Histopathology* 1993 **22**: 565–568.

39. Wake N, Fujino T, Hoshi S *et al.* The propensity to malignancy of dispermic heterozygous moles. *Placenta* 1987 **8**: 318–326.

40. Mutter GL, Pomponio RJ, Berkowitz RS, Genest DR. Sex chromosome composition of complete hydatidiform mole: relationship to metastasis. *Am J Obstet Gynecol* 1993 **168**: 1547–1551.

41. Robertson WB, Brosens I, Dixon HG. Uteroplacental vascular pathology. *Eur J Obstet Gynecol Reprod Biol* 1975 **5**: 47–65.

42. Pijnenborg R, Bland JM, Robertson WB, Dixon HG, Brosens I. The pattern of interstitial trophoblastic invasion of the myometrium in early human pregnancy. *Placenta* 1981 **2**: 303–316.

43. Fox H. Placenta accreta, 1945–1969. *Obstet Gynecol Surv* 1972 **27**: 475–490.

44. Hertig AT. Hydatidiform mole and chorionepithelioma. In Meigs JB, Sturgis SH (eds) *Progress in Gynecology*, Vol 2. New York: Grune & Stratton, 1950: 372–394.

45. Elston CW. The histopathology of trophoblastic tumours. *J Clin Pathol* 1976 **29** (**Suppl. 10**): 11–131.

46. Ring AM. The concept of benign metastasizing hydatidiform moles. *Am J Clin Pathol* 1972 **58**: 111–117.

47. Johnson TR, Comstock CH, Anderson DG. Benign gestational trophoblastic disease metastatic to pleura: unusual cause of hemothorax. *Obstet Gynecol* 1979 **53**: 509–511.

48. Mueller UW, Hawes CS, Wright AE *et al.* Isolation of fetal trophoblast cells from peripheral blood of pregnant women. *Lancet* 1990 **336**: 197–200.

49. Attwood HD, Park WW. Embolism to the lungs by trophoblast. *J Obstet Gynaecol Br Cmmwlth* 1961 **68**: 611–617.

50. Dawood MY, Teoh ES, Ratnam SS. ABO blood group in trophoblastic neoplasia. *Am J Obstet Gynecol* 1971 **78**: 918–923.

51. Bagshawe KD. Recent observations related to chemotherapy and immunology of gestational choriocarcinoma. *Adv Cancer Res* 1973 **18**: 231–263.

52. Bagshawe KD. Risk and prognostic factors in trophoblastic neoplasia. *Cancer* 1976 **38**: 1373–1385.

53. Buckley JD, Henderson BE, Morrow CP *et al.* Case-control study of gestational choriocarcinoma. *Cancer Res* 1988 **48**: 1004–1010.

54. Chaganti RSK, Koduru PRK, Chakraborty R, Jones WB. Genetic origin of a trophoblastic choriocarcinoma. *Cancer Res* 1990 **50**: 6330–6333.

55. Azuma C, Saji F, Nobunaga T *et al.* Studies of the pathogenesis of choriocarcinoma by analysis of restriction fragment length polymorphisms. *Cancer Res* 1990 **50**: 488–491.

56. Osada H, Kawata M, Yamada M, Okumura K, Takamizawa H. Genetic identification of pregnancies responsible for choriocarcinoma after multiple pregnancies by restriction fragment length polymorphism analysis. *Am J Obstet Gynecol* 1991 **165**: 682–688.

57. Fisher RA, Newlands ES, Jeffreys AJ *et al.* Gestational and non-gestational trophoblastic tumors distinguished by DNA analysis. *Cancer* 1992 **69**: 839–845.

58. Suzuki T, Goto S, Nawa A, Kurauchi D, Saito M, Tomoda Y. Identification of the pregnancy responsible for gestational trophoblastic disease by DNA analysis. *Obstet Gynecol* 1993 **82**: 629–634.

59. Driscoll SG. Choriocarcinoma: an 'incidental finding' within a term placenta. *Obstet Gynecol* 1963 **21**: 96–102.

60. Brewer JL, Gerbie AB. Early development of choriocarcinoma. *Am J Obstet Gynecol* 1966 **94**: 692–710.

61. Brewer JL, Mazur MT. Gestational choriocarcinoma: its origin in the placenta during seemingly normal pregnancy. *Am J Surg Pathol* 1981 **5**: 267–277.

62. Tsukamoto N, Kashimura Y, Sano M, Salto T, Kanda T, Taki I. Choriocarcinoma occurring within the normal placenta with breast metastasis. *Gynecol Oncol* 1981 **11**: 348–363.

63. Fox H, Laurini RN. Intraplacental choriocarcinoma: a report of two cases, *J Clin Pathol* 1988 **41**: 1085–1088.

64. Hallam LA, McLaren KM, El-Jabbour JN, Helm CW, Smart GE. Intraplacental choriocarcinoma: a case report. *Placenta* 1990 **11**: 247–251.

65. Christopherson WA, Kanbour A, Szulman AE. Choriocarcinoma in a term placenta with maternal metastases. *Gynecol Oncol* 1992 **46**: 239–245.

66. Lage GM, Roberts DJ. Choriocarcinoma in a term placenta: pathologic diagnosis of tumor in an asymptomatic patient with metastatic disease. *Int J Gynecol Pathol* 1993 **12**: 80–85.

67. Heifetz SA, Csaja J. *In situ* choriocarcinoma arising in partial hydatidiform mole: implications for risk of persistent trophoblastic disease. *Pediatr Pathol* 1992 **12**: 601–611.

68. Acosta-Sison H. Can the implanting trophoblast of the fertilized ovum develop immediately into choriocarcinoma? *Am J Obstet Gynecol* 1955 **69**: 442–444.

69. Fox H. Biology of teratomas. In Anthony PP, MacSween RNM (eds) *Recent Advances in Histopathology*, vol 13. Edinburgh: Churchill Livingstone, 1987: 33–43.

70. Lage JM, Young RH. Pathology of trophoblastic disease. In Clement PB, Young RH (eds) *Tumors and Tumorlike Lesions of the Uterine Corpus and Cervix.* New York: Churchill Livingstone, 1993: 419–475.

71. Young RH, Kuraman RJ, Scully RE. Proliferations and tumors of the placental site. *Semin Diagn Pathol* 1988 **5**: 223–237.

72. Eckstein RP, Paradinas FJ, Bagshawe KD. Placental site trophoblastic tumour (trophoblastic pseudotumour): a study of four cases requiring hysterectomy, including one fatal case. *Histopathology* 1982 **6**: 221–226.

73. How J, Scurry J, Sapountzis K, Ostor A, Fortune D, Armes J. Placental site trophoblastic tumor: report of three cases and review of the literature. *Int J Gynecol Cancer* 1995 **5**: 241–249.

Molecular Analysis in Gynecological Pathology

M Wells

INTRODUCTION

As we approach the turn of the century the rapid developments in molecular biology are being increasingly felt in the diagnostic histopathology laboratory. This chapter will focus on aspects of molecular pathology relevant to a variety of gynecological malignancies.

CURRENT CONCEPTS

Oncogenes

Oncogenes are genes governing the neoplastic behavior of cells and were originally discovered in oncogenic RNA retroviruses. These viruses contain the enzyme, reverse transcriptase, which enables their RNA to be transcribed into complementary DNA which is then incorporated into the genome of the infected cell. It was subsequently discovered that DNA sequences identical to oncogenes in these viruses are present in the genome of normal cells (cellular or proto-oncogenes). These cellular oncogenes produce proteins which are essential for normal cell and tissue growth and differentiation. It is when they are aberrant or inappropriately expressed that they result in the growth of a tumor.[1]

Oncogenes can be classified into five groups according to the function of the gene product (oncoprotein):

1. Growth factors;
2. Growth factor receptors (e.g. *erb*B coding for epidermal growth factor receptor);
3. Intracellular transducers of growth factor signals (tyrosine kinase activity);
4. Nuclear-binding oncoproteins involved in the regulation of cellular proliferation (e.g. *myc*);
5. Cyclic nucleotide binding activity disrupting intracellular signaling (e.g. *ras*).

Oncogene activation may occur by one of the following mechanisms:

1. Translocation – this is often evident from the karyotype; part of one chromosome which is known to bear an oncogene may be translocated to another chromosome where a gene known to be actively 'read' is situated.
2. Mutation
3. Amplification – this can be recognized in chromosome preparations from tumor cells by the presence of homogeneously staining regions and double minute chromosomes.

Altered oncogene expression can result in either (a) normal quantities of the oncoprotein molecule altered by mutation in such a way that it is abnormally active or (b) normal oncoprotein produced in excessive quantities because of gene amplification or enhanced transcription.

Mutant oncoproteins may have lesser or greater biological activity than the normal molecule. This can have profound effects on receptor function and intracellular signaling. Increased expression of oncogenes has been found in many tumors and may be detected by: (a) the presence of more of the oncogene product (oncoprotein) within the cells; (b) increased production of mRNA transcripts of the oncogene; or (c) increased numbers of copies of the oncogene in the genome. It is important to remember that no single oncogene is capable of promoting and inducing all of the biological properties required for tumor formation by itself. Oncogenes may cooperate with each other and multiple oncogene abnormalities are usually present within a single tumor. A distinction must be drawn between molecular analysis and the use of antibodies (monoclonal or polyclonal) to the oncogene protein product.

Tumor suppressor genes (anti-oncogenes)

Anti-oncogenes or tumor suppressor genes are important in the negative control of cell growth.[2-4] Mutations causing a loss, rather than gain, of function are associated with malignant development. Both copies of the gene must be inactivated for neoplastic effect (i.e. they act recessively at a cellular level). Retinoblastoma (Rb-1) and p53 are members of this group of genes. There continues to be intense interest in the molecular pathology of p53.

p53 is a nuclear phosphoprotein, the gene for which has been cloned and localized to chromosome 17p13. The p53 gene was originally considered to be an oncogene, but is now believed to have the properties of a tumor suppressor gene.[5] The current view regards the role of wild-type p53 as the 'guardian of the genome', responsible for halting progression through the G1/S boundary of the cell cycle to allow time for repair or, if cellular damage is too severe, to induce apoptosis. The association of p53 with human carcinogenesis is now well established with mutations in the tumor suppressor gene representing the most common genetic abnormality observed. Such mutations cause loss of suppressor function and induction of growth-promoting potential. Its role may also depend on the level of remaining wild type p53 protein in the cell.[6]

Cervical neoplasia

Human papillomavirus

Certain 'high risk' types of human papillomaviruses (particularly HPV 16 and 18 but also HPV 31, 33, 35, and others) occur more frequently in high-grade cervical intraepithelial neoplasia (CIN) and invasive cervical squamous carcinoma.[7] The most important application for HPV typing is in cervical cytology and, in particular, in the assessment of women with mildly abnormal (dyskaryotic) smears. Two things are becoming increasingly clear; first, women with a mildly abnormal smear in the presence of HPV type 16 are at greater risk of harboring a more severe histological lesion.[8] Second, there is a greater risk of neoplastic progression from mild dyskaryosis in the presence of HPV type 16.[9] Integration of the viral genome into host DNA is usual in these lesions and the protein coding sequences of the viral early (E) or late (L) open reading frames appear to have a major role in oncogenesis.[7] Viral infection with integration usually occurs specifically, disrupting the genome between the E2 and L2 or L1 open reading frames, resulting in loss of the E2 regulatory protein and late regions associated with structural proteins, but increased expression of the transforming E6 and E7 regions.[10] The cell target appears to be basal squamous epithelial cells and in normal proliferating cells, transcription of the viral genes is regulated by host inhibitory factors which must be inactivated before transformation can occur.

p53

The E6 protein of HPV 16 is capable of binding to cellular p53 protein to form a complex which neutralizes the normal function of p53. Binding capacity correlates with the *in vivo* transforming activity of different papillomavirus types. E6 protein from the 'benign' or 'low-risk' HPV

types 6 and 11 for example does not appear to form a complex with p53.[11] Replicative DNA repair after damage requires wild-type p53 and HPV 16 E6 has been shown to disrupt the normal response of cervical epithelial cells to DNA damage mediated by p53 and may thereby also allow the accumulation of genetic abnormalities associated with cervical oncogenesis.[12]

Mutation of the *p53* gene does not appear to be a common event in cervical carcinogenesis. Several studies have now reported an inverse relationship between the presence of HPV DNA and that of *p53* gene mutation both in primary cervical carcinomas[13] and cell lines.[14] The attractive hypothesis is therefore that p53 is inactivated in cervical carcinoma, either by complexing with HPV 16 protein (in HPV-positive tumors), or by *p53* gene mutation in those that are HPV-negative. This has not, however, been a consistent finding and other workers have shown that inactivation of the *p53* gene by allelic loss or by point mutation is infrequent in cervical cancer, irrespective of the presence or absence of HPV infection.[15–17] Such discrepancies raise the possibility of different pathogenetic factors being involved. Crook and Vousden[18] have identified p53 point mutations in metastases arising from HPV-positive cervical carcinomas suggesting that acquisition of *p53* mutation may play a role in the progression of some HPV associated primary cancers.

The results from immunohistochemistry have been somewhat confusing. Overexpression of p53 protein in tissues has generally been assumed to reflect p53 mutation, since wild-type protein is not usually demonstrable by immunohistochemistry. Recent reports suggest that p53 immunoreactivity does not correlate with mutation but may reflect the change of wild-type p53 from a suppressor to a promoter form during the cell growth response, or a longer half-life of the protein due to binding by another protein.[19,20]

The prognostic significance of an established invasive cervical carcinoma being positive for human papillomaviruses is controversial. There is evidence in the literature that human papillomavirus detection in squamous cell carcinomas confers a better prognosis though a worsened prognosis for HPV type 18 positive tumors has been reported.[21–23] Recently, it has been suggested that there is a low risk group of tumors with HPV type 31, 16 and 'unknown' and a high-risk group consisting of HPV type 33 and 18 and HPV negative cases.[24]

Human papillomaviruses are possibly also implicated in the etiology of adenocarcinoma of the cervix though the relationship is less clear than is the case for squamous carcinoma since most studies show a lower incidence of infection than squamous neoplasia in both *in situ* and invasive adenocarcinoma. Types 16, 18 and 33 may be identified and type 18 seems to be predominant.[25–28]

Smoking has been associated on epidemiological grounds with an increased risk of cervical neoplasia. Characteristic smoking-related DNA additional products have been demonstrated in cervical tissue and a significant difference in their levels detected between current and non-current smokers.[29,30] Such findings suggest a causal relationship between smoking and cervical neoplasia. The carcinogenic constituents of cigarettes are likely to be important co-factors along with high risk human papillo-mavirus types in the etiology of cervical neoplasia.

Oncogenes

The *ras* gene family has three main members; Harvey (*Ha-ras*), Kirsten (*Ki-ras*) and neuroblastoma (*N-ras*), which each code for a 21 kDa protein product termed p21. p21 functions as a signal transducer relaying messages from the plasma membrane to intracytoplasmic effectors. The *ras* gene has been associated with a number of malignancies through various mechanisms including overexpression, mutation and amplification.

The oncogenes of the *myc* family code for products which localize to the nucleus, are elevated upon stimulation by mitogenic stimuli or growth factors, and probably affect transcription by binding to regulatory DNA regions or small ribonucleoproteins. The *myc* gene may be activated by rearrangement or amplification. It codes for a gene product known as p62 which may also be overexpressed.

H-ras is amplified as well as overexpressed in the major-ity of cervical carcinomas.[1] It has been suggested that over-expression of *c-myc* is a significant independent indicator of the risk of overall relapse and distant metastases, even in early stage cervical carcinoma.[31]

Endometrial neoplasia

Endometrial carcinomas have been shown to have muta-tions of *Ki-ras*, amplification of *myc*, c-*erb*-B2 and p53 mutation. Several reports have suggested that point muta-tions in codon 12 of *Ki-ras* are significant events in the eti-ology of adenocarcinoma of the endometrium.[32–36] Other reports have failed to confirm this and have argued that the presence of *Ki-ras* does not contribute to the differential diagnosis of hyperplasia and carcinoma or predict the bio-logical behavior of established endometrial cancer.[37] The *fms* oncogene encodes the receptor for macrophage colony-stimulating factor (CSF-1). *fms* mRNA has been identified in proliferative but not secretory endometrium as well as in endometrial adenocarcinoma. In general much higher lev-els of mRNA were observed in malignant as compared to benign tissues and were associated with disease of high stage and grade.[38]

A high degree of c-*myc* amplification has been reported in advanced stage disease, poorly differentiated lesions and serous papillary adenocarcinoma.[39] In a study of *erb*-B2 amplification in endometrial adenocarcinomas,[39] 11/16 had multiple copies of the gene and those patients with amplification had more advanced stage disease and poorly differentiated lesions; a finding supported by others.[40] Sasano *et al.*[41] studied serous papillary carcinomas of the endometrium but observed no *erb*-B2 amplifications. At present such abnormalities are not established as prognos-tic indicators in endometrial cancer.

p53 mutations have also been demonstrated in human endometrial lesions.[42–44] A recent report has shown p53 mutation in atypical endometrial hyperplasias identical to those seen in some endometrial cancers. Such mutations were not seen in endometrial hyperplasia without cytolog-ical atypia.[45] These findings have not, however, been sup-ported by others.[46]

Ovarian germ cell neoplasms

Germ cells undergo meiosis, a process of chromosomal crossover, and reductive divisions that leaves its mark on the genome of progeny cells. By comparing heterozygous host markers with those markers seen in tumors, the stage of meiotic development that the tumor stem cell attained prior to neoplastic transformation can be determined.[47]

The extent to which the tumor stem cell has progressed through meiotic development prior to neoplastic transfor-mation correlates with histological subtype and natural his-tory. When applied to mature ovarian teratomas, marker studies indicate various stages of neoplastic transforma-tion.[48–50] The majority of ovarian mature cystic teratomas arise from an oocyte that has completed the first meiotic division, in a manner analogous to parthenogenesis. Although essentially all postmeiosis 1 (M1)-derived female germ cell tumors are benign, mature cystic teratomas or low-grade immature teratomas, pre-M1 lesions fall into several discrete subsets:

1. Pre-M1 immature teratomas tend to have worse prog-nostic features, such as aneuploidy compared with euploidy in post-M1 cases;
2. Multiple mature teratomas tend to be pre-M1;
3. Malignant tumors of embryonic histology (dysgermi-noma, embryonal carcinoma, yolk sac tumor, mixed germ cell tumor) are always pre-M1. These, like their testicular counterparts frequently have specific chromo-somal abnormalities.[51]

A non-random marker chromosome composed of two attached short arms of chromosome 12, an isochromosome of 12p or i(12p) is frequently present in ovarian dysgermi-nomas[52] and yolk sac tumors.[53,54]

Patients with dysgenetic gonads have a greatly increased risk of developing some types of germ cell tumors, especially gonadoblastoma. The risk for developing gonadoblastoma in a dysgenetic setting is highest when Y chromosome sequences can be documented directly by karyotype or indirectly by detection of Y chromosome-derived proteins such as HY antigen. Molecular methods for identification of Y chromosome sequences in paraffin embedded, fresh, or fixed tissues include PCR[55] and fluo-rescent *in situ* hybridization (FISH). Fresh tissue may be suitable for karyotypic analysis. However, some patients who exhibit no cytological evidence of a Y chromosome have small portions of the Y chromosome if studied by more sensitive and specific molecular techniques.[56]

Gestational trophoblastic disease

Complete moles

Most techniques confirm that complete moles are diploid and of paternal origin, having arisen by androgenesis with loss or inactivation of the oocyte nucleus. Fertilization may occur by a haploid sperm which duplicates or a diploid sperm which fails to undergo meiotic division resulting in a diploid homozygous complete mole (46XX, with 46YY apparently non-viable). A third method is synchronous fertilization by two haploid sperm resulting in diploid heterozygous complete mole (46XX or 46YY). Cases of triploidy or tetraploidy are also considered to lack the maternal contribution.[57]

Partial moles

These arise with diploid fertilization of the oocyte but with retention of the female nucleus. They are XXX or XXY, rarely XYY and are homozygous or heterozygous for the paternal contribution.[57]

It seems likely that the excess paternal contribution therefore contributes to the development of molar disease, particularly if the maternal influence is completely lost as in complete mole. It would be expected that choriocarcinoma following complete mole would arise from paternally derived DNA. However, using restriction fragment length polymorphism analysis it has been shown that either maternal or paternal contributions are present.[58]

The relative DNA content of molar disease has been investigated by cytogenetic analysis, flow cytometry, and AgNORs. Although giving valuable assessment of ploidy, only cytogenetics gives the relative maternal : paternal contribution but this may be problematic in routine diagnosis. There is a requirement for fresh tissue and specialist centers with occasional difficult interpretation of some chromosomal patterns and lack of growth in culture.

DNA fingerprinting has been used on fresh molar material to confirm the androgenetic origin of complete moles or to make the diagnosis in difficult cases.[59-62] These assessments have confirmed the previous cytogenetic analyses of DNA parental contributions of complete and partial mole. The pieces of DNA required, however, are too large for extraction from archival material.

The smaller microsatellites can be detected in material extracted from fresh or routinely processed specimens. These polymorphisms have alleles which may differ in length by only two base pairs and are not detectable by gel electrophoresis or Southern blotting. They can be amplified using the PCR technique so that they may be detected on a sequencing gel, using radioactive or fluorescent probes.[63,64]

With both these techniques, if only paternal alleles are present, the gestation is confirmed as a complete mole. If unique maternal sequences are present, then complete mole is excluded.

This latter situation may arise however with partial mole, hydropic abortion or in cases where the polymorphisms are not unique to either parent and further investigation is necessary. Peripheral blood may be used for comparison to confirm that maternal and paternal alleles are the same and not diagnostic. A panel of highly polymorphic sequences will give a higher probability of finding unique, diagnostic alleles.

Quantitative PCR using fluorescent probes and gene scanning equipment will determine the relative contribution of each allele and thus give the ploidy and parental contribution with the same test. This should be a rapid and useful method, not only of confirming the diploid androgenetic complete mole, but also of investigating the nature of triploid partial moles and hydropic abortuses and cases of tetraploidy.

FUTURE PERSPECTIVES

Molecular pathology will radically change the way we diagnose disease in the 21st century. There are a number of clinical reasons why the molecular genetic analysis of tumors may prove important:

1. Assigning a primary diagnosis;
2. Staging the tumor;
3. Determining prognosis;
4. Monitoring the effects of therapy or directing therapy;
5. Evaluating the risk of cancer particularly in familial syndromes.

There seems little doubt that molecular analysis of certain tumors will become routine. The development of techniques such as *in situ* hybridization which work on formalin-fixed, paraffin-embedded sections has increased the scope of molecular investigation enormously and means that the histopathology laboratory will retain its pivotal role in patient management.

SUMMARY

- The application of molecular biological techniques to formalin-fixed, routinely processed and paraffin-embedded tissue means that there is a vast archive of potential research material within diagnostic histopathology laboratories.
- Extraction of DNA from tissues, Southern blotting and hybridization with specific probes does not allow the topographical localization of the signal within tissues.

- This may be achieved by *in situ* hybridization, where the hybridization signal is viewed down the microscope.
- The exquisite sensitivity of the polymerase chain reaction means that very careful practical steps must be taken to avoid cross-contamination and resulting false-positive results.
- The results of immunohistochemical studies should, ideally, always be supported by molecular

pathological data. This is particularly true when investigating overexpression or mutations of onco-genes and tumor suppressor genes.

- There is already a strong case for the application of human papillomavirus typing in routine practice.
- There is also a case for the routine molecular pathological analysis of hydatidiform mole to assist in the distinction between complete (of paternal origin) and partial mole.
- Molecular pathological studies have, in some

areas, produced contradictory findings with regard to their clinical or prognostic significance. This is particularly true of the prognostic significance of oncogene overexpression.

- With the exceptions noted in points 5 and 6 there is little, at present, that can be reliably applied in day to day diagnostic practice.
- The identification of genetic abnormalities has, nevertheless, enormous potential in terms of screening, diagnosis and prognosis.

REFERENCES

1. Curling M, Watson JV. Oncogenes in gynaecological cancer. In Lowe D, Fox H (eds) *Advances in Gynaecological Pathology* Edinburgh: Churchill Livingstone, 1992: 63–68.
2. Tidy JA, Wrede D. Tumor suppressor genes: new pathways in gynecological cancer. *Int J Gynecol Cancer* 1992 2: 1–8.
3. Marshall CJ. Tumor suppressor genes. *Cell* 1991 64: 313–326.
4. Weinberg RA. Tumor suppressor genes. *Science* 1991 254: 1138–1146.
5. Levin AJ, Momand J, Finlay CA. The *p53* tumor suppressor gene. *Nature* 1991 351: 453–456.
6. Vogelstein B, Kinzler KW. p53 function and dysfunction. *Cell* 1993 70: 523–526.
7. Scurry J, Wells M. Viruses in anogenital cancer. *Epithel Cell Biol* 1992 1: 138–145.
8. Bavin PJ, Giles JA, Deery A *et al.* Use of semi-quantitative PCR for human papillomavirus type 16 to identify women with high grade cervical disease in a population presenting with a mildly dyskaryotic smear report. *Br J Cancer* 1993 67: 602–605.
9. Gaarenstroom KN, Melkert P, Walboomers JMM *et al.* Human papillomavirus DNA and genotypes: prognostic factors for progression of cervical intraepithelial neoplasia. *Int J Gynecol Cancer* 1994 4: 73–78.
10. Thierry F. Proteins involved in the control of HPV transcription. *Papillomavirus Rep* 1993 4: 27–32.
11. Werness BA, Levine AJ, Howley PM. Association of human papillomavirus types 16 and 18 E6 proteins with p53. *Science* 1990 248: 76–79.
12. Kessis TD, Slebos RJ, Nelson WG *et al.* Human papillomavirus 16 E6 expression disrupts the p53-mediated cellular response to DNA damage. *Proc Natl Acad Sci USA* 1993 90: 3988–3992.
13. Crook T, Wrede D, Tidy JA, Mason WP, Evans DJ, Vousden KH. Clonal p53 mutation in primary cervical cancer: association with human papillomavirus-negative tumours. *Lancet* 1992 239: 1070–1073.
14. Scheffner M, Munger K, Byrne JC, Howley PM. The state of the *p53* and retinoblastoma genes in human cervical carcinoma cell lines. *Proc Natl Acad Sci USA* 1991 88: 5523–5527.
15. Fujita M, Inoue M, Tanizawa O, Iwamoto S, Enomoto T. Alterations of the *p53* gene in human primary cervical carcinoma with and without human papillomavirus infection. *Cancer Res* 1992 52: 5323–5328.
16. Paquette RL, Lee YY, Wilczynski SP *et al.* Mutations of p53 and human papillomavirus infection in cervical carcinoma. *Cancer* 1993 72: 1272–1280.
17. Busbyearle RMC, Steel CM, Williams ARW, Cohen B, Bird CC. *p53* mutations in cervical carcinogenesis: low frequency and lack of correlation with human papillomavirus status. *Br J Cancer* 1994 69: 732–737.
18. Crook T, Vousden KH. Properties of p53 mutations detected in primary and secondary cervical cancers suggest

mechanisms of metastasis and involvement of environment carcinogens. *EMBO J* 1992 11: 3935–3940.
19. Cooper K, Herrington CS, Evans MF, Gatter KC, McGee JO'D. p53 antigen in cervical condylomata, intraepithelial neoplasia and carcinoma: relationship to HPV infection and integration. *J Pathol* 1993 171: 27–34.
20. Helland A, Hollm R, Kristensen G *et al.* Genetic alterations of the TP53 gene, p53 protein expression and HPV infection in primary cervical carcinomas. *J Pathol* 1993 171: 105–107.
21. Riou G, Farue M, Jeannel D, Bourhis J, Le Doussal V, Orth G. Association between poor prognosis in early stage invasive cervical cancer and non-detection of HPV-DNA. *Lancet* 1990 335: 1171–1174.
22. Higgins GD, Davy M, Roder D, Uzelin DM, Philips GE, Burrell CH. Increased age and mortality associated with cervical carcinomas negative for human papillomavirus RNA. *Lancet* 1991 338: 910–913.
23. Girardi F, Fuchs P, Haas J. Prognostic importance of human papillomavirus type 16 DNA in cervical cancer. *Cancer* 1992 69: 2502–2504.
24. Hagmar B, Platz-Christensen J-J, Johansson B *et al.* HPV type in cervical squamous cell carcinoma; implications for survival. *Int J Gynecol Cancer* (in press).
25. Griffin NR, Dockley D, Lewis FA, Wells M. Demonstration of low frequency of human papillomavirus DNA in cervical adenocarcinoma and adenocarcinoma in situ by the polymerase chain reaction and in situ hybridization. *Int J Gynecol Pathol* 1991 10: 36–43.
26. Duggan MA, Benoit JL, McGregor SE, Nation JG, Inoue M, Stuart GCE. The human papillomavirus status of 114 endocervical adenocarcinoma cases by dot blot hybridization. *Hum Pathol* 1993 24: 121–125.
27. Milde-Langosch K, Schreiber C, Becker G. Human papillomavirus detection in cervical adenocarcinoma by polymerase chain reaction. *Hum Pathol* 1993 24: 590–594.
28. Duggan MA, Benoit JL, McGregor SE, Inoue M, Nation JG, Stuart GCE. Adenocarcinoma in situ of the endocervix: human papillomavirus determination by dot blot hybridisation and polymerase chain reaction amplification. *Int J Gynecol Pathol* 1994 13: 143–149.
29. Simons AM, Phillips DH, Coleman DV. Damage to DNA in cervical epithelium related to smoking tobacco. *Br Med J* 1993 306: 1444–1448.
30. Ali S, Astley SB, Sheldon TA, Peel KR, Wells M. Detection and measurement of DNA adducts in the cervix of smokers and non-smokers. *Int J Gynecol Cancer* 1994 4: 188–193.
31. Riou G, Le M G, Favre M, Jeanell D, Bourhis J, Orth G. Human papillomavirus-negative status and c-*myc* gene overexpression: independent prognostic indicators of distant metastasis for early stage invasive cervical cancers. *J Natl Cancer Inst* 1992 84: 1525–1526.
32. Enomoto T, Inoue M, Perantoni A *et al.* K-*ras* activation in premalignant and malignant epithelial lesions of the human uterus. *Cancer Res* 1991 51: 5304–5314.
33. Ignar-Trowbridge D, Risinger JI, Dent GA *et al.* Mutations

of the Ki-*ras* oncogene in endometrial carcinoma. *Am J Obstet Gynecol* 1992 **167**: 227–232.

34. Imamura T, Arima T, Kato H, Miyamoto S, Sasazuki T, Wake N. Chromosomal deletions and K-*ras* gene mutations in human endometrial carcinomas. *Int J Cancer* 1992 **51**: 47–52.

35. Sasaki H, Nishii H, Takahashi H *et al.* Mutation of the Ki-*ras* protooncogene in human endometrial hyperplasia and carcinoma. *Cancer Res* 1993 **53**: 1906–1910.

36. Duggan BD, Felix JC, Muderspach LI, Tsao J-L, Shibata DK. Early mutational activation of the c-ki-*ras* oncogene in endometrial carcinoma. *Cancer Res* 1994 **54**: 1604–1607.

37. Sato S, Ito K, Ozawa N *et al.* Analysis of point mutations at codon 12 of k-*ras* in human endometrial carcinoma and cervical adenocarcinoma by dot blot hybridization and polymerase chain reaction. *Tohoku J Exp Med* 1991 **165**: 131–136.

38. Kacinski B M, Carter D, Mittal K *et al.* High level of expression of *fms* proto-oncogene mRNA is observed in clinically aggressive human endometrial adenocarcinomas. *Int J Rad Oncol Biol Phys* 1989 **15**: 823–829.

39. Borst MP, Baker VV, Dixon D, Harch KD, Shingleton HM, Miller DM. Oncogene alterations in endometrial carcinoma. *Gynecol Oncol* 1990 **38**: 364–366.

40. Berchuk A, Rodriguez G, Kinney RB *et al.* Overexpression of HER-2/*neu* in endometrial cancer is associated with advanced stage disease. *Am J Obstet Gynecol* 1991 **164**: 15–21.

41. Sasano H, Comerford J, Wilkinson DS *et al.* Serous papillary adenocarcinoma of the endometrium: proto-oncogene amplification, flow cytometry, estrogen and progesterone receptors and immunohistochemical analysis. *Cancer* 1990 **65**: 1545–1551.

42. Okamoto A, Sameshima Y, Yamada Y *et al.* Allelic loss of chromosome 17p and p53 mutations in human endometrial carcinoma of the uterus. *Cancer Res* 1991 **51**: 5632–5636.

43. Kohler MF, Berchuck A, Davidoff AM *et al.* Overexpression and mutation of p53 in endometrial carcinoma. *Cancer Res* 1992 **52**: 1622–1627.

44. Honda T, Kato H, Imamura T *et al.* Involvement of p53 gene mutations in human endometrial carcinomas. *Int J Cancer* 1993 **53**: 963–967.

45. Enomoto T, Fujita M, Inoue M *et al.* Alterations of the p53 tumor suppressor gene and its association with activation of the c-K-*ras*-2 protooncogene in premalignant and malignant lesions of the human uterine endometrium. *Cancer Res* 1993 **53**: 1883–1888.

46. Kohler MF, Nishii H, Humphrey PA, Saski H, Marks J, Bast RC *et al.* Mutation of the p53 tumor-suppressor gene is not a feature of endometrial hyperplasia. *Am J Obstet Gynecol* 1993 **169**: 690–694.

47. Mutter GL. Germ cell neoplasia: molecular genetics. Course notes: The Molecular Biology of Women's Health: Breast and Reproductive Tract, Harvard Medical School 1992.

48. Dahl N, Gustavson K-H, Rune C, Gustavsson I, Pettersson U. Benign ovarian teratomas: an analysis of their cellular origin. *Cancer Genet Cytogenet* 1990 **46**: 115–123.

49. Deka R, Chakravarti A, Surti U *et al.* Genetics and biology of human ovarian teratomas. II. Molecular analysis of origin of nondisjunction and gene-centromere mapping of chromosome I markers. *Am J Hum Genet* 1990 **47**: 644–655.

50. Surti U, Hoffner L, Chakravarti A, Ferrell RE. Genetics and biology of human ovarian teratomas. I. Cytogenetic analysis and mechanism of origin. *Am J Hum Genet* 1990 **47**: 635–643.

51. Gibas Z, Talerman A. Analysis of chromosome aneuploidy in ovarian dysgerminoma by flow cytometry and fluorescence in situ hybridization. *Diagn Mol Pathol* 1993 **2**: 50–56.

52. Atkin NB, Baker MC. Abnormal chromosomes including small metacentrics in 14 ovarian cancers. *Cancer Genet Cytogenet* 1987 **26**: 355–361.

53. Speleman F, De Potter C, Dal Cin P *et al.* i(12p) in a malignant ovarian tumor. *Cancer Genet Cytogenet* 1990 **45**: 49–53.

54. Vos A, Oosterhuis JW, de Jong B *et al.* Karyotyping and DNA flow cytometry of metastatic ovarian yolk sac tumor. *Cancer Genet Cytogenet* 1990 **44**: 223–228.

55. Mutter GL, Pomponio RJ. Molecular diagnosis of sex chromosome aneuploidy using quantitative PCR. *Nucleic Acids Res* 1991 **19**: 4203–4207.

56. Shah KD, Kaffe S, Gilbert F, Dolgin S, Gertner M. Unilateral microscopic gonadoblastoma in a prepubertal Turner mosaic with Y chromosome material identified by restriction fragment analysis. *Am J Clin Pathol* 1988 **90**: 622–627.

57. Lane SA, Taylor GR, Quirke P. The diagnosis of molar disease. In Lowe D, Fox H (eds) *Advances in Gynaecological Pathology.* Edinburgh: Churchill Livingstone, 1992: 235–260.

58. Azuma C, Saji F, Nobunaga T *et al.* Studies on the pathogenesis of choriocarcinoma by analysis of restriction fragment length polymorphisms. *Cancer Res* 1990 **50**: 488–491.

59. Saji F, Tokugawa Y, Kimura T *et al.* A new approach using DNA fingerprinting for the determination of androgenesis as a cause of hydatidiform mole. *Placenta* 1989 **10**: 399–405.

60. Fisher RA, Povey S, Jeffreys AJ, Martin CA, Patel I, Lawler SD. Frequency of heterozygous complete hydatidiform moles, estimated by locus-specific minisatellite and Y chromosome-specific probes. *Hum Genet* 1989 **82**: 259–263.

61. Nobunaga T, Azuma C, Kimura T *et al.* Differential diagnosis between complete mole and hydropic abortus by deoxyribonucleic acid fingerprints. *Am J Obstet Gynecol* 1990 **163**: 634–638.

62. Takahashi H, Kanazawa K, Ikarashi T, Sudo N, Tanaka K. Discrepancy in the diagnosis of hydatidiform mole by macroscopic and microscopic findings and the deoxyribonucleic acid fingerprint method. *Am J Obstet Gynecol* 1990 **163**: 112–113.

63. Fisher RE, Newlands ES. Rapid diagnosis and classification of hydatidiform moles with polymerase chain reaction. *Am J Obstet Gynecol* 1993 **168**: 563–569.

64. Lane S, Taylor GR, Ozols B, Quirke P. Diagnosis of complete molar pregnancy by microsatellites in archival material. *J Clin Pathol* 1993; **46**: 346–348.

4.9

Principles of Radiotherapy

RP Symonds

INTRODUCTION

Radiotherapy is the art of using ionizing radiation to destroy malignant tumors with no or minimal damage to normal tissues. Accurate estimates of the contribution of the various modalities to cure cancer are somewhat arbitrary but the estimates of De Vita *et al.*[1] in the USA and Souhami and Tobias[2] in the UK agree very closely. Excluding non-melanomatous skin cancer and *in situ* carcinoma of cervix about 40% of patients with cancer are cured. About 40% of these cures follow radiation treatment. Radiotherapy is an important treatment modality in the management of gynecological cancer. Younger fitter patients with Stage Ib cervical cancer are usually selected for radical surgery and older less fit patients often with bigger tumors are given radiotherapy. Yet overall cure rates with either treatments are similar at about 80%.[3] Complete tumor elimination is possible in a significant portion of patients with locally advanced tumors. About 40% of those with Stage IIIb disease (extending to the pelvic side wall) can be cured.[4] Adjuvant radiotherapy can be given after primary surgery. Small tumor foci, such as occult metastases in pelvic lymph nodes or small deposits left after surgery can be sterilized by a lower radiation dose needed to control bulky disease. Radiation used in selected cases after hysterectomy for endometrial cancer can markedly reduce the chance of local recurrence and increase the chance of cure.[5] Radiotherapy may be integrated with both surgery and chemotherapy. The most common instance is in the treatment of breast cancer. There is an increasing tendency towards breast conservation. Following removal of the breast lump, megavoltage radiation is given to the breast and if necessary the local lymph nodes. Radiation treatment can be followed or preceded by chemotherapy if there is a significant risk of occult micrometastasis.

When cure is impossible, palliation with minimal side effects may follow a short course of radiotherapy. Pain from bone metastasis can be eased in 80% and abolished in 50% of patients receiving a single X-ray treatment.[6] Similarly symptom relief in lung cancer is an important indication for radiotherapy.[7]

CURRENT CONCEPTS

Ionizing radiation has been used for almost 90 years to treat a variety of diseases. Initially treatment was very haphazard but increasingly knowledge was applied more rationally. Fifty years ago the majority of patients treated by radiation at Stobhill General Hospital Glasgow did not have cancer. The only common benign disease now treated by ionizing radiation is thyrotoxicosis. The use of radiotherapy to produce an artificial menopause fell markedly following the work of Doll and Smith[8] who examined the records of patients suffering from benign menorrhagia treated in Edinburgh, Dundee and Aberdeen. There was a small increase in late radiation-induced malignancies particularly leukemia. However, there is still a role for radiotherapy in highly selected cases of benign menorrhagia when conventional treatment has failed and the risks of surgery outweigh the very small cancer risk.

Radiotherapy is very largely confined to the treatment of malignant disease. The majority of radiation treatment schedules are the result of clinical experience rather than laboratory research but increasingly radiobiology and allied disciplines are influencing patient management. The success of radiotherapy as a local curative modality depends on a concept called the therapeutic ratio. This has been defined as the relationship between the desired and the undesired effects of therapy.[9] It is possible to destroy a malignant tumor with little damage to normal tissue. This is the major advantage of radiotherapy over surgery which is typified in the treatment of laryngeal cancer. Early laryngeal cancer can be cured in at least 90% of cases with minimal damage to the larynx.[10] The surgical alternative would be laryngectomy depriving the patient of the power of speech.

Radiation particles

Ionizing radiation is energy that during absorption causes ejection of an orbital electron. Radiation treatment may be given using either subatomic particles or electromagnetic photons. Alpha particles are of no therapeutic value but may be an important health hazard if ingested. Neutron and proton beam treatments have a very limited clinical role but the use of electrons is increasing. Most radiation treatment is given using X or gamma ray photons. They differ only in the way they are produced. Gamma rays originate from the nucleus, X-rays from the orbiting electrons. In practice gamma rays are produced by the decay of radioactive isotopes and X-rays by machines. Small gamma ray-emitting sources may be inserted or implanted in tumors (brachytherapy).

Clinical radiobiology

The reasons why tumors are destroyed and normal tissues recover following radiotherapy are complex and poorly understood. Radiation kills cells by the production of secondary charged particles and free radicals which interact with the nucleus. Cellular lethality seems to be related to the number of double-strand DNA breaks produced in the nucleus. The intensity of ionization along a particle track varies between different forms of radiation. Megavoltage X-rays produce relatively few ionization events per unit length as they pass through tissue. By comparison particles such as neutrons produce much more dense ionization per unit length for a given dose. Alpha particles may only travel a few millimeters in tissue but may impart all their energy over a very small distance producing very intense ionization. The term linear energy transfer (LET) is used to describe the intensity of ionization in particle tracks. Gamma and X-rays are low LET forms of radiation, neutrons, protons and alpha particles are high LET. Cellular lethality is increased per unit of radiation as LET increases. The differing cell killing effects of high and low LET radiation can be presented as a ratio: the relative biological effect (RBE). The RBE can vary at different dose levels. High LET radiation is also more likely to produce a non-lethal event such as a mutation leading perhaps to cancer. At low doses, differences in RBE are most marked. In 1985 the International Commission on Radiation Protection recommended that the 'safe' maximum dose of neutrons received during occupation exposure should be 20 times less than the biologically equivalent gamma ray dose.[11]

Repair of radiation damage

Differences in repair of radiation damage may explain success or failure of radiation damage. There are three major types of radiation damage, lethal, sublethal and potentially lethal. Sublethal damage has been studied by Elkind *et al.*[12] who observed the survival of Chinese hamster cells after a single radiation dose or the same dose given as two equal fractions separated by varying periods of time. Cell kill was less after two fractions compared with the same dose given as a single treatment. This suggested that there had been significant repair between fractions. Sublethal damage repair in Elkind's experiments was complete in 3 hours.

Potentially lethal damage (PLD) under certain conditions leads to cell death. However, if postradiation conditions are modified to allow repair, cells can recover. In the laboratory, storage of cells at 4°C for a few hours[13] or plating in balanced salt solution[14] can provide a suitable environment for cells to recover from radiation injury. Such maneuvres stop progression through the cell cycle and allow cells to repair radiation-induced damage to DNA. Similar conditions may exist in some malnourished areas of tumors where cells are not dividing rapidly and are able to repair PLD. Osteogenic sarcomas are often quite radioresistant. This radioresistance has been ascribed to an increased capacity to repair potentially lethal damage compared to more radioresponsive tumors.[15]

The oxygen effect

Numerous chemical and pharmacological agents are known to modify the effects of radiation on tissue. The most important is oxygen. As early as 1921 Holthusen[16] noted that *Ascaris* eggs were relatively resistant to radiation if irradiated under hypoxic conditions. At that time this resistance was ascribed to lack of cellular division under hypoxia. Hypoxic mammalian cells are more resistant to the lethal effects of ionizing radiation than well oxygenated cells.[17] The ratio of doses needed to produce the same biological effect when hypoxic and well-aerated cells are irradiated is called the oxygen enhancement ratio (OER). For a given type of radiation the OER is independent of dose and level of cell killing. For low LET radiation the OER in most tissues is between 2.5 and 3.0. As tumors grow, new blood vessels develop to feed the neoplasm (angioneogenesis). By and large the new vessels are primitive in nature and the blood supply is inadequate to meet all the needs of the growing tumor. The classical study of Thomlinson and Gray[18] generated great interest in the oxygen effect which dominated radiobiology and experimental radiobiology for almost 30 years. In this study fresh specimens of bronchial carcinoma were cut into thin sections and examined histologically. Tumors of this type grow as infiltrating solid cords of malignant tissue often with a necrotic centre. No tumor cord with a radius greater than 200 μm was seen without a necrotic center, but no necrosis was seen in tumors less than 160 μm. However great the radius of the necrotic center was, the thickness of actively growing tumor sheath was never more than 180 μm. Thomlinson and Gray subsequently carried out calculations to find the oxygen tension at various distances from a capillary. The distance at which oxygen tension is essentially zero was 150–200 μm from a capillary. The agreement between calculated diffusion gradients for oxygen and the size of active growing tumor sheaths was regarded as evidence that oxygen was one of the critical nutrients for tumor growth. It was argued that poorly oxygenated viable cells at the edge of necrotic areas were a source of radioresistance and a major reason for treatment failure.

In order to destroy this subpopulation of hypoxic cells held responsible for treatment failure, a number of approaches were tried. Patients were irradiated in hyperbaric oxygen. A trial organized by the British Medical Research Council demonstrated increased local control and survival when patients suffering from Stage III carcinoma of cervix were irradiated in hyperbaric oxygen rather than air.[19] However other studies failed to confirm this and treatment in hyperbaric oxygen has been discontinued. Research efforts switched to the nitroimidazole group of drugs which mimic oxygen sensitizing hypoxic cells to ionizing radiation. Spectacular sensitization was demonstrated in murine tumors treated by single X-ray fractions but the effects in man have been less impressive. Clinical trials of misonidazole[20] and more recently pimonidazole[21] have shown no improvement in local control and survival in cervical cancer.

Following a large single dose of X-rays most of the sensitive, well oxygenated cells in a tumor will be killed. The cells that survive will be predominately hypoxic. However, following alterations in blood flow in the tumor, decreased cellular respiration of damaged cells and cell death, the portion of hypoxic cells falls over a period of hours and days. This process is called reoxygenation. Reoxygenation has important implications for clinical radiotherapy. Treatment is usually divided into 15–30 individual fractions. If reoxygenation occurs between fractions, killing of initially hypoxic cells will be greater and hypoxic cells will have less effect on ultimate treatment outcome.

Re-oxygenation may be more efficient in human rather than murine tumors and may partially explain the lack of efficacy in humans of the nitroimidazole hypoxic cell sensitizers.

Radiosensitivity and the cell cycle

The radiosensitivity of cells varies throughout the cell cycle. Cells are most sensitive at or close to mitosis and resistance is usually greatest at the end of S-phase. If the G1 phase is of appreciable length, a resistant period can be demonstrated in early G1 followed by a more sensitive period towards the end of G1. Cells in G2 are almost as radiosensitive as in mitosis.[22] In clinical practice it has not proved possible to take advantage of the variation in sensitivity during the cell cycle. Cellular arrest in the sensitive G2 phase of the cell cycle by hydroxyurea is possible experimentally[23] but the concentration of this drug that would produce this effect *in vivo* is toxic and could not be tolerated by patients if given systemically.

Radiotherapy machines

The workhorse of the modern radiotherapy department is the linear accelerator which is used to produce X-rays of energies of 4–20 million electron volts (MeV) (Fig. 4.9.1). Such X-rays have major clinical advantages over low energy X-rays generated by older kilovoltage machines. Megavoltage X-rays are relatively 'skin sparing'. It is fairly easy to treat deep-seated tumors with a homogeneous radiation dose and the radiation dose in bone is no higher than surrounding tissue. Older kilovoltage apparatus generates X-rays of 100–300 thousand electron volts (keV). These machines look similar to diagnostic X-ray units and produce X-rays which are only two or three times more energetic than those used to take diagnostic radiographs. The maximum energy of kilovoltage X-rays is deposited on the skin surface and moist desquamation of the skin was often the dose-limiting effect. The dose received by bone is higher than soft tissue. It is difficult to treat deep-seated tumors as these rays are rapidly attenuated, therefore at present kilovoltage machines are relegated to low dose palliative treatments or the treatment of superfical tumors.

An alternative to a linear accelerator is a highly radioactive cobalt-60 source which produces a gamma ray with similar physical characteristics to a 3 MeV X-ray beam. Cobalt machines are much simpler than linear accelerators but the source requires replacement about every 3 years. In the past cobalt was viewed as a cheaper, simpler, more reliable alternative to a linear accelerator. However, linear accelerators are gradually becoming more reliable and cheaper. On the other hand the cost of replacement cobalt sources is rising, therefore increasingly, cobalt machines are viewed as obsolescent or obsolete.

The absorption of photons

Gamma and X-ray photons are absorbed in tissues by two major processes, the photoelectric effect and the Compton process.

The photoelectric effect predominates at low (kilovoltage) energies. A photon of electromagnetic energy interacts with the highly bound electron shell of an atom leading to the ejection of an electron. The photon gives up all its energy overcoming the binding energy of the electron and imparting kinetic energy to the particle. The vacancy in the atomic shell is filled by another electron from the outer shell of the same atom or from outside the atom. The magnitude of the photoelectric effect varies with the cube of the atomic number. This is why dense material such as lead is such an effective shield and why bones absorb significantly more radiation than soft tissue. The differential absorption of radiation by photoelectric interactions is the basis of conventional diagnostic radiology.

In the Compton process a photon interacts with a distant orbital electron with a low binding energy, giving up only part of its energy. A significant proportion reappears as a secondary photon to interact with further electrons. The probability of a Compton type interaction does not depend so much on the atomic number but the electron density. At megavoltage energies the Compton effect predominates. This explains the skin sparing of megavoltage radiation as the maximum effect is not seen on the skin surface, but owing to the 'build-up' effect of tissue some distance subcutaneously. In order to protect staff and the public against radiation exposure, linear accelerators are

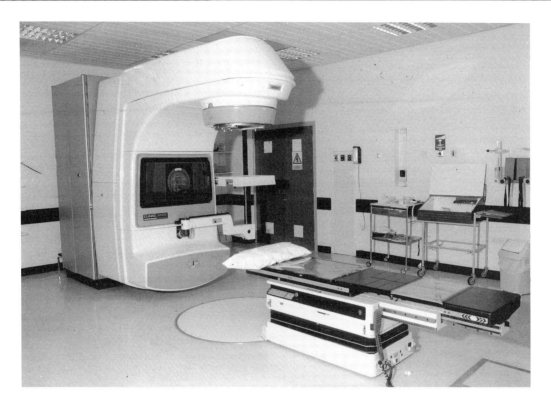

Fig. 4.9.1 *Varian Clinac 2100 Linear Accelerator. This machine produces 6 and 10 MeV X-rays. Tumors situated in a very large pelvis can be irradiated homogeneously. As well as producing X-rays this machine can produce electrons of 6, 9, 12, 16 and 20 MeV. For electron treatments an applicator is fitted to the machine which is in contact with the patient's skin.*

housed in thick-walled rooms made of barium concrete up to 1 meter in thickness. By contrast owing to the predominance of photoelectric interactions kilovoltage X-ray units can be shielded by a few millimeters of lead.

Electrons

As well as producing high energy X-rays, linear accelerators can produce megavoltage electrons (Fig. 4.9.1). The attenuation of this particle in tissues is entirely different to X or gamma ray photons. Electrons can irradiate homogeneously a slab of tissue the thickness of which depends on the electron energy. The dose received beneath this slab rapidly falls to zero. This allows the irradiation of fairly superficial lesions such as lymph nodes in the neck with sparing of deeper tissues such as the spinal cord.

Fast neutrons

Neutrons generated by the cyclotron in Berkeley, California were used by Stone in the 1940s to treat patients with a variety of advanced cancers.[24] Virtually all long-term survivors had severe late radiation complications. In the 1950s radiobiological studies revealed new facts about high LET radiation and differences in relative biological effects compared with photons. Clinical trials at the Hammer-

smith Hospital, London led to claims of marked superiority of neutron therapy compared to standard treatment.[25] Patients receiving photon treatment received rather low doses which may account for better survival of neutron-treated patients. A large very thorough trial comparing fast neutron therapy and good photon treatment of squamous cancer of head and neck in Edinburgh showed that local control rates were similar in both groups with markedly increased incidence of complications with neutron treatment.[26] A clinical trial of neutron treatment for pelvic cancers in Liverpool was stopped owing to increased mortality in the neutron arm.[27] Neutron radiotherapy was always experimental and does not seem to have any role in routine practice.

Protons

Protons are also produced by a cyclotron. These particles have a preferential deposition of energy and the maximum effect is often near the end of their path through tissues. By using appropriate proton energies this sharp ionization peak (the Bragg peak) can be made to correspond to the target volume. Precision high dose proton studies are in progress in selected malignancies such as melanomas of the uveal tract of the eye and tumors lying close to the spinal cord or base of brain (cordomas, chondrosarcomas or meningiomas).

Radiation dosage

The interaction of radiation with tissues is measured as the absorbed dose which is the quantity of energy absorbed per unit mass. In the SI system of units this is measured as joules per kilogram. One joule per kg is one Gray (Gy). One hundred rad equals 1 Gy. In radiotherapy practice doses may also be expressed in centigray.

What limits the radiation dose given in an attempt to cure a tumor is the risk of normal tissue damage. This damage is initially seen as acute radiation effects in rapidly proliferating cells such as skin epithelium, the mucosal lining of the upper digestive tract or the surface lining of the small bowel. This may manifest itself as moist desquamation of skin, mucositis inside the mouth or diarrhea caused by damage to jejunal crypt cells. This damage usually heals. What is potentially more worrying is risk of late damage appearing 9 months to 5 years after treatment owing to effects on slowly proliferating tissue particularly vascular endothelium. This is expressed as progressive fibrosis and endarteritis leading to necrosis, fistula or stricture.

Fractionation

One method to reduce the risk of normal tissue injury and increase the therapeutic ratio is to fractionate treatment. The total radiation dose is divided into 20–30 separate treatments and given daily over 4–6 weeks. Fractionation was made popular by Regaud[28] who carried out a series of experiments on rams testicles in the early 1920s. When a large single treatment was given the animal was not sterilized but there was marked moist desquamation of the overlying skin. When the treatment was spread out over a number of sessions the animal was rendered sterile without damage to the scrotal skin. Coutard then showed the value of fractionation in the treatment of squamous cancers of pharynx and larynx.[29] Fractionation takes advantage of the differing abilities of malignant tumors and normal tissues to repair radiation damage and proliferate to replace cells killed by radiation. Fractionation also allows reoxygenation, rendering cells initially hypoxic and potentially radioresistant to become well oxygenated and more radiosensitive. In many parts of the world, radiotherapy is given in 2 Gy fractions. The advantage of this regimen is that the severity of acute reactions predict the development of severe late complications particularly in skin and oral mucosa. If there is only moderate desquamation of skin or moderate mucositis, late fibrosis scarring, and necrosis is extremely unlikely.

Brachytherapy

Another method of increasing the therapeutic ratio is the use of continuous low dose rate radiation. Suitable radionuclides, traditionally radium, now caesium-137 or iridium-192 can be implanted in tumors (brachytherapy) These nuclides may be in tubes, needles or in the form of wire. Radium has a very long half-life (1620 years) and therefore provides a stable long-lived source of gamma irra-

diation. The major source of the gamma rays is the gaseous daughter product radon. Radium tubes or needles must be gas tight and frequently checked for leaks. The gamma rays produced (range 0.05–2.45 MeV) are very penetrating and very thick lead shields are required to provide adequate radiation protection. Caesium-137 which has no gaseous daughter products, a useful half-life of 30 years and a somewhat less penetrating 660 KeV gamma ray has largely replaced radium for gynecological work (Fig. 4.9.2). Iridium in the form of flexible wire has many advantages over traditional radium or caesium needles. Thin wire (0.3 mm in diameter) can be supplied in long lengths and can be inserted into flexible nylon tubes or afterloading needles implanted into tumors. Thicker wire (0.6 mm in diam.) in the form of 'hairpins' can be inserted directly into tumors through suitable introducers. Iridium produces a gamma ray of 330 KeV and lead shields only 2 cm in thickness provide very good protection. The only major disadvantage of iridium is the short half-life (74 days) therefore fresh material must be ordered for each implant.

The major advantage of brachytherapy is that a high dose is given to the tumor with minimal irradiation of surrounding normal tissues. Constant low dose irradiation takes advantage of the different rates of repair and repopulation of normal and malignant tissue to produce differential cell killing. Reoxygenation may occur during low dose rate radiotherapy with initially resistant hypoxic cells becoming well aerated and sensitive. Iridium sources are implanted and the dose to tissues calculated using a set of rules called the Paris system.[30] A typical dose would be 65 Gy given over 6–7 days.

Manually inserted radium or cesium is still an excellent treatment for early cervical cancer. The most well-known methods were developed in Manchester and Stockholm.[31] The disadvantage of these techniques is the radiation dose received by operating theatre staff and nurses. In order to reduce staff radiation exposure, various afterloading devices have been introduced.[32] The most popular in Europe is the Selectron. Stainless-steel pellets containing caesium in glass move backwards and forwards pneumatically from a computer controlled lead-lined safe into intrauterine and vaginal applicators (Figs 4.9.3 and 4.9.4). This allows the nurses to leave the room before starting treatment. If a

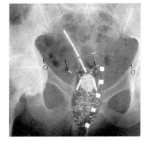

Fig. 4.9.2 *AP radiograph of a manually inserted cesium insertion in an elderly patient suffering from carcinoma of cervix (note osteoarthritic changes in right hip). Such patients tend to tolerate manually inserted cesium better than afterloading. The A and O points (dose to obturator node) are marked.*

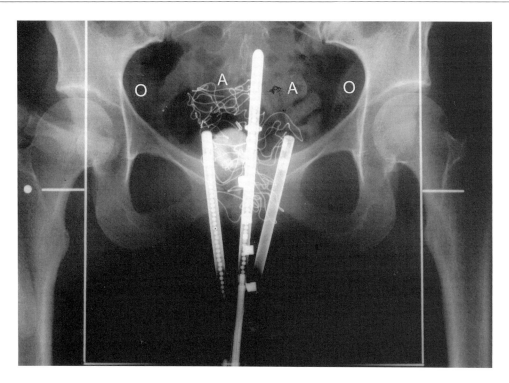

Fig. 4.9.3 *Anterior radiograph of a selectron afterloading cesium insertion. Cesium pellets in glass can be moved pneumatically in and out of the applicators in the uterus and vagina. The position of the A points and O points (the position of the obturator node) are marked.*

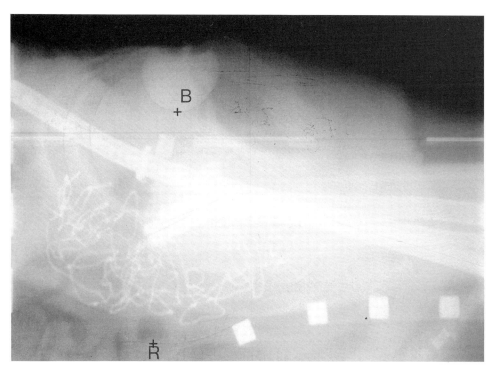

Fig. 4.9.4 *Lateral radiograph of a selectron afterloading insertion. Gauze containing a radiopaque 'raytex' thread was packed beneath the ovoids to reduce the dose to the rectum. A marker was placed in the rectum and the bladder position was delineated by contrast medium ('Conray') used to expand to the Foley catheter balloon. Points B and R are the points where the dose to the bladder and rectum are measured.*

nurse needs to re-enter the room, at a touch of a button the radioactive sources can be rapidly returned to the safe.

Radiation dosimetry

Most radiation treatment plans aim to deliver a homogeneous dose to the target volume (Fig. 4.9.5). For instance in the treatment of head and neck cancer the dose variation through the target volume is usually only + or −2% and rarely more than + or −5%. The converse is true in the treatment of carcinoma of cervix where treatment dosage is very dishomogeneous. This is because the tolerance of the various pelvic organs to radiation is markedly different. The first attempt to define a point in the pelvis where the measured dose was a predictor of normal tissue damage was in 1938.[33] The dose at a point where the uterine artery crossed the ureter proved to be a good predictor of damage to the ureter and also the bladder and rectum. This was called 'point A' and is defined as the point 2 cm lateral to the uterine canal and 2 cm above the cervical os. Often both brachytherapy and external beam treatment are combined in the treatment of this cancer. Typical doses to point A from brachytherapy alone or a combination of brachytherapy and external radiation are in the order of 75 Gy. Much higher doses (up to 200 Gy) can be delivered to parts of cervical tumors very close to interstitial sources. In order to prevent late damage the dose to rectum, bladder and small bowel should be less than at point A. Small bowel is the most vulnerable pelvic organ. A fixed loop of small bowel in the pelvis following previous surgery or pelvic inflammatory disease is particularly at risk. To avoid small bowel injury pelvic sidewall dose is usually limited to 40–50 Gy.

FUTURE PERSPECTIVES

Improved diagnostic accuracy

In order to ensure cure after radiotherapy all tumor must be included in the treated volume. Improvements in diagnostic imaging have reduced the possibility of inadvertently missing part of the cancer. A good example is the treatment of bladder cancer. Traditionally treatment was planned by instiling contrast medium into the bladder and, taking account of the cystoscopic findings, drawing a treatment volume on orthogonal radiographs. The accuracy of this method has been compared to planning using computerized tomography (CT). In one study[34] 18% of tumors treated received in part significantly less than the prescribed dose. The same group have shown that the prognosis of bladder cancer patients has been improved by CT assisted treatment planning.

Neither ultrasound nor CT scanning has proved satisfactory in the detection of small pelvic lymph node metastasis. Magnetic resonance imaging (MRI) looks more promising. A comparison of MRI with surgical staging in early cervical cancer has shown MRI has a 76% accuracy in the detection of lymph nodes spread.[35] The latest MRI machines have better resolving power and the ability to detect lymph nodes should improve further. The inclusion of previously unsuspected lymph node metastases into the irradiated volume may improve survival for some patients.

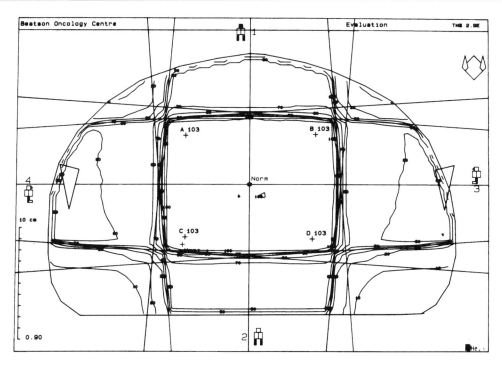

Fig. 4.9.5 *A four-field radiation treatment plan for the external beam treatment of a cervical tumor including pelvic lymph nodes. The dose variation across the target volume is 3%.*

Interaction of chemotherapy and radiotherapy

Radiotherapy is primarily a local treatment, chemotherapy is mainly used to treat systemic disease. However, chemotherapy may be combined with radiotherapy in three main ways, adjuvant, induction (neo-adjuvant) or as combination treatment when both modalities are given together. In the treatment of common solid tumors, chemotherapy is most effective against a small tumor burden such as occult metastasis. Adjuvant chemotherapy before or after radiotherapy has been shown to produce a modest increase in survival in node positive premenopausal breast cancer patients.[36] Induction (neo-adjuvant) chemotherapy is given prior to radiotherapy to reduce the size of the primary tumor therefore making radiotherapy more effective. Response rates of up to 80% were seen after cisplatin and 5-fluorouracil chemotherapy was given prior to radiotherapy in advanced squamous cancer of head and neck. However, controlled trials have failed to show any improvement in survival by this approach.[37] Response rates of at least 50% have followed cisplatin-based chemotherapy prior to radiation in cervical cancer. Although chemotherapy responders can be shown to have statistically better survival than non-responders[38] the results of large randomized trials are keenly awaited.

Giving chemotherapy along with radiation is in theory one way of killing radioresistant cells. Two recent studies in locally advanced head and neck cancer[39,40] of cisplatin along with radiation show this approach seems to give an impressive improvement in survival with very little additional toxicity. Certainly further studies seem warranted.

Individualization of therapy schedules

At present all patients with the same tumor stage and histology are treated using the same schedule, usually a fractionation regimen that has been shown to produce reasonable results. It is presently believed that surviving cells in some tumors undergo rapid repopulation during fractionated radiotherapy which partially offsets the tumoricidal effects of treatment.[41] It is possible that rapidly repopulating tumors may be identified as having a short potential doubling time (the theoretical doubling time with a fixed growth fraction in the absence of cell loss). Potential doubling time can be calculated by flow cytometric analysis of tumor biopsy specimens taken from patients given bromodeoxyuridine (Budr) as a cell phase marker.[42] In a group of 72 head and neck patients treated by 2 Gy fractions over 7 weeks, those with a potential doubling time (T_{pot}) of less than four days had inferior local control compared to those with longer doubling times.[43] Accelerated radiotherapy when treatment is given twice or three times daily usually using a fraction of less than 2 Gy is being tried throughout the world mainly to treat head and neck cancer. A French collaborative group treating oropharyngeal cancer have demonstrated improved local control rates for twice daily treatment compared with orthodox fractionation.[44]

No novel fractionation studies for cervical cancer are currently in progress. However, cell kinetic studies suggest that control rates could be improved by this approach. The study by Bolger et al.[45] showed a progressive elevation of calculated labeling index (an indicator of increased growth rate) with advancing stage (Spearman rank correlation $r=0.27$, $P=0.005$). The median potential doubling time (T_{pot}) of the series was 4.4 days. If T_{pot} reflects population kinetics these results imply that a substantial group of patients may benefit from accelerated fractionation if such a regimen was used selectively.

One of the most important factors governing outcome following radiotherapy is intrinsic tumor radiosensitivity. The intrinsic radiosensitivity of biopsies taken from patients with carcinoma of cervix was investigated in Manchester.[46] Cell suspensions were exposed to a test dose of 2 Gy and the surviving fraction (SF2 value) assayed using the Courtney Mills technique (a clonogenic assay growing colonies on semi-solid agar). There was a strong correlation between survival and SF2 value. One of the disadvantages of this method is that the Courtney Mills technique is laborios and 5 weeks must elapse before meaningful results are available. More rapid methods such as pulsed gel electrophoresis[47] and the cell adhesive matrix (CAM) assay are under investigation.[48]

As well as assessing radiation sensitivity of tumors, it is important to recognize individuals who have abnormal normal tissue radiosensitivity. The treatment schedule and total dose used to treat any tumor is a compromise between curing the patient and the risks of damaging normal tissues. A serious complication rate of 5% in the treatment of cervical cancer is usually accepted as the dose-limiting level.[32] In 1980 a child was treated at St Bartholomew's Hospital in London for Hodgkin's disease by a standard and well-tolerated radiotherapy schedule. Unfortunately this child developed very severe postradiation sequelae that proved to be fatal.[49] Post radiotherapy this child was found to be suffering from the ataxia–telangiectasia syndrome (A-T). Taylor et al.[50] found that fibroblasts and lymphocytes from patients suffering from A-T were about three times more sensitive to the lethal effects of radiation than normal cells. A-T is inherited as an autosomal recessive disorder and is rare, with an incidence of only 1 in 40 000 of the population. Heterozygous carriage of the gene is common and the prevalence of A-T carriage in a western population is estimated to be 1–3%.[51] Radiobiological studies suggest that A-T heterozygotes exhibit abnormal cellular repair of DNA.[52] As it is estimated that A-T heterozygotes have a 2–6-fold risk of dying from cancer this group of people may be a significant proportion of those receiving radiotherapy. The small minority of patients developing serious complications after radiotherapy may include a substantial number of A-T heterozygotes. There are an increasingly large number of DNA repair deficiency diseases that show abnormal radiosensitivity.[53] Identification of these individuals may result in a reduction in late radiation injuries and perhaps a clinically significant increase in the dose to the majority of normal patients. This could offer a worthwhile increase in local control and cure.

SUMMARY

- Radiotherapy is responsible for about 40% of all cures from cancer. It can offer patients beyond cure significant palliation.
- The art of radiotherapy is to destroy a malignant tumor with little or no damage to normal tissues.
- Successful radiotherapy depends on the optimal exploitation of the therapeutic ratio, which is the relationship between the desired and undesired effects of treatment. What limits the radiation dose given in an attempt to cure a tumor is the risk of normal tissue damage.
- Fractionation, dividing a course of treatment into 20 or 30 daily doses is an important device to increase the therapeutic ratio.
- Differential cell killing is probably due to differences in repair of radiation damage, differential repopulation of malignant and normal cells and reoxygenation of initially hypoxic and consequently radioresistant cells.
- Megavoltage X-rays generated by a linear accelerator are used in modern external beam radiotherapy. Unlike kilovoltage X-rays from older apparatus megavoltage X-rays are 'skin sparing' and can easily reach deep-seated tumors.
- Continuous low dose radiation from sources implanted into the tumor give a high dose to the lesion with minimal irradiation of surrounding tissues. Such treatments exploit differences in repair and repopulation between malignant and normal cells, and allow hypoxic cells to reoxygenate.
- Interstitial radiotherapy using manually inserted radium or cesium is an important treatment method for cervical and some cases of endometrial cancers. Remote afterloading systems such as the Selectron are being introduced to reduce staff radiation exposure.
- Improvements in diagnostic imaging such as CT or MRI scanning have improved cure rates by ensuring previous unsuspected tumor spread is included in the irradiated volume.
- In the future, novel fractionation schemes, in which treatment is given twice or three times daily, may improve local control rates. Already, accelerated hyperfractionated regimens are producing improved results in the treatment of head and neck cancer. It may be possible to use individual patient data such as tumor cell kinetics, normal tissue and tumor radiosensitivity to design 'tailormade' fractionation schedules.

REFERENCES

1. De Vita VT, Goldin A, Olivera VT et al. The drug development and clinical trials programs of the Division of Cancer Treatment, National Cancer Institute. Cancer Clinical Trials 1979 2: 195–216.
2. Souhami R, Tobias J. Cancer and Its Management, Oxford: Blackwell, 1988: 86.
3. Bissett DB, Symonds RP, Lamont DW et al. The treatment of stage 1 cancer of cervix in the West of Scotland 1980–1987. Br J Gynaecol Obstet 1994 101: 615–620.
4. Davidson SE, Symonds RP, Lamont DW, Watson ER. Does adenocarcinoma of uterine cervix have a worse prognosis than squamous carcinoma when treated by radiotherapy? Gynecol Oncol 1989 33: 23–26.
5. Joslin CA, Vaishampayan GV, Mallik A. The treatment of early cancer of the corpus uteri. Br J Radiol 1977 50: 38–45.
6. Price P, Hoskin PJ, Easton D et al. Prospective randomised trial of single and multi-fraction schedules in the treatments of bone metastasis. Radiother Oncol 1986 6: 247–255.
7. Lung Cancer Working Party of the Medical Research Council. Inoperable non-small cell lung cancer (HSCLC). A Medical Research Council randomised trial of two or ten fractions. Br J Cancer 1991 63: 265–270.
8. Doll RD, Smith PG The long term effects of X irradiation in patients treated for metropathia haemorrhagica. Br J Radiol 1968 41: 362–368.
9. Fingl E, Woodbury DM. General principals. In Goodman LS, Gilman A (eds) The Pharmacological Basis of Therapeutics London: MacMillan, 1975: 28.
10. Robertson AG, Boyle P, Symonds RP et al. The effects of differing radiotherapeutic schedules on response of glottic carcinoma of larynx. Eur J Cancer 1993 29A: 501–510.
11. Sowby FD Statement of the 1985 Paris meeting of the International Commission on Radiation Protection. Phys Med Biol 1985 30: 863–864.
12. Elkind MM, Sutton H, Moses WB et al. Radiation response of mammalian cells in culture V. Temperature dependence of the repair of X-ray damage in surviving cells (aerobic and hypoxic) Radiat Res 1965 25: 359–376.
13. Whitmore GF, Gulyas S. Studies on the recovery processes in mouse L cells. Natl Cancer Inst Monogr 1967 24: 141–156.
14. Belli JA, Shelton M. Potentially lethal radiation damage repair by mammalian cells in culture. Science 1969 165: 490–492.
15. Weichselbaum R, Little JB, Nove J. Response of human osteosarcoma in vitro to irradiation: evidence for unusual cellular repair activity. Int J Radiat Biol 1977 31: 295–299.
16. Holthusen H. Beitrage zur biologie der strahlenwirkung. Pflugers Archiv 1921 187: 1–24.
17. Grady LH, Conger AD, Ebert M. The concentration of oxygen dissolved in tissues at the time of irradiation as a factor in radiotherapy. Br J Radiol 1953 26: 638–648.
18. Thomlinson RH, Gray LH. The histological structure of some human lung cancers and the possible implications for radiotherapy. Br J Cancer 1955 9: 539–549.
19. Watson ER, Halnan KE, Dische S et al. Hyperbaric oxygen and radiotherapy. A Medical Research Council trial in carcinoma of cervix. Br J Radiol 1978 51: 879–887.
20. Medical Research Council trial of Misonidazole in carci-

noma of cervix. A report of the MRC working party on misonidazole for cancer of cervix. *Br J Radiol* 1984 **57**: 491–499.

21. Dische S, Chassange D, Hope-Stone HF *et al.* A trial of Ro 03–8799 (pimonidazole) in carcinoma of the uterine cervix: An interim report from the Medical Research Council working party on advanced carcinoma of cervix. *Radiother Oncol* 1993 **26**: 93–103.

22. Terasima R, Tolmach LJ. X-ray sensitivity and DNA synthesis in synchronous populations of Hela cells. *Science* 1963 **140**: 490–492.

23. Withers HR, Mason K, Reid BO *et al.* Response of mouse intestine to neutrons and gamma rays in relation to dose, fractionation and division cycle. *Cancer* 1974 **34**: 39–47.

24. Stone RS. Neutron therapy and specific ionisation. *Am J Roent Genol* 1948 **59**: 771–785.

25. Catherall M, Bewley DK, Sutherland I. Second report of a randomised clinical trial of fast neutrons with x or gamma rays in the treatment of advanced cancer of the head and neck. *Br Med J* 1977 **1**: 194–195.

26. Macdougall RH, Orr JA, Kerr GR *et al.* Fast neutron treatment for squamous carcinoma of the head and neck: final report of the Edinburgh randomised trial. *Br Med J* 1990 **301**: 1241–1242.

27. Errington RD, Ashby D, Gore SM *et al.* High energy neutron treatments for pelvic cancers: study stopped because of increased mortality. *Br Med J* 1991 **302**: 1045–1051.

28. Regaud C. Influence de la duree de radiation sur les effects determines dans le testicle par le radium. *C R Soc Biol (Paris)* 1922 **86**: 878–890.

29. Coutard H. Roentgen therapy of epitheliomas of the tonsillar region, hypopharynx and larynx from 1920–1926. *Am J Roent Genol* 1932 **28**: 313–331.

30. Pierquin B, Dutreix A, Paine CH *et al.* The Paris system of interstitial radiation therapy. *Acta Radiol Oncol* 1978 **17**: 33–48.

31. Kjellgren O. Clinical invasive carcinoma of the cervix: place of radiotherapy as primary treatment. In Coppleson M (ed.) *Gynecologic Oncology* Edingburgh: Churchill Livingstone, 1992: 673–695.

32. Jones RD, Symonds RP, Habeshaw T *et al.* A comparison of remote afterloading and manually inserted caesium in the treatment of carcinoma of cervix. *Clin Oncol* 1990 **2**: 193–198.

33. Meredith WJ. *Radium Dosage: The Manchester System.* Livingstone: Edinburgh, 1967: 42–49.

34. Rothwell RI, Ash D V, Thorogood J. An analysis of the contribution of computed tomography to treatment outcome in bladder cancer. *Clin Radiol* 1985 **36**: 369–372.

35. Greco A, Mason P, Leung WL *et al.* Staging of carcinoma of uterine cervix: MRI-surgical correlation. *Clin Radiol* 1989 **40**: 401–405.

36. Early Breast Cancer Trials Collaborative Group. Systemic treatment of early breast cancer by hormonal, cytotoxic or immune therapy. *Lancet* 1992 **339**: 1–15 and 71–85.

37. Vokes EE, Weichelbaum RR, Lipman SM *et al.* Head and neck cancer. *N Engl J Med* 1993 **328**: 184–194.

38. Symonds RP, Burnett RA, Habershaw T *et al.* The prog-

nostic value of a response to chemotherapy given before radiotherapy in advanced cancer of cervix. *Br J Cancer* 1989 **59**: 473–475.

39. Slotman GJ, Doolitle CH, Glicksman AS. Preoperative combined chemotherapy and radiation therapy plus radical surgery in advanced head and neck cancer. *Cancer* 1992 **69**: 2736–2743.

40. Merlano M, Vitale V, Rosso R *et al.* Treatment of advanced cancer of head and neck with alternating chemotherapy and radiotherapy. *N Engl J Med* 1992 **327**: 1115–1121.

41. Fowler JF. Modelling altered fractionation schedules. *Br J Radiol* 1992 **Suppl 24**: 187–192.

42. Begg AC, McNally NJ, Shrieve DC *et al.* A method to measure the duration of DNA synthesis and the potential doubling time from a single specimen. *Cytometry* 1985 **6**: 620–626.

43. Begg AC. Predictive value of potential doubling time for radiotherapy of head and neck tumour patients: results from EORTC Cooperative Trial 22851. *Semin Radiat Oncol* 1992 **2**: 1–3.

44. Horiot JC, Le Fur R, N'Guypen T *et al.* Hyperfractionated compared with conventional radiotherapy in oropharyngeal carcinoma. An EORTC randomised trial. *Eur J Cancer* 1990 **26**: 779–780.

45. Bolger BS, Cooke TG, Symonds RP *et al.* Measurement of cell kinetics in cervical tumours using bromodeoxyuridine. *Br J Cancer* 1993 **68**: 168–171.

46. West CML, Davidson SE, Roberts SA *et al.* Intrinsic radiosensitivity and prediction of patient response to radiotherapy for carcinoma of cervix. *Br J Cancer* 1993 **68**: 819–823.

47. Giacca AJ, Schwatz J, Shieh J *et al.* The use of assymetric field inversion gel to predict tumour cell radiosensitivity. *Radiother Oncol* 1992 **24**: 231–238.

48. Girinsky T, Lubin R, Pignon JP *et al.* Predictive value of *in vitro* radiosensitivity parameters in head and neck cancers and cervical carcinomas: preliminary correlation with local control and overall survival *Int J Radiat Oncol Biol Phys* 1992 **25**: 3–7.

49. Pritchard J, Sandland MR, Breatnach FB, Pincott JR, Cox R, Husband P. The effects of radiation therapy for Hodgkin's disease in a child with ataxia telangiectasia. *Cancer* 1984 **50**: 877–886.

50. Taylor AMR, Harnden DG, Arlett CR *et al.* Ataxia–telangiectasia, a human mutation with abnormal radiosensitivity. *Nature* 1975 **258**: 427–429.

51. Nagasawa H, Kraemer KH, Shiloh Y, Little JB Detection of telangiectasia heterozygous cell lines by post irradiation cummulative labelling measurements with coded samples. *Cancer Res* 1987 **47**: 398–402.

52. Blocher D, Sigut D, Hannah MA Fibroblasts from ataxia telangiectasia (AT) and AT heterozygotes show an enhanced level of residual DNA double-strand breaks after low dose rate gamma irradiation as assayed by pulsed field gel electrophoresis. *Int J Radiat Biol* 1991 **60**: 803–818.

53. Cartwright R, McMillan TJ. Isolation of DNA repair genes. In Yarnold J, Stratton M, McMillan TJ (eds) *Molecular Biology for Oncologists*. Amsterdam: Elsevier, 1993: 199–211.

4.10

Principles of Chemotherapy

J Cassidy and SB Kaye

INTRODUCTION

The use of cytotoxic chemotherapy in hematological malignancies revolutionized the survival pattern of these diseases. This promise has not so far been continued into most common solid tumors. However, even in those patients not curable by currently available chemotherapy, useful palliation and extension of life span can be achieved.

In the field of gynecologic cancers most attention has been focused on ovarian and cervical carcinoma, and for that reason the drugs described in this chapter will be those which have found clinical utility in these diseases.

In addition, we will attempt to give the reader enough conceptual framework on which to be able to judge new drug developments in the field, or to critically assess new therapeutic strategies.

CURRENT CANCERS

Basic principles

In experimental systems the growth of neoplastic cells is initially exponential and slows later as contact inhibition occurs *in vitro*, or as the tumor outgrows its nutrient and oxygen supply *in vivo*. This pattern of growth is also influenced by local hormonal and growth factor concentrations as well as interaction between tumor cells, host cells and stromal components.

Since most anticancer drugs act on DNA or the mechanics of cell division they tend to be most effective when the tumor is growing rapidly with a short doubling time. In highly aggressive tumors the total cell cycle duration may be as short as 12 h; conversely indolent tumors

may have many G_0 cells which are generally insensitive to anticancer drugs. Various mathematical models have been constructed to try to model the interaction between cell kinetics and cytotoxic drugs.[1]

In understanding the principles behind cytotoxic drug usage it is necessary to review three hypotheses which influence our rationale in this area.

In 1964, Skipper et al.[2] using a rodent leukemia model showed that:

1. A single cell is capable of replication to kill the host;
2. There is a relationship between dose and the fraction of cell kill;
3. Survival of the host is inversely related to tumor cell burden.

This work has a number of clinical implications; from (1) it would appear that cytotoxic therapy should be continued until *all* tumor cells have been killed, and from (3) the inference is that one should treat tumors at an early stage when tumor burden is smallest.

In 1979, Goldie and Coldman[3] produced a model to explain the development of drug resistance in tumor cells. They suggested that spontaneous random mutation, occurring at a rate of 10^{-6} or higher, in a clinically detectable tumor of 10^9 cells, was likely to produce resistant cells capable of clonal expansion. This model explains the inverse relationship between curability and tumor mass independent of tumor growth kinetics. It also serves as the clinical rationale for the use of combination rather than single agent chemotherapy.

In 1977, Norton and Simon[4] hypothesized that to overcome the acceleration of cell turnover that occurs as a tumor is debulked it was necessary to increase treatment intensity as the tumor became smaller. This has led to the clinical strategies of 'late-intensification' in hematological and some solid tumors, and forms part of the rationale for the current use of high-dose therapy with bone marrow or peripheral blood stem cell transplantation.

Specific classes of anticancer drugs relevant to gynecological malignancy (Table 4.10.1)

Alkylating agents

As the name suggests, these exert a cytotoxic action by linking alkyl groups covalently to proteins and nucleic acids. Although capable of binding to a variety of subcellular components the impairment of DNA replication is felt to be the major mechanism of cytotoxicity.[5] There are a large number of clinically available alkylators which vary in toxicity and activity profiles. These variations between members of the group can be largely explained by the relative efficiency of alkylation. Alkylators which can give two bifunctional alkylation products (e.g. thiotepa) can produce within-strand or between-strand bonding, and tend to be more efficient than so-called monofunctional drugs. The large choice of clinically available agents within this group allows selection of appropriate 'aggressiveness' in therapy. In elderly ovarian cancer patients the less toxic (and less effective) drugs such as chlorambucil are often employed, whereas in younger patients cyclophosphamide or ifosfamide may be more appropriate as first-line therapy. Both cyclophosphamide and ifosfamide require metabolic activation by hepatic metabolism and both produce an acrolein metabolite which can cause hemorrhagic cystitis.[6]

Cisplatin

The development of cisplatin in the mid-1970s revolutionized the therapy of certain malignancies such as testicular teratoma and ovarian carcinoma, and has made a significant impact in many others. As the molecule diffuses into cells because of the 30-fold difference in chloride concentration between intracellular and extracellular fluid the chloride ions are lost from its structure and the compound then forms DNA cross-links by an action similar to a bifunctional alkylating agent.[7] The DNA lesions induced are frequent and difficult to repair, thus leading to a high cell kill. Cisplatin is the single most active drug in cervical carcinoma and arguably (vs. carboplatin) in ovarian cancer.[8] The clinical utility is, however, reduced by its toxicity profile, which in turn is largely explained by its tissue distribution and clearance.

Cisplatin which is highly bound to plasma proteins and is taken up avidly into tissues produces a terminal excretion half-life of about 60 h. The main route of excretion is renal and the use of high doses necessitates monitoring of renal function and induction of a forced diuresis to minimize renal toxicity. The occurrence of a peripheral neuropathy and ototoxicity is common and limits cumulative doses. In addition cisplatin is capable of producing profound nausea and vomiting and a particular syndrome of 'delayed emesis' which can last for 7–10 days post-administration.

Synergy of cisplatin with antimetabolites and topoisomerase II inhibitors has been demonstrated in vitro and in clinical trials. The full mechanism underlying this synergy is not clear but enhancement of the affinity of cisplatin for DNA binding sites, alterations in the mode of DNA damage and disruption in DNA repair mechanisms have all been suggested.[7]

This toxicity profile of cisplatin prompted a search for less toxic analogs and led to the development of carboplatin. Although the cytotoxic lesions induced by both agents are similar they should not be considered as interchangeable in clinical practice. In particular, although carboplatin does not (in standard dosage) produce neurotoxicity or renal toxicity, it does cause myelosuppression (particularly thrombocytopenia) which reduces the dose-intensity of platinum which can be administered. This is of most importance when considering combination therapy with other myelosuppressive drugs.

Controversy still exists as to which of these platinum agents is optimal in ovarian carcinoma, but a recent consensus meeting recommended that carboplatin should not routinely replace cisplatin.[9]

Antimetabolites

Methotrexate

Methotrexate is an antifolate, the cytotoxic effects of which are dependent on a number of interrelated biochemical events including membrane transport of the drug, polyglutamation, saturation of dihydrofolate reductase binding sites, and depletion of intracellular tetrahydrofolate pools. The net result is to produce a block in thymidylate monophosphate synthesis which inhibits RNA and DNA synthesis.

The metabolic blockade induced by methotrexate can be reversed by administration of reduced folates. The most common form being 'folinic acid rescue'.[10] This agent is particularly useful in cases of unexpected delay in clearance of methotrexate or in planned rescue from high-dose methotrexate therapy.

In gynecological practice methotrexate is most often used in cervical cancer patients, and less often in pelvic

Table 4.10.1 Classification of anticancer drugs use in gynecological cancer

Alkylating agents	Cyclophosphamide
	Ifosfamide
	Treosulphan
	Chlorambucil
	Thiotepa
Platinum compounds	Cisplatin
	Carboplatin
Antimetabolites	Methotrexate
	5-fluorouracil
Antitumor antibiotics	Adriamycin
	Bleomycin
Vinca alkaloids	Vincristine
	Vinclesine
	Vinblastine
Topiosomerase inhibitors	Etoposide (VP-16)
Miscellaneous	Hexamethylmelanine
	Taxanes

sarcoma. In these instances particular care must be taken to ensure adequate renal function and to maintain diuresis throughout the treatment.

Methotrexate is also capable of forming a 'reservoir' in biological fluids such as ascites or pleural effusion. This can lead to the 'third space effect' whereby the drug excretion follows a prolonged, delayed pattern leading to extreme toxicity in the form of diarrhea, mucositis and myelosuppression.

Methotrexate is approximately 50% bound to serum albumin and can produce clinically significant interactions with drugs which alter or compete for protein binding e.g. the non-steroidal anti-inflammatory drugs.

5-Fluorouracil

Substitution of fluorine for a hydrogen atom on uracil yields 5FU. Intracellularly the drug is metabolized to fluorouridine monophosphate (FUMP) and subsequently to fluorodeoxyuridine monophosphate (FdUMP). In most experimental systems FdUMP inhibition of thymidylate synthetase appears to be the prime cytotoxic action. However, incorporation into RNA and DNA has also been demonstrated and may be important in some tumor types.[11]

Thymidylate synthase (TS) is the only *de novo* source of thymidylate in the cell and, as such, is a key enzyme in mammalian DNA synthesis. The inhibition of TS can be increased by changes in 5FU administration schedule (prolonged infusion) or by co-medication with biochemical modulators such as folinic acid or alpha-interferon.

5FU has single agent activity in ovarian cancer, but is most often used in palliation of recurrent malignant ascites or effusions, because of its low systemic toxicity. When used intravenously toxicity includes nausea, diarrhea, mucositis and myelosuppression.

Antitumor antibiotics

Anthracyclines

The prototypes of this class; daunomycin and adriamycin are derived from species of *Streptomyces* fungus. A number of semi-synthetic analogs have been introduced (e.g. epirubicin) with similar activity but some improvements in toxicity profile.

The mechanism of action of anthracyclines is still unclear despite the clinical importance of these drugs. Most would support a nuclear site of action, with DNA as the prime target.[12] Important aspects of drug action include:

1. production of free radicals;
2. direct intercalation of DNA through the aglycone moiety;
3. binding through ternary complexes of iron, anthracycline and DNA;
4. stabilization of topoisomerase II–DNA complexes.

As a class these are the most widely used cytotoxic agents, with activity in multiple tumor types. Adriamycin has single agent activity in ovarian cancer, but is more usually used in combination with an alkylator or platinum compound. For first-line therapy, cisplatin combinations which include an anthracycline may lead to minor benefits compared with those without an anthracycline, but this may well be outweighed by greater toxicity. As a group, anthracyclines possess the greatest single agent activity in sarcoma (approximately 20–30% response rate) and they are now in use in many research protocols in this area.

Toxicity of anthracyclines is mainly manifest as alopecia, nausea and vomiting and myelosuppression. In addition, high cumulative doses are associated with a risk of cardiomyopathy. The newer analogs (epirubicin) have a reduced risk of this toxicity.

Bleomycin

Bleomycin consists of a mixture of glycopeptides originally isolated from *Streptomyces verticillus*, but it is now chemically synthesized. Bleomycin produces strand scission of DNA, primarily single-strand breaks. Fragmentation of DNA may be enhanced by concurrent irradiation of the target cells.[13] Studies have also demonstrated that bleomycin can damage mitochondrial DNA with impact on the respiratory chain enzymes.[14] It is active in a wide spectrum of diseases and is used as part of curative therapy of germ cell tumors (including ovarian germ cell tumors) or palliative therapy of cervical carcinoma. In addition, partly because of its sclerosant nature it is frequently used in intracavitary therapy (pleura, pericardium, peritoneum).

The toxicities of bleomycin are manageable and allow inclusion of this drug in myelosuppressive combinations. Common toxicities include; chills, fevers, allergic reactions, mucositis and skin pigmentation.

Vinca alkaloids

The vinca alkaloids are extracted from the periwinkle *Catharanthus roseus*. They induce cytotoxicity by binding to tubulin and preventing the function of microtubules, including formation of the mitotic spindle. Although mitotic arrest is considered the prime mode of action, there is evidence to support a direct cytotoxic effect of vinca alkaloids[15] but the clinical significance of this is not clear.

Three vinca alkaloids are in clinical use, vincristine, vindesine and vinblastine. Although they share the same mechanism of action they differ in respect of spectra of activity and toxicity. In gynecological practice, vinblastine is most commonly used in germ cell tumors and choriocarcinoma. Vincristine is used in uterine or pelvic sarcomas (in combination with other agents), and in combination with cisplatin for cervical cancer.

Toxicities include peripheral neuropathy, alopecia and myelosuppression.

Podophyllotoxins

Podophyllotoxins are semi-synthetic derivatives of extracts of the American mandrake *Podophyllin peltatum*. Although capable of tubulin binding these drugs do not inhibit microtubule assembly at clinically relevant concentrations. They do induce a blockade of cells in the premitotic phase, and produce both single and double-strand breaks in DNA, probably as a result of the formation of a stable ternary complex with DNA and the key nuclear enzyme topoisomerase II.[16]

Etoposide (VP-16) is the most widely used member of this class to date, and has high activity in germ cell tumors and some sarcomas when given in IV schedules. Recent data have emerged to show significant activity for low-dose oral etoposide administered chronically in refractory ovarian carcinoma.[39]

Myelosuppression is the dose-limiting toxicity, with nausea and vomiting more frequently observed with oral than IV administration.

Hexamethylmelamine

Hexamethylmelamine was originally thought to be an alkylating agent but is active in human tumors which are alkylator-resistant.[17] Its exact mechanism is unknown but it has been suggested that inhibition of incorporation of precursors into DNA and RNA may be important.[18]

Hexamethylmelamine has very poor aqueous solubility and is therefore only available for oral use. However, it is rapidly and reliably absorbed, and undergoes hepatic metabolism to a number of active derivatives. It is most commonly used in combination with other agents in management of ovarian carcinoma,[19] but its use is limited because of troublesome nausea and vomiting.

Taxol

Taxol was discovered in the 1960s in a screen of plant extracts for antitumour activity carried out by the National Cancer Institute in the USA.[20] Taxol was isolated from the bark of the western yew (*Taxus brevifolia*). Problems of formulation and the necessary use of a large number of trees for each dose led to the interruption of drug development for about a decade. The recognition of a unique mechanism of action; promotion of polymerization of microtubules,[21] as well as a good spectrum of activity in preclinical models[22] led to greater efforts to secure supplies and improve extraction of taxol from yew trees.

In the 1980s several phase I trials were initiated in the USA, but many did not reach a conclusion because of the incidence of unforeseen severe type I hypersensitivity reactions. In those phase I studies which were completed the dose-limiting toxicity was short-lived, non-cumulative, neutropenia.[23,24] In addition, investigators introduced a cocktail of prophylactic medication as an 'anti-allergic' regimen. This consisted of steroids and both H_1 and H_2 receptor antagonists. In subsequent clinical trials the adoption of this routine has significantly reduced both severity and frequency of anaphylactic reactions to taxol.

Other toxicities encountered were alopecia, peripheral neuropathy and transient myalgias and arthralgias. None of these have proven to be dose-limiting in subsequent studies. In these phase I studies responses were seen in several tumor types including ovarian cancer. A variety of dose-schedules were tested in phase I trials, but the 24 hour infusion schedule was selected for the initial US phase II trials.

Several phase II trials have confirmed a clinically useful level of activity for taxol in patients with refractory ovarian cancer (reviewed in reference 25). Responses have been seen in approximately 20–30% of heavily pretreated patients, but they have been relatively short-lived. The next logical step was to perform studies incorporating taxol into first-line combination therapy. In the USA the Gynecology Oncology Group (GOG).[26] showed a higher response rate for a taxol/cisplatin combination (54%) versus cyclophosphamide/cisplatin (33%). A statistically significant difference in progression-free survival has also emerged in favor of the taxol arm.

This important finding requires confirmation; in addition exploration of alternative dose schedules will continue to define optimum conditions for taxol usage in ovarian cancer.

Taxotere is derived from the needles of the European yew tree (*Taxus baccata*) and therefore has fewer supply problems than taxol.[27] It exerts cytotoxic activity in a manner similar to taxol. Clinical studies in a wide variety of malignancies have confirmed activity for this agent. In particular, encouraging levels of antitumor effect have been demonstrated in ovarian cancer.[28]

Principles of treatment

Dose

In the laboratory it is easy to demonstrate a dose–response relationship for cytotoxic drugs (Fig. 4.10.1). Similarly it is easy to demonstrate a dose–toxicity response in a clinical setting. The intrinsic heterogeneity of drug delivery and tumor response, as well as the difficulty in assessing response in deep-seated tumors makes it much more difficult to demonstrate dose–response in a patient population. Nevertheless a positive dose–response relationship has been demonstrated in both retrospective[29] and prospective studies,[30] and is part of the rationale of the current use of intensive high dose regimens in many tumor types.

It is believed that tumor 'drug exposure' as measured by the area under the concentration–time curve (AUC) is the crucial determinant of drug activity (Fig. 4.10.2). Clearly, both the concentration and duration of exposure can be

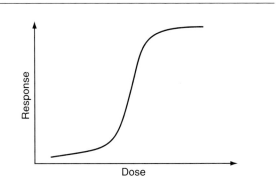

Fig. 4.10.1 *Dose–response for a typical cytotoxic drug.*

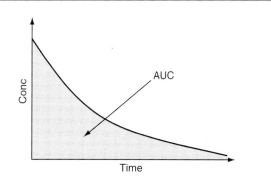

Fig. 4.10.2 *Area under the time–concentration curve (AUC).*

altered by changes in dose and schedule of administration. At present much of clinical pharmacology in this area is focused on optimization of these parameters, to achieve maximum antitumor effect.

The maximum dose of a cytotoxic is limited by normal tissue toxicity. In most instances this is manifest as damage to rapid turnover tissues such as the mucous membranes, hair follicles, skin and bone marrow. In some specific cases toxicity to other organs is limiting, particularly in use of high dose or high cumulative doses, e.g. lung toxicity with bleomycin, cardiomyopathy with anthracyclines.

The exploration of dose as an important parameter in determination of response in female genital tract cancer has been focused on cisplatin, with controversial and sometimes contradictory results from clinical trials.

The GOG in the USA conducted a series of single agent cisplatin studies in over 800 patients with squamous cell carcinoma of the cervix. They concluded that higher dose schedules did produce slight advantages.[31] However, it should be noted that high dose cisplatin is not always a feasible option for such patients with a propensity to renal dysfunction or urinary outflow obstruction.

The question of dose (and dose–intensity) in ovarian cancer is still controversial. Levin and Hrynuik[32] in a meta-analysis of ovarian cancer trials demonstrated a positive correlation between dose intensity of cisplatin and both response and survival. This led us to a Scottish study comparing 100 mg m^{-2} of cisplatin vs 50 mg m^{-2} in combination with 750 mg m^{-2} of cyclophosphamide. This randomized trial demonstrated conclusively that 100 mg m^{-2} was superior.[30] However, the dose of 100 mg m^{-2} of cisplatin was associated with troublesome neuropathy. Further escalation of 'platinum' intensity is being investigated using carboplatin in conjunction with hematological growth factors to abrogate marrow toxicity.

Route of administration

Most cytotoxic drugs are administered by the IV route for ease of administration and purposes of compliance with therapy. Pharmaceutical considerations of stability, molecular size, charge and lipid/aqueous solubility must be taken into consideration for all drugs, but have particular relevance in the field of oncology.

Few cytotoxics are administered by mouth because of problems of variable bioavailability leading to wide differences in 'drug exposure' of both the tumor and the host normal cells.

Cytotoxic drugs do lend themselves to loco-regional delivery, which tends to increase the drug concentration at the tumor site but reduce systemic exposure and hence reduce systemic toxicity. Examples include intracavitary administration, intrathecal use, isolated limb perfusion and intra-arterial therapy.

In gynecology, the use of intraperitoneal chemotherapy has been extensively explored. In ovarian cancer the opportunity exists to bathe most of the tumor bulk directly in cytotoxic solutions, since ovarian cancer spreads in a transcelomic fashion and remains localized to the peritoneal cavity for most of its natural history. A number of agents have been shown to have a 'pharmacokinetic' advantage for IP use, i.e. the peritoneal cavity/plasma AUC ratio is greater than one. This advantage ranges from 10–15 for cisplatin to 1408 for mitoxantrone. Cisplatin has an established single agent activity in ovarian cancer and has good local tolerability with no vesicant or irritant potential, and most studies have used this drug. A number of phase II studies have been performed which demonstrate significant antitumor effect, occasionally in cases of resistance to IV cisplatin.[33] The use of IP cisplatin also allows further exploration of dose–intensity with doses as high as 200 mg m^{-2} being reported. However, only one clinical trial supports IP over IV use for ovarian cancer chemotherapy. Although IP treatment does seem to produce some long-term survivors, it is unclear if this is more or less common than equivalent IV therapy.[34] At present it remains experimental therapy and the very limited penetration into tumor modules which has so far been demonstrated may prove to be a major obstacle.

Trials have also been conducted to investigate IP use of biologicals, antibodies, radionuclides or immune adjuvants in ovarian cancer; all with small patient numbers insufficient to demonstrate any possible advantages.

Combination chemotherapy

An ideal combination of cytotoxic drugs should have: (a) good single activity in that disease; (b) different mechanisms of action and phase specificity; and (c) minimally overlapping toxicity to allow maximal dosage of each agent. Such an ideal combination has not yet been defined for most solid cancers, and this has led to a profusion of trials using a multitude of combinations. Biological and cell kinetic principles should influence potential choices of combinations, and if applied will reduce the empiricism evident in some 'cookery class' designs.

Although there appear good theoretical reasons for the use of combination rather than single agents, it has often proven difficult to show conclusively any benefit in the clinical context. In particular it is unclear whether any combination is superior to single agent cisplatin in cervical carcinoma.[8] Combination treatment has been proven superior in germ cell tumors and probably in ovarian carcinoma.[35-37] This has led to a widespread acceptance of cisplatin plus cyclophosphamide as standard therapy in ovarian cancer.

The introduction of taxol has led to its inclusion in combination with cisplatin for ovarian carcinoma. As already mentioned a GOG study[26] demonstrated advantages for this combination over cisplatin–cyclophosphamide, and two large trials are currently underway to try to confirm and extend these observations.

Schedule

The therapeutic index of cytotoxic drugs is typically low. In preclinical testing many agents will show clear-cut schedule dependency, which may then influence the design of ensuing clinical trials. However, a number of existing cytotoxic agents have not yet found an optimum schedule of administration; good examples being 5FU and etoposide.

The advent of simple, safe access devices for intravenous infusions; together with major technical advances in ambulatory pump design has led to an upsurge in interest using prolonged IV infusion of drugs. This has clear theoretical advantages for drugs which have a short-plasma half-life, or display marked phase specificity (such as 5FU). Early results of continuous ambulatory 5FU trials in colonic cancer are very promising. If confirmed this may lead to a re-appraisal of the role of 5FU in cervical cancer.[38]

As well as increasing efficacy, continuous low-dose infusions can be used to reduce toxicity, e.g. bleomycin. Some drugs have particular toxicity associated with high peak plasma levels; thus use of divided doses or infusions reduced peak levels and reduces the risks of side-effects, e.g. adriamycin cardiomyopathy, cisplatin neurotoxicity.

It may even be possible to reduce toxicity and increase activity by changing the schedule of administration of some drugs, prolonged oral administration of etoposide being one example.[39]

Multimodality treatments

Chemotherapy is rarely if ever used as a single modality of therapy for malignant disease. Almost all patients will have had surgery of a diagnostic or therapeutic nature prior to treatment, and particularly in gynecological malignancies radiotherapy may be combined at some stage of therapy.

'Adjuvant' chemotherapy is given in a setting where all macroscopic and known microscopic disease has been excised. Such an approach is of proven benefit in breast cancer, but remains unproven in any female genital tract carcinoma.

'Neoadjuvant' chemotherapy is a term used to describe chemotherapy given prior to definitive surgery in an attempt to down-stage the disease or allow more limited surgery. No convincing benefits have yet been demonstrated for this approach, although breast cancer may soon prove to be the first tumor type to show such benefits.

The efficacy of chemotherapy is usually reduced where tissues have been exposed to prior irradiation, e.g. salvage treatment for relapsed cervical cancer. This effect is probably due to reduction in vasculature of the tumor, and hence gives penetration problems for cytotoxic drugs. This has led some investigators to explore the use of chemotherapy prior to planned potentially curative radiotherapy. Such trials have been confounded by problems with increased local and normal tissue toxicity caused by radiosensitization induced by certain chemotherapy drugs (5FU, cisplatin, adriamycin, bleomycin).

Optimal timing of chemotherapy, surgery and radiotherapy is an active area of research in many tumor types, but it is not currently possible to draw conclusions from this research.

Treatment of relapse

Ovarian cancer provides a good example of a disease in which courses of chemotherapy can be given on more than one occasion to the patient's benefit. The main factor which guides repeated chemotherapy is the time interval since previous treatment was used. Where this amounts to less than 4 months, repeat treatments (with cis- or carboplatin) is probably fruitless and any further chemotherapy should probably comprise experimental agents. For patients with longer treatment-free intervals, courses of chemotherapy with the same agents as used previously can yield responses in up to 50% of cases, and although these are generally shorter in duration, significant palliation can still be obtained in ovarian cancer patients[40] (occasionally in conjunction with further surgery).

Drug interactions

Significant drug interactions occur in all areas of therapeutics, but because of the low therapeutic index of cytotoxics, such interactions can have life-threatening consequences. Interactions can occur between cytotoxics or between cytotoxics and non-cytotoxic drugs. Most patients will be co-administered analgesics, antiemetics (including steroids), anxiolytics and antidepressants. The scope for interaction is self-evident.

In addition, cytotoxic drug anabolism and catabolism can be altered by co-administered drugs or by repeated administration of the cytotoxic itself (auto-induction).

Some drugs should not be combined with cytotoxics because of the risk of additive toxicity, e.g. gentamicin and cisplatin, both of which can cause nephrotoxicity and ototoxicity.

The only way to avoid catastrophic interactions is to regularly review concomitant medication, and maintain a high level of vigilance in this patient population.

Organ dysfunction and dose

Liver dysfunction

Those drugs which are excreted as active compounds into the bile should be used with caution in the presence of impaired liver function since the half-life of the active components will be prolonged, resulting in increased toxicity. The dose of the drugs in Table 4.10.2 should be modified

Table 4.10.2 Drugs to be used with caution when serum bilirubin elevated

Daunorubicin
Doxorubicin
Epirubicin
Mitozantrone
Vinblastine
Vincristine
Vindesine

in the presence of biliary obstruction. The precise dosage reduction is uncertain, but usually the dose is reduced by 50% for serum bilirubin levels up to two times normal and the drug omitted if the bilirubin is higher than this.[41]

Renal dysfunction

Drugs which are cleared by the kidney may cause increased toxicity in patients with impaired renal function. Forced diuresis enhances the excretion of methotrexate and cisplatin; urinary alkalinization also helps to increase methotrexate excretion. Full doses of the drugs listed in Table 4.10.3 should be given only when the creatinine or EDTA clearance is greater than 60 ml min⁻¹.

Drug resistance

What are the obstacles to more successful treatment with currently available drugs, particularly with reference to gynecological cancers such as ovarian cancer? Essentially, the major factor is the development of drug resistance, manifest by a decreasing likelihood of tumor response to repeated exposure to cytotoxic agents. How can this be overcome?

The first issue is dose. As mentioned, a positive dose–response relationship can be demonstrated both experimentally and clinically for the key drugs but dose-escalation is limited by normal tissue effects. Recently, the use of peripheral blood stem cells which are harvested from patients after stimulation with exogenous colony-stimulating factors and then reinfused following high-dose chemotherapy, has indicated that agents whose major organ toxicity is myelosuppression, e.g. carboplatin and cyclophosphamide, can in fact be given safely at doses which are up to 10-fold higher than standard doses. However, there are no data available yet from randomized trials in any tumor type to indicate that this approach carries a positive survival benefit, and for the present it remains an experimental procedure.

Table 4.10.3 Drugs requiring dosage modification when renal function deranged

Bleomycin
Carboplatin
Cisplatin
Cyclophosphamide
Thiotepa
Methotrexate

Second, a range of cellular biochemical changes has been noted in experimental models of drug resistance. For cisplatin/carboplatin and alkylating agents, increased cellular levels of metallothionein and glutathione have been identified as being responsible for enhanced detoxification and reduced sensitivity to these agents. Clinical trials have now begun with an agent which will reduce cellular levels of glutathione, i.e. buthionine sulfoximine (BSO) the aim being to establish whether this will lead to attenuation of clinical drug resistance to these drugs.

An increased capacity to repair damage to DNA has also been suggested as a mechanism through which tumor cells develop resistance to platinum compounds and alkylating agents, and a range of potential methods for circumventing cisplatin resistance has been proposed.[42] For taxol, the development of drug resistance experimentally relates to increased expression of a drug efflux pump in the cell membrane, known as P-glycoprotein (P-gp); the interest here is the evidence at least in the laboratory that this can be overcome by a wide range of non-cytotoxic agents which competitively inhibit P-gp, preventing drug efflux and rendering resistant cells sensitive to natural products such as taxol.[43]

New drug development

Unfortunately current therapy can cure only a minority of patients with cancer. In fact, the numbers cured by chemotherapy are small, particularly in regard to the common solid tumors (lung, breast, colon). This situation may be improved upon by development of newly discovered anticancer drugs.

New compounds of interest are defined by a combination of random screening, serendipity, analog development and rational design. Once the compound has shown antitumor activity in model systems, with no untoward toxicity in animal tests it is considered for clinical trials.

When the compound reaches clinical testing, this is planned in three phases:

1. Phase I: the aim here is to establish the maximum tolerated dose in patients with cancer, and detailed information on toxicity is accumulated at this time. Any antitumor activity seen in phase I studies is useful in planning further studies, although that is not the primary aim at this stage.
2. Phase II: using an appropriate dose and schedule, the new drug is then tested in groups of patients with selected tumors and measurable lesions; these patients may or may not have received prior chemotherapy according to tumor type. If a drug proves to be active at this stage, it may then proceed to phase III testing.
3. Phase III: at this stage an attempt is made to establish whether the new agent has a significant role in cancer therapy, by comparing it in randomized studies (sometimes in drug combination) with so-called standard

chemotherapy in those tumor types in which activity was detected.

This sequence of events has yielded a few agents which have promising levels of clinical activity in gynecological cancer, good examples being taxol and taxotere.[44] Other promising drugs include topoisomerase I inhibitors (topotecan and CPT-11), gemcitabine (a fluorinated analog of cytosine arabinoside) and new more potent thymidylate synthase inhibitors.

FUTURE PERSPECTIVES

Future cytotoxic drug development looks set to move away from the traditional target of DNA towards some of the new targets which are emerging from our increasing understanding of the molecular and biochemical differences between tumor cells and their normal counterparts.[45]

SUMMARY

- Current cytotoxics act at the level of DNA synthesis or on the mechanics of cell division.
- Agents are divided by their biochemical actions into various classes.
- Multidrug combinations utilizing agents from different classes are superior to single agent therapy in most diseases.
- Dose–intensity is important in determining antitumor response.
- Cytotoxic drugs are generally given intravenously, but intraperitoneal use in ovarian cancer is an area of active research.

- Smaller tumor masses theoretically respond better to chemotherapy.
- New agents (like the taxanes) hold great promise for the future of cancer therapy.
- The narrow therapeutic index of cytotoxics necessitates great care in dosage calculation.
- All chemotherapy treatment is attended by significant side-effects and therefore should be used only by appropriately trained doctors.
- Chemotherapy is rarely curative on its own and should be viewed as part of a multimodality approach to cancer.

REFERENCES

1. Birkhead BG, Rankin EM, Gallivan S *et al.* A mathematical model of the development of drug resistance to cancer chemotherapy. *Eur J Cancer Clin Oncol* 1987 23: 1421–1427.
2. Skipper HE, Schabel FM, Jay R *et al.* Experimental evaluation of potential anti-cancer agents. XIII on the criteria and kinetics associated with availability of experimental leukaemia. *Cancer Chemother Rep* 1964 35: 1–11.
3. Goldie JH, Coldman AJ. A mathematical model for relating the drug sensitivity of tumours to their spontaneous mutation rate. *Cancer Treat Rep* 1979 63: 1727–1733.
4. Norton L, Simon R. Tumour size, sensitivity to therapy and design of treatment schedules. *Cancer Treat Rep* 1977 61: 1307–1317.
5. Hermminki K, Ludlum DM. Covalent modification of DNA by antineoplastic agents. *J Natl Cancer Inst* 1984 73: 1021–1028.
6. Brock N, Phol J, Stekar J. Studies on the urotoxicity of oxazaphorine cytostatics and its prevention. I. Experimental studies on the urotoxicity of alkylating agents. *Eur J Cancer Clin Oncol* 1981 17: 596–607.
7. Loehrer PJ, Einhorn LH. Cisplatin. *Ann Intern Med* 1984 100: 704–713.
8. Park RC, Thigpen JT. Chemotherapy in advanced and recurrent cervical cancer. A review. *Cancer* 1993 71: 1446–1450.
9. Vermorken JB, ten Bokkel Huinink WW, Eisenhauer EA, Faualli G, Befponine D, Conte PF, Kaye SB. Carboplatin versus cisplatin. *Ann Oncol* 1993 4: 541–548.
10. Matherly LH, Barlowe CK, Phillips VM *et al.* The effects of 4-amino-antifolates on 5-formyltetrahydrofolate metabolism in L1210 cells. A biochemical basis for the selectivity of leucovorin rescue. *J Biol Chem* 1987 262: 710–717.
11. Evans RM, Laskin JD, Hakala MT. Assessment of growth limiting events caused by 5-fluorouracil in mouse cells and human cells in culture. *Cancer Res* 1979 39: 383–390.

12. Capranico G, Deisabella P, Penco S, Tunelli S, Zumino F. Role of DNA breakage in cytotoxicity of doxorubicin, 9-deoxydoxorubicin, and 4-demethyl-6-deoxydoxorubicin in murine leukaemia P383 cells. *Can Res* 1989 49: 2022–2027.
13. Sikic BI. Biochemical and cellular determinants of bleomycin cytotoxicity. *Cancer Surv* 1986 5: 81–91.
14. Lim LO, Neims AH. Mitochondrial DNA damage by bleomycin. *Biochem Pharmacol* 1987 36: 2769–2774.
15. Strychmans PA, Lurie PM, Manaster J, Vameco G. Mode of action of chemotherapy in vivo on human acute leukaemia. II. Vincristine. *Eur J Cancer* 1973 9: 613–620.
16. Van Maanen JMS, Retel J, de Vries J, Pinedo HM. Mechanism of action of antitumour drug etoposide, a review. *J Natl Cancer Inst* 1988 80: 1526–1533.
17. Dorr RT, Fritz WL. *Cancer Chemotherapy Handbook.* New York: Elsevier, 1980: 362–367.
18. Hahn PA. Hexamethylmelamine and pentamethylmelamine: an update. *Drug Intell Clin Pharm* 1983 17: 418–424.
19. Foster BJ, Clagett-Carr K, Marsoni S *et al.* Role of hexamethylmelamine in the treatment of ovarian cancer: Where is the needle in the haystack? *Cancer Treat Rep* 1986 70: 1003–1014.
20. Rowinsky EK, Cazenave LA, Donehower RC. Taxol: A novel investigational antimicrotubule agent. *J Natl Cancer Inst* 1990 82: 1247–1259.
21. Schiff PB, Font J, Horwitz SB. Promotion of microtubule assembly in vitro by taxol. *Nature* 1979 22: 665–667.
22. National Cancer Institute. Clinical Brochure: Taxol (NSC 125973) Bethesda, MD: Division of Cancer Treatment. NCI September, 1983: 6–12.
23. Wiernik PH, Schwartz EL, Strauman JJ *et al.* Phase I clinical and pharmacokinetic study of taxol. *Cancer Res* 1987 47: 2486–2493.
24. Kris MG, O'Connell JP, Gralla RJ *et al.* Phase I trial of taxol given as a 3 hour infusion every 21 days. *Cancer Treat Rep* 1986 70: 605–607.

25. Hansen HH, Eisenhauer EA, Hansen M *et al.* New cyto-toxic drugs in ovarian cancer. *Ann Oncol* 1993 4: S63–S70.

26. McGuire WP, Hoskins WJ, Brady MF *et al.* A phase II comparing cisplatin/cytoxan and cisplatin/taxol in advanced ovarian cancer. *Proc Am Soc Clin Oncol* 1993 12: 255.

27. Harris H, Irvin R, Kuhn J *et al.* Phase I clinical trial of tax-otere administered as either a 2 hour or 6 hour intravenous infusion. *J Clin Oncol* 1993 11: 950–958.

28. Kavanagh JJ, Kudelka AP, Freedman RS *et al.* A phase II trial of taxotere (RP56976) in ovarian cancer patients refractory to cisplatin/carboplatin therapy. *Proc Am Soc Clin Oncol* 1993 12: 823.

29. Hryniuk WM, Levine MN. Analysis of dose intensity for adjuvant chemotherapy trials. *J Clin Oncol* 1986 4: 1162–1170.

30. Kaye SB, Lewis CR, Paul J *et al.* Randomised study of two doses of cisplatin with cyclophosphamide in epithelial ovarian cancer. *Lancet* 1992 340: 329–333.

31. Bononi P, Blessing J, Stehman F *et al.* Randomised trial of three cisplatin dose schedules in squamous cell carcinoma of the cervix: a Gynecologic Oncology Group Study. *J Clin Oncol* 1985 3: 1079–1085.

32. Levin L, Hyrnuik W. Dose intensity analysis of chemother-apy regimens in ovarian carcinoma. *J Clin Oncol* 1987 5: 756–767.

33. Hacker NF, Berek JS, Pretorius RG, Zuckerman J, Eisenhop S, Lagasse LD. Intraperitoneal cisplatinum as salvage therapy for refractory epithelial ovarian cancer. *Obstet Gynecol* 1987 60: 759–764.

34. Howell SB, Zimm S, Markman M *et al.* Long term survival of advanced refractory ovarian carcinoma patients with small volume disease treated with intraperitoneal chemo-therapy. *J Clin Oncol* 1987 5: 689–695.

35. Omura G, Blessing J, Erlich C *et al.* A randomised trial of cyclophosphamide and doxorubicin with or without cis-platin in advanced ovarian carcinoma. *Cancer* 1986 57: 1725–1730.

36. Omura G, Morrow P, Blessing J *et al.* A randomised com-parison of melphalan versus melphalan plus hexamethyl-melamine versus adriamycin plus cyclophosphamide in ovarian cancer. *Cancer* 1983 51: 783–789.

37. Omura G, Bundy B, Wilbanks G *et al.* A randomised trial of cyclophosphamide plus cisplatin with or without adrimyacin in ovarian carcinoma. *Proc Am Soc Clin Oncol* 1987 6: 112.

38. Bonomi P, Blessing J, Ball H *et al.* A phase II evaluation of cisplatin and 5-fluorouracil in patients with advanced squamous cell carcinoma of the cervix: a Gynaecologic Oncology Group Study. *Gynecol Oncol* 1989 34: 357–359.

39. Greco FA. Etoposide: seeking the best dose and schedule. *Semin Oncol* 1992 19: 59–63.

40. Markman M, Rothman R, Hakes T *et al.* Second-line plat-inum therapy in patients with ovarian cancer previously treated with cisplatin. *J Clin Oncol* 1991 9: 389–393.

41. Kaye SB, Cummings J, Kerr D. How much does liver disease affect the pharmacokinetics of adriamycin. *Eur J Cancer* 1985 21: 893–895.

42. Timmer-Bosscha H, Mulder NH, de Vries EG. Modulation of cisplatin resistance: a review. *Br J Cancer* 1992 66: 227–238.

43. Sikic BI. Modulation of multidrug-resistance: at the thresh-old. *J Clin Oncol* 1993 11: 1629–1635.

44. Bissett D, Kaye SB. Taxol and taxotere – current status and future prospects. *Eur J Cancer* 1993 29A: 1228–1231.

45. Workman P (ed.) New approaches in cancer pharmacology: drug design and development. I. *European School of Oncology Monograph.* Berlin: Springer-Verlag, 1992.

Section 5

Applied Science

5.1

Clinical Trials

A Grant and D Elbourne

INTRODUCTION

This first chapter in the section on applied science discusses the use of scientific principles in the evaluation of clinical practice. In particular, it addresses the question of how clinical research can be conducted to ensure that the effects of therapies, both beneficial and adverse, are identified as reliably as possible. The potent treatments of modern medicine can cause harm as well as benefit, and it is beholden on those who give or advocate giving the treatments to ensure that they are doing more good than harm.

In simple terms, the challenge of a clinical trial is to allow any effects of alternative treatments to be distinguished reliably from other inherent differences between the groups being compared in the trial ('bias'), and from any chance differences between the trial groups ('imprecision'). With this in mind, we shall first describe the principal sources of bias and of random (chance) differences, and the ways they may be minimized.

Definition of 'clinical trial'

The research method used to evaluate therapies is the clinical trial. We have to admit to some unease about using this term as the title for this chapter because it is commonly used to mean widely different things by different people. For the purposes of this chapter, we shall not consider the description of the use of a new treatment given to a single patient (case report) or to an isolated group of patients (a case series) as a clinical trial. A trial must include a comparison group, and we shall be arguing that almost invariably the groups to be compared should be generated by random treatment allocation; we shall return to this later.

Meaning of blinding and placebo treatment

At this stage, two other terms that are commonly associated with clinical trials are mentioned. The first is 'blind-ing', perhaps more properly called 'masking'. (A related concept, 'concealment', is discussed later.) This means keeping all or some of those involved in the trial in ignorance of the nature of the treatments given. Blinding may be restricted to the patient alone in which case the trial is said to be 'single-blind'; or it may apply to both the patient and the clinician giving treatment, in which case it is 'double-blind'. Sometimes the reliability of a trial can be increased if the people assessing outcome and performing the statistical analysis are also kept blind.

Often, the only way to hide the true nature of the treatments given is by means of a 'placebo' therapy. This is a dummy treatment which seems identical to the active treatment. Placebos are most common in drug trials; an inert substance presented in an identical fashion to the active substance, with the same color and taste, is given to the comparison or 'control' group. Placebos are also used in other types of clinical trial, such as in the evaluation of some physical treatments. But there are some circumstances where the provision of a placebo treatment is either extremely difficult, or impossible or inappropriate (for example, when the administration itself is hazardous or painful), and this applies in particular to many surgical interventions.

The value of blinding and placebo treatments will be discussed in more detail later in this chapter.

CURRENT CONCEPTS

Bias

The term bias means an inherent (as opposed to chance) difference between the groups being compared in the context of a clinical trial, other than any differences in the nature of the treatments being compared. There are three principal sources of potential bias: first arising from the method of selecting the groups for comparison; second arising from the method of assessing the outcome of treatment; and third due to differences in the management of the groups other than in the way intended. We shall discuss each of these in turn.

Choice of comparison group

There are three broad ways in which comparison groups have traditionally been derived in clinical trials. Two of these are, however, so likely to generate a comparison group which is fundamentally different from the group receiving the experimental treatment and thereby introduce bias, as to be too unreliable to provide a basis for subsequent clinical practice.

The first of these unreliable approaches is the use of 'historical controls'. At first sight it may seem obviously sensible to compare the experience of a current group treated in a new way with that of an apparently similar group treated differently in the past. Leaving aside the problems commonly encountered in collecting clinical data retrospectively, historical controls treated in the past may be fundamentally different from currently managed patients in at least two ways. First, they may differ in important respects which may influence outcome. The types of patients referred for treatment may alter or the natural history of the condition change. The second source of bias in historically controlled studies is changes in other aspects of treatment over time which alter (usually improving) outcome.

The obvious way to get round changes over time is to compare two groups managed concurrently. In the past, it was not uncommon for groups managed in a new way to be compared with other patients to whom the clinician chose not to give the new treatment. These studies using 'concurrent, non-randomized controls' are also prone to bias because these controls too may be fundamentally different from those receiving the new treatment, reflecting the clinician's decision whether or not to use the experimental management. The basis for some of these comparisons has sometimes been an assumption that the group getting the new treatment was at higher risk than the group who did not receive the new treatment, and so any equivalence in outcome was considered to demonstrate benefit. However, closer examination of the comparison groups in such studies often reveals that these assumptions were not justified. For example, in studies of electronic fetal monitoring during labor which used concurrent, non-randomized controls, the control group was commonly found to contain extremely immature babies whose viability was thought so unlikely as not to warrant any monitoring at all.

The problem is that the sizes of the biases that may be introduced by the use of historical or concurrent, non-randomized controls are very likely to be of the same magnitude as any effects of the new treatment, and so may either hide or grossly exaggerate any true treatment effect.

The only way of ensuring that the groups compared in a clinical trial are truly comparable, only differing by chance, is by random treatment assignment. That is, the decision about which trial treatment a particular person receives is taken not by the clinician responsible for care nor by the patient, but by a chance process, such that every participant has a known chance of being allocated to the treatment options being compared. The use of random allocation acknowledges that individual patients differ, but that these differences are evened out between the groups being compared by random assignment. The larger the numbers of people recruited the more successful will be this evening out.

Selection bias introduced at the time of analysis

The basis for random allocation of treatments is that the two groups created only differ by chance at the time they are generated. A consequence is that the comparison only remains unbiased if the two groups are compared in total. Withdrawals after trial entry may introduce bias, particularly if the reason for withdrawal is related to one or other of the treatments being compared. It is easy to envisage ways in which those who do not comply with their trial allocation are atypical. Patients may choose not to follow a course of treatment for a variety of reasons, including that they feel particularly well, or particularly ill, or that the treatment actually makes them feel unwell. Clearly, removing such people from the analysis would lead to a serious distortion of the results. In practice, to avoid bias due to withdrawal after trial entry, the statistical analysis should be based on the groups according to their original random allocation regardless of subsequent management, rather than according to the treatment that they actually received. In other words, those participants who stop treatment or start to take the alternative treatment should, for the purpose of the trial, be considered as part of the group to which they had originally been assigned. The implication of such 'intention to treat' analyses in trials is that the comparison is between two policies for treatment (recognizing that not all participants received the treatment to which they were allocated) rather than a comparison in which all members of a group received the same actual treatment. This general rule applies in most trials, although we shall discuss later the occasional circumstances where analysis based on the actual treatment received may be useful and appropriate.

Bias introduced during the measurement of outcome

The second area of the trial where large biases may be introduced is during the measurement of outcome. This is potentially a major problem in trials where the assessment of outcome may be influenced by knowledge of the allocated treatment or the actual treatment received. It is well recognized that patients are more likely to report the symptoms of a possible side-effect if they have already been warned that such a side-effect may occur. Preconceived ideas about the differential effects of treatments compared in a trial may lead to similar suggestibility. This potential for bias may be reduced, but not excluded entirely, by using 'hard' endpoints, such as death. For example, it is easy to imagine how knowledge of whether or not a particular patient was taking active treatment in a trial of low-dose aspirin to prevent the complications of pre-eclampsia might influence the decision whether or not a perinatal death is ascribed to pre-eclampsia. A similar argument applies to nearly all measures of outcome.

The most satisfactory way to avoid this problem is to ensure that the assessment of outcome is made in ignorance of ('blind' or 'masked' to) the trial allocation or the treatment actually received. This should, of course, always apply in a trial where there is double or triple blinding through the use of a placebo treatment, as described earlier. However, it is also possible to blind the assessment of outcome in a trial where the use of placebo and blinding of the clinician and participant is not possible, as for example in a trial of a surgical procedure. One way is to ensure that the person assessing outcome is not involved in the earlier stages of the trial and is kept in ignorance of the actual management received. A second approach to minimizing assessment bias is to ensure that the method used for measuring outcome is truly objective. For example, there are methods available for measuring blood pressure which minimize the subjective component of the readings.

Intervention bias

The third area of a trial where the possibility of a bias should be considered is around the time of the interventions compared. As will be described, this is less straightforward than the other sources of bias described above because arguably, a problem here may not be a true 'bias'. As mentioned earlier, comparisons between the groups as randomized are not in the strict sense biased. Clearly, however, the interpretation of results needs to take into account what constituted the actual treatments received. The first issue here is whether there were differences between the comparison groups in the other treatments received ('co-interventions') which might alter outcome independently of the treatments of interest. Clearly, if a large number of participants in one group receive a co-intervention that is known to be effective while few, if any, in the other trial group received it, this may make interpretation of the results difficult; some commentators have viewed this as a bias. A related problem is 'contamination', where despite a particular allocation, participants in the trial receive the alternative treatment regimen. Again, comparisons based on the groups as allocated may not be viewed as strictly biased, but serious contamination may blur the distinctions between the managements being compared which in extreme circumstances may mean little differences between the trial groups in the treatment they actually received. The potential for contamination is greatest in open trials and it should not occur in a fully blind study. Appropriate steps should be taken in the protocol to ensure that the managements compared are kept appropriately separate, and the effect of any contamination should be considered when interpreting the results of a completed trial. One form of trial design that may be used when the risk of contamination is serious is discussed below.

The third issue around the time of the interventions is compliance with the allocated management more generally. Once again, provided the analyses are based on 'intention to treat' with those who choose not to persist with the allocated treatment retained in the group to which they were randomized, non-compliance does not introduce bias – indeed it may be seen as an 'outcome' for a particular policy. Nevertheless, if large proportions of participants choose not to comply, this could seriously reduce the chances of observing a difference between the groups as allocated in respect of outcome, even if one or other treatment was in fact truly superior. In a blinded trial, it would be expected that non-compliance would be similar in the two trial groups (unless one treatment causes side-effects that lead to discontinuation). In an open trial, knowledge of the actual treatment received may lead to a differential rate of compliance, irrespective of whether or not there are side-effects, particularly when one or other treatment is suspected to have side-effects or is thought to be ineffective or inferior. The issue of compliance therefore needs to be considered seriously when developing a protocol for a trial, particularly an open trial. Its implications should also be considered carefully when appraising the results of a completed study.

Random errors

A trial is conducted on a sample of those people who might be suitable for the treatments being compared. As such, it gives an estimate of any differential effects that really exist. Just by chance, the trial result may be an overestimate or underestimate of this true value.

It is always possible that an observed difference may just reflect chance. This is the reason why it is commonly recommended that a trial's objective should be expressed as a 'null hypothesis' (that there is no clinically significant difference between two alternative treatments). In some circumstances the observed differences are so unlikely to reflect random errors that a chance difference can in effect be ruled out and the null hypothesis rejected with considerable confidence. When differences are less extreme, the issue is at what level (probability) is the likelihood considered to be so extreme that it is safe to assume that the observed difference is real. Standard statistical tests derive a figure for the probability that the observed difference reflects chance, and traditionally a probability of less than 0.05 (1 in 20) has been taken, somewhat arbitrarily, as a basis for rejecting the null hypothesis. Nevertheless, whatever level of 'statistical significance' is chosen the possibility always exists that the conclusion that there is a real difference between the groups may be wrong, and this is called a 'type I error'; this issue is discussed further later.

Random errors or the possibility that they may exist, also leads to the complementary problem of concluding that there is no real difference between the groups, when one does in fact exist, a type II error. By chance, any differences between the trial treatments may be underestimated such that the smaller difference observed is falsely ascribed to chance, or the differential effect may be correctly estimated but the data are too few to distinguish this from a chance difference, again leading incorrectly to acceptance of the null hypothesis when in truth there is a real difference between the treatments.

These errors are presented schematically in Fig. 5.1.1. Generally speaking, the larger the size of the trial, particularly the larger the frequency of the primary outcome, the less likely are type I and type II errors. Clearly, trials have to be a finite size and the basis of sample size calculations is an appropriate level of protection against such problems. Reflecting this, there are four parameters that must be considered when deciding a trial's sample size. These are:

1. The size of any true difference in respect of the primary measure of outcome that would be considered sufficiently important clinically to warrant the introduction of the experimental management into clinical practice;
2. The expected frequency of the primary outcome measure amongst the group receiving the standard management (or alternatively some measure of the average value and its spread (variability) such as standard deviation, if the outcome is a continuous rather than categorical variable);
3. The level of probability that would be considered sufficiently low to accept the results as indicating a true difference; that is, a decision about what would be an acceptable level for a type I error (the trial's alpha level, also called the level of statistical significance);
4. The level of certainty that a true difference of the size stipulated in (1) above, would be identified at the level of statistical significance chosen (in 3, above), taking into account the fact that the trial result may by chance be an underestimate of the true effect; the chosen level for a type II error is commonly referred to as its beta level and the degree of protection against a type II error is commonly expressed as a trial's 'statistical power' (1 − beta, discussed again on p. 559).

		TRUTH	
		Difference Exists	Difference Does Not Exist
Trial Result	Difference Exists	A	B
	Difference Does Not Exist	C	D

In situations A and D the trial results reflect the truth.

In situation B the trial results suggest a difference although, in truth, no difference exists (Type I error).

In situation C the trial results do not detect a difference although, in truth, a difference does exist (Type II error).

Fig. 5.1.1 *Type I and type II statistical errors.*

Once decisions have been made about these four parameters, it is usually relatively easy to calculate a sample size estimate. For example, in a trial assessing the value of extracorporeal membrane oxygenation (ECMO) compared to conventional ventilatory care for mature babies with severe respiratory failure,[1] the primary end-point is death or survival with severe disability. On the assumption that the likely event rate for this outcome among babies in the conventionally ventilated group would be approximately 43%, and that a reduction to 24% would be considered clinically significant, a sample size of about 300 would be required to be reasonably confident (80% power) of identifying this difference at the 1% level of statistical significance. Although formulae for these calculations are available in standard statistical textbooks, we would, nevertheless, recommend discussion and active collaboration with a statistician about this and indeed other aspects of trial design.

Protection against type I errors

One method of protecting against type I errors is to only accept relatively extreme probabilities as statistically significant. Reflecting this, there is an increasing tendency, particularly in large trials, to stipulate that differences observed will only be accepted as real if the likelihood of a chance difference is less than 1 in 100 (P less than 0.01) rather than, as conventionally, less then 1 in 20 (P less than 0.05). The practical implication of this is that the required sample size is increased by a factor of about 50%.

Choice of appropriate levels of statistical significance in sample size calculations is not the only method for protection against type I errors, however. Technically, the chosen alpha level applies only to the analysis of the principal measure of outcome at the completion of the trial. Each time an additional statistical test is performed there is an additional risk of a type I error. In other words, the larger the number of statistical tests performed the greater the probability that one will be 'statistically significant' just by chance. If 20 statistical tests are performed, for example, it should not be surprising if one generates a P value of less than 0.05. The problems caused by multiple statistical testing have been exacerbated by the ease with which modern computer-based statistical packages can generate large numbers of probability values in a single analysis. For these reasons, we would argue for a clear distinction to be drawn between prestated hypotheses based on predefined outcomes and 'statistically significant' differences observed in secondary exploratory analyses. The former may be considered as formal hypothesis testing, whereas the latter at best are merely hypothesis generating requiring confirmation or refutation in further research. The same issues apply when repeated significance testing is applied to multiple interim analyses during the conduct of the trial. Table 5.1.1 indicates how importance attached to a 'significant result' should be modified in this context. For example, a finding of a probability of 0.05 in 1 of 10 repeated tests, in fact, has a significance level equivalent to 0.19; in other words, such a finding should not be surprising. The issues around the monitoring of accumulating data in a trial are beyond the scope of this chapter, but the implication is that only

Table 5.1.1 The effect on the overall significance level of repeated significance tests on accumulating data[a]

No. of repeated tests at the 5% level	Overall significance level
1	0.05
2	0.08
3	0.11
4	0.13
5	0.14
10	0.19
20	0.25
50	0.32
100	0.37
1000	0.53
∞	1.0

[a]For two treatments, a normal response with known variance and equally spaced analyses, though broadly similar results for other types of data.
Modified in reference 7 from reference 8.

relatively extreme probabilities should be accepted as the basis for changing a protocol in the context of repeated interim analyses, so as to avoid a type I error.

A particular kind of type I error may result from what has become know as 'publication bias'; that is, the selective publication of trials which seem to show differences between the two groups at the expense of other trials that seem to show no such effect. This problem is considered later in the chapter.

Protection against type II errors

The principal protection against a type II error is a large sample size. Conventionally, statistical power has been set at 80% which has the practical meaning that if the trial were to be repeated 10 times and the differential effect was exactly as hypothesized, the result would be statistically significant 80% of the times, that is 8 of the 10. There is a view that is increasingly often held, that a 20% risk of a false negative result is unacceptable. But the practical implications of stipulating 90% (instead of 80%) power, for example, is an increase in the sample size by a factor of about 30%. In practice, trials with adequate protection against both type I and type II errors are not infrequently beyond the scope of a single center, particularly when the final outcome is definitive and 'hard', such as death or childhood disability in the context of a perinatal trial, because these are statistically uncommon. It is these considerations that have led to an increasing number of multicenter trials, particularly in perinatal medicine and gynecological oncology. However, most current trials are not large enough to give sufficiently precise estimates of treatment effects on the most important measures of outcome and the recognition of this has led to the increased use of overviews (meta-analyses) of similar trials. In this way, more data become available, thereby allowing the derivation of more precise estimates of treatment effects; this is discussed further later in the chapter.

Issues in trial design

Explanatory and pragmatic trials

In the context of trial design, a useful distinction can be drawn between trials that address the question 'Can a treatment have a particular effect in an ideal setting?' (an explanatory trial) and 'Is a treatment effective in an everyday clinical setting?' (pragmatic trial). Explanatory trials are characterized by being relatively small, tightly controlled with high or perfect compliance, concentrating on a short-term measure which is commonly a surrogate for the final outcome. In contrast, pragmatic trials are characterized by being large, less strictly controlled to reflect the realities of everyday clinical practice, and concentrating on a definitive longer-term end-point, such as death or serious morbidity. There is a spectrum of trial design between these two extremes. Arguably, it is sensible first to derive evidence of efficacy for a new treatment in the context of explanatory trials before embarking on a large pragmatic field trial. On the other hand, it is important that it is acknowledged that the actual performance of an intervention in a real clinical setting may be different from its performance in an explanatory trial, and also that an effect on a surrogate measure may not necessarily be reflected in an effect on a definitive outcome. Ideally, pragmatic trials should therefore be required before the introduction of the new treatment approach into routine practice.

We have already argued that, as a matter of principle, analyses in randomized controlled trials should be on an intention-to-treat basis, that is on the groups as randomly allocated. One situation where an analysis based on the actual treatment received may be more appropriate, however, is in an explanatory trial where just about every participant receives the allocated management, but one or two do not for reasons beyond the control of the investigators. 'Error' introduced by the extra variance (random error) from including non-compliers may then be greater than any selection bias that results from excluding them. Nevertheless, analyses based on actual treatment received should be interpreted with caution, particularly if there are more than a few non-compliers.

Uncertainty principle and eligibility

The eligibility criteria in explanatory trials are tightly defined. In contrast, these criteria in pragmatic trials are looser, with the person giving care taking greater responsibility. Reflecting this, it is increasingly common in large pragmatic trials to base eligibility on 'uncertainty'. A particular patient is eligible for the trial if the clinician responsible for care is uncertain which of the alternative treatment strategies to recommend. Trial eligibility then dovetails more easily into clinical practice, by acknowledging that individual clinicians will have varying degrees of uncertainty about the place of the particular treatment or treatments in their practice. For example, some may only be uncertain about the place of the new treatment for high-risk patients, whereas others may be uncertain about patients at more moderate risk. There are clear advantages of this approach. First, all patients who might meet more rigid criteria should be recruited to a trial based on uncertainty but, in addition, other patients will also be recruited with the effect that larger numbers of patients of the types that clinicians would be considering for treatment if the new management was introduced into clinical practice, will be available for analysis. Secondly, there is also the possibility of exploring differential effects within predefined subgroups of patients.

Secure randomization

We have already implied that the groups compared in clinical trials should, where possible, be derived by random treatment assignment. Selection bias is, however, only avoided if the randomization is secure. The key principles are that the assignment should not be predictable nor changeable once the assignment is known. In practice, this means clear trial entry before formal treatment assignment, and for the purpose of analysis the retention of a particular patient in the allocated group, regardless of subsequent management and outcome. Methods of quasi-randomization such as 'alternation', allocation based on date of birth, hospital number, or day of the month are not satisfactory because the allocation can be predicted in advance. An investigator's decision whether or not to recruit a particular patient may be influenced by this, and this would introduce selection bias. Methods which are not preceded by clear trial entry are also unsatisfactory, because an investigator may choose to withdraw a patient from a trial once the treatment allocation is known, again introducing bias. We are even unhappy about using the sealed envelope approach unless there is strict monitoring. It is surprisingly easy to see through many such envelopes with the aid of a bright light. Certainly, if envelopes are used, we recommend they are held by a third party such that there is clear trial entry signaled, for example, by entry of the participant's name in a trial register, before the envelope is opened. Furthermore, involving a third party who is not involved in treatment decisions, also protects against subsequent withdrawals or allocation changes (because it would require an unlikely conspiracy!). In locally based trials, the use of a personal computer may obviate the need for a third party (provided that none of those involved in the trial is a computer hack!). In larger trials, the safest approach is to use distance randomization by telephone, fax or E-mail to a central randomization service. The use of computer allocation, irrespective of whether the coordination is local or distant, has the extra advantage of allowing the allocation to be balanced within particular types of patients ('stratification' or 'minimization').

Large, simple multicenter trials

We have already argued that decisions about policy and practice should ideally be based on pragmatic trials. The principal measures of outcome in these trials, such as death or serious morbidity, are, however, statistically uncommon. Furthermore, the size of effect of a new treatment can only be expected to be moderate, say, a 20% propor-

tional reduction. For these reasons, trials have to be surprisingly large, commonly involving some thousands of people. Such trials must therefore involve large numbers of centers. These trials can only be successful if they are kept very simple in design with data collection limited to those items which are absolutely essential.

Factorial designs

Given the work involved in conducting clinical trials, it is always sensible to consider whether more than one question can be addressed in a particular study. A good and statistically efficient way is by using a factorial design. The trial includes all the various combinations of the treatments being compared. For example, if the intention is to have two different comparisons (A versus B, and Y versus Z), each comparing two different treatment modalities, there are four assignment groups as illustrated in Fig. 5.1.2. When the total group receiving A, as opposed to B are considered, it can be seen that the numbers receiving the other treatments (Y and Z) are evenly balanced. Looking vertically, the same applies to the comparison of Y and Z. In other words, data from all the patients are used in each of the two principal trial analyses; in addition, however, it is also possible to look to see whether the combination of any two treatments has an effect over and above any individual effects of A over B or Y over Z.

Cluster and other quasi-experimental designs

There are circumstances where simple random allocation of individuals to alternative management policies may not be possible or sensible. This would apply, for example, where the intervention is clearly aimed at a group of people, such as in some health promotion interventions. It also applies when the intervention is at the level of the health

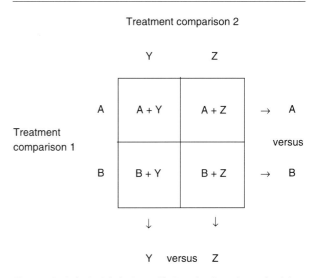

Fig. 5.1.2 *A factorial design with two treatments, each at two levels (2 × 2 design).*

professional who provides care for a group of patients. An example is the evaluation of clinical guidelines for a particular complaint or problem. The most common reason why simple randomization is not appropriate is a high risk of 'contamination'. For example, when a trial to assess the value of teaching women to formally count fetal movements was considered, it was thought that women would be influenced by knowing that other women attending the same clinic were following a different policy if there was random allocation of individual women to the alternative policies. In particular, women asked not to count movements formally might decide to start counting after hearing from a woman at the same clinic that she was recording her movement count each day. The randomization was therefore performed at the level of the consultant obstetrician, with all women booked for care from a particular consultant following the same policy either to count or not to count movements. Allocation in groups as in this trial is called cluster randomization. Whereas this design is simpler than using individual randomization and may be particularly attractive for participating clinicians, it may have serious trade-offs in terms of loss of statistical power, because the analysis should be based on the clusters rather than individual participants.

Generalizability

Description of the groups at trial entry

The ultimate aim of clinical trials is to produce results which will have clear implications which can then be translated into clinical practice. To put this another way, a clinician must be able to judge whether the results of a trial are applicable (generalizable) to a particular patient, or to particular groups of patients. To allow this, there must be clear description of the types of people recruited to a trial, particularly in respect of the most important prognostic variables.

Description of exclusions

The value of collecting information to describe those eligible for a trial but excluded, is less obvious. Those recruited to a trial are always selected in some way (even if all people eligible in the trial's setting are successfully recruited). A purist might argue that the results are therefore only generalizable to this group of people, but clearly they are likely to be similar or very similar to people who meet the same eligibility criteria elsewhere. Furthermore, whereas the size of effect may vary somewhat among people eligible for a trial, there are very few examples where the direction of effect varies (that is, a treatment is beneficial in one group but has a harmful effect in another). One such rare example seems to be cervical cerclage for suspected cervical incompetence. The operation is beneficial for women at high risk of very early delivery (for example, as judged on a history of three or more previous preterm deliveries). The insertion of a cervical suture may itself occasionally precipitate second trimester miscarriage, however, and so may increase the risk of early delivery in women at relatively low

risk. Information about those eligible people who do not participate may therefore occasionally aid interpretation. Knowledge of their outcome might help to gauge whether they were at particularly high risk or particulary low risk.

A description of those eligible but who were not included may also give insights that aid generalizability in other ways. For example, in a trial comparing medical with surgical termination of pregnancy, it was noted that those women who lived some distance from the hospital were particularly likely to choose the surgical approach. The reason was that this required a single visit to hospital whereas the medical approach required a return visit a few days after the procedure.

There are then occasions when information about eligible people who are excluded can aid interpretation and hence generalizability. Nevertheless, in our experience this is not common. Certainly, collection of detailed information about exclusions should not be allowed to jeopardize recruitment to the trial proper.

Generalizability of the interventions

Incorporation of the results of a trial into clinical practice would not be possible unless the interventions are described in sufficient detail to allow replication. There also needs to be a clear description of the treatment policies actually used, in addition to the maneuvres allocated. The more complex the interventions the less easy is generalization. Complex maneuvres are also less likely to be widely applicable; and for these two reasons interventions evaluated in trials should, ideally, be relatively simple. Questions may also be raised about the generalizability of the results of a trial conducted in a single center, because they may reflect the particular skills or attributes of those who worked there. Another great advantage of multicenter trials is therefore that their results are more widely generalizable.

Estimation rather than hypothesis testing

In a previous section, hypothesis testing was discussed in the context of sample size calculations. In deciding whether or not to generalize the results of the trial to clinical practice, an estimate of the size of any effects is more useful than simply knowing whether or not there is an effect. For this reason, the results of trials should be presented as an estimate of the treatment effect, with a range (the confidence interval) within which the true size of effect is likely to lie. The confidence interval may be very helpful in judging generalizability. If the lower estimated effect is still judged to be clinically useful, the results can be confidently implemented into practice; similarly, where the estimate of maximum effect is still less than what would be judged to be a sufficient benefit to be clinically useful it can be safely concluded that the experimental treatment is not superior and so should not be incorporated into practice. Confidence intervals do in fact incorporate a hypothesis testing element. If a 95% confidence interval excludes no difference between the two treatments, the result is in fact statistically significant at the 5% level ($P<0.05$); a 99% confidence interval excluding 'no difference' indicates that the difference is statistically significant at the 1% level ($P<0.01$).

Number needed to treat

Treatment effects are usually presented as a proportional reduction in risk. This may be as a relative risk, that is the rate in the experimental group divided by the rate in the control group, or as an odds ratio, the odds of the outcome in the experimental group divided by the odds of the outcome in the control group. The basis for this is an assumption that the proportional reduction is fixed such that those who are at higher risk derive greater absolute benefit. As has been indicated already, this assumption is not always valid; occasionally, the direction of effect may vary in different risk groups, and sometimes the benefit or risk may be fixed in absolute terms. For example, a procedure may carry an absolute risk which is not influenced by the type of patient treated.

From a clinical point of view it is the absolute risk applied to a particular patient (or patient group) which is most relevant. This may be presented as the absolute difference between the groups, that is the rate in the experimental group minus the rate in the control group. The reciprocal of the absolute rate difference multiplied by one hundred may be particularly informative clinically. This gives an estimate of the number of patients needed to be treated to prevent one case of the principal outcome. Confidence intervals can be derived easily by calculating the reciprocal of the confidence interval values expressed as absolute rate differences, and multiplying by one hundred. If the clinical view is that a patient should receive the experimental treatment even if the number needed to treat is near the upper end of the confidence interval, then the new management is clearly appropriate. The clinical decision becomes more a matter of judgement when the limit for the number needed to be treated is somewhere within the confidence interval. Numbers needed to treat are, then, merely an alternative way of expressing the absolute benefit, but may be preferable because they are clinically more meaningful.

Systematic review of controlled trials

Earlier we discussed the problems caused by random errors, and particularly the danger of falsely concluding that there was no treatment effect, when there really is one (type II error). The only reliable protection against this is relatively large amounts of data to provide a sufficiently precise estimate of any treatment effects. This commonly requires multicentre collaboration. An alternative or additional approach is to combine data from similar controlled trials in overviews (meta-analyses). The statistical techniques for combining data from trials of a particular intervention are described elsewhere.[2] In brief, differences within individual trials are weighted according to the size of the trial, principally on the number of participants with the outcome of interest. An overall, 'typical' estimate of any treatment effect is then derived. Obviously, the confidence interval of the typical estimate is usually narrower than the estimate from individual

trials, and this is the greatest strength of overviews. The typical estimate is most commonly expressed as an odds ratio because this is the easiest statistic to derive, but new computer programs have now made it easy to derive typical estimates for relative risks, absolute differences, and numbers needed to treat.

The other potential advantage of overviews of similar controlled trials is to increase generalizability. If a consistent effect is seen across a number of trials conducted in a range of settings this is obviously persuasive evidence that there is a real treatment effect and that the treatment is likely to be widely applicable.

Cochrane Collaboration – pregnancy and childbirth database

The Cochrane Collaboration is a movement to identify all controlled trials leading to systematic reviews. This is not as easy as it sounds. Relevant publications are widely dispersed throughout the medical literature, over a 40 year period. Computer searches are not sufficiently reliable, and may identify only 50% of trial reports. For this reason, particularly for earlier years before recent improvement in indexing within Index Medicus, it is necessary to back-search journals by hand, a cumbersome and time-consuming process.

The element of the Cochrane Collaboration that is furthest advanced is that related to maternity care. The Cochrane Collaboration Pregnancy and Childbirth Database (which arose out of the Oxford Database of Perinatal Trials) is a computerized portfolio of systematic reviews of controled trials in perinatal medicine. Back-searching is complete and the database is constantly updated as new trial reports are published. The advanced stage of development of this aspect of the Cochrane Collaboration reflects the fact that early development was coordinated by Iain Chalmers when he was Director of the National Perinatal Epidemiology Unit in Oxford, before he established the Cochrane Collaboration. This sophisticated software provides an immediate summary of current evidence on a particular intervention in the perinatal period; it is highly recommended.

Publication bias

Identification of all relevant controlled trials should lead to an unbiased, yet more precise, estimate of any treatment effects. As indicated above, however, identification of trials is not easy and it is essential to use systematic methods to maximize this. Despite best attempts, some trials will remain unidentified because their results are never formally published. These unpublished reports would not cause a problem if they were a random sample of relevant trials, but as might be expected, they tend to be those that are judged to be 'uninteresting', for example because they suggest no difference between the treatments. To put this another way, there is evidence that trials that suggest clear treatment effects are more likely to be published than trials that do not. This is a particularly common problem for small trials, which is exacerbated by the fact that differences in small trials tend to be statistically significant only if they are an exaggeration of the true treatment effect. The 'publication bias' that this causes therefore tends to overestimate any treatment effects and is therefore a form of Type I error. Striking evidence of publication bias has recently come from trials of low-dose aspirin in pregnancy.[3,4] Data from as many as 18 small controlled trials suggested a very large protective effect against pre-eclampsia and other measures of adverse outcome. Recently published larger, multicenter trials have indicated that this was a gross overestimate, with the true effect being much more moderate. Publication bias is certainly less of a problem in relation to large trials. It is important, therefore, when interpreting systematic reviews of controlled trials to gauge the extent to which the data come from small trials and to ascertain whether analyses restricted to larger trials (with, say, more than 200 participants) show the same pattern of results. The fact is that most reviews in the Cochrane Collaboration Pregnancy and Childbirth Database are based on small trials. This is the reason why, ideally, the effects of promising treatments should be confirmed in further, larger trials.

Bias caused by undue emphasis on particular outcomes

A problem with systematic reviews that is related to publication bias is bias introduced by undue emphasis within individual trials on particular outcomes. This is not a problem due to failure to report a trial at all, rather it is a failure to publish data on particular outcomes that leads to bias. There is an understandable tendency to report data on outcomes that show 'interesting' differences, at the expense of other outcomes that show no such differences. Overviews can only show data that are available and this can obviously introduce important bias. The optimal way of performing a systematic review is to choose the outcome measures that will be used in advance and then to seek a complete dataset for these. Ideally, individual patient data are acquired for each trial and overviews derived using these data. To our knowledge, this approach has not been used in the field of reproductive medicine, although it has been used very successfully in other areas of medical care.[5,6] Failing this, additional aggregated data may be sought from individual investigators, where these are not available in the trial report. Acquiring additional data is often not easy, particularly where an investigation was conducted some years previously and the principal investigator may have moved or the data been destroyed. Nevertheless, our experience is that this process is often extremely useful in protecting against such bias.

Multidisciplinary approach

So far in this chapter we have tended to concentrate on more clinical aspects of evaluation and this is reflected in the title of this chapter. However, this restrictive view does not take into account the wider dimensions of evaluation which are relevant to all branches of medicine, but particularly to maternity care where the majority of the 'patients' have nothing clinically wrong with them.

Psychosocial perspective

Women's views of the alternative forms of care that they receive may make an important contribution to subsequent decisions about clinical practice. This more qualitative approach to research may identify particular concerns that are hidden in a more traditional evaluation. For example, this approach identified the discomfort felt by women when intermittent fetal heart rate auscultation is performed using a traditional Pinard stethoscope; intermittent auscultation with a hand-held Doppler machine is less uncomfortable. In other situations, women's overall view of their care and outcome may be the determining factor in deciding management. This may apply where other outcomes are similar in the two groups or where there are competing risks and benefits.

Health economics

There is an increasing emphasis within health care evaluation on estimating the costs of health care and ensuring that interventions are cost-effective. Resources for health care are limited and should be used as efficiently as possible. Health economics is not simply the study of costs, however (this is accountancy), rather it is the valuation of resources in relation to health outcomes. Cost-effectiveness, for example, is usually expressed as the extra cost (or saving) required to achieve a unit of specified health gain. The cost-effectiveness of antenatal corticosteroid administration, for example, has been expressed as the cost per death or case of respiratory distress syndrome averted.

Consumer involvement in the evaluation

An extension of the psychosocial perspective is the incorporation of the broader views of consumers of health care. Representatives of users of maternity services have been particularly vocal in expressing their views. They have identified aspects of maternity care that are unpopular with women, and problems, such as those experienced during the postnatal period, that have been relatively neglected by clinical researchers. The research agenda, which includes clinical trials, should take into account the priorities identified by such groups, and incorporate aspects of evaluation that are judged to be particularly important by women themselves. The active involvement of consumer groups in recent large-scale trials has been very beneficial in ensuring that information is given to women sensitively and that a broader perspective is taken in the evaluation. This in turn has helped to encourage women to join these trials.

FUTURE PERSPECTIVES

Large simple trials, widespread collaboration, collaborative groups

Many measures of serious adverse outcome are now thankfully uncommon in developed countries. The implication of this is that surprisingly large trials will be required to identify the sorts of treatment effects that are clinically plausible. Such questions can therefore usually only be addressed reliably through widespread collaboration in multicenter trials. There is a limit to the number of such large trials that can be conducted and the choice of interventions for evaluation may prove difficult. We believe that trials should concentrate on the problems that are the most important, as judged by the number of people affected, or the seriousness of the complications, or the costs involved. Ideally, promising treatments to ameliorate or prevent such problems should be identified through systematic reviews of available evidence, concentrating on randomized controlled trials. Collaboration in multicenter trials requires unusual unselfishness and ways must be found to reward those who do participate. Our view is that local coordination of a multicenter trial is a major contribution to research and should be more widely acknowledged as such, for instance by job selection committees. There is a tension between the need to take a broad view of evaluation, which implies more complex data collection, and the need for really large numbers which necessitate simplicity. In practice, we envisage in-depth studies being limited to subsamples of people taking part in large simple-in-design trials with the numbers in these components reflecting formal sample size calculations.

Trials of procedures and policies

Whereas the methodology for evaluating drug treatments in placebo-controlled trials in now established, there are outstanding challenges in the evaluation of procedures and policies. The performance of a procedure may reflect technical ability in respect of skill and learning, and there is debate about how these issues should be addressed in a controlled clinical trial. Policies often involve a complex of actions and interactions whose independent effects may be hard to disentangle. This may also raise questions about the appropriateness of generalizing results of trials of policies to other health care settings.

Critical appraisal and evidence-based medicine

Clinical trials are of no value unless they influence clinical practice appropriately. This requires the ability to appraise evidence critically, in terms of potential for bias, the likelihood of problems caused by random errors, and the generalizability of the results, both for individual trials and for systematic reviews. This process is part of a broader move towards basing clinical practise on reliable evidence, so called 'Evidence-based Medicine'.

SUMMARY

- The challenge of a clinical trial is to distinguish real differences between the treatments being compared from bias (systematic errors), and from chance differences (random errors).
- Bias is introduced most commonly first, when the groups for comparison are being selected; secondly, when the outcome of treatment is being assessed; and thirdly, by differences in management other than in the way intended.
- The only way to ensure that the groups in a clinical trial are truly comparable is by random allocation of the participants to the alternative treatments; the allocations must remain 'concealed' until after formal trial entry. To avoid selection bias introduced by withdrawal after trial entry, the statistical analysis should be based on the groups according to their original treatment allocation (intention to treat analysis).
- Outcome should be assessed, where possible, 'blind' to the trial allocation and to the treatment actually received.
- Contamination, co-interventions, and crossovers from one treatment to another, may reduce the value of the trial results.
- There are two main types of statistical error;

type I errors occur when the results suggest a difference although, in truth, no difference exists; type II errors occur when the results do not detect a difference although, in truth, a difference does exist. The principal protection against type I and II errors is a larger sample size.
- The sample size for randomized controlled trial depends on what size of difference in the primary end-point is sought; the expected frequency of the primary outcome; and the likelihood of type I and II errors that are judged to be acceptable.
- A useful distinction can be drawn between 'explanatory' and 'pragmatic' trials; an explanatory trial addresses the question 'can a treatment have a particular effect in an ideal setting?', whereas a pragmatic trial addresses the question 'is a particular treatment effective in an everyday clinical setting'. Pragmatic trials take a broad view of evaluation, often incorporating psychosocial, health economics and consumers' perspectives.
- The generalizability of a trial's results depends on the types of people studied and on the interventions compared.

● Systematic reviews of similar trials reduce the risks of statistical errors, particularly type II errors, and increase generalizability, but every attempt should be made when conducting a systematic review to reduce the risk of bias introduced by selective publication (publication bias), or undue emphasis on variables that differ between the groups in published reports of trials.

REFERENCES

1. Elbourne D. The UK Collaborative ECMO Trial. *Midwives Chron Nurs Notes* 1994: 312–316.
2. Chalmers I, Hetherington J, Elbourne D, Keirse MJNC, Enkin M. Materials and methods used in synthesizing evidence to evaluate the effects of care during pregnancy and childbirth. In: Chalmers I, Enkin M, Keirse MJNC (eds) *Effective Care in Pregnancy and Childbirth.* Oxford: Oxford University Press, 1989: 39–65.
3. CLASP (Collaborative Low-dose Aspirin Study in Pregnancy) Collaborative Group. CLASP: a randomised trial of low-dose aspirin for the prevention and treatment of pre-eclampsia among 9364 pregnant women. Lancet 1994 **343**: 619–629.
4. Collins R. Antiplatelet agents for IUGR and pre-eclampsia. In Enkin MW, Keirse MJNC, Renfrew MJ, Neilson JP (eds) *Pregnancy and Childbirth Module* Cochrane Database of Systematic Reviews: Review No. 04000, 12 March 1994. Published through 'Cochrane Update on Disk'. Oxford: Update Software 1994, Disk issue 3.
5. Antiplatelet Trialists' Collaboration. Collaborative overview of randomised trials of antiplatelet treatment. I. Prevention of death, myocardial infarction, and stroke by prolonged antiplatelet therapy in various categories of patients. *Br Med J* 1994 **308**: 81–106.
6. Early Breast Cancer Trialists' Collaborative Group. Systematic treatment of early breast cancer by hormonal, cytotoxic, or immune therapy: 133 randomised trials involving 31,000 recurrences, and 24,000 deaths among 75,000 women. Lancet 1992 339: 1–15 (part I); 71–85 (part II).
7. Pocock SJ. Clinical Trials. Chichester: Wiley, 1983.
8. Armitage P, McPherson K, Rowe BC. Repeated significance tests on accumulating data. *J R Statist Soc* 1969 **132**: 235–244.

FURTHER READING

Bradford Hill A. The clinical trial. *N Engl J Med* 1952; **247**: 113–119
Chalmers I. Evaluating the effects of care during pregnancy and childbirth. In Chalmers I, Enkin M, Keirse MJNC (eds) *Effective Care in Pregnancy and Childbirth.* Oxford: Oxford University Press, 1989: 3–38.
Enkin MW, Keirse MJNC, Renfrew MJ, Neilson JP (eds) *Pregnancy and Childbirth Module.* 'Cochrane Database of Systematic Reviews'. Cochrane Updates on Disk, Oxford: Update Software.
Grant A. Reporting controlled trials. *Br J Obstet Gynaecol* 1989 **96**: 397–400.

5.2

Statistics

D Ashby

INTRODUCTION

In advancing the understanding of reproductive medicine, the design, analysis and interpretation of both observational and experimental studies play an important role.

To understand the importance of cytomegalovirus infection in pregnancy, for example, it is useful to know which women are likely to have antibodies, so that it is then clear who is at risk of a primary infection. This involves collecting data on the likely risk factors, and analysing the data to see which of these are (jointly) associated with their prevalence. In trying to decide whether ultrasound is beneficial in pregnancy, randomized controled trials have been carried out. The analysis of a single trial illustrates many of the principal elements of a statistical analysis, but to really make progress in this area, the results from several trials may need to be looked at simultaneously.

Similarly, understanding the epidemiology of cancers such as those of the ovary and cervix require the collection, analysis and interpretation of routine data, as well as scientific studies. The most usual design for looking at treatment options is again the randomized trial, but for looking at some aspects, for example some of the rarer longer-term consequences of treatment, observational studies may also be necessary.

In the related area of urodynamics, it is interesting to understand which factors are associated with a woman's urine flow rate, and if these are well enough understood, to use this knowledge in the clinical situation to determine whether a patient has a flow rate that is in some sense abnormal.

All of these examples, and many, many more, involve the collection, analysis and interpretation of data. Although the clinical situations vary, and the final interpretation of a study will depend on the particular context, there are principles of design and analysis that are common to all of them. In this chapter, some of the examples given above and others will all be discussed in more detail to illustrate these principles. The elements of good design

are briefly reviewed. Graphical methods for the display of data are illustrated, and the commonly used tools of statistical inference are described, first in simple situations, to establish the key elements, but then in more complex situations to show their versatility. Regression analysis underpins much statistical analysis, and multiple regression, logistic regression and survival analysis will all be described. Systematic overviews, whether in the area of clinical trials or of epidemiology are being used more commonly, and the technique of meta-analysis will be described. The use of tests and charts for clinical diagnosis will be outlined. A brief introduction to sample size determination follows, and finally a few words will be offered to guide the reader into the jungle of statistical packages now available.

The purpose of this chapter is not to provide a step-by-step guide on how to perform these statistical techniques: references will be made to some of the textbooks written with that in mind. Rather the aim is to give an overview of the range of statistical options now coming into regular use in the medical field, so that their rationale can be understood, and their potential contribution to furthering the field of reproductive medicine appreciated.

CURRENT CONCEPTS

Study design

The importance of good study design cannot be overemphasized. A study should have clear objectives, whether descriptive or to test specific hypotheses. The design of the study should be appropriate to this. Data collection should be well planned, using appropriate data-collection instruments, be these a regularly calibrated set of weighing scales, or a questionnaire on depression validated for use in that setting. A plan of analysis can be specified at the study design stage. The purpose of this is partly to have a record of the primary outcomes, so that more speculative analysis can be seen as hypothesis generation, but it also plays a useful role in making sure data are being collected in an appropriate format, and in inhibiting the temptation to collect data on every variable in sight 'just in case'. Perhaps the most difficult aspect to plan is the appropriate sample size, but if the study needs to justify its funding, this can be one of the most critical aspects. The principles are outlined on p. 571.

Clinical trials are discussed in Chapter 5.1: suffice to say that the primary analysis of a well-designed randomized controlled trial is usually very straightforward, at least in the case of two parallel groups. In a trial to explore the effect of ultrasound screening on perinatal mortality, we are essentially comparing the proportions of dead in the control group and the screened group. The same principles can be applied to other experiments. Whether the units of study are cells or animals or anything else in the laboratory, the comparability of the control group and the treated groups is of paramount importance, and the most efficient way of trying to achieve this is randomization.

There are, however, many situations where randomization is either not feasible or not ethical, and then an observational study is required. If anything, the importance of design is even greater. In the field of epidemiology, the understanding of the causes of disease from a population perspective, there are several key designs. Routine data such as cancer registration give valuable information on the distribution of, say, cancer of the cervix by age, region and time period. Surveys can yield useful information on risk factors such as sexual behavior. Prospective studies of women's patterns of contraceptive use and their subsequent morbidity are a long-term investment to help inform choice for future generations. A quicker type of study is the case control study which compares, for example, women with breast cancer with those without the disease to see if those with breast cancer were more likely to have been exposed to, say, particular types of contraception, or to have experienced different child-bearing patterns. These latter two designs have been well described in the context of cancer by Breslow and Day,[1,2] but are equally useful in other areas.

A growing area of interest is that of audit. Again, all the principles of good study design apply, and most of the general considerations which apply to other observational studies.

Descriptive plots

'A picture speaks a thousand words', and this is particularly true when it comes to understanding a data set. For a small data set, each individual observation can be displayed on a suitable plot. For a single set of continuous (measured) observations, this might involve plotting crosses along a single axis to display the spread of values, or for a slightly larger data set a histogram can be a useful summary. A useful graphical summary is the box-whisker plot. To carry this out, for each group, first rank the data, then determine the median (the middle value, or the average of the two middle values), the two interquartile values (those which have 25% and 75% respectively of the data above them) and the minimum and maximum. A box is then formed

from the quartiles, with the median marked in the box, and the whiskers are formed to the minimum and maximum. For several groups being compared, the box–whisker plots demonstrate clearly differences in average values, differences in variability, and any skewness in the data. Box and whisker plots can be formed with different quartiles, depending on the emphasis of the analysis. Milman et al.[3] carried out a randomized, double-blind, placebo-controlled trial of the effect of iron supplementation during pregnancy. Fig. 5.2.1 shows very clearly the serum ferritin levels in the pregnant women at term and in the newborn infants. Note the use of the logarithmic scale, to deal with widely varying values.

For two continuous variables measured on the same set of individuals, a scatterplot shows whether there seems to be a relationship, and if so, whether it is approximately linear, or whether it has some other shape. A study of fetal measurements, shows the relationship of ulnar length with gestational age.[4] Fig. 5.2.2 illustrates the strong association

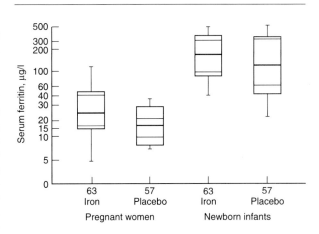

Fig. 5.2.1 *Serum ferritin levels in pregnant women at term and in their newborn infants according to supplementation with 66 mg ferrous iron daily from the 16th week of gestation. From below, horizontal bars indicate the following percentiles: 1st, 5th, 10th, median, 90th, 95th, 99th. (From reference 3.)*

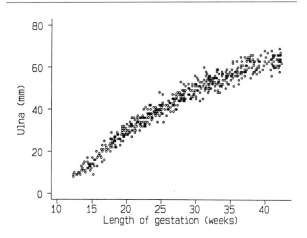

Fig. 5.2.2 *572 measurements of ulna length by length of gestation (courtesy of DG Altman).*

between the two, but also clearly shows a curvilinear relationship, and variability which increases with gestational age, which are important features for further analysis of the data.

There are many other plots that can be useful. With recent developments in computing, it is possible to try different plots, both to explore the data, and to choose the most appropriate for presentation. Always look carefully at other people's presentations to collect good ideas. The book by Altman[5] is a good source of inspiration.

Confidence intervals

When looking at a set of data, we are often interested not so much in that set of patients, but in generalizing to a much wider set of patients. Some of these judgments will be subjective, based on general scientific considerations (can we generalize from men to women, older to younger patients, patients in one country to those in another?). Some of the judgments are rather narrower and mainly concern sampling variation. If the sample is a properly chosen random sample from some larger group, or if it may reasonably be regarded as such, then *confidence intervals* help quantify the size of the likely population mean (or proportion etc.), based on the information from the sample in hand.

In a study to look at maternal nutritional status in pregnancy and blood pressure in childhood,[6] the systolic blood pressures of 77 children aged between 10 and 12 years in Kingston, Jamaica were measured. Their mean blood pressure was 94.8 mmHg, with a standard deviation of 8.5 mmHg. We may be interested in knowing the average blood pressure of children from Kingston. If we can regard these children as a random sample of all the children of that age in the town, we can calculate the 95% confidence interval for the mean blood pressure as 92.9–96.7. We are then 95% confident that the true mean blood pressure for 10–12 year olds in Kingston is no less than 92.9 and no greater than 96.7.

This is an example of a confidence interval for a mean. Very often we are interested in making statements about the differences between two groups. In a clinical trial which measured the effect of Doppler ultrasound on perinatal death, McParland and Pearce[7] observed six deaths out of 254 births in the treated group, compared to 20 deaths out of 255 births in the control group. The odds ratio can be calculated as 0.32, which implies that a baby in the treated group has a risk of dying which is one-third of that in the control group. However, the 95% confidence interval is 0.15–0.71, which means that the true odds ratio could be a half or double that which was estimated.

For any statistic that can be estimated, such as a mean, a proportion, differences in means, relative risks, regression coefficients and so on, uncertainty in the estimation can be quantified using a confidence interval. For the simple cases the calculations are very straightforward, whereas others are more complex, and for a comprehensive review of rationale and methods, the reader is referred to Gardner and Altman.[8]

Classical hypothesis testing

Sometimes data are collected to test a particular hypothesis, and this is most clearly illustrated by considering the clinical trial. In its simplest form it is set up to establish whether one treatment is better than another. To formalize this, a *null hypothesis* is set up that the two treatments are equally effective in the relevant population. It is then possible to calculate, under this assumption, how likely it is to observe results at least as extreme as those obtained in a particular trial. The resulting *P value* can then be regarded as a measure of evidence against the null hypothesis, and if this is strong enough, the null hypothesis can be rejected and the conclusion drawn that one treatment is better than another.

In the trial of Doppler ultrasound described above, we could set up a null hypothesis that there is no difference in the perinatal death rate between the two trial groups. To carry out a test of this hypothesis, we first have to choose an appropriate test of significance. Because the data are categorical, and come from two independent samples we can use a chi-squared test. We calculate a test statistic of 7.12, which is then referred to tables of the chi-squared distribution. These tell us that the probability of getting such an extreme result, were the null hypothesis true, is less than one in a hundred, and on the basis of this we would reject the null hypothesis. It is worth noting that this rather convoluted procedure really tells us very little more than could be obtained from the 95% confidence interval: the fact that the interval did not contain the value, 1.0 tells us that it is unlikely that the two groups are equivalent in terms of perinatal death rates.

There are many different hypothesis tests for different kinds of data. For comparing two groups with respect to a continuous measurement such as blood pressure the two-sample *t*-test is often used. If the data are paired because of some feature of the design of the study, the analogous tests to the chi-squared test and the two-sample *t*-test are McNemar's test and the paired (one-sample) *t*-test. There are tests for ranked observations known as *non-parametric tests*. For full details and worked examples, the reader is referred to the standard introductory texts by Campbell and Machin[9] or Bland.[10]

If there are more than two groups, for continuous measurements the *t*-tests can be generalized in various ways to Analysis of Variance. These and the analogous procedures for categorical measurement are closely linked to regression analysis, and for further explanations, the reader is referred to the excellent book by Altman.[5]

Hypothesis testing sounds attractive in that superficially it matches the clinical decision-making process, but it has several pitfalls. The *P* value (sometimes called the statistical significance) is determined by both the magnitude of the difference, the variability of the observations (for continuous data) and the size of the samples. It follows that small studies can miss important differences, and very large studies can detect even clinically meaningless differences as being 'statistically significant'. A more informative summary of a trial is to calculate a relevant summary measure, such as a difference in proportions, or an odds-ratio, and to present confidence intervals for it. This shows how large or small the difference between the groups might plausibly be, and, in particular, whether a clinically relevant difference has been ruled out.

Simple linear regression

In many studies, the purpose is to understand what causes variation in a particular characteristic, and then to model this in such a way that it is then useful for clinical purposes. Examples might be modeling variation in birthweight as a function of gestational age and sex, or looking at urine flow rates as a function of volume urinated. The key technique is known as *regression analysis*. In its simplest form this is equivalent to drawing a scatter plot of one measurement against another, and fitting a straight line to the points. The usual assumption is linearity, but by use of transformations, a variety of curvilinear and other relationships can be incorporated into this framework. The importance of plotting data to check assumptions cannot be over-emphasized.

In the study of Jamaican children already described, the blood pressures at age eleven were related to the mother's triceps skinfold thickness at 15 weeks of gestation. Plots of the data indicate a linear relationship with log triceps skinfold thickness, rather than the original measurement. By fitting a straight line, the authors estimated that each log mm decrease in skinfold thickness was associated with a 5.8 mmHg increase in the child's systolic blood pressure. However, the 95% confidence interval went from −0.3 mmHg to 11.9 mmHg, which indicates that whereas the relationship is almost certainly positive, the magnitude was known only imprecisely.

Multiple regression

Multiple regression extends the ideas of simple linear regression to cope with several factors simultaneously associated with a continuous outcome measure. The factors used to 'explain' or 'predict' variations in the outcome measure can be either continuous or categorical. Hypothesis tests can be used to help determine whether a particular variable has an effect, once other variables have been accounted for.

In the above example maternal skinfold thickness was not the only factor associated with the child's blood pressure. The child's own weight and sex both have an influence, and the authors were also interested in the effects of the lowest maternal hemoglobin, and maternal weight gain during pregnancy.

The authors checked the assumption of linearity, and then fitted the model shown in Table 5.2.1.

We can see, for example, that the child's blood pressure increases, on average by 1 mmHg for every kilogram of bodyweight, that boys on average have blood pressures 2.9 mmHg lower than girls, when other factors are simultaneously taken into account. There is no association with hemoglobin, but for each kg of weight increase in the mother during pregnancy, the blood pressure is lower by 0.6 mmHg. Once all these adjustments have taken place, the triceps association is strengthened, from a drop of 5.8 mmHg per log mm, to a drop of 10.7 mmHg. The 95% confidence intervals express the uncertainty in the estimation, and the *P* values test the hypothesis that there is no association of that particular variable with the child's blood pressure, once other factors have been taken into account. For example, we are very sure that the associations with the child's weight and the maternal triceps thickness are not chance findings, and the association with maternal weight gain is also unlikely to be due to chance. However the association with sex may well be chance variation, and the coefficient for maternal hemoglobin is just what we would expect if no association exists.

A final point is that regression can tell us a great deal about *association* between variables. We must be very careful not to interpret these relationships causally: that inference always rests on wider judgments. Bradford Hill[11] describes some very helpful criteria that can be useful in establishing whether a relationship is causal.

Regression with a categorical outcome: logistic regression

With a categorical outcome, a simple summary of the relationship between the outcome and one or two variables is usually possible. Griffiths *et al.*[12] give plots to show the prevalence of cytomegalovirus (CMV) infection by race and age, and by social class and age in a group of 1000

Table 5.2.1 Simultaneous effects of the child's sex and weight at 11 years and maternal influences expressed as continuous variables, on systolic pressure

	Regression slope	95% C.I.	P
Weight at 11 years (kg)	1.0	(0.7 to 1.2)	<0.0001
Male sex	−2.9	(−5.9 to 0.2)	0.07
Maternal influences			
Lowest maternal hemoglobin (d/dl)	0.0	(−1.9 to 1.8)	1.0
Maternal triceps thickness at 15 weeks of gestation (log mm)	−10.7	(−15.5 to −5.8)	0.0001
Maternal weight gain 15–35 weeks of gestation (kg)	−0.6	(−1.0 to −0.1)	0.02

From reference 6

pregnant women. To assess formally the influence of these and other confounding variables on the prevalence and to predict the chances of a future woman being CMV positive, we need an analogy of ordinary regression. It is usual to work with the *log-odds* of the proportion, rather than the proportion itself, and the resulting model is called the *logistic regression model*. Griffiths *et al.* showed that the strongest effects were race and age, but that social class still had some independent effect. No other variables had any effect.

The computation needed for this model is more complex than for ordinary regression, but logistic regression is widely available in standard statistical packages. Logistic regression can seem strange to start with, but by reading a book such as Altman[5] and by discussing early attempts with a statistician many clinical researchers are discovering the power and wide applicability of this model.

Survival

In many situations, data are of the form *time to an event*. In a clinical trial this could be time to death, or time to recurrence of cancer. Interest is usually focused on which variables are predictive of time to an event. In a clinical trial the primary focus is usually the treatment variable, whereas in an observational study we may need to disentangle the effects of several potential variables. As with most other kinds of data, the first step is usually to plot the data, using Kaplan–Meier curves.

A trial of Ro 03–8799 (pimonidazole) was performed in patients undergoing radiotherapy for Stage II and Stage III squamous cell carcinoma of the uterine cervix.[13] There were two important end-points: local tumor control, and survival. Figs 5.2.3 and 5.2.4 shows the Kaplan–Meier plots for each of these end-points, clearly showing that the radiosensitizer group had worse outcomes.

For a more formal inference to take place we require a regression-type model that can handle *censored* data, i.e. patients for whom the relevant outcome had not occurred at the time of analysis. One of the most commonly used techniques is *Cox's proportional hazards model*. This assumes that for two similar patients, who differ in only one characteristic, who have both survived to a given day, their risks of dying on that day will be proportional, and furthermore, whatever day we consider, their relative chances of dying remain constant. The ratio of the two risks is called the *hazard ratio*. For the radiosensitizer trial the hazard ratio for local tumor control for the radiosensitizer group compared to control is 2.1 (95% confidence interval 1.2–3.7), and for survival is 1.6 (95% confidence interval 1.0–2.5). This means that a patient in the radiosensitizer group had twice the chance of a recurrence being diagnosed on a particular day, and a 60% excess risk of dying, compared to the control group.

For a clinical trial there is often just one important characteristic, the treatment. For more complex clinical trials, and for observational studies with many factors, Cox's proportional hazards model extends in a way analogous to the previous regression models considered. Although Cox's proportional hazards model is widely used, it does make reasonably strong assumptions, and there are other possible models for dealing with survival data.

Meta-analysis

The techniques used so far all relate to the analysis of individual studies. However the scientific process is concerned with making inferences across studies. This may be a set of epidemiological studies, or a set of clinical trials. The most difficult tasks are the identification and extraction of the trials and their results. A simple tabulation of the study characteristics and the key results contains most of the information, but sometimes a more formal estimate of the overall effect is required. The technique known as *meta-*

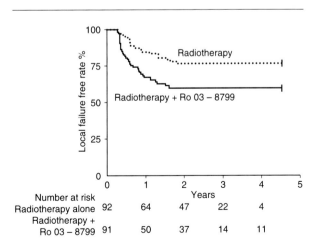

Fig. 5.2.3 *Lifetable showing failure to control tumor within the irradiated area for the radiosensitizer plus radiotherapy group versus the radiosensitizer alone group. (From reference 13.)*

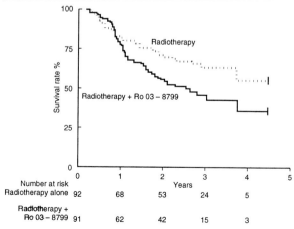

Fig. 5.2.4 *Lifetable showing overall survival for the radiosensitizer plus radiotherapy group versus the radiosensitizer alone group. (From reference 13.)*

analysis[14] can provide this. Essentially this summarizes firstly within each study, and secondly across studies.

The Cochrane Collaboration aims to collate systematically the evidence from randomized trials in all areas of medicine, and the module in Pregnancy and Childbirth is well established. In a review of all trials of Doppler ultrasound in pregnancy, Neilson[15] reviewed 12 trials with respect to 14 outcomes, ranging from antepartum admission to hospital to various indices of mortality. The results on perinatal deaths are shown in Table 5.2.2. The best estimate of the odds ratio is 0.64, and we are reasonably sure that ultrasound reduces deaths by at least 15%, and maybe as much as 52%.

Diagnostic tests

In reproductive medicine it is often necessary to make a decision on the basis of a test. In the obstetric field an example is screening for neural tube defects on the basis of alpha-fetoprotein levels. In the cancer field, screening for breast cancer carries a similar problem of balancing the risks of falsely diagnosing the disease in a healthy situation, versus declaring a woman cancer-free when she is not.

These ideas can be formalized, and to look at the performance of a diagnostic test, three measures are useful. The sensitivity of a test is calculated as the proportion of all truly diseased individuals who actually screen positive. The specificity of a test is the proportion of all truly non-diseased individuals who screen negative, and the positive predictive value is the proportion of all those who screen positive who actually have the disease in question.

Piggott *et al.*[16] evaluated the use of the triple test – measurement of α fetoprotein, unconjugated estriol and human gonadotropin concentration – in antenatal screening for Down's syndrome in two health districts. Of eleven pregnancies with Down's syndrome present, eight had screened positive, and three negative. Of the 6979 pregnancies without Down's syndrome, 203 had screened positive, and 6776 negative. This gives a sensitivity of 73%

and a specificity of 97%. However, the positive predictive value, i.e. the probability of carrying a child with Down's, given a positive result on screening, is only 2.8%.

Sometimes a test reports either 'positive' or 'negative', but more often a cut-off needs to be chosen for a continuous measure. The three measures outlined can be very valuable in determining the appropriate cut-off in a particular situation.

Reference ranges

In reproductive medicine we are often concerned with whether a measurement is in a 'normal' or acceptable range. This might be a fetal measurement, a baby's weight, or a urodynamic measurement. Usually, reference ranges are derived from measurements on a large group of individuals. In a simple example quantiles of the distribution might provide an adequate comparison, but for many measurements in reproductive medicine, the measurement varies with some characteristic, such as gestational age, and charts are needed. The derivation of these charts can depend on extensions of regression methodology outlined above, but have often been poorly done on inadequate size samples. Altman and Chitty[4] give a good description of methodology, and they then apply this[17–19] to measures of fetal size. They show that it is important to model both the mean and the variability. For the ulna data shown in Fig. 5.2.1, Fig. 5.2.5 shows the derived chart with fitted 5th, 50th and 95th centiles. They have also used the methodology to derive charts for head measurements, abdominal measurements and fetal lengths.

Sample size considerations

One of the questions most often asked of statisticians is 'How large should my sample be?' Books such as Altman[5] give details of calculations, Pocock[20] has a very good section for those planning clinical trials, and Machin and

Table 5.2.2 The effect of Doppler ultrasound (all trials) on perinatal death

Reference key	No. Events/No. Entered Treatment	Control	Odds ratio	95% CI LO	HI
Pattinson+ 1992	1/61	6/63	0.23	0.05	1.05
Newnham+ 1991	9/275	9/270	0.98	0.38	2.51
Tyrrell+ 1990	3/250	3/250	1.00	0.20	4.99
Hanretty	3/1642	8/1344	0.33	0.10	1.07
Biljan+ 1992	1/338	4/336	0.30	0.05	1.72
Marsal+ 1991	0/214	3/212	0.13	0.01	1.28
Davies+ 1992	17/1246	7/1229	2.29	1.02	5.11
Johnstone	12/1128	16/1196	0.79	0.38	1.67
McParland+ 1988	6/254	20/255	0.32	0.15	0.71
Trudinger+ 1987	1/127	5/162	0.32	0.06	1.65
Omtzigt 1990	16/825	28/815	0.56	0.31	1.03
Mason+ 1993	4/1015	5/1001	0.79	0.21	2.92
Total (95% CI)	73/7375	114/7133	0.64	0.48	0.85
χ^2 (11) for heterogeneity: 20.43					

From reference 15

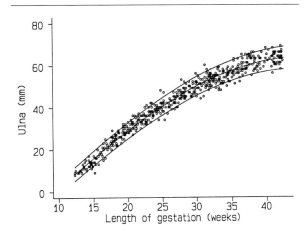

Fig. 5.2.5 *Ulna length measurements with fitted 5th, 50th and 95th centiles (from reference 4.)*

Campbell[21] contains tables for all the sample size calculations in common use. For the details of the calculations readers are referred to these texts, but the key features can be summarized briefly.

To describe one group with respect to a continuous measurement, the key information needed is some idea of the variability of the measurement in the population, and how accurately the average needs to be known. The larger the sample, the more accuracy is possible. For a proportion, the variability of its estimate depends on its value, but if in doubt, err towards 50%, as this gives a conservative estimate.

If we wanted to estimate the mean blood pressure of a second group of Jamaican children we might be prepared to assume the standard deviation to be about the same as the children from Kingston. If we wished to know the blood pressure of the new group to within 1 mmHg, we would need a representative sample of 280 children.

For a two-group comparison, which covers most clinical trials, we need to decide how big a difference between groups is clinically worth detecting. There are two kinds of errors to be balanced. One is the possibility that there is no real difference between the groups, but that we mistakenly say there is. The second is the possibility that a difference exists, but the trial fails to establish it. The first error is called the type I error, the second the type II error. The power of a study can be calculated as $1-$ (type II error), and is the probability of detecting a difference should it exist. If we can specify the difference that it would be clinically worthwhile to detect, and the type I and II errors, then we can determine the sample size. In addition, as before we need some idea of the variability, for a continuous measure, or the proportion expected in the control group for categorical outcomes.

For example, in planning a trial of ultrasound to look at perinatal death, we expect a control group rate of 10%, and would be interested in detecting an improvement to 5% in the screened group. With a type I error of 5%, and a power of 90%, we would need 582 women in each group. To increase the power to 95%, 719 women in each group would be needed.

Sample size determination is never easy, and sometimes pilot studies will be required to get estimates of some of the quantities. However, studies are expensive to mount, and an appreciation of the likely benefits for a given sample size are an essential component of the decision to embark on a study.

Computing

Many of the statistical techniques outlined above can be carried out on a hand calculator, but many people concerned with the collection and analysis of even moderate sized data-sets will need to learn about statistical computing. This is a difficult area to address in detail in a book, as computing is a rapidly advancing field, but a few general points are worth making.

The first is that computers do not undermine the need for good study design, planning of data collection, or careful thought given to a plan of analysis, but in conjunction with these, can be very powerful. Personal computers can store and manipulate very large quantities of data, and for those with access to work-stations and mainframes, there is effectively no limit on size. For most analysis, the hard work is in the sorting of data into groups, and the calculation of basic summary statistics for those groups such as means, standard deviations, and counts. Many spreadsheets and databases can do these tasks very well, and the final niceties of confidence interval calculations and so on can be done using a hand-calculator. There are any number of statistical packages available. Good packages include EPI-INFO, which is freely available, and is useful for surveys and other studies, MINITAB, and SPSS and SAS, which come in versions to suit most kinds of computers. Time spent in learning to use any of these is an investment, as they are all well-tested and widely available. Perhaps one of the greatest contributions of computing to statistics is the ease with which good quality graphics can be prepared.

FUTURE PERSPECTIVES

In one sense, statistics as applied to medicine is not a rapidly moving subject. There are certain key principles, and they stay constant, although the details of the studies may change. However, in another sense, changes have been apparent, and will continue to be so. There are two main influences. The first is the progression in medicine in general, and in reproductive medicine in particular, to making decisions based on rigorous evidence. This demands good studies, which in turn emphasizes the role of statistics. The second influence is the explosion of computing power, which has far-reaching implications for the collection and analysis of data. This means, among other things, that more complex statistical techniques, such as logistic regression and meta-analysis, are becoming more widely accessible, and hence are appearing more regularly in the journals. Clinicians increasingly will need familiarity at reading about, if not actually doing, these techniques.

For those who find themselves potentially needing to use unfamiliar techniques, it is worth getting to know your local statistician. Although few can take on analyses, many are prepared to talk with a doctor for an hour or so, and this can be very valuable. Occasionally such conversations can result in collaborations: it is noticeable that most of the examples of good practice in this chapter have arisen from such collaborations. Statisticians, in turn, continue to

develop their methodology, and many current developments in epidemiology, clinical trials methodology and other areas are arising from the challenges presented by their clinical colleagues. It would be a difficult task to outline these developments in a short space. For most doctors involved in reproductive medicine, familiarity with the ideas outlined in this chapter will suffice, and will stand them in good stead for much of their working lives. Most doctors' appreciation of statistics comes from analysing their own studies, or thinking hard and critically about other people's work.

SUMMARY

- Good analysis cannot rescue bad design.
- Always plot the data, to help you understand it, and to explain your data to others.
- Calculate appropriate descriptors that are clinically meaningful.
- Confidence intervals help show how accurate your estimates are.
- Hypothesis testing should be used sparingly.
- Regression helps to understand and quantify the relationship between variables.

- Collating evidence systematically is a key scientific activity.
- Computing power can make life easier, although your hand calculator can be your best friend.
- Sample size estimation requires hard thought, but is an essential part of planning any study.
- Most doctors' appreciation of statistics comes from analysing their own studies, or thinking hard and critically about other people's work.

REFERENCES

1. Breslow NE, Day NE. *Statistical Methods in Cancer Research I: The Analysis of Case-Control Studies.* International Agency for Research on Cancer, Scientific Publication No 32, Lyon, 1980.
2. Breslow NE, Day NE. *Statistical Methods in Cancer Research II: The Design and Analysis of Cohort Studies.* International Agency for Research on Cancer, Scientific Publication No 32, Lyon, 1987.
3. Milman N, Agger AO, Nielson OJ. Iron status markers and serum erythropoietin in 120 mothers and newborn infants. *Acta Obstet Gynecol Scand* 1994 **73**: 200–204.
4. Altman DG, Chitty LS. Charts of fetal size: 1. Methodology. *Br J Obstet Gynaecol* 1994 **101**: 29–34.
5. Altman DG. *Practical Statistics for Medical Research.* London: Chapman and Hall, 1991.
6. Godfrey KM, Forrester T, Barker DJP, Jackson AA, Landman JP, Hall JStE *et al.* Maternal nutritional status in pregnancy and blood pressure in childhood. *Br J Obstet Gynaecol* 1994 **101**: 398–403.
7. McParland P, Pearce JM. Doppler blood flow in pregnancy. *Placenta* 1988 **9**: 427–450.
8. Gardner MJ, Altman DG. *Statistics with Confidence.* London: British Medical Journal, 1989.
9. Campbell MJ, Machin D. *Medical Stastistics: a Commonsense Approach.* 2nd edn. Chichester; Wiley, 1993.
10. Bland JM. *An Introduction to Medical Statistics.* Oxford: Oxford University Press, 1987.
11. Bradford Hill A. *A Short Textbook of Medical Statistics.* 11th edn. London: Hodder and Stoughton, 1984.
12. Griffiths P, Baboonian C, Ashby D. The demographic characteristics of pregnant women infected with cytomegalovirus. *Int J Epidemiol* 1985 **14**: 447–452.
13. MRC Working Party on Advanced Carcinoma of the Cervix. A trial of Ro 03–8799 (pimonidazole) in carcinoma of the uterine cervix: an interim report from the Medical Research Council Working Party on advanced cancer of the cervix. *Radiother Oncol* 1993 **26**: 93–103.
14. Collins R, Gray R, Godwin J, Peto R. Avoidance of large biases and large random errors in the assessment of moderate treatment effects: the need for systematic overviews. *Statist Med* 1987 **6**: 245–250.
15. Neilson JP. Doppler ultrasound (all trials). In Enkin MW, Keirse MJNC, Renfrew MJ, Neilson JP (eds) *Pregnancy and Childbirth Module, 'Cochrane Database of Systematic Reviews'*: Review No 07337, 26 February 1993. Cochrane Updates on Disk, Oxford: Update Software, 1993, Disk Issue 2, 1992.
16. Piggott M, Wilkinson P, Bennett J. Implementation of an antenatal serum screening programme for Down's syndrome in two districts (Brighton and Eastbourne). *J Med Screen* 1994 **1**: 45–49.
17. Chitty LS, Altman DG, Henderson A, Campbell S. Charts of fetal size: 2. Head measurements. *Br J Obstet Gynaecol* 1994 **101**: 35–43.
18. Chitty LS, Altman DG, Henderson A, Campbell S. Charts of fetal size: 3. Abdominal measurements. *Br J Obstet Gynaecol* 1994 **101**: 125–131.
19. Chitty LS, Altman DG, Henderson A, Campbell S. Charts of fetal size: 4. Femur length. *Br J Obstet Gynaecol* 1994 **101**: 132–135.
20. Pocock SJ. *Clinical Trials – a Practical Approach.* Chichester; Wiley, 1983.
21. Machin D, Campbell MJ. *Statistical Tables for the Design of Clinical Trials.* Oxford: Blackwell, 1987.

Index

Entries in **bold** are main discussions; entries in *italics* indicate reference to illustrations and tables.